Volume III

CORNEA

Surgery of the Cornea and Conjunctiva

VOLUME III

CORNEA

Surgery of the Cornea and Conjunctiva

EDITORS

JAY H. KRACHMER, M.D.

Professor and Chairman, Department of Ophthalmology
University of Minnesota, Minneapolis, Minnesota

MARK J. MANNIS, M.D.

Professor and Director, Cornea, External Disease, and Refractive Surgery, Department of Ophthalmology
University of California, Davis, Sacramento, California

EDWARD J. HOLLAND, M.D.

Professor and Director of Cornea and External Disease Service, Department of Ophthalmology
University of Minnesota, Minneapolis, Minnesota

MEDICAL ILLUSTRATOR

MARTIN FINCH

Mosby

St. Louis Baltimore Boston Carlsbad Chicago Naples New York Philadelphia Portland
London Madrid Mexico City Singapore Sydney Tokyo Toronto Wiesbaden

Mosby
Dedicated to Publishing Excellence

A Times Mirror Company

Publisher: Anne Patterson
Acquisition Editor: Laurel Craven
Managing Editor: Kathryn H. Falk
Project Manager: Linda McKinley
Production Editor: Rich Barber
Manufacturing Supervisor: Theresa Fuchs
Designer: Elizabeth Fett

Printed in the United States of America
Composition by: Graphic World, Inc.
Printing/binding by: Maple-Vail Book Manufacturing Group

Mosby–Year Book, Inc.
11830 Westline Industrial Drive
St. Louis, Missouri 63146

International Standard Book Number 0-8151-5249-3

96 97 98 99 00 / 9 8 7 6 5 4 3 2 1

Contributors

Richard L. Abbott, MD
Professor and Co-Director
Corneal and Refractive Surgery
Beckman Vision Center and Francis I. Proctor Foundation
Department of Ophthalmology
University of California, San Francisco
San Francisco, California

Patricia Aiken-O'Neill
President and Chief Executive Officer (CEO)
Eye Bank Association of America
Washington, DC

Eduardo C. Alfonso, MD
Associate Professor
Bascom Palmer Eye Institute
University of Miami
Miami, Florida

Hassan Alizadeh, PhD
Assistant Professor
Department of Ophthalmology
The University of Texas Southwestern Medical Center at Dallas
Dallas, Texas

Claron Douglas Alldredge, MD
University of Utah
Salt Lake City, Utah

O. Claron Alldredge, Jr, MD
Professor
Department of Ophthalmology
University of Utah
Salt Lake City, Utah

Juan J. Arentsen, MD
Medical Director
Centro Oftalmologico Reconquista
Department of Cornea, Anterior Segment
Centro Oftalmologico Reconquista
Casilla 253-9, Correo 9, Providencis
Santiago, CHILE

Penny A. Asbell, MD
Professor
Director, Cornea Service
Department of Ophthalmology
Mount Sinai Medical Center
New York, New York

Kerry K. Assil, MD
Medical Director and CEO
Sinskey Eye Institute
Santa Monica, California

Dimitri T. Azar, MD
Director
Refractive Surgery Service
Department of Ophthalmology
Wilmer Ophthalmological Institute
Johns Hopkins University Hospital
Baltimore, Maryland

Neal P. Barney, MD
Assistant Professor
Department of Ophthalmology and Visual Sciences
University of Wisconsin Medical School
Madison, Wisconsin

Jules Baum, MD
Research Professor
Department of Ophthalmology
Tufts University School of Medicine
Boston, Massachusetts

Michael W. Belin, MD, FACS
Associate Professor
Director of Cornea, External Disease, and Refractive Surgery
Department of Ophthalmology
Albany Medical College-Lions Eye Institute
Albany Stratton Veteran Administration Medical Center
Albany, New York

Richard J. Bensinger, MD
Medical Director
Pacific Eye Foundation
Seattle, Washington

William H. Benson, MD
Assistant Professor
Department of Ophthalmology
Medical College of Virginia
Virginia Commonwealth University
Richmond, Virginia

Charles S. Bouchard, MD
Associate Professor of Ophthalmology
Director, Cornea Service
Department of Ophthalmology
Loyola University Medical Center
Maywood, Illinois

Robert E. Brass, MD
Group Practice–Eye Department
Allina Health Care
St. Paul, Minnesota

William Z. Bridges, Jr, MD
Department of Ophthalmology
Emory University
Atlanta, Georgia

Frederick S. Brightbill, MD
Professor
Head Corneal Service
Department of Ophthalmology and Visual Science
University of Wisconsin Medical School
Madison, Wisconsin

Terry E. Burris, MD
Northwest Corneal Services
Portland, Oregon

J. Douglas Cameron, MD
Associate Professor
Departments of Ophthalmology and Laboratory Medicine and Pathology
Hennepin County Medical Center
University of Minnesota
Minneapolis, Minnesota

Robert C. Campbell, MD
Medical Director
Department of Ophthalmology
Park Nicollet Contact Lens Clinic and Research Center
Park Nicollet Clinic HealthSystem Minnesota
Minneapolis, Minnesota

Emmett F. Carpel, MD
Clinical Professor
Department of Ophthalmology
University of Minnesota
Staff Physician
Hennepin County Medical Center
Minneapolis, Minnesota

H. Dwight Cavanagh, MD, PhD
The W. Maxwell Thomas Professor and Vice Chairman
Department of Ophthalmology
University of Texas Southwestern Medical Center at Dallas
Dallas, Texas

John William Chandler, MD
Chief
Department of Ophthalmology
University of Illinois Hospital
Professor and Head
Department of Ophthalmology and Visual Sciences
University of Illinois at Chicago
Chicago, Illinois

Kevin C. Chang, MD
Corneal Consultants of Indiana
Indianapolis, Indiana

Steven D. Chang, MD
Cornea and External Disease Service
Department of Ophthalmology
University of California, Davis
Sacramento, California

Kenneth C. Chern, MD
Chief Resident
Department of Ophthalmology
The Cleveland Clinic Foundation
Cleveland, Ohio

Steven S.T. Ching, MD
Associate Professor
Department of Ophthalmology
University of Rochester
Rochester, New York

Christopher Y.C. Chow, MD
Clinical Instructor
Department of Ophthalmology
William Belmont Hospital
Royal Oak, Michigan

Elisabeth J. Cohen, MD
Attending Surgeon
Wills Eye Hospital
Co-Director Cornea Service;
Professor
Department of Ophthalmology
Jefferson Medical College
Philadelphia, Pennsylvania

Judith B. Coran, MD
Staff Surgeon
Department of Ophthalmology
Ophthalmology Inc.
Brown University—Rhode Island Hospital
Providence, Rhode Island

Scott W. Cousins, MD
Associate Professor
Department of Ophthalmology
Bascom Palmer Eye Institute
University of Miami School of Medicine
Miami, Florida

John W. Cowden, MD, FACS
Professor and Chairman
Department of Ophthalmology
University of Missouri—Columbia
Columbia, Missouri

Christopher R. Croasdale, MD
Clinical Instructor
Department of Ophthalmology
University of Wisconsin
Madison, Wisconsin

Vincent P. Dahringer, MD
Cornea-Refractive-External Disease
Southeastern Eye Center
Raleigh, North Carolina

Jan Daniel, MD
Department of Ophthalmology
Emory University
School of Medicine
Atlanta, Georgia

Mary Beth Danneffel, BSN, RN
Executive Director/Manager
Sierra Regional Eye and Tissue Bank
University of California Davis, Medical Center
Sacramento, California

Richard M. Davis, MD
Assistant Professor
Department of Ophthalmology
Wake Forest Eye University Eye Center
Bowman Gray School of Medicine
Winston-Salem, North Carolina

Marc D. de Smet, MD, CM, FRCSC, FRC.Ophth
Clinical Immunology Section
Laboratory of Immunology
National Eye Institute
Bethesda, Maryland

Luciene B. de Sousa, MD
Assistant Professor
Department of Ophthalmology
Paulista School of Medicine
Federal University of Sao Paulo
Sao Paulo, BRAZIL

Claes H. Dohlman, MD, PhD
Professor
Department of Ophthalmology
Harvard Medical School
Massachusetts Eye and Ear Infirmary
Boston, Massachusetts

Eric D. Donnenfeld, MD
Co-Chairman, Cornea and External Disease
Department of Ophthalmology
Manhattan Eye, Ear, and Throat Hospital
Assistant Professor
North Shore University Hospital
Cornell University Medical College
New York, New York

Richard K. Dortzbach, MD
Professor
Department of Ophthalmology and Visual Sciences
University of Wisconsin Medical School
Madison, Wisconsin

Donald J. Doughman, MD, FACS
Professor
Department of Ophthalmology
University of Minnesota
Medical Director
Minnesota Lions Eye Bank
Minneapolis, Minnesota

William T. Driebe, Jr, MD
Associate Professor
Cornea and External Diseases
Director, Contact Lens Service
Department of Ophthalmology
University of Florida
Gainesville, Florida

Paul Driver, MD
Clinical Instructor
Department of Ophthalmology
Georgetown University Medical Center
Washington, DC

Paul J. Dubord, MD, FRCSC
Clinical Associate Professor
University of British Columbia
Vancouver, British Columbia
CANADA

Richard J. Duffy, MD
Department of Ophthalmology
Mobile Eye, Ear, Nose and Throat Clinic
Mobile, Alabama

Marcia J. Dunn, MD
Voluntary Clinical Instructor
Department of Ophthalmology
Mount Sinai Medical Center
New York, New York

STEVEN P. DUNN, MD
Director
Cornea Service
Department of Ophthalmology
William Beaumont Hospital
Royal Oak, Michigan

DANIEL S. DURRIE, MD
Assistant Clinical Professor
Department of Ophthalmology
University of Missouri
Kansas City, Missouri

RICHARD A. EIFERMAN, MD, FACS
Clinical Professor
Department of Ophthalmology
University of Louisville;
Chief
Department of Ophthalmology
VA Medical Center
Louisville, Kentucky

JOSEPH A. ELIASON, MD
Chairman
Division of Ophthalmology
Santa Clara Valley Medical Center
Associate Professor
Ophthalmology (Clinical)
Stanford University
Stanford, California

VICTOR M. ELNER, MD, PHD
Associate Professor
Department of Ophthalmology
University of Michigan
Ann Arbor, Michigan

ANNA F. FAKADEJ, MD
Department of Ophthalmology
University of Rochester
Rochester, New York

EMILE J. FARGE, PHD, MPH
Executive Director
Lions Eye Bank of Texas;
Associate Professor
Department of Ophthalmology
Cullen Eye Institute
Baylor College of Medicine;
President
Pan-American Association of Eye Banks
Houston, Texas

R. LINSY FARRIS, MD
Professor
Department of Clinical Ophthalmology
College of Physicians and Surgeons
Columbia, University;
Director
Department of Ophthalmology
Harlem Hospital Center
New York, New York

WILLIAM J. FAULKNER, MD
Cincinnati Eye Institute
Cincinnati, Ohio

ROBERT S. FEDER, MD, MBA
Associate Professor
Department of Ophthalmology
Director, Cornea and External Disease Service
Northwestern University Medical School
Chicago, Illinois

SANDY T. FELDMAN, MS, MD
Associate Professor in Residence
Department of Ophthalmology
University of California, San Diego
School of Medicine
La Jolla, California

M. ELIZABETH FINI, PHD
Director, Developmental Biology
Associate Professor
Departments of Ophthalmology, Dermatology,
and Anatomy and Cellulic Biology
New England Medical Center
Tufts University School of Medicine
Boston, Massachusetts

GEORGE J. FLORAKIS, MD
Assistant Professor
Department of Clinical Ophthalmology
Edward S. Harkness Eye Institute
Columbia University College of Physicians and Surgeons
New York, New York

RICHARD K. FORSTER, MD
Professor
Department of Ophthalmology
Bascom Palmer Eye Institute
University of Miami School of Medicine
Miami, Florida

C. STEPHEN FOSTER, MD, FACS
Professor
Department of Ophthalmology
Massachusetts Eye & Ear Infirmary
Harvard Medical School
Boston, Massachusetts

F. Stuart Foster, PhD
Professor
Department of Medical Biophysics
University of Toronto
Toronto, Ontario
CANADA

Gary N. Foulks, MD, FACS
Professor
Department of Ophthalmology
Director
Cornea Service
Duke University Medical Center
Durham, North Carolina

Bradley D. Fouraker, MD
Associate Professor of Ophthalmology
Cornea & External Disease
Department of Ophthalmology
University of South Florida
Tampa, Florida

Mitchell H. Friedlaender, MD
Director
Cornea and Refractive Surgery
Department of Ophthalmology
Scripps Clinic
La Jolla, California

Richard L. Fuller, BA, MSW
President/CEO U.S. Division
Tissue Banks International
Baltimore, Maryland

Lawrence A. Gans, MD, FACS
Assistant Professor of Clinical Ophthalmology
Department of Ophthalmology & Visual Sciences
Washington University
St. Louis, Missouri

Joel A. Geffin, MD
Private Practice
Windham Community Memorial Hospital
Willimantic, Connecticut

Jeffrey P. Gilbard, MD
Clinical Assistant Professor
Department of Ophthalmology
Harvard Medical School;
Clinical Associate Scientist
Schepens Eye Research Institute
Boston, Massachusetts;
Medical Director
The Cornea Center
Woburn, Massachusetts

Steven M. Gilberg, MD, FRCS(C)
Assistant Professor
Department of Ophthalmology
University of Ottawa Eye Institute
Ottawa, Ontario
CANADA

Peter Gloor, MD
Associate Professor and Director of the Cornea and External Disease Service
Department of Ophthalmology and Visual Science
Yale University School of Medicine
New Haven, Connecticut

Marc Andrew Goldberg, MD
Assistant Professor
Department of Ophthalmology
New York Eye and Ear Infirmary
New York, New York

Andrew Neil Goodfriend
Department of Ophthalmology
University of Rochester
Rochester, New York

John D. Goosey, MD
Clinical Assistant Professor
Department of Ophthalmology
University of Texas Medical School
Houston, Texas

R. Bruce Grene, MD
Assistant Clinical Professor
Department of Surgery
The University of Kansas School of Medicine
Wichita, Kansas

Michael R. Grimmett, MD, FACP
Cornea and External Disease
Lexington, Kentucky

Erich B. Groos, Jr, MD
Private Practice
Cornea and External Disease
Nashville, Tennessee

Robert H. Gross, MD
Shaw Eye Center
Phoenix, Arizona

William D. Gruzensky, MD
Assistant Professor
Department of Ophthalmology
The Wilmer Ophthalmological Institute
Johns Hopkins University School of Medicine
Baltimore, Maryland

Yan Guex-Crosier, MD
Department of Ophthalmology
Hopital Jules Gonin
University of Lausanne
Lausanne, SWITZERLAND

M. Bowes Hamill, MD
Associate Professor
Department of Clinical Ophthalmology
Deputy Chief of Service
Ben Taub General Hospital
Baylor College of Medicine
Houston, Texas

Ellen L. Heck, MT(ASCP), MA
Director
Transplant Services Center
University Southwestern Medical Center
Dallas, Texas

David G. Heidemann, MD
Clinical Instructor
Department of Ophthalmology
William Beaumont Hospital
Royal Oak, Michigan

Michael E. Hettinger, MD, MS
Clinical Assistant Professor
Department of Ophthalmology
Kansas University Medical Center
Kansas City, Kansas;
Kansas City Eye Clinic
Overland Park, Kansas

William G. Hodge, MD, MPH, FRCS(C)
Clinical Instructor
Department of Ophthalmology
Francis I. Proctor Foundation
University of California
San Francisco, California;
Faculty of Medicine
Department of Ophthalmology
McGill University
Montreal, CANADA

Carol J. Hoffman, MD
Department of Ophthalmology
Medical Center of Delaware
Wilmington, Delaware

Edward J. Holland, MD
Professor
Director of Cornea and External Disease Service
Department of Ophthalmology
University of Minnesota
Minneapolis, Minnesota

Gary N. Holland, MD
Professor
Department of Ophthalmology
UCLA School of Medicine
Director
UCLA Ocular Inflammatory Disease Center
Jules Stein Eye Institute
Los Angeles, California

Marc A. Honig, MD
Department of Cornea Service
Wills Eye Hospital
Department of Ophthalmology
Thomas Jefferson University School of Medicine
Philadelphia, Pennsylvania

Sandeep Jain, MD
The Wilmer Institute
Johns Hopkins University
Baltimore, Maryland

Frederick A. Jakobiec, MD, DSc (Med)
Henry Willard Williams Professor
Department of Ophthalmology
Professor
Department of Pathology
Chairman
Department of Ophthalmology
Harvard Medical School
Chief
Department of Ophthalmology
Massachusetts Eye and Ear Infirmary
Boston, Massachusetts

James V. Jester, PhD
Professor
Department of Ophthalmology
University of Texas Southwestern Medical School
Dallas, Texas

Florence M. Johnston, RN, MS
Vice President
Midwest Eye-Bank and Transplantation Center
Ann Arbor, Michigan

David R. Jordan, MD
Associate Professor
Oculoplastic, Orbital and Lacrimal Service
University of Ottawa Eye Institute
Ottawa, Ontario
CANADA

Anastasios John Kanellopoulos, MD
North Shore University Hospital
Cornell University Medical College
New York, New York

Carol L. Karp, MD
Assistant Professor
Department of Clinical Ophthalmology
Bascom Palmer Eye Institute
University of Miami
Miami, Florida

Hassan M. Kattan, MD
Private Practice
Amman, Jordan

Kenneth R. Kenyon, MD
Associate Clinical Professor
Department of Ophthalmology
Harvard Medical School, Cornea Service
Massachusetts Eye and Ear Infirmary
Senior Scientist
The Schepens Eye Research Institute
Boston, Massachusetts

Robert C. Kersten, MD
Associate Professor
Department of Ophthalmology
University of Cincinnati
College of Medicine
Cincinnati, Ohio

David W. Kielty, MD
Clinical Instructor
Department of Ophthalmology
Vanderbilt University
Nashville, Tennessee

Terry Kim, MD
Chief Resident
Emory Eye Center
Atlanta, Georgia

Soohyung Kim, BS
Department of Ophthalmology
University of Vermont College of Medicine
Burlington, Vermont

Colin M. Kirkness, MBChB, FRCS(Ed & Glas), FRCOphth, DEBO
Tennent Professor and Head
Department of Ophthalmology
Tennent Institute
University of Glasgow
Glasgow, SCOTLAND

Steven Klyce, PhD
Professor
Department of Ophthalmology
Louisiana State University Medical Center School of Medicine
Adjunct Professor
Department of Biomedical Engineering
Tulane University
Lions Eye Research Laboratories
LSU Eye Center
Louisiana State University Medical Center School of Medicine
New Orleans, Louisiana

Timothy O. Koch, COT, FCLSA
Director of Eye Care Services
Department of Ophthalmology
Park Nicollet Clinic
St. Louis Park, Minnesota

Jay H. Krachmer, MD
Professor and Chairman
Department of Ophthalmology
University of Minnesota
Minneapolis, Minnesota

Peter R. Laibson, MD
Director
Cornea Service
Wills Eye Hospital;
Professor
Department of Ophthalmology
Thomas Jefferson University School of Medicine
Philadelphia, Pennsylvania

Ronald Laing, PhD
Research Professor
Department of Ophthalmology
Boston University School of Medicine
Boston, Massachusetts

Sheridan Lam, MD
Assistant Professor
Department of Ophthalmology
University of Illinois at Chicago
College of Medicine
Chicago, Illinois

Stephen S. Lane, MD
Associate Clinical Professor
Department of Ophthalmology
University of Minnesota
Minneapolis, Minnesota

Roger H.S. Langston, MD, CM, FACS
Cornea Service
Eye Institute
Cleveland Clinic Foundation
Cleveland, Ohio

Jacques G.H. Lasudry, MD
Department of Ophthalmology and Visual Sciences
University of Wisconsin Medical School
Madison, Wisconsin

Stephen Y. Lee, MD
Instructor
Cornea Service
Department of Ophthalmology
Wills Eye Hospital
Philadelphia, Pennsylvania

Bradley N. Lemke, MD, FACS
Associate Clinical Professor
Department of Ophthalmology and Visual Sciences
University of Wisconsin Medical School
Madison, Wisconsin

Michael A. Lemp, MD
Clinical Professor
Department of Ophthalmology
Georgetown University Medical Center
Washington, DC

Thomas J. Liesegang, MD
Chairman and Professor
Department of Ophthalmology
Mayo Clinic Jacksonville
Jacksonville, Florida

Marilyn R. Lindenauer, MPH
President and Chief Executive Officer
Midwest Eye-Banks and Transplantation Center
Ann Arbor, Michigan

Thomas D. Lindquist, MD, PhD
Professor
Director, Cornea and External Disease Service
Department of Ophthalmology
University of Washington
Medical Director
Lions Eye Bank Serving Washington, Alaska, and Northern Idaho
Seattle, Washington

David Litoff, MD
Opticare
Norwalk, Connecticut

Careen Yen Lowder, MD, PhD
Professional Staff
Department of Uveitis
Division of Ophthalmology
Cleveland Clinic Foundation
Cleveland, Ohio

Anthony J. Lubniewski, MD
Assistant Professor
Cornea and External Disease Service
Chief
Ophthalmology Section, St. Louis VAMC
Department of Ophthalmology and Visual Sciences
Washington University
St. Louis, Missouri

Damien C. Macaluso, MD
Oregon Health Sciences University
Portland, Oregon

Jeffrey J. Machat, MD, FRCSC, DABO
Medical Director
The Laser Center, Inc.
Windsor, Ontario
CANADA

Robert J.S. Mack, MD
Assistant Professor
Department of Ophthalmology
Rush University
Chicago, Illinois

Marian S. Macsai, MD
Associate Professor
Director, Cornea & External Disease Service
Department of Ophthalmology
West Virginia University
Morgantown, West Virginia

Thomas H. Mader, MD
Director
Department of Ophthalmology
Madigan Army Medical Center
Tacoma, Washington

Ezra Maguen, MD
Ophthalmology Research Laboratories
Cedars-Sinai Medical Center
Associate Clinical Professor
Jules Stein Eye Institute
University of California School of Medicine
Los Angeles, California

Leo J. Maguire, MD
Associate Professor
Department of Ophthalmology
Mayo Clinic
Rochester, Minnesota

Mark R. Mandel, MD
Medical Director
Optima Ophthalmic Medical Association
Hayward, California

Mark J. Mannis, MD
Professor
Director, Cornea and External Disease Service
Department of Ophthalmology
University of California, Davis
Sacramento, California

Pierre G. Mardelli, MD
Department of Ophthalmology
University of Missouri-Kansas City
Eye Foundation of Kansas City
Kansas City, Missouri

Csaba L. Mártonyi, COPRA
Associate Professor and Director
Ophthalmic Photography
Department of Ophthalmology
W.K. Kellogg Eye Center
University of Michigan
Ann Arbor, Michigan

William D. Mathers, MD
Associate Professor of Ophthalmology
Director of Corneal Service
Department of Ophthalmology
University of Iowa Hospitals and Clinics
Iowa City, Iowa

Alice Y. Matoba, MD
Chief
Ophthalmology Service
Houston Veterans Affairs Medical Center
Associate Professor
Department of Ophthalmology
Baylor College of Medicine
Houston, Texas

Camille S. Matta, MD
Professor
Department of Ophthalmology
University of Missouri-Kansas City
Eye Foundation of Kansas City
Kansas City, Missouri

Ruth Marie Mattern, MD, PhD
Department of Ophthalmology
The University of Texas Southwestern Medical Center at Dallas
Dallas, Texas

James P. McCulley, MD, FACS, FRCOphth(U.K.)
The David Bruton, Jr. Chair in Ophthalmology
Professor and Chairman
Department of Ophthalmology
University of Texas
Southwestern Medical Center at Dallas

Peter J. McDonnell, MD
Professor
Department of Ophthalmology
Doheny Eye Institute
University of Southern California
Los Angeles, California

Ian W. McLean, MD
Chairman
Department of Ophthalmic Pathology
Armed Forces Institute of Pathology
Washington, DC

James I. McNeill, MD
Professor
Department of Ophthalmology
Loma Linda University
Loma Linda, California

David M. Meisler, MD
Consultant in Corneal and External Diseases
Department of Ophthalmology
Cleveland Clinic Foundation
Cleveland, Ohio

Corey A. Miller, MD
Chairman
Division of Ophthalmology
LDS Hospital
Clinical Associate Professor
Department of Ophthalmology
University of Utah
Salt Lake City, Utah

Royce Mohan, MS, PhD
Research Associate
Department of Ophthalmology
New England Eye Center
New England Medical Center
Boston, Massachusetts

Bartly J. Mondino, MD
Chairman
Department of Ophthalmology
Director
Jules Stein Eye Institute
Los Angeles, California

Andrew Lee Moyes, MD
Clinical Instructor
Department of Ophthalmology
University of Kansas Medical Center
Kansas City, Kansas

Reza M. Mozayeni, MD
Department of Ophthalmology
University of Minnesota
Minneapolis, Minnesota

Fernando Murillo-Lopez, MD
Cornea Department
Department of Ophthalmology
Bascom Palmer Eye Institute
University of Miami School of Medicine
Miami, Florida

Michael Murphy, MD
Department of Ophthalmology
University of Iowa
Iowa City, Iowa

Samuel E. Navon, PhD, MD
Massachusetts Eye & Ear Infirmary
The Schepens Eye Research Institute
Department of Ophthalmology
Harvard Medical School
Cornea Consultants
Boston, Massachusetts

J. Daniel Nelson, MD, FACS
Chairman
Department of Ophthalmology
HealthPartners-Ramsey Clinic
HealthPartners-St. Paul-Ramsey Medical Center
St. Paul, Minnesota;
Associate Professor
Department of Ophthalmology
University of Minnesota
Minneapolis, Minnesota

Jeffrey A. Nerad, MD
Professor of Ophthalmology
Director, Oculoplastic, Orbital and Oncology Service
Department of Ophthalmology
University of Iowa Hospitals and Clinics
Iowa City, Iowa

Bruce D. Nichols, BSc, MD, FRCSC, FACS
Assistant Professor
Department of Ophthalmology
University Hospital
University of Western Ontario
London, Ontario
CANADA

Jerry Y. Niederkorn, PhD
Professor
Director, Ophthalmic Research
Department of Ophthalmology
The University of Texas Southwestern Medical Center at Dallas
Dallas, Texas

Teruo Nishida, MD, DSc
Professor and Chairman
Department of Ophthalmology
Yamaguchi University School of Medicine
Ube-City, Yamaguchi
JAPAN

Robert A. Nozik, MD
Co-Director Uveitis Clinic
Proctor Foundation
University of California at San Francisco
San Francisco, California

Robert B. Nussenblatt, MD
Scientific Director
National Eye Institute
National Institutes of Health
Bethesda, Maryland

Terrence P. O'Brien, MD
Director, Ocular Microbiology Laboratory
Department of Ophthalmology
The Wilmer Eye Institute
Johns Hopkins University School of Medicine
Baltimore, Maryland

David George O'Day, MD
Assistant Professor
Department of Ophthalmology
Cornea Service
Case Western Reserve University
Cleveland, Ohio

Mary Jane O'Neill
Executive Director
The Eye-Bank for Sight Restoration, Inc.
New York, New York

Donna Oiland
Director
Lions Eye Bank Serving Washington, Northern Idaho, and Alaska
Department of Ophthalmology
University of Washington School of Medicine
Seattle, Washington

Karen W. Oxford, MD
Assistant Clinical Professor
Department of Ophthalmology
California Pacific Medical Center
San Francisco, California

David A. Palay, MD
Assistant Professor
Department of Ophthalmology
Emory University
Atlanta, Georgia

Alan G. Palestine, MD
Clinical Associate Professor
Department of Ophthalmology
Georgetown University
Washington, DC

Florentino E. Palmon, MD
Eye Centers of Florida
Fort Myers, Florida

Noorjahan Panjwani, PhD
Associate Professor
Department of Ophthalmology
New England Eye Center
Department of Ophthalmology
Tufts University School of Medicine
Boston, Massachusetts

Thanassis Papaioannou, MS
Research Scientist
Laser Research & Technology Development Program
Cedars-Sinai Medical Center
Los Angeles, California

Matthew R. Parsons, MD
Assistant Clinical Professor
Department of Ophthalmology
University of Utah
Salt Lake City, Utah

Charles J. Pavlin, MD, FRCS (Can)
Associate Professor
Department of Medicine
University of Toronto
Toronto, Ontario
CANADA

Eric S. Pearlstein, MD
Assistant Attending
Department of Ophthalmology
The Long Island College Hospital
Brooklyn, New York

Jay S. Pepose, MD, PhD
Bernard Becker Professor
Department of Ophthalmology and Visual Sciences
Washington University School of Medicine
St. Louis, Missouri

W. Matthew Petroll, PhD
Associate Professor of Ophthalmology
Member, Joint Graduate Studies Committee
in Biomedical Engineering
Department of Ophthalmology
University of Texas
Southwestern Medical Center at Dallas
Dallas, Texas

Daryl A. Pfister, MD
Department of Ophthalmology
University of Minnesota
Minneapolis, Minnesota

Roswell R. Pfister, MD
Past Chairman
Clinical Professor
Department of Ophthalmology
University of Alabama
Director
The Eye Research Laboratories
Brookwood Medical Center
Birmingham, Alabama

Stephen C. Pflugfelder, MD
Associate Professor
Department of Ophthalmology
Bascom Palmer Eye Institute
University of Miami School of Medicine
Miami, Florida

Christine T. Pham, MD
Department of Internal Medicine
Division of Rheumatology
Washington University
St. Louis, Missouri

Larry W. Piebenga, MD
Clinical Professor
Director of Cornea Service
Department of Ophthalmology
University of Missouri-Kansas City
Eye Foundation of Kansas City
Kansas City, Missouri

Ronald D. Plotnik, MD
Assistant Professor
Department of Ophthalmology
University of Rochester School of Medicine and Dentistry
Rochester, New York

Peter J. Polack, MD
Cornea & External Disease
Department of Ophthalmology
University of South Florida
Tampa, Florida

Francis W. Price, Jr, MD
Corneal Consultants of Indiana
Indianapolis, Indiana

Louis E. Probst, MD
Assistant Professor
University of Western Ontario
London, Ontario
CANADA

Julian A. Procope, MD
Corneal Consultants of Indiana
Indianapolis, Indiana

John J. Purcell, Jr, MD, FACS
Associate Professor
Department of Ophthalmology
St. Louis University School of Medicine;
Director
Department of Ophthalmology
St. Mary's Health Center
St. Louis, Missouri

Andrew A. E. Pyott, BSc, MB, FRCS (Glasgow), FRC.Ophth
Senior Registrar
Department of Ophthalmology
Tennent Institute
University of Glasgow
Glasgow, SCOTLAND

Michael B. Raizman, MD
Director
Cornea and Anterior Segment Service
New England Eye Center
Assistant Professor
Department of Ophthalmology
Tufts University School of Medicine
Boston, Massachusetts

Christopher J. Rapuano, MD
Attending Physician
Cornea Service
Wills Eye Hospital
Assistant Professor
Thomas Jefferson University School of Medicine
Philadelphia, Pennsylvania

C. Derek Ratliff, MD
Attending Ophthalmologist
Cornea and External Disease
Department of Ophthalmology
Bassett Healthcare
Cooperstown, New York

Charles S. Reing, MD
Clinical Instructor
Mount Sinai Medical Center
Attending Physician
New York Eye and Ear Infirmary
New York, New York;
Attending Physician
Wayne General Hospital
Wayne, New Jersey;
Attending Physician
St. Joseph's Hospital and Medical Center
Peterson, New Jersey;
Attending Physician
Chilton Memorial Hospital
Pompton Plains, New Jersey

William J. Reinhart, MD
Associate Professor
Department of Ophthalmology
Director, Cornea Service
Case Western Reserve University
Cleveland, Ohio

John Jacob Requard, III, BS
Director
Eye Bank Operations
Mid-America Transplant Services
St. Louis, Missouri

Larry F. Rich, MD, MS
Associate Professor
Department of Ophthalmology
Director
Cornea and External Disease Service
Casey Eye Institute
Oregon Health Sciences University
Portland, Oregon

Robert H. Rosa, Jr, MD
Assistant Professor
Bascom Palmer Eye Institute
University of Miami
Miami, Florida

J. James Rowsey, MD
Professor and Chairman
Department of Ophthalmology
University of South Florida
Tampa, Florida

Roy Scott Rubinfeld, MD
Clinical Associate Professor
Department of Ophthalmology
Georgetown University Medical Center
Attending Surgeon
Washington Hospital Center
Private Practice
Washington, DC

David I. Sabir, MD
Department of Ophthalmology
University of Minnesota
Minneapolis, Minnesota

Alan E. Sadowsky, MD
Clinical Assistant Professor
Department of Ophthalmology
University of Minnesota;
Practice Affiliation: Columbia Park Medical Group
Minneapolis, Minnesota

James J. Salz, MD
Clinical Professor
Department of Ophthalmology
University of Southern California
Los Angeles, California

John R. Samples, MD
Director
Glaucoma Services
Casey Eye Institute
Portland, Oregon

Steven C. Schallhorn, MD
Doheny Eye Institute
University of Southern California
Los Angeles, California

Bradley H. Scharf, MD
Private Practice
The New York Eye and Ear Infirmary
New Rochelle Hospital Medical Center
New Rochelle, New York

Miriam Schteingart, MD
Ophthalmologist–Cornea Uveitis
Anderson Eye Center
Saginaw, Michigan

Gregory S. Schultz, PhD
Professor
Department of Obstetrics/Gynecology
Adjunct Professor
Department of Ophthalmology
University of Florida
Gainesville, Florida

Ivan R. Schwab, MD
Professor of Ophthalmology
University of California, Davis
Department of Ophthalmology
Sacramento, California

Brian L. Schwam, MD
Clinical Instructor
Department of Ophthalmology
University of Pittsburgh School of Medicine
Pittsburgh, Pennsylvania;
Department of Ophthalmology
Wheeling Eye Institute
Wheeling, West Virginia;
Former Cornea Fellow and Clinical Instructor
Department of Ophthalmology
New England Eye Center
Tufts University School of Medicine
Boston, Massachusetts

Gary S. Schwartz, MD
Clinical Instructor
Department of Ophthalmology
University of Minnesota
Minneapolis, Minnesota

Gaurav K. Shah, MD
Department of Ophthalmology
University of Minnesota
Minneapolis, Minnesota

Michael B. Shapiro, MD
Cornea Specialist
Department of Ophthalmology
Davis Duehr-Eye Association and University of Wisconsin
Madison, Wisconsin

John W. Shore, MD
Assistant Clinical Professor
Department of Ophthalmology
Harvard Medical School
Department of Ophthalmology
Eye Plastics and Orbit Service
Ophthalmic Consultants of Boston
Boston, Massachusetts

Janine A. Smith, MD
National Eye Institute
National Institutes of Health
Bethesda, Maryland

Eugene M. Smith, Jr, MD
Clinical Lecturer
Department of Ophthalmology
University of Arizona
Tucson, Arizona

H. Kaz Soong, MD
Associate Professor of Ophthalmology
Department of Ophthalmology
University of Michigan Medical School
Ann Arbor, Michigan

Sarkis H. Soukiasian, MD
Director
Cornea and External Diseases
Department of Ophthalmology
Lahey Clinic Medical Center
Assistant Clinical Professor
Tufts University School of Medicine
Burlington, Massachusetts

Mark G. Speaker, MD, PhD
Director of Corneal & Refractive Surgery
Department of Ophthalmology
New York Eye and Ear Infirmary
New York, New York

John F. Stamler, MD, PhD
Clinical Instructor
Department of Ophthalmology
University of Iowa
Iowa City, Iowa

Walter Stark, MD
Professor
Department of Ophthalmology
Director, Corneal Service
The Johns Hopkins Hospital
The Wilmer Institute
Baltimore, Maryland

George A. Stern, MD
Professor
Department of Ophthalmology
Director
Corneal and External Disease Service
University of Florida College of Medicine
Gainesville, Florida

Scott X. Stevens, MD
Assistant Professor of Ophthalmology
Cornea & External Disease
Department of Ophthalmology
University of South Florida
Tampa, Florida

E. Lee Stock, MD
Director
Cornea & External Eye Disease Laboratory
VA Lakeside Medical Center
Associate Professor
Department of Ophthalmology
Northwestern University
Chicago, Illinois

Glenn L. Stoller, MD
Department of Ophthalmology
Harkness Eye Institute
Columbia Presbyterian Hospital
New York, New York

Barbara W. Streeten, MD
Professor
Departments of Ophthalmology and Pathology
State University of New York Health Science Center at Syracuse
Syracuse, New York

R. Doyle Stulting, MD, PhD
Professor
Department of Ophthalmology
Emory University School of Medicine
Atlanta, Georgia

Alan Sugar, MD
Professor
Department of Ophthalmology
W.K. Kellogg Eye Center
University of Michigan Medical School
Ann Arbor, Michigan

Joel Sugar, MD
Professor and Director of Cornea Service
Department of Ophthalmology
University of Illinois at Chicago
Chicago, Illinois

Joseph Tauber, MD
Associate Professor
Department of Ophthalmology
University of Missouri at Kansas City
Kansas City, Missouri

Howard H. Tessler, MD
Professor
Department of Ophthalmology
University of Illinois at Chicago
University of Illinois Eye and Ear Infirmary
Chicago, Illinois

Keith P. Thompson, MD
Assistant Professor
Department of Ophthalmology—Cornea and External Diseases
The Emory Clinic
Atlanta, Georgia

Elias I. Traboulsi, MD
Associate Professor
Departments of Ophthalmology and Pediatrics
The Johns Hopkins Center for Hereditary Eye Diseases
The Wilmer Ophthalmological Institute
Baltimore, Maryland

Julie C. Tsai, MD
Cornea & External Disease
Department of Ophthalmology
University of South Florida
Tampa, Florida

David T. Tse, MD, FACS
Professor
Department of Ophthalmology
Bascom Palmer Eye Institute
University of Miami School of Medicine
Miami, Florida

Woodford Van Meter, MD
Associate Clinical Professor
Department of Ophthalmology
University of Kentucky
Lexington, Kentucky

Gary A. Varley, MD
Cincinnati Eye Institute
Cincinnati, Ohio

David D. Verdier, MD
Associate Clinical Professor
Michigan State University College of Human Medicine
Grand Rapids, Michigan

Michael P. Vrabec, MD, FACS
Assistant Clinical Professor
Department of Ophthalmology and Visual Sciences
University of Wisconsin
Madison, Wisconsin

Michael D. Wagoner, MD
Medical Director
King Khaled Eye Specialist Hospital
Riyadh, Saudi Arabia;
Department of Ophthalmology
Harvard Medical School
Cornea Service
Massachusetts Eye and Ear Infirmary
The Schepens Eye Research Institute
Boston, Massachusetts

R. Christopher Walton, MD
Laboratory of Immunology
National Eye Institute
National Institutes of Health
Bethesda, Maryland

George O. Waring, III, MD, FACS, FRC.Ophth
Professor of Ophthalmology
Director Refractive Surgery
Department of Ophthalmology
Emory University School of Medicine
Atlanta, Georgia

Michael A. Warner, MD
Harvard Medical School
Department of Ophthalmology
Massachusetts Eye & Ear Infirmary
Boston, Massachusetts

Guy F. Webster, MD, PhD
Associate Professor
Department of Dermatology
Jefferson Medical College
Philadelphia, Pennsylvania

Robert G. Webster, Jr, MD
Consultant
Cornea-External Disease
Department of Ophthalmology
California Pacific Medical Center
San Francisco, California

Robert W. Weisenthal, MD
Clinical Assistant Professor
Chief—Veterans Administrator
Department of Ophthalmology
State University of New York Health Science Center at Syracuse
Syracuse, New York

Scott M. Whitcup, MD
Clinical Director
National Eye Institute
National Institutes of Health
Bethesda, Maryland

William E. Whitson, MD
Corneal Consultants of Indiana
Indianapolis, Indiana

Kirk R. Wilhelmus, MD
Professor
Department of Ophthalmology
Cullen Eye Institute
Baylor College of Medicine
Houston, Texas

Joseph M. Williams, MD, PhD
Instructor
Department of Ophthalmology and Visual Sciences
Washington University Medical Center
St. Louis, Missouri

Rebecca M. Willis, MD
Department of Ophthalmology
Marshfield Clinic
Marshfield, Wisconsin

Darrell E. Wolfley, MD
Director of Orbital and Ophthalmic Plastic Surgery
Department of Ophthalmology
Yale School of Medicine
New Haven, Connecticut

Douglas A. Young, MD
Cornea & External Disease
Department of Ophthalmology
University of South Florida
Tampa, Florida

Gerald W. Zaidman, MD
Associate Professor of Ophthalmology
Director, Cornea and External Disease Service
Department of Ophthalmology
New York Medical College
Westchester County Medical Center
Valhalla, New York

To

my Wife, Kathryn
our Children, Edward, Kara, and Jill
our Parents, Paul and Rebecca Krachmer
and Louis and Gertrude Maraist
with great love and appreciation.

Jay H. Krachmer

To

these dedicated Men of Medicine,
Elia M. Ayoub
Hugh M. Hill
Melvin L. Rubin
Gerold L. Schiebler
Morton E. Smith
who inspired me to teach.

Mark J. Mannis

To

my Wife, Melissa
our Son, Edward Colson
my Mother, Joan
and my Father, John
who have provided me with the love, understanding,
and support that enabled me to complete this project.

Edward J. Holland

Preface

Who would believe that so small a space (the eye) could contain the images of all the universe?

Leonardo da Vinci

Two years ago, when we were first approached by Mosby–Year Book to edit a comprehensive set of volumes on cornea and external disease, we asked ourselves if there was truly a need for another text on the cornea. There are already several fine books currently available on the subject. As our mission began to define itself, however, we realized that there was no single compendium of information that covered basic science, primary and secondary corneal disease, disorders of the external eye, and the broad variety of surgery that falls into the purview of the corneal specialist—including refractive surgery.

We accepted the challenge with some trepidation, spurred on by the tantalizing possibility of assembling the very best of our subspecialty to provide a resource that would yield useful information at every level of interest. To this end, we have made a concerted effort to construct this book in a way that we feel will be most useful to a variety of readers.

Volume One reviews the basic science of the cornea and external eye. Also included in this volume is a lengthy section on examination techniques and clinical approaches to common problems in cornea and external disease; this section is designed to help organize the reader's clinical thinking rather than to present clinical entities in the usual annotated textbook format. Relying on the clinical experience of seasoned experts in the field, this section is aimed at fostering clinical acumen rather than summoning scholarly erudition. The first volume also contains a section on state-of-the-art eye banking. In a more traditional fashion, Volume II catalogs the clinical diagnosis and management of the broad variety of diseases that affect the lids, conjunctiva, cornea, sclera, and anterior uvea. Volume III is devoted to surgery of the cornea and conjunctiva, including related anterior segment, oculoplastic, and refractive surgery.

Producing a "single source" text of this type that truly adds something to the ophthalmic library is an enormous challenge. Our goal was to provide a book that teaches but that also serves as an encyclopedic resource. In addition, because ophthalmology is an essentially graphic specialty of medicine in which diagnosis and treatment are based on what one sees rather than what one infers or deduces, the graphic elements of this book were as important as the text. In the same way in which we edited text to maximize information and clarity, we employed computer enhancement technology to produce "edited" photographic images that clearly illustrate salient clinical features.

The demands on our contributing authors were significant. But thanks to their zeal and hard labor, we were able to produce this work in a relatively short time in order to provide the reader with the most current information in the field. The collective knowledge of our contributors represents an enormous body of information, and it has been our great privilege to attempt to organize it in a way that will be of use to our colleagues in ophthalmology.

Our desire to produce this text has been fueled by our fellows and residents, who have continued to give us both the challenge and the satisfaction of teaching what is surely the most beautiful aspect of the most noble of medical specialties. Da Vinci's wonder of the eye is echoed by those of us who have spent our professional lives with the transparent disc through which all visible light passes and from which emanates so much fascination.

Acknowledgments

It is clear that a work of this size is the product of many individuals. First and foremost, our thanks must go to our contributing authors without whose expertise this effort would not have been possible. Their drive to provide the very best and their resilience in response to the difficult process of editing has been exceptional. We also thank the often unsung contributors to projects of this scope. Our special thanks go to Kari Graham, who served as the "central dispatcher" of this text, carefully coordinating the tracking and editorial progress of 178 chapters over many months to ensure the timely and efficient management of each contribution. Likewise, we would like to thank Nancy Robinson, who handled and coordinated the transfer of manuscripts between Minneapolis and Sacramento. Our appreciation is also extended to Joanna Krahn at the University of Minnesota and to Linda McKinley and Kathy Falk at Mosby for their attention to the book during the editing process. To our professional colleagues and to our fellows and residents who suffered our obsession with this book, we express our appreciation both for their patience and for the many ideas they gave us. And finally, we thank our families who nurtured our enthusiasm and gave us the time taken from them to accomplish this task.

Contents

Volume I

Fundamentals of Cornea and External Disease

Part I BASIC SCIENCE AND PATHOPHYSIOLOGIC RESPONSES

SECTION 1 *Basic Science: Cornea, Sclera, and Ocular Adnexa Anatomy, Biochemistry, Physiology, and Biomechanics*

1. Cornea, 3
TERUO NISHIDA
2. Sclera, 29
NOORJAHAN PANJWANI
JOYCE MOHAN
3. The Conjunctiva: Anatomy and Physiology, 41
J. DANIEL NELSON
J. DOUGLAS CAMERON
4. Tear Film, 49
CHRISTOPHER Y.C. CHOW
JEFFREY P. GILBARD
5. Eyelids, 61
DARRELL E. WOLFLEY

SECTION 2 *Pathologic Responses of the Cornea, Sclera, and Ocular Adnexa*

6. The Ocular Immune Response, 68
CHARLES S. BOUCHARD
7. Corneal Responses to Infection, 129
JOSEPH M. WILLIAMS
M. ELIZABETH FINI
SCOTT W. COUSINS
JAY S. PEPOSE
8. Corneal Reaction to Injury, 163
J. DOUGLAS CAMERON
9. Modulation of Corneal Wound Healing, 183
GREGORY S. SCHULTZ
10. Pathogenesis of Sterile Corneal Erosions and Ulcerations, 199
DAMIEN C. MACALUSO
SANDY T. FELDMAN

Part II EXAMINING AND IMAGING THE CORNEA AND EXTERNAL EYE

SECTION 1 *The Anterior Refracting Surface of the Cornea*

11. Refraction of the Abnormal Cornea, 215
DAVID W. KIELTY
12. Keratometry, Photokeratoscopy, and Computer-assisted Topographic Analysis, 223
LEO J. MAGUIRE

SECTION 2 *Basic Evaluation and Photography of the Cornea and External Eye*

13. Examination of the Lids, 237
WILLIAM D. MATHERS
14. Slit Lamp Examination, 243
CSABA L. MÁRTONYI
15. Tear Film Evaluation, 269
R. LINSY FARRIS
16. Corneal Diagnostic Techniques, 275
WILLIAM J. FAULKNER
GARY A. VARLEY
17. Photography of the Cornea and External Eye, 283
CSABA L. MÁRTONYI

SECTION 3 *Microbiologic and Cytologic Testing*

18. Laboratory Investigation: Microbiologic and Cytologic Testing, 305
ALICE Y. MATOBA

SECTION 4 *High Magnification Techniques*

19. Specular Microscopy, 313
RONALD LAING
20. Confocal Microscopy, 335
W. MATTHEW PETROLL
H. DWIGHT CAVANAGH
JAMES V. JESTER

21. High Resolution Ultrasound, 351
CHARLES J. PAVLIN
F. STUART FOSTER

SECTION 5 *Routine Examination*
22. Points of Emphasis, 361
JAY H. KRACHMER

PART III APPROACH TO THE DIAGNOSIS AND MANAGEMENT OF SELECTED CORNEA AND EXTERNAL EYE DISEASE PROBLEMS

23. Congenital Corneal Opacities: Diagnosis and Management, 367
JUDITH B. CORAN
EUGENE M. SMITH, JR.
JUAN J. ARENTSEN
24. Peripheral Corneal Disease, 387
GEORGE A. STERN
25. The Corneal Ulcer, 403
CAROL L. KARP
RICHARD K. FORSTER
26. Corneal Edema, 409
JOEL A. GEFFIN
ROBERT G. WEBSTER, JR.
27. Corneal Deposits, 417
WILLIAM Z. BRIDGES, JR.
DAVID A. PALAY
28. Corneal Infiltrates in the Contact Lens Patient, 429
CAROL J. HOFFMAN
CHRISTOPHER J. RAPUANO
ELISABETH J. COHEN
29. The Red Eye: A Clinical Guide to a Rapid and Accurate Diagnosis, 437
MICHAEL B. SHAPIRO
CHRISTOPHER R. CROASDALE
30. Minimal Visual Loss: Determining the Role of the Cornea, 447
DAVID LITOFF
31. The Patient with Itching and Burning, 457
E. LEE STOCK

PART IV EYE BANKING

SECTION 1 *Organization of Eye Banks*
32. Structure and Function of Eye Banks, 463
MARY BETH DANNEFFEL
33. The Eye Bank Association of America: Purpose, Organization, Medical Standards, and Certification, 469
ELLEN L. HECK
34. The Evolution, Structure, and Function of Eye Bank Networks, 475
JOHN JACOB REQUARD, III
35. International Eye Banking Structure and Function, 481
PAUL J. DUBORD

SECTION 2 *Eye Banking Methods and Standards*
36. Medical Standards for Eye Banking, 485
WILLIAM J. REINHART
37. Tissue Removal, 493
DONNA OILAND
38. Tissue Evaluation, 501
RICHARD M. DAVIS
39. Tissue Storage, 509
DONALD J. DOUGHMAN
40. Tissue Distribution, 519
MARILYN R. LINDENAUER
FLORENCE M. JOHNSTON

SECTION 3 *Special Eye Banking Issues*
41. Governmental Relations, 525
PATRICIA AIKEN-O'NEILL
42. Ethics and Eye Banking, 531
EMILE J. FARGE
43. Medical Legal Issues, 537
RICHARD L. FULLER
44. Fundraising and Financial Issues, 543
MARY JANE O'NEILL
45. Public Relations and Education, 547
MARY JANE O'NEILL
46. The Role of Eye Banking in Vision Research, 553
RUTH MARIE MATTERN
H. DWIGHT CAVANAGH

VOLUME II

Cornea and External Disease: Clinical Diagnosis and Management

PART V THE OCULAR ADNEXA

SECTION 1 *Diseases of the Lid: Anatomic Abnormalities*
47. Entropion, Ectropion, and Trichiasis, 561
JACQUES G. H. LASUDRY
RICHARD K. DORTZBACH
BRADLEY N. LEMKE
48. Lagophthalmos and Other Malpositions of the Lid, 571
ROBERT C. KERSTEN

SECTION 2 *Diseases of the Lid: Tumors*
49. Benign Lid Tumors, 581
MICHAEL L. MURPHY
JEFFREY A. NERAD

50. Malignant Lid Tumors, 601
DAVID T. TSE
STEVEN M. GILBERG

SECTION 3 *Diseases of the Lid: Inflammation and Infections*

51. Blepharitis: Overview and Classification, 621
JOSEPH A. ELIASON
52. Seborrhea and Meibomian Gland Dysfunction, 625
PAUL DRIVER
MICHAEL A. LEMP
53. Bacterial Eyelid Infections, 633
LOUIS E. PROBST
54. Viral Eyelid Infections, 641
BRADLEY H. SCHARF
55. Fungal and Parasitic Eyelid Infections, 653
ANDREW LEE MOYES
VICTOR M. ELNER

SECTION 4 *Disorders of Tear Production and the Lacrimal System*

56. Dry Eye, 663
FERNANDO MURILLO-LOPEZ
STEPHEN C. PFLUGFELDER
57. Dacryoadenitis, Dacryocystitis, and Canaliculitis, 687
DAVID R. JORDAN
58. Epiphora, 695
RICHARD J. BENSINGER

SECTION 5 *Conjunctival Disease: Tumors*

59. Squamous Neoplasms of the Conjunctiva, 701
MICHAEL A. WARNER
FREDERICK A. JAKOBIEC
60. Melanocytic Neoplasms of the Conjunctiva, 715
IAN W. MCLEAN
61. Subepithelial Neoplasms of the Conjunctiva, 723
MICHAEL A. WARNER
FREDERICK A. JAKOBIEC

SECTION 6 *Conjunctivitis*

62. Conjunctivitis: An Overview and Classification, 745
THOMAS D. LINDQUIST
63. Bacterial Conjunctivitis, 759
SARKIS H. SOUKIASIAN
JULES BAUM
64. Viral Conjunctivitis, 773
JOHN F. STAMLER
65. Chlamydial Infections, 779
JOHN WILLIAM CHANDLER
66. Ophthalmia Neonatorum, 789
THOMAS D. LINDQUIST
67. Parinaud's Oculoglandular Syndrome, 797
WILLIAM D. GRUZENSKY
68. Allergic Conjunctivitis, 805
MITCHELL H. FRIEDLAENDER
69. Vernal and Atopic Keratoconjunctivitis, 811
NEAL P. BARNEY
70. Giant Papillary Conjunctivitis, 819
STEVEN P. DUNN
DAVID G. HEIDEMANN
71. Cicatricial Pemphigoid, 827
C. STEPHEN FOSTER
72. Erythema Multiforme, Stevens-Johnson Syndrome, and Toxic Epidermal Necrolysis, 835
FLORENTINO E. PALMON
GUY F. WEBSTER
EDWARD J. HOLLAND
73. Toxic Conjunctivitis, 847
STEVEN D. CHANG
74. Superior Limbic Keratoconjunctivitis, 857
WILLIAM T. DRIEBE, JR.
75. Ligneous Conjunctivitis, 863
EDWARD J. HOLLAND
GARY S. SCHWARTZ

PART VI DISEASES OF THE CORNEA

SECTION 1 *Developmental Abnormalities of the Cornea*

76. Developmental Corneal Anomalies of Size and Shape, 871
TERRY KIM
DAVID A. PALAY
77. Anterior Chamber Cleavage Syndromes, 885
JOHN R. SAMPLES

SECTION 2 *Corneal Manifestations of Systemic Disease and Therapies*

78. Corneal Manifestations of Metabolic Diseases, 897
KENNETH R. KENYON
SAMUEL E. NAVON
79. Skeletal and Connective Tissue Disorders with Anterior Segment Manifestations, 925
ELIAS I. TRABOULSI
HASSAN M. KATTAN
80. Inflammatory Bowel Disease and Other Systemic Inflammatory Diseases, 943
GEORGE J. FLORAKIS
GLENN L. STOLLER
81. Nutritional Disorders, 955
ANDREW A.E. PYOTT
COLIN M. KIRKNESS
82. Hematologic Disorders, 967
MICHAEL R. GRIMMETT
83. Endocrine Disease and the Cornea, 979
REBECCA M. WILLIS
84. Dermatologic Disorders, 989
ALAN E. SADOWSKY
85. Infectious Disease: Corneal Manifestations, 1003
GAURAV K. SHAH
JAY H. KRACHMER
86. Corneal and External Ocular Infections in Acquired Immunodeficiency Syndrome (AIDS), 1017
DAVID M. MEISLER
CAREEN Y. LOWDER
GARY N. HOLLAND

87. Corneal Manifestations of Local and Systemic Therapies, 1023
CAROL J. HOFFMAN
PETER R. LAIBSON

SECTION 3 *Corneal Dystrophies, Ectatic Disorders, and Degenerations*

88. Anterior Corneal Dystrophies, 1033
PETER R. LAIBSON

89. The Stromal Dystrophies, 1043
MARK J. MANNIS
LUCIENE B. DE SOUSA
ROBERT H. GROSS

90. Posterior Membrane Dystrophies, 1063
ROBERT W. WEISENTHAL
BARBARA W. STREETEN

91. Noninflammatory Ectatic Disorders, 1091
ROBERT S. FEDER

92. Iridocorneal Endothelial Syndrome, 1107
EMMETT F. CARPEL

93. Corneal and Conjunctival Degenerations, 1119
ANDREW NEIL GOODFRIEND
STEVEN S.T. CHING

SECTION 4 *Corneal Infections*

94. Bacterial Keratitis, 1139
TERRENCE P. O'BRIEN

95. Herpes Simplex Keratitis, 1191
EDWARD J. HOLLAND
REZA M. MOZAYENI
GARY S. SCHWARTZ

96. Herpes Zoster Keratitis, 1225
THOMAS J. LIESEGANG

97. Less Common Viral Corneal Infections, 1243
KENNETH C. CHERN
DAVID M. MEISLER

98. Fungal Keratitis, 1253
EDUARDO C. ALFONSO
ROBERT H. ROSA, JR.

99. Acanthamoeba Keratitis, 1267
HASSAN ALIZADEH
JERRY Y. NIEDERKORN
JAMES P. MCCULLEY

SECTION 5 *Interstitial Keratitis*

100. Syphilitic Interstitial Keratitis, 1275
KIRK R. WILHELMUS

101. Nonsyphilitic Interstitial Keratitis, 1307
SCOTT M. WHITCUP
JANINE A. SMITH

SECTION 6 *Noninfectious Keratopathy*

102. Recurrent Erosion Syndromes, 1317
ROY SCOTT RUBINFELD

103. Filamentary Keratitis, 1327
ANNA F. FAKADEJ
RONALD D. PLOTNIK

104. The Superficial Punctate Keratitis of Thygeson, 1333
IVAN R. SCHWAB

105. Neurotrophic Keratitis, 1339
ERICH B. GROOS, JR.

106. Factitious Keratoconjunctivitis, 1349
MATTHEW R. PARSONS

SECTION 7 *Immunologic Disorders of the Cornea*

107. Corneal Disease in Rheumatoid Arthritis, 1359
MARC ANDREW GOLDBERG
CHRISTINE T. PHAM
ANTHONY J. LUBNIEWSKI

108. Corneal Disease Associated With Non-rheumatoid Collagen-vascular Disease, 1377
JOEL SUGAR

109. Phlyctenular Keratoconjunctivitis and Marginal Staphylococcal Keratitis, 1389
REZA M. MOZAYENI
SHERIDAN LAM

110. Mooren's Ulcer, 1397
GERALD W. ZAIDMAN
BARTLEY J. MONDINO

SECTION 8 *Corneal Trauma*

111. Corneal Injury, 1403
M. BOWES HAMILL

112. Surgical Trauma: Pseudophakic and Aphakic Corneal Edema, 1423
ALAN SUGAR

113. Acid Injuries of the Eye, 1437
DARYL A. PFISTER
ROSWELL R. PFISTER

114. Alkali-Injuries of the Eye, 1443
ROSWELL R. PFISTER
DARYL A. PFISTER

SECTION 9 *Contact Lenses*

115. Indications for Contact Lens Use, 1453
ROBERT C. CAMPBELL
TIMOTHY O. KOCH

116. Fitting the Abnormal Cornea, 1457
PENNY A. ASBELL
MARCIA J. DUNN

117. Complications of Contact Lens Wear, 1461
JOHN F. STAMLER

PART VII THE SCLERA AND ANTERIOR UVEA

SECTION 1 *Disorders of the Sclera*

118. Episcleritis, 1473
ERIC S. PEARLSTEIN

119. Scleritis, 1479
BRIAN L. SCHWAM
MICHAEL B. RAIZMAN

SECTION 2 *Anterior Uveitis*

120. Classification and Diagnosis of Anterior Uveitis, 1493
R. CHRISTOPHER WALTON
ROBERT B. NUSSENBLATT

121. Idiopathic Uveitis, 1505
WILLIAM G. HODGE
ROBERT A. NOZIK

122. HLA-B27–Related Uveitis, 1515
MARC D. DE SMET
YAN GUEX-CROSIER

123. Sarcoidosis, 1523
MIRIAM SCHTEINGART
HOWARD H. TESSLER

124. Behçet's Disease, 1529
DAVID I. SABIR
ALAN G. PALESTINE

125. Fuchs' Heterochromic Iridocyclitis, 1537
SHERIDAN LAM
HOWARD H. TESSLER

126. Juvenile Rheumatoid Arthritis, 1541
JOSEPH TAUBER

VOLUME III

Surgery of the Cornea and Conjunctiva

PART VIII PENETRATING KERATOPLASTY

SECTION 1 *Preoperative Considerations*

127. Indications and Outcomes, 1551
JAMES I. MCNEILL

128. Preoperative Evaluation of the Keratoplasty Patient, 1563
FREDERICK S. BRIGHTBILL
ROBERT E. BRASS

129. Instrumentation for Corneal Transplant Surgery, 1571
MARK R. MANDEL

SECTION 2 *Penetrating Keratoplasty: Technique*

130. Penetrating Keratoplasty, 1581
DAVID D. VERDIER

131. Penetrating Keratoplasty and Cataract Extraction, 1593
CLARON DOUGLAS ALLDREDGE
C. CLARON ALLDREDGE, JR.

132. Penetrating Keratoplasty and Intraocular Lens Exchange, 1603
LOUIS E. PROBST
EDWARD J. HOLLAND

133. Suturing Techniques, 1627
WOODFORD VAN METER

134. Intraoperative Complications of Penetrating Keratoplasty, 1639
JOHN J. PURCELL, JR.

SECTION 3 *Penetrating Keratoplasty: Postoperative Management*

135. Routine Management, 1645
COREY A. MILLER

136. Early Postoperative Complications, 1659
BRADLEY H. SCHARF

137. Postkeratoplasty Astigmatism, 1675
CHARLES S. REING
MARK G. SPEAKER

138. Clinical Aspects of Corneal Allograft Rejection, 1687
GARY N. FOULKS

139. Infections after Penetrating Keratoplasty, 1697
KAREN W. OXFORD
RICHARD L. ABBOTT

140. Retrocorneal Membranes, 1709
STEPHEN Y. LEE
CHRISTOPHER J. RAPUANO

141. Glaucoma after Penetrating Keratoplasty, 1719
DAVID GEORGE O'DAY

SECTION 4 *Complicated Penetrating Keratoplasty*

142. Pediatric Penetrating Keratoplasty, 1731
PETER GLOOR

143. High-Risk Penetrating Keratoplasty, 1757
THOMAS H. MADER
R. DOYLE STULTING

144. Large Diameter Corneal Grafts, 1773
JOHN W. COWDEN

145. Penetrating Keratoplasty in Ocular Surface Disease, 1781
H. KAZ SOONG

146. Surgery for Peripheral Corneal Thinning Disorders, 1789
RICHARD A. EIFERMAN
VINCENT P. DAHRINGER

147. Penetrating Keratoplasty in Herpes Simplex Disease, 1799
ROGER H. S. LANGSTON

PART IX THERAPEUTIC AND RECONSTRUCTIVE PROCEDURES

SECTION 1 *Corneal Surgery*

148. Management of Corneal Perforations, 1815
MARC A. HONIG
CHRISTOPHER J. RAPUANO

149. Lamellar Keratoplasty, 1833
WILLIAM H. BENSON
JOHN D. GOOSEY

150. Therapeutic Keratoplasty, 1843
ERIC D. DONNENFELD
ANASTASIOS JOHN KANELLOPOULOS

151. Keratoprosthesis, 1855
CLAES H. DOHLMAN

152. Corneal Surgery for Ocular Surface Disease, 1865
LARRY F. RICH

SECTION 2 *Conjunctival Surgery*

153. Management of Pterygium, 1873
MICHAEL R. GRIMMETT
EDWARD J. HOLLAND

154. Ocular Surface Transplantation, 1887
KENNETH R. KENYON
MICHAEL D. WAGONER
JOHN W. SHORE

155. Conjunctival Flaps, 1903
BRUCE D. NICHOLS

156. Management of Conjunctival and Corneal Neoplasia, 1911
GARY S. SCHWARTZ
EDWARD J. HOLLAND

SECTION 3 *Anterior Segment Surgery*

157. Surgical Management of Anterior Segment Trauma, 1925
MARIAN S. MACSAI

158. Anterior Segment Rehabilitation after Trauma, 1947
MICHAEL W. BELIN
C. DEREK RATLIFF

159. Cyclectomy and Iridocyclectomy, 1957
LAWRENCE A. GANS

160. Management of Scleral Perforation, 1965
M. BOWES HAMILL

PART X REFRACTIVE SURGERY

SECTION 1 *History and Overview of Refractive Surgery*

161. Refractive Surgery: Past, Present, and Future, 1977
STEVEN C. SCHALLHORN
PETER J. MCDONNELL

SECTION 2 *Preoperative Considerations*

162. Patient Selection and Evaluation, 2007
LARRY W. PIEBENGA
CAMILLE S. MATTA
PIERRE G. MARDELLI

163. Refractive Keratotomy—Assistive Technology and Instrumentation, 2013
KERRY K. ASSIL

164. Predictive Formulas for Refractive Surgery, 2025
THANASSIS PAPAIOANNOU
JAMES J. SALZ
EZRA MAGUEN

165. Role of Corneal Topography in Keratorefractive Surgery, 2039
STEPHEN D. KLYCE

SECTION 3 *Radial Keratotomy*

166. Radial Keratotomy Surgical Techniques, 2059
STEPHEN S. LANE

167. Results of Radial Keratotomy, 2083
MICHAEL P. VRABEC
SOOHYUNG KIM

168. Complications of Radial Keratotomy, 2101
SCOTT X. STEVENS
DOUGLAS A. YOUNG
PETER J. POLACK
JULIE C. TSAI
BRADLEY D. FOURAKER
J. JAMES ROWSEY

169. Postoperative Complications of Radial Keratotomy, 2117
RICHARD J. DUFFEY

SECTION 4 *Astigmatic Keratotomy*

170. Congenital Astigmatism, 2143
R. BRUCE GRENE

171. Astigmatism and Cataract Surgery, 2155
MICHAEL E. HETTINGER

SECTION 5 *Lamellar Refractive Procedures*

172. Automated Lamellar Keratoplasty, 2165
WILLIAM E. WHITSON
KEVIN C. CHANG
JULIAN A. PROCOPE
FRANCIS W. PRICE, JR.

SECTION 6 *Laser Corneal Surgery*

173. Laser Refractive Keratoplasty: Instrumentation and Techniques, 2181
DANIEL S. DURRIE
ROBERT J.S. MACK

174. Results and Complications of Photorefractive Keratoplasty, 2191
EZRA MAGUEN
JEFFREY J. MACHAT
JAMES J. SALZ

175. Phototherapeutic Keratectomy, 2211
DIMITRI T. AZAR
SANDEEP JAIN
WALTER STARK

SECTION 7 *Corneal Devices and Beyond*

176. Intrastromal Devices, 2225
TERRY E. BURRIS

177. Synthetic Epikeratoplasty, 2233
KEITH P. THOMPSON
JAN DANIEL

178. The Future of Refractive Surgery: Searching for the Ideal Procedure and Method of Delivery, 2243
GEORGE O. WARING, III

PART VIII

PENETRATING KERATOPLASTY

SECTION ONE *Preoperative Considerations*

CHAPTER 127

JAMES I. McNEILL

Indications and Outcomes

Corneal transplantation is a forever fascinating surgical procedure because of the many indications for its use and the many ways that it may need to be performed—often in combination with other challenging procedures. New indications arise, but old indications rarely disappear. Expectations only increase, as new ideas and understandings displace old ones.

The preparation for penetrating keratoplasty is unique in eye surgery because of the need for live human donor tissue. A corneal transplant surgeon simply cannot operate without tissue. Providing this tissue in quality, quantity, and location sufficient to meet needs has led to the evolution of a complex eye banking industry.

Corneal tissue for transplantation comes from a wide variety of donors and situations, often with unpredictable variables. The outcome of the surgery depends on many tissue-associated variables and the success of the procedure is truly remarkable. Host conditions also constitute important variables of success. The patient's condition before surgery may vary from blurred vision to frank perforation. The surgical procedure must not cause greater problems than it is expected to relieve. Expectations are not always realized despite great intentions.

The long-term outcome of corneal transplantation depends on skilled long-term care. The need for a lifetime of skilled care is common in the transplantation field in contrast to the care required after most ophthalmic procedures. Penetrating keratoplasty is still the only ophthalmic procedure in which rejection is a consideration, and rejection can occur as long as the host is alive and foreign tissue is present. A lifetime of care for the patient undergoing transplantation, is therefore, necessary to ensure an optimal outcome, and the corneal transplant surgeon can expect to experience an extra measure of challenge, commitment, and satisfaction.

Number of Penetrating Keratoplasties

The number of penetrating keratoplasty cases reported by the Eye Bank Association of America (EBAA) has increased each year since 1980. Some of the recent growth is from the addition of several overseas members, but more than 98% of the EBAA member's activity is in the United States and Canada. Figure 127-1 shows the number of cases reported by the EBAA between 1980 and 1994. Since 1990, more than 40,000 penetrating keratoplasties have been performed each year. The greater rate of growth in the earlier years probably represents more complete reporting with time, as well as increased activity. The growth in the number of penetrating keratoplasties performed each year, however, appears to have slowed considerably in recent years.

General Considerations

Corneal transplantation is not performed just because a corneal problem exists. This bit of simple philosophy may seem obvious, but it can be overlooked. The transplanting surgeon must reasonably expect significant eventual improvement in the patient's condition as a result of the surgical procedure. If not the indication is suspect medically, ethically, and possibly legally.

Reasonably expected improvement is based on past experience or logical and timely steps toward a new treatment method. Significant improvement in vision is two or more smaller lines on a Snellen reading chart (until a better way is accepted). Significant improvement also may be less pain, the ability to see with glasses instead of contact lenses, restoration of binocularity, decreased glare, and other improvements in

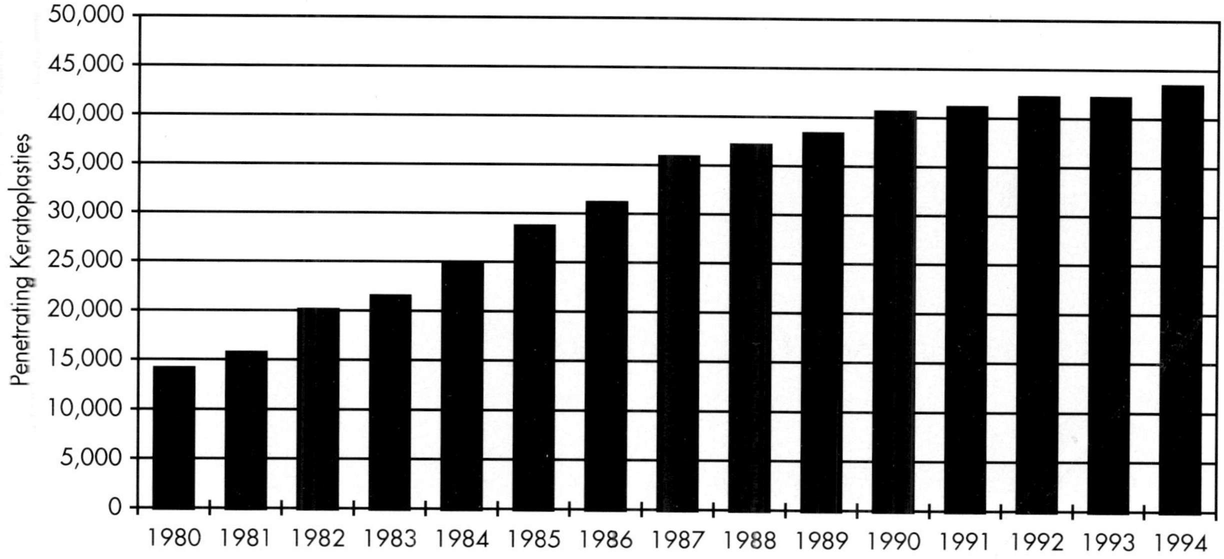

FIGURE 127-1 EBAA reported penetrating keratoplasties, 1980-1994, Total = 477,820. (From the 1994 Statistical Report, Eye Bank Association of America, 1001 Connecticut Ave, NW, Suite 601, Washington, DC 20036.)

function and lifestyle. Eventual improvement may take more than a year.

Many reports have detailed the indications for penetrating keratoplasty during the past few decades.[1-15] Because of the many reasons for penetrating keratoplasty, the indications are covered in this chapter in three general categories: anatomic, functional, and clinical. Considering each of these categories helps to validate the surgical decision process and form reasonable expectations.

Anatomic Indications for Penetrating Keratoplasty

Anatomic indications involve optics, structure, therapy, and cosmesis. An anatomic indication must be present for penetrating keratoplasty to be considered ethically. However, not all anatomic situations may be ethical indications (for example, transplanting an opaque cornea in a nonseeing eye). Multiple anatomic indications may be present.

OPTICAL INDICATIONS

The anatomy of the eye determines its optical properties. An optical indication for penetrating keratoplasty is directed to vision correction and is rarely the sole anatomic indication.

Disparate graft sizing can affect the optical result, although it is debatable.[16-18] When performing a penetrating keratoplasty on a patient with hypermetropia, an attempt can be made to obtain a "steep" graft that will have greater converging optical power. Using a donor button that is more than 0.5 mm larger than the host incision sometimes makes the corneal transplant steeper than it would otherwise be, if the suture is not too tight. However, this approach is not very predictable, and its range is probably less than 2 diopters. A better plan is to use a steep donor cornea, but no method is available for measuring the donor corneal shape. Lens implants currently have the best predictability and range for the correction of hypermetropia with penetrating keratoplasty.

The optical correction of aphakia or high degrees of hyperopia at the time of penetrating keratoplasty has at times been approached with the use of infant donor corneas.[19-23] Donor corneas less than 1 year of age are much more elastic than an adult cornea. The normal intraocular pressure in a recipient eye will cause these young elastic corneas to bulge. A sufficient graft bulge can correct for 10 or more diopters of aphakia or hypermetropia. Unfortunately, young donors are scarce, the tissue is difficult to handle in surgery, and the optical outcome is highly variable. The availability of suitable intraocular lenses has made the use of infant corneas for penetrating keratoplasty largely of historical interest.

When operating on a patient with myopia, an attempt can be made to obtain a "flat" graft. One approach is to use a donor button that is smaller than normal. For most surgeons, this would be a "same size" donor or one that is slightly undersized. Tight suturing will temporarily flatten a graft. The limit of this

technique is probably about 2 diopters and is not very predictable. This technique is most commonly used in patients with keratoconus and axial myopia, in which a flat graft can optically reduce the remaining myopia from a long eye.[24]

Large amounts of astigmatism, regular or irregular, can produce an optically nonfunctional eye. A distorted cornea from trauma, a keratoconic cornea that is otherwise clear but cannot be corrected with lenses, and a badly warped corneal transplantation are the most likely cases requiring penetrating keratoplasty for optical reasons alone. However, optical considerations are a part of the decision-making process in most corneal transplants.

RECONSTRUCTIVE INDICATIONS

Reconstructive penetrating keratoplasty, also called tectonic keratoplasty, is performed to improve the structure of the cornea and not primarily for visual purposes. Corneal thinning and perforation are common indications. These situations are usually advanced so that the continued integrity of the eye is compromised. Ulceration, trauma, and keratoconus are the most common clinical situations. A reconstructive graft also may improve the patient's visual function, or an optical graft may be possible at a later time.

THERAPEUTIC INDICATIONS

Therapeutic indications (i.e., the treatment of diseases) are the most common of the general indications for penetrating keratoplasty. Edema, scarring, dystrophy, degeneration, infection, and various deposits in the cornea can be therapeutic indications. Corneal edema after previous eye surgery is the most common therapeutic indication for penetrating keratoplasty

Medically unresponsive infections may require penetrating keratoplasty. These cases are usually fungal or *Acanthamoeba* keratitis. These infections can be difficult to diagnose and limited medical treatment is available for them. An adequate excisional biopsy of the infection site by penetrating keratoplasty can be curative.

Pain may be a significant factor in advanced corneal swelling with bullous epithelial changes. Penetrating keratoplasty is effective in reducing, and usually eliminating, the pain of bullous keratopathy.

COSMETIC INDICATIONS

Penetrating keratoplasty can be performed to remove unsightly corneal scars or deposits. Usually a better cosmetic result can be obtained with a cosmetic contact lens, corneal tattooing, enucleation, or evisceration with a skillfully prepared prosthesis. Cosmesis alone is not a good indication for penetrating keratoplasty, although it is often considered with other indications.

Functional Indications for Penetrating Keratoplasty

Functional indications are often the most important factors in the final surgical decision-making process. Functional indications for penetrating keratoplasty consider the patient's current capabilities, potential capabilities, and willingness to risk change.

A logical approach is needed for many different and sometimes complex situations. The following protocol will handle most cases: If the patient has an anatomic indication for penetrating keratoplasty that (1) cannot be adequately corrected medically or with lenses, or (2) the correction cannot be tolerated, then penetrating keratoplasty is reasonable to recommend to the patient.

For example, a person with keratoconus will initially have a clear, but distorted, cornea that can be optically corrected with a contact lens. This is the appropriate treatment while the cornea remains clear enough to provide adequate acuity and the contact lens is tolerated long enough to meet that individual's visual requirements. When the acuity or the tolerance is no longer adequate, penetrating keratoplasty is reasonable to consider. Incidentally, this type of approach also applies to most other surgical procedures.

Although poor visual acuity is the most common functional indication for penetrating keratoplasty, the control of disabling pain associated with bullous keratopathy may be a primary functional indication, with improvement in visual acuity a secondary goal. Restoration of binocularity is an important, but less common, functional indication for penetrating keratoplasty.

Clinical Indications for Penetrating Keratoplasty

Clinical indications for penetrating keratoplasty are the diseases and situations for which penetrating keratoplasty is performed. The EBAA has adopted a set of 16 clinical indication categories for penetrating keratoplasty.[25] Table 127-1 lists these categories, along with specific examples and relative frequencies between 1991 and 1993. These data are the largest (more than 77,000 cases) and most geographically diverse available (eye banks throughout the United States and Canada), but are limited to North America, and only

Table 127-1. EBAA's clinical indications for penetrating keratoplasty, 1991-1993 with relative frequencies

	Frequency by year (%)		
Indication	**1991 n = 20,038**	**1992 n = 27,332**	**1993 n = 29,72[illegible]**
1. Pseudophakic corneal edema	25.09%	23.04%	21.44%
pseudophakic bullous keratopathy with epithelial bullae associated with anterior chamber lens, iris-fixated lens, posterior chamber lens			
2. Aphakic corneal edema	8.53%	7.91%	[illegible].71%
aphakic bullous keratopathy with epithelial bullae			
vitreoendothelial touch			
3. Stromal corneal dystrophies	4.09%	5.10%	[illegible].75%
granular stromal dystrophy			
lattice stromal dystrophies			
macular stromal dystrophy			
central crystalline dystrophy of Schnyder			
central cloudy dystrophy of François			
4. Primary corneal endotheliopathies	11.08%	13.99%	1[illegible].98%
Fuchs' endothelial dystrophy			
congenital hereditary endothelial dystrophy			
posterior polymorphous dystrophy			
iridocorneal endothelial syndromes			
Chandler's syndrome			
5. Ectasias/thinnings	11.40%	11.78%	14.48%
anterior keratoconus			
keratoglobus			
posterior keratoconus			
6. Congenital opacities	0.56%	0.67%	0.92%
Peter's anomaly			
sclerocornea			
congenital glaucoma/buphthalmos			
aniridia			
7. Viral/postviral keratitis	1.47%	1.25%	1.29%
herpes simplex virus			
varicella zoster virus			
adenovirus			
epidemic keratoconjunctivitis			
measles			
infectious mononucleosis			
Epstein-Barr virus			
8. Microbial/postmicrobial keratitis	0.92%	0.64%	0.73%
bacterial			
Infectious crystalline keratopathy			
fungal			
chlamydial			
trachoma			
parasitic			
Acanthamoeba			
9. Spirochete-associated keratitis	0.39%	0.49%	0.[illegible]7%
luetic interstitial keratitis			
Lyme disease keratitis			

Continued.

about two thirds of the cases in North America are reported in this manner. The more general term *corneal edema* is used instead of *bullous keratopathy.*[26] Multiple indications are only beginning to be tracked. These categories are followed by the EBAA to identify important trends for its member eye banks. This list is dynamic and changes, especially additions, are expected. Pseudophakic corneal edema (PCE) is the most common clinical indication.

The clinical indications for penetrating keratoplasty

Table 127-1. EBAA's clinical indications for penetrating keratoplasty, 1991-1993 with relative frequencies*—cont'd

	Frequency by year (%)		
Indication	**1991 n = 20,038**	**1992 n = 27,332**	**1993 n = 29,729**
10. Noninfectious ulcerative keratitis or perforation	3.13%	3.38%	3.78%
keratoconjunctivitis sicca			
Sjögren's syndrome			
neuroparalytic/neurotrophic keratopathy			
exposure keratopathy			
systemic vasculitides			
bullous oculocutaneous diseases			
Mooren's ulcer			
thyroid eye disease			
rheumatoid disease			
rheumatoid arthritis			
11. Corneal degenerations	4.23%	3.72%	3.48%
Terrien's marginal degeneration			
calcific band keratopathy			
polymorphic amyloid degeneration			
12. Chemical injuries	0.47%	0.42%	0.27%
alkaline			
acid			
petroleum based			
tear gas			
13. Mechanical trauma, nonsurgical	2.62%	1.58%	1.65%
traumatic opacity/irregular astigmatism			
traumatic corneal edema			
14. Regraft related to allograft rejection	4.67%	2.24%	3.09%
15. Regraft unrelated to allograft rejection	2.41%	4.64%	4.76%
primary tissue failure			
optical			
pseudophakic corneal edema			
microbial			
viral			
vitreoendothelial touch			
recurrent stromal dystrophy			
trauma/rupture			
glaucoma			
16. Other causes of corneal opacification/distortion	18.92%	19.13%	21.29%
uveitis			
detached Descemet's membrane			
glaucoma			
radial/astigmatic keratotomy			
failed epikeratoplasty			
thermal injury			
postlaser			
silicone oil keratopathy			
epithelial downgrowth			

*From the Corneal Transplant Recipient Diagnosis Report 1993, 1993 Statistical Report, Eye Bank Association of America, 1001 Connecticut Ave., NW, Suite 601, Washington, DC 20036.

can show considerable variation by site. Table 127-2 describes the experience in an academic referral center in Southern California between 1980 and 1992. The percentages in this data are higher in some categories than most other reports, partly because of the tabulation of multiple indications in about 20% of cases. This experience shows a peak in PCE at 48% in 1987 with a percentage of over twice that reported by the EBAA with their peak of PCE (27.4%) in 1989. Southern California experienced early and heavy use of implant technology with cataract surgery. The regrafting rate is higher (18.1%) than the EBAA data (6.9% to 8.8%, Table 127-1), but similar to the large group reported by Tissue Banks International (17%).[13]

Reports of indications for penetrating keratoplasty from other parts of the world are often quite different from those in North America.[27-45] Pseudophakic corneal edema (PCE) has been relatively uncommon

Table 127-2. Author's clinical indications for penetrating keratoplasty, 1979-1992, with relative frequencies*

Total number of operated eyes = 1410 Indication	Eyes†	%†	Range (year)
1. Pseudophakic corneal edema	457	32.4%	18%(1980) – 48%(1987)
2. Aphakic corneal edema	160	11.3%	2%(1992) – 22%(198[illegible])
3. Stromal corneal dystrophies	18	1.3%	0%-3%(1989)
4. Primary corneal endotheliopathies	185	13.1%	7%(1992) – 20%(199[illegible])
5. Ectasias/thinnings	137	9.7%	5%(1981) – 14%(198[illegible])
6. Congenital opacities	17	1.2%	0%-4%(1986)
7. Viral/postviral keratitis	115	8.2%	5%(1984) – 12%(198[illegible])
8. Microbial/postmicrobial keratitis	77	5.5%	2%(1984) – 11%(197[illegible])
9. Spirochete-associated keratitis	54	3.8%	1%(1992) – 7%(1985)
10. Noninfectious ulcerative keratitis/perforation	75	5.4%	1%(1985) – 9%(1990)
11. Corneal degenerations	11	0.5%	0%-2%(1992)
12. Chemical injuries	20	1.4%	0%-4%(1982)
13. Mechanical trauma, nonsurgical	79	5.6%	1%(1987) – 13%(198[illegible])
14. Regraft related to allograft rejection	90	6.4%	2%(1979,80,83) – 11%(1992)
15. Regraft unrelated to allograft rejection	165	11.7%	5%(1982) – 23%(197[illegible])
16. Other causes of corneal opacification/distortion	27	1.9%	0%-6%(1991)

*Loma Linda University, Loma Linda, California.
†The sum of all the eyes (1,687) is greater than the total number of eyes (1,410) and the sum of the corresponding percentages (119.4%) is greater than 100% because of multiple indications in about 20% of cases (e.g., pseudophakic corneal edema with Fuchs' dystrophy).

outside North America, and keratoconus and regrafts are usually the most common clinical indications for penetrating keratoplasty abroad. Where donor corneal tissue is difficult to obtain, there is a selection bias in favor of patients with the best prognosis.[43]

Trends in Clinical Indications for Penetrating Keratoplasty

Some interesting trends in the clinical indications for penetrating keratoplasty have been observed over the last two decades. Before 1980, keratoconus and aphakic corneal edema were the most common indications, and pseudophakic corneal edema (PCE) was just appearing. In the 1980s, PCE rapidly became the most common indication for penetrating keratoplasty in the United States. The emergence of PCE as the most common cause for penetrating keratoplasty correlated well with the dramatic increase in the number of cataract extractions with lens implantation performed since the mid-1970s in the United States.[4]

EBAA data demonstrated in Figure 127-2 shows the rapid increase in PCE frequency in the late 1980s with a peak in 1989 and a slow decrease since then. PCE may continue to be the leading indication for penetrating keratoplasty as more cataract surgeries are performed in people with longer life expectancies.[7,46] An expected decrease in aphakic corneal edema has been slow to occur.

Figure 127-2 also shows the EBAA data for repeat penetrating keratoplasty and keratoconus. Keratoconus can be considered as a "biologic" control group because there are no known clinical or environmental causes or cures for the disease. The percentage of penetrating keratoplasties performed for keratoconus has not changed much in recent years, although the total number has increased as the number of penetrating keratoplasties performed has increased.

It might be expected that the relative number of regrafts would increase as the pool of keratoplasties in the population increased.[47] This increase has not occurred. The percentage of penetrating keratoplasties for regrafts in the EBAA data has only varied between 7% and 9%, with the percentage in recent years being lower than in the past.

The combination of pseudophakic and aphakic corneal edema includes most of the penetrating keratoplasties performed on eyes after previous eye surgery. The EBAA data in Figure 127-3 show that this combination peaked in the late 1980s and has been decreasing steadily since then. This decrease probably reflects improved cataract surgery technique.

Indications for Associated Procedures

About half of penetrating keratoplasty cases are combined with a variety of other surgical procedures. Cataract surgery and various lens implant manipulations are the most common.

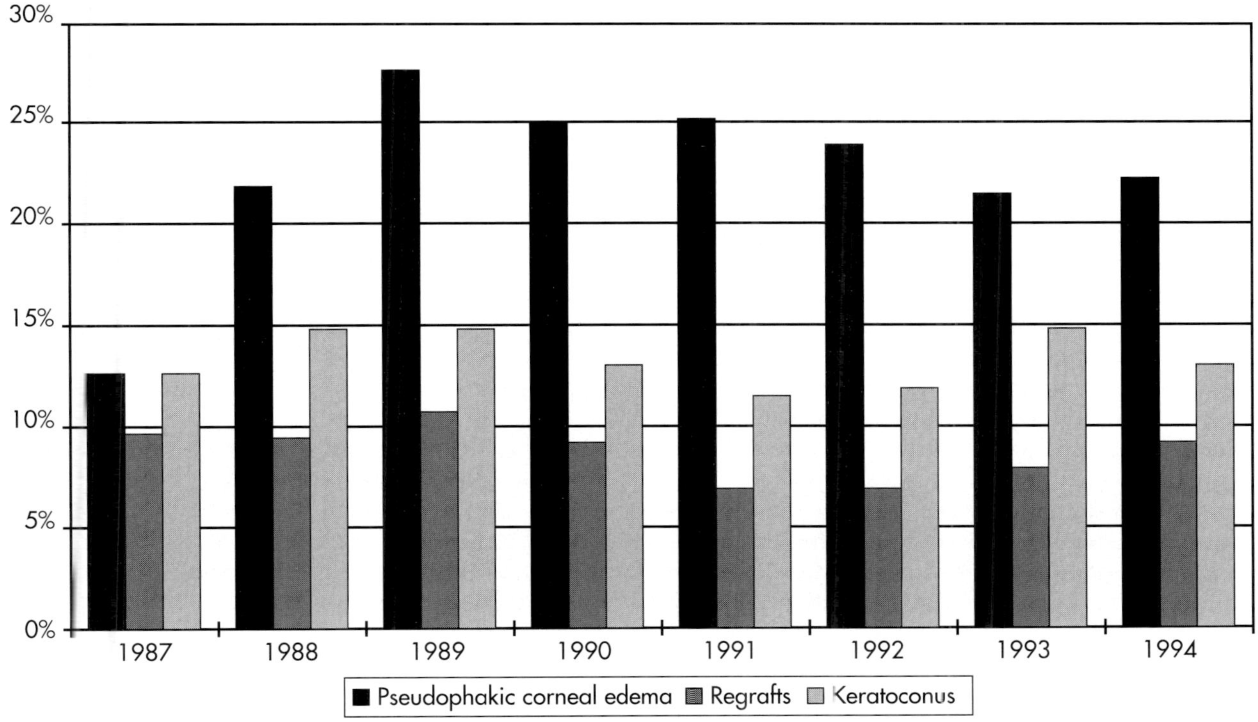

FIGURE 127-2 Trends in clinical indications for penetrating keratoplasty. (Data from the Corneal Transplant Recipient Diagnosis Reports 1987-1994, Eye Bank Association of America, 1001 Connecticut Ave, NW, Suite 601, Washington, DC 20036.)

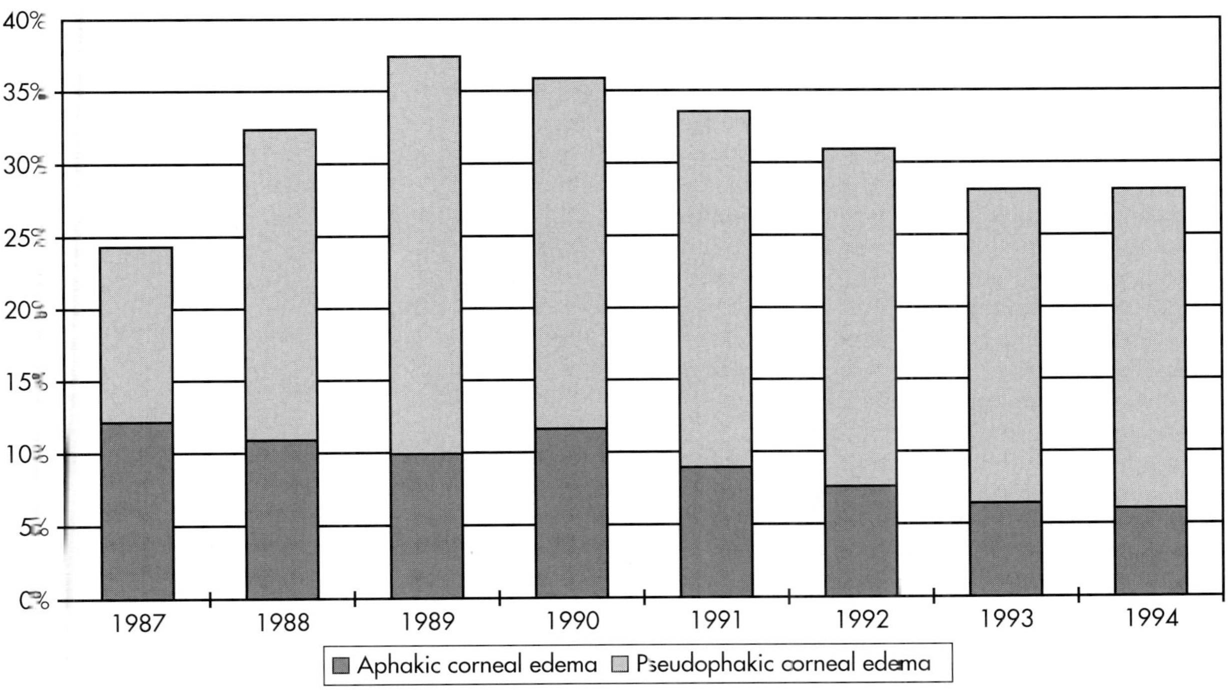

FIGURE 127-3 Trends in clinical indications for penetrating keratoplasty. (From the Corneal Transplant Recipient Diagnosis Reports 1987-1994, Eye Bank Association of America, 1001 Connecticut Ave, NW, Suite 601, Washington, DC 20036.)

THE CORNEAL "TRIPLE PROCEDURE"

The corneal "triple procedure" combines penetrating keratoplasty with cataract extraction and lens implantation in about 20% of cases.[48] "Open-sky" extracapsular cataract extraction is quite different from routine cataract extraction performed through the corneal limbus. A smooth capsulorhexis ensures long-term, in-the-bag lens placement. A soft eye is essential. Implant power calculation is not precise because of the need to estimate postoperative keratometry and axial length. Ideally, the penetrating keratoplasty would be performed alone and allowed to completely heal and stabilize. The lens implant power for cataract surgery could then be accurately determined. However, timing becomes a significant consideration because the corneal suture is now often left for several years.

Most patients undergoing the corneal triple procedure are older, and they often prefer the chance of better vision sooner rather than later despite some optical risk. Most corneal surgeons will evaluate a series of similar surgeries they have performed and use the average postoperative keratometry for calculating new cases. Axial length is usually measured directly, and occasionally the measurement for the fellow eye is used when the operated eye has significant anterior segment distortion.

REMOVAL OF LENS IMPLANTS

Virtually all iris and capsule fixated lens implants are removed when present at the time of penetrating keratoplasty. These lenses are associated with chronic cystoid macular edema.

Most anterior chamber lens implants probably should be removed.[49] Problems with anterior chamber lenses are well known and include chronic inflammation and pain, peripheral anterior synechiae, angle-closure and pupillary block glaucoma, iris and pupillary distortions, and cystoid macular edema. Only lenses with proper power and no associated problems should be considered for retention.

Few posterior chamber lenses need to be removed. Having the wrong optical power is the most common reason for removing posterior chamber lenses at the time of penetrating keratoplasty. Dislocated lenses usually can be relocated and stabilized by rotation, replacement with a different type of lens, or suturing of the lens to the sclera or iris.

ANTERIOR VITRECTOMY

Vitrectomy has given aphakic penetrating keratoplasty a reasonable prognosis. Loose vitreous in the anterior chamber can compromise the endothelium of a new corneal graft. Vitreous to the transplant wound can aggravate macular edema. A thorough anterior vitrectomy is indicated whenever vitreous is encountered during penetrating keratoplasty.[50] About 20% of penetrating keratoplasties—all aphakic and many pseudophakic grafts—are performed in association with anterior vitrectomy.[48]

SECONDARY PLACEMENT AND REPLACEMENT OF LENS IMPLANTS

Good pseudophakic vision is preferable to aphakic vision. Placing secondary anterior chamber lenses is debatable, but at times can be a good consideration. Several suggestions might be helpful. An anterior chamber lens is placed only if the anterior chamber angle has opposite quadrants that are completely open, as is usually the case in aphakic eyes and after removal of iris and capsule fixated implants. Open quadrants are not common after removal of anterior chamber lenses, especially those with three looped fixation points 120 degrees apart.

An anterior chamber lens should not be used to "hold the angle open." Bad things tend to get worse. Most important, anterior chamber lenses must be carefully sized so that they are not too long. A lens that is too long puts constant pressure on the angle structures, causing chronic inflammation that leads to erosion and synechia formation.

Whenever an anterior chamber lens is placed in an eye, a patent iridectomy is essential. An anterior chamber lens is a pupillary block glaucoma eager to happen. If a vitrectomy is performed (and it should be), the vitrectomy instrument should be inserted through the iridectomy, and it should be verified that fluid can be drawn down through the pupil.

Posterior chamber lenses usually can be placed in the ciliary sulcus if at least three quadrants of the patient's lens capsule remains intact. A sulcus lens needs to be approximately 13 mm long. Sutured posterior chamber lenses can be considered when insufficient lens capsule remains and an anterior chamber lens is not appropriate. Whether the lens is fixed by suturing to the iris or sclera is debatable, but the trend seems to be toward transscleral fixation. Sutured posterior chamber lenses are more successful than many originally expected; however, it is difficult to evaluate them because eyes in which they are placed are often compromised in multiple ways.

SYNECHIOLYSIS

Most synechia are not fixable, but it is challenging to try. Using the blunt end of closed, curved microsurgical scissors is convenient. A No. 3 dental mouth mirror allows direct visualization of the angle through the corneal incision. It is important to remember that the image is reversed in one dimension, and that dimension rotates with the lens.

Timing of Penetrating Keratoplasty

The best vision after penetrating keratoplasty usually does not occur until 4 to 8 months after surgery. Before this time, vision may be worse than before surgery. For this reason, the better eye should be operated with reluctance, and the fellow eye should not be operated for 6 months. It is rare for eyes to require surgery within 6 months of each other. On the other hand, if both eyes are similar and progressive, as in Fuchs' endothelial dystrophy, the first eye should be operated before the second eye deteriorates too significantly.

Complicating Factors

Many diverse factors can complicate the outcome of penetrating keratoplasty and are important considerations in surgical planning. These factors include poor eyelid anatomy or function, severe sicca, chemical burns especially alkaline, previous radiation, the presence of an anterior chamber or iris-supported intraocular lens, young recipient age, elevated intraocular pressure, intraocular inflammation, number of previous grafts, quadrants of anterior synechiae, quadrants of stromal blood vessels, blood group ABO incompatibility, fewer grafts performed by the surgeon, very large and very small grafts, and previous corneal incisions such as radial keratotomy.[42,51-57]

Expected Outcomes for Penetrating Keratoplasty

A definite improvement in outcomes for penetrating keratoplasty has been witnessed over the last few decades. Vitrectomy has greatly improved the prognosis in aphakic and pseudophakic grafts. Microsurgical techniques, instruments, and materials have allowed unprecedented operating precision. Strong and inert materials such as nylon allow stable wound closures. An appreciation of the function of the corneal endothelium has contributed immeasurably to preventing and treating preoperative and postoperative corneal problems. Finally, corticosteroids have provided the means to suppress and reverse the foreign tissue rejection phenomenon in the great majority of cases.

The following description of outcomes is divided into four major categories patterned after the method used by Buxton et al.[15,58-62] Surgeons performing corneal transplants for patients in the better categories need to realize that these patients reasonably have the greatest expectations for a result that includes fine visual acuity. Their postoperative course must include the skills required to deal with early detection and treatment of rejection and the treatment of early (suture in) and late (suture out) astigmatism. Failed grafts usually have a poorer prognosis than their primary diagnosis group.

DEFINITION OF SUCCESS

It used to be enough to say that a successful graft was clear and thin. Today we must include a significant improvement in the patient's condition to claim success for penetrating keratoplasty. Significant improvement in vision is two or more lines on a Snellen reading chart (until a better way is accepted). Significant improvement also may be less pain, the ability to see with glasses instead of contact lenses, restoration of binocularity, decreased glare, and other improvements in function and lifestyle.

GROUP 1—EXCELLENT PROGNOSIS

This group consists of corneas with avascular central corneal thinning, scarring, or edema surrounded by healthy peripheral cornea. Examples include keratoconus, central or paracentral inactive scars, lattice or granular stromal dystrophies, and early central Fuchs' dystrophy. The prognosis in this group is excellent, with over 90% success expected. Group 1 also tends to have the highest expectations.

GROUP 2—VERY GOOD PROGNOSIS

This group includes corneal lesions that involve part or all of the corneal periphery with adequate surgical surface and only mild to moderate vascularity involving no more than two quadrants. Examples are advanced Fuchs' dystrophy, aphakic and pseudophakic corneal edema and bullous keratopathy, inactive herpetic keratitis, the iridocorneal endothelial syndromes, interstitial keratitis, and macular stromal dystrophy. The prognosis in this group is very good, with an 80% to 90% success rate expected. Group 2 includes the largest number of corneal transplantations.

GROUP 3—FAIR PROGNOSIS

The corneas in this group are characterized by extremes of corneal thickness, perforations, peripheral descemetoceles, and active infectious or inflammatory disease. Examples of this group include active bacterial keratitis, active herpetic keratitis, congenital hereditary endothelial dystrophy, grafts on young children, active fungal keratitis, mild chemical injury, and moderate sicca. The prognosis in this group is only fair, with a success rate ranging from 50% to 80%.

GROUP 4—POOR PROGNOSIS

The eyes in this group have one or more of the following characteristics: severe fibrovascular replacement of the cornea, conjunctival ischemia, anterior chamber obliteration, and advanced dry eye. Examples from this group are severe chemical injury, radiation injury, ocular pemphigoid, Stevens-Johnson syndrome, Lyell's disease, neuroparalytic disease, congenital glaucoma, epithelial downgrowth, anterior chamber cleavage syndromes, and multiple graft failures. The prognosis in this group is very poor, with a success rate of less than 50%, often much less. Most eyes in group 3 should not be operated, but there is often little to lose and even small improvements in visual function may be important to the patient when the disease is bilateral or involves an only eye.

REFERENCES

1. Arentsen JJ, Morgan B, Green WR: Changing indications for keratoplasty, *Am J Ophthalmol* 81:313-318, 1976.
2. Chandler JW: Indications for penetrating keratoplasty and management of cases, *Trans Pac Coast Oto-Ophthalmol Soc* 59:97-104, 1976.
3. Smith RE, McDonald HR, Nesburn AB, Minckler DS: Penetrating keratoplasty: changing indications, 1947-1978, *Arch Ophthalmol* 98:1226-1229, 1980.
4. Robin JB et al: An update of the indications for penetrating keratoplasty, 1979-1983, *Arch Ophthalmol* 104:87-89, 1986.
5. Stanley JA: Indications for corneal transplant surgery, *Int Ophthalmol Clin* 28:5-13, 1988.
6. Brady SE et al: Clinical indications for and procedures associated with penetrating keratoplasty, 1983-1988, *Am J Ophthalmol* 108:118-122, 1989.
7. Mohamadi P et al: Changing indications for penetrating keratoplasty, 1984-1988, *Am J Ophthalmol* 107:550-552, 1989.
8. Morris RJ, Bates AK: Changing indications for keratoplasty, *Eye* 3:455-459, 1989.
9. Damji KF et al: Changing indications for penetrating keratoplasty in Vancouver, 1978-1987, *Can J Ophthalmol* 25:243-248, 1990.
10. Lindquist TD, McGlothan JS, Rotkis WM, Chandler JW: Indications for penetrating keratoplasty: 1980-1988, *Cornea* 10:210-216, 1991.
11. Mamalis N et al: Penetrating keratoplasty 1981-1988: clinical indications and pathologic findings, *J Cataract Refract Surg* 17:163-167, 1991.
12. Baker RS, Sasey R, Lee DA, Wilson MR: Epidemiology of penetrating keratoplasty, ARVO Abstracts (#2581), *Invest Ophthalmol Vis Sci* 33(4, suppl):1211, 1992.
13. Hyman L, Wittpenn J, Yang C: Indications and techniques of penetrating keratoplasties, 1985-1988, *Cornea* 11:573-576, 1992.
14. Mamalis N et al: Changing trends in the indications for penetrating keratoplasty, *Arch Ophthalmol* 110:1409-1411, 1992.
15. Buxton JN, Buxton DF, Westphalen JA: Indications and contraindications. In Brightbill RD (ed): *Cornea surgery: theory, technique, and tissue,* ed 2, St Louis, 1993, Mosby.
16. Olson RJ, Mattingly TP, Waltman SR, Kaufman HE: Refractive variation and donor tissue size in aphakic keratoplasty: a prospective randomized study, *Arch Ophthalmol* 97:1480-1481, 1979.
17. Perl T, Charlton KH, Binder PS: Disparate diameter grafting, astigmatism, intraocular pressure, and visual acuity, *Ophthalmology* 88:774-780, 1981.
18. Bourne WM, Davison JA, O'Fallon WM: The effects of oversize donor buttons on postoperative intraocular pressure and corneal curvature in aphakic penetrating keratoplasty, *Ophthalmology* 89:242-246, 1982.
19. Wood TO, Nissenkorn I: Infant donor corneas for penetrating keratoplasty, *Ophthalmic Surg* 12:500-502, 1981.
20. Koenig S, Graul E, Kaufman HE: Ocular refraction after penetrating keratoplasty with infant donor corneas, *Am J Ophthalmol* 94:534-539, 1982.
21. Pfister RR, Breaud S: Aphakic refractive penetrating keratoplasty using newborn donor corneas: a preliminary report on an alternative approach to refractive correction, *Ophthalmology* 90:1207-1212, 1983.
22. Gloor P, Keech RV, Krachmer JH: Factors associated with high postoperative myopia after penetrating keratoplasties in infants, *Ophthalmology* 99:775-779, 1992.
23. Chen JQ: Refractive evaluation of donor corneas from the newborn in aphakic penetrating keratoplasty, *Chung Hua Yen Ko Tsa Chih* 29:224-226, 1993.
24. Javadi MA, Mohammadi MJ, Mirdehghan SA, Sajjadi SH: A comparison between donor-recipient corneal size and its effect on the ultimate refractive error induced in keratoconus, *Cornea* 12:401-405, 1993.
25. Lindquist TD, McNeill JI, Wilhelmus KR: Indications for keratoplasty (editorial), *Cornea* 13:105-107, 1994.
26. Waring GO III: The 50-year epidemic of pseudophakic corneal edema, *Arch Ophthalmol* 107:657-659, 1989.
27. Boke W: Perforating keratoplasty: preconditions, indications, complications, follow-up treatment, *Klin Monatsbl Augenheilkd* 171:657-677, 1977.
28. Kok-van Alphen CC, Volker-Dieben HJ: Indications and contra-indications for perforating keratoplasty, *Doc Ophthalmol* 44:[illegible]5-38, 1977.
29. Bordiugova GG, Gundorova RA, Iluridze SL: Indications for keratoplasty taking into account immunological reactions, *Vestn Oftalmol* 59-63, 1978.
30. Krey H, Jacobi KW: Indication for keratoplasty in keratoconus, *Buch Augenarzt* 73:109-110, 1978.
31. Michaud PA: A study of the indications and results of 1[illegible]5 keratoplasties undertaken at the University Eye Clinic of Geneva, *Schweiz Rundsch Med Prax* 67:469-474, 1978.
32. Pouliquen Y: Keratoplasty: indications, *Annee Ther Clin Ophtalmol* 29:125-132, 1978.
33. Weekers R et al: Indications for keratoplasty in the treatment of corneal perforation, *Bull Soc Belge Ophtalmol* 184:8[illegible]-89, 1979.
34. Naumann GO, Eisert S, Volcker HE: Indications for lamellar and perforating keratoplasty, *Buch Augenarzt* 9-26, 1982.
35. Collum LM, McGettrick PM: Indications for and complications of keratoplasty, *Bull Soc Belge Ophtalmol* 211:15-20, 1984.
36. Gong XM, Chen JQ, Feng CM, Du NZ: Changes in indications for keratoplasty, *Yen Ko Hsueh Pao* 1:142-147, 1985.
37. Gorgiladze TU: Classification of corneal opacities and indications for keratoplasty, *Oftalmol Zh* 23-27, 1985
38. Brooks AM, Weiner JM: Indications for penetrating keratoplasty: a clinicopathological review of 511 corneal specimens, *Aust N Z J Ophthalmol* 15:277-281, 1987.
39. Collum LM et al: A comparative analysis over a decade of the changing indications for penetrating keratoplasty in Ireland, *Br J Med Sci* 156:262-264, 1987.
40. Burk R, Bohnke M, von Domarus D, Abramo F: Penetrating keratoplasty—indications with special reference to artificial lens keratopathy, *Klin Monatsbl Augenheilkd* 192:191-19[illegible], 1988.
41. Lang GK, Wilk CM, Naumann GO: Changes in the indications status for keratoplasty, *Fortschr Ophthalmol* 85:255-258, 1988.

42. The Australian Corneal Graft Registry, 1990 to 1992 report: *Aust N Z J Ophthalmol* 21(2 Suppl):1-48, 1993.
43. Legeais JM et al: Indications for penetrating keratoplasty: a retrospective study of 2,962 cases over 11 years, *J Fr Ophtalmol* 16:516-522, 1993.
44. Sharif KW, Casey TA: Changing indications for penetrating keratoplasty 1971-1990, *Eye* 7:485-488, 1993.
45. De Cock R: Penetrating keratoplasty in the West Bank and Gaza, *Eye* 8:29-34 1994.
46. Stark WJ, Leske MC, Worthen DM, Murray GC: Trends in cataract surgery and intraocular lenses in the United States, *Am J Ophthalmol* 96:304-310, 1983.
47. Robinson CH: Indications, complications and prognosis for repeat penetrating keratoplasty, *Ophthalmic Surg* 10:27-34, 1979.
48. Aiello LP, Javitt JC, Canner JK: National outcomes of penetrating keratoplasty: risks of endophthalmitis and retinal detachment, *Arch Ophthalmol* 111:509-513, 1993.
49. Price FW Jr, Whitson WE, Collins K, Johns S: Changing trends in explanted intraocular lenses: a single center study, *J Cataract Refract Surg* 18:470-474, 1992.
50. Meyer HJ: Indications for vitrectomy in keratoplasty, *Fortschr Ophthalmol* 79:113-115, 1982.
51. Kirkness CM, Ezra E, Rice NSC, McG Steele AM: The success and survival of repeat corneal grafts, *Eye* 4:58-64, 1990.
52. McNeill JI, Wilkins DL: A purse-string suture for penetrating keratoplasty following radial keratotomy, *Refract Corneal Surg* 7:392-394, 1991.
53. Kirkness CM, Ficker LA: Risk factors for the development of postkeratoplasty glaucoma, *Cornea* 11:427-432, 1992.
54. Williams KA et al: Factors predictive of corneal graft survival: report from the Australian Corneal Graft Registry, *Ophthalmology* 99:403-414, 1992.
55. Boisjoly HM et al: Risk factors of corneal graft failure, *Ophthalmology* 100:1728-1735, 1993.
56. Maguire MG et al: Risk factors for corneal graft failure and rejection in the collaborative corneal transplantation studies, *Ophthalmology* 101:1536-1547, 1994.
57. Vail A et al: Corneal graft survival and visual outcome, A multicenter study, Corneal Transplant Follow-up Study Collaborators, *Ophthalmology* 101:120-127, 1994.
58. Polack FM: *Corneal transplantation,* New York, 1977, Grune & Stratton.
59. Arentsen JJ, Laibson PR: Surgical management of pseudophakic corneal edema: complications and visual results following penetrating keratoplasty, *Ophthalmic Surg* 13:371-373, 1982.
60. Sugan A: An analysis of corneal endothelial and graft survival in pseudophakic bullous keratopathy, *Trans Am Ophthalmol Soc* 87:762, 1990.
61. Wilson SE, Kaufman HE: Graft failure after penetrating keratoplasty, *Surv Ophthalmol* 34:325-356, 1990.
62. Price FW, Whitson WE, Marks RG: Graft survival in four common groups of patients undergoing penetrating keratoplasty, *Ophthalmology* 98:322-328, 1991.

CHAPTER 128

FREDERICK S. BRIGHTBILL   ROBERT E. BRASS

Preoperative Evaluation of the Keratoplasty Patient

Importance of Preoperative Evaluation

A thorough preoperative evaluation should consider the factors making each case unique, allowing the surgeon to identify and avoid potential problems during and after keratoplasty. A systemic history will often indicate the feasibility of performing the proposed procedure and may dictate the type of anesthesia to be used. The slit lamp examination and ocular history provide the cornerstone of diagnosis and management. Proper patient selection and preoperative evaluation maximize the potential for a favorable outcome.

General History

The main questions to be answered when obtaining the patient's history and review of systems relate to the ability of the patient to undergo the proposed operative procedure. In considering local anesthesia for example, the ability of the patient to lie flat for the duration of the procedure could be compromised by pulmonary or cardiac abnormalities. Severe arthritis may make it impossible for the patient to remain comfortably in any one position for an extended time and may warrant general anesthesia. Preexisting medical problems such as hypertension and diabetes should be stabilized in concert with the patient's primary care physician before the keratoplasty. Because preoperative anxiety is common, patients should be advised to take their normal dose of antihypertensive medication on the morning of surgery. Persons with insulin-dependent diabetes should undergo surgery early in the day if possible and use one half their normal dose before surgery, with the other one half given postoperatively along with breakfast. Cardiopulmonary disease may limit use of β-blockers postoperatively. Allergies to medications such as antibiotics, systemic medications, and anesthetics should be directly questioned, noted in the chart, and reviewed to avoid subsequent complications. In regard to topical medications, patients may be allergic to the preservative in the medication rather than the medication itself. In such cases, allergies to preservatives can be identified by skin testing before excluding an entire class of medications.

Patients taking aspirin, nonsteroidal antiinflammatory drugs, and other medications that interfere with blood coagulability deserve special preoperative consideration. It has been traditional practice to discontinue anticoagulants 10 to 14 days before surgery in consultation with the prescribing physician, with or without heparinization perioperatively. Recently, relative safety has been demonstrated in patients undergoing intraocular procedures who have remained on medications that affect their coagulation. McCormack et al[1] demonstrated that procedures such as extracapsular cataract extraction with intraocular lens insertion, vitreoretinal, and trabeculectomy surgery can be performed safely without changing the anticoagulation status of the patient. Gainey et al.[2] concluded that "if anticoagulants are necessary for a patient's well-being, they should not be discontinued for cataract surgery." When prothrombin times are in reasonably good range, we have had good success simply discontinuing anticoagulation 48 hours before keratoplasty and resuming treatment on the first postoperative day.

The patient's social and family support system also need to be reviewed. Because consistent follow-up and proper use of postoperative medications are needed, patient reliability and compliance are important to the ultimate success of the graft. The patient's compliance with appointments and preoperative testing will have a direct bearing on his or her postoperative compliance. History of substance abuse or abrupt changes in family conditions that may interfere with patient follow-up may be a relative contraindication to surgery until conditions stabilize.

Ocular History

When contemplating keratoplasty, the ophthalmologist must have complete understanding of the events that have led to the patient's current status. The nature of the patient's ocular complaints in the history often leads to the diagnosis and helps guide the physician during the ocular examination. A careful history that reveals good visual acuity in the affected eye at some time before the current condition carries a better prognosis (e.g., good acuity after cataract surgery in eyes later developing pseudophakic bullous keratopathy). The presence of a corneal scar since childhood may have resulted in amblyopia, limiting potential visual acuity in the affected eye. Information should be obtained pertaining to the onset of visual disturbance, whether it was preceded by a prior intraocular procedure or infection, or whether it simply deteriorated over time. The presence of pain should be questioned, and if present, quantified as to occurrence and severity. Changes in quality of vision as the day progresses also should be ascertained; for example in Fuchs' dystrophy, vision is often worse immediately upon awakening, with gradual improvement as the day progresses.

Evaluation for Keratoplasty

Myriad factors affect the timing of keratoplasty. The patient's subjective complaints are important when evaluating a patient for surgery. An 80-year-old patient with 20/100 visual acuity and no pain and who is functioning well in his or her home environment with probable Fuchs' dystrophy, may be less in need of intervention than a 24-year-old keratoconus patient with an enlarging cone, diplopia, contact lens intolerance, and difficulty with night vision. The rheumatoid patient with acute corneal melting and impending perforation may require emergency patch grafting. At times the status of the other eye must be considered. For example, a patient with pseudophakic bullous keratopathy in one eye, poor visual acuity, and the same closed loop anterior chamber lens in the other eye is in greater need of a keratoplasty than the keratoconus patient with asymmetric involvement and good contact lens tolerance.

When available, old records are invaluable and can alert the physician to potential operative problems and confirm important information such as prior best corrected visual acuity, past intraocular pressure control, and previous intraocular lens powers. Patients often carry intraocular lens identification cards with the desired information we find useful in computing the replacement intraocular lens power. A history should be ascertained of prior ophthalmic surgical procedures such as cataract extraction, filtering procedures, or Nd:YAG laser for posterior capsular opacification. Knowledge of complications during the preceding case will help prevent potential surprises during keratoplasty.

Glaucoma and its control must be carefully questioned and evaluated. Intraocular pressure should be stabilized before keratoplasty is performed, since elevated postoperative pressure can have deleterious effects on graft survival.[3] Investigators have demonstrated that elevated intraocular pressure leads to thinning of the corneal endothelium, morphologic signs of damage, and decreased endothelial cell count.[4,5]

Prognosis for successful outcome is ultimately linked to a knowledge of the patient's preoperative history. A corneal leukoma in the visual axis has important implications worthy of consideration. Is the leukoma the result of bacterial keratitis in a soft contact lens wearer, or is it of viral origin (i.e., herpes simplex), with potential for graft rejection and perhaps requiring topical antiviral or oral acyclovir[6] postkeratoplasty.

Examination

VISUAL ACUITY

Good history taking should confirm when in the past visual acuity was better. One should rule out any amblyopia secondary to anisometropia, strabismus, or corneal scarring during childhood. The patient's best corrected visual acuity should be determined initially. Standard Snellen testing is the normal mode of visual acuity testing. If the patient cannot read the chart at 20 feet, poorer acuity such as counting fingers, hand motions, light perception, or no light perception needs to be documented. One of the most important acuity factors involves the careful testing of an eye for light projection. In eyes with corneal opacity and light perception vision, the ability of the patient to discern the direction from which a light is projected is an important indicator of retinal and optic nerve function. A patient with good retinal function should be able to appreciate the light emitted from a standard muscle lamp in all quadrants (Figure 128-1). In some eyes with severe central visual loss, light emitted from the indirect ophthalmoscope may be required. Testing visual acuity in a darkened room to compensate for light scattering and glare also may be beneficial.

The importance of a good refraction cannot be overemphasized. In keratoconus for example, where retinoscopy may be impossible because of scissoring light reflexes, it may be prudent to check keratometry and to refract the patient by dialing in the high astigmatic components (e.g., +3.00 first at 90 degrees, then 180 degrees and refining) and then progressively

A B

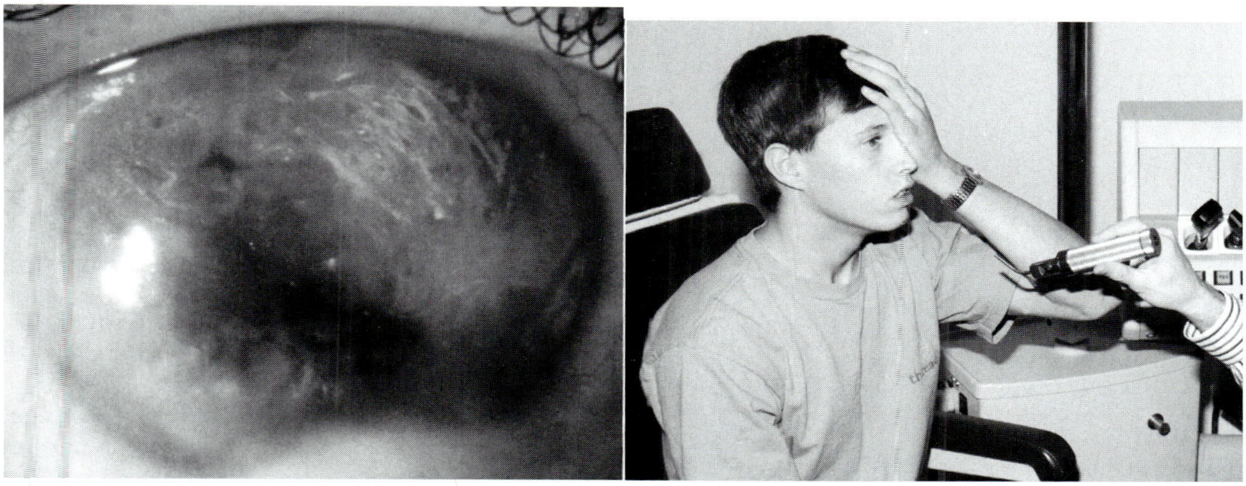

FIGURE 128-1 **A,** Slit lamp photo of severe corneal scarring and band keratopathy in a 17-year-old man referred for evaluation for penetrating keratoplasty. **B,** Evaluation of light projection in same patient. Note patient looking straight ahead with other eye completely covered. Central visual acuity was hand movements with temporal light projection only.

changing the sphere. It is also helpful to test for visual acuity with a rigid gas-permeable lens on the eye after instilling topical anesthetic. Even if not practical for long-term management, a contact lens can often eliminate irregular corneal astigmatism and provide an indication of better corrected visual acuity and visual potential. Pinhole visual acuity, potential acuity meter, and glare testing in our experience have limited value in predicting best visual acuity, probably because of severe light scattering from corneal pathology. One study suggests that the placement of a hard contact lens over the cornea before performing potential acuity meter testing[7] may be beneficial.

In cases in which there is a question as to whether there will be improvement in visual acuity after keratoplasty in eyes with corneal edema, instilling topical glycerine after anesthesia and waiting 20 to 30 minutes for corneal clearing may improve acuity and facilitate retinal viewing. Epithelial debridement and intravenous fluorescein study also may be used preoperatively for evaluating preexisting cystoid macular edema[3] (Figure 128-2).

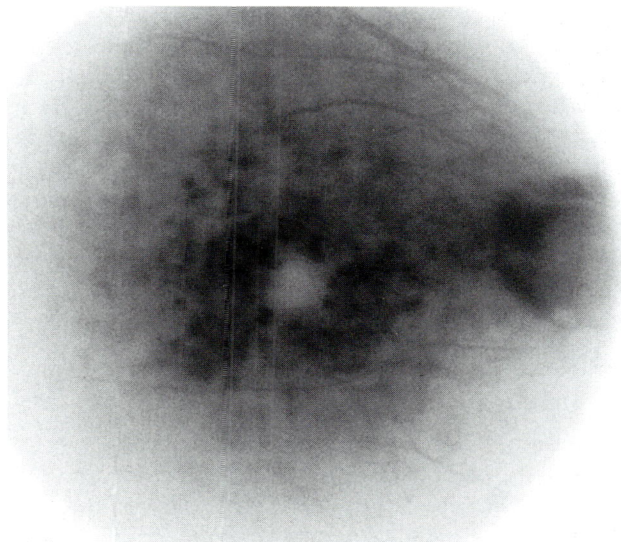

FIGURE 128-2 Cystoid macular edema viewed through cornea with Fuchs' endothelial dystrophy 20 minutes after topical glycerine was applied.

EXTERNAL EXAMINATION

A preoperative evaluation of the bony structures of the orbit and prominence of the brow should be undertaken. If the patient has deep set eyes or abnormally thin palpebral fissures, the need for proper positioning of the patient's head and choice of appropriate lid speculum at the time of surgery can be planned in advance. If the patient has active acne rosacea with staphylococcal blepharitis, appropriate treatment should be instituted for stabilization of the disease process before the procedure. Herpes zoster, trauma, and radiation may account for lid scarring or neurotrophic keratitis and ultimate graft failure.

SLIT LAMP EXAMINATION

Lids, lashes, lacrimal gland

The presence of lid disease such as blepharitis or meibomitis should be identified and controlled before keratoplasty. If the patient has an ectropion, entropion, or trichiasis, all of which can lead to epithelial scarring, permanent correction, usually surgical, before the

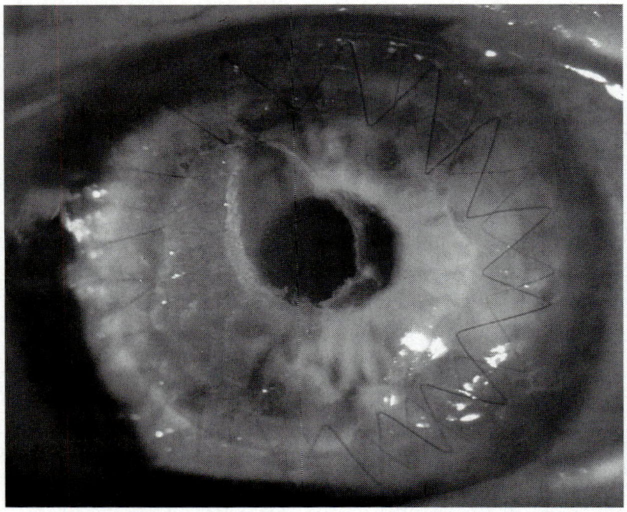

FIGURE 128-3 Nonhealing epithelial defect in corneal graft of patient with dry eye.

keratoplasty is advised. Mild spastic entropion is frequently subclinical until surgery and should be treated rapidly when noted postoperatively.

Because normal tear production is crucial to graft reepithelization, the examiner must note tear film abnormalities and dryness during the preoperative examination. The use of fluorescein and/or rose bengal and Schirmer testing gives the ophthalmologist an indication as to the extent of dryness and epitheliopathy. With significant evidence of dryness, consideration should be given to partial or complete punctal occlusion preoperatively or at keratoplasty, sometimes in combination with partial medial or lateral tarsorrhaphy, particularly when exposure keratitis is suspected.

Conjunctiva

A history of Stevens-Johnson syndrome, ocular cicatricial pemphigoid, or chemical burn should alert the ophthalmologist to look for scarring and symblepharon. These patients are at significant risk for dry eyes, nonhealing epithelial defects (Figure 128-3), and infections postoperatively as the normal external immune defense mechanisms of IgA and lysozyme are compromised. Procedures such as punctal occlusion or limbal transplantation performed before keratoplasty may increase prognosis for graft survival in these high-risk patients. On the day of surgery, the patient should be evaluated for blepharitis and conjunctivitis. If these conditions are present, the surgery should be cancelled and undertaken only after treatment and complete resolution.

Cornea

The underlying corneal problem necessitating transplantation is of obvious importance in planning keratoplasty. The causes of corneal dysfunction requiring transplantation can be divided broadly into ectatic disorders such as keratoconus and stromal dystrophies such as lattice, granular, and macular dystrophy; postinfectious corneal scarring with or without corneal vascularization, such as bacterial or viral ulcers; endothelial dysfunction with secondary stromal and/or epithelial edema, such as Fuchs' dystrophy and endothelial degeneration such as pseudophakic bullous keratopathy (box).

The diameter of the graft will be determined in part by the diameter of the corneal irregularity and its proximity to the central visual axis. For example, if possible the diameter of the cone in keratoconus should be surrounded completely by the trephine to avoid thick to thin edge suturing and progressive recipient bed thinning postoperatively. Cone diameter is best determined by direct ophthalmoscopic viewing at +6.00 diopters following maximum mydriasis or viewing the Fleisher ring intraoperatively. Leukoma need not be totally surrounded except in scars caused by herpes simplex virus where removal of possible latent virus is desirable.

Consideration also must be given to the condition of the host graft bed, its corneal thickness or peripheral thinning. Ultrasonic pachymetry should be performed to quantify thinning or thickening. The presence of corneal vascularity dictates graft sizing and suturing technique to best minimize the propensity toward vascularization of the graft and possible rejection. In eyes with a postinfectious leukoma without vascularization, or in corneal edema either secondary to Fuchs' or bullous keratopathy the central visual axis should be the center of the donor button, with average diameters ranging from 7.5 to 8.5 mm. A diameter of 8 mm, is usually a good average size for trephination, but total corneal diameter must be considered, and when overall corneal diameter is large, the surgeon should consider larger graft sizes. In most of our patients, the donor cornea is oversized by 0.25 mm. In the patient with keratoconus, some surgeons will not oversize the donor button and may even use a smaller donor cornea.[9,10] In cases with postinfectious scarring with thinning and vascularization, or displaced corneal ectasias as in pellucid marginal degeneration, sizing and placement of the graft may be less straightforward and some decentering may be required. The surgeon needs to decide the optimal sizing of the graft while avoiding areas of vascularization and peripheral thinning. Interrupted sutures may be indicated to allow for selected suture removal in cases in which the areas of vascularization are aggravated by the sutures (Figure 128-4). In cases of corneal edema, an increased depth of trephination and deep suturing into the host bed to allow Descemet membrane to Descemet membrane graft-host approximation is important.

Prognosis for graft clarity

Excellent prognosis 90% or more
Diagnosis:
- Keratoconus
- Central Fuchs' dystrophy (early)
- Granular dystrophy
- Central or paracentral inactive scars
- Rotating grafts or autografts

Very good prognosis 80%-90%
Diagnosis:
- Advanced Fuchs' dystrophy
- Pseudophakic bullous keratopathy
- Aphakic bullous keratopathy
- Inactive herpes simplex keratitis
- Macular dystrophy
- Interstitial keratitis
- Iridocorneal endothelial syndromes

Fair prognosis 50%-80%
Diagnosis:
- Active bacterial keratitis
- Active herpes simplex keratitis
- Congenital hereditary endothelial dystrophy and breaks in Descemet's membrane associated with birth trauma
- Active fungal keratitis
- Mild chemical burns
- Moderate keratitis sicca
- Lattice dystrophy
- Congenital glaucoma

Poor prognosis 0-50%
Diagnosis:
- Severe chemical burns
- Radiation burns
- Ocular pemphigoid
- Stevens-Johnson syndrome
- Neuroparalytic disease

Poor prognosis 0-50%
Diagnosis:
- Epithelial downgrowth
- Anterior chamber cleavage syndromes
- Multiple graft failures

From Buxton JN, Buxton DF, Westphalen JA: Penetrating Keratoplasty; indications and contraindications. In Brightbill FS: *Corneal surgery: theory, technique, and tissue,* ed 2, St Louis, 1993, Mosby (with slight modifications). This information is meant as a guideline and is certainly not absolute. The prognosis for each group is worsened by the presence of elevated intraocular pressure, intraocular inflammation, lid and conjunctival defects, and other ocular surface disorders. Failed grafts are generally considered to possess the prognosis for the group of their primary diagnosis, or slightly less.

Anterior segment/iris

Perhaps most important in this part of the ocular examination is to rule out active inflammation. In cases of elective transplantation, the chance for the best outcome is in a quiet, noninflamed eye. Presence of a ciliary flush, keratic, or intraocular lens precipitates; anterior synechiae; and iridocorneal adhesions are all signs of past or present inflammation and should be noted. If an anterior chamber lens is present, it must be identified as either an open-looped or closed-loop lens. Iris-supported and closed-loop anterior chamber lenses should be replaced as should any open-looped anterior chamber lens when movement is suspected[11,12] (Figure 128-5). Gonioscopy should be considered to examine iridocorneal adhesions and peripheral iridectomies and to locate the position of lens haptics if an anterior chamber lens is present. If the anterior chamber lens needs to be replaced, consideration of the patient's anterior chamber anatomy (e.g., location of posterior and anterior synechiae and residual lens capsule) will play a role in deciding the appropriate lens replacement type. A thorough evaluation of the iris is important. Presence of rubeosis, fibrovascular membranes obscuring the pupil, and location of peripheral iridectomies needs to be noted.

If the pupil can be visualized well, the presence or absence of a relative afferent pupillary defect should be documented. Presence of color visual perception also helps to rule out optic nerve damage.

Lens

Before keratoplasty, the patient's lens should be examined with the slit lamp microscope. The lens may have weakened zonules and exhibit phakodinesis. In many elderly patients, especially eyes with Fuchs' dystrophy, the lens may exhibit early cataractous changes, which may signal the need for a combined keratoplasty and cataract extraction. We believe that keratoplasty, perhaps aided by high-dose postoperative corticosteroids, is frequently a cataractogenic procedure. Triple procedures (penetrating keratoplasty, cataract extraction, and intraocular lens implantation) should be performed when even minimal lens opacities are present to avoid the need for future cataract extraction that may damage the endothelium and threaten the integrity of the graft.

Patients with inactive leutic interstitial keratitis and scarring frequently do not present to the corneal surgeon until progressive cataract occurs, which when combined with the leukoma, produces significant inability to function necessitating a combined procedure.

A

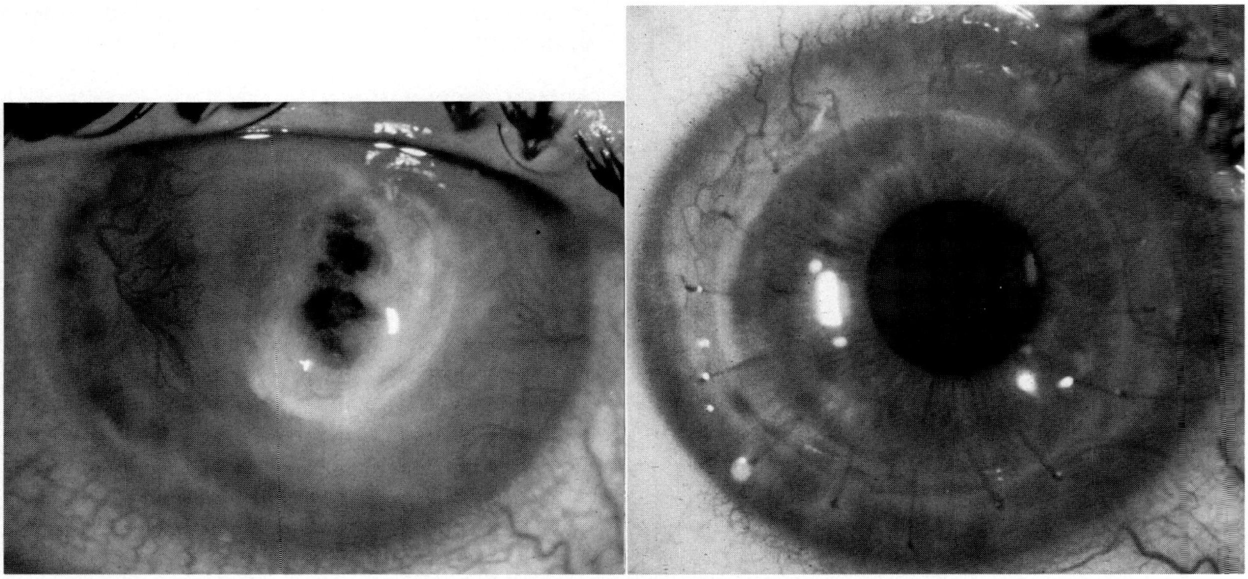

B

FIGURE 128-4 **A,** Stromal necrotizing keratitis secondary to herpes simplex infection with descemetocele and deep vascularization. **B,** Same eye 6 months after penetrating keratoplasty demonstrating clear graft with interrupted suture placement. Note absence of vessels in donor tissue.

A

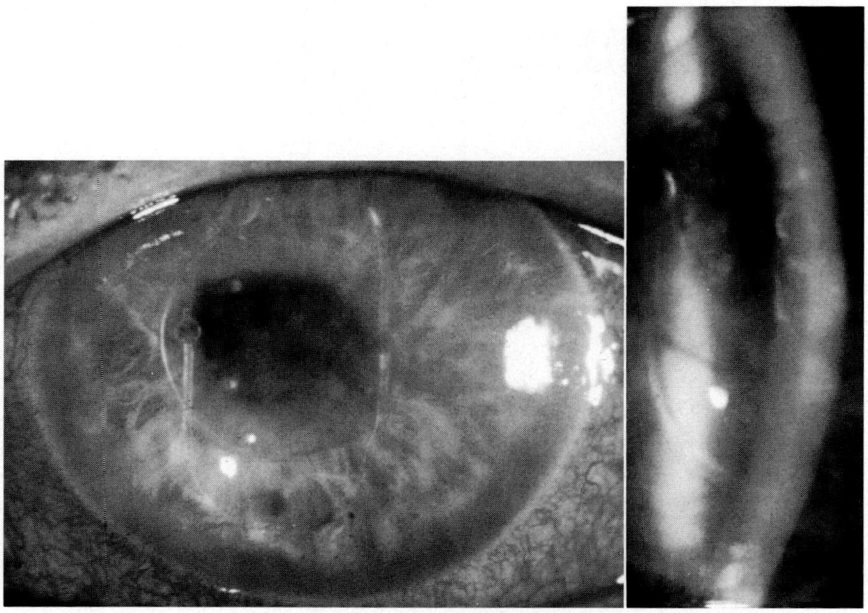

B

FIGURE 128-5 **A,** Patient with iris-supported lens and pseudophakic bullous keratopathy. **B,** Magnified slit beam view of same eye demonstrating stromal edema.

In eyes that have undergone prior cataract extraction, knowledge of intraocular lens design (anterior chamber, iris-supported, or posterior chamber) or aphakia is critical to operative planning. The type of lens implanted will dictate whether it should be replaced. Is there a clear, intact posterior capsule, or has Nd:YAG capsulotomy been performed?

Intraocular pressure

The presence of borderline controlled or uncontrolled glaucoma is a contraindication to keratoplasty. Accurate applanation pressures in corneas with epithelial edema are difficult to obtain and falsely low readings may be generated. The use of a Tono-Pen, pneumotonometer, or MacKay-Marg tonometer is considered to be more accurate.[13,14] We believe that intraocular pressure should be no higher than the low twenties on no more than two topical medications. If it is not, primary filtering or combined filtering and penetrating keratoplasty should be considered. Because all keratoplasty patients receive intraoperative viscoelastics to coat donor endothelium, aid in control of bleeding, and help prevent synechiae,[15] eyes with preexistent glaucoma usually require immediate postoperative oral ocular hypotensives and topical aqueous inhibitors to control intraocular pressure. The use of a lower viscosity viscoelastic and removal or dilution with balanced salt solution in the anterior chamber before button placement and suturing is recommended. The long-term use of topical steroids to prevent rejection may lead to steroid-induced glaucoma and requires careful intraocular pressure monitoring for the entire postoperative period. In our experience, longstanding chronic glaucoma with intraocular pressures in the low to mid twenties is a common cause of slow graft failure.

RETINA/VITREOUS

An evaluation of retinal function and the vitreous is required to ensure that decreased vision is secondary to problems with the cornea alone. Macular degeneration, cystoid macular edema, macular holes, and an opaque or hazy vitreous among other maladies are all factors that will not improve after keratoplasty. Knowledge of such conditions before keratoplasty will help in prognostication and can often be obtained in examination of old records and discussions with the referring ophthalmologist. In cases where there is a question, potential acuity meter testing, laser inferometry, or electrophysiologic testing may be tried, but have limited sensitivity. If the retina and vitreous cannot be visualized by direct or indirect ophthalmoscopy, ultrasonography should be undertaken to rule out a retinal detachment, retinal mass, or vitreous hemorrhage.

Communication with Patient

Once the evaluation has been completed, the diagnosis and plans for keratoplasty should be discussed with the patient. The procedure should be clearly explained using handouts, models, and videotapes as indicated. The risks of the procedure specifically regarding the long healing time, need for antiglaucoma treatment, and rejection rates should be addressed. The patient should be given realistic expectations for potential visual acuity and the time it may take to reach that acuity. The possible use of a contact lens, relaxing incisions, or wedge resection to reach best visual acuity should be understood by the patient before the procedure to ensure patient satisfaction in the postoperative period. The patient who undergoes keratoplasty is entering into a lifelong doctor/patient relationship. Sound preoperative planning and explanation between the surgeon and patient will help make this relationship productive.

REFERENCES

1. McCormack P, Simcock PR, Tullo AB: Management of the anticoagulated patient for ophthalmic surgery, *Eye* 7:749-750, 1993.
2. Gainey S et al: Ocular surgery on patients receiving long term warfarin therapy, *Am J Ophthalmol* 108:142-146, 1989.
3. Maguire MG et al: Risk factors for corneal graft failure and rejection in the collaborative corneal transplant studies. Collaborative Corneal Transplantation Studies Research Group, *Ophthalmology* 101:1536-1547, 1994.
4. Svedbergh B: Effects of artificial intraocular pressure elevation on corneal endothelium in the vervet monkey, *Acta Ophthalmol (Copenh)* 53:839, 1975.
5. Vannag A, Setala K, Ruusuvaana P: Endothelial cells in capsular glaucoma, *Acta Ophthalmol (Copenh)* 55:951, 1977.
6. Barney NP, Foster CS: A prospective randomized trial of oral acyclovir after penetrating keratoplasty for herpes simplex keratitis, *Cornea* 13:231-236, 1994.
7. Smiddy WE et al: Potential acuity meter for predicting postoperative visual acuity in penetrating keratoplasty: a new method using a hard contact lens, *Ophthalmology* 94:12-16, 1987.
8. Brightbill FS, Dudley SS: Aphakic bullous keratopathy: preoperative fluorescein angiographic screening for macular edema, *Contact Intraocul Lens Med J* 7:144-149, 1981.
9. Lanier JD, Bullington RH Jr, Prager TC: Axial length in keratoconus, *Cornea* 11:250-254, 1992.
10. Girard LJ et al: Use of grafts smaller than the opening for keratoconic myopia and astigmatism: a prospective study, *J Cataract Refract Surg* 18:380-384, 1992.
11. Doren GS, Stern GA, Driebe WT: Indications for and results of intraocular lens explantation, *J Cataract Refract Surg* 18:79-85, 1992.
12. Kornmehl EW et al: Penetrating keratoplasty for pseudophakic bullous keratopathy associated with closed-loop anterior chamber lenses, *Ophthalmology* 97:407-412, 1990.
13. Rootman DS et al: Accuracy and precision of the Tono-Pen in measuring intraocular pressure after keratoplasty and epikeratophakia and in scarred cornea, *Acta Ophthalmol (Copenh)* 106:1600-1700, 1988.
14. Wind CA, Irvine AR: Electronic applanation tonometry in corneal edema and keratoplasty, *Invest Ophthalmol* 8:620-624, 1969.
15. Liesegang TJ: Viscoelastics, *Int Ophthalmol Clin* 33:127-147, 1993.

CHAPTER 129

MARK R. MANDEL

Instrumentation for Corneal Transplant Surgery

During the last two decades, the number of surgical instruments available to the corneal surgeon has increased dramatically. Many of the newer instruments are often subtle variations on earlier designs. Every corneal surgeon has a favorite toothed and tying forceps, scissors, and speculum, each with slightly different modifications. The suitability of these instruments is based primarily on surgeon preference rather than on specific use requirements.

The selection of instrumentation for corneal transplantation surgery is largely a personal choice. Many options are available. Certain instruments facilitate more than a single maneuver and increase the efficiency of the entire procedure. The chapter is organized according to instrument categories.

Instrumentation for corneal transplant surgery can be divided into four categories:

1. Instruments specifically designed to create a circular incision of the recipient cornea and to prepare the donor cornea, such as trephines/handles, punches, and blocks.
2. Instruments used to secure the donor cornea and to remove and replace lens implants such as forceps, scissors, and needle holders.
3. Instruments used to assist in the maintenance and reconstruction of the anterior segment such as cannulae, spatulas, and hooks.
4. Qualitative keratometers used intraoperatively to assess corneal toricity.

Preparation of the Recipient Globe

After surgical preparation of the operative field, the eye should be draped to conceal the lashes beneath the reflected ends of the drape when the speculum is placed. A solid plastic drape such as the 3M 1060 or equivalent, is ideal.

SPECULUM

The transplant surgeon must have several speculae available in order to meet the needs of the various different anatomic configurations frequently encountered. The speculum should be light weight and have a minimum of extraneous parts onto which suture can become entangled. A wire lid speculum such as the Barraquer or Kratz-Barraquer is ideal for most cases (Figure 129-1). A Maumenee-Park speculum (with or without canthus bar) should be available for those cases in which the eyelids impose excessive pressure on the globe. (Figure 129-2). The adjustable blades can be elevated to diminish pressure on the globe. The disadvantage of this speculum is that there are areas both on the blades of the speculum and on the large lateral end that can snag suture. If a Maumenee-Park speculum is used, it should be supported by folding gauze pads between the lateral edge of the speculum and the drape to avoid undue torsion and globe pressure from the weight of the speculum.

GLOBE SUPPORTING RINGS

The Flieringa ring or any of its modifications is useful for maintaining the architecture of the globe once the corneal button has been removed. Although the surgeon should have an array of available sizes, most commonly the 17 and 18 mm sizes are used (Figure 129-3). Some surgeons prefer the McNeill-Goldmann blepharostat ring, which incorporates a scleral fixation ring and wire lid retractor. Fixation rings are generally secured with interrupted 5-0 or 7-0 sutures in each of the four quadrants using a medium curved, spatulated needle.

LARGE NEEDLE HOLDER

For securing the ring or, if preferred, for the placement of superior and inferior rectus sutures for stabilization of the globe, a spring action needle holder with standard jaws is used. The fine needle holder for placing 10-0 nylon sutures is not suited to this function because the larger needles will damage the jaws, the

1
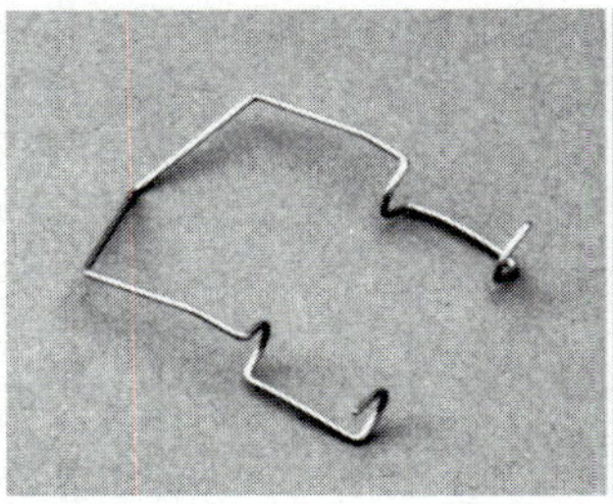

2
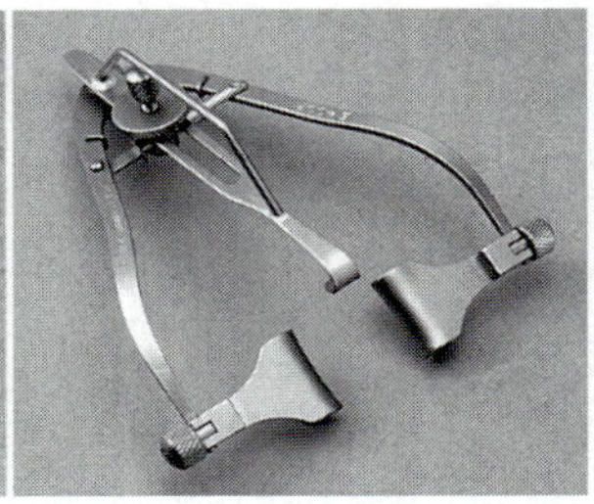

FIGURE 129-1 Kratz-Barraquer eye speculum.
FIGURE 129-2 Maumenee-Park speculum with canthus bar.

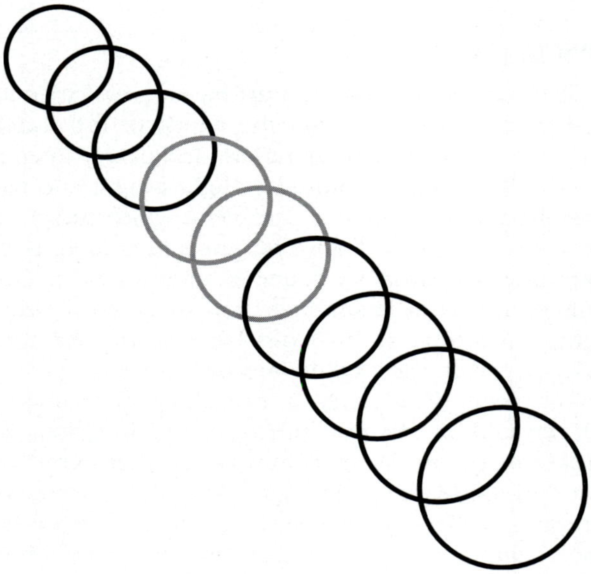

FIGURE 129-3 An array of Flieringa rings. The gray rings are 17 and 18 mm, the most commonly used sizes.

joint, and the spring action of the needle holder. A curved, nonlocking, spring action, rounded handled needle holder with standard jaws should be used. The Barraquer holder is ideal for this maneuver (Figure 129-4).

FORCEPS (LARGE TOOTHED)

To secure the globe while placing the ring or rectus sutures, large toothed (0.3 or 0.5 mm) Castroviejo forceps should be used. The 0.12 mm forceps used to manipulate donor tissue would be damaged by the large gauge stainless steel of the Flieringa ring and would not provide the surgeon adequate globe fixation when placing the rectus or ring suture if used directly on the conjunctiva/episclera.

Preparation of Recipient Bed

A trephine is a seamless, cylindrical scalpel blade, which, when rotated, creates a circular corneal incision. The trephine blade is usually attached to a handle for greater stability, leverage, and control. Although most commonly hand held, the trephine can be secured to the cornea using a vacuum system. Vacuum-assisted trephines use either a circular metal trephine blade or a single point diamond blade to create the keratotomy.

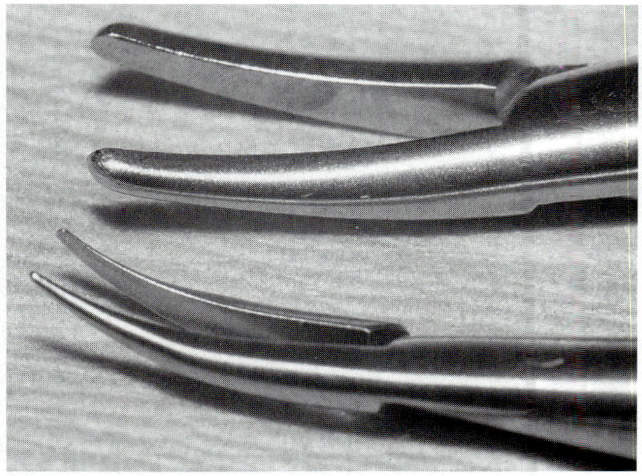

FIGURE 129-4 Barraquer needle holder with standard jaws compared to Barraquer needle holder with fine jaws.

Trephine blades range in size from 5 to 17 mm and, except for the very small and very large sizes, fit on a handle (Figure 129-5). The handle secures the trephine and confers a mechanical advantage over simply holding the trephine blade by hand. The trephine handle may have a hollow core to allow the surgeon to observe the central cornea through the center of the trephine (Figure 129-6), or it may have a central obturator with or without a calibrated nut, which can be set so as to adjust the depth of the trephination to avoid inadvertent entry into the anterior chamber (Figure 129-7). The advantage of the handle obturator is that it is adjustable and allows for fairly accurate depth determination. The disadvantage of the obturator is that it reduces the surgeon's view of the central cornea. The disadvantage of both the hollow core and the solid obturator-type of handle is that each size trephine must be matched to the handle size, necessitating the purchase of many different handles to accommodate different trephine sizes. "Universal" trephine handles, which accommodate various blade sizes (Figure 129-8), are available from several surgical manufacturers. The advantage of this type of handle is that this single instrument will secure trephine sizes used in the great majority of transplantation surgeries. The disadvantage is that it is neither hollow for optimal visualization nor does it provide protection against precipitous entry into the anterior chamber.

Another type of trephine system is the vacuum-assisted system. The Hessburg-Barron vacuum tre-

5 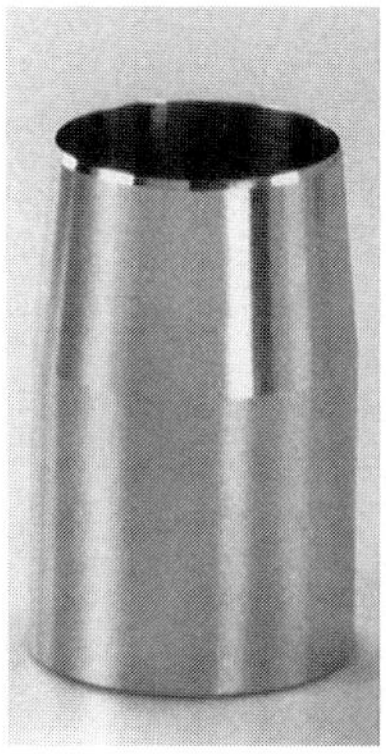 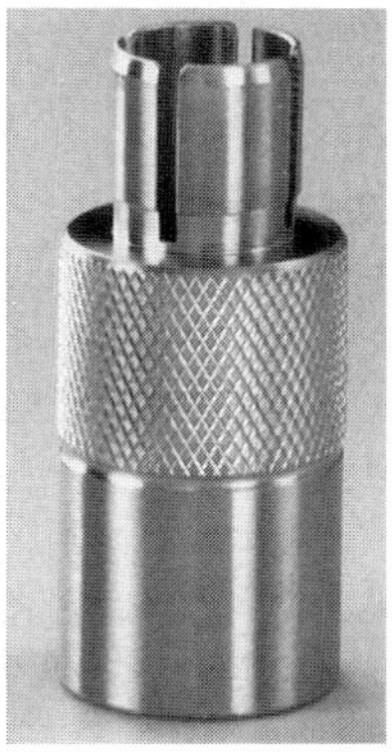 6

FIGURE 129-5 A disposable trephine blade.
FIGURE 129-6 Hollow core single-size trephine blade handle.

7 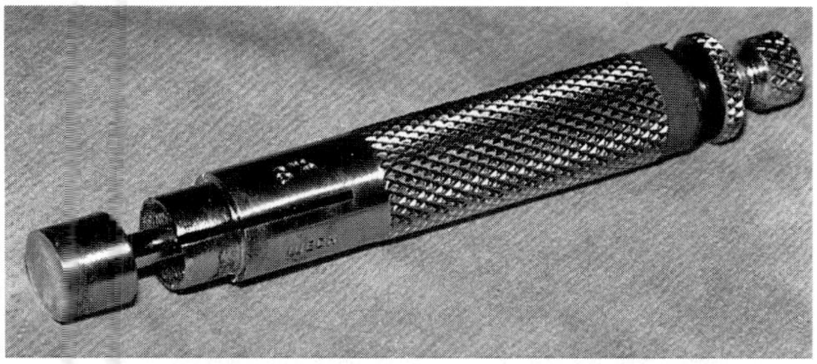

8 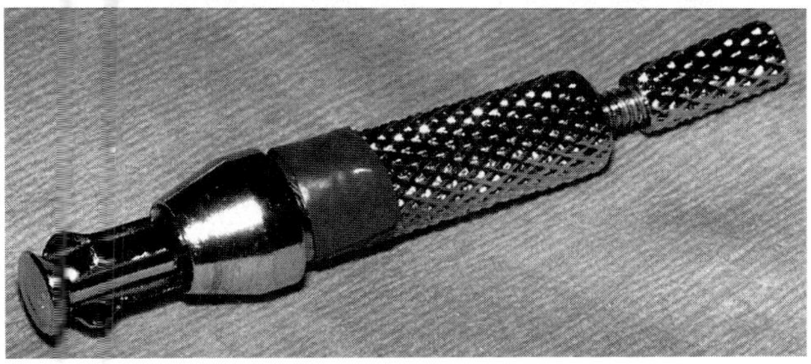

FIGURE 129-7 Single size handle with central obturator without a calibration.
FIGURE 129-8 Universal trephine handle (7 to 9 mm).

phine, the Hanna, the Krumeich, and the Lieberman systems are examples (Table 129-1). The advantage of the suction trephine is that it stabilizes the globe and diminishes tilt of the trephine and possible resultant overcutting or undercutting of the incision bevel. For some cases they are useful in soft, perforated globes. The disadvantage of these systems is that they aresomewhat bulky and cumbersome to use and, other than the Hessburg-Barron system, are extremely expensive.

The disposable Hessburg-Barron trephine has an outer 360-degree suction chamber activated by a spring-loaded 6 ml syringe that creates negative pressure. The suction in the chamber facilitates attachment of the trephine to the peripheral cornea establishing fixation and stability during trephination. The inner trephine blade is advanced by a manual rotating mechanism, which allows the surgeon to advance the blade 250 μm for each 360-degree rotation of the handle (Figure 129-9). This system is particularly advantageous in the perforated globe, which is soft and extremely difficult to trephine using the free hand technique. The trephine is available in 16 to 9 mm sizes in half-millimeter increments. The newer units have 16 evenly spaced markers along the outer suction ring, which can be moistened with a sterile marking pen to provide a symmetric pattern on the recipient cornea to assist in suture placement.

The Hanna trephine system for penetrating keratoplasty also incorporates a syringe-driven 360-degree outer chamber, which is part of the trephine unit. This secures the trephine to the limbus. A disposable steel trephine blade, which is available in 7 to 11 mm sizes, is advanced by turning a knurled knob that extends obliquely from the upper edge of the trephine. One turn of the knob extends the blade 88 μm. A "gunsight" alignment system helps ensure centration. The trephine is approximately the same size and shape of a Goldmann 3-mirror contact lens (Figure 129-10).

The Krumeich-guided trephine system incorporates a separate Barraquer-style suction ring, that affixes to the limbus. Centration of the suction ring is achieved using a crosshair device. The footplate of the trephine guide fits into a track in the center of the suction ring. A disposable Weck trephine is held in place with a central hollow cylinder that fits into the trephine guide. The trephine is advanced by a top screw that controls its descent in approximately 100 μm increments while viewing the central cornea through a clear obturator placed in the shaft of the hollow cylinder.

Lieberman has developed a cam-guided single point diamond blade trephine that fashions either round or oval shaped openings. An outer suction ring secures the body of the trephine to the limbus. As the surgeon rotates the cutting insert, the single point diamond knife is lowered onto the surface of the cornea. The knife follows the shape and dimensions of the internal cam to produce the desired diameter and configuration of the corneal incision. There are two cutting inserts. One holds the blade vertically or 90 degree to the limbus, and a second holds the blade at 20 degrees to the limbus. The 20-degree insert creates a significant bevel. The donor cornea is incised with the same system using an artificial anterior chamber to secure the corneoscleral rim (Figure 129-11).

Back Table: Preparation of the Donor Cornea

In corneal transplantation surgery, unlike other forms of anterior segment surgery, a separate back

Table 129-1. Comparison of current commercially available vacuum trephine systems

Blade type	System	Limbal vacuum attachment	Donor cornea punch
Circular steel trephine blade	Barron	Outer chamber of trephine body	Separate disposable blade Manual punch from endothelial side
	Krumeich	Separate Barraquer-style suction ring	Artificial anterior chamber
	Hanna	Outer chamber of trephine body	Suction-assisted block to punch from endothelial side or Artificial anterior chamber to incise from epithelial surface
Single point diamond blade cam-guided for circular or oval incision	Lieberman	Outer chamber of trephine body	Artificial anterior chamber

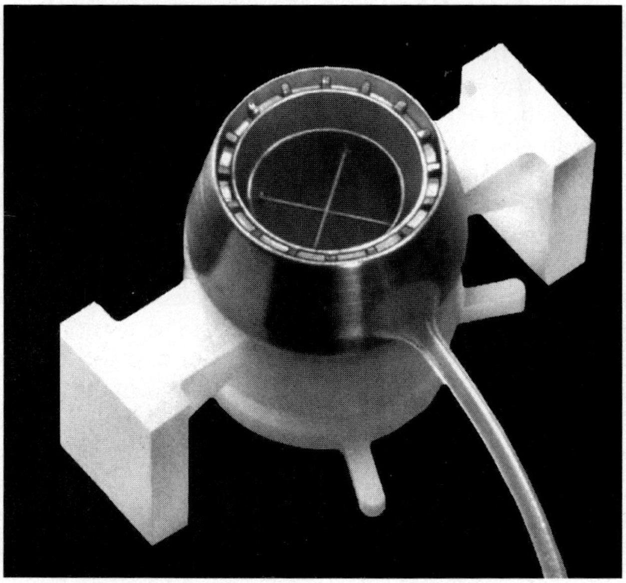

FIGURE 129-9 Barron radial vacuum trephine.

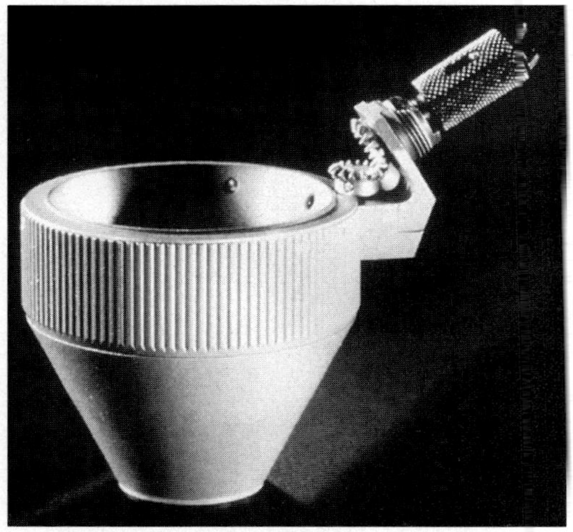

FIGURE 129-10 Hanna corneal trephine system

table setup is required to prepare the donor tissue. Because the entire cornea and a few millimeters of sclera is commonly preserved in tissue culture medium, a circular corneal button is created from the center of the donor cornea by punching from the endothelial surface using a trephine-loaded punch system. Less commonly, the central button is excised from the epithelial side using an artificial anterior chamber such as the Krumeich, Hanna, or Lieberman systems (Figure 129-12). A punch system consists of a cutting block onto which the donor corneoscleral complex is placed and centered; a piston to secure, center, stabilize, and advance the trephine blade; and a piston guide.

Cutting blocks are constructed from either Teflon, nylon, or polycarbonate. Although these blocks are disposable, they can be used multiple times. Most modern blocks are designed with a compound-curved concave "well," which approximates the central, midperipheral, and peripheral curvature of the donor cornea and sclera. This stabilizes the cornea and helps to ensure a central round cut. Many blocks incorporate a central air vent and some, such as the Brightbill Teflon cutting block, the Iowa punch block, and the Tanne block, have a colored centering target (Figure 129-13).

The Troutman corneal punch is a simple system incorporating a centered block and a piston carrier with a central piston. Three pistons are available to fit different blade diameters. The most frequently used piston accommodates the 7 to 9 mm blades. This straightforward system relies on pressure from the surgeon's thumb to incise the donor cornea.

The Iowa punch (manufactured by Weck and Storz) incorporates a spring-loaded piston with an expandable retaining edge to accommodate 6 to 9.5 mm trephines (Storz unit) or 6.5 to 9 mm (Weck unit). The piston is inserted into the carrier guide, and, using pressure from the surgeon's thumb, advanced to punch from the endothelial side (Figure 129-14).

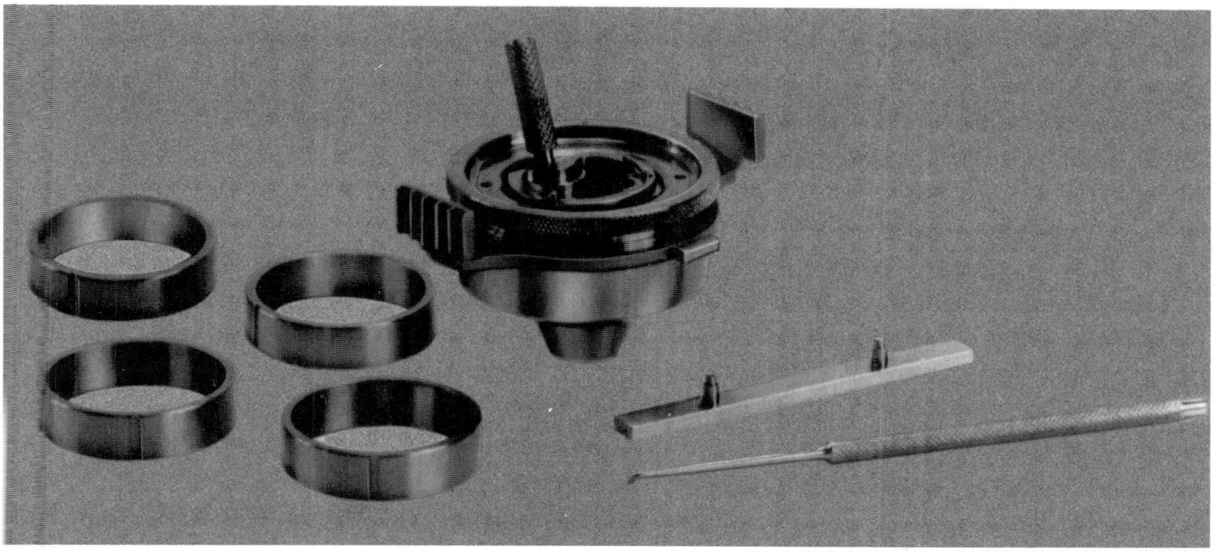

FIGURE 129-11 Lieberman system.

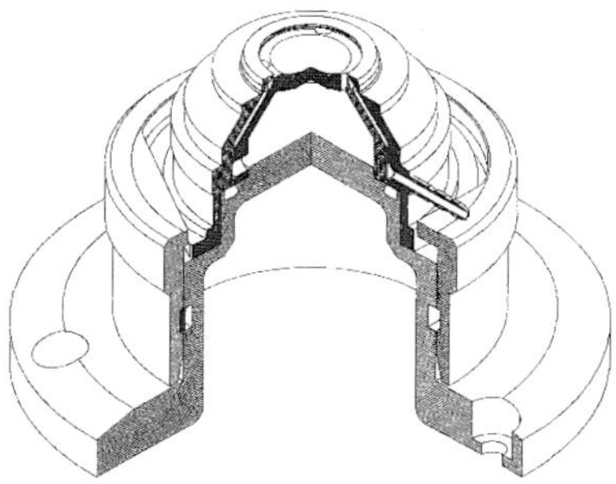

FIGURE 129-12 Hanna artificial anterior chamber.

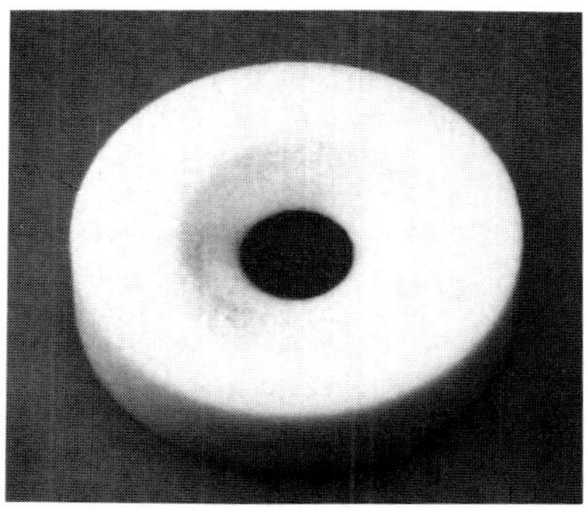

FIGURE 129-13 Example of a Teflon cutting block with multicurved well and centering target.

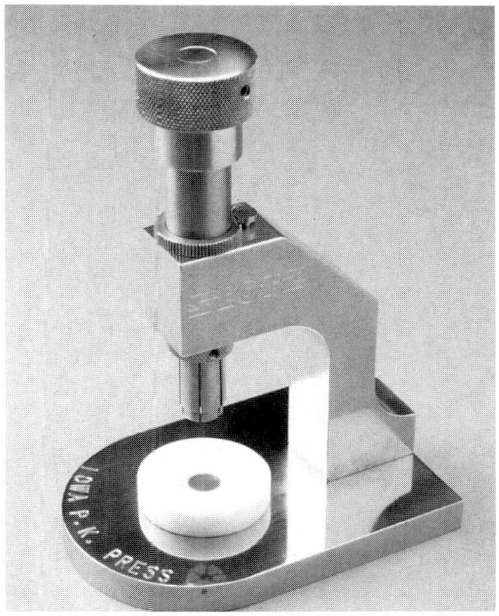

FIGURE 129-14 Iowa corneal punch.

The Lieberman gravity-action corneal donor punch (Katena K2-8200) is a guillotine-style punch with a weighted head that uses the force of gravity rather than the surgeon's power to incise the corneal button.

The Rothman-Gilbard cornea punch (Storz E3051) uses a piston that is not spring loaded. It differs from the other units in that the block incorporates eight evenly spaced suction holes that are used to secure the corneal button firmly to the block, minimizing movement during trephination. Additionally, these holes can be inked with a sterile pen to place marks on the donor cornea to facilitate suturing (Figure 129-15).

The Barron corneal donor button punches are disposable sharp block/trephine assemblies. The trephine blade is permanently mounted in a white nylon housing with four steel alignment posts. The punch base/block incorporates a compound-curved well with a central air vent. The base and trephine housing are assembled by aligning the posts into corresponding holes in each corner of the base. This automatically centers the trephine over the donor cornea (Figure 129-16).

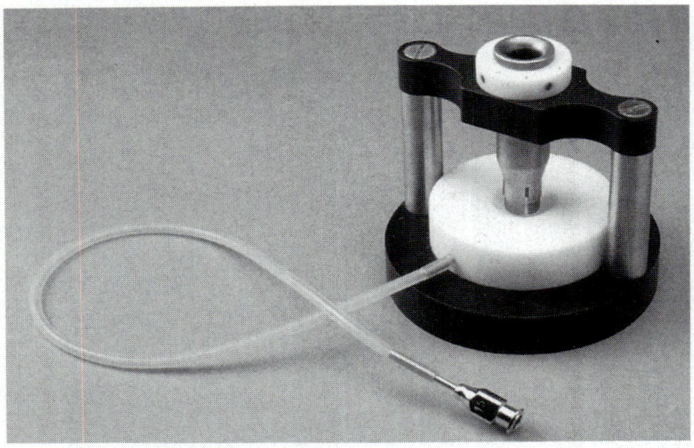

FIGURE 129-15 **Rothman-Gilbard corneal punch.**

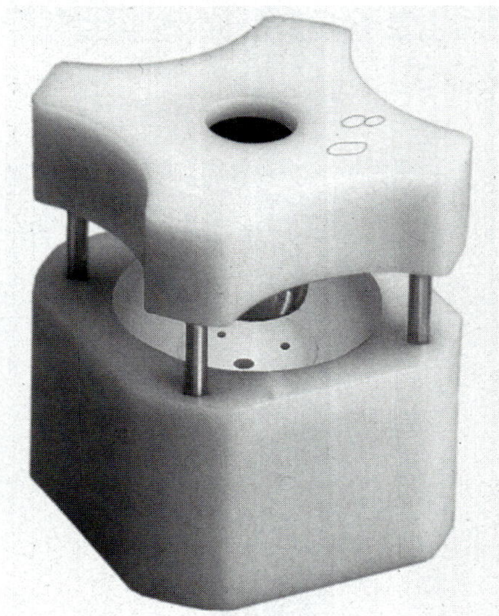

FIGURE 129-16 **Barron corneal donor button punch.**

The Krumeich, Hanna, and Lieberman systems incorporate the use of an artificial anterior chamber. Although the design and mechanics of each anterior chamber device differ among systems, the overall strategy involves incising the donor cornea from the epithelial, rather than the endothelial side. This is achieved by placing the donor corneoscleral button over a support system, which secures and centers the preserved button shell and creates a pressurized environment, allowing trephination from the anterior surface. Pressure within the artificial anterior chamber is adjusted to approximate the normal intraocular pressure by attaching the chamber to an infusion system. The Hanna and Krumeich systems use a disposable steel trephine blade, and the Lieberman system uses a single-point diamond blade to effect the keratotomy.

There are many systems of trephines and punches. Like most instruments for corneal surgery, the system used depends on training, personal experience, availability, and cost effectiveness. Each has subtle advantages and disadvantages. The main goal of trephination of either the recipient cornea or the donor button is to achieve a central cut with minimal tissue distortion and avoidance of endothelial damage.

Instruments Used in Securing Donor to Recipient Cornea and in Anterior Segment Tissue and Implant Manipulations

FORCEPS

Perhaps the most important forceps in the armamentarium of the corneal surgeon is the 0.12 mm fine-toothed forceps. A Colibri-style forceps is particularly well suited for corneal transplant surgery. Its design not only lends itself to grasping corneal tissue from all angles, but when combined with a tying platform, it can be used to grasp, control, and tie the 10-0 nylon suture (Figure 129-17). Although not an uncommon practice among corneal surgeons, grasping the needle with the Colibri forceps is not advised because of its very fine teeth, platforms, jaws, and its delicate spring action. The Colibri forceps is an ideal example of an instrument that, if used to its full advantage, can offer the surgeon economy of time and space. Specifically, if used as both a forceps to grasp tissue and to tie suture, it is unnecessary to put down the forceps and needle holder to pick up the tying forceps. The successful use of the Colibri forceps for tying suture depends on the use of a needle holder with a gently curved shaft and jaws fine enough to accurately grasp and manipulate the suture.

The Colibri-style Polack double corneal forceps is specifically designed for placement of the first corneal suture. A pair of smooth forceps such as straight and angled McPherson-type forceps are useful not only for tying suture but also for manipulating tissue such as iris and retropupillary membranes, the placement of anterior and posterior chamber intraocular lenses, and the removal of previously placed anterior chamber and iris-supported lenses. Longer-shafted Kelman-McPherson forceps are ideal for "hand-over-hand" maneuvers like those associated with removal of closed loops flexible anterior chamber lense. The straight McPherson forceps are also useful for completing the open sky capsulorrhexis during extracapsular cataract surgery combined with corneal transplant surgery. MacPherson forceps are used for tying 10-0 polypropylene suture inside the chamber angle when recon-

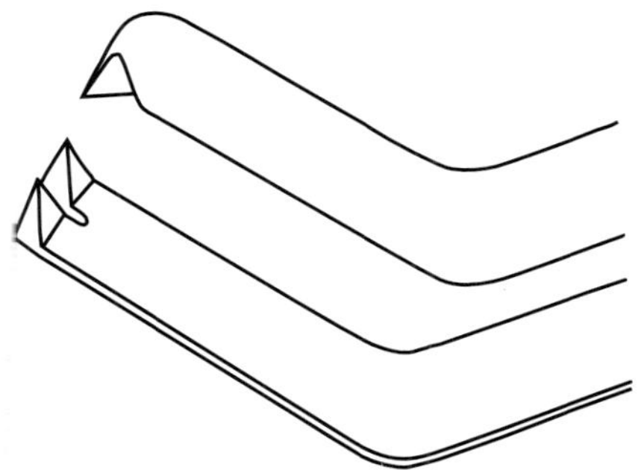

FIGURE 129-17 Tip and tying platform of the Colibri-style forceps.

structing the iris and for manipulating the delicate and often friable iris tissue.

NEEDLE HOLDER

Although a large-nosed standard Barraquer needle holder is useful for securing the Flieringa ring or placing bridle sutures, its heavy gauged working end will bend the delicate needles of 10-0 and 11-0 nylon and polypropylene suture. Therefore, a delicate or fine-tipped needle holder is necessary. Curved jaws provide the mechanical advantage of working in many hand positions. Additionally, the curve facilitates tying fine suture. The needle holder should be nonlocking to avoid tissue distortion when attempting to unlock the needle holder during each suture pass. The Barraquer needle holder with delicate curved jaws without a lock is recommended. The surgeon also should have a fine needle holder with an acute "hockey stick" configuration such as the Troutman-Barraquer needle holder (Weck 4161). This needle holder is particularly useful when working in the superior nasal quadrant of the left eye in an individual with a deep set globe.

SCISSORS

A pair of blunt tip direct action "iris" or tenotomy scissors are useful for cutting the drape and the large-gauge bridle or Flieringa ring sutures. The Westcott scissors also can be used to cut the suture securing the Flieringa ring or bridle sutures, to cut vitreous strands and fibrous retropupillary membranes, and to perform a sectoral or circumferential conjunctival resection in the case of a dense pannus. The Shepard-Westcott scissors with a serrated edge (Storz E3320-RS) is useful for cutting the closed loop PMMA anterior chamber lenses and iris-supported lens haptics before removal.

Vannas scissors are manufactured in many sizes and shapes that differ in handle and blade lengths and configuration. The corneal surgeon should have at least one straight and one curved-blade Vannas scissors for cutting tissues inside the anterior chamber and the suture used to secure the donor tissue to the recipient cornea. The Vannas scissors are useful for creating an iridectomy or reconstructing the iris diaphragm, incising and excising more diaphanous retropupillary membranes, and trimming an uneven or excessively beveled posterior corneal ledge following trephination.

The most important and transplant-specific scissors on the surgical tray are those used to excise the recipient corneal button. Although there are many subtle variations in design, these scissors cannot be substituted by the standard corneoscleral scissors because of the difference in blade curvature, configuration, and size. The corneoscleral scissors used for perilimbal sections in cataract surgery have more gradually curved blades, with the lower blade outside of the upper blade to create the beveled incision necessary for cataract surgery. Conversely, corneal transplantation scissors have the lower blade inside the upper blade to create the slightly beveled, but more perpendicular incision critical for a tight wound in penetrating keratoplasty. Additionally, the blades have a shorter radius of curvature and are differently angled to follow the trephination groove. Many different handle and blade lengths, configurations, and curvatures are available (Figure 129-18).

SPATULAS AND HOOKS

A selection of spatulas and hooks for use in the maintenance and reconstruction of the anterior chamber, the manipulation of the iris, and assistance in the placement of anterior and posterior chamber intraocular lenses should be available.

The double-ended square-handled Castroviejo, or round-handled single-bladed Barraquer cyclodialysis spatula is useful for lysis of synechiae between the iris and lens capsule, dissection of iris from retrocorneal membranes and iris-supported implants, lysis of broad-based anterior synechiae, and sweeping the anterior chamber through a side-port incision once the cornea has been secured in cases where intraoperative iridocorneal apposition has occurred.

Intraocular lens manipulators such as the Sinskey and Lester hooks are very useful. The greatest mechanical advantage is achieved with an angled shaft for each of these instruments. One of each type of manipulator should be on the set to allow the greatest flexibility for selection. Occasionally, it is necessary to use an implant manipulator in each hand when placing and stabilizing an anterior chamber lens.

A useful, multipurpose iris/implant manipulator is the Hirschman iris hook (Storz E0549H). This hook is used not only to retract the iris in cases of small pupil open sky cataract extraction and/or examination of the posterior chamber, but also in the stabilization of the anterior chamber intraocular lens during implantation and while dialing a posterior chamber lens while retracting the edge of the iris or capsulorrhexis.

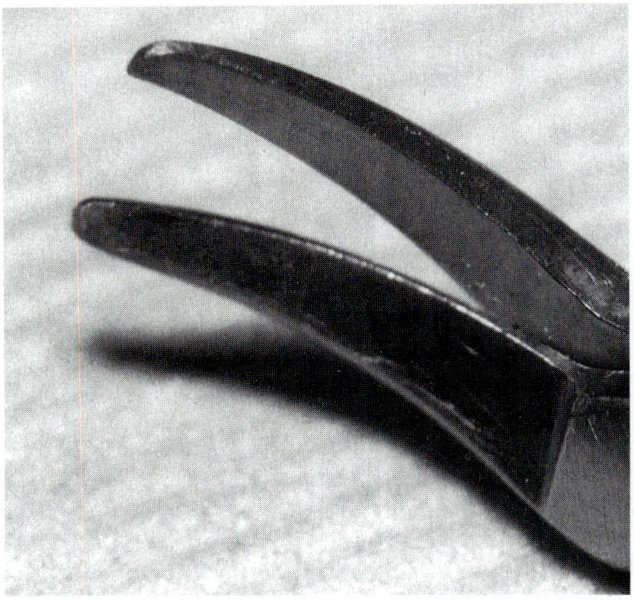

FIGURE 129-18 Blades of the Katzin corneal scissors.

A Paton spoon/spatula can be used to transfer the corneal button from the cutting block to the surgical field. Alternatively, the peripheral anterior stroma of the donor button can be grasped with the Colibri forceps to facilitate transfer.

A useful, but seldom discussed instrument is the twist hook. Although not frequently used in routine corneal transplant surgery, this instrument can prove extremely helpful for scleral fixation in a soft perforated globe, which is difficult to grasp and stabilize using toothed forceps. It can be used during the trephination phase and to secure the globe when free-hand dissection of the trephination groove is required.

BLADES

A 15-degree disposable blade is useful for entrance into the anterior chamber through the trephination groove and in making peripheral side-port incisions. These blades are also used to create sclerotomies in cases with excessive posterior vitreous pressure, for the pars plana aspiration of fluid vitreous, and to drain suprachoroidal fluid and blood if a suprachoroidal hemorrhage is encountered. An unguarded diamond or other gem blade also can be used for this function.

The unguarded diamond or gem blade is useful for the free-hand dissection of the host groove that is often required for the soft globe of a perforated cornea. In these cases, if a suction trephine cannot be used, it is often impossible to create a deep corneal incision with a standard trephine because of the soft globe. After superficial trephination is accomplished, the diamond/gem blades are used to complete the incision. A guarded blade, such as those used for radial keratotomy, would not be as useful in this instance because the footplates may obscure the surgeon's view and may hinder delicate maneuvers that are often necessary in free-hand dissection.

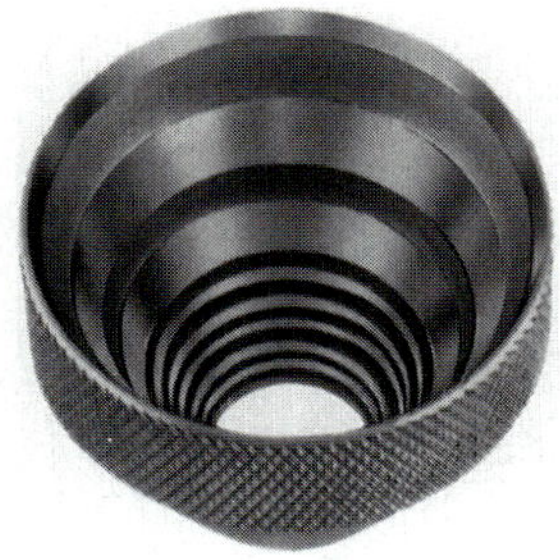

FIGURE 129-19 Maloney intraoperative qualitative keratometer.

CANNULAE

A set of cannulae is necessary. For the reconstitution of the anterior chamber once the corneal button is in place, a 30-gauge cannula can be placed through a peripheral side port or between host and donor cornea. Additionally, a viscoelastic cannula and a 23- or 25-gauge cannula for hydrodissection should be on the tray. Eitherr the phacoemulsification irrigation and aspiration hand piece or a curved Simcoe cannula (Storz E4969) with the opening on the top of the cannula is useful for removing cortex. In cases of mild posterior pressure in which the capsular bag is collapsed and space is limited, this Sinicoe cannula can be useful for removing residual cortical material.

QUALITATIVE KERATOMETERS

Once the cornea has been sutured into position, the anterior chamber reconstituted, and intraocular pressure normalized, it is often helpful to assess qualitatively the degree of corneal toricity.

Surgical keratometers that physically attach to the surgical microscope and work by reflecting projected light off of the surface of the cornea can be useful for assessing corneal curvature. A number of units such as the Smirmaul, Troutman, and the Varidot are available. The disadvantages of these units are that they are physically fixed to a given microscope and are not portable, they require a regular smooth refracting surface off of which to reflect their image, and they are quite expensive.

Simpler, more cost-effective, and portable instruments work by reflecting a circle from corneal surface. Any observed ovality of the reflection indicates excessive curvature in the axis of the shortest diameter of the oval. Several inexpensive instruments, all of which are hand-held, portable, and reusable, are available for

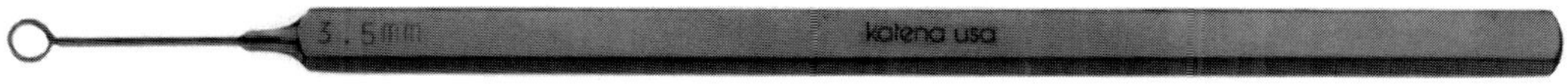

FIGURE 129-20 **Mandel intraoperative keratometer.**

qualitative measurement using this principle. (Figure 129-19 and Figure 129-20).

Although the number of instruments available to the transplantation surgeon is legion, each surgeon will develop a set based on initial training and surgical experience. Many of the instruments used in transplantation surgery are the same as those used for other anterior segment procedures. Some such as corneal scissors, however, are unique to transplantation and cannot be substituted.

SECTION TWO *Penetrating Keratoplasty: Technique*

CHAPTER 130

DAVID D. VERDIER

Penetrating Keratoplasty

Penetrating keratoplasty is the corneal transplant procedure in which full-thickness host corneal tissue is replaced with donor corneal tissue. The objectives of penetrating keratoplasty, depending on the corneal pathology present, may include one or more of the following: (1) establish a clear central cornea/visual axis, (2) minimize refractive error, (3) provide tectonic support, (4) alleviate pain, and (5) eliminate infection.

Approximately 41,000 penetrating keratoplasties are performed in the United States each year.[1] Success rates defined by grafts remaining clear at 1 year approach or exceed 90% in numerous series.[2-4] Thus it is an attractive but mistaken notion to consider this procedure common, simple, or undemanding. Although a clear graft with watertight closure may be accomplished by many surgeons, an essential goal is to strive for minimal refractive error. A meticulous approach to corneal transplant surgery is likely to reward the surgeon and patient with the best visual results.

History

"Could not a small piece of cornea be excised with a trephine the size of a small bristle or a large quill and would it not heal with a transparent scar?"*

—Erasmus Darwin, 1796

Erasmus Darwin, (Figure 130-1) grandfather of Charles Darwin, is credited for his vision of restoring a scarred cornea to its transparent state. This idea helped lead to our present corneal transplantation procedure.[5] This evolution did not come easily.

Frans Reisinger first experimented with corneal transplantations in rabbits and chickens in 1818.[6,7] In 1837 Bigger[8] reported a successful homograft procedure on a pet gazelle. Von Hippel[9] favored lamellar transplantation, performing the first successful human corneal transplant in 1886, in which a full thickness rabbit cornea was placed into a human recipient corneal lamellar bed.[9] It was not until the twentieth century, in 1905, that Zirm[10-12] performed the first successful human penetrating keratoplasty. Until mid-century, penetrating keratoplasty was considered a procedure of last resort.[13,14] The success of penetrating keratoplasty has accelerated in the last 50 years as a result of advances in the following areas: surgical instrumentation including microscopes and suture, tissue preservation and understanding of corneal endothelial function, antiinflammatory agents and their role in graft rejection; and surgical training and techniques.

Patient Selection

Patient selection is sometimes beyond the surgeon's control, but several key points should be emphasized. (For a more detailed review, please refer to Chapter 127: Indications and Outcomes; and Chapter 143: High Risk Penetrating Keratoplasty.)

AGE

One of the advantages of advancing age is that the immune system is less likely to mount a graft-destroying rejection.[15-17] Most elderly patients are surprised and pleased to learn that because of their age, they have a much better chance than a child of maintaining a clear graft. It is important to let the patient know that he or she is not wasting time, yours or theirs, and that people 70 years old deserve to see just as much as people who are 7.

*From Darwin E: *Zoonomia or the laws of organic life,* vol II, London, 1796, J Johnson.

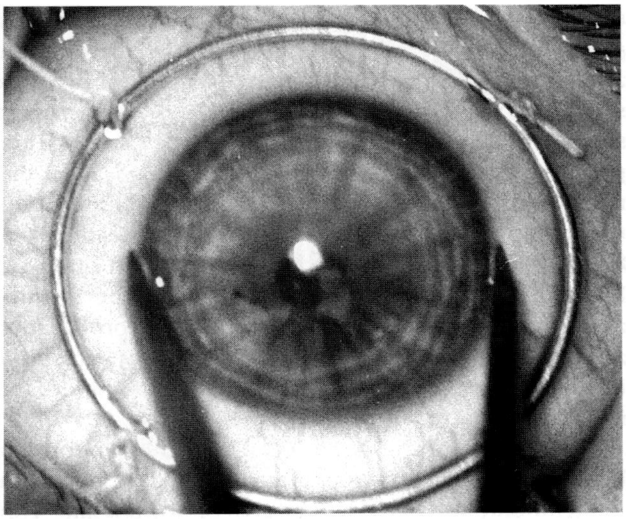

FIGURE 130-2 Scleral fixation ring well positioned. The corneal horizontal diameter is measured with calipers.

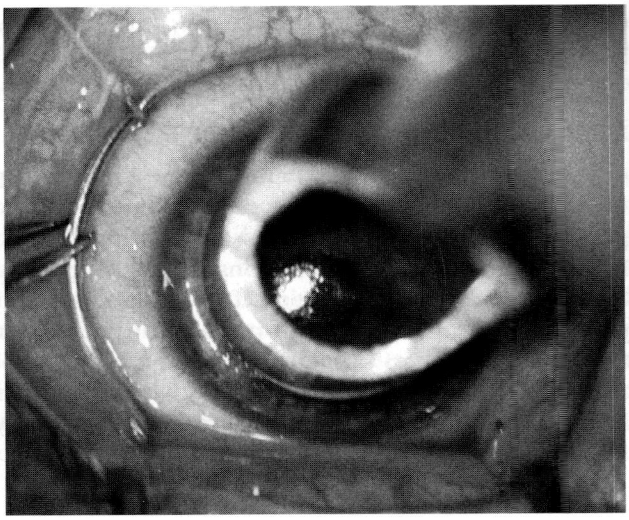

FIGURE 130-3 Marking host cornea.

the eye, which I prefer, or cut close to the knot at the ring. The ring should be sutured with only enough force to rest gently on but not be pressured against the sclera, and with minimal traction applied to the sutures if they are used to position the eye, to avoid distorting the globe. The ring should be just loose enough to be easily rotated with a tying forceps. The ring functions as a potential scaffold to maintain scleral support, exerting its influence once the eye is opened if scleral rigidity is insufficient.

Some surgeons prefer to use fixation sutures rather than a fixation ring, especially in phakic penetrating keratoplasty in which scleral collapse is unlikely to occur. Another option is to proceed without using a fixation ring or fixation sutures, to avoid associated globe distortion and astigmatism.[40,42] Many surgeons therefore have abandoned the use of fixation rings except in pediatric and aphakic patients.

MARKING OF HOST CORNEA

The optical axis is marked by the surgeon, using where possible the center of the pupil (Figure 130-3). The donor graft is usually centered on the host cornea or over the pupillary axis, which is often displaced slightly nasal. If there is much disparity between the pupillary axis and center of the cornea, a compromise position midway between the two may be chosen. The host cornea is marked by applying brief gentle pressure with a hand-held trephine. The mark may be difficult to see if the corneal surface is wet, but becomes readily apparent if dried with a cellulose sponge (Figure 130-4). The mark is checked for centering and size and repositioned if unsatisfactory. The cornea is then

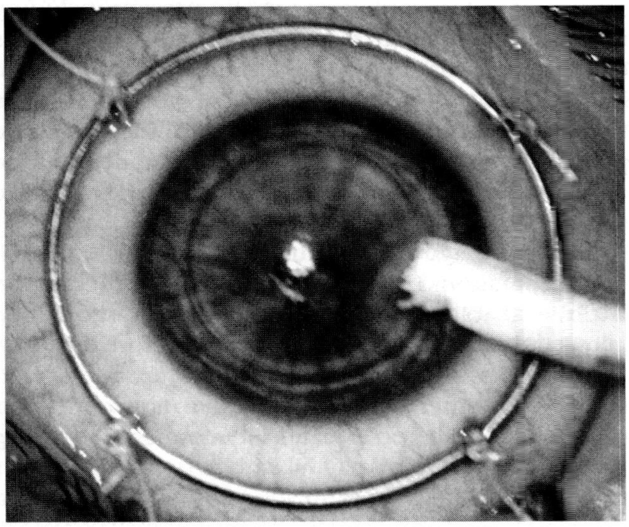

FIGURE 130-4 Mark on host cornea accentuated by drying with cellulose sponge.

covered with a wet cellulose sponge to avoid light toxicity from the operating microscope,[42,44] while attention is directed to preparing the donor button. Before trephination, some surgeons use a 12- or 16-prong radial marker to assist in donor-host suture symmetry and alignment.

Sizing of the host trephine depends on several factors including host corneal size, pathology, and risk of rejection. The donor tissue trephine is routinely sized 0.25 millimeter larger than the host trephine because using current techniques, donor corneal tissue cut with a trephine from the endothelial surface measures approximately 0.25 mm smaller in diameter than host corneal tissue cut with the same diameter

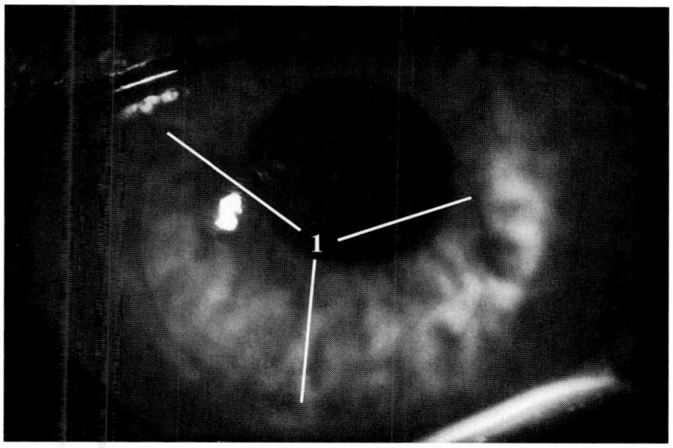

FIGURE 130-5 Fleischer ring *(1)* accentuated with cobalt blue light.

trephine from the epithelial surface.[45,46] For patients with a larger-than-average corneal horizontal diameter (limbal white-to-white measurement ≥ 12.5 mmeters) an 8.25 or 8.5 mm host trephine is often used, and for patients with a smaller-than-average corneal diameter (white-to-white measurement ≤ 11.5 mm), a 7.5 or 7.75 mm trephine is often used.

The graft may need to be decentered and occasionally oversized to encompass pathology, as can occur with severe peripheral corneal thinning, active infection, or most commonly with keratoconus. Mildly decentered grafts are well tolerated, but severely decentered grafts can be associated with high astigmatism.[47] Patients with poor endothelial cell counts or function, as in Fuchs' corneal dystrophy or pseudophakic bullous keratopathy, may benefit from the increased number of healthy endothelial cells in a larger graft. However, the risk of rejection increases with grafts larger than 8.5 mm in diameter and as the graft-host junction moves closer to the limbus.[48,49] Oversize grafts may be relatively contraindicated for patients with increased risk factors for rejection such as stromal neovascularization, previous graft failure, and age less than 50 years old.[15,17,50]

In keratoconus, the cone is often inferiorly displaced and should be fully removed to avoid residual or recurrent disease.[51,52] The extent of cone formation should be well known before surgery, as this will be difficult to discern with the operating microscope. Assessment is best made at the slit lamp, with the slit beam used to map out thinning and the cobalt blue light helpful in delineating Fleischer iron ring formation that may circumscribe the cone (Figure 130-5). Computerized corneal topography often cannot resolve the inferior extent of cone formation and should not be relied on for this purpose. Keratoconus patients also may benefit from using same diameter trephines

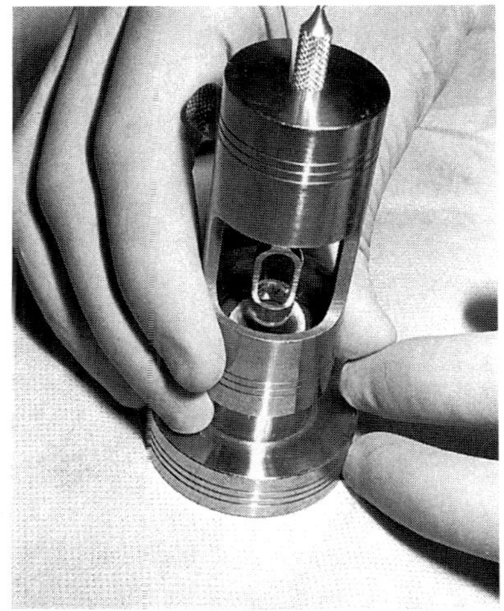

FIGURE 130-6 Trephining donor cornea.

for both the donor and host tissue, which in effect undersizes the donor button and helps reduce postoperative myopia.[53] The surgeon should be mindful, that obtaining watertight wound closure with an undersized donor tissue can be challenging and may require additional sutures.

TREPHINATION OF DONOR CORNEA

The donor cornea is trephined with the endothelial side facing up using a sharp disposable blade in a guillotine punch block apparatus (Figure 130-6). Obtaining a well-cut, round donor button with perpendicular edges and little trauma to the endothelium is achieved with most modern mechanical punch devices.[40,54-56] Donor tissue should be kept submerged in the storage medium and protected by a cover while the surgeon is preparing the host corneal bed.

TREPHINATION OF HOST CORNEA

The host cornea is trephined using a hand-held disposable trephine held perpendicular to the cornea. Minimal pressure is exerted against the cornea as the trephine is progressively rotated, allowing its sharp edges to penetrate gently to pre-Descemet's membrane or until the anterior chamber is entered. This is usually signaled by a drop of aqueous at the corneal surface, or if excess pressure is being applied, some shallowing of the anterior chamber. Because the cornea is not of uniform thickness, even if the trephine is held absolutely perpendicular during trephination, the initial opening will usually be less than one clock hour. Some surgeons prefer to trephine almost to full thickness, then enter with a sharp blade, a maneuver that adds an extra measure of control and allows for the formation of a posterior wound ledge. Carbachol is

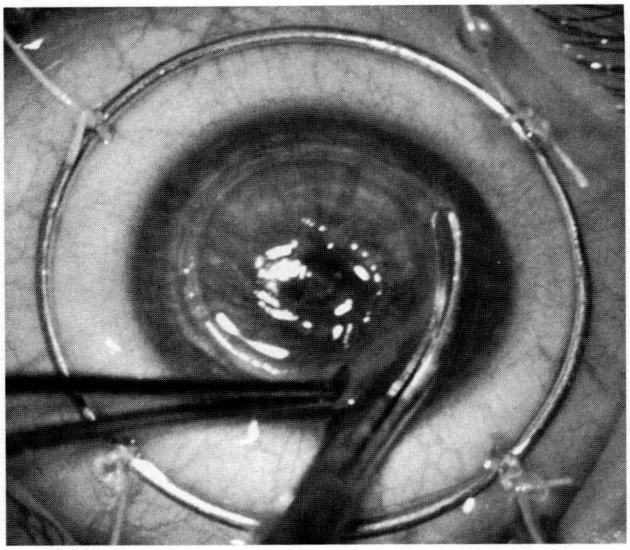

FIGURE 130-7 Cutting host cornea with corneal scissors.

injected through the initial opening to constrict the pupil and protect the crystalline lens unless a combined lens or posterior segment procedure is planned.

Recipient site preparation is completed with beveled corneal scissors, aided by maintaining host button alignment with fine-toothed forceps 45 to 90 degrees away (Figure 130-7). Scissor tips should be visualized at all times and neutral or slightly upward pressure maintained to avoid inadvertent iris damage. To minimize astigmatism, completion of the cut is best made perpendicular to the corneal plane; however, a slightly inward beveled cut allows for the formation of a posterior wound ledge that may facilitate a watertight closure.

Remaining tags of tissue can be trimmed with curved corneal or Vannas scissors, but with great discretion and care, because any excess trimming may easily lead to wound leak and apposition problems. The enemy of good is perfect.

Tissue disparity between the host corneal bed and donor cornea is considered to be a major cause of astigmatism.[45,57,58] It results in part from preexisting donor corneal astigmatism and topographic mismatch with the host tissue. However, errors resulting from trephination, especially of the host cornea, play a major role. Suction trephines such as the Hessberg-Barron and Hanna trephine system are used by many surgeons and may offer the advantage of making less tilted and more uniform cuts.[56,59-63] Sharpness, cutting characteristics, and incision diameter produced by different trephines vary to the extent that surgeons may obtain unexpected results when switching products.[64,65]

PLACEMENT OF VISCOELASTIC MATERIAL IN ANTERIOR CHAMBER

The anterior chamber is filled with a viscoelastic. Viscoelastic helps maintain donor button orientation for accurate suture placement and provides inexpensive endothelial protection.

PLACEMENT OF THE DONOR CORNEAL TISSUE IN THE HOST BED

The tissue is gently grasped with fine-toothed forceps at the junction of the epithelium and stroma and transferred onto the recipient bed where it rests on viscoelastic material. Care should be taken when handling the tissue to avoid any contact of the endothelium with instruments or surfaces.

Belmont et al.[66] report that rotating the donor tissue in the host bed until the most spherical reflex is obtained with an intraoperative keratometer, before placing sutures, may help reduce astigmatism even after all sutures are out.

PLACEMENT OF FOUR INTERRUPTED RADIAL 10-0 NYLON CARDINAL SUTURES

The first 10-0 nylon interrupted suture is placed at the 12 o'clock position. The donor cornea is grasped with fine-toothed, double-pronged forceps at the epithelial-stromal junction, and the suture is passed directly under the forceps teeth, through the donor and aligned host tissue. Suture depth is approximately 90% to prevent wound gape.[67] The suture is tied snugly using an initial triple loop followed by two additional single loops or using a slipknot that allows precise modulation of tension. Additional viscoelastic is placed in the anterior chamber as needed to help maintain proper graft orientation and anterior chamber depth. The second suture, placed 180 degrees away at 6 o'clock, is the most critical in terms of tissue alignment and subsequent astigmatism. It should be placed so that an equal amount of tissue is distributed on either side. This can be fine-tuned as the suture is passed through the donor cornea and is about to be passed through the host, by moving the inferior donor rim several degrees in either direction until tissue distribution appears equal, and then completing the pass (Figure 130-8). After the suture is tied, the anterior chamber should be re-formed and tissue alignment checked once again. If indicated, the 6 o'clock suture should be replaced at that point. The 3 o'clock suture is placed and tied, followed by the 9 o'clock suture. Once again tissue alignment should be checked and any aberrant cardinal sutures replaced.

COMPLETE SUTURING

Eight to 12 additional radial interrupted 10-0 nylon sutures are placed snugly to ensure adequate tissue

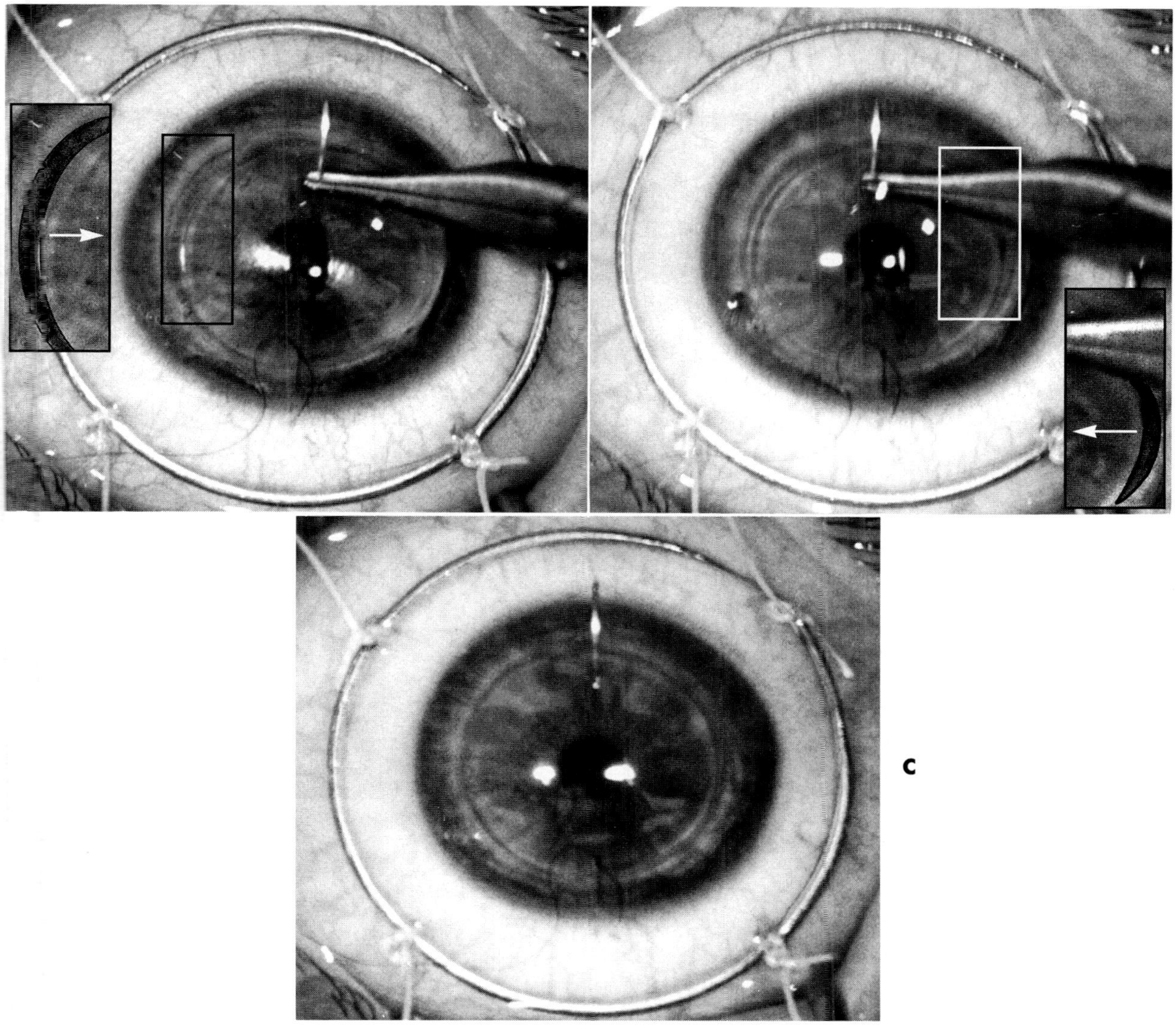

FIGURE 130-8 Placement of critical second cardinal suture. **A,** Suture aligned too temporal (to viewer's right), with disproportionate medial wound gape (*inset*). **B,** Suture aligned too medial (to viewer's left), with disproportionate temporal wound gape (*inset*). **C,** Suture correctly aligned, with equal medial and temporal wound apposition.

apposition, but not tightly (Figures 130-9 through 130-12). The anterior chamber is re-formed with viscoelastic or balanced salt solution as needed. The knots are buried on either the donor side (my preference) or host side, facilitated by a quick flicking motion and a tightly formed chamber. The wound is closed with an additional 10-0 nylon running suture with 90% stromal depth radial bites, with the knot buried at the 12:30 donor side. Running suture tension is evenly distributed by estimating and adjusting the tension of each bite with tying forceps. The wound is checked with a cellulose sponge for leaks, and any microleaks are closed with additional 10-0 or 11-0 nylon interrupted sutures or replacement of existing sutures. An "X" suture can be effectively used to close a stubborn leak (Figure 130-13).

A variety of suturing techniques exist: interrupted sutures only, combined interrupted/running suture techniques, and double running sutures, all of which are valid approaches to wound closure. However, several points regarding suturing deserve special emphasis. First, the most prevalent suturing error in corneal transplantation surgery is tying sutures too tight, which seems to be an almost irresistible urge for many surgeons, and therefore, one must always be on guard. Tight sutures can lead to surface healing problems, cheese wiring and associated loss of wound integrity, flat corneal curvature and hyperopia, and

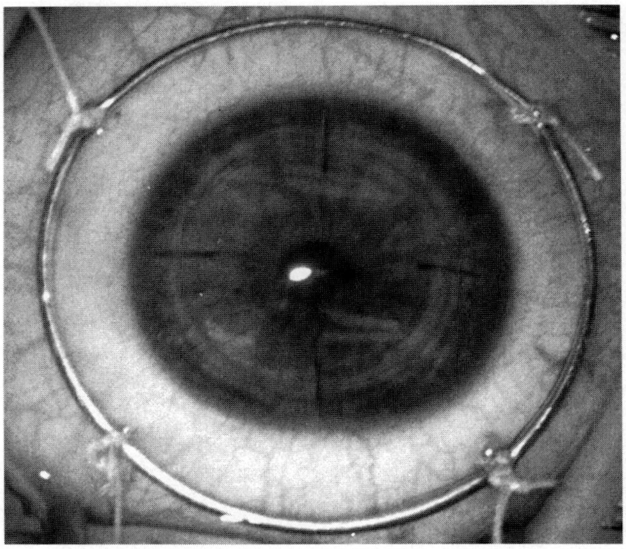

FIGURE 130-9 Four cardinal sutures in place.

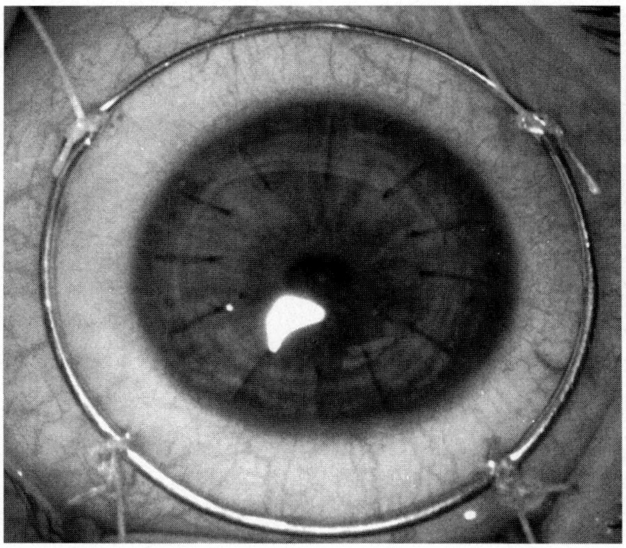

FIGURE 130-10 All 12 interrupted sutures in place.

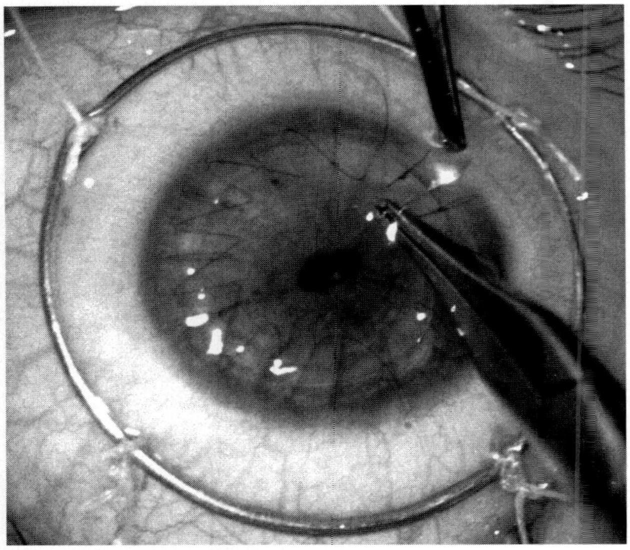

FIGURE 130-11 Placing running suture.

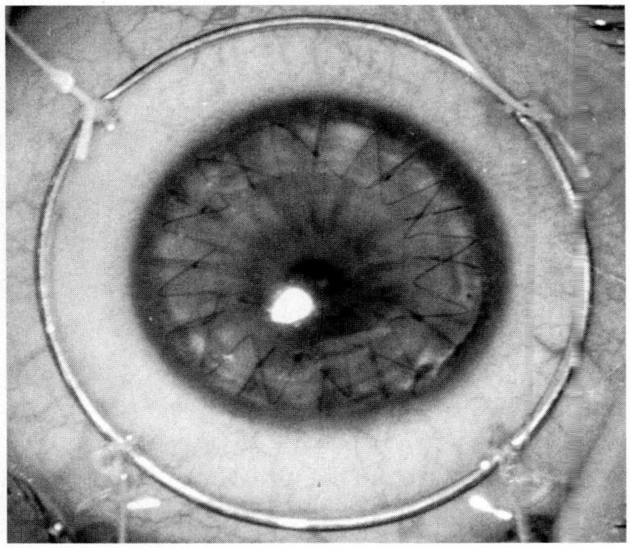

FIGURE 130-12 Sutures in, knots buried.

severe astigmatism. Because sutures may need to remain in place for many months, these problems often become chronic and difficult to deal with. Second, corneal suture knots should be buried. Exposed knots are a well-known source of irritation and giant papillary conjunctivitis.[68] Third and more controversial is how best to align donor with host tissue. Epithelial rather than endothelial approximation, may be more important because far more surface than endothelial problems occur with misalignment. Astigmatism is also more of a problem with epithelial misalignment.[69,70] As a practical matter, override of the donor tissue at the graft-host junction is far more common than host tissue override, even when attempts are made to prevent it.

Some surgeons believe that an antitorque running suture is helpful in reducing astigmatism,[70,71] whereas others have not appreciated any significant effect.[72] The torquing effect of the radial suture technique versus the nonradial antitorque technique is demonstrated in Figure 130-14.[70]

As noted earlier, many different corneal suturing patterns for penetrating keratoplasty are used today (see also Chapter 133). No single technique has been proven superior. The combination interrupted/running suture technique has the advantage of allowing selective removal of interrupted sutures for astigma-

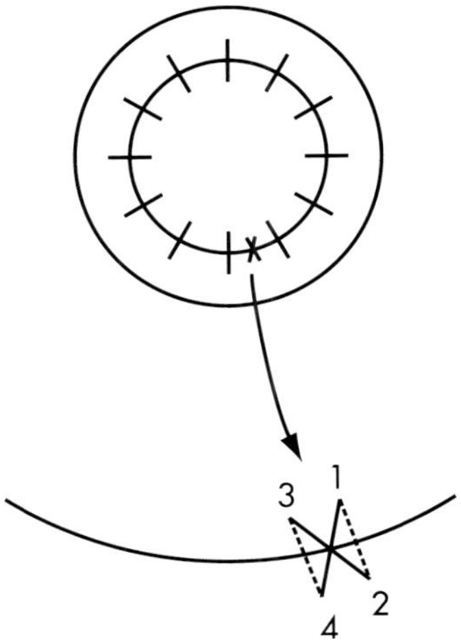

FIGURE 130-13 "X" suture.

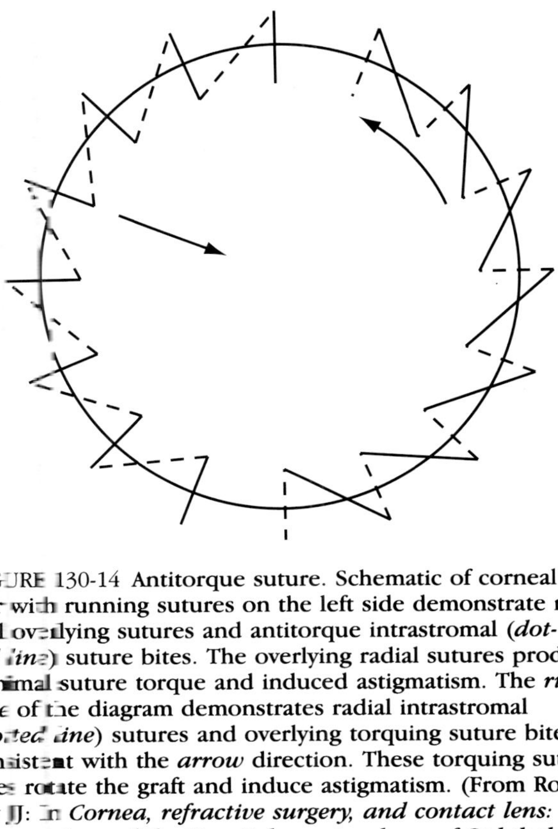

FIGURE 130-14 Antitorque suture. Schematic of corneal donor with running sutures on the left side demonstrate radial overlying sutures and antitorque intrastromal (*dotted line*) suture bites. The overlying radial sutures produce minimal suture torque and induced astigmatism. The *right side* of the diagram demonstrates radial intrastromal (*dotted line*) sutures and overlying torquing suture bites consistent with the *arrow* direction. These torquing suture bites rotate the graft and induce astigmatism. (From Rowsey JJ: In *Cornea, refractive surgery, and contact lens: Transactions of the New Orleans Academy of Ophthalmology,* New York, 1987, Raven Press.)

tism control while still preventing wound dehiscence.[73-76] Corneal wound healing can take many years, and dehiscences are common if most sutures are removed before 9 to 12 months postoperatively.[77,78] All interrupted sutures are best suited to corneas that are likely to have uneven or premature wound healing (and associated loosening of the running suture if used), usually when stromal neovascularization or ongoing inflammation at the graft-host junction is present. Other suture pattern options include single-running suture,[79] double-running suture,[2,76,80] single-running suture with postoperative adjustment,[81,82] and double-running suture with postoperative adjustment.[83]

Whatever suture technique is used, final astigmatism cannot be predicted until all sutures are out. Visual acuity often improves once all sutures are out because of a decrease in irregular astigmatism.

READJUSTMENT OF SUTURES TO MINIMIZE ASTIGMATISM

Some surgeons use a surgical or hand-held keratometer to check for astigmatism. This step should be performed after removal of the fixation ring. An inexpensive, plastic ring (Karickhoff keratoscope, DORC keratoscope, or the like) or even the round end of a safety pin can be used effectively for this purpose. Before measuring astigmatism, the anterior chamber should be reinflated to normal intraocular pressure with balanced salt solution. Astigmatism can be decreased by adjusting segments of the running suture on the operating table from the flat meridian into the steep meridian, as in the postoperative technique described by McNeill and Wessels.[42,81] Offending tight interrupted sutures can be replaced.

ADMINISTERING MEDICATIONS

Subconjunctival dexamethasone, 4 mg; subconjunctival gentamicin, 20 mg; and subconjunctival cefazolin, 25 mg, or another suitable antibiotic are injected. Two drops of timolol 0.25% are placed unless contraindicated by heart or respiratory problems.

PERFORM A TEMPORARY SUTURE TARSORRHAPHY IF SURFACE HEALING PROBLEMS ARE ANTICIPATED

Tarsorrhaphy is an underused option. A suture tarsorrhaphy can be performed with double-armed silk, nylon, or polypropylene suture in a mattress fashion with 3 mm bites passing through the eyelid gray lines and tied with or without a bolster.[84,85] A lateral or central tarsorrhaphy can be performed. These sutures remain effective for several weeks during the critical reepithelialization process, then are easily removed without sequelae. Punctal occlusion also should be considered in such patients. A patch and shield are placed and secured with adhesive tape.

Special Circumstances

THE POSTRADIAL KERATOTOMY PATIENT

The radial keratotomy patient in need of a penetrating keratoplasty presents a challenging problem. Radial

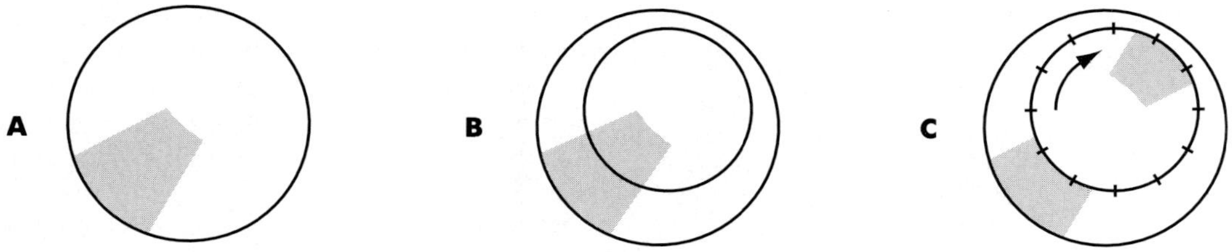

FIGURE 130-15 Rotating autograft. **A,** Central opacity. **B,** Eccentric trephination of host cornea. **C,** Host button rotated and sutured.

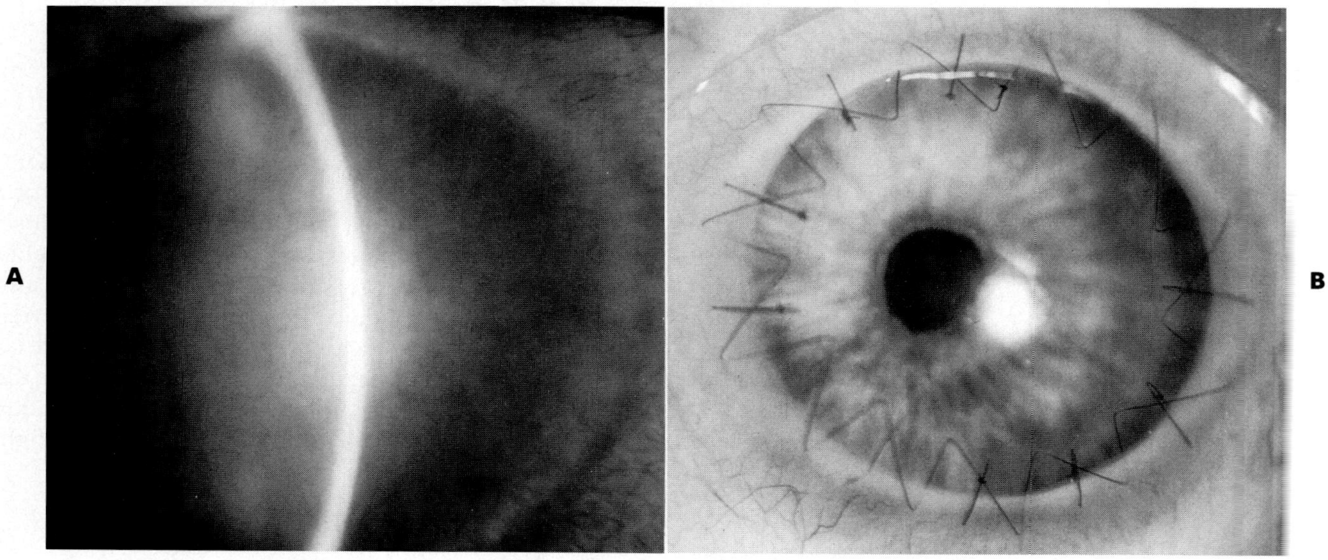

FIGURE 130-16 **A,** Before penetrating keratoplasty. **B,** After penetrating keratoplasty.

keratotomy wounds do not fully heal, and as long as 9 years later can splay open during the trephination or suturing steps in penetrating keratoplasty.[86-90] Before trephination, placing either interrupted sutures or a running purse string suture transversely across the radial keratotomy scars just peripheral to the graft-host junction can stabilize the cornea and help keep the radial keratotomy incisions from splitting open.[91,92]

ROTATING AUTOGRAFT

An ipsilateral autograft can be considered for the patient with a nonprogressive scar that violates the central visual axis from the periphery (Figure 130-15). Given enough area of clear cornea, the scarred cornea can be eccentrically trephined, rotated to remove the scar from the central visual axis, and sutured.[93-95] This procedure avoids the risk of rejection and is especially suited for the pediatric or high rejection risk patient.

A carefully crafted penetrating keratoplasty can yield many rewards. Few sights in medicine are more beautiful than the slit lamp view of a clear corneal transplant, with its surface glistening and sutures a study in symmetry (Figure 130-16). Achieving this result requires a carefully planned and meticulously executed surgical procedure.

REFERENCES

1. Eye Bank Association of America: *1994 statistical report,* Washington DC, 1995, Eye Bank Association of America.
2. Davison JA, Bourne WM: Results of penetrating keratoplasty using a double running suture technique, *Arch Ophthalmol* 99:1591-1595, 1981.
3. Price FW Jr, Whitson WE, Marks RG: Graft survival in four common groups of patients undergoing penetrating kerato-plasty, *Ophthalmology* 98:322-328, 1991.
4. Price FW Jr et al: Five-year corneal graft survival. A large, single-center patient cohort, *Arch Ophthalmol* 111:797-805, 1993.
5. Coster DJ: Doyne lecture: influences on the development of corneal transplantation, *Eye* 8:1-11, 1994.
6. Forstot SL, Kaufman HE: Corneal transplantation, *Annu Rev Med* 28:21-35, 1977.
7. Mannis MJ, Krachmer JH: Keratoplasty: a historical perspective, *Surv Ophthalmol* 25:333-338, 1981.
8. Bigger S: Inquiry into the possibility of transplanting the cornea, with the view of relieving blindness (hitherto deemed incurable) caused by several diseases of that structure, *Dublin J Med Sci* 11:408-417, 1837.
9. Von Hippel A: Eine neue methode der hornhauttransplantation, *Archiv Ophthalmologie* 34:I, 1888.

10. Zirm E: Eine erfolgreiche totale Keratoplastik, *Graefes Arch Ophthalmol* 64:580-593, 1906.
11. Zirm EK (*v. Graefe's Archiv fur Ophthalmologie,* 1906): Eine erfolgreiche totale keratoplastik (a successful total keratoplasty), *Refract Corneal Surg* 5:258-261, 1989.
12. Zirm ME: Eduard Konrad Zirm and the "wondrously beautiful little window", *Refract Corneal Surg* 5:256-257, 1989.
13. Leigh AG: *Corneal transplantation,* Oxford, England, 1966, Blackwell Scientific.
14. Laibson PR: Max Fine's contribution to keratoplasty, *Refract Corneal Surg* 7:105-109, 1991.
15. Alldredge OC, Krachmer JH: Clinical types of corneal transplant rejection. Their manifestations, frequency, preoperative correlates and treatment, *Arch Ophthalmol* 99:599-604, 1981.
16. Boisjoly HM et al: Effect of factors unrelated to tissue matching on corneal transplant endothelial rejection, *Am J Ophthalmol* 107:647-654, 1989.
17. Maguire MG et al: Risk factors for corneal graft failure and rejection in the collaborative corneal transplantation studies, *Ophthalmology* 101:1536-1547, 1994.
18. Christy NE, Lall P: Postoperative endophthalmitis following cataract surgery: effects of subconjunctival antibiotics and other factors, *Arch Ophthalmol* 90:361-366, 1973.
19. Starr MB: Prophylactic antibiotics for ophthalmic surgery, *Surv Ophthalmol* 27:353-373, 1983.
20. Hughes DS, Hill RJ: Infectious endophthalmitis after cataract surgery, *Br J Ophthalmol* 78:227-232, 1994.
21. Chitkara DK et al: Lack of effect of preoperative norfloxacin on bacterial contamination of anterior chamber aspirates after cataract surgery, *Br J Ophthalmol* 78:772-774, 1994.
22. Sherwood DR et al: Bacterial contamination of intraocular and extraocular fluids during extracapsular cataract extraction, *Eye* 3:308-312, 1989.
23. Speaker MG et al: Role of external bacterial flora in the pathogenesis of acute postoperative endophthalmitis, *Ophthalmology* 98:639-649, 1991.
24. Apt L et al: Chemical preparation of the eye in ophthalmic surgery. III. Effect of povidone-iodine on the conjunctiva, *Arch Ophthalmol* 102:728-729, 1984.
25. Isenberg SJ et al: Chemical preparation of the eye in ophthalmic surgery. IV. Comparison of povidone-iodine on the conjunctiva with a prophylactic antibiotic, *Arch Ophthalmol* 103:1340-1342, 1985
26. Speaker MG, Menikoff JA: Prophylaxis of endophthalmitis with topical povidine-iodine, *Ophthalmology* 98:1769-1775, 1991.
27. Kirsch RE, Steinman W: Digital pressure, an important safeguard in cataract surgery, *Arch Ophthalmol* 54:697-703, 1955.
28. Quist LH, Stapleton SS, McPherson SD Jr: Preoperative use of the Honan intraocular pressure reducer, *Am J Ophthalmol* 95:536-538, 1983.
29. Lay WM et al: Effect of applying the Honan intraocular pressure reducer before cataract surgery, *Am J Ophthalmol* 100:523-527, 1985
30. Bourne WM: Reduction of endothelial cell loss during phakic penetrating keratoplasty, *Am J Ophthalmol* 89:787-790, 1980
31. Hwang DG et al: Combination antibiotic supplementation of corneal storage medium, *Am J Ophthalmol* 115:299-308, 1993.
32. Ingraham HJ, Donnenfeld ED, Perry HD: Massive suprachoroidal hemorrhage in penetrating keratoplasty, *Am J Ophthalmol* 108:670-675, 1989.
33. Speaker MG et al: A case-control study of risk factors for intraoperative suprachoroidal expulsive hemorrhage, *Ophthalmology* 98:202-209, 1991.
34. Price FW Jr et al: Suprachoroidal hemorrhage in penetrating keratoplasty, *Ophthalmic Surg* 25:521-525, 1994.
35. Purcell JJ Jr et al: Expulsive hemorrhage in penetrating keratoplasty, *Ophthalmology* 89:41-43, 1982.
36. Taylor DM: Expulsive hemorrhage, *Am J Ophthalmol* 78:961-966, 1974.
37. Arnold PN: Study of acute intraoperative suprachoroidal hemorrhage, *J Cataract Refract Surg* 18:489-494, 1992.
38. Kay MD, Epstein RJ, Torczynski E: Histopathology of acute intraoperative suprachoroidal hemorrhage associated with transscleral intraocular lens fixation, *J Cataract Refract Surg* 19:83-87, 1993.
39. Maumenee AE, Schwartz MF: Acute intraoperative choroidal effusion, *Am J Ophthalmol* 100:147-154, 1985.
40. Olson RJ: The effect of scleral fixation ring placement and trephine tilting on keratoplasty wound size and donor shape, *Ophthalmic Surg* 12:23-26, 1981.
41. Warwick R: *Eugene Wolff's anatomy of the eye and orbit,* ed 7, Philadelphia and Toronto, 1976, WB Saunders.
42. Serdarevic ON, Renard GJ, Pouliquen Y: Randomized clinical trial comparing astigmatism and visual rehabilitation after penetrating keratoplasty with and without intraoperative suture adjustment, *Ophthalmology* 101:990-999, 1994.
43. McDonald HR, Irvine AR: Light-induced retinopathy from the operating microscope in extracapsular cataract extraction and intraocular lens implantation, *Ophthalmology* 90:945-951, 1983.
44. Stamler JF et al: Microscope light-induced maculopathy in combined penetrating keratoplasty, extracapsular cataract extraction, and intraocular lens implantation, *Ophthalmology* 95:1142-1146, 1988.
45. Troutman RC: Astigmatic considerations in corneal graft, *Ophthalmic Surg* 10:21-26, 1979.
46. Olson RJ: Variation in corneal graft size related to trephine technique, *Arch Ophthalmol* 97:1323-1325, 1979.
47. van Rij G et al: Postoperative astigmatism after central versus eccentric penetrating keratoplasties, *Am J Ophthalmol* 99:317-320, 1985.
48. Sharif KW, Casey TA: Penetrating keratoplasty for keratoconus: complications and long-term success, *Br J Ophthalmol* 75:142-146, 1991.
49. Tuft SJ, Gregory WM, Davison CR: Bilateral penetrating keratoplasty for keratoconus, *Ophthalmology* 102:462-468, 1995.
50. Wilson SE, Kaufman HE: Graft failure after penetrating keratoplasty, *Surv Ophthalmol* 34:325-356, 1990.
51. Krachmer JH, Feder RS, Belin MW: Keratoconus and related noninflammatory corneal thinning disorders, *Surv Ophthalmol* 28:293-322, 1984
52. Kremer I et al: Histologic evidence of recurrent keratoconus seven years after keratoplasty, *Am J Ophthalmol* 119:511-512, 1995.
53. Wilson SE, Bourne WM: Effect of recipient-donor trephine size disparity on refractive error in keratoconus, *Ophthalmology* 96:299-304, 1989.
54. Brightbill FS, Polack FM, Slappey T: A comparison of two methods for cutting donor corneal buttons, *Am J Ophthalmol* 75:500-506, 1973.
55. Clinch TE, Fung KL, Laibson PL: Corneal endothelial cell loss following trephination, *Ophthalmic Surg* 19:703-705, 1988.
56. Pflugfelder SC et al: Photogrammetric analysis of corneal trephination, *Arch Ophthalmol* 110:1160-1166, 1992.
57. Olson RJ: Corneal curvature changes associated with penetrating keratoplasty: a mathematical model, *Ophthalmic Surg* 11:838-842, 1980.
58. Swinger CA: Postoperative astigmatism, *Surv Ophthalmol* 31:219-248, 1987.
59. Hessburg PC, Barron M: A disposable corneal trephine, *Ophthalmic Surg* 11:730-733, 1980.

60. Pouliquen Y et al: New trephine for keratoplasty (Hanna trephine), *Dev Ophthalmol* 11:99-102, 1985.
61. Krumeich J, Binder PS, Knulle A: The theoretical effect of trephine tilt on postkeratoplasty astigmatism, *CLAOJ* 14:213-219, 1988.
62. van Rij G, Waring GO III: Configuration of corneal trephine opening using five different trephines in human donor eyes, *Arch Ophthalmol* 106:1228-1233, 1988.
63. Waring GO III, Hanna KD: The Hanna suction punch block and trephine system for penetrating keratoplasty, *Arch Ophthalmol* 107:1536-1539, 1989.
64. Olson RJ: Variation in disposable corneal trephine sharpness, *Ophthalmic Surg* 15:590-591, 1984.
65. Perlman EM: Unusual refractive errors induced by interchanging trephines during penetrating keratoplasty, *Refract Corneal Surg* 5:271-273, 1989.
66. Belmont SC, Troutman RC, Buzard KA: Control of astigmatism aided by intraoperative keratometry, *Cornea* 12:397-400, 1993.
67. Eve FR, Troutman RC: Placement of sutures used in corneal incisions, *Am J Ophthalmol* 82:786-789, 1976.
68. Sugar A, Meyer RF: Giant papillary conjunctivitis after keratoplasty, *Am J Ophthalmol* 91:239-242, 1981.
69. Lang GK, Green WR, Maumenee AE: Clinicopathologic studies of keratoplasty eyes obtained post mortem, *Am J Ophthalmol* 101:28-40, 1986.
70. Rowsey JJ: Prevention and correction of corneal transplant astigmatism. In *Cornea, refractive surgery, and contact lens: transactions of the New Orleans Academy of Ophthalmology,* New York, 1987, Raven Press.
71. Troutman RC: *Microsurgery of the anterior segment of the eye,* vol 2, St Louis, 1977, Mosby.
72. Olson RJ: Prevention of astigmatism in corneal transplant surgery, *Int Ophthalmol Clin* 28:37-45, 1988.
73. Stainer GA, Perl T, Binder PS: Controlled reduction of postkeratoplasty astigmatism, *Ophthalmology* 89:668-676, 1982.
74. Binder PS: Selective suture removal can reduce postkeratoplasty astigmatism, *Ophthalmology* 92:1412-1416, 1985.
75. Binder PS: The effect of suture removal on postkeratoplasty astigmatism, *Am J Ophthalmol* 105:637-645, 1988.
76. Musch DC et al: Corneal astigmatism after penetrating keratoplasty: the role of suture technique, *Ophthalmology* 96:698-703, 1989.
77. Brown SI, Tragakis MP: Wound dehiscence with keratoplasty: complication of the continuous-suture technique, *Am J Ophthalmol* 72:115-116, 1971.
78. Binder PS et al: Keratoplasty wound separations, *Am J Ophthalmol* 80:109-115, 1975.
79. Boruchoff SA, Jensen AD, Dohlman CH: Comparison of suturing techniques in keratoplasty for keratoconus, *Ann Ophthalmol* 7:433-436, 1975.
80. McNeill JI, Kaufman HE: A double running suture technique for keratoplasty: earlier visual rehabilitation, *Ophthalmic Surg* 8:58-61, 1977.
81. McNeill JI, Wessels IF: Adjustment of single continuous suture to control astigmatism after penetrating keratoplasty, *Refract Corneal Surg* 5:216-223, 1989.
82. Van Meter WS et al: Postkeratoplasty astigmatism control: single continuous suture adjustment versus selective interrupted suture removal, *Ophthalmology* 98:177-183, 1991.
83. Clinch TE et al: An adjustable double running suture technique for keratoplasty, *Am J Ophthalmol* 116:201-206, 1993.
84. Koenig SB, Harris GJ: Temporary suture tarsorrhaphy after penetrating keratoplasty, *Cornea* 10:121-122, 1991.
85. Gossman MD, Bowe BE, Tanenbaum M: Reversible suture tarsorrhaphy for eyelid malposition and keratopathy, *Ophthalmic Surg* 22:237-239, 1991.
86. Deg JK, Binder PS: Wound healing after astigmatic keratotomy in human eyes, *Ophthalmology* 94:1290-1298, 1987.
87. Binder PS et al: An ultrastructural and histochemical study of long-term wound healing after radial keratotomy, *Am J Ophthalmol* 103:432-440, 1987.
88. Binder PS et al: Histopathology of traumatic corneal rupture after radial keratotomy, *Arch Ophthalmol* 106:1584-1590, 1988.
89. Jester et al: Variations in corneal wound healing after radial keratotomy: possible insights into mechanisms of clinical complications and refractive effects, *Cornea* 11:191-199, 1992
90. McNeill JI: Corneal incision dehiscence during penetrating keratoplasty nine years after radial keratotomy, *J Cataract Refract Surg* 19:542-543, 1993.
91. Beatty RF, Robin JB, Schanzlin DJ: Penetrating keratoplasty after radial keratotomy, *J Refract Surg* 2:207-214, 1986.
92. McNeill JI, Wilkins DL: A purse-string suture for penetrating keratoplasty following radial keratotomy, *Refract Corneal Surg* 7:392-394, 1991.
93. Gundersen T, Calnan A: Corneal autografts, ipsilateral and contralateral, *Arch Ophthalmol* 73:164-168, 1965.
94. Stocker FW: Rotating autokeratoplasty, *South Med J* 62:1183-1184, 1969.
95. Groden LR, Arentsen JJ: Ipsilateral rotating autokeratoplasty, *Ann Ophthalmol* 15:899-90, 1983.

CHAPTER 131

CLARON DOUGLAS ALLDREDGE O. CLARON ALLDREDGE, JR

Penetrating Keratoplasty and Cataract Extraction

Whenever penetrating keratoplasty (PK) is indicated, the status of the crystalline lens must be assessed; conversely, whenever cataract extraction is indicated, the status of the cornea must be assessed. In some cases the cornea is the primary cause of decreased visual acuity, a cataract is present, and a PK is clearly indicated. In these cases, the question arises, should the cataract also be removed? Cataract formation is more common in cases with Fuchs' dystrophy (Figure 131-1) or in cases in which inflammation or trauma have been a factor. Cataract formation is less common in younger patients requiring PK such as in keratoconus. However, whenever penetrating keratoplasty is considered and a cataract is present, one must decide whether to remove the cataract at the same time as corneal transplantation.

The indication for removing the cataract along with penetrating keratoplasty is determined by the visual significance of the opacity. This variable is often more difficult to determine than when the cornea is normal because the evaluation of the cataract is impaired when there is a loss of corneal clarity. Nevertheless, a reasonable estimation of the visual significance of the cataract can usually be obtained before penetrating keratoplasty is performed. A general rule-of-thumb for removal of nuclear sclerotic cataracts is a cataract of more than 2+ (on a scale of 1+ to 4+). A guideline for removal of posterior subcapsular cataracts is a cataract of 1+ or more. However, each case must be individualized, considering the visual needs of the patient, the status of the rest of the eye, and the patient's overall health. One must bear in mind that corneal transplantation can hasten the development of cataract.[1,2]

Let us consider those situations in which a patient has a significant cataract in the presence of corneal pathology. It is not uncommon to have a patient requiring cataract surgery who also has significant corneal guttata. The surgeon must decide when cataract surgery alone should be performed and when corneal transplantation combined with cataract extraction with an intraocular lens (triple procedure) should be performed. If stromal edema is not seen with the slit lamp and/or the central corneal pachymetry reading is 0.60 mm or less, cataract surgery alone can usually be performed without resulting corneal decompensation. If cataract surgery is performed in the face of significant cornea guttata, a viscoelastic that gives maximum protection to the endothelium (such as Viscoat) should be used.[3,4] If a patient has frank stromal edema with pachymetry readings greater than 0.62 to 0.65 mm, it is advisable to consider a triple procedure. If corneal scarring is present and cataract extraction is indicated, one must bear in mind that the anterior corneal surface is the largest contributor to the refractive power of the eye. On the other hand, significant stromal corneal scarring can be present that has little effect on visual acuity, as exists with interstitial keratitis. Assessing the smoothness of the anterior corneal surface with keratometry or computerized topography can be useful in deciding whether to perform a PK with the cataract extraction.

When corneal transplantation and cataract surgery need to be performed for visual rehabilitation, a key strategic question is whether the procedures should be performed in one operation or as two separate procedures. The arguments suggesting an advantage to a combined procedure are (1) the need for only one procedure, (2) less expense for one combined procedure than for two separate procedures, (3) less risk to the endothelium of the transplanted cornea from subsequent cataract surgery,[5-7] and (4) evidence suggesting that posterior capsual opacification occurs less often when a combined procedure is performed than in primary cataract extraction.[8] The primary advantage of performing two separate operations is that the intraocular lens power calculation can be performed more accurately. It is disheartening to carry out a combined cornea transplantation and cataract procedure only to find that the patient has a high degree of myopia or hyperopia. The difficulty of accurately predicting the intraocular lens power in a combined procedure stems from the fact that the postoperative keratometric readings can only be estimated, and estimates can be quite inaccurate. If the decision is

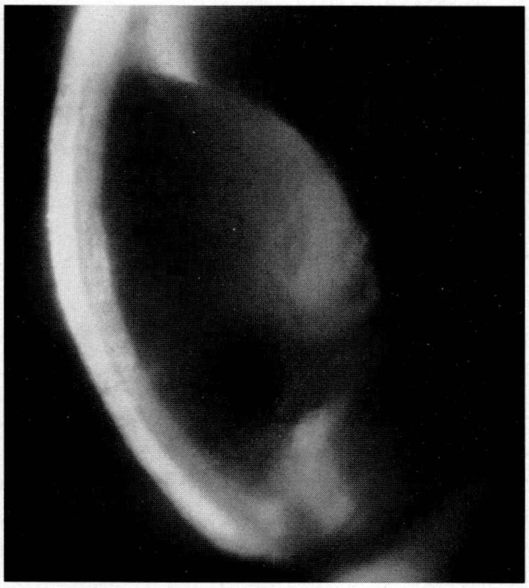

FIGURE 131-1 Fuchs' dystrophy and cataract.

made to perform the transplantation first, followed by a cataract procedure at a later date, the second procedure should be performed at least 2 or 3 months after the PK to allow for stabilizaton of the keratometric readings. The corneal curvature will not be fully stabilized until all the PK sutures have been removed.

Preoperative evaluation of the patient scheduled for a combined PK/cataract extraction includes a complete eye examination, with special attention given to the intraocular pressure and the retinal evaluation. Performing a corneal transplant in a patient with uncontrolled intraocular pressure can greatly complicate the postoperative course, especially in this context. It is best to control intraocular pressure before proceeding with penetrating keratoplasty.[9,10] This approach may require the use of topical or systemic antiglaucoma medications, argon laser trabeculoplasty, or even trabeculectomy. An assessment of macular function also should be performed so that the patient can be counseled as to postoperative visual acuity expectations. Devices such as a potential acuity meter (PAM) can be helpful. In the presence of both a corneal and a lenticular opacity, a favorable PAM reading is less likely; however, when a favorable reading is obtained, a reasonably good visual outcome can be expected. The converse (poor PAM reading = poor visual outcome) is not always true. Sometimes, therefore, macular function is more reliably assessed on the basis of the appearance of the macula rather than functional testing.

Because most combined cataract and transplantation procedures are performed in older patients, it is important to have a good assessment of general medical health, with special attention given to blood pressure and blood abnormalities. These patients may be at greater risk for choroidal hemorrhage.

Axial length determination should be performed and intraocular lens power determined. The axial length of both eyes should be measured as a cross-check for accuracy. Various methods of determining the keratometry readings for use in intraocular lens calculations are used by different surgeons.[11] One technique is to average the keratometric readings for a particular surgeon based on a large series of his or her own patients who have undergone penetrating keratoplasty. Some surgeons modify this reading based on preoperative keratometric readings of the operative or fellow eye. Others assume that if a patient has a relatively steep cornea, the results may be steeper than average keratometric readings. If they have a relatively flat cornea, they may experience flatter keratometry postoperatively. Still other surgeons try to use an average change in keratometric readings, using the preoperative readings from the operated eye or the fellow eye if accurate keratometry is not possible in the operated eye, and then adding or subtracting the average change in keratometric readings determined by averaging the change of keratometric readings in a large series of cases. Consideration also has been given to keratometry of the donor before the donor cornea was removed. McCulley has shown a fairly high correlation of keratometric readings in the recipient cornea postoperatively. This finding merits further study and may ultimately be useful in selecting the appropriate keratometric readings to use for intraocular lens power calculations in combined procedures.

It is also appropriate to have alternate intraocular lenses available. If in-the-bag or ciliary sulcus placement of the intraocular lens is not possible, it is important to determine preoperatively which lens would be used to be sutured transsclerally or to the iris or which anterior chamber intraocular lens would be appropriate. Even when the posterior capsule has been torn, however, it is rare that enough capsular remnant cannot be found to place a lens in the ciliary sulcus.[12]

Cataract Extraction Techniques

The conventional method of removing a cataract with the corneal transplantation procedure is to use an "open sky" extracapsular cataract extraction (ECCE). The intraocular lens is placed in the capsular bag, and the donor corneal button is sutured in place. Another alternative is to perform the cataract extraction first using the technique of small-incision phacoemulsification and then proceeding with corneal transplantation as in a phakic eye. Cataract extraction by phacoemulsification followed by the keratoplasty has advantages.[13-15] First and foremost, the operation is accomplished in a closed system, which makes cataract surgery much safer. The risk of ruptured capsule and posterior vitreous pressure is much less, the procedure much more controlled, and the risk of choroidal hemmorrhage and other complication certainly much less.[16-20] All corneal surgeons who perform cataract extractions along with corneal transplantation know that the most worrisome time during the procedure is the "open sky" removal of the cataract and placement of the intraocular lens in position because of posterior vitreous pressure and possible posterior-capsular rupture. Phacoemulsification is not always possible because not all corneas are clear enough to allow visualization of the cataract clearly enough to remove it using this technique. A surprising number of procedures, however, can be performed this way. By focusing the microscope down through the scarred or cloudy cornea, an adequate view of the cataract and the capsule can usually be obtained. Also, in edematous corneas, the epithelium can be removed, which improves the view. This technique should not be used by surgeons who are inexperienced in phacoemulsification procedures, because it is more difficult than procedures performed with a clear cornea.

Phacoemulsification with Penetrating Keratoplasty

The combined procedure with phacoemulsification can be performed under local anesthesia, using a longer acting anesthetic such as bupivicaine for longer anesthesia time and for relief of some postoperative discomfort. Some surgeons prefer to use a peribulbar anesthetic,[21,22] although the degree of anesthesia is more variable. A seventh nerve block is also important because it is undesirable to have any orbicularis function during the corneal transplantation.

The patient is prepped and draped in the usual fashion. A small incision should be made at the superior limbus in the conjunctiva and the conjunctiva reflected slightly back away from the limbus. Any bleeding of episcleral vessels should be lightly cauterized. It is important not to cauterize too much because the sclera can actually shrink, causing some difficulties with the wound. A scleral tunnel incision is then completed. A clear corneal approach is not appropriate when a transplant is also being performed. An incision 1.5 to 2 mm posterior to the limbus is performed using a steel or diamond knife to half thickness of the sclera. A frown incision is most efficient at reducing incision-related astigmatism. A lamellar dissection is then carried into the peripheral cornea. It is important not to tunnel too far into clear cornea because this may interfere with the subsequent transplant. However, for the wound to seal properly, the dissection does need to be carried into the peripheral cornea just beyond the limbal vascular palisades.

A stab incision is then performed at the limbus to facilitate placement of a second instrument and syringes for injecting fluids. The most common location of the stab incision is two clock hours to the left of the scleral tunnel for a right-handed surgeon. The internal incision of the scleral tunnel is then completed using a 3 or 3.2 mm keratome. A viscoelastic substance is injected into the anterior chamber. A continuous-tear capsulotomy is then performed. This step in the procedure can be more difficult because of decreased visibility.

After the capsulotomy has been made, hydrodissection is carried out. Phacoemulsification of the nucleus is then accomplished in the usual fashion. A fractionation technique works well in this setting. By using a low phacoemulsification power, such as 50% or 60%, along with zero vacuum and an aspiration flow rate of approximately 20 to 25, one can perform the grooves with much less risk of posterior capsule rupture, since visualization can sometimes be decreased.[23] When it comes to removing the four nuclear fragments, one can use fairly high vacuum powers, particularly with the newer machines, which have fluids that allow the anterior chamber to be properly maintained.

After the nuclear fragments are removed, irrigation and aspiration of the remaining cortical material are accomplished in the usual fashion. The posterior capsule is polished with a diamond-dusted capsule polisher; this helps prevent opacification of the posterior capsule. After this step has been completed, a foldable intraocular lens can then be used through a 3 mm incision. If the posterior capsule has been ruptured and vitreous loss occurs, the vitreous must be dealt with appropriately.[24] A vitrectomy should be performed, and vitreous must be meticulously cleaned from the iris and anterior chamber. A posterior chamber intraocular usually can be used, but if there is a significant tear in the posterior capsule, intraocular lens is placed in the sulcus. Next the pupil is constricted with acetylcholine chloride (Miochol). A single interrupted 10-0 Vicryl suture is used in a horizontal mattress fashion to close the wound. With the pupil constricted and the in-

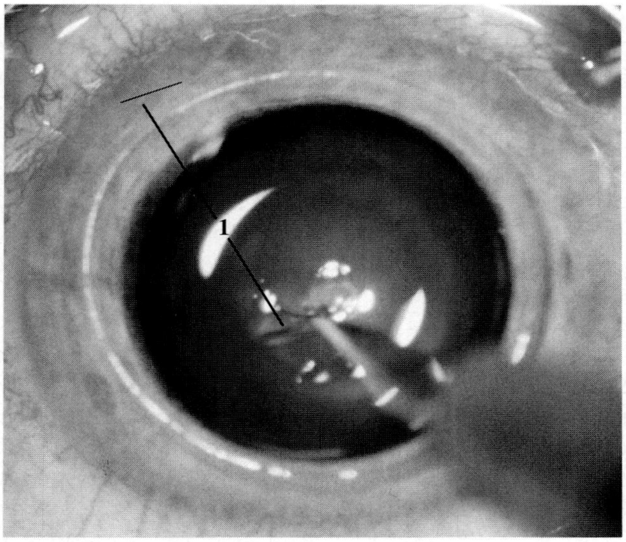

FIGURE 131-2 Horizontal incision (1) in anterior capsule. Surgeon's view.

traocular lens in good position, transplantation surgery can then proceed (see Chapter 130).

Penetrating Keratoplasty with ECCE

If phacoemulsification is not advisable or possible, ECCE is performed during the transplantation procedure. Preoperative softening of the eye is important and is achieved using a super-pinky, Honan balloon, or digital massage to minimize posterior pressure. Combined PK and cataract surgery can be made infinitely more difficult when there is significant vitreous pressure. If excessive posterior pressure is encountered after entering the anterior chamber but before removing the corneal button, it is best to perform a posterior sclerotomy 4 mm posterior to the limbus with aspiration of liquid vitreous to allow the iris-lens diaphragm to fall back. Alternatively, intravenous mannitol may be administered, which will effectively reduce the vitreous pressure. If cataract removal is attempted in the face of significant posterior pressure, posterior capsular rupture may result with its attendant complications. For the ECCE, it is still advantageous to perform a continuous-tear capsulotomy to begin the cataract removal. This is more difficult than under a closed system, but with some practice it can be completed successfully.[25,26] A curved rent should be made in the anterior capsule fairly near the center (Figures 131-2 and 131-3, *A*), and a tear at one edge initiated. A curved incision has much less tendency than a straight incision to autoextend peripherally, resulting in a torn posterior capsule. The capsular flap can next be turned over to be grasped by the forceps (Figure 131-3, *B*).

With a Utrata forceps (Figure 131-4), a continuous-tear capsulotomy can be performed. This should be performed as far as possible into the periphery (Figure 131-3, *C*), but one must bear in mind that the tendency for a capsule to tear out toward the equator is greater using the open-sky approach. The technique for performing a continuous-tear capsulotomy in an open-sky fashion is to begin the capsular tear and then to fold the flap of the torn capsule over the portion of the capsule to be torn next. The tear proceeds along the line made by the torn edge of the capsule (Figure 131-3, *D*) If the capsule begins to tear out toward the periphery, that tear should be stopped and one should begin again from the starting point in the opposite direction. The use of a Vannas scissors to start the tear in the other direction can facilitate this maneuver. Because it is an open-sky approach, it is possible to perform a circular capsulotomy using only scissors. Even though this maneuver theoretically may appear easy, however, the continuous-tear method is much more reliable. In some cases there is too much posterior pressure, with the nucleus of the lens pushing forward; regardless of the approach, the capsule tends to tear toward the periphery. If this happens, scissors can be used to complete the capsulotomy with as smooth an edge as possible. Another useful technique to reduce tension on the capsulorrhexis caused by vitreous pressure is to push the lens back with a blunt instrument such as a cyclodialysis spatula in one hand while completing the capsulotomy with the other hand.

Once a capsulotomy has been performed, the nucleus is simply expressed. It is often helpful to perform hydrodissection by injecting balanced salt solution (BSS) just under the anterior capsular edge; in some cases, the nucleus will almost deliver itself after the hydrodissection has been performed (Figure 131-5). Pressure with one instrument at the limbus and counterpressure with a second instrument applied 180 degrees from the first 4 mm posterior to the limbus will facilitate lens delivery. If the nucleus is too large to pass through the capsular opening, one must perform a relaxing incision out toward the periphery of the capsule. It is best to have only one relaxing incision because this facilitates in-the-bag intraocular lens placement.

Following expression of the nucleus, the cortical material is removed using either the automated irrigating aspirating (I/A) machine or by using a manual aspiration system. With an automated instrument approach, little or no irrigation can be used and the cortical material can be removed by engaging the anterior aspect of the material and then peeling out the residual

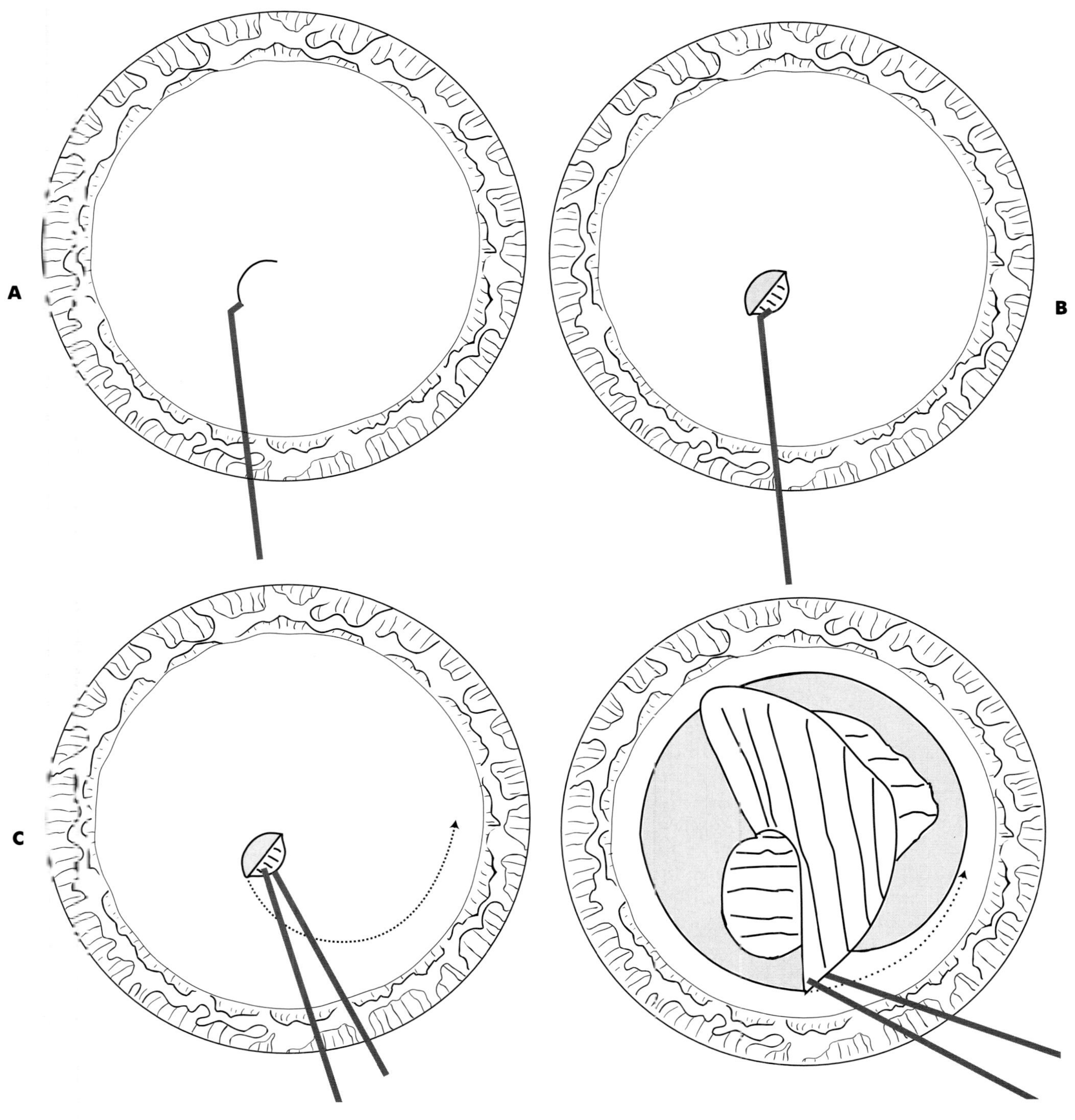

FIGURE 131-3 **A,** A curved rent is made in the capsule with a sharp instrument. Surgeon's view. **B,** The flap of the capsule is turned over in preparation for the forceps. **C,** The edge of the tear is grasped with a Utrata forceps. The capsule is torn toward the periphery in a curved fashion, stopping to regrasp close to the torn edge. **D,** The continuous tear is made by pulling the torn edge around a continuation of the curvilinear line made by the already torn edge of the capsule. The tear is complete when the new edge reaches the point at which the beginning tear began its uniform peripheral location. The edge must be regrasped several times a slight distance from the site of new tearing.

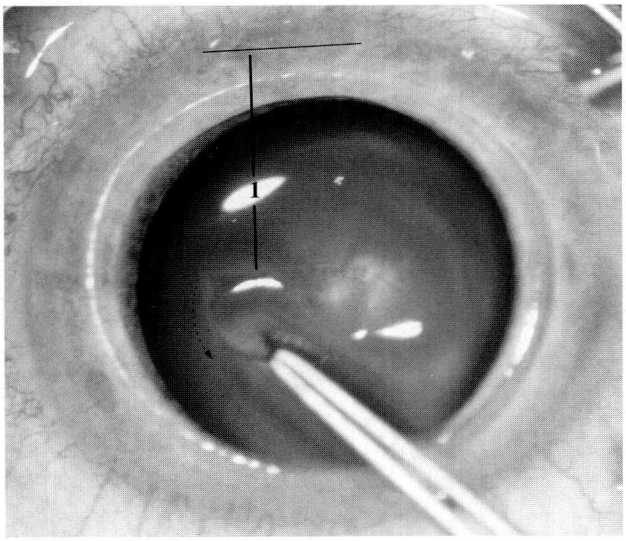

FIGURE 131-4 Beginning of capsular tear with a Utrata forceps. After initial incision *(1)*, a tear is begun in the direction of the arrow. Surgeon's view.

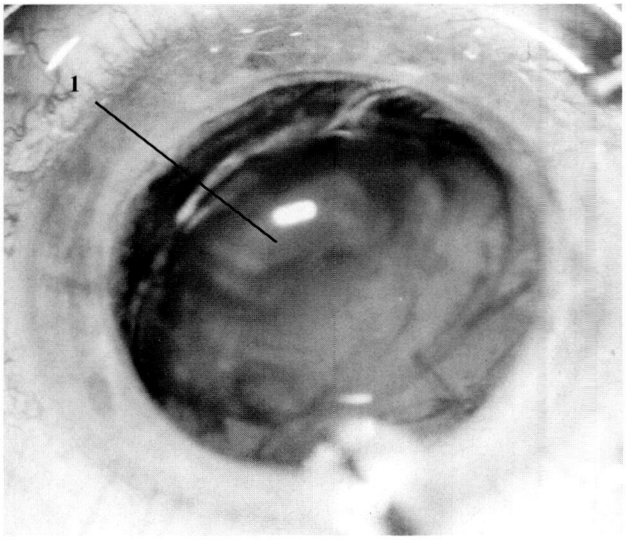

FIGURE 131-5 Nucleus *(1)* being "delivered" after hydrodissection alone. Surgeon's view.

cortex (Figure 131-6). It is often helpful to place the I/A tip against the posterior cortex and posterior capsule, pushing it slightly away from the anterior cortex, facilitating engagement of the anterior cortex, which will then strip out nicely. This procedure also can be performed with the manual aspiration approach. However, one must use a tip that has the opening on the side and not on the end of the tip.

After all cortical material has been removed, the posterior capsule is polished using a diamond-dusted capsule polisher. Other capsule polishers or even a Weck sponge can be used. At this point, the capsule should be filled with a viscoelastic substance, and the inferior haptic of the posterior chamber intraocular lens can be introduced into the capsular space. Care must be taken to make sure that the haptics go into the capsular bag. This can be ensured by placing the haptic against the posterior capsule centrally and then gently pushing the intraocular lens inferiorly. After the inferior haptic is in place, the optic of the lens should be introduced through the capsular opening (Figure 131-7). With a second instrument, pressure can be maintained on the optic of the intraocular lens to prevent it from moving, and the trailing haptic of the intraocular lens can then be grasped with a forceps. With a pronation movement of the wrist, one introduces the trailing haptic into the capsular bag superiorly. Once the intraocular lens is in the capsular bag, it is worthwhile to "dial" the lens slightly to make sure that it is securely in the capsular bag (Figure 131-8).

If significant tears have been in the anterior capsule, or if difficulty is encountered in determining how much of the anterior capsule is present, it is preferable to insert the intraocular lens in the ciliary sulcus. It is much better to have the haptics in the ciliary sulcus than to have one in the bag and one out of the bag. Such positioning will result in decentration of the intraocular lens. Holland et al. demonstrated that the average diameter of the ciliary sulcus allows a 12.5 mm intraocular lens to center nicely. If one decides to put the implant in the ciliary sulcus, a viscoelastic substance should be injected just under the iris. The cannula tip of the viscoelastic can be used to lift up the edge of the iris and the viscoelastic is injected directly under the iris, making sure that the anterior capsule or any remnants from it are pushed back. The haptics are placed in a fashion similar to that used for capsular fixation. Once the lens is in good position, either in the capsular bag or the ciliary sulcus, acetylcholine chloride should be used to constrict the pupil. I have found that (Miostat) is useful, because the pupillary constriction will be maintained through the rest of the procedure.

If the posterior capsule tears during any part of the procedure, it must be managed. If the tear is fairly central and small, the tear can be converted to a continuous tear in the same manner as previously described for the anterior capsule. If vitreous presents through the tear, a limited vitrectomy should be performed. If the tear is larger and extends toward the periphery, it is not usually possible to convert it to a circumscribed continuous tear. In this case, care must be taken to preserve as much of the posterior capsule as possible. A vitrectomy is almost always required, and an automated vitrectomy will usually preserve more of the capsule. The vitreous must be completely removed from the anterior chamber, and no vitreous strands can

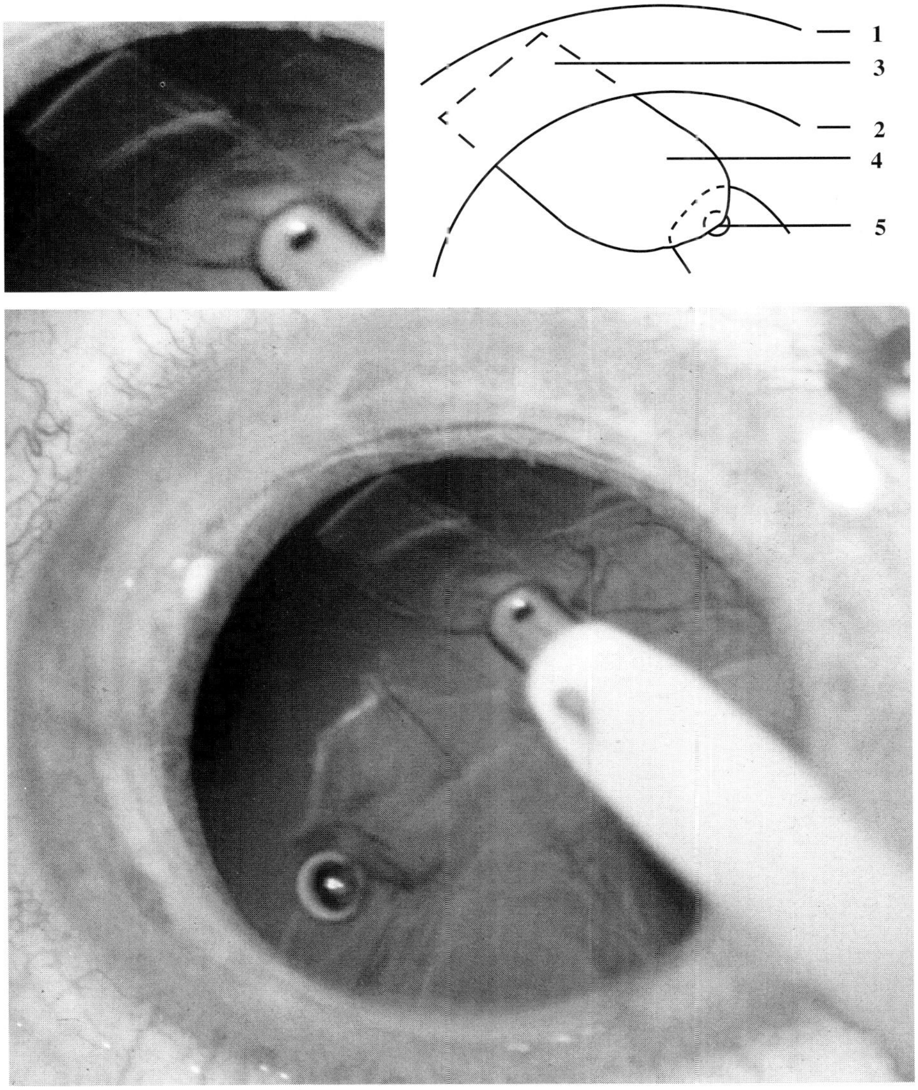

FIGURE 131-6 Stripping out cortex with irrigation and aspiration handpiece. Surgeon's view. Iris *(1)*. Edge of smooth capsular tear *(2)*. Cortex under anterior capsule *(3)*. Cortex in capsular opening *(4)*. Cortex being aspirated into handpiece *(5)*.

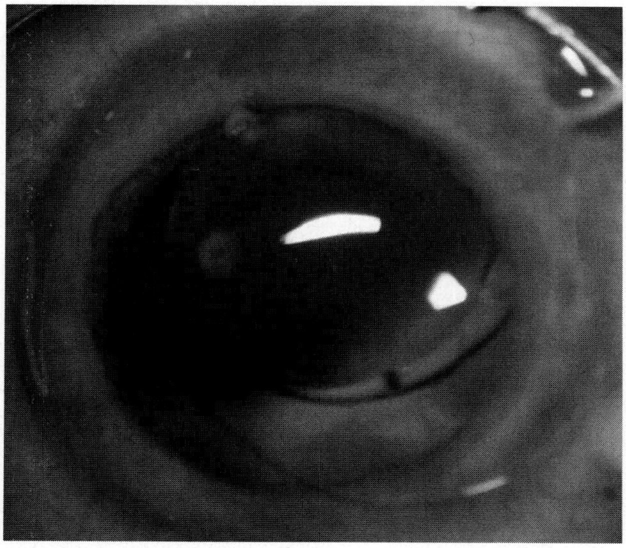

FIGURE 131-7 Inferior haptic in the capsular bag. Surgeon's view.

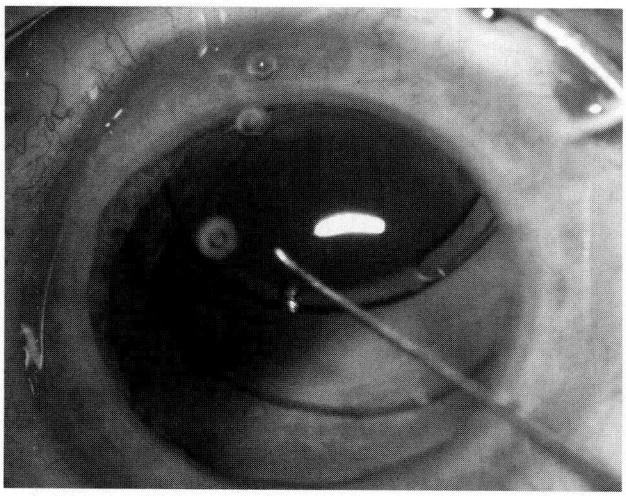

FIGURE 131-8 IOL being "dialed." Surgeon's view.

be left coming through the capsular tear. Once all the vitreous is removed from the anterior chamber and around the iris and capsular tear, the capsule that remains must be inspected. This can be done by gently retracting the iris. It is rare that there is not enough capsule to support a posterior chamber intraocular lens. When a larger posterior capsular tear is present, it is best to place the haptics in the ciliary sulcus in areas where there is more capsular support. A continuous tear anterior capsulotomy is a great advantage in those cases in which the posterior capsule tears, because invariably a posterior chamber intraocular lens can be placed in the ciliary sulcus. In such instances where most or all of the capsule is lost or where there is little zonular support, a posterior lens can be sutured into the sulcus transsclerally or can be sutured to the iris. Alternatively, an anterior chamber intraocular lens can be used. Once the intraocular lens is in good position and the cataract extraction has been completed, corneal transplantation can proceed as described in Chapter 130.

REFERENCES

1. Martin TP et al: Cataract formation and cataract extraction after penetrating keratoplasty, *Ophthalmology* 101:113-119, 1994.
2. de Charnace B, Guidi M, Valiere-Vialeix JP: Short, medium and long-term post-operative complications in 150 patients undergoing penetrating keratoplasty after one year, *Ophtalmologie* 3:11-12, 1989.
3. Craig MT, Olson RJ, Mamalis N: Air bubble endothelial damage during phacoemulsification in human eye bank eyes: the protective effects of Healon and Viscoat, *J Cataract Refract Surg* 16:597-602, 1990.
4. Koch DD et al: A comparison of corneal endothelial changes after use of Healon or Viscoat during phacoemulsification, *Am J Ophthalmol* 115:188-201, 1993.
5. Bourne WM, Nelson LR, Hodge DO: Continued endothelial cell loss ten years after lens implantation, *Ophthalmology* 101:1014-1022, 1994.
6. Zacks CM, Abbott RL, Fine M: Long-term changes in corneal endothelium after keratoplasty, *Cornea* 9:92-97, 1990.
7. Binder PS: Intraocular lens implantation after penetrating keratoplasty, *Refract Corneal Surg* 5:224-230, 1989.
8. Dangel ME, Kirkham SM, Phipps MJ: Posterior capsule opacification in extracapsular cataract extraction and the triple procedure, *Ophthalmic Surg* 25:82-87, 1994.
9. Yamagami S et al: Statistic evaluation of prognostic risk factors in penetrating keratoplasty using Cox multiple regression model. *Nippon Geka Gakkai Zasshi* 98:777-781, 1994.
10. The Australian Corneal Graft Registry: 1990 to 1992 report, *Aust N Z J Ophthalmol* 21:1-48, 1993.
11. Vajpayee RB, Angra SK, Honavar SG: Combined keratoplasty, cataract extraction, and intraocular lens implantation after corneolenticular laceration in children, *Am J Ophthalmol* 17:507-511, 1994.
12. Donnenfeld ED et al: Soemmering's ring support for posterior chamber intraocular lens implantation during penetrating keratoplasty. Changing trends in bullous keratoplasty, *Ophthalmology* 99:1229-1233, 1992.
13. Keates RH, Rothchild EJ, Bloom R: Endocapsular triple procedure—a new triple procedure technique, *J Cataract Refract Surg* 15:332-335, 1989.
14. Malbran ES, Malbran E, Buonsanti J, Adroque E: Closed-system phacoemulsification and posterior chamber implant combined with penetrating keratoplasty, *Ophthalmic Surg* 24:403-406, 1993.
15. Gloor B, Kalman A: Choroidal effusion and expulsive hemorrhage in penetrating interventions—lessons from 26 patients, *Klin Monatsbl Augenheilkd* 202:224-237, 1993.
16. Aiello LP, Javitt JC, Canner JK: National outcomes of penetrating keratoplasty: risks of endophthalmitis and retinal detachment, *Arch Ophthalmol* 111:509-513, 1993.
17. Egger SF et al: Bacterial contamination during extracapsular cataract extraction: prospective study on 200 consecutive patients, *Ophthalmologica* 208:767-781, 1994.
18. Boke W: Phacoemulsification. Why? *Klin Monatsbl Augenheilkd* 197:100-105, 1990.
19. Ohrloff C: Comparison of phacoemulsification and planned

extracapsular cataract extraction, *Klin Monatsbl Augenheilkd* 203:93-98, 1993.

20. Loots JH, Venter JA: Posterior peribulbar anaesthesia for intra-ocular surgery, *S Afr Med J* 74:507-509, 1988.
21. Davis DB, Mandel MR: Posterior peribulbar anesthesia: an alternative to retrobulbar anesthesia, *J Cataract Refract Surg* 12:182-184, 1986.
22. Johnson SH: Split and lift: nuclear quadrant management for phacoemulsification, *J Cataract Refract Surg* 19:420-424, 1993.
23. Wang HS: Management of a posterior capsule rupture in planned extracapsular cataract extraction and posterior chamber lens implantation, *J Cataract Refract Surg* 12:73-76, 1986.
24. Galand A: Capsulorrhexis and manual extracapsular extraction, *Bull Soc Belge Ophtalmol* 247:43-5, 1993.
25. Groden LR: Continuous tear capsulotomy and phacoemulsification cataract extraction combined with penetrating keratoplasty, *Refract Corneal Surg* 6:458-459, 1990.
26. Orgul SI, Daicker B, Buchi ER: The diameter of the ciliary sulcus; a morphometric study, *Graefes Arch Clin Exp Ophthalmol* 231:487-490, 1993.

CHAPTER 132

LOUIS E. PROBST EDWARD J. HOLLAND

Penetrating Keratoplasty and Intraocular Lens Exchange

Cataract surgery has undergone remarkable improvements over the last two decades, primarily due to the popularization and refinement of intraocular lens (IOL) implantation. Unfortunately, pseudophakic corneal edema (PCE) has emerged as a significant complication of this advancement. The treatment of PCE offers a number of challenges to the ophthalmic surgeon. Intensive surgical planning and meticulous anterior segment surgery are required with several options of IOL replacement. While anatomical success has been achieved in approximately 90% of cases, results of functional visual acuity have been inconsistent.[1]

Waring described the epidemic of PCE that began with the implantation of rigid or flexible loop anterior chamber lenses in the early 1950s.[1] PCE was the most common indication for penetrating keratoplasty (PK) until 1989[2] when most studies reported an incidence of 21% to 23%.[2-6] Since 1987, the number of PCE cases has decreased, and in 1990, keratoconus surpassed PCE as the most common indication for PK.[2] An FDA study conservatively estimated the incidence of PCE at 1 year after cataract surgery to be 1.2% with anterior chamber IOL (ACIOLs), 1.5% with iris supported IOL, and 0.6% with posterior chamber IOL (PCIOLs).[7] Since it has been estimated that approximately 1.4 million cataract surgeries were performed on Medicare beneficiaries alone in 1991,[8] it would appear that PCE will continue to be a major indication for surgery in the future.

Interestingly, the average postoperative interval between IOL implantation and the onset of PCE varies depending on the type of IOL involved. Postoperatively, ACIOLs tend to develop PCE after 24 months, whereas iris supported IOLs develop PCE after 47 months.[9-11] PCIOLs develop corneal edema quite acutely, often within 4 months after surgery.[9,11] This is most often due to preoperative endothelial dystrophy[12] and/or excessive intraoperative endothelial trauma and is not related to the PCIOL itself.

Indications and Goals of Surgery

The indications for PK and/or IOL exchange can be divided into three groups. The first group includes patients with obvious corneal pathology, including PCE or frank painful bullous keratopathy, caused by the IOL and those who have failed medical therapy. These eyes will require PK and replacement of the IOL to improve vision and relieve the ocular pain. The second group of patients have borderline PCE, which often occurs over the peripheral cornea in the area of endothelial touch to an ACIOL. Specular microscopy can determine the residual endothelial cell function in these cases; counts less than 500 cells/mm^2 are usually associated with corneal edema. Pachymetry can assess the extent of the corneal edema. We use a pachymetry value of 0.62 mm to 0.65 mm as an indicator of clinical edema. The clinical examination and the results of these investigations must be correlated to determine whether a PK and IOL exchange or an IOL exchange alone should be performed in these patients. The third group has clinically normal corneas and lens-related problems including displacement of the IOL, endothelial touch, the uveitis-glaucoma hyphema (UGH) syndrome, erosion of the uveal tissue, iris neovascularization, angle fibrosis, and persistent anterior chamber inflammation.[10] These patients only require an IOL exchange without PK. There are no specific contraindications to surgery because potential transplant rejection can be handled with aggressive topical and systemic steroids, and the location and technique of IOL placement can be modified according to the preoperative ocular pathology.

The goals of surgery include the restoration of the optical integrity of the cornea with minimal postoperative astigmatism, atraumatic removal of the intraocular lens from its fibrous attachments in the delicate uveal tissue, and removal of intraocular vitreal attachments. Other considerations include restoration of

will allow the surgeon to maintain position of the IOL temporarily until it is removed.[44]

Intraocular Lens Explantation

The management of the IOL at the time of surgery for PCE has changed dramatically in recent years. In 1983, Speaker et al. reported that the IOL was removed or exchanged at the time of surgery for PCE in 26% of cases.[45] Studies performed in the early 1980s by Samples and Binder[46-48] recommended retention of the implant because of equal or better visual prognosis with the reduced hazards of removing the lens. In 1987, Waring suggested that the IOL can be retained when it is the correct diopter power; in a stable, desirable position that will not contact the corneal endothelium; and not associated with inflammation, progressive peripheral anterior synechiae (PAS), vitreous in the anterior chamber, or CME.[20]

Since the late 1980s, there has been an obvious trend in the literature towards IOL exchange in PK for PCE. By 1990, the incidence of IOL exchange with PK for PCE had increased to 68%.[45] Speaker et al. summarized the indications for removal of the IOL during PK and they are: any unstable IOL; the presence of significant uveitis, poorly controlled glaucoma or recurrent hyphema (UGH syndrome); metal clips or loops on the IOL, and any closed-loop ACIOL such as the Leiske, Azar 91Z, Stableflex, Americal 100-AC, Optiflex, Hessburg, Coopervision 600, Dannheim, or rigid Choyce style IOL; and most iris supported IOLs with the optic in front of the iris.[14,49] The presence of CME and incorrect IOL power have also been reported as indications for IOL removal.[50-52] The goals of surgery are to remove the IOL atraumatically, preserve iris tissue, minimize intraocular hemorrhaging, and minimize vitreous traction.

The indication for removal of the semiflexible closed-loop ACIOL from the anterior chamber is well supported by several studies demonstrating greater rates of graft failure if the IOL is retained.* The management of modern flexible open-loop ACIOLs are more controversial. If they are well fixated in a quiet eye with a deep chamber they can be left in place.[45] However, ACIOLs that are loose, dislocated, or associated with shallow anterior chambers in inflamed, tender eyes should be exchanged.[14]

While it has been suggested that iris-supported PCIOLs be retained during the surgery for PCE,[45] most surgeons now remove these lenses. PCIOLs with capsular support should be left in place except when the PCIOL has dislocated, when vitreous is in the anterior chamber, or when very large capsular tears are present.[9]

*References 24, 31, 45, 49, 53-56

TECHNIQUE

Removal of the IOL from the eye is a delicate procedure that must be approached cautiously if the complications of iridodialysis, cyclodialysis, tears to the iris, traction on the zonules and vitreous, and intraocular hemorrhage are to be avoided. Waring suggested maneuvers to elucidate the status of the IOL including an angle to directly inspect the surface of the iris, gentle tugging to determine how firmly the haptics are attached to the iris, retraction of the iris to inspect the haptics in the posterior chamber, inspecting the angle with a dental mirror, and eversion of the limbus.[20] The haptics of the ACIOL are often encased in a "cocoon" in the anterior chamber angle. Iris-supported PCIOLs typically do not have adherent synechiae[20] and therefore are more easily removed.

Amputating one of the haptics while inserting the optic lens has been recommended because it creates a long amputated segment that allows easy visualization of the cut end of the haptic and provides a firm handle to grasp.[20,56-61] The opposite end of the haptic can also be amputated at the optic base or at its entrance into the angle; this would minimize the size of the haptic segment to pull through the ciliary body.[58] Amputation can be performed with the Westcott, Grieshaber, Vannas, or Rappozzo scissors. The haptic should be cut as cleanly as possible since a crushed haptic can be very difficult to remove through the tunnel of fibrosis.[21]

Using a McPherson or Pierse-Colibri forceps around the long exposed end of the haptic as it emerges from the iris root, apply gentle traction while keeping the forceps parallel to the iris plane. The haptic should then be rotated along its arc of curvature from the tunnel of adhesions.[59] With careful manipulation the haptic can be removed from the ciliary body without creating an iridodialysis.[56] Particular attention should be paid to any vitreous adhesions to the IOL; amputate with the Westcott scissors before removing the IOL from the anterior chamber to avoid traction on the vitreous (Figure 132-1).

Bleeding from the iris often occurs during removal of the ACIOL from its iris attachments or during anterior segment reconstruction, and can usually be controlled with the application of 1 to 10,000 epinephrine. Other choices for hemostasis include intraoperative application of thrombin 100 units per ml of balanced salt solution,[60] viscoelastic tamponade to trap the blood in the angle and compress the bleeding vessels, direct coagulation of the vessels with fine tipped underwater diathermy, or bipolar cautery.[20] When the bleeding is controlled, the viscoelastic can be removed from the anterior chamber with the vitrectomy instruments.

The Stableflex semiflexible closed-loop ACIOL offers a particular challenge for removal from the anterior chamber. This IOL has two double loop haptics that

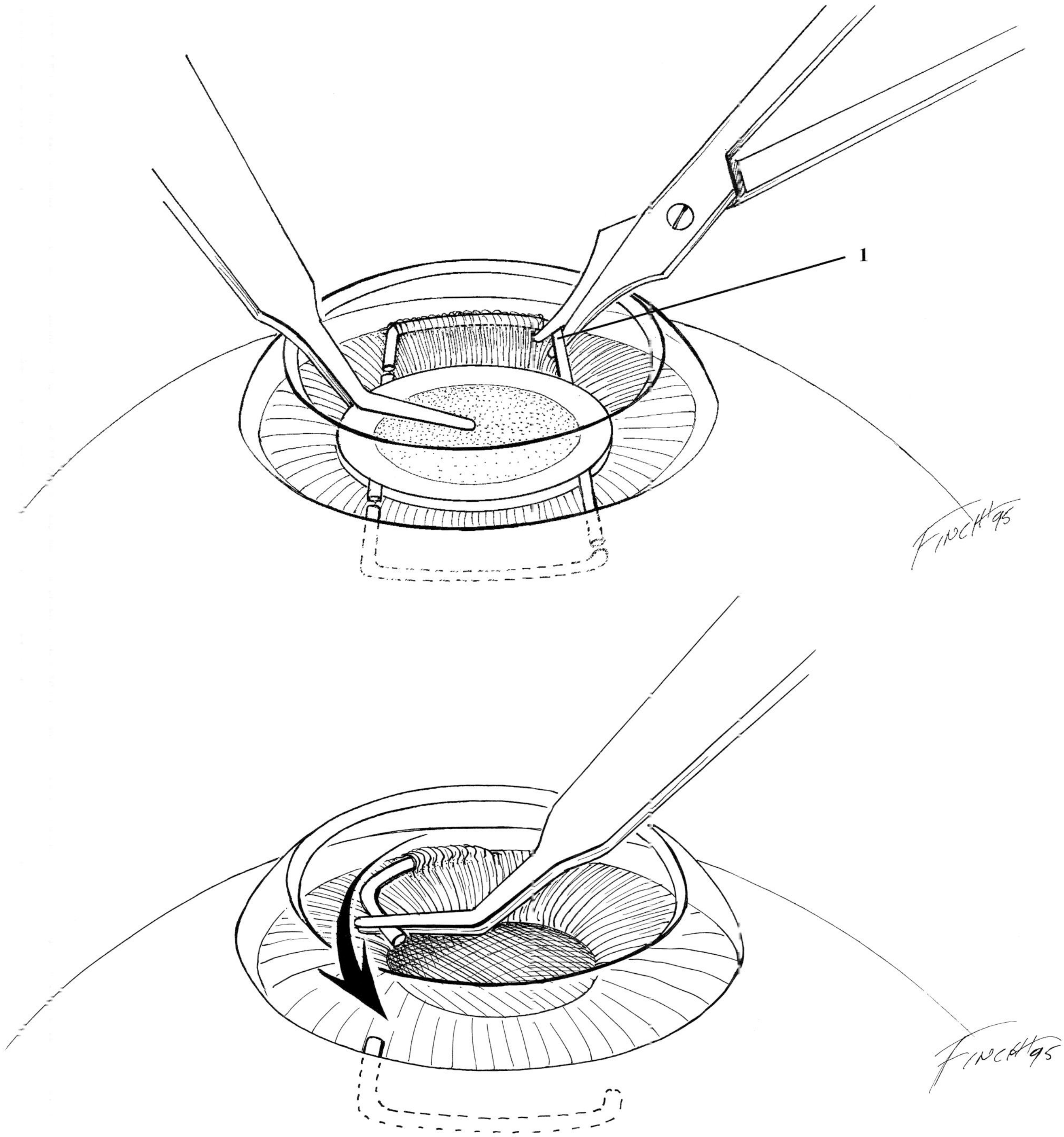

A

B

FIGURE 132-1 **A,** Removal of closed-loop anterior chamber IOLs is complicated by the fibrous adhesions to the haptics in the angle. The closed-loop implant is stabilized with forceps and one haptic is amputated *(1)* at its entrance into the angle. The other haptic of the closed-loop implant is amputated at the optic base to provide a portion to grasp. Once the haptics have been cut free, the IOL optic can be removed. **B,** The haptics are then removed by grasping the long, visible end of the cut haptic and rotating it out of the fibrous encasement of ciliary tissue.

become encased in fibrous tissue in the angles. The technique for the removal of this IOL includes amputation of both double haptics on either side of the IOL at their origin from the optic. The amputated proximal portion of the haptic is then gently manipulated so that the haptic can be removed by gently traction[56,59,62,63] (Figure 132-2).

In the rare circumstance that a PCIOL requires removal, the haptic configuration should be identified through a dilated pupil to determine the orientation of the optic. Using a Sinskey hook at the haptic origin, the IOL is rotated clockwise to release the superior haptic from the adhesions to the lens capsule, iris, ciliary body, or residual cortical tissue.[20] Once the superior haptic is freed, the inferior haptic can be released in a similar manner. If the IOL haptic cannot be removed from the fibrous encasement due to an enlargment on the end of the haptic, it should be amputated as close to the ciliary sulcus as possible.[52]

Open-Sky Subtotal Vitrectomy

Open-sky subtotal vitrectomy is indicated when the vitreous is adherent to the IOL, capsule remnants, or posterior iris, and when placement of a transsclerally sutured PCIOL is anticipated. A vitrectomy is not necessary when the replacement of a PCIOL supported by the capsule or an ACIOL is selected and the anterior hyaloid face is intact, or when the vitreous is behind the iris plane.[64] The vitreous should be handled with extreme care and meticulous clean-up.

The goals of vitrectomy are to remove as much vitreous as possible. During IOL removal, vitrectomy can reduce vitreous traction and it is used postoperatively when retinal detachment or macular edema can develop.[65]

TECHNIQUE

We cut any vitreous strands adherent to the IOL cautiously with Westcott scissors before complete explantation to minimize traction. We recommend that an open-sky subtotal vitrectomy be performed after the IOL is removed using a disposable hand-held vitrector with the cutting set at 400 to 600 cuts per minute and the aspiration set at 100 to 200 mm Hg. We have described using a fiber optic light pipe as a second instrument that can function in iris retraction and vitreous illumination when the tip of the attached membrane pick is bent to produce an iris retraction hook[27] (Figure 132-3). This technique provides direct visualization of the vitreous strands,

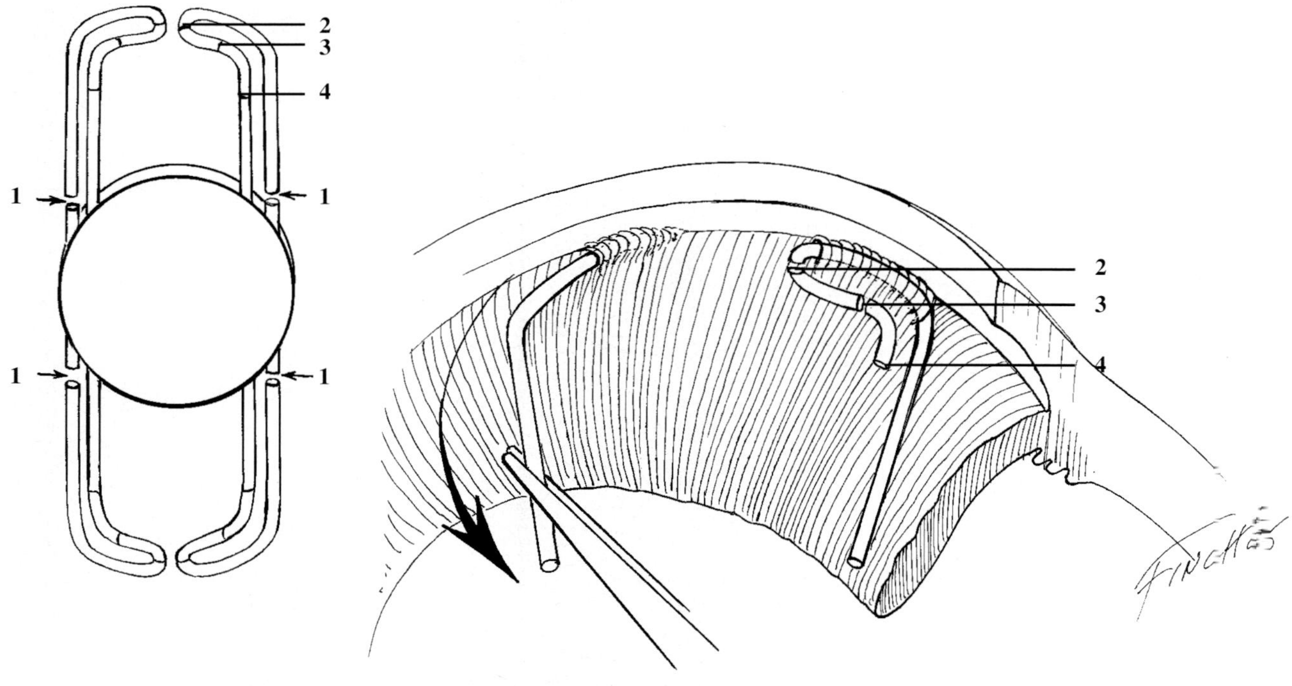

FIGURE 132-2 Removal of the Stableflex IOL begins with amputation of one side of each haptic at the optic *(1)* and the other side as close to the angle as possible. Possible sites include the optimum *(2)*, next optimum *(3)*, and usual *(4)*. The distal loop of the haptic is then removed from the tunnel of synechiae.

which allows for complete removal of the anterior half of the vitreous.[66] Vitrectomy should be performed through the pupil as well as through any iris defects such as iridectomies to ensure patency and prevent any postoperative vitreous blockage.[64] Injection of balanced salt solution during vitrectomy hydrates the hydrophilic vitreous strands, floating them anteriorly and allowing for a more complete vitrectomy.[20] If sufficient Soemmering's ring is present, the surgeon may elect to leave this in place to provide partial or complete support for ciliary sulcus placement of the IOL.[21,67] If a transsclerally sutured PCIOL is being used, any potential vitreous attachments to the posterior iris and ciliary sulcus in the areas of the fixation sutures should be removed. When automated vitrectomy is completed, the pupil and the iridectomy sites should be probed with a cellulose sponge to identify any residual vitreous that should then be excised with Westcott scissors.

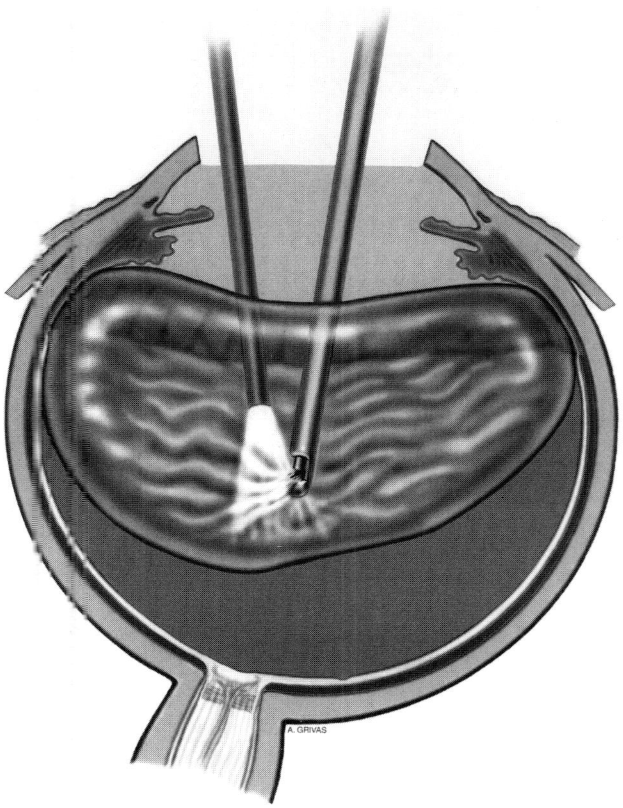

FIGURE 132-3 Open-sky subtotal vitrectomy is performed using the hand-held vitrector with cutting set at 400 to 600 cuts per minute and the aspiration set at 100 to 200 mm Hg. The fiber optic light pipe provides illumination of the vitreous strands.

Anterior Segment Reconstruction

Anterior segment reconstruction is frequently required during PK and IOL exchange due to the trauma and distortion to the anterior segment, which occurs preoperatively from ACIOLs and iris sutured PCIOLs, or intraoperatively with difficult IOL explantation. More recently, PCIOLs have also been associated with PCE. Since PCIOLs are generally not associated with anterior segment trauma, reconstruction is usually not required. Preoperative damage to the angle structures can lead to the progressive formation of peripheral anterior synechiae (PAS) with partial angle closure postoperatively, resulting in new onset glaucoma unless this process can be arrested. A solid platform of iris is required for both ACIOL and iris sutured PCIOL fixation to ensure that the IOL remains well supported and the risks of lens decentration or dislocation are minimized. The goals of anterior segment reconstruction are to restore the anatomy to as near normal as possible and reduce the visually disabling postoperative problems of CME and glaucoma.[20]

TECHNIQUE

The angle is examined with a dental mirror adjacent to the keratoplasty opening to identify any PAS that would place the patient at risk for glaucoma or graft rejection.[68] For further examination viscodissect the peripheral iris.

Gonioplasty

Gonioplasty can repair the damaged angle. Iris adhesions to the cornea can be reduced by gently stroking the iris radially towards the pupil with a cellulose sponge, pulling the iris radially with smooth forceps, sweeping the cyclodialysis spatula through the angle, and then cutting the PAS using the goniotomy technique or Vannas scissors.[20] Large iridocorneal adhesions that cannot be separated should have iridotomies on either side of the lesion[20] to prevent progression of angle closure postoperatively. Bleeding is controlled as previously described for IOL explantation.

Iridoplasty

Iridoplasty is performed to pull the iris from the angle thus reducing the potential for the reformation of PAS. Reconstruction of the pupil reduces glare, improves optical function, improves cosmesis, reduces entrapment of the iris around the replacement IOL,[20] and supports the new IOL in the correct position. This technique uses 9-0 or 10-0 polypropylene sutures on a tapered needle to minimize iris tearing. Miosis can be

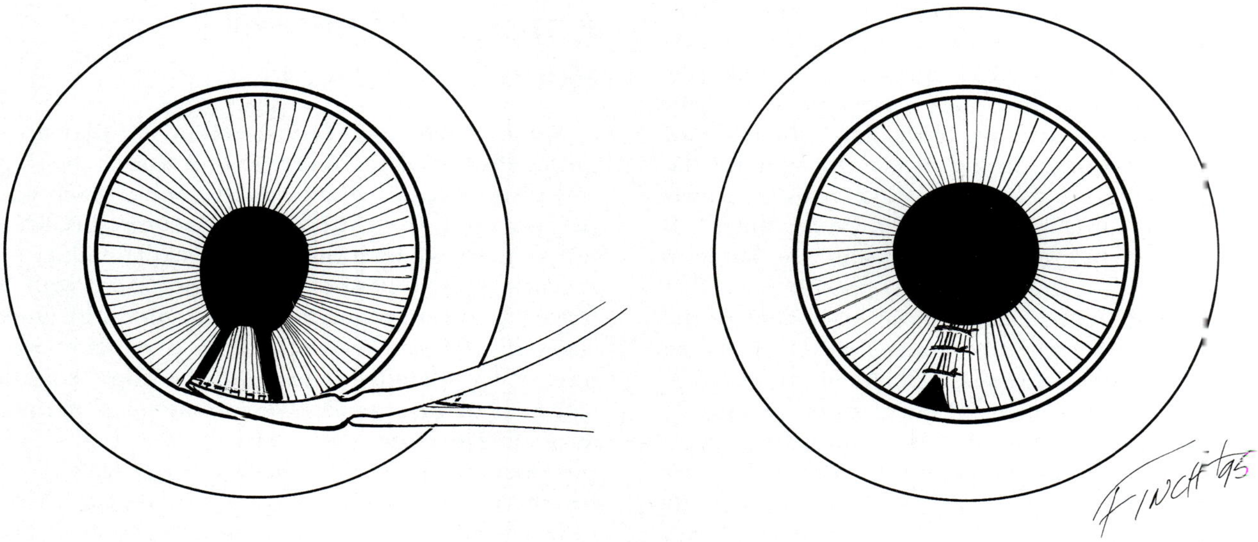

FIGURE 132-4 Iridoplasty reconstructs the pupil and pulls the iris away from the anterior chamber angle. *Left,* If the area of synechiae is not large, a small sector iridectomy is performed. *Right,* 10-0 polypropylene sutures on a tapered needle are used to approximate the edges of the iris.

induced pharmacologiocally to reduce tension and help create a central pupil. Iridectomies and sphincterotomies are closed with interrupted sutures that are started peripherally and continued inward toward the pupil. The sutures are tied tight enough to approximate the iris, but not so tight as to cause iris ischemia and atrophy (Figure 132-4).

In areas of extensive PAS, which have a high risk of recurrence, we use a *sector iridoplasty* technique. A sector iridectomy is performed to remove completely the area of adhesive iris and to minimize the possibility of recurrent iris adhesions to the donor cornea that may thereby be compromised. The sector iridectomy may need to be enlarged to achieve a taut iris once the defect is closed. Interrupted polypropylene sutures on a tapered needle are then used to close the defect starting at the pupil and continuing peripherally, leaving a small basal peripheral iridectomy in the area of the previous PAS to prevent recurrence (Figure 132-5).

Restoration of a central pupil from an eccentric pupil can be accomplished by performing regular relaxing sphincterotomies at the advancing edge of the pupil and placing interrupted sutures starting peripherally along the sphincterotomy defect.[14] Purse string sutures have been used along the pupillary margin to assist further in creating a circular, central pupil.[20]

Intraocular Lens Implantation

There are four options for replacing the IOL at the time of PK and IOL exchange. These include placement of a PCIOL in the ciliary sulcus supported by the remnants of the capsular bag (CS-PCIOL), placement of a flexible, open-loop ACIOL in the anterior chamber angle, iris suture fixation of a PCIOL (IS-PCIOL), and a transslerally sutured PCIOL (TS-PCIOL) in the ciliary sulcus.

There has been considerable debate in the literature regarding the best option for IOL replacement from both theoretical and practical standpoints. Numerous series have been reported on the success and complication rate of each IOL replacement option.* Unfortunately, it is impossible to compare the results of these studies because they generally include small numbers of patients with varying degrees of follow-up, have different indications for surgery, and use different reporting strategies.[15]

We recommend complete or partial CS-PCIOL placement if sufficient posterior capsular support is identified. If insufficient support is available, the other methods of IOL fixation are considered. ACIOLs are recommended in eyes with minimal anterior chamber pathology when reduced operating time is desirable. IS-PCIOLs are considered when significant anterior chamber pathology is identified preoperatively and sufficient iris tissue is available for IOL fixation. TS-PCIOLs are recommended for surgeons experienced with this technique, particularly in eyes with anterior chamber pathology and limited iris tissue (Figure 132-6).

*References 11, 20, 23-29, 50, 52, 69-79

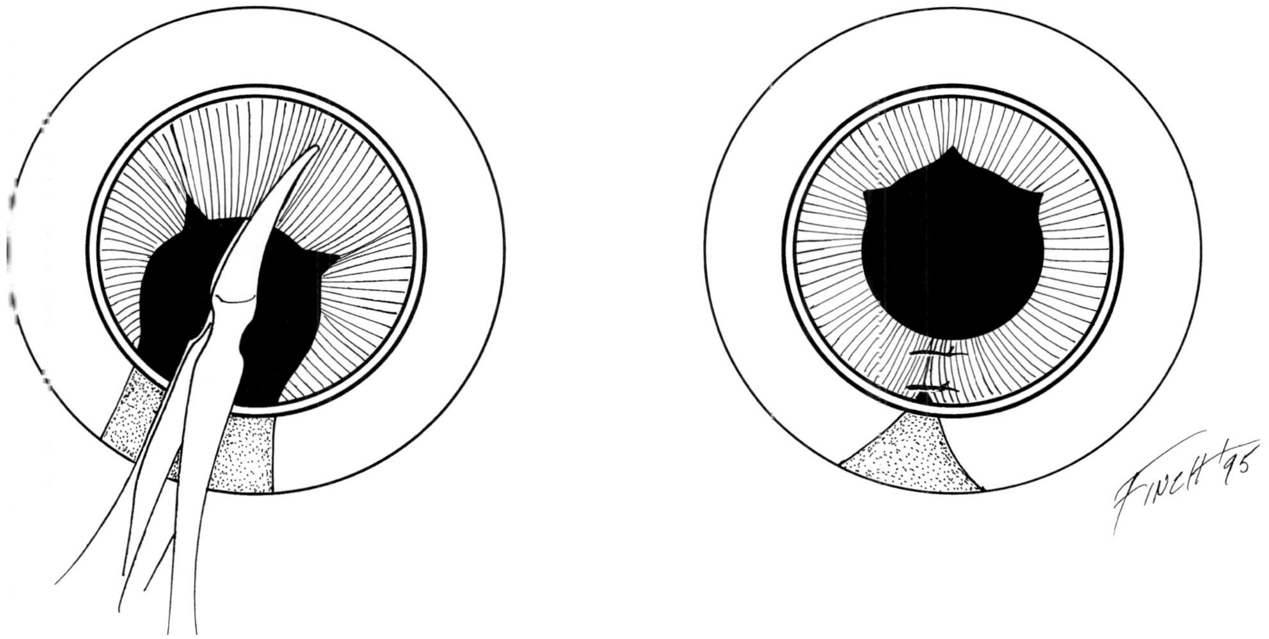

FIGURE 132-5 A large sector iridoplasty technique is used in an area of extensive peripheral anterior synechiae. *Left,* The sector iridectomy is performed in the area of the synechiae to completely remove all adhesions. Additional iris may be removed to achieve a taut iris once the edges are approximated. Sphincterotomies are added to keep the pupil centered. *Right,* Interrupted polypropylene sutures on a tapered needle are then used to close the defect starting at the pupil and continuing peripherally.

CAPSULAR SUPPORTED POSTERIOR CHAMBER INTRAOCULAR LENSES

Since modern day cataract surgery involves either extracapsular cataract extraction or phacoemulsification, both of which aim to preserve the posterior capsule, complicated cataract surgery with ACIOL placement will commonly leave posterior capsular remnants or a Soemmering's ring. If sufficient amounts of these tissues are available, implantation of the PCIOL into the ciliary sulcus with posterior support is possible during PK and IOL exchange.[67] This technique is not technically demanding, requires less surgical time than with an open globe, avoids the complications of ACIOL on the anterior chamber angle structures, and the need for scleral fixation sutures and their reported complications allows placement of the IOL closer to the nodal point of the eye, and offers the least number of postoperative complications with comparable visual results.[21,67] A vitrectomy is required if the posterior capsule is ruptured and the vitreous face is not intact. Caution is warranted since insufficient capsular support can allow the IOL to become decentered or to dislocate into the vitreous cavity.[21]

Technique

Once corneal trephination is completed and the previous IOL is removed, a careful inspection is made for residual posterior capsule by retracting the iris with an iris retractor or Sinsky hook. A combination of blunt dissection with the cyclodialysis spatula, viscodissection,[14] and sharp dissection,[67] can be used to dissect the posterior iris free from the remaining posterior capsule, which may include dissection of the adherent iris pigment epithelium from the remaining iris stroma. Only small amounts of capsule or Soemmering's ring are required for successful PCIOL placement because the capsule becomes stiff a few months after the original cataract surgery.[14] We recommend that a least three clock hours of posterior capsule or Soemmering's ring be present in the region of haptic insertion to ensure adequate support. If insufficient support is available for both haptics, often one haptic can be supported by the residual capsule remnants while the other is fixated transsclerally.[80] Vitrectomy is carried out through the break in the posterior capsule with the light pipe, as described previously, to ensure that the vitreous is well away from the capsular remnants. Residual Soemmering's ring should not be removed at the time of vitrectomy because this provides additional support for the IOL without enacting additional ocular inflammation.

Generally, a one piece, all polymethylmethacrylate (PMMA) PCIOL with a 7.0 mm optic and a 13.4 to 14.0 mm haptic diameter is used, although successful

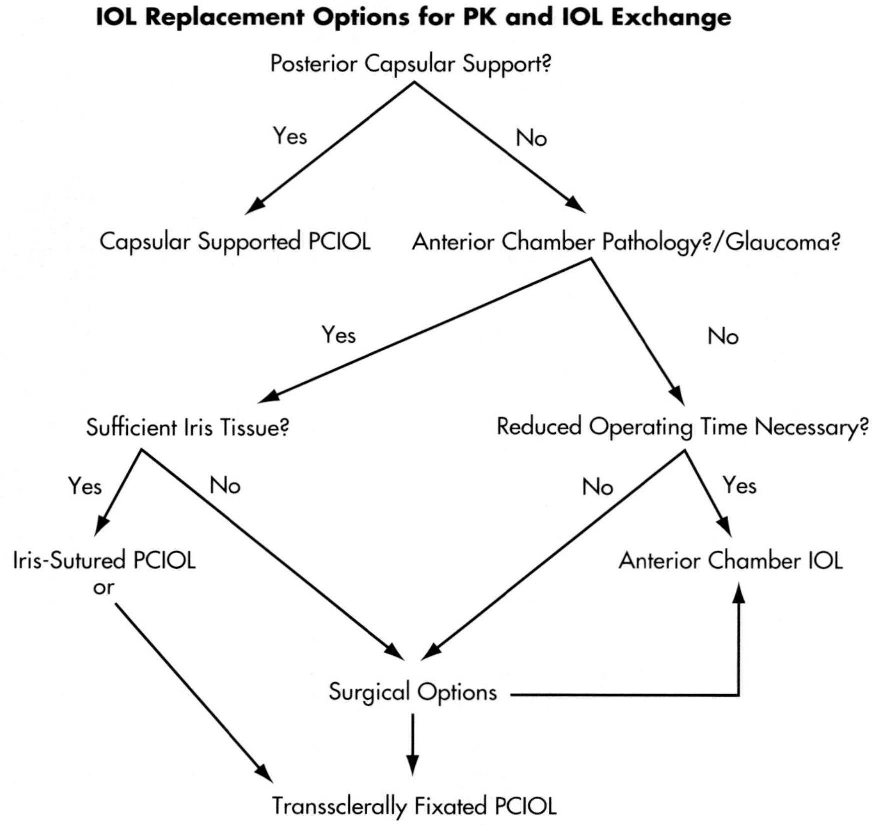

FIGURE 132-6 There are four IOL replacement options at the time of penetrating keratoplasty and IOL exchange. The selection of the best option for each patient is based on the ocular history, the intraoperative findings, and patient factors such as age and ability to tolerate a long operative time.

implantation of a PCIOL with 12.5 mm diameter haptics has also been reported with good fixation in the ciliary sulcus.[67] Great care must be taken to gently form a space for the IOL by using a spatula to separate iridecapsular adhesions. (For details of this procedure, see the study by Smith et al.[21]) The IOL is gently rotated to the region of greatest capsular support. The stability of the IOL is tested by assessing the immediate recentration of the IOL after the optic is displaced toward each haptic with a hook.[14]

ANTERIOR CHAMBER INTRAOCULAR LENSES

ACIOLS have several advantages over the other methods of IOL replacement. The ease of insertion and lack of suturing results in a shorter operating time with an open globe. New lens designs have corrected the previous problems of the rigid closed-loop ACIOLs.[31] Modern ACIOLs have an excellent finish that makes them very biocompatible, an oval haptic cross-section that prevents anterior vaulting, solid footplates without positioning holes that limit the formation of goniosynechiae, and flexible haptics that eliminate sizing problems.[14] Most commonly, the Kelman style ACIOL is recommended. This lens has an 6.0 to 6.5 mm optic diameter that allows for easy introduction through the keratoplasty wound. The use of ACIOLs have been discouraged when there is greater than 90 degrees of PAS in the anterior chamber angle,[36] intractable glaucoma, shallow anterior chamber, or insufficient iris tissue either due to an iris coloboma or extensive peripheral iridectomies and sphincterotomies.

Technique

The patient should have the horizontal limbal diameter, white to white, measured prior to the attachment of the Flieringa's ring. One millimeter is then added to this measurement to determine the size of the new IOL.[11,22]

The insertion of the flexible ACIOL has been described by Insler and Caldwell.[81] Acetylcholine chloride (Miochol) is first instilled into the anterior chamber to constrict the pupil and minimize the incidence of peripheral iris tuck. Then a small amount of viscoelastic is injected into the peripheral angle to minimize any trauma to the trabecular meshwork during the IOL insertion. The ACIOL is grasped along

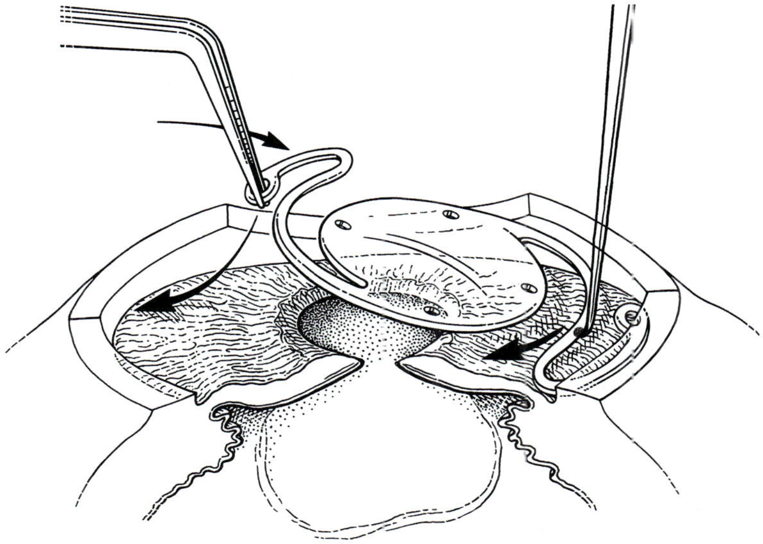

FIGURE 132-7 Anterior Chamber IOLs (ACIOLs) are gently inserted into the angle under viscoelastic control after the pupil has been constricted. Once the other haptic has been flexed into the angle, the two haptics are simultaneously compressed in an accordian-like manner to minimize iris tuck and allow for IOL rotation. (Modified with permission from Waring GO III: Management of pseudophakic corneal edema with reconstruction of the anterior ocular segment, *Arch Ophthalmol* 105: 709-714, 1987.)

the edge of the haptic or the superior edge of the optic and inserted into the angle using the smallest angle of insertion to minimize entrapment of the peripheral iris. Using a positioning hook on the inserted haptic to minimize the pressure and trauma to the inferior angle, the other haptic is grasped, flexed, and lowered into the keratoplasty opening and then released. Then, using an accordion-like technique, the two haptics are compressed simultaneously until the lens is in its final position. The pupil should be monitored to ensure that it is round without any oval distortion that would indicate entrapment of the peripheral iris. If entrapment of the iris is suspected, the involved haptic can be grasped with the Kelman MacPherson forceps and gently pulled back from the angle, lifted slightly anteriorly, and reinserted until displacement of the pupil is no longer visualized (Figure 132-7).

While some authors have suggested placing the haptics of the replacement ACIOL in the same orientation as in the explanted IOL,[15,35] most have recommended that ACIOLs be placed 90 degrees opposite to the orientation of the explanted IOL, away from the goniosynechiae, damaged angle, or peripheral iridectomies.[4,23,26] Orienting the replacement ACIOL away from the location of the explanted ACIOL avoids the areas of abnormal angle that may erode, hemorrhage, or become a source of persistent inflammation. The major disadvantage of this orientation is the potential of creating new sites of PAS, thereby reducing the amount of normal angle available for filtration and possibly increasing the incidence of postoperative glaucoma.[26]

IRIS-SUTURED POSTERIOR CHAMBER INTRAOCULAR LENSES

IS-PCIOLs were popular until the late 1980s[59] when interest in the TS-PCIOL method of IOL fixation increased. Recently, the results of the first prospective, randomized, multicenter trial of IOL implantation in PK and IOL exchange has renewed interest in the IS-PCIOL method because of the lower number of complications reported.[15] IS-PCIOL fixation is a technically straightforward procedure that involves minimal operating time with an open globe, avoids the anterior chamber structures, and places the IOL closer to the nodal point of the eye. Minimal postoperative IOL movement occurs due to the mid-iris sutures, peripheral haptic contact in the ciliary sulcus, and wide-based contact of the IOL to the posterior iris surface.[72] This technique also avoids the potential complications of the transscleral fixation sutures of the TS-PCIOL.

The disadvantages of this technique are due to the large area of uveal contact with the IOL and the suture,[82] which increases the risk of suture-induced uveitis, iris atrophy, and possible dislocation of the IOL. IS-PCIOLs can only be used for PK and IOL exchange because they require open-sky placement. Insufficient iris from previous iridectomies or iris colobomas may not allow iris fixation, and a vitrectomy is required in all cases. The iris sutures may also cause an ellipsoid dilation of the pupil.[28] A survey of corneal surgeons in 1990 revealed that TS-PCIOL (56.7%) was the preferred method of IOL implantation during PK and IOL exchange, although IS-PCIOL (43.2%) was still a very popular method of fixation.[83]

Technique

Initially the iris is inspected to ensure that there is adequate tissue to determine whether anterior segment reconstruction is required to repair the damaged iris, or to decide whether the TS-PCIOL technique should be selected. An anterior vitrectomy is required in all cases. Three techniques of IS-PCIOL have been described and include the two point fixation technique, four point fixation technique, and McCannell suture technique. Most surgeons now use the four point fixation technique.[83]

Soong et al. described the four point fixation technique using a PCIOL with four positioning holes. Either planar or angled haptics can be used to suture the optic to the iris.[28] A 13 to 14 mm haptic diameter allows good fixation of the haptics in the ciliary sulcus. A double armed 9-0 to 10-0 polypropylene (Prolene) suture is passed through the centering holes in a mattresslike fashion. Koch designed an IOL with the positioning holes slightly closer together and located distally in a clockwise direction from the haptic insertion on the optic to allow for easier insertion.[84] The polypropylene suture is then passed through the mid-iris. The PCIOL is slipped behind the iris with each haptic directed into the ciliary sulcus. A dental mirror can be used to ensure correct placement. The sutures are then tied snugly[28,59,73] (Figure 132-8). Placement of the suture knot between the optic and the iris has been recommended to reduce the area of uveal contact.[82,85] Two point fixation uses one positioning hole on either side of the optic with the suture tied around the edge of the optic and through the iris.[20,72,85] In the McCannell technique, one haptic is placed into the ciliary sulcus, which is then sutured to the peripheral iris with a polypropylene suture. This is then repeated for the other haptic.[83]

TRANSSCLERALLY FIXATED POSTERIOR CHAMBER INTRAOCULAR LENSES

The use of TS-PCIOLs in PK and IOL exchange has become increasingly popular as an alternative to ACIOL and IS-PCIOL placement. This technique involves suturing the haptics into the ciliary sulcus, which then places the IOL in the anatomic position of the lens. It has greater surgical flexibility because it does not require iris or posterior capsular support. TS-PCIOLs are particularly indicated when preoperative glaucoma or PAS place the eye at risk for further angle damage with an ACIOL, and insufficient iris precludes the use of a IS-PCIOL. The posterior location limits endothelial damage, and the lack of iris sutures allows full pupillary dilation. A decreased incidence of CME and endothelial cell loss has also been suggested with TS-PCIOLs.[36] The firm suture attachment and the haptic support to the ciliary sulcus allow for less pseudophacodonesis.[27] However, this technique involves placing fixation sutures through the ciliary sulcus, which is in close proximity to the major arterial circle of the iris and to the long posterior ciliary nerves. In addition, this technique creates a potential route for bacteria spread into the eye along the suture tract.

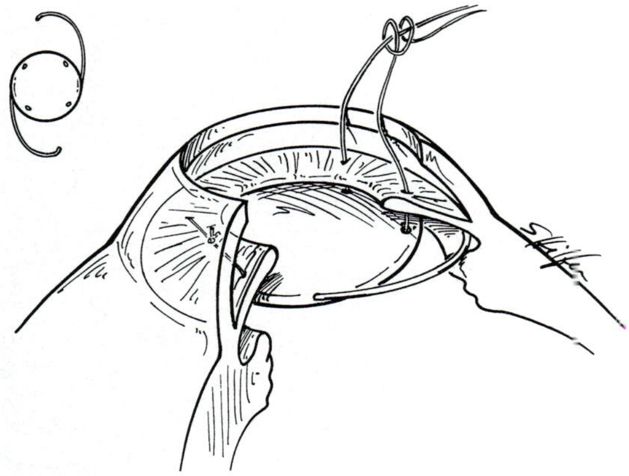

FIGURE 132-8 Iris-sutured PCIOLs (IS-PCIOLs) are useful when anterior chamber pathology has been identified. Two double-armed 10-0 polypropylene sutures are passed through the positioning holes of the implant and through the iris. The haptics are flexed into the ciliary sulcus, and the PCIOL is secured with the sutures. (From Davis RM, Best D, Gilbert GE: Comparison of intraocular lens fixation techniques performed during penetrating keratoplasty, *Am J Ophthalmol* 111: 743-744, 1991. Used with permission.)

In the TS-PCIOL procedure, accurate placement of the polypropylene sutures into the ciliary sulcus is a challenging component because it is generally performed blindly behind the iris. Anatomical studies have demonstrated that the ciliary sulcus is located 0.46 mm horizontally and 0.83 mm vertically from the limbus.[86] Postoperative investigations of ciliary sulcus suture placement have shown that it is generally very inaccurate.[87,88] In an histological study of two eyes that were placed with TS-PCIOLs before identifying the exact location of the ciliary sulcus, only one of the four haptics was actually in the ciliary sulcus.[87] Ultrasound biomicroscopy examination of 17 eyes with TS-PCIOLs found that only 38.2% of haptics were in the ciliary sulcus, whereas an equal number were anterior to the ciliary sulcus,[88] a location that places these eyes at risk for localized angle closure.[89] This study also found that the size of the ciliary sulcus is variable; it tends to be narrower in eyes without a posterior capsule.[88]

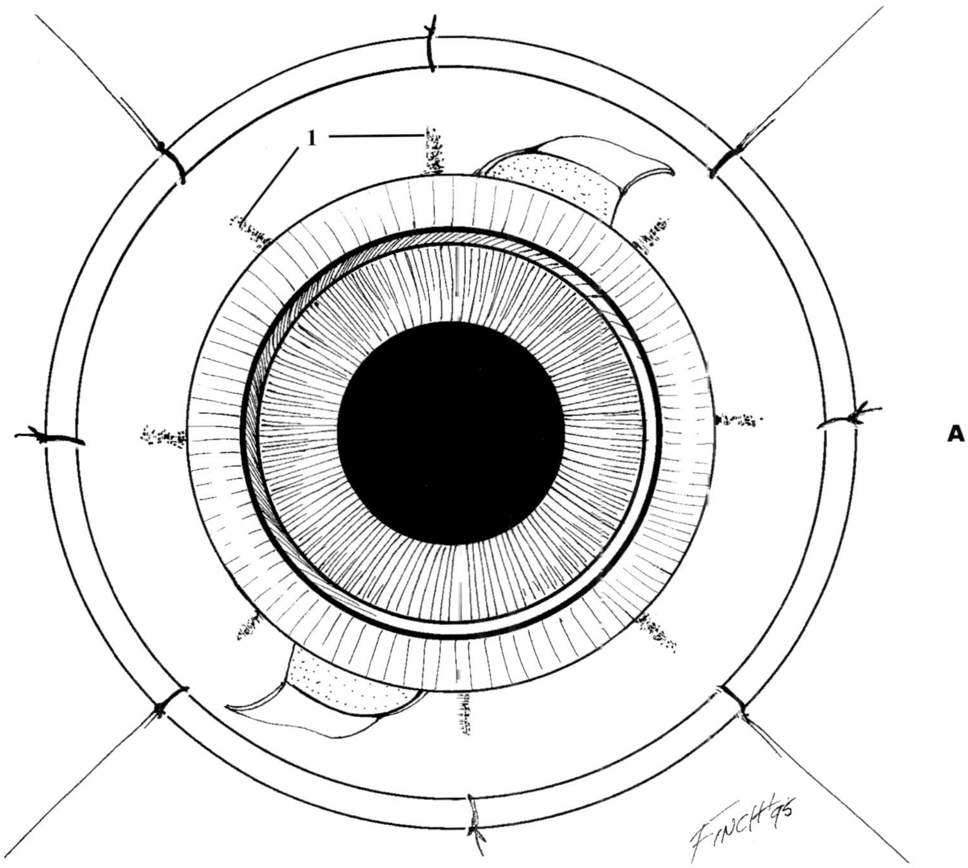

FIGURE 132-9 **A,** Transsclerally-sutured PCIOLs (TS-PCIOLs) are used by experienced surgeons when anterior chamber pathology is identified and iris tissue is deficient. Marks *(1)* are made using a radial keratotomy instrument so that if the anterior segment collapses the surgeon will still know when sutures are 180° apart. A Flierenga ring is sutured into place with eight 7-0 polygalactin sutures. Of the eight sutures, four are oblique sutures and are used to fixate the globe. *Continued.*

In 1990, Sen and Smith reported that TS-PCIOLs had become the favored method of fixating the PCIOL during PK and IOL exchange.[83] Since then, the popularity of this procedure has increased substantially. Recently, the results of a randomized, multicenter trial of PK and various IOL exchange techniques challenged the advantages of TS-PCIOLs by finding a significantly higher risk for CME in the TS-PCIOL group when compared to the ACIOL and IS-PCIOL groups.[15]

Technique

The surgical approach for the TS-PCIOLs has evolved since it was first described in 1981.[90] Before PK is performed and while the globe is still firm, two conjunctival peritomies over two clock hours are made 180 degrees apart, usually centered at the 1 o'clock and the 7 o'clock positions. A radial keratotomy marker can be used to mark the cornea and limbus in order to accurately place the fixation sutures 180 degrees apart and to allow symmetrical suture placement for the graft. Scleral flaps can be constructed to cover the fixation sutures; however, erosion of sutures through these flaps often occurs and most surgeons no longer perform this step.[83]

Previously a single piece, PMMA IOL with a haptic length of 13.3 to 14.0 mm and a 5 to 10 degree angulation was the most common lens reported.[27] However, we now use PMMA PCIOL with a 12.5 mm haptic length, which provides good fixation clinically. A 7.0 mm biconvex optic is recommended to minimize the effects of any lens decentration that could occur postoperatively.[28] The IOL has modified "C" loops that contain an eyelet on the inner curve of the "C." A 10-0 polypropylene suture with double-armed needles is passed through the eyelet. The surgeon should ensure that both ends of the suture pass on the same side of the haptic to avoid any torque effect that could result in IOL tilt.

B

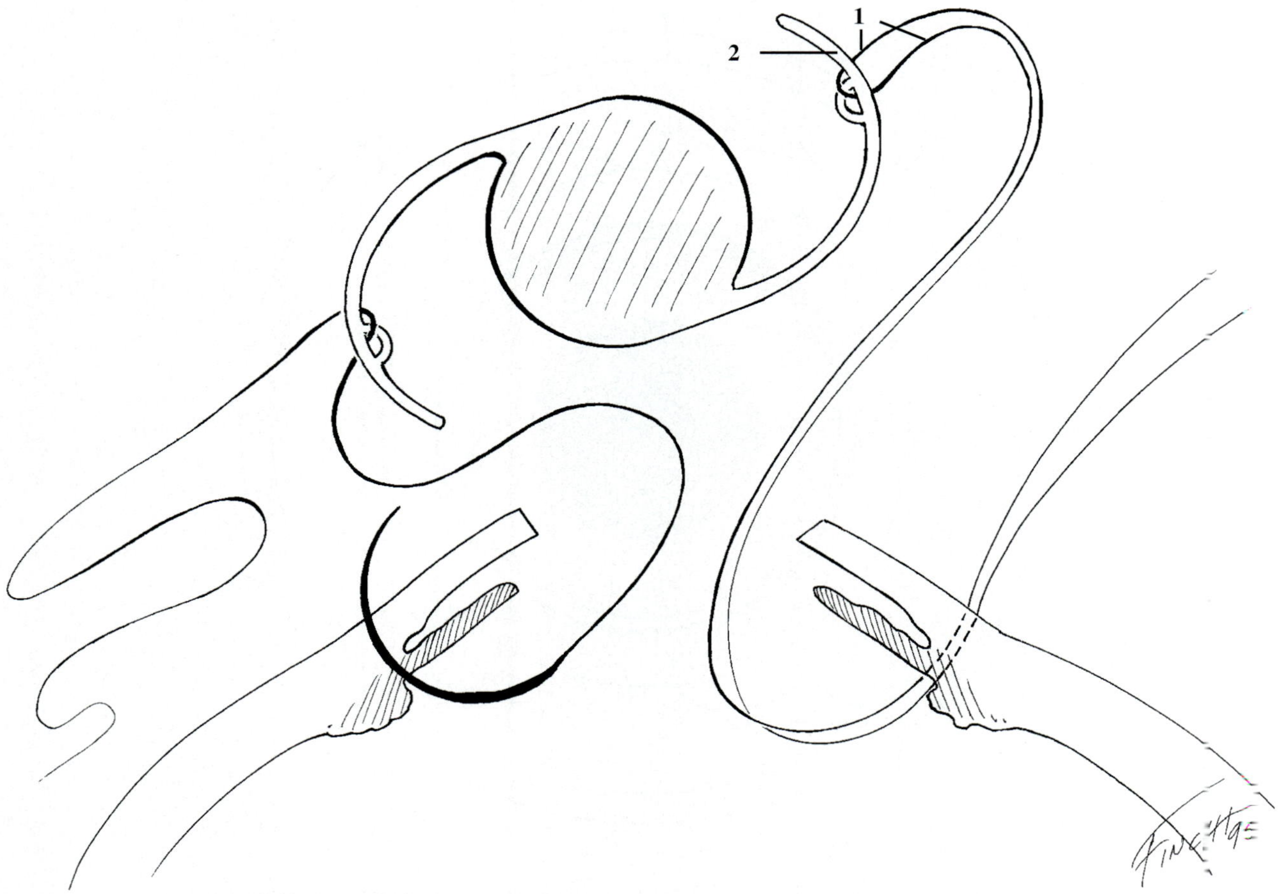

FIGURE 132-9 cont'd. **B,** The polypropylene sutures are passed through the eyelets so that both ends of the suture *(1)* pass on the same side of the haptic *(2)*. **C,** The needles are then gently walked back along the iris and placed in the ciliary sulcus so that they exit the sclera 0.75 mm back from the surgical limbus and 3.00 mm *Continued.*

We do not tie the suture on the haptic since this does not permit rotation of the suture to bury the knot at the end of the procedure. Prior to the modifications of the "C" loop, a "girth hitch" knot was used to firmly attach the IOL haptic and minimize tilt.[91] Three point[77] and a four point fixation techniques[92] with two sutures tied onto one of the haptics to prevent rotation and allow firm adhesion to the scleral wall have also been described.

The transscleral fixation can be approached internally by the ab interno or externally by the ab externo procedure. The ab interno approach uses two polypropylene sutures on a short tapered needle[24,75] (Figure 132-9, *A-F*). A 10-0 polypropylene monofilament suture is available in 2 and 3 inch lengths, which helps avoid the inevitable tangle of sutures during IOL placement with longer polypropylene sutures. The tip of the needle is held parallel to the iris and gently "walked" back along the posterior surface of the iris until the ciliary sulcus is entered approximately 0.75 mm back from the surgical limbus.[86] Both ends of the double-ended suture are passed through the ciliary sulcus approximately 3 mm apart. The IOL haptics are gently placed into the ciliary sulcus while the fixation sutures are alternately tightened to avoid any tangling of the excess suture and to ensure symmetrical placement of the TS-PCIOL. The IOL is then checked for adequate central fixation and tilt by gentle retraction of the pupil. The sutures are then pulled taut and tied to themselves. The knots are buried by gently rotating the sutures. Enlargement of the needle tract by side to side movement during the initial placement of the needle can facilitate burying the knot. In cases when the knot becomes exposed or when it cannot be buried, corneal autografts have been described using the patient's own corneal button cut with a 3 mm trephine and split through the stroma.[93] With Descemet's membrane side up, these buttons can be sutured over exposed polypropylene sutures using two interrupted 10-0 nylon sutures.

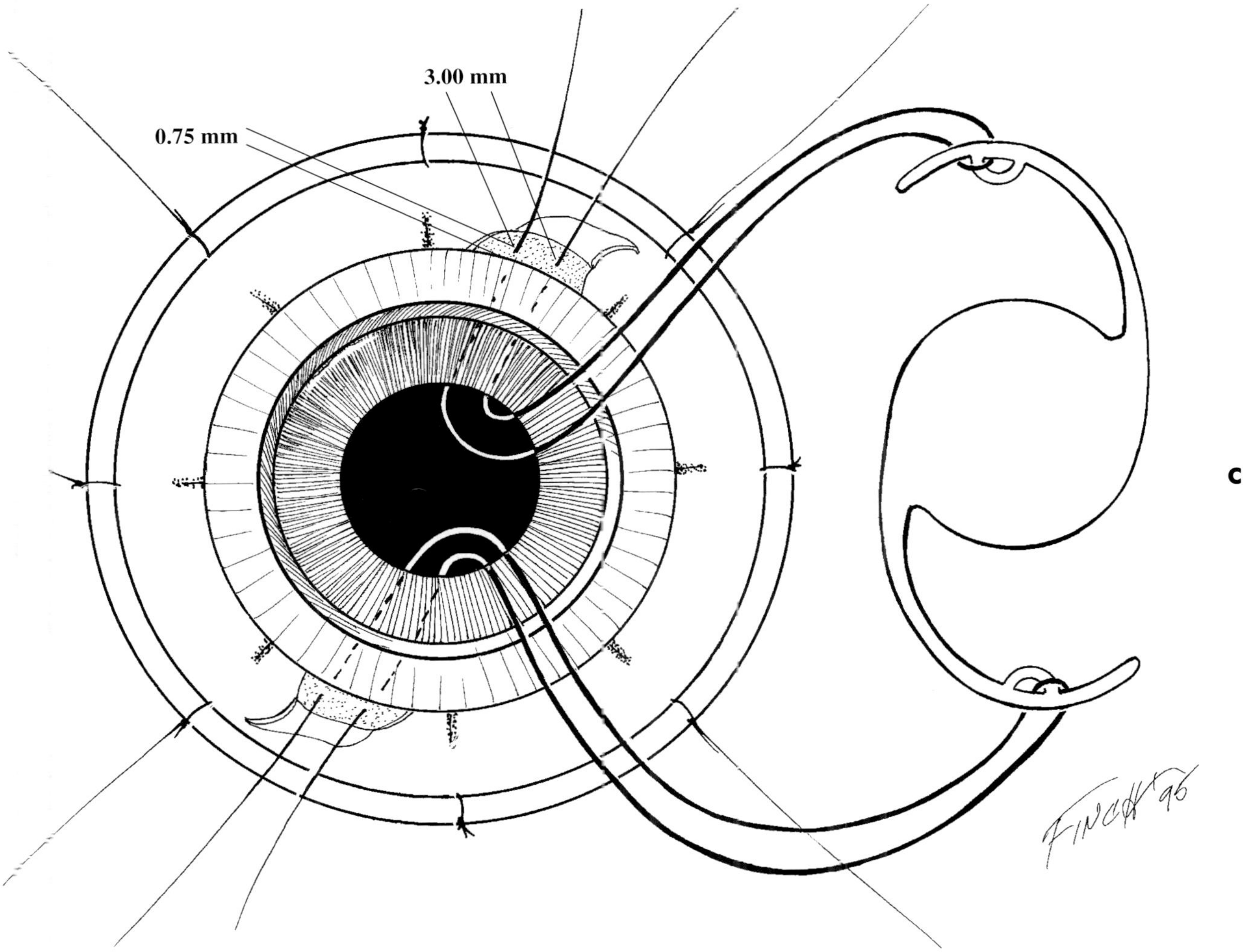

FIGURE 132-9 cont'd. C, The needles are then gently walked back along the iris and placed in the ciliary sulcus so that they exit the sclera 0.75 mm back from the surgical limbus and 3.00 mm apart. *Continued.*

The ab externo approach uses four 27-gauge needles that enter the eye 1.5 mm back from the surgical limbus before trephination of the cornea when the globe is still firm. The polypropylene suture is then fed through the lumen of the needles that are then removed, and the sutures are tightened.[92]

The accuracy of placing the scleral fixation sutures by the ab interno approach can be improved by using an intraoperative dental mirror to monitor the suture placement in the sulcus; however, these are cumbersome to use.[77] Transillumination of the ciliary sulcus with a fiber optic light through the pupil[94] and an intraoperative endoscope[14] have been used to guide suture placement. Direct visualization with temporary operating keratoprosthesis and scleral indentation have also been described; this allows for a thorough vitrectomy and accurate ab externo suture placement.[95]

Suturing of the Donor Cornea

If areas of corneal neovascularization, thinning, or inflammation are present, wound healing can be asymetrical. In this situation, we prefer to use 12 to 24 interrupted sutures, which would allow selective postoperative suture removal. If no peripheral corneal pathology is identified, we use 12 10-0 interrupted nylon sutures followed by a 12 bite 10-0 nylon running suture. Other options for the corneal suturing include 4 interrupted sutures followed by a 24 bite running suture or a double running suture. Knots are buried just underneath Bowman's layer on the donor side of the graft-host junction to facilitate removal. Protection of the corneal donor button epithelium and endothe-

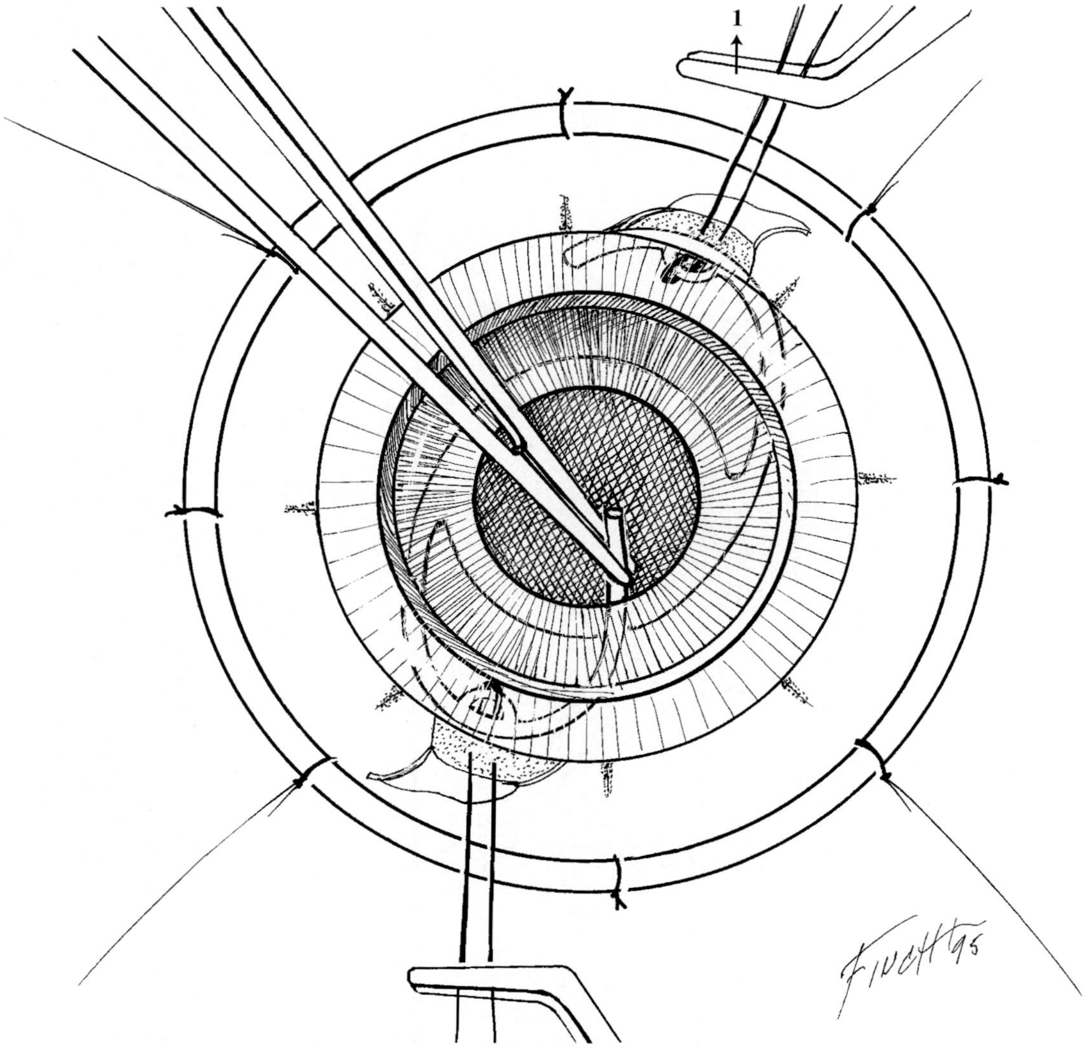

D

FIGURE 132-9 cont'd. **D,** The haptics of the TS-PCIOL are then gently inserted into the ciliary sulcus with constant traction on the fixation sutures *(1)*. Once in position, both fixation sutures are fed back and forth through the sclera to facilitate burying the knots.

Continued.

lium during suturing is crucial. This is accomplished by minimizing intraoperative trauma and the generous use of viscoelastic agents to provide a protective barrier around the cornea throughout the procedure.

Postoperative Care

After a PK and IOL exchange, patients need to be monitored in the same way that phakic PK eyes are followed postoperatively, with additional considerations given to the traumatized nature of these eyes and the advanced age of the patients. Intraocular pressure elevations need to be followed carefully and controlled in order to preserve the function of a compromised optic nerve. For the first few postoperative weeks, we generally do not treat intraocular pressure (IOP) elevations less than 30 mm Hg in eyes with a healthy optic nerve, since the detrimental effects of these potentially toxic topical medications on the healing epithelium outweigh the benefits of the treatment. If IOP elevation persists, topical and oral medications are given, and if necessary, trabeculectomy or shunt surgery are performed to lower the IOP.

Frequent lubrication with nonpreserved viscous artificial tears is required to combat the ocular surface/epithelial disease that is often present due to the diminished tear production, the irregular corneal surface, and the decreased lid function. Persistent dry eyes may require punctal occlusion or tarsorrhaphy to

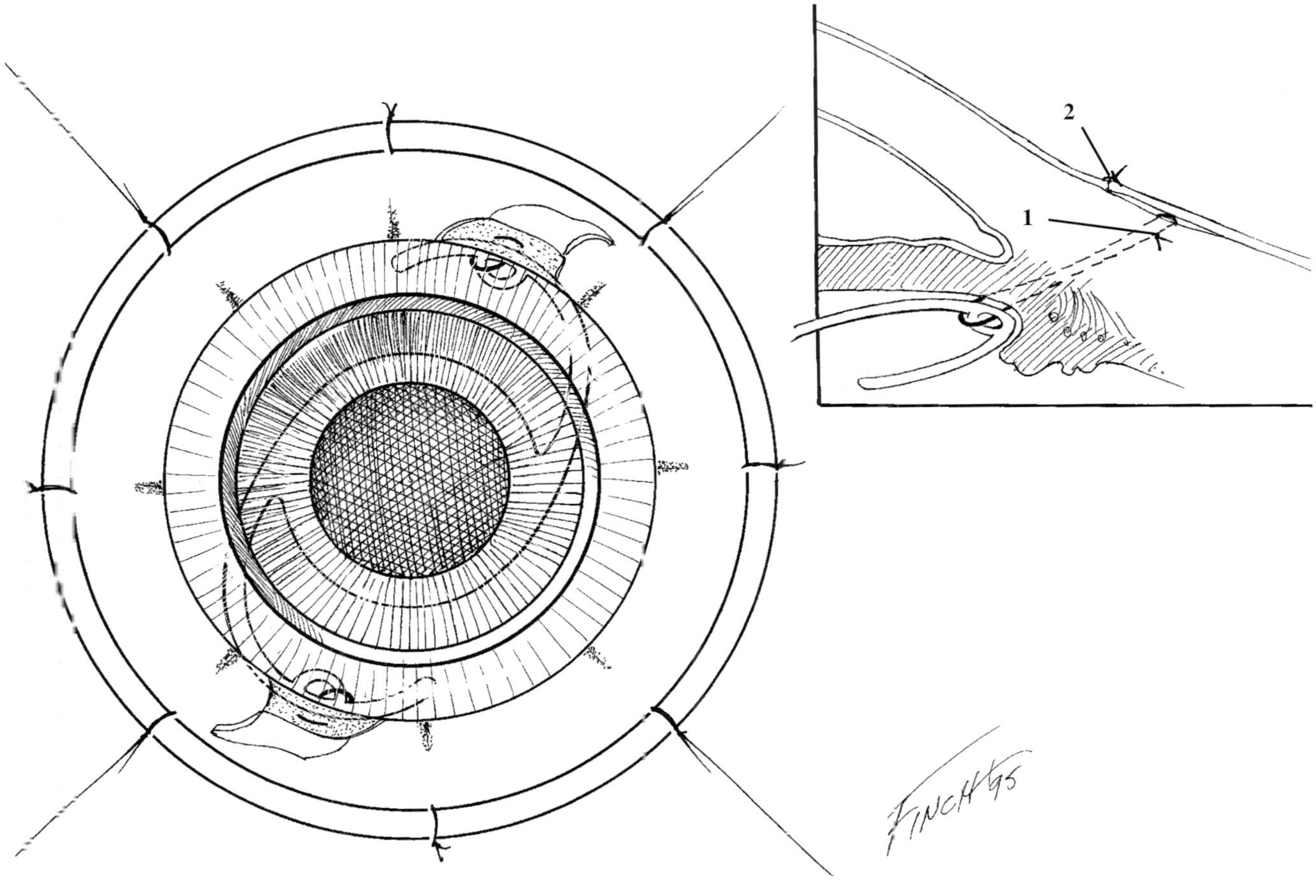

E

FIGURE 132-9 cont'd **E,** The fixation sutures are then tied snugly so that the TS-PCIOL remains in a stable position. Gentle rotation of the sutures usually allows the knots to be easily buried *(1)*. The conjunctiva is then closed over the top of the fixation sutures *(2)*.

Continued.

restore the corneal surface. If chronic nonhealing epithelial defects develop, tarsorrhaphy may be required to allow healing of the epithelium.

Evaluation of Penetrating Keratoplasty and Intraocular Lens Exchange

PENETRATING KERATOPLASTY

While graft clarity is achieved in approximately 90% of cases following PK and IOL exchange, graft failures, graft rejections, epithelial defects, corneal ulceration, and filamentary keratitis have all been significant corneal complications of this procedure.[27,76,77,85] Graft surface-related problems are the cause of about 30% of graft failure, and keratitis sicca has been responsible for the graft failure in about one half of these cases.[96]

The management of the IOL at the time of PK will affect the incidence of graft failure. The graft failure rate 2 years after PK has been 9% to 29% for retained iris supported PCIOLs, 34% to 60% for retained ACIOLs, 6% to 20% for retained PCIOLs, 9% to 20% for explanted IOLs, and 16% to 20% for exchanged ACIOLs.[31,45] When the results of PK and IOL exchange for PCE are compared to the other indications for PK, such as keratoconus or Fuchs' dystrophy, the rate of graft failure, graft rejection, and endothelial decompensation are much higher in the PK and IOL exchange group.[96]

INTRAOCULAR LENS EXPLANTATION

Apple et al have provided a thorough review of IOL complications from a historical and histopathological perspective.[97] The most commonly explanted IOLs have been found to be (in order of frequency): the ACIOLs, 52.8% to 56.2%; the iris supported PCIOLs, 10.7% to 33.7%; and the PCIOLs, 17.4% to 20.9%.[3,4,49] The most common ACIOLs associated with explantation have been (in order of frequency), the Leiske,

F

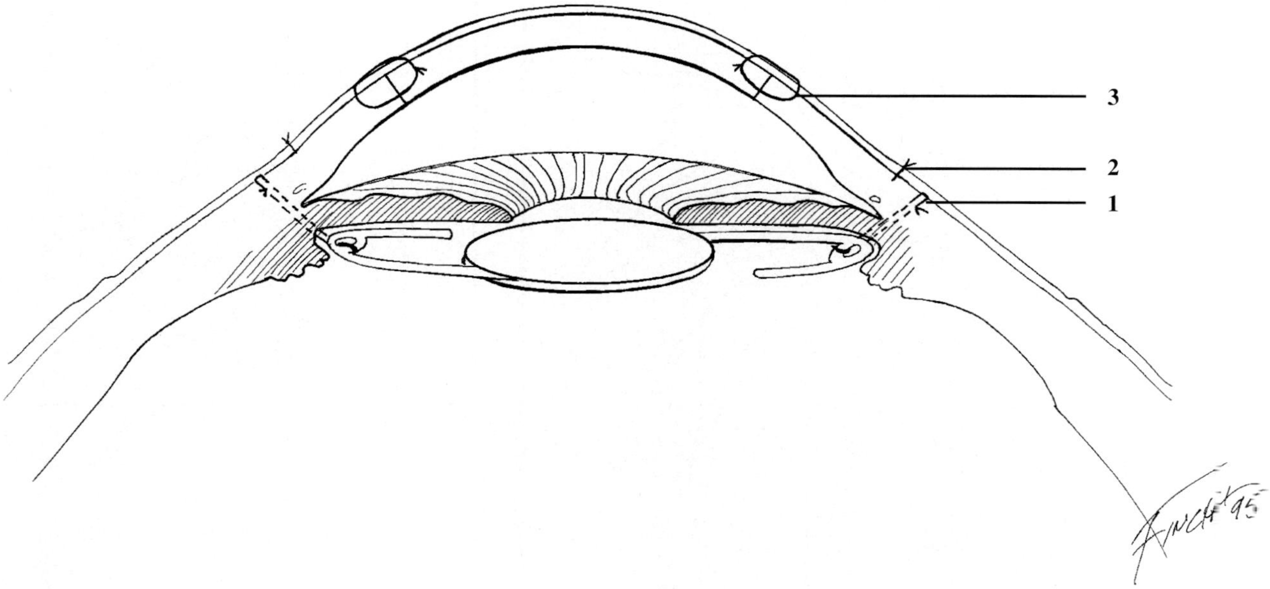

FIGURE 132-9 cont'd **F,** A profile view shows the completed operation with buried transscleral sutures *(1),* closed conjunctiva *(2),* and sutured donor cornea with buried knots *(3).*

Stableflex, Azar 91Z, and the Choyce. All of these ACIOLs have a small diameter, and rigid, round, closed loops except for the Choyce, which has solid footplates.[3,5,49,98]

Doren et al found that the results of IOL explantation vary depending on the indications for surgery.[49] The best results were found in cases of IOL exchange alone for IOL instability with all patients achieving a visual acuity of 20/40. PK and IOL explantation, with or without IOL replacement, achieved the same level of vision in 41% of cases. The UGH syndrome group had the worst prognosis with none of the patients achieving a visual acuity of 20/40, and 83% having a visual acuity of 20/200 or worse after IOL explantation alone.[49]

When the results of retained IOL, explanted IOL, and exchanged IOL with PK were compared, there was no significant difference in the incidence of graft clarity, visual acuity, or specular microscopy between the three groups.[31] Sugar et al used specular microscopy to demonstrate an increased rate of endothelial cell loss with retained iris-supported PCIOLs (39.2%) and retained ACIOLs (37.2%), when compared to exchanged ACIOLs (27.1%).[71] Alpar has shown that long-term results of graft survival are improved if iris-supported IOL and ACIOL are replaced during surgery for PCE.[54]

OPEN-SKY SUBTOTAL VITRECTOMY

The concern that vitrectomy increases postoperative macular edema has been alleviated by several studies that have demonstrated postoperative improvement of CME and visual acuity.[28,51,67] Price and Whitson were able to demonstrate resolution of clinical and angiographic CME after PK, vitrectomy, and IOL exchange in 75% of their PCE cases.[51]

ANTERIOR SEGMENT RECONSTRUCTION

With careful reconstruction of the anterior segment, restoration of anterior segment anatomy is generally possible except in those cases with a significant deficiency in iris tissue. While no study has been reported on the results of anterior segment reconstruction alone, we feel that it increases graft survival by reducing the incidence of postoperative glaucoma, endothelial cell loss, and IOL dislocation by providing a stable platform of iris support.

INTRAOCULAR LENS REPLACEMENT

Capsular-supported posterior chamber intraocular lenses

There have been only two series in the literature regarding the implantation of PCIOLs in the ciliary sulcus with posterior capsular support and these are summarized in Table 132-1. A total of 21 cases have been reviewed with 2 to 56 months of follow-up, which achieved a visual acuity of at least 20/40 in 36% to 43% of cases and clear grafts in 100% of cases.[31,67] The incidence of new onset glaucoma (30%) was similar to that of other techniques. The incidence of CME was very low (0%) when compared to the results for other types of IOL insertion, perhaps due to the minimal operative manipulation and the avoidance of the anterior chamber angle structures during IOL placement. This technique provides the simplest, most effective method of IOL replacement in cases

Table 132-1. Results of penetrating keratoplasty and intraocular lens exchange

IOL type, authors, and year of publication	No. of eyes	Follow-up (months)	Clear grafts (%)	Visual acuity ≥ 20/40 (%)	New glaucoma (%)	New CME (%)	Graft rejection (%)	Intraoperative hemorrhage (%)	Retinal detachment (%)	Endoophthalmitis (%)
Capsular-supported PCIOLs										
Smith et al (1987)	7	5-15	100	43	0	0	NR	NR	NR	NR
Donnenfeld et al (1992)	14	2-56	100	36	14	NR	NR	NR	NR	NR
Total or range (%)	***21***	***2-56***	***100***	***36-43***	***0-14***	***0***				
Open-loop ACIOLs										
Waring et al (1987)	25	12-38	88	32	28	36	NR	NR	NR	4
Polack (1988)	99	12-60	96	10	NR	NR	1	NR	NR	NR
Insler et al (1989)	32	4-42	84	9	16	25	22	3	3	3
Koenig et al (1989)	20	4-45	100	75	25	25	NR	15	NR	5
Kornmehl et al (1990)	40	7-59	95	58	18	10	5	3	NR	NR
Lass et al (1990)	25	12	88	24	0	NR	4	NR	NR	NR
Hassan et al (1991)	40	3-51	95	50	23	33	13	NR	3	NR
Total or range (%)	***281***	***4-60***	***84-100***	***9-75***	***0-28***	***10-36***	***1-22***	***3-15***	***3***	***3-5***
Iris-fixated PCIOLs										
Hall and Muenzler (1985)	53	6-63	88	38	6	4	12	2	2	NR
Price and Whitson (1989)	233	12-68	96	60	NR	NR	1	NR	1	5
Soong et al (1989)	133	3-24	97	64	12	24	4	NR	2	2
Van der Schaft et al (1989)	29	12-56	76	41	NR	10	10	3	3	NR
Busin et al (1990)	14	13-18	93	7	29	21	7	NR	NR	NR
Lass et al (1990)	24	12	96	29	4	NR	NR	NR	NR	NR
Gaster et al (1991)	21	2-19	100	19	24	15	10	NR	NR	NR
Muenzler and Hall (1994)	67	32-60	88	42	9	NR	8	NR	NR	NR
Total or range (%)	***574***	***3-68***	***76-100***	***7-64***	***4-29***	***4-24***	***1-12***	***2-3***	***2-3***	***2-5***
Transsclerally-fixated PCIOLs										
Johnson et al (1989)	47	5-30	98	27	NR	NR	0	9	0	0
Hill (1992)	36	9-36	NR	44	3	11	14	8	0	0
Holland et al (1992)	105	6-43	97	28	30	10	14	1	4	0
Heidemann et al (1992)	112	4-47	NR	24	30	4	6	12	3	NR
Total or range (%)	***300***	***4-47***	***97-98***	***24-44***	***3-30***	***4-11***	***6-14***	***1-12***	***0-4***	***0***

NR, not reported.

where sufficient posterior capsular support render it possible.

Anterior chamber intraocular lenses

Sugar et al reported poor results when the ORC Stableflex closed-loop ACIOL was used in PK and IOL exchange, with a 31% graft failure at an average of 29.5 months after PK, and an endothelial cell loss of 40% 1 year postoperatively.[70] This IOL is no longer available.

The results of 281 cases of open-loop flexible ACIOLs exchanged after PK for PCE are summarized in Table 132-1. The follow-up of these cases ranged from 4 to 60 months. Clear grafts were found in 84% to 100% of cases. Visual acuity of at least 20/40 was found in 9% to 75% of cases. Postoperative complication rates included new glaucoma requiring medication or surgery (0% to 28%), new CME (10% to 36%), and graft rejection (1% to 22%). Intraoperative hemorrhage occurred in 28% of cases in one study involving anterior segment reconstruction.[20] However, most studies did not mention this complication. Retinal detachment (3%) was reported in only two studies.[23,24] Hassan et al. documented a 28% incidence of new goniosynechiae in one to four quadrants 3 to 51 months postoperatively when flexible, open-loop, ACIOLs were implanted; however, all synechia formation occurred in the meridians corresponding to the location of the haptics of the previous ACIOL.[23]

A selection bias may influence the results of the ACIOL studies since these eyes may have less anterior chamber pathology preoperatively.[36] Many authors have recommended ACIOLs as a feasible alternative to other techniques of IOL replacement in eyes without anterior chamber angle pathology because they are technically less demanding and have comparable results.*

Iris sutured posterior chamber intraocular lenses

The results of 574 cases of IS-PCIOL with 3 to 68 months of follow-up are summarized in Table 132-1. A visual acuity of at least 20/40 was achieved in 7% to 64%, and graft clarity was achieved in 76% to 100% of cases. Postoperative complications included glaucoma (4% to 29%), macular edema (4% to 24%), and graft rejection (1% to 12%). Retinal detachment and endophthalmitis were rarely reported.† Sugar and Lass analyzed the endothelial cell and graft survival after PK and IOL exchange for PCE and found no difference between the ACIOL and the IS-PCIOL results.[31,69] Since the method of IS-PCIOL placement is technically intermediate in difficulty and provides comparable results compared to the other fixation techniques, ISPCIOLs should be considered when anterior chamber angle pathology is present and sufficient iris tissue is available.

*References 11, 22, 23, 26, 45, 68, 82, 99

†References 28, 69, 72-74, 86, 100

Transsclerally sutured posterior chamber intraocular lenses

The results of 300 cases of TS-PCIOLs with follow-up from 4 to 47 months are summarized in Table 132-1.[25,27,75-77] A visual acuity of at least 20/40 was obtained in 24%-44% of cases. Clear grafts were reported in 97%-98% of cases. The postoperative complications included glaucoma (3% to 30%), macular edema (4% to 11%), graft rejection (6% to 1?%), intraoperative hemorrhage (1% to 12%), and retinal detachment (0% to 4%).

The results from using TS-PCIOLs as a secondary IOL in the surgical correction of aphakia are remarkably better than those for PK and IOL exchange.[17-19,78,101-104] Early results of secondary TS-PCIOL implantation achieved a visual acuity of at least 20/40 in up to 100% of cases.[18,19,31] The only complication noted in these reports was intraoperative vitreous bleeding.[18] No macular pathology has been reported. The results of *IOL exchange* with a TS-PCIOL without PK are intermediate. Short-term studies with follow-ups from 4 to 20 months have achieved visual acuities of at least 20/40 in 50% to 62% of eyes.[31,101] A study with slightly longer follow-up found only 13% of the IOL exchanges achieved this level of visual acuity. The less successful visual results in these patients is due primarily to the preoperative CME or the UGH syndrome necessitating the IOL rmoval.[101] Since the eyes selected for PK and IOL exchange by the TS-PCIOL technique generally have the greatest ocular pathology of the PCE group, there may be a case selection basis against the results of this method of IOL replacement.

Exposure of the polypropylene fixation sutures through the conjunctiva has been reported in 20% of cases of TS-PCIOLs, prior to the development of the techniques to bury the suture knot.[27] Inadvertent removal of the fixation sutures can result in IOL dislocation as the haptics are often not fibrosed into the ciliary sulcus.[88,105] Suture-wick endophthalmitis has been purported to be caused by the erosion of the conjunctival covering of a polypropylene fixation suture, providing a track for bacteria to gain entrance to the eye.[106,107] Necrotizing scleritis of the scleral flaps in a patient with rheumatoid arthritis, which caused loosening of the fixation suture and lens decentration, has also been reported.[108]

The incidence of other IOL complications include decentration (4%) and tilt (11%). Early postoperative astigmatism has been found to be oriented perpendicular to the meridian of the TS-PCIOL in the majority of patients.[109,110] Intraoperative hemorrhages in the form of hyphema or vitreous hemorrhages have been reported in approximately 10% of cases.[25,75,77] Other less commonly reported complications include those of retinal detachment,[25,27,75] choroidal hemorrhages,[27,111] and choroidal detachments.[72] Despite these complications, the short-term results of TS-PCIOL appear acceptable in experienced hands. They are particularly useful in cases with anterior segment pathology and limited iris tissue.

Comparison of intraocular lens fixation techniques

A number a retrospective, uncontrolled, series have compared the results of ACIOLs with IS-PCIOLs, CS-PCIOLs, and TS-PCIOLs.[69,82,109,112] These studies are limited by their retrospective design, small numbers of patients, and bias in treatment assignment, whereby patients with significant glaucoma or PAS were excluded from the ACIOL group. None of these studies was able to detect a significant difference in the clinical or the endothelial morphometric results between the different types of IOL replacement.[23,35,69,110,113] While there has been an obvious trend toward the insertion of TS-PCIOLs, the use of an open-loop ACIOL during PK is clearly a simpler procedure in selected circumstances. The use of IS-PCIOLs has fluctuated in popularity due primarily to the theoretical concerns of iris irritation inducing iris atrophy, uveitis, and lens dislocation with intermittent pupillary dilation.[114]

Schein et al recently reported the first prospective, randomized, multicenter, comparison of three IOL insertion and fixation techniques.[15] The 176 patients were randomized into one of three types of IOL replacement methods; CS-PCIOLs were not included in the study. Standard evaluations were performed up to 18 months postoperatively. The selection of each group was completely random with no assignment bias based on anterior chamber pathology. The results were reported in a survival analysis format, which allows a comparison of results with different rates of follow-up at different time intervals. This format reports a higher crude rate and cumulative risk, since patients with complications are more likely to keep their follow-up visits.[15] An overall visual acuity of at least 20/40 was found in only 17.4% for cases, 40% achieved a visual acuity of 20/50 to 20/100, and 42.6% of cases achieved visual acuity of 20/200 or worse. These results were based on best corrected spectacle acuity, rather than best hard contact lens acuity. Therefore they may be an underestimate.

When the survival analysis was applied to the outcomes of interest, it was found that the likelihood of an adverse outcome was greatest with TS-PCIOL in all the outcomes measured except for graft failure when it was least likely. IOL dislocation and CME occurred least with IS-PCIOLs. The rates of CME were statistically different between the three groups with less CME in the ACIOL and IS-PCIOL groups. When a complication index was constructed by combining the results of the adverse outcomes, including glaucoma treatment escalation, graft failure, IOL dislocation, and CME, it was found that the likelihood of a complication was least likely in the IS-PCIOL group. It was felt that the complication index for the ACIOLs was intermediate, and that the TS-PCIOL group had the highest likelihood of complications.[17]

Despite the prospective randomized nature of this trial, a number a criticisms have been raised regarding various aspects of the study. Fluorescein angiograms were not performed on the patients preoperatively.[115] Since the identification of CME would be extremely difficult through edematous corneas,[23] it is likely that many cases were not identified preoperatively, yet this was the only significant difference between the outcomes of the treatment groups, and played a major role in finding the IS-PCIOL superior by the cumulative risk method. The technique of inserting the new ACIOL in the same orientation as the previous ACIOL was implicated as a cause of the increased inflammation and CME in this group. It was suggested that the new ACIOL should be oriented orthogonally to the old ACIOL.[116] The poor results of the scleral fixation technique can be applied only to the technique used during this study, which has since evolved with potentially improved results.[117] While the survival analysis and cumulative risk techniques of data presentation allow excellent comparisons between the groups, they cannot be compared to the results of other studies. Unfortunately this study did not include the CS-PCIOL group. Despite these criticisms, this is clearly the best comparison of the IOL replacement options in the surgery for PCE. This study has demonstrated that ACIOLs and IS-PCIOLs are still viable options for IOL replacement, and that TS-PCIOLs can involve significant postoperative complications.

Summary

PK and IOL exchange can alleviate the ocular pain and improve the impaired visual function associated with PCE. Advanced microsurgical techniques and a multi-stepped approach are required to adequately address each component of this procedure. Intense and frequent postoperative care is required to ensure adequate healing of the corneal epithlium and combat the associated dry eye disease. The recent advances in ophthalmic microsurgical techniques have given the ophthalmologist the opportunity to surgically rectify PCE, an ocular disease that began during the evolution of ophthalmic surgery.

REFERENCES

1. Waring GO III: The 50-year epidemic of pseudophakic corneal edema, *Arch Ophthalmol* 107:657-659, 1989.
2. Mamalis N et al: Changing trends in the indications for penetrating keratoplasty, *Arch Ophthalmol* 110:1409-1411, 1992.
3. Mamalis N et al: Penetrating keratoplasty 1981-1988: clinical indications and pathologic findings, *J Cataract Refract Surg* 17:163-167, 1991.
4. Hyman L, Wittpenn J, Yang C: Indications and techniques of penetrating keratoplasties, 1985-1988, *Cornea* 11(6):573-576, 1993.
5. Lindquist TD et al: Indications for penetrating keratoplasty: 1980-1988, *Cornea* 10(3):210-216, 1991.
6. Brady SE et al: Clinical indications for and procedures associated with penetrating keratoplasty, 1983-1988, *Am J Ophthalmol* 108:118-122, 1989.
7. Satrk WJ, Worthen DM, Holladay JT et al: The FDA report on intraocular lenses, *Ophthalmology* 90(4):311-317, 1983.
8. Steinberg EP et al: The content and cost of cataract surgery, *Arch Ophthalmol* 111:1041-1049, 1993.
9. Arentsen JJ et al: Penetrating keratoplasty for the treatment of pseudophakic corneal edema associated with posterior chamber lens implantation, *Ophthalmic Surg* 18(7):514-517, 1987.
10. Wilson SE, Kaufman HE: Graft failure after penetrating keratoplasty, *Surv Ophthalmol* 34(5):325-356, 1990.
11. Polack FM: Results of keratoplasty for aphakic and pseudophakic corneal edema with intraocular lens implantation of exchange, *Cornea* 7(4):239-243, 1985.
12. Lugo M, Cohen EJ, Eagle RC et al: The incidence of preoperative endothelial dystrophy in pseudophakic bullous keratopathy, *Ophthalmic Surg* 19:16-19, 1988.
13. Waring GO III, Stulting RD: Triple procedure for intraocular lens exchange, *Arch Ophthalmol* 105:609-610, 1987.
14. Speaker MG, Laibson PR, Cohen EJ: Penetrating keratoplasty for pseudophakic bullous keratopathy. In Brightbill FS, editor: *Corneal surgery. Theory, technique and tissue,* ed 2, St Louis, 1994, Mosby, pp. 151-163.
15. Schein OD, Kenyon KR, Steinert RF et al: A randomized trial of intraocular lens techniques with penetrating keratoplasty, *Ophthalomology* 100(10): 1437-1443, 1993.
16. Price FW, Whitson WE, Marks RG: Progression of visual acuity after penetrating keratoplasty, *Ophthalmology* 98(8):1177-1185, 1991.
17. Stark WJ et al: Posterior chamber intraocular lens implantation in the absence of posterior capsular support, *Ophthalmic Surg* 19:240-243, 1988.
18. Kora Y, Fukado Y, Yaguchi S: Sulcus fixation of posterior chamber lenses by transscleral sutures, *J Cataract Refract Surg* 17:636-639, 1991.
19. Hu BV et al: Implantation of posterior chamber lens in the absence of capsular and zonular support, *Arch Ophthalmol* 106:416-420, 1988.
20. Waring GO III: Management of pseudopkakic corneal edema with reconstruction of the anterior ocular segment, *Arch Ophthalmol* 105:709-715, 1987.
21. Smith RE, Beatty RF, Clifford WS: Pseudophakic keratoplasty posterior chamber lens implantation in the presence of ruptured capsule, *Ophthalmic Surg* 18(5):344-348, 1987.
22. Zaidman GW, Goldman S: A prospective study on the implantation of anterior chamber intraocular lenses during keratoplasty for pseudophakic and aphakic bullous keratopathy, *Ophthalmology* 97(6):757-762, 1990.
23. Hassan TS et al: Implantation of Kelman-style open-loop anterior chamber lenses during keratoplasty for aphakic and pseudophakic bullous keratopathy. A comparison with iris-sutured posterior chamber lenses, *Ophthalmology* 98 875-880, 1991.
24. Insler MS, Kook MS, Kaufman HE: Penetrating keratoplasty for pseudophakic keratopathy associated with semiflexible, closed-loop anterior chamber intraocular lenses, *Am J Ophthalmol* 107:252-256, 1989.
25. Heidemann DG, Dunn SP: Transclerally sutured intraocular lenses in penetrating keratoplasty, *Am J Ophthalmol* 113:619-625, 1992.
26. Kornmehl EW et al: Penetrating keratoplasty for pseudophakic bullous keratopathy associated with closed loop anterior chamber intraocular lenses, *Ophthalmology* 97(4):407-414, 1990.
27. Holland EJ, Daya SM, Evangelista A et al: Penetrating keratoplasty and transscleral fixation of posterior chamber lens, *Am J Ophthalmol* 114:182-187, 1992.
28. Soong HK, Meyer RF, Sugar A: Techniques of posterior chamber lens implantation without capsular support during penetrating keratoplasty: review, *Refract Corneal Surg* 5:249-255, 1989.
29. Gaster RN, Ong HV: Results of penetrating keratoplasty with posterior chamber intraocular lens implantation in the absence of a lens capsule, *Cornea* 10(6):498-506, 1991.
30. Kok-VanAlphen CC, Volker-Dieben HJM: Corneal dystrophy following lens implantation, *Doc Ophthalmol* 48:243-250, 1979.
31. Sugar A: An analysis of corneal endothelial and graft survival in pseudophakic bullous keratopathy, *Trans Am Ophthalmol Soc* 87:762-801, 1989.
32. Chien AM, Schmidt CM, Cohen EJ et al: Glaucoma in the immediate post-operative period after penetrating keratoplasty, *Am J Ophthalmol* 115:711-714, 1993.
33. Abdel-Hakim AS, Khalil A: Intraocular lens power calculations in the triple procedure, *Br J Ophthalmol* 73:709-713, 1989.
34. George J, Doughman DJ, Holland EJ: Comparison of refractive results for the combined PK/TS-SPCL procedure and the triple procedure, Unpublished manuscript, 1996.
35. Davis RM, Best D, Gilbert GE: Comparison of intraocular lens fixation techniques performed during penetrating keratoplasty, *Am J Ophthalmol* 111:743-749, 1991.
36. Lass JH: Lens replacement in pseudophakic bullous keratopathy. Anterior chamber intraocular lenses. In Brightbill FS, editor: *Corneal surgery. Theory, technique and tissue,* ed 2, St Louis, 1994, Mosby, pp. 163-167.
37. Geggel HS: Intraocular lens implantation after penetrating keratoplasty. Improved unaided visual acuity, astigmatism and safety in patients with combined corneal disease and cataract, *Ophthalmology* 97(11):1460-1467, 1990.
38. Hoffer KJ: Triple procedure for intraocular lens exchange, *Arch Ophthalmol* 105:609, 1987 (letter).
39. Binder PS: Secondary intraocular lens implantation during or after corneal transplantation, *Am J Ophthalmol* 99:515-520, 1985.
40. Binder PS: Intraocular lens implantation after penetrating keratoplasty, *Refract Corneal Surg* 5:224-230, 1989
41. Waring GO III et al: Results of penetrating keratoplasty in 123 eyes with pseudophakic or aphakic corneal edema, *Ophthalmology* 90(1):25-33, 1983.
42. Nelson JD: Epithelial problems. In Brightbill FS, editor: *Corneal surgery. Theory, technique and tissue,* ed 2, St Louis, 1994, Mosby, pp. 235-246.
43. Meyer RF, Bobb KC: Corneal epithelium in penetrating keratoplasty, *Am J Ophthalmol* 90:142-147, 1980.
44. McCartney DL, Gottsch JD, Stark WJ: Managing posterior pressure during pseudophakic keratoplasty, *Arch Ophthalmol* 107:1384-1386, 1989.
45. Speaker MG, Lugo M, Laibson PR et al: Penetrating keratoplasty

for pseudophakic bullous keratopathy. Management of the intraocular lens, *Ophthalmology* 95(9):1260-1268, 1988.

46. Samples JR, Binder PS: Visual acuity, refractive error, and astigmatism following corneal transplantation for pseudophakic bullous keratopathy, *Ophthalmology* 92(11):1554-1560, 1985.
47. Kozarsky AM, Stopak S, Waring GO III et al: Results of penetrating keratoplasty for pseudophakic corneal edema with retention of intraocular lens, *Ophthalmology* 91(10):1141-1146, 1984.
48. Roper-Hall MJ, Watts MT: Retention of iris supported intraocular lenses at the time of penetrating keratoplasty for pseudophakic corneal edema, *Br J Ophthalmol* 73:407-409, 1989.
49. Doren GS, Stern GA, Driebe WT: Indications for and results of intraocular lens explantation, *J Cataract Refract Surg* 18:79-85, 1992.
50. Busin M et al: Intraocular lens removal during penetrating keratoplasty for pseudophakic bullous keratopathy, *Ophthalmology* 94(5):505-509, 1987.
51. Price FW, Whitson WE: Natural history of cystoid macular edema in pseudophakic bullous keratopathy, *J Cataract Refract Surg* 16 163-169, 1990.
52. Smith SG, Lindquist TD, Lindstrom RL: Removal of intraocular lenses. In Lindquist TD, Lindstrom RL, editors: *Ophthalmic surgery,* St Louis, 1990, Mosby, pp. IH0-IH11.
53. Haggan JC III: Intraocular lens removal during penetrating keratoplasty for pseudophakic bullous keratopathy, *Ophthalmology* 94(12):1672, 1987 (letter).
54. Alpar JJ: Long-term results of keratoplasty in eyes with intraocular lenses, *Ophthalmic Surg* 17(10):650-654, 1986.
55. Noecker RJ, Branner WA, Cohen KL: Intraocular lens explantation with and without penetrating keratoplasty, *Ophthalmic Surg* 20(12):849-854, 1989.
56. Koenig SB, Solomon JM: Removal of closed-loop anterior chamber intraocular lenses during penetrating keratoplasty, *Cornea* 6(3):207-208, 1987.
57. Hunkeler JD: Longer haptic allows for better manipulation, *Ophthalmic Surg* 20(3):171-172, 1989 (letter).
58. Terry AC, Stark WJ: Removal of closed loop anterior chamber lens implants, *Ophthalmic Surg* 15(7):575-577, 1984.
59. Morrison LK, Waltman SR: Management of pseudophakic bullous keratopathy, *Ophthalmic Surg* 20(3):205-210, 1989.
60. Mannis MJ et al: Uses of thrombin in ocular surgery: effect on the corneal endothelium, *Archives of Ophthalmology* 106:251-253, 1988.
61. Spigelman AV et al: Management of the pseudophakos during penetrating keratoplasty. In Lindquist TD, Lindstrom RL, editors: *Ophthalmic surgery,* St Louis, 1990, Mosby, pp. IIF0-IIF10.
62. Epstein RJ, Vastine DW, Fried WI: Removing the Stableflex intraocular lens during penetrating keratoplasty, *Ophthalmic Surg* 20(3):171-172, 1989.
63. Epstein RJ, Vastine DW, Fried WI: Refining the technique for the removing the Stableflex lens, *Ophthalmic Surg* 20(3):599, 1989 (letter).
64. Arentsen JJ: Penetrating keratoplasty techniques, *Int Ophthalmol Clin* 28(1):14-23, 1988.
65. Fung WE: Vitrectomy for chronic aphakic cystoid macular edema. Results of a national, collaboarative, prospective, randomized investigation, *Ophthalmology* 92(8):1102-1111, 1985.
66. Probst LE, Holland EJ: Open-sky subtotal vitrectomy during penetrating keratoplasty and IOL exchange, Manuscript in preparation, 1996.
67. Donnenfeld ED, Ingraham HJ, Perry HD et al: Soemmering's ring support for posterior chamber intraocular lens implantation during penetrating keratoplasty. Changing trends in bullous keratopathy, *Ophthalmology* 99(8):1229-1233, 1992.
68. Tragakis MP, Brown SI: The significance of anterior synechiae after corneal transplantation, *Am J Ophthalmol* 74(3):532-533, 1972.
69. Lass JH, Desantis DM, Reinhart WJ et al: Clinical and morphometric results of penetrating keratoplasty with one-piece anterior-chamber or suture-fixated posterior-chamber lenses in the absence of lens capsule, *Arch Ophthalmol* 108:1427-1431, 1990.
70. Sugar A, Bhugra M, Felbeck P et al: Follow-up of closed-loop anterior chamber intraocular lenses inserted at penetrating keratoplasty, *Trans Am Ophthalmol Soc* 88:255-262, 1990.
71. Sugar A et al: Specular microscopic follow-up of corneal grafts for pseudophakic bullous keratopathy, *Ophthalmology* 92(3): 325-330, 1985.
72. Hall JR, Muenzler WS: Intraocular lens replacement in pseudophakic bullous keratopathy, *Trans Ophthalmol Soc UK* 104:541-545, 1985.
73. Soong HK, Meyer RF, Sugar A: Posterior chamber IOL implantation during keratoplasty for aphakic or pseudophakic corneal edema, *Cornea* 6(4):306-312, 1987.
74. Muenzler WS, Hall JR: Posterior chamber intraocular lenses-iris fixated. In Brightbill FS, editor: *Corneal surgery. Theory, technique and tissue,* ed 2, St Louis, 1994, Mosby pp. 167-171.
75. Heidemann DG, Dunn SP: Visual results and complications of transsclerally sutured intraocular lenses in penetrating keratoplasty, *Ophthalmic Surg* 21(9):609-614, 1990.
76. Hill JC: Transsclerally-fixated posterior chamber intraocular implants without capsular support in penetrating keratoplasty, *Ophthalmic Surg* 23(5):321-324, 1992.
77. Johnson SM: Results of exchanging anterior chamber lenses with sulcus-fixated posterior chamber IOLs without capsular support in penetrating keratoplasty, *Ophthalmic Surg* 20(7): 465-468, 1989.
78. McCluskey P, Harrisberg B: Long-term results using scleral-fixated posterior chamber intraocular lenses, *J Cataract Refract Surg* 20:34-39, 1994.
79. Van Der Scaft TL et al: Results of penetrating keratoplasty for pseudophakic bullous keratopathy with the exchange of an intraocular lens, *Br J Ophthalmol* 73:704-708, 1989.
80. Shin DH: Implantation of a posterior chamber lens without capsular support during penetrating keratoplasty or as a secondary lens, *Ophthalmic Surg* 19(10):755-756, 1988.
81. Insler MS, Caldwell DR: Techniques of flexible intraocular lens insertion during keratoplasty, *Am Intra-Ocular Implant Soc J* 11:487-488, 1985.
82. Steinert RF: Visual results of suture-fixated posterior chamber lenses during penetrating keratoplasty, *Ophthalmology* 96: 1239-1240, 1989 (discussion).
83. Sen HA, Smith PW: Current trends in suture fixation of posterior chamber intraocular lenses, *Ophthalmic Surg* 21:689-695, 1990.
84. Koch DD: New optic hole configuration for iris fixation of posterior chamber lenses (letter), *Arch Ophthalmol* 106:163-164, 1988 (letter).
85. Price FW, Whitson WE: Visual results of suture-fixated posterior chamber lenses during penetrating keratoplasty, *Ophthalmology* 96:1234-1240, 1989.
86. Duffey RJ et al: Anatomic study of transclerally sutured intraocular lens implantation, *Am J Ophthalmol* 108:300-309, 1989.
87. Lubniewski AJ, Holland EJ, Van Meter WS et al: Histologic study of eyes with transsclerally sutured posterior chamber intraocular lenses, *Am J Ophthalmol* 110(3):237-243, 1990.

88. Pavlin CJ, Rootman D, Arshinoff S et al: Determination of the haptic position of transclerally fixated posterior chamber intraocular lenses by ultrasound biomicroscopy, *J Cataract Refract Surg* 19:573-577, 1993.
89. Obstbaum SA: Post-iridial implantation revisited, *J Cataract Refract Surg* 19:571, 1993 (editorial).
90. Girard LJ: Pars plana phacoprosthesis (aphakic intraocular implant), a preliminary report, *Ophthalmic Surg* 12:19, 1981.
91. Cowden JW, Hu BV: A new surgical technique for posterior lens fixation during penetrating keratoplasty in the abscence of capsular or zonular support, *Cornea* 7(3):231-235, 1988.
92. Mannarino AP, Hannush SB: A new technique for transcleral fixation of a posterior chamber intraocular lens in the absence of capsular support during penetrating keratoplasty, *Refract Corneal Surg* 6:353-356, 1990.
93. Bucci FA, Holland EJ, Lindstrom RL: Corneal autografts for external knots in transclerally sutured posterior chamber lenses, *Am J Ophthalmol* 112(3):353-354, 1991.
94. Horiguchi M et al: Identifying the ciliary sulcus for suturing a posterior chamber intraocular lens by transillumination, *Arch Ophthalmol* 111:1693-1695, 1993.
95. Menapace R: Temporary keratoprosthesis for transscleral fixation of posterior chamber intraocular lenses with penetrating keratoplasty, *J Cataract Refract Surg* 19:747-754, 1993.
96. Price FW, Whitson WE, Marks RG: Graft survival in four common groups of patients undergoing penetrating keratoplasty, *Ophthalmology* 98(3):322-328, 1991.
97. Apple DJ, Mamalis N, Loftfield K et al: Complications of intraocular lenses. A historical and histopathological review, *Surv Ophthalmol* 29(1):1-54, 1984.
98. Apple DJ, Hansen SO, Richards SC et al: Anterior chamber lenses. A laboratory study, *J Cataract Refract Surg* 13:175-189, 1987.
99. Koenig SB, McDermott ML, Hyndiuk RA: Penetrating keratoplasty and intraocular lens exchange for pseudophakic bullous keratopathy associated with closed-loop anterior chamber intraocular lens, *Am J Ophthalmol* 108:43-48, 1989.
100. Busin M et al: Complications of sulcus-supported intraocular lenses with iris sutures, implanted during penetrating keratoplasty after intracapsular cataract extraction, *Ophthalmology* 97(4):401-406, 1990.
101. Lindquist TD, Agapitos PJ, Lindstrom RL et al: Transscleral fixation of the posterior intraocular lenses in the absence of capsular support, *Ophthalmic Surg* 20:769-775, 1989.
102. Stark WJ, Gottsch JD, Goodman DF et al: Posterior chamber intraocular lens implantation in the absence of capsular support, *Arch Ophthalmol* 107:1078-1083, 1989.
103. Shapiro A, Leen MM: External transscleral posterior chamber lens fixation, *Arch Ophthalmol* 109:1759-1760, 199[illegible].
104. Agapitos PJ, Lindstrom RL: Transcleral ciliary sulcus fixation of posterior chamber intraocular lens implants, *Aust N Z J Ophthalmol* 17(2):169-172, 1989.
105. Cahane M, Chen V, Avni I: Dislocation of a scleral-fixated, posterior chamber intraocular lens after fixation suture removal, *J Cataract Refract Surg* 20:186-187, 1994.
106. Schechter RJ: Suture-wick endophthalmitis with sutured posterior chamber intraocular lenses, *J Cataract Refract Surg* 16:755-756, 1990.
107. Heilskov T et al: Late endophthalmitis after transcleral fixation of a posterior chamber intraocular lens, *Arch Ophthalmol* 107:1427, 1989.
108. Glasser DB, Bellor J: Necrotizing scleritis of the scleral flaps after transscleral suture fixation of an intraocular lens, *Am J Ophthalmol* 113:529-532, 1992.
109. Hardten DR et al: Early postkeratoplasty astigmatism following placement of anterior chamber lenses and transsclerally sutured posterior chamber lenses, *CLAO J* 18(2):108-111, 1992.
110. Hardten DR, Holland EJ, Doughman DJ et al: Clinical and anatomical study of the effect of transscleral fixation of posterior chamber lenses on early postkeratoplasty astigmatism, *Cornea* 12(4):282-288, 1993.
111. Price FW, Whitson WE: Suprachoroidal hemorrhage after the placement of a scleral fixated lens, *J Cataract Refract Surg* 18:514-515, 1990.
112. Insler MS, Cooper D, Caldwell DR: Analysis of corneal thickness and endothelial cell density in pseudophakic and aphakic patients undergoing penetrating keratoplasty, *Arch Ophthalmol* 103:390-393, 1985.
113. Koenig SB, Apple DJ, Hyndiuk RA: Penetrating keratoplasty and intraocular lens exchange: open-loop anterior chamber lenses versus sutured posterior chamber lenses, *Cornea* 13(4):418-421, 1994.
114. Rapoza PA: Posterior chamber intraocular lenses-sclera fixated. In Brightbill FS, editor: *Corneal surgery. Theory, technique and tissue,* ed 2, St Louis, 1994, Mosby, pp. 171-176.
115. Friedberg MA: IOL fixation techniques at keratoplasty, *Ophthalmology* 101(5):797-798, 1994 (letter).
116. Koenig SB, Hyndiuk RA: IOL fixation techniques at keratoplasty, *Ophthalmology* 101(5):798-799, 1994 (letter).
117. Cykiert RC: IOL fixation techniques at keratoplasty, *Ophthalmology* 101(5):799, 1994 (letter).

CHAPTER 133

WOODFORD VAN METER

Suturing Techniques

The purpose of suturing is to secure the donor cornea in place. A stable wound is the first and foremost goal. The ideal suturing technique would secure the wound, induce no optical aberration, and provide consistent and constant tension throughout the life of the sutures. Ideally, sutures would not necessarily have to be removed, or, if so, there would be no or minimal change following suture removal. Unfortunately, the perfect suture material and the perfect suturing technique do not currently exist. Anecdotal cases exist of emmetropia before and after suture removal, but large spherical errors and astigmatism today remain postoperative problems that corneal surgeons frequently face. Careful attention to suturing, however, can minimize postoperative astigmatism and facilitate rapid visual rehabilitation following keratoplasty surgery.

Obtaining a clear graft in penetrating keratoplasty has become almost expected, with a clear cornea resulting from keratoplasty surgery in over 90% of cases in the past 25 years.[1] Current suturing techniques have improved with microsurgical skills due to the operating microscope, improved instruments, and corneal storage media, and enhanced appreciation of the vital importance of the corneal endothelium. This chapter will cover a variety of suturing techniques and suturing materials that are appropriate in different situations.

Castroviejo's original suturing technique used a continuous silk suture coursing across the external surface of a square graft, holding the graft in place using intraocular pressure to support the graft against the suture (Figure 133-1). Many of his square grafts fared extremely well and provided good acuity for many years (Figure 133-2). However, as surgical techniques have improved, patients now expect early visual rehabilitation with minimal morbidity. Because excellent results can be obtained with a variety of suturing techniques, it is advantageous for the surgeon to be familiar with multiple techniques and to apply these techniques to different clinical situations where indicated.

There are four categories of suturing techniques in keratoplasty:

1. Interrupted sutures
2. Combined interrupted and continuous sutures
3. Single continuous suture
4. Double continuous suture

Initial intraoperative steps are comparable for all four techniques.

Once the trephined donor is brought to the field for suturing into the host site, the wound is secured with four cardinal sutures that may or may not be removed. Cardinal sutures can be placed with 8-0 silk for security and ease of tying if they are going to be removed, but 10-0 nylon can also be used and left in place. By the time the four cardinal sutures have been placed, wound apposition and configuration have largely been determined and most of the script has already been written on the effectiveness of the suturing. All suturing techniques work better if the wound is even and there are no extraneous stress vectors distorting smooth and gentle apposition of donor and host tissue. The initial sutures determine the efficacy of those that follow and can ultimately determine what the patient's final topographic profile will be.

Forceps with double 0.12 fixation teeth are helpful for stabilizing the donor cornea for the initial suture at 12 o'clock. The needle is passed initially through the donor cornea and then through the host at 12 o'clock. The ideal bite is approximately 90% depth, or as close to Descemet's membrane as possible. Donor corneas can be thick due to the hyperosmolarity of glycosaminoglycans in the preservation medium, thus rendering suturing to a thin host (e.g., keratoconus) difficult. Conversely, if fresh donor tissue is used in patients with severe corneal edema, the donor might actually be thinner than the host cornea.

The second cardinal suture is the most important suture for reducing corneal astigmatism. The second suture is placed using a 0.12 forceps as the tissue is slightly stretched 180 degrees to place the needle exactly opposite of the initial suture (Figure 133-3, *A*). The area of donor/host overlap should be equal on both sides of the second suture so that tissue distribution is even for placement of all subsequent sutures. The first or second cardinal suture can be removed and replaced to provide appropriate tension. The third and fourth sutures are placed by grasping the donor cornea and placing the suture at 3 o'clock and 9 o'clock

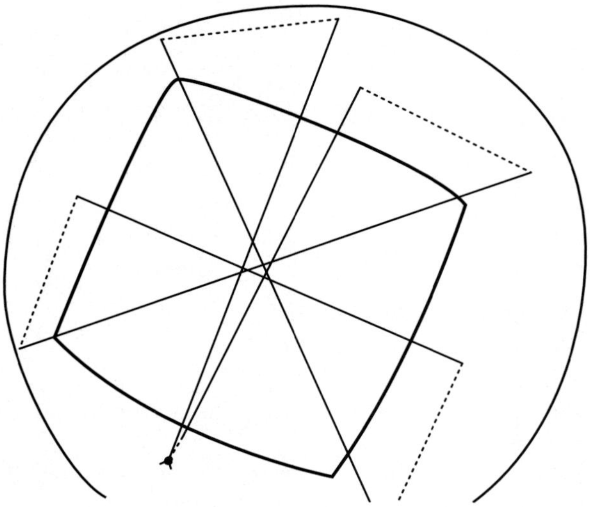

FIGURE 133-1 Schematic diagram of Castroviejo's original suturing technique used for square grafts. This figure illustrates the method of suturing the graft pictured in Figure 133-2.

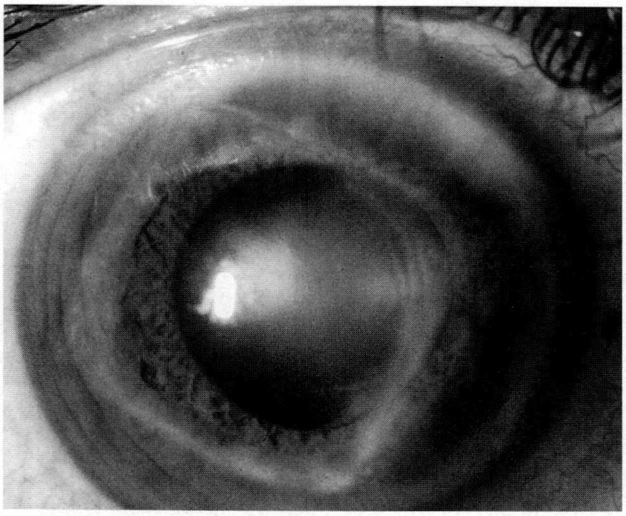

FIGURE 133-2 Clear square graft within an opaque host bed. Many of these grafts are still clear today, more than 25 years postoperatively.

equidistant from the first two cardinal sutures. Frequently, a diamond shaped pattern of corneal striae will appear in the donor cornea (Figure 133-3, *B*).

Nylon, because of its elasticity, strength, and biocompatibility in the cornea is the most effective suture material for keratoplasty. Polypropylene and Mersilene suture cause more stromal fibrosis and reaction than nylon.[2] Nylon permits postoperative adjustment of a continuous 10-0 suture, whereas nonelastic sutures result in loss of suture tension once corneal edema resolves.

The anterior chamber should be kept inflated during suture placement to protect the endothelium. After four cardinal sutures have been placed, the anterior chamber can usually be inflated with balanced salt solution if there is no posterior pressure and the wound is symmetric. A viscoelastic substance of choice can be used to re-form the chamber if posterior pressure exists or there is a wound leak from irregularity in wound approximation. Irregularities in wound approximation can be fixed at this time by replacement of one or more cardinal sutures. In pediatric keratoplasty, keratoconus, or instances of significant posterior pressure and or thin donor or host tissue, four additional sutures for a total of eight can be placed to secure the wound. In general the wound should be watertight at this stage.

Single Interrupted Sutures

Interrupted sutures are easiest to place because they can be put in and taken out as many times as necessary to secure a satisfactory bite, knot, or tension. Interrupted sutures permit partial or complete suture removal in one region of the graft if necessary. Interrupted sutures are indicated for pediatric keratoplasty so that partial suture removal may be performed at different times in the postoperative course. Vascularization in the host cornea, multiple previous rejections, or inflammatory conditions that may predispose to localized vascularization, rejection, or ulceration are indications for interrupted sutures.

Interrupted sutures are generally placed with 10-0 nylon using a 160 degree single curve 6 ml needle, such as the Ethicon CS160-6 needle. In general, compound curve needles do not provide any advantage over single curve needles, because larger bites are helpful in holding the wound together without excessive tension, whereas smaller bites require more bites and tighter sutures.

Eight sutures in general is the minimal number required to keep the wound watertight, and 16 sutures is the average number for an interrupted suture wound closure (Figure 133-4). If a suture becomes loose, it can be removed without disrupting the wound. Additional sutures, up to a total of 24 or 32, may be necessary in pediatric grafts, keratoconus patients, or if there is same size donor/host sizing.

After all interrupted sutures have been placed and securely knotted, the loose ends are cut short using a microsharp blade such as a Beaver 75 blade and the knots are buried. The knots should be buried by rotating them through the graft to the host tissue so that the cut ends on the knot are not pointing away from the surface like barbs to impair removal. This author prefers to bury knots in the host tissue so that

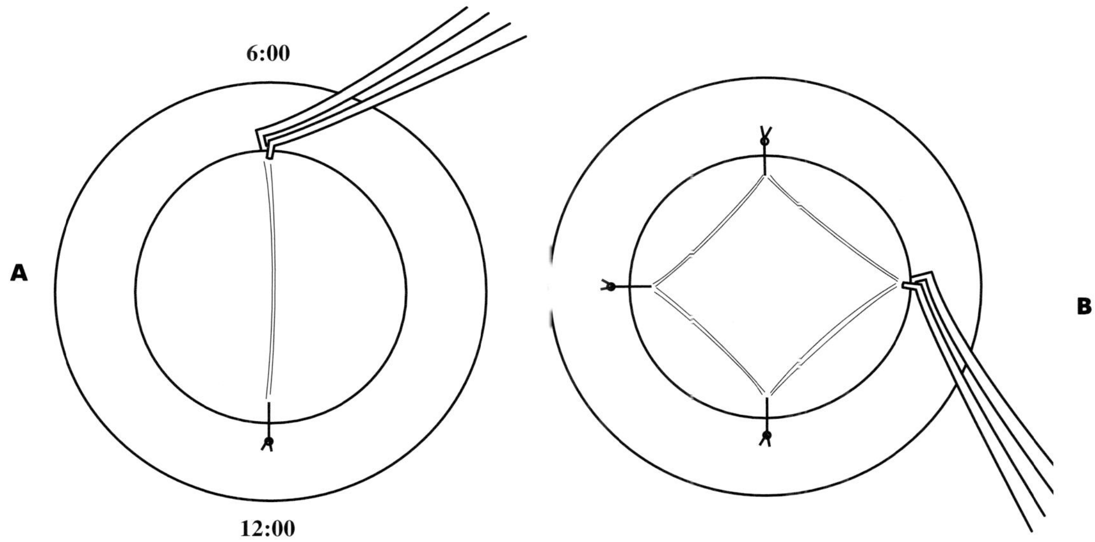

FIGURE 133-3 **A,** The second suture is 180 degrees from the first suture so that the donor tissue and wound are divided equally into temporal and nasal halves. **B,** The third and fourth sutures also divide the donor tissue and wound evenly.

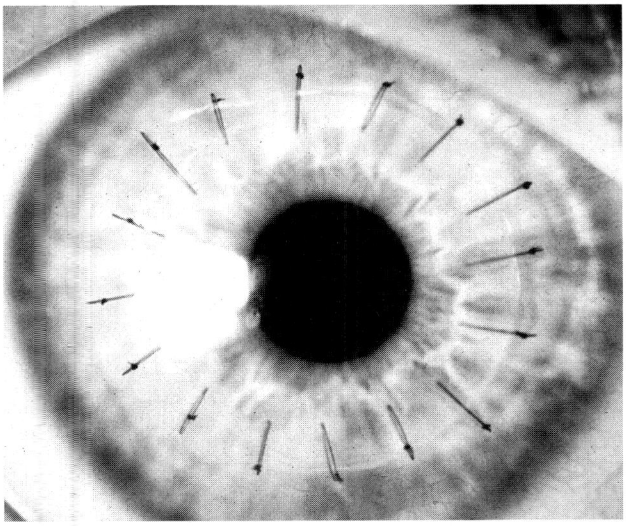

FIGURE 133-4 Keratoplasty wound closure with 16 interrupted 10-0 nylon sutures.

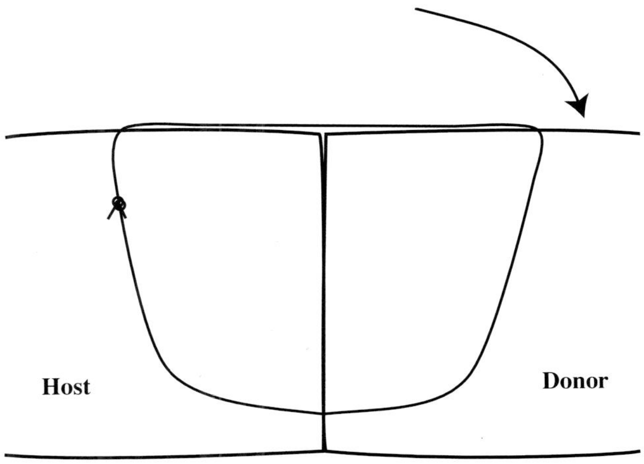

FIGURE 133-5 Sutured knots pulled through donor cornea into host, aligning small barbs on suture to facilitate suture removal. Arrow shows direction of knot rotation.

after the knots are cut and the suture is pulled, there is less tension on the graft-host junction, reducing the chance of dehiscence should the sutures be removed during the early stages of wound healing[3] (Figure 133-5).

Special considerations are required for pediatric grafts because of the high scleral elasticity of the host eye and the very thin donor tissue. Pediatric grafts may require twice the number of sutures expected for an adult cornea. Although pediatric graft size is frequently smaller than adults, a minimum of 24 and sometimes as many as 32 sutures may be required to close the graft. A continuous suture is inadvisable for pediatric grafts because the tissue is so soft that imperfect suture bites can result in wound leaks. Suture adjustment is, in most cases, impossible. Partial suture removal may commence as early as 3 weeks postoperatively, and complete suture removal is usually completed by 3 months. Because of the heightened inflammatory response and the higher incidence of rejection, all interrupted sutures may be removed from one region of the graft before another (Figure 133-6).

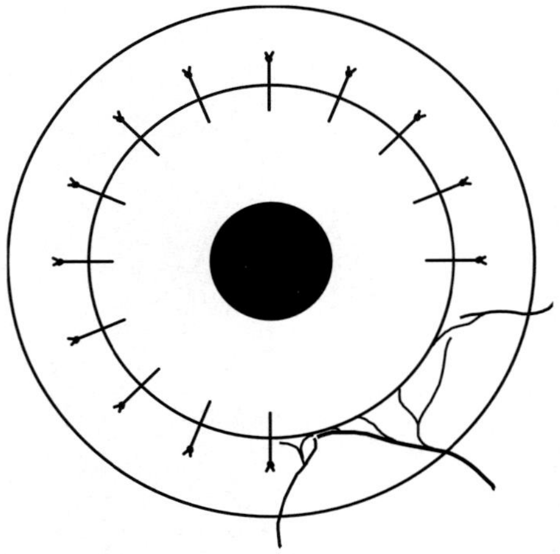

FIGURE 133-6 Postoperatively, interrupted sutures may be removed from one region of the graft for vascularization or inflammation without affecting integrity of wound closure in other regions of graft.

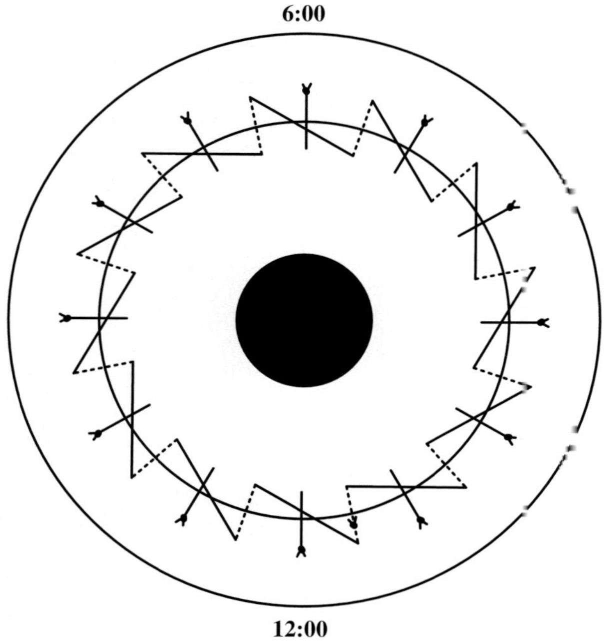

FIGURE 133-7 Keratoplasty closure using combined continuous and interrupted sutures (CCIS). The continuous suture can be either 10-0 or 11-0 nylon. In this example, 12 interrupted sutures and a 12 bite running suture are used.

Combined Continuous and Interrupted Suture Technique

The combined continuous interrupted suturing technique (CCIS) uses a continuous suture in addition to interrupted sutures to stabilize the wound so that the interrupted suture can be removed earlier than if interrupted sutures were used alone (Figure 133-7). The combined continuous interrupted suture technique is most often performed using 12 interrupted 10-0 nylon sutures and a 12 bite continuous 10-0 or 11-0 nylon running suture with bites of the continuous suture placed between each of the interrupted sutures. The superficial portion of the continuous suture approximates Bowman's layer. Consequently, the needle pass of the continuous suture bites should be made close to the interrupted suture so that the epithelial portion of the continuous suture lies across the wound between the interrupted sutures to help stabilize Bowman's layer. If suture bites are made halfway between the interrupted sutures, the superficial segment will lie across the interrupted sutures, making the interrupted sutures more difficult to remove without cutting the continuous suture and providing little additional wound support. An 11-0 nylon is less likely to alter corneal topography than 10-0 nylon suture, but it is more difficult to use; whether to use 10-0 or 11-0 continuous suture is a matter of surgeon preference.

Twelve interrupted 10-0 nylon sutures can be placed evenly using a 12 blade RK marker as a guide. The knots are secured, the loose ends are cut short, and the knots are buried. An 11-0 or 10-0 nylon continuous suture is then run with 12 bites for 360 degrees, temporarily knotted at 12 o'clock, and tightened sufficiently to take up slack. The purpose of the continuous suture is to simply maintain wound apposition whenever the interrupted sutures are removed.

The combined continuous and interrupted suture technique should not be used if there is possible need for suture removal in some portions of the wound before others. If removal of all sutures from one quadrant is a possibility, for example, because of corneal vascularization, interrupted sutures alone are indicated. The techniques for selective suture removal for control of astigmatism are discussed in the section following on suture adjustment.

Single Continuous Suture

Antitorque suturing is not necessary for continuous sutures with 12 or more bites. Meticulous care should be taken to place deep, even bites in a continuous keratoplasty suture with multiple identical passes using the same needle. A single continuous suture (SCS) is technically more difficult than interrupted sutures, because one irregular bite can impair the integrity of the closure and cannot be removed without removing the entire suture (Figure 133-8). If the needle is bent,

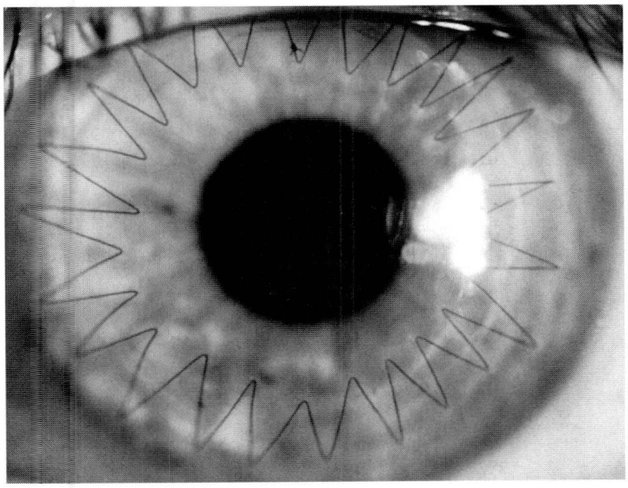

FIGURE 133-8 Single continuous 10-0 nylon suture keratoplasty closure. The elasticity of nylon suture permits tension even after the resolution of edema in the donor or host tissue postoperatively.

dulled, or the suture pulled off, the entire suture may have to be repeated or a new needle spliced onto the existing suture. If irregular spacing of sutures fails to close the wound, additional interrupted sutures may be necessary.

After the four cardinal sutures have been placed, a continuous 10-0 nylon suture with at least 24 bites is placed using a 12 blade RK marker as a guide: two suture bites placed between each line of the RK marker results in six bites per quadrant. Meticulous care should be taken to avoid dulling the point of the needle. The sutures are placed as radially and evenly spaced as possible, with the ideal depth of each suture bite 95%. Suture perforations, that occur by engaging the host tissue on the endothelial surface rather than in the stroma, will generally be Seidel positive the following day but eventually heal without additional intervention. Suture perforations can be made worse with excessive tightening of the continuous suture, and the asymmetry caused by one irregularly placed suture through the endothelial surface may indeed induce sufficient tightening to make a suture perforation problematic for more than 24 hours. A single suture bite that is too short or too shallow can permanently distort wound morphology.

After the 24 bite continuous suture has been placed, the suture is knotted temporarily at 12 o'clock while the four interrupted cardinal sutures are carefully removed. Inadvertent division of the continuous suture while trying to cut the cardinal sutures can be repaired by splicing or replacing the continuous suture. After the cardinal sutures have been cut, the anterior chamber is inflated with BSS plus. If the continuous suture is tightened when the eye is soft, "barrel topping" of the graft with a topographically flat donor cornea results.

After the chamber has been inflated to physiologic intraocular pressure (or slightly higher), the continuous interrupted suture is tightened, stitch by stitch, in clockwise fashion 360 degrees to achieve the desired tension, and is then permanently knotted at 12 o'clock. The knot is secured, the loose ends are cut short, and the knot is then buried. Tightening of the suture, bite by bite, should commence on the second or third bite to allow some laxity for the knot to be buried in the host cornea at 12 o'clock. The suture is then adjusted using an intraoperative keratometer or other keratoscopic instrument for intraoperative assessment of corneal sphericity; the cornea should be as spherical as possible. Intraoperative suture adjustment is not entirely reliable because the intraocular pressure may be different postoperatively, due to alterations in corneal astigmatism from the lid speculum or patient posture and because the donor epithelium may be smooth. Most importantly, the donor cornea will become thinner postoperatively and reduce the suture tension 360 degrees so that the wound may shift. However, intraoperative suture adjustment is helpful and is especially useful when combined with postoperative adjustment at the slit lamp.

Inadvertent breakage of the continuous suture during procedure is managed by splicing the suture, burying the knots, and tightening the suture on both sides of the splice knot back toward 12 o'clock. If the running suture is broken in the first quadrant, it should be removed and restarted because the time required for splicing the suture often exceeds the time required to replace the first few sutures. Breakage of the suture in the second or third quadrant can be alleviated by splicing a new 10-0 nylon suture to the old suture and continuing with the new needle. For instance, if the needle is pulled off the suture and a sufficient length of the original suture is left, another small segment of suture can be tied to the old segment. The continuous suture can be completed with the new needle, resulting in a single knot at 12 o'clock as originally planned. If the suture is divided so that there is no additional length of suture left to proceed, a longer portion of new suture is spliced to the old suture, the new suture is continued to complete the 360 degree closure, and then the spliced knot is buried. Once a spliced knot is buried, the suture can be tightened from either side of the buried knot toward the final termination of the suture at 12 o'clock to avoid exposure of the spliced knot. The 12 o'clock knot is then buried. Suture adjustment is, in general, difficult through a knot because the knot serves as an anchor. When two knots are buried, the suture should be adjusted in two separate portions without trying to move the knots.

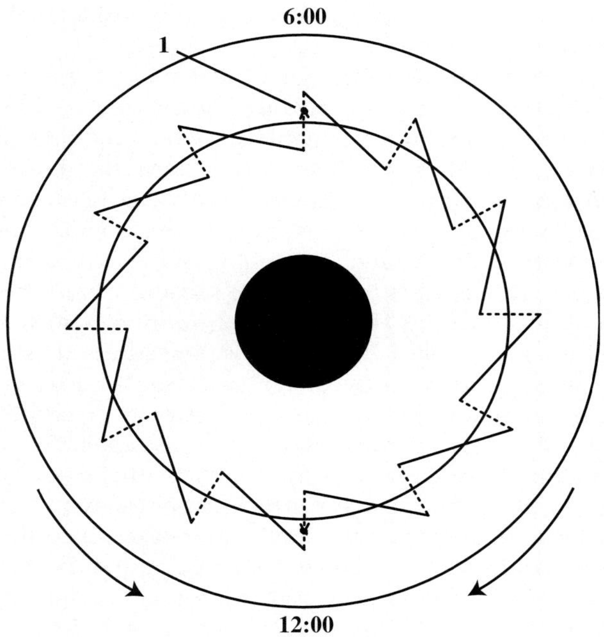

FIGURE 133-9 If a continuous suture is inadvertently broken after partial closure, a new suture can be spliced on and the spliced knot buried. The suture can be continued 360 degrees, and then advanced toward the 12 o'clock knot from the inferior knot *(1)* to avoid exposure of the spliced knot. Slack is taken up from both sides of the spliced knot. The 12 o'clock knot is then buried.

Attempting to move the knots can result in suture breakage (Figure 133-9).

Double Continuous Suture

A double continuous suture provides the advantage of a single continuous suture with the additional safety of having an extra suture in place should one suture break or have to be removed early.

After the four cardinal sutures are placed, a 12 bite 10-0 nylon suture is placed with bites at approximately 80% depth, using an RK marker to measure the interval for the sutures. The suture is then knotted superiorly; the knot is buried in the host cornea tissue under the lid, and the tension can be adjusted as described for a single continuous suture. A second continuous suture (either 10-0 or 11-0 nylon) is then placed with bites alternating between each 10-0 bite for 360 degrees. The second 11-0 suture is placed approximately 50% to 60% the corneal depth, and is tied with only enough tension to take up slack in the suture. An 11-0 nylon suture permits early removal of the 10-0 nylon suture for astigmatism control in 2 or 3 months, whereas the 11.0 suture is generally removed in 12 to 18 months postoperatively (Figure 133-10). A 10-0 nylon suture,

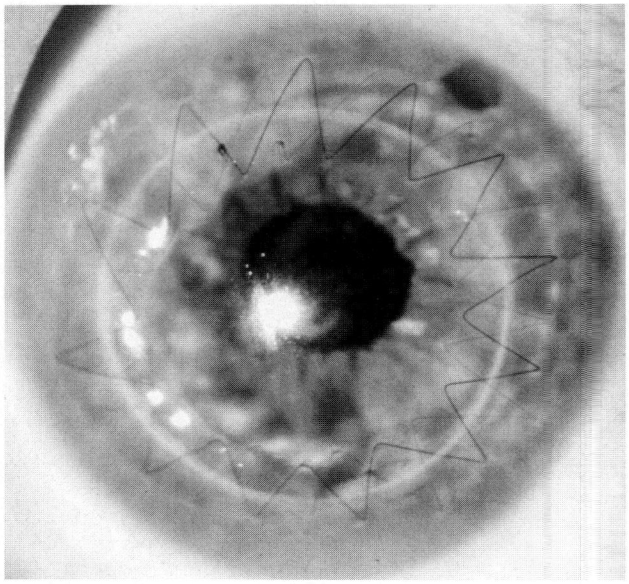

FIGURE 133-10 Double continuous keratoplasty closure using a 10-0 continuous suture and an 11-0 continuous suture. The 10-0 suture can be adjusted for astigmatism control, or removed after 3 months to improve corneal topography.

placed with superficial bites and less tension, can also stabilize the wound and permit adjustment of one or both sutures.

Both of the double continuous suture techniques require more technical expertise than interrupted sutures. Whereas interrupted sutures can be replaced as many times as needed to achieve a satisfactory stitch, a continuous suture is only as strong as its weakest segment and is only as regular as its most irregular bite. Suture adjustment is described in the next section.

Suture Adjustment

Postoperative suture adjustment for astigmatism control has become common practice in modern keratoplasty. A patient with a clear graft who has a large ametropia is still significantly disadvantaged. Ametropias can include spherical refractive error and astigmatism. The purpose of suture adjustment is to minimize postoperative astigmatism. Postoperative suture adjustment can effectively reduce postoperative astigmatism with sutures in place, but is less effective in reducing spherical refractive errors. Large amounts of myopia can result from thin corneas that stretch postoperatively, oversized donor/host disparity, or loose sutures. A flat cornea, which can result from sutures too tight or same size graft/host disparity, can also be refractory to any adjustment, although in general the corneal curvature steepens postoperatively.

Corneal astigmatism following keratoplasty can be due to suturing technique or a variety of other factors that are discussed in Chapter 137. Wound morphology, irregular, angled, or oral trephination of the donor or host, localized scarring or vascularization, or misplacement of cardinal and/or permanent sutures can result in corneal astigmatism refractory to suture adjustment. Although specific suturing techniques are dictated by the expertise of the surgeon and by the presence or absence of localized disease, all suturing techniques in some form or another lend themselves to adjustment for reduction of keratoplasty astigmatism, even if the "adjustment" means removing the sutures following wound stabilization.

Suture adjustment plays an important role in postoperative visual rehabilitation following keratoplasty. It should be performed as early as feasible before wound healing is complete so that collagen remodeling follows the vectors altered by suture adjustment. Suture adjustment can be performed as soon as the corneal surface is completely epithelialized to permit quantitative and qualitative evaluation of topography. In addition, postoperative thinning of the donor cornea should be well under way because adjustment with a thick cornea may not be effective when the donor cornea subsequently thins and alters the tension of the elastic nylon suture in the wound.

Topographical analysis using keratometry, photokeratoscopy, or videokeratography, individually or in combination, are helpful in planning suture adjustment and measuring the effects of adjustment on the cornea.

SUTURE REMOVAL

Suture adjustment can take the form of removal of all sutures, partial suture removal, or adjustment in the tension of a continuous 10-0 nylon running suture. Astigmatism following suture removal is variable. Therefore, if corneal astigmatism is satisfactory with sutures in place, sutures should remain until there is some indication for removal, such as increased risk of rejection (scarring, vascularization), patient discomfort (suture breakage), or decreased vision (residual astigmatism). Leaving sutures in place as long as possible for controls astigmatism. At the time of suture placement, therefore, surgeons should avoid excessive trauma to the nylon sutures with tying forceps, needle holders, and scissors that might lead to early breakage.

SINGLE INTERRUPTED SUTURES

Postoperative adjustment of interrupted sutures is simplest in concept but self-limiting in function: the only adjustment possible with an interrupted suture is removal. With silk sutures, early removal was necessary to prevent inflammation and vascularization; such early removal reduced the effect of suture on astigmatism. However, clear grafts were not as common with silk as with the less reactive sutures currently available today. There is a narrow interval between the stage at which the wound will dehisce after suture removal and the point at which healing has progressed so that suture removal will effect no change in topography. Loose, interrupted sutures provide no structural support and can be removed at any time without affecting the wound.

Because flattening is the only possible outcome, the adjustment in topography from interrupted sutures is limited in scope. Once the interrupted suture is removed, if too little or too much flattening is obtained, nothing else can be done in that axis with suture manipulation. Consequently, qualitative and quantitative measurement of corneal topography should be obtained before and after suture removal. Tight interrupted sutures can be removed earlier. For instance, with 16 interrupted sutures, one suture can be removed as early as 6 weeks if it is too tight, although no adjacent sutures should be removed for at least 6 more weeks. Occasionally earlier suture removal is indicated at the discretion of the surgeon, as long as it can be reliably determined that the wound is sufficiently healed to withstand suture removal without adverse effect.

Once the suture(s) to be removed are identified, a drop of topical antibiotic is placed in the eye and the eye is anesthetized with topical anesthesia. The suture is cut and removed with a tying forceps. A sudden jerk is more effective at removing the interrupted suture than slower, less forceful pressure. Some surgeons then patch the eye for 18 to 24 hours with topical antibiotic ointment.

COMBINED CONTINUOUS AND INTERRUPTED SUTURES

At approximately 3 to 4 weeks after keratoplasty, corneal topography is evaluated. Tight interrupted sutures are identified using keratometry or photokeratoscopy, and then removed (Figure 133-11). One to three weeks later, the patient's corneal topography is remeasured to assess changes induced by removal of the suture and to determine whether or not additional removal is indicated. Subsequent sutures are removed as described until corneal astigmatism is reduced to less than 3 diopters or until there are no more interrupted sutures to remove in the tight meridian. If the astigmatism is acceptable, the sutures remain in place indefinitely or until removal is dictated by breakage, erosion, or scarring.[4-8]

A limitation of CCIS suture adjustment is that only the tight suture can be removed; accordingly, only the steep axis can be reduced. A cornea that is excessively

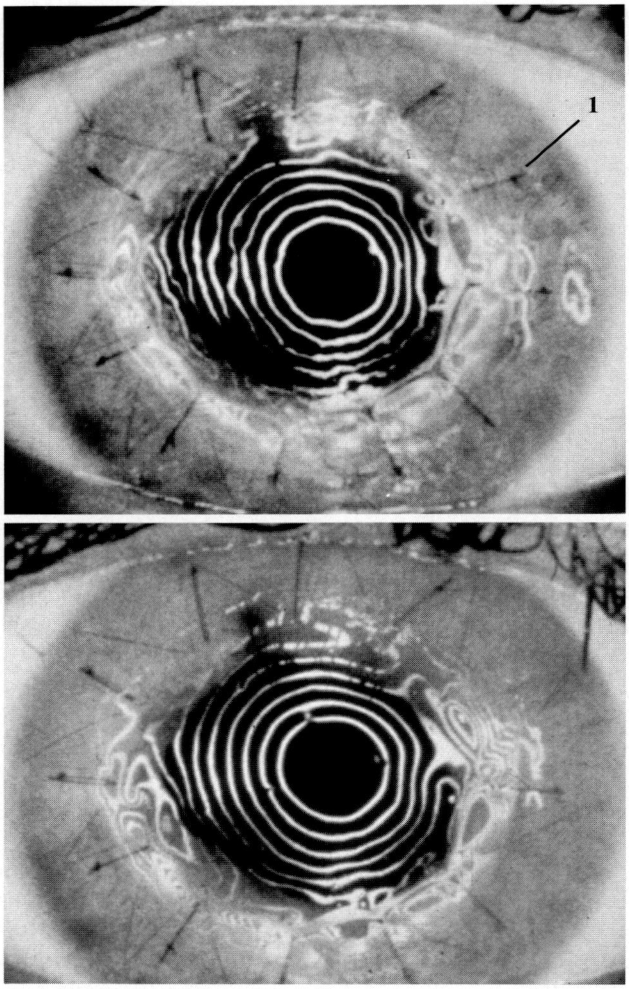

FIGURE 133-11 **A,** Tight interrupted suture *(1)* identified with photokeratoscopy. **B,** The suture in the tight axis is removed to reduce corneal astigmatism.

flat in one axis cannot be steepened by removing sutures. If removing sutures from the tight meridian does not reduce the corneal cylinder, adjustment is not effective, and additional alteration is not possible when there are no more sutures left to remove. The patient and physician must then wait until all sutures can be removed and address corneal astigmatism with surgical methods.

One disadvantage of the CCIS technique is that interrupted sutures are very difficult to remove after several years. Sutures that are partially eroded, loose, or break years after surgery may be difficult to remove due to fibrosis around buried knotted segments. However, once acceptable corneal astigmatism has been achieved, the suture should be left in place until there is an indication for removal.

Patients sutured with the CCIS technique have a reduction in corneal astigmatism from an average of 7.5 diopters with sutures in to 2.6 diopter at 1 year when stable. The ability to adjust astigmatism suture by suture is advantageous over removal of a continuous suture.[9] Average astigmatism with sutures out regresses to approximately 4 diopters.

SINGLE CONTINUOUS SUTURE

Suture adjustment can effectively reduce astigmatism as long as the astigmatism is due to uneven tension in the sutures and the wound is symmetric.

The single continuous suture is an effective technique for keratoplasty wound closure but is problematic because removal of a single continuous suture is an all or none phenomenon. However, adjustment of the single continuous suture can change corneal topography and still support the wound, and adjustment can be repeated more than once if desired. McNeill first described adjustment of a single continuous suture to reduce postkeratoplasty astigmatism in 1988.[10] Large amounts of corneal astigmatism can be reduced by adjusting the tension of a continuous suture using forceps at the slit lamp.[11] Multiple surgeons have confirmed the effectiveness of this technique.[12,13] A continuous suture should be placed with meticulous attention for proper suture depth and tension, because short or shallow bites are refractory to adjustment and leave the cornea steep where bites are shallow.

The single continuous suture is adjusted using sterile typing forceps. The forceps are used to divide Bowman's layer by carefully burying one end of the forceps into the cornea stroma, taking care not to advance in beyond 50% corneal depth. The suture is very carefully advanced from the flat toward the steep meridian, simultaneously flattening the steep meridian and steepening the flat meridian. Carefully advance the suture along a line parallel to the suture bite and do not twist the suture over the edge of the tying platform or divide the suture by pinching it too tightly (Figure 133-12). The suture is advanced loop by loop with the goal of equal distribution of suture tension around the wound (Figure 133-13). If the suture is tied too tightly, adjustment should not be pursued because attempts to move a very tight suture will result in suture breakage. In general, once the epithelium is broken, the suture can be grasped and easily advanced in the direction desired by 0.5 to 1 mm. If the suture appears too tight to adjust, adjustment should be deferred, and attempts to resolve astigmatism should follow suture removal.

Frequent remeasurement with the keratometer during the adjustment procedure provides quantitative and qualitative feedback on the effectiveness of adjustment. Some regression of the astigmatism generally occurs following adjustment because of wound destabilization; slight overcorrection in the adjustment endpoint to account for regression may be helpful. For

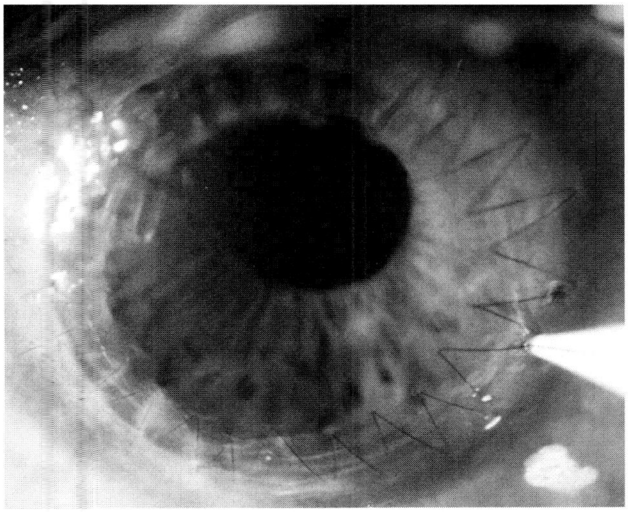

FIGURE 133-12 Adjustment of a single continuous 10-0 nylon suture at the slit lamp using tying forceps. The suture is advanced from the flat meridian toward the tight meridian to equally distribute suture tension around the wound.

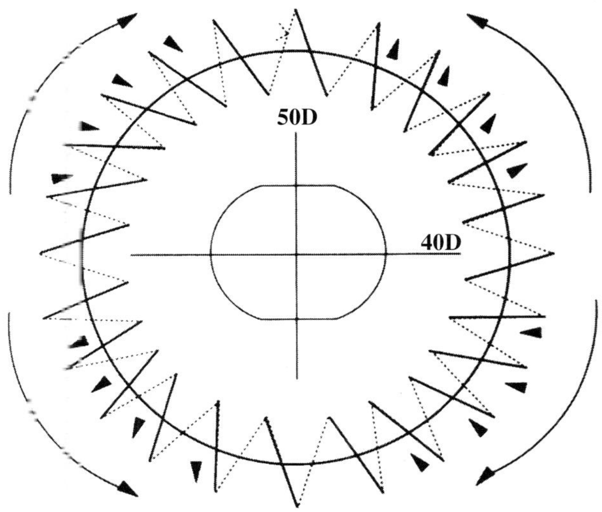

FIGURE 133-13 The direction of suture adjustment is shown. The suture is moved from the area of flat topography toward steep topography, thus steepening the flat meridian and flattening the steep meridian.

example, a patient with 8 diopters of cylinder at 9 o'clock might have the suture adjusted to provide 2 diopters of cylinder at 90° in order to allow for some regression. When using the keratometer, the image viewed is inverted, so that a flat keratometric image at 10 o'clock corresponds to a flattening of the corneal wound at 4 o'clock.

The continuous suture adjustment technique is similar to adjusting the tension in the shoe laces of high-top basketball shoes once they have been tied. The shoe laces are tightest superiorly near the ankle and are loose near the toes. To even the tension on the laces, the laces are grasped near the toes and worked superiorly, tightening the toes and at the same time shifting the laxity toward the ankle. Figure 133-12 demonstrates the suture adjustment in a cornea with theoretic K-readings of 40.00 × 180/50.00 × 90. The suture in each quadrant is advanced from the flattest toward the steepest meridian, leaving a spherical cornea.

An example of corneal mires before and after suture adjustment is shown in Figure 133-14. Corneal mires can be changed from an elliptic reflex on a toric cornea to a circular reflex from a spherical cornea as shown in Figure 133-14, *A*. Figure 133-14, *B* demonstrates suture adjustment from a teardrop pattern, in which the suture is advanced from the loose region, or point of the teardrop, and evenly distributed around the spherical portion. Figure 133-14, *C* demonstrates suture adjustment of a D-shaped pattern, in which the suture is advanced from the loose region to the tighter regions to equalize tension 360 degrees.

Postoperative suture manipulation permits reduction of astigmatism to an acceptable level in a majority of patients. Acceptable astigmatism with sutures in allows the patient to achieve early visual rehabilitation and is gratifying for the surgeon. Sutures should be left in place as long as possible when astigmatism is acceptably corrected because topography following suture removal varies tremendously, and once astigmatism is adjusted to an acceptable range, little improvement can be gained by taking sutures out. Because astigmatism is multifactorial, acceptable corneal topography with sutures in place usually means that sutures are compensating for some other nonsuture factors and the nonsuture factors may contribute to a increased astigmatism factor when sutures are removed.[14] However, multiple problems have been reported from leaving sutures in too long. Erosion of broken or loosened corneal sutures through the epithelium has been identified as a leading risk factor for postkeratoplasty (PK) graft infections.[15-19] Suture erosion is also a risk factor for the development of endophthalmitis[16,18] because suture abscesses after PK can lead to endophthalmitis. The spontaneous rupture or erosion of corneal sutures is associated with visually disabling astigmatism[5,6,20-22] and sutures in long after keratoplasty have caused foreign body sensation, conjunctival ulceration, giant papillary conjunctivitis, filamentary keratitis, blepharoptosis, uveitis, granuloma formation, and corneal neovascularization.[23-29] Dana et al. reported that 71% of patients who had corneal sutures removed had broken sutures, and breakage occurred an average of 36 months postoperatively;

A

B

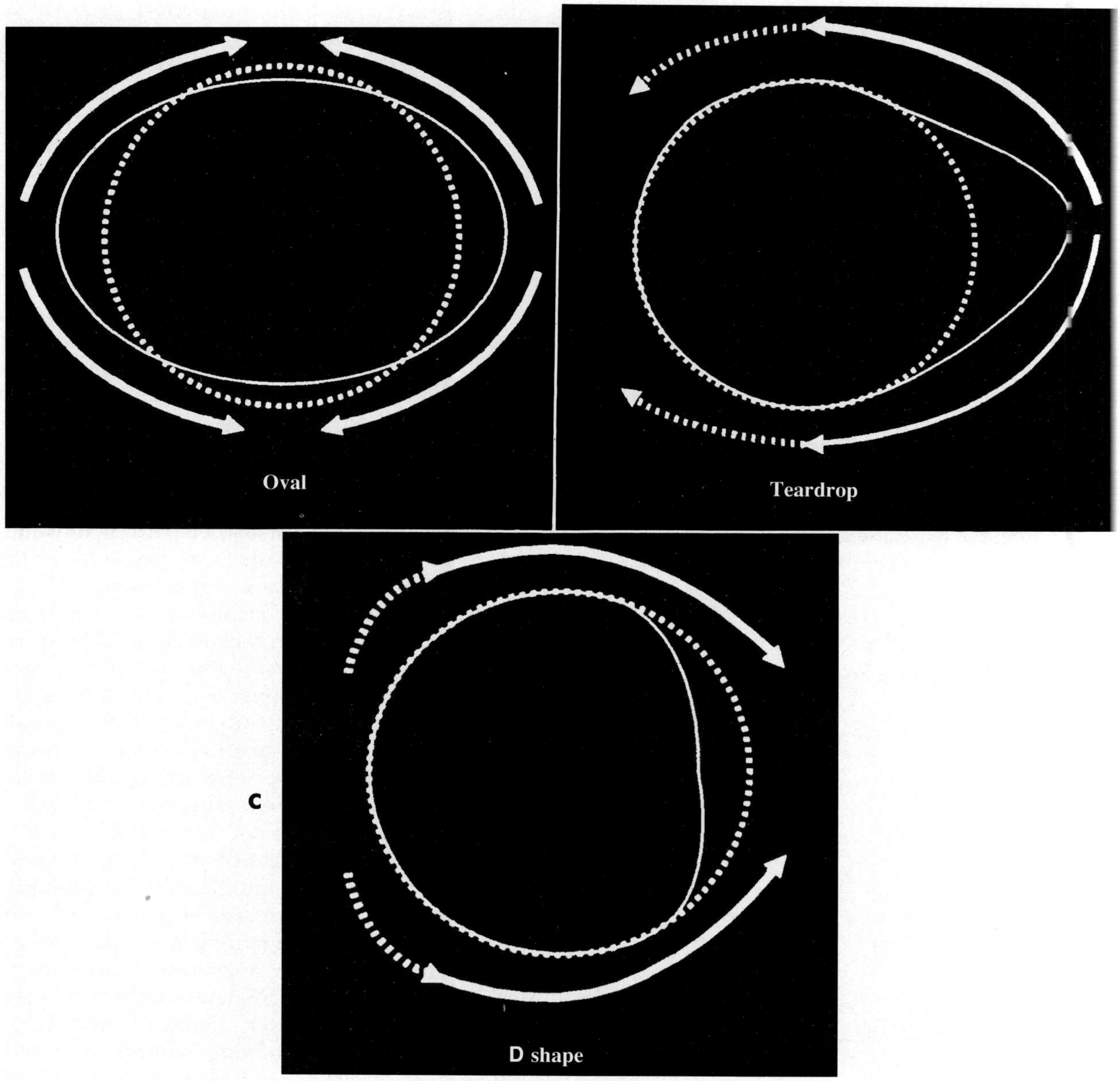

C

FIGURE 133-14 The principles of suture adjustment are illustrated by different topographic mires. **A**, An elliptical reflex requires adjustment in all four quadrants in the direction of the arrows. **B**, Adjustment of a teardrop pattern, in which the sutures are advanced from the loose region and evenly distributed around the tighter spherical portion. **C**, The adjustment of a D-shaped pattern requires the suture taken up from the round regions and redistributed toward the flat side of the "D."

29% had intact but loosened eroded sutures an average of 25 months postoperatively.[30]

Indications for suture removal include loose interrupted sutures, tight interrupted sutures with obvious focal compression demonstrating hemimeridional steepening, highly vascularized interrupted sutures, and broken sutures. Highly vascularized suture tracts, pronounced inflammation, or infiltration around sutures can necessitate the removal of all interrupted sutures or a continuous suture. The question of whether to remove a suture from a patient with a clear graft who is seeing well must be weighed against the risk of leaving the suture in place. Eyes that have clinically demonstrated a propensity in the past for suture breakage and erosion should have sutures removed from an intact wound to minimize the risk of subsequent suture breakage. Careful handling of the nylon suture intraoperatively with minimal trauma to the corneal wound can reduce the incidence of long-term suture complications.

The risk of suture breakage during the adjustment procedure is real and should be considered a potential risk, because the wound is not stable enough to remain intact without suture support during the early postoperative period, when suture adjustment can most effectively be performed. Suture breakage can result in wound dehiscence and requires prompt repair in the operating room. Consequently, suture adjustment of the single continuous suture should not be attempted unless facilities are available to make the repair.

Regression after the second or third suture adjustment is a poor prognostic sign. Because residual postkeratoplasty astigmatism is multifactorial, other factors causing astigmatism such as wound morphology or gross imsplacement of sutures may prevent adjustment from being effective. If suture adjustment is not effective, the patient can be fitted with glasses or contact lenses when possible and should have final suture removal when the wound has stabilized, at which point other procedures such as relaxing incisions or wedge resections can be useful.

Suture adjustment can effectively reduce astigmatism as long as the astigmatism is due to uneven tension in the sutures and the wound is symmetric. Suture adjustment can produce small individual variations in suture tension to alleviate astigmatism due to uneven tension in the suture. Larger variations, such as those necessary to overcome disparity in the wound in unusual features of the donor on host tissue, do not work or are temporary at best. If wound abnormalities are not present, suture adjustment is effective.

The effectiveness of a single continuous suture adjustment depends on a relatively even wound, for 360 degrees, with no unusual or uneven features. Some variability in corneal topography should be expected following suture removal due to variable features of the wound.

Following suture removal, epithelial disruption around the wound is common. Some surgeons instruct their patients to patch the eye overnight after applying a polymyxin/bacitracin ointment the patch may be removed the following day. Often surgeons treat their patients with antibiotic drops for 3 to 4 days after suture removal. Reevaluation of topography to determine the effects of suture removal can be completed within 2 to 3 weeks.

DOUBLE CONTINUOUS SUTURES

Adjustment of the double continuous sutures initially involved removing one of the two 10-0 continuous sutures.[13,31] This technique was modified using a 10-0 and an 11-0 nylon suture.[32] The 10-0 nylon suture was removed at 2 to 3 months and the 11-0 suture remained for 12 months. [Removal of the deeper, tighter 10-0 nylon suture reduced astigmatism due to the tightness suture.[33]] The 11-0 nylon suture was left in place to secure the wound and prevent dehiscence. (See Figure 133-10.)

Recently Waring used a double 10-0 running suture. He adjusted the deeper, tighter 10-0 nylon suture so that it altered corneal topography, and left the shallower suture in place as a safety net. Both sutures can be left in place postoperatively if the patient is optically stable, but if the patient requires adjustment, the deep 10-0 nylon suture can be adjusted to flatten or steepen irregular meridians to reduce corneal astigmatism. The second 10-0 nylon suture remains as a safety net if the suture is broken or if one suture needs to be removed.

Final Considerations

Three important points regarding suture adjustment should be emphasized:

1. Corneal astigmatism is multifactorial and suture adjustment or removal can only correct astigmatism that is due to uneven suture tension in a reasonably approximated wound. If the wound is unevenly approximated, adjustment of suture tension does little to reduce astigmatism.

   If uniform tension in a regular wound is present, and vector forces are even across the wound, continuous sutures work well. However, continuous sutures do not protect a wound from locally applied forces and they are poorly suited for irregularly-shaped wounds that require vastly different amounts of tension at different sites in the wound. Such irregularly-shaped wounds are better served by interrupted sutures. Consequently, astigmatism with all sutures out postoperatively may reflect donor trephination, use of scissors, and or placement of the initial interrupted cardinal sutures.
2. Once the suture has been adjusted to achieve suitable topography, the sutures should be left in place until they have to be removed. Patients should be advised that sutures can be left in place as long as there is no inflammation. Some fibrosis can be expected around the suture tract but usually this is not an indication for removal. The most common indication for removal of a single continuous suture is suture breakage.
3. After several years, continuous sutures are easier to remove than interrupted sutures. If sutures are left in the cornea for more than 2 years, continuous sutures cause less inflammation and less

likelihood of residual buried remnants than interrupted sutures.

REFERENCES

1. Bourne WM: Current techniques for improved visual results after penetrating keratoplasty, *Ophthalmic Surg* 12:321, 1981.
2. Holland E et al: A comparison of suture types in the stimulation of corneal inflammation, *Invest Ophthalmol Vis Sci,* (Suppl) 31(4):270, 1990.
3. Melles GRH, Binder PS: A comparison of wound healing in sutured and unsutured corneal wounds, *Arch Ophthalmol* 108:546-548, 1980.
4. Binder PS: Selective suture removal can reduce postkeratoplasty astigmatism, *Ophthalmology* 92:1412-1416, 1985.
5. Binder PS: The effect of suture removal on postkeratoplasty astigmatism, *Am J Ophthalmol* 105:637-645, 1988.
6. Binder PS: Reduction of postkeratoplasty astigmatism in selective suture removal, *Dev Ophthalmol* 11:86-90, 1984.
7. Feldman ST, Brown SI: Reduction of astigmatism after keratoplasty, *Am J Ophthalmol* 103:477-478, 1987.
8. Burk LL et al: The effect of selective suture removal on astigmatism following penetrating keratoplasty, *Ophthalmic Surg* 19:849-854, 1988.
9. McNeill JI, Kaufman HE: A double running suture technique for keratoplasty: early visual rehabilitation, *Ophthalmic Surg* 8(4): 58-61, 1977.
10. McNeill JI: Eliminating astigmatism in PKP. The adjustable Suture, *Video J Ophthalmol* 4(3):Vol. IV, No 3, 1988.
11. McNeill JI, Wessels IF: Adjustment of single continuous suture to control astigmatism after penetrating keratoplasty, *Refract Corneal Surg* 5:216-223, 1989.
12. Van Meter WS et al: Postkeratoplasty astigmatism control. Single continuous suture adjustment versus selective interrupted suture removal, *Ophthalmology* 98:177-183, 1991.
13. Lin TC et al: An adjustable single running suture technique to reduce postkeratoplasty astigmatism, *Ophthalmology* 97:934-938, 1990.
14. Mader TH, Rumei Y, Lynn MJ et al: Changes in keratometric astigmatism after suture removal more than one year after penetrating keratoplasty, *Ophthalmology* 100:119-127, 1993.
15. Fong LP et al: Microbial keratitis complicating penetrating keratoplasty, *Ophthalmology* 95:1269-1275, 1988.
16. Bates AK, Kirkness CM, Ficker LA et al: Microbial keratitis after penetrating keratoplasty, *Eye* 4:74-78, 1990.
17. Tuberville AW, Wood TO: Corneal ulcers in corneal transplants, *Curr Eye Res* 1:479-485, 1981.
18. Harris DJ et al: Late bacterial and fungal keratitis after corneal transplantation, *Ophthalmology* 95:1450-1457, 1988.
19. Varley GA, Meisler DM: Complications of penetrating keratoplasty: graft infections, *Refract Corneal Surg* 7:62-66, 1991.
20. Stainer GA, Perl T, Binder PS: Controlled reduction of postkeratoplasty astigmatism, *Ophthalmology* 89:668-676, 1982.
21. Harris DJ, Waring GO III, Burk LL: Keratography as a guide to selective suture removal for the reduction of astigmatism after penetrating keratoplasty, *Ophthalmology* 96:1597-1607, 1989.
22. Frueh BE, Feldman ST, Feldman RM et al: Running nylon suture dissolution after penetrating keratoplasty, *Am J Ophthalmol* 113:406-411, 1992.
23. Shaw EL, Brighbill FS: Suture removal. In Brightbill FS, editor: *Corneal surgery. Theory, technique, and tissue,* ed 2, St Louis, 1993, Mosby.
24. Nirankari VS, Karesh JW, Richards RD: Complications of exposed monofilament sutures, *Am J Ophthalmol* 95:515-519, 1983.
25. Skyrpuch OW, Willis NR: Giant papillary conjunctivitis from an exposed prolene suture, *Can J Ophthalmol* 21:189-192, 1986.
26. Sugar A, Meyer RF: Giant papillary conjunctivitis after keratoplasty, *Am J Ophthalmol* 91:239-242, 1981.
27. Shahinian L, Brown SI: Postoperative complications with protruding monofilament nylon sutures, *Am J Ophthalmol* 83:546-548, 1977.
28. Weiss JL et al: Bacterial endophthalmitis following penetrating keratoplasty suture removal, *Cornea* 3:278-280, 1984/1985.
29. Forstot SL, Abel R Jr, Binder PS: Bacterial endophthalmitis following suture removal after penetrating keratoplasty, *Am J Ophthalmol* 80:509-512, 1975.
30. Dana MR, Goren MB, Gomes JAP et al: Suture erosion after penetrating keratoplasty, *Cornea* 14(3):243-248, 1995.
31. McNeill JI, Kaufman HE: A double running suture technique for keratoplasty: early visual rehabilitation, *Ophthalmic Surg* 8(4): 58-61, 1977.
32. Davison JA, Bourne WM: Results of penetrating keratoplasty using a double running suture technique, *Arch Ophthalmol* 99:1591-1595, 1981.
33. Musch DC, Meyer RF, Sugar A: The effect of removing running sutures on astigmatism after penetrating keratoplasty, *Arch Ophthalmol* 106:488-492, 1988.

CHAPTER 134

JOHN J. PURCELL, JR

Intraoperative Complications of Penetrating Keratoplasty

Intraoperative complications during keratoplasty are rarely reported, primarily because most of the complications that can occur are technical and with proper training and meticulous attention to detail, can usually be avoided. Many of the technical problems associated with shallowing of the anterior chamber or bulging anterior segment contents are now easier to deal with since the advent of viscoelastic materials[1] and preoperative massage, or compression techniques for lowering intraocular pressure.[2] Expulsive hemorrhage is the only catastrophic complication that may be considered nontechnical in nature. Consequently a review of intraoperative complications of keratoplasty will be divided into technical and nontechnical complications.

Technical Complications of Penetrating Keratoplasty

SCLERAL PERFORATION WITH FIXATION SUTURES

Many corneal surgeons employ fixation of the globe to prevent scleral collapse. The need for fixation is especially true in children who have elastic sclera and in aphakic or pseudophakic patients. Generally, phakic patients and extracapsular pseudophakic patients have excellent scleral support and require no fixation. Flieringa's rings, the McNeill-Goldman blepharostat[3] (Figure 134-1) and silk sutures beneath the superior and inferior recti have been used for stabilization of the globe and scleral support.

When placing sutures beneath the superior and inferior recti, the sclera can be perforated resulting in a retinal hole and possible retinal detachment. Care should be taken to use a rounded rather than cutting needle. When a perforation is recognized, cryotherapy should be applied to the area of suspected perforation[4] and the patient should be closely observed postoperatively.

Sutures for Flieringa's rings or a McNeill-Goldman blepharostat are placed at or anterior to the pars plana. If scleral perforation occurs during placement of these sutures, damage to the ciliary body may occur and hemorrhage may be observed at the angle in this region. This is usually self limited and is not generally problematic. Some surgeons employ prophylactic cryoplexy even in this anterior location.

IMPROPER TREPHINATION

Oversized donor grafts (0.25 mm) are commonly used in keratoplasty.[5,6] If the trephines are inadvertently reversed and the donor button is smaller than the recipient site, it may be difficult to suture the button in place and secure a water-tight wound. In addition, hyperopia would be induced.[7] The tightened sutures may collapse the trabecular meshwork and cause elevations in intraocular pressure.[8]

If the host has not been trephined or only partially trephined without entering the anterior chamber and it is recognized that the donor button has been prepared with the smaller trephine, a trephine 0.25 mm smaller than used on the donor may be used on the host if it adequately encompasses the pathology. If the donor has been prepared and the host anterior chamber entered, the smaller button may be used. If an intraocular lens is being placed, the power of the lens must be adjusted to account for 2 to 3 diopters of induced hyperopia. Great care must be taken to monitor the intraocular pressure postoperatively.

Eccentric trephination

Improper, eccentric placement of the trephine can result in large amounts of postoperative astigmatism. If the host has been only trephined to partial depth, a larger trephine, appropriately centered, may be used for completion of the trephination to correct this error.

DAMAGED DONOR BUTTON

Donor corneas must be handled with extreme care to prevent damage to the endothelium. Endothelial cell loss is greater in phakic than aphakic grafts.[9] This is thought to be due to endothelial-iris contact during

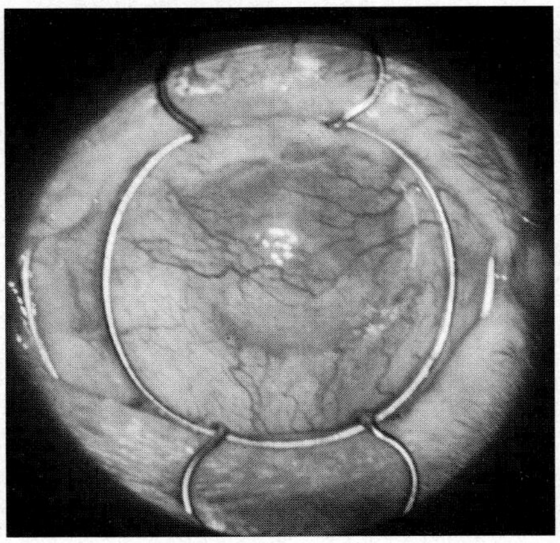

FIGURE 134-1 Globe fixation and lid retraction with a McNeill-Goldman blepharostat.

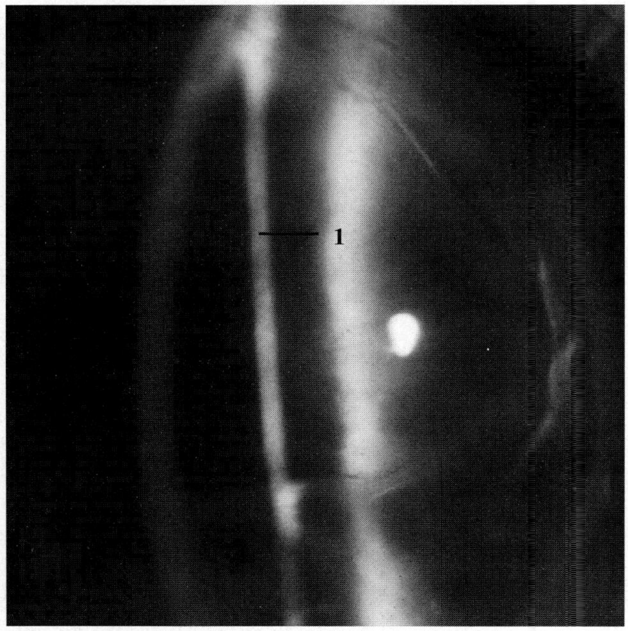

FIGURE 134-2 Postkeratoplasty retained host Descemet's membrane *(1)* creating a false anterior chamber. (Photo courtesy of Peter Laibson, MD.)

surgery, and is lessened by softening the eye preoperatively.[10] Viscoelastics have greatly enhanced protection of the endothelium, and when layered over these materials prior to suturing the donor cornea in place, prevent iris, lenticular, or intraocular lens touch.

The donor cornea may be severely damaged if the initial punch of the trephine has not completely cut the donor. If the partially cut donor button adheres to the trephine and is slightly displaced, repunching will cut the donor cornea. The donor cornea may be dropped during transfer to the donor eye, damaging the endothelium and contaminating the donor material.

It is important to prepare the donor cornea before removing the host tissue, so that if the donor is damaged or contaminated, surgery may be canceled if another cornea is unavailable.

RETAINED DESCEMET'S MEMBRANE

When removing the host cornea, the corneal scissors may inadvertently be placed anterior to Descemet's membrane and the membrane may be stripped and left in place (Figure 134-2). This is particularly easy to do with edematous corneas and in cases of interstitial keratitis in which Descemet's membrane is thickened. This can easily be missed and will create a false anterior chamber. Grafts placed over a retained Descemet's membrane fail from endothelial damage. Retained Descemet's membrane is often difficult to see, and if it has been left, must be carefully dissected free and removed. The iris architecture should be carefully inspected and the iris should be able to be gently picked up with forceps.[11] Viscoelastic placed behind retained Descemet's membrane will elevate it from the iris and facilitate removal.

IRIS-LENS DAMAGE

Trephination that is full thickness in one area or for 360 degrees may damage the iris or the lens. This type of trephination is more likely to occur in thinned or perforated corneas. To prevent this, some have recommended filling the entire anterior chamber with a viscoelastic via paracenteses before trephination.[12] This can also be easily accomplished by partial depth trephination, a small scratch down incision, and deepening of the anterior chamber with viscoelastic. Softening the eye preoperatively with massage or a compression device may facilitate proper technique.[13]

To prevent excision of the iris in perforated globes, viscoelastic re-formation of the anterior chamber combined with a cyanoacrylate adhesive can be used to restore the anterior chamber before trephination.[14]

Significant iris damage during trephination should be repaired (Figure 134-3). The iris may also be damaged or partially excised with scissors during removal of the host button. An iridodialysis may also occur. Iridodialysis is most common when removing embedded intraocular lens (IOL) material. The iridodialysis is repaired with 10-0 polypropylene suture and pupilloplasty is performed if necessary.

Trephination damage to the anterior lens capsule is a serious intraoperative complication that must be identified and dealt with immediately. Fortunately it is extremely rare. If the capsule has been opened, an extracapsular cataract extraction should be performed. A posterior chamber intraocular lens should be placed. It may be prudent to measure phakic patients for IOL powers in case this complication should occur, particularly in patients in whom posterior pressure and

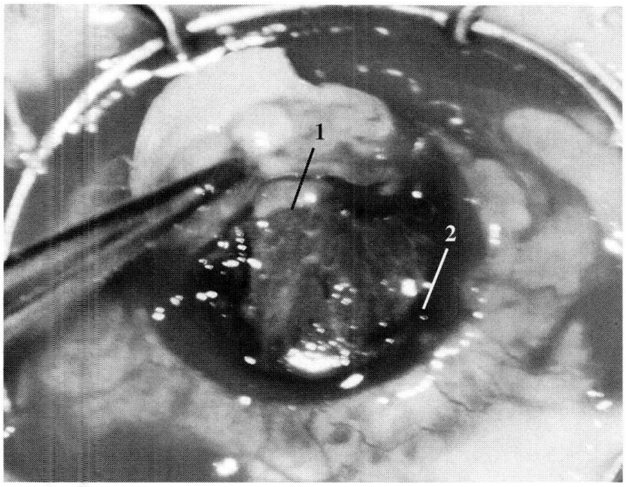

FIGURE 134-3 Iris adherent to perforated ulceration *(1)* leading to iridodialysis *(2)* as cornea is removed.

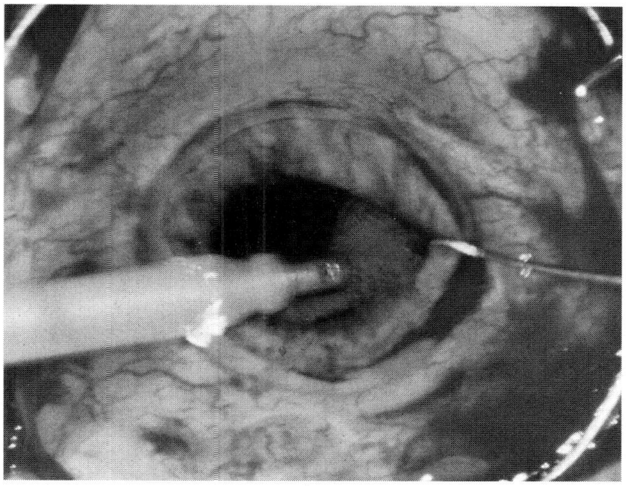

FIGURE 134-4 During cortical clean-up the posterior capsule may be inadvertently torn.

forward displacement of the anterior segment is expected.

TORN POSTERIOR CAPSULE

During combined keratoplasty extracapsular cataract extraction, the posterior capsule may be torn (Figure 134-4). Small tears without vitreous loss are usually of little significance, and careful placement of a posterior chamber intraocular lens with sulcus or in-the-bag fixation is possible.

Capsular rupture with vitreous loss is a different matter. Incidence has been reported at 0%,[15] 1.1%,[16] 4%,[17] and up to 16%.[18]

If posterior capsular rupture with vitreous loss occurs, an anterior vitrectomy must be performed. This should be performed with an automated system, clearing the anterior chamber, posterior chamber, and anterior vitreous cavity. An open loop anterior chamber intraocular lens or a sutured posterior chamber intraocular lens can be used. Many surgeons do not routinely perform a peripheral iridectomy with posterior chamber IOLs. However, if vitreous loss has occurred or if the posterior capsule is open without vitreous loss, a peripheral iridectomy should be performed in order to prevent postoperative pupillary block.

ANTERIOR CHAMBER HEMORRHAGE

Anterior chamber hemorrhage most commonly occurs in surgery on inflamed or perforated eyes from iris vessel leakage (Figure 134-5). It is usually minimal. Minimal hemorrhage can usually be ignored; it will stop after the wound is closed and intraocular pressure is restored.

Severe intraocular hemorrhage may occur when

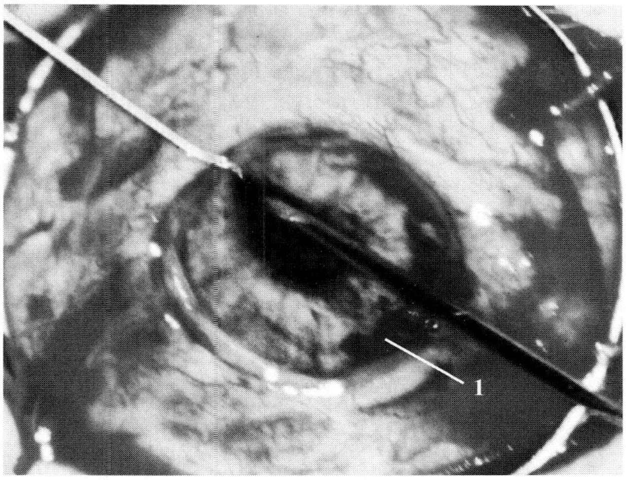

FIGURE 134-5 Persistent oozing anterior chamber hemorrhage *(1)* from the iris vessels and angle during extracapsular cataract extraction in an eye with a perforated cornea.

explanting closed-looped anterior chamber intraocular lenses[19] (Figure 134-6). Lens haptics are frequently embedded in synechial sheaths, and if these haptics are pulled, they will rip the iris or may even cause an iridodialysis that may result in severe anterior chamber bleeding. The haptics of closed-looped anterior chamber intraocular lenses must be severed from the optic and carefully slid through the synechial sheaths to prevent bleeding or iris damage.[20] Haptics tightly embedded in the angle or in the cataract incision site may be severed from the optic, trimmed, and left in place.[21]

Bleeding may be controlled with cautery, compression with viscoelastic, or tamponade with Weck cell

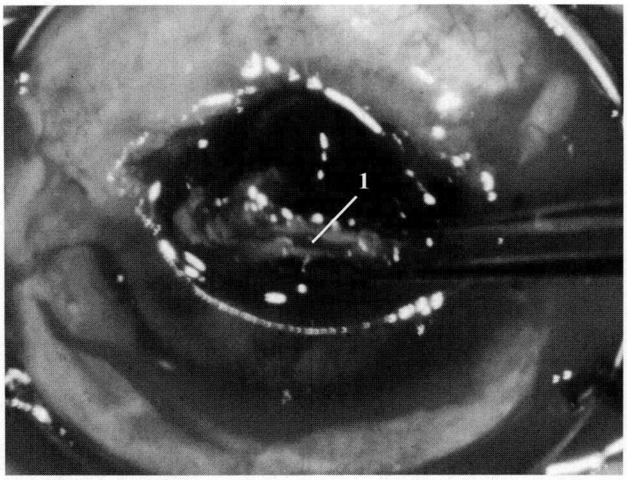

FIGURE 134-6 Intraocular lens *(1)* embedded in iris and scar tissue.

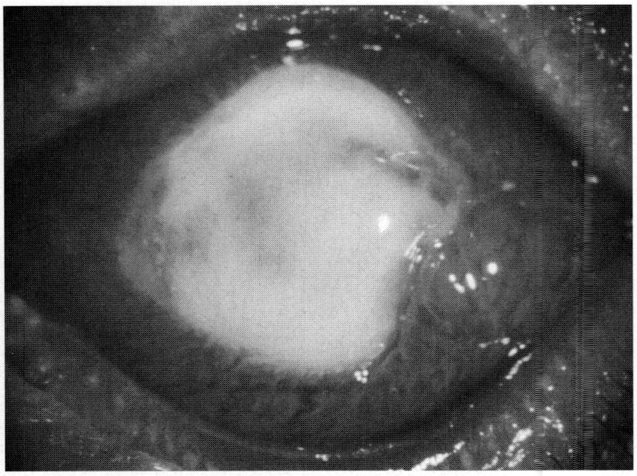

FIGURE 134-7 A perforated *Pseudomonas* ulcer in a severely inflamed eye is more likely to undergo expulsive choroidal hemorrhage.

sponges soaked with epinephrine 1:1,000, or thrombin 1:100. If bleeding cannot be controlled, the restoration of intraocular pressure by suturing the donor in place will usually stop the hemorrhage. It should be noted, however, that the anterior segment blood that seeps into the vitreous usually clears very slowly. An iridodialysis should be repaired with nylon or Prolene sutures.

Nontechnical Complications

EXPULSIVE CHOROIDAL HEMORRHAGE

The one "nontechnical" complication that may occur during keratoplasty is expulsive choroidal hemorrhage. The incidence of expulsive hemorrhage has been reported from 0.47%[22] to 3.3%.[15] Early reports were of isolated cases[23,24] until a collaborative report of 14 cases[25] reviewed the subject. Predisposing factors are advanced age,[26] myopia,[27] glaucoma,[28] inflammation (Figure 134-7), hypotonia or previous trauma. This is a devastating complication that may lead to blindness because of the extrusion of intraocular contents. With more aggressive attempts to repair perforated, infected, or severely traumatized eyes, one must be prepared to deal with expulsive hemorrhage.

Theoretically, preoperative reduction in intraocular pressure and shrinkage of aqueous and vitreous volume with decreased choroidal blood flow should help decrease the probability of an expulsive hemorrhage. This can be achieved with massage or a compression apparatus.[22] Trephination should be performed gently so that the intraocular pressure is not markedly elevated by downward pressure with the trephine and then rapidly reduced when the anterior chamber is opened.

During the open-sky phase of keratoplasty, choroidal detachments or effusions may occur and can be observed through the microscope. These are dark shadows or actual brown masses that may be seen in the red reflex. They do not mean that an expulsive hemorrhage is imminent. Expulsive hemorrhage may occur rapidly with sudden extrusion of intraocular contents (Figure 134-8) and hemorrhage or may be a gradual hemorrhage that slowly extrudes the iris, lens, or vitreous and then begins bleeding.

In our series, Valsalva maneuvers by two patients during keratoplasty led to expulsive hemorrhage.[25] Since blood flow in the choroid is the highest per unit volume of any tissue and since the capillary diameter is 4 times that of the normal capillaries,[29] one would expect that Valsalva maneuvers with open-sky keratoplasty would further engorge these vessels and predispose them to hemorrhage.

The management of expulsive hemorrhage depends on the immediate recognition of its development and prompt action. The rationale of management is to redirect the hemorrhage posteriorly and to restore normal ocular architecture anteriorly. How this is done depends on when the hemorrhage occurs. If the hemorrhage occurs immediately or shortly after entering the globe, an immediate posterior sclerotomy via a stab incision through the conjunctiva and sclera is performed. The inferotemporal quadrant is the most readily accessible. The sclerotomy should be large enough to allow blood and clots to be expressed as needed. Multiple sclerotomies may be required. Number 9-0 or 10-0 nylon or Prolene sutures will not usually be sufficient to secure the wound, and 6-0 or 7-0 silk sutures should be used. Once the wound is closed, the anterior segment structures should be restored to their proper anatomical configuration.

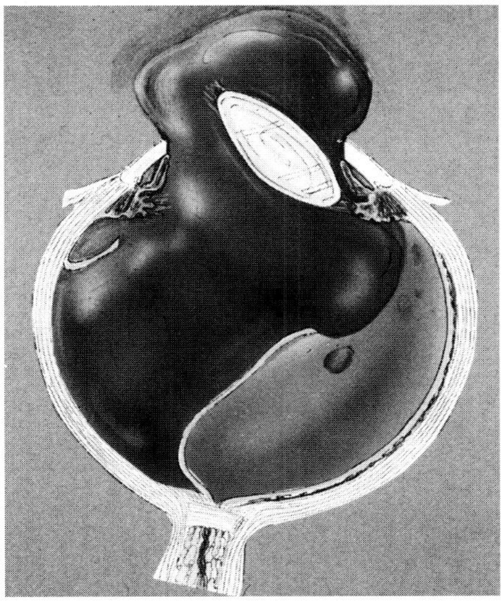

FIGURE 134-8 Expulsive choroidal hemorrhage during keratoplasty with extrusion of lens, iris, vitreous, and retina.

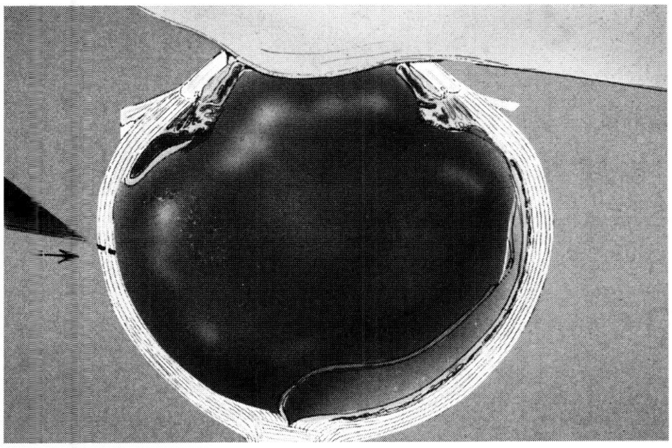

FIGURE 134-9 Occlusion of "open sky" with finger and posterior sclerotomy to stop extrusion of intraocular cataracts and to redirect the hemorrhage posteriorly.

If the hemorrhage occurs during the open-sky phase of keratoplasty, management is more difficult. The surgeon should immediately occlude the wound with the thumb or finger, perform a posterior sclerotomy, (Figure 134-9), and replace the recipient (or the donor cornea if it has been prepared) with interrupted silk sutures. The sclerotomy may need to be reopened several times in order to restore anterior segment integrity. If the cornea is secured and the hemorrhage is directed posteriorly, management of the lens, vitreous, iris, and anterior chamber re-formation are then appropriately handled.

Intraoperative complications during keratoplasty often result from technical errors and can be avoided with attention to detail. These complications should be corrected at the time of surgery. If they occur and are promptly recognized and dealt with, the likelihood of a successful outcome is greater.

REFERENCES

1. Alpar JJ: The use of Healon in corneal transplant surgery with and without intraocular lenses, *Ophthalmic Surg* 15:757, 1984.
2. Kirsch RE: Further studies on the use of digital pressure in cataract surgery. 1. Optimal length of time for application of digital pressure, *Arch Ophthalmol* 58: 641, 1957.
3. McNeill JI, Goldman KN, Kaufman HE: Combined scleral ring and blepharostat, *Am J Ophthalmol* 83: 592-593, 1977.
4. Waltman SR, Krupin T: *Complications in Ophthalmic Surgery,* Philadelphia, 1980, *J P Lippincott,* p 140.
5. Olson RJ: Variation in corneal graft size related to trephine technique, *Arch Ophthalmol* 97: 1323-1325, 1979.
6. Perl T, Charlton KH, Binder PS: Disparate diameter grafting, astigmatism, intraocular pressure, and visual acuity, *Ophthalmology* 88: 774-781, 1981.
7. Wilson SE, Bourne WM: Effect of recipient-donor trephine size disparity or refractive error in keratoconus, *Ophthalmology* 96: 299-304, 1989.
8. Zimmerman T, Olson R, Waltman S et al. Transplant size and elevated intraocular pressure post keratoplasty, *Arch Ophthalmol* 96: 2231-2233, 1978.
9. Bourne WM, O'Fallon Wm: Endothelial cell loss during penetrating keratoplasty, *Am J Ophthalmol* 85: 760-766, 1978.
10. Bourne WM: Reduction of endothelial cell loss during phakic penetrating keratoplasty, *Am J Ophthalmol* 89: 787-790, 1980.
11. Casey TA, Mayer DJ: *Corneal grafting - principals and practice;* London, 1984, WB Saunders, p 291.
12. Gruber PF, Schipper I, Kerr R: Use of Healon for corneal trephination in penetrating keratoplasty, *Ophthalmol Surg* 15: 773, 1984.
13. Gills JP: Constant mild compression of the eye to produce hypotension, *J Am Intraocular Implant Soc* 5: 52-53, 1979.
14. Hirst LW, DeJaun E Jr: Sodium Hyaluronate and tissue adhesives in treating corneal perforation, *Ophthalmology* 89: 1250, 1982.
15. Taylor DM, Stern AL, McDonald P: The triple procedure: 2 to 10 year follow-up, *Trans Am Ophthalmol Soc* 84: 221-249, 1986.
16. Hunkeler JD, Hyde LL: The triple procedure: combined penetrating keratoplasty, extracapsular cataract extraction: an expanded experience, *Am Intraocular Implant Soc J* 9:20-24, 1983.
17. Meyer RF, Musch DC: Assessment of success and complications of triple procedure surgery, *Trans Am Ophthalmol Soc* 85: 350-367, 1987.
18. Crawford GJ, Stulting RD, Waring Geo et al: The triple procedure, *Ophthalmology* 93: 817-824, 1986.
19. Koenig SB, McDermott ML, Hyndiuck RA: Penetrating keratoplasty and intraocular lens exchange for pseudophakic bullous keratopathy associated with a closed loop anterior chamber intraocular lens, *Am J Ophthalmol* 108: 43, 1989.
20. Koenig SB, Solomon JM: Removal of closed loop anterior chamber intraocular lenses during penetrating keratoplasty, *Cornea* 6: 207, 1987.
21. Lass JH: Lens replacement in pseudophakic bullous keratopathy: *Corneal surgery, theory, technique and tissue;* ed2, St. Louis, 1993, Mosby, pp 163-166.
22. Purcell JJ Jr: Expulsive hemorrhage. In Brightbill F, editor: *Corneal surgery, theory, technique and tissue,* ed2, St Louis, 1993, Mosby, pp. 221-224.
23. Girard LJ et al: Expulsive hemorrhage during intraocular surgery, *Trans Am Acad Ophth Otolaryngal* 77: 119-125, 1973.

24. Taylor DM: Expulsive hemorrhage: some observations and comments, *Trans Am Ophthalmol Soc* 92: 33-35, 1974.
25. Purcell JJ Jr et al: Expulsive hemorrhage in penetrating keratoplasty, *Ophthalmology* 89: 41-43, 1982.
26. Samuels B: Postoperative non-expulsive subchoroidal hemorrhage, *Arch Ophthalmol* 8: 842-851, 1931.
27. Gressel MG, Parrish RK, Heuer DK: Delayed non-expulsive suprachoroidal hemorrhage, *Arch Ophthalmol* 102: 1757-1760, 1984.
28. Manschot WA: Glaucoma-vascular necrosis expulsive hemorrhage, *Acta Ophthalmol (Copenh)* 23: 309-342, 1945
29. Alm A, Bill A: Ocular and optic nerve blood flow at normal and increased intraocular pressures in monkeys (macaca irus): a study with radioactively labeled microsphere including flow determinations in brain and some other tissues, *Exp Eye Res* 15: 15-29, 1973.

SECTION THREE *Penetrating Keratoplasty: Postoperative Management*

CHAPTER 135

COREY A. MILLER

Routine Management

Penetrating keratoplasty has become the most common tissue transplant procedure with more than 40,000 cases performed annually in the United States.[1] The success of this procedure has usually been gauged by a resultant clear graft in greater than 90% of first corneal transplants.[1,2] Graft survival in high risk corneal transplants at 3 years follow-up is reduced to approximately 65%.[3]

The greater success of corneal transplants compared to other organ transplants has been attributed to the cornea's avascularity and immunologic privilege. Advances in corneal preservation techniques, storage media, and antibiotics have created more viable donor material. Newer surgical methods and technology have improved the initial results and reduced intraoperative complications. This chapter will focus on the routine postoperative care of the corneal transplant patient from the time of surgery until stabilization of the graft and visual rehabilitation. Managing complications of penetrating keratoplasty will be covered more in depth in Chapter 136.

The risk factors unique to the particular patient and transplant procedure need to be noted by the surgeon and the recipient preoperatively when planning the postoperative visual rehabilitation.[4,5] Emphasis should be placed on avoidance, early recognition, and treatment of complications through frequent postoperative evaluations, management of associated ocular and systemic conditions, and effective, routine postoperative care.

Most corneal surgeons recognize that there are many problems and challenges that may arise in the postoperative corneal transplant patient even in low risk categories and after uncomplicated surgery. The indications for penetrating keratoplasty have changed over time, with a higher relative percentage of patients with prior ocular surgery and previous failed grafts, as compared to corneal transplants in previously unoperated eyes[2,3,5,6] (box). The associated problems with these previously operated eyes create new risks and challenges in postoperative management.[7,8] Recent collaborative studies in the United States have standardized the treatment regimen and clarified outcomes in these higher risk patients.[9]

Routine postoperative care varies greatly even among subspecialist corneal surgeons in the United States.[10] Standardized care regimens facilitate study and comparison of methods and patient groups but do not allow for the individual differences seen in transplanted patients. The suggested treatment parameters in this chapter should be used as reference guidelines to be modified by the individual surgeon. The goal is to combine the anatomic success of a clear graft with the functional result of good vision.[11,12]

This chapter is divided into five sections: Immediate postoperative care (first 24 hours), early postoperative care (1 week), postoperative care, (1-12 weeks), postoperative care after 3 months, and postoperative care in infants and children.

Immediate Postoperative Care

FIRST 24 HOURS

Care during the first 24 hours following completion of surgery for penetrating keratoplasty should focus on maintenance of wound integrity, prevention of infection, control of possible elevations of intraocular pressure, and patient comfort. The medications administered will depend on the type and nature of the procedure performed and the occurrence of intraoperative complications.

Antibiotics should be given to prevent wound contamination and to treat possible microbial inocu-

Indications for penetrating keratoplasty

- Pseudophakic corneal edema
- Keratoconus
- Aphakic corneal edema
- Failed graft
- Fuchs' corneal dystrophy
- Herpes simplex keratopathy
- Inflammation
- Trauma
- Stromal dystrophies

lation at the time of surgery. The ideal antibiotic is broad spectrum with low toxicity and allergic potential, in addition to high potency, solubility, and the ability to sustain tear film levels after administration. Currently, the fluoroquinolones offer the best combination of these characteristics in the commercially available topical medications. Ofloxacin 0.3% penetrates the eye better than ciprofloxacin 0.3% or norfloxacin 0.3% and may provide significant anterior chamber levels of antibiotic following topical administration. Ofloxacin also has better activity against alpha-hemolytic streptococci. The author currently prefers to use topical ofloxacin or ciprofloxacin in the perioperative period following a subconjunctival injection of cefazolin immediately following surgery.[13] Subconjunctival tobramycin and topical tobramycin ointment are administered with cefazolin in cases in which topical fluoroquinolones are not used. Collagen shields may enhance drug delivery to the postsurgical eye and promote early epithelial healing and wound protection.[14,15] Donor rim cultures should be performed routinely since there is a high correlation between causative organisms in early postoperative endophthalmitis and the results of rim cultures.[16,17]

Oral fluoroquinolone administration may also be considered in addition to topical application in high risk cases such as those with preexisting external eye infections, prosthesis use in the fellow eye, penetrating trauma, and combined procedures, especially with vitrectomy or the use of intraocular lenses, notably those with proline haptics. Ciprofloxacin 500 to 750 milligrams or ofloxacin 200 to 400 milligrams taken twice daily perioperatively and for 3 to 5 days following surgery may achieve and maintain significant intraocular levels of antibiotic in these cases.[18-21]

Prophylactic antiglaucoma medication should be given particularly in penetrating keratoplasties combined with cataract surgery, vitrectomies, lysis of synechiae or the use of large amounts of sodium hyaluronate.[22] Patients with a history of glaucoma are at a higher risk for postoperative intraocular pressure elevation and should have their medications continued or augmented with intracameral miotics or systemic carbonic anhydrase inhibitors. Significant intraocular pressure increases may occur in the first few hours following surgery and high-risk patients or patients with significant postoperative pain and nausea may need to be evaluated on the day of surgery.[22]

Other topical medications used at the end of surgery include cycloplegics, especially in phakic patients. Traditionally, corneal surgeons have avoided using atropine in keratoconus due to the reported occurrence of long-term mydriasis. More recent data has refuted this claim.[23] Shorter acting agents such as cyclopentoltate 1% may be administered safely in these patients for early postoperative pain and inflammation control. Approximately one half of corneal surgeons administer subconjunctival steroids following keratoplasty in both routine and high-risk categories.[10]

A pressure patch and Fox shield should be placed following the medications mentioned above. The patient may resume a normal diet and most routine activities depending on the type of anesthesia used for the surgery. Most of the traditional warnings about activities such as bending over, stooping, straining and position of sleep are probably outmoded in routine modern cases. Moderation should be encouraged and avoidance of direct eye trauma should be emphasized to both the patient and family members.

Pain in the early postoperative period has been greatly reduced by the use of long-acting retrobulbar anesthetic agents such as bupivacaine. Treatment of postoperative pain should be undertaken with acetaminophen and oral nonsteroidal antiinflammatory medications and, in more severe cases, with narcotic medication. Aspirin-containing medications should probably be avoided due to the higher potential for bleeding, especially in more complicated anterior segment reconstructions. Extreme, early pain should alert the operating surgeon to the possibility of unexpected complications and should prompt early examination of the patient.[22] Systemic steroids are commonly administered in high-risk keratoplasty in the early postoperative period, usually at a dose of 1 milligram per kilogram per day over the first 5 to 7 days. Acyclovir in a prophylactic dose of 400 milligrams twice daily is given perioperatively in some cases of herpetic keratitis.[24,25]

Early Postoperative Care

1 TO 7 DAYS

Treatment of the postkeratoplasty patient in the first week following surgery should focus on reestablishing the corneal epithelium, controlling inflammation, preventing infection, treating any operative complications, and continuing good patient and family education. Often the corneal surgeon will view the first postoperative visit as a quick check-up focused on the presence or absence of immediate complications. This examination brings the surgeon together with a more alert patient, usually in the company of family and friends. It is a good opportunity for initiating therapy in a context that assumes better patient compliance and follow-up, and insures an improved postoperative course.

The postkeratoplasty patient should be examined in the first 36 hours following surgery. Often it is helpful to remove the pressure patch and give the patient a few minutes to adapt before proceeding with the evaluation. The level of uncorrected, or at least pinhole acuity should be documented. The status of the pupil is assessed. Extraocular motility may still be affected depending on the type of anesthesia administered.

Careful attention must be given to the presence of concomitant external eye and eyelid disease including blepharitis, lagophthalmos, spastic entropion, or trichiasis. These conditions may not be significant to the normal eye but can be a notable impairment to return of function in the postkeratoplasty eye. Vigorous eyelid scrubbing should be avoided in the postoperative period, and patients with blepharitis may be treated with nighttime antibiotic ointment applied to the lid margins or with systemic tetracycline or doxycycline.

Lagophthalmos may be exaggerated by recovery from anesthesia, conjunctival chemosis, and periocular swelling. The application of preservative-free tears and or ointments may be sufficient in milder cases Reapplication of the pressure patch may be necessary for a short period of time. More severe cases of exposure should be treated with tarsorrhaphy. This can be accomplished by application of cyanoacrylate glue, botulinum toxin injections, or by suture techniques.[26-28] Generally, a lateral tarsorrhaphy is performed first with a medial tarsorrhaphy performed later if needed. Intraoperative tarsorrhaphy is preferred in patients with known preoperative lid pathology and in neurotrophic conditions such as herpes zoster keratopathy.[29]

Examination with the slit lamp should be performed initially without topical fluorescein to assess the surgical wound, level of corneal edema, anterior chamber reaction, and overall status of the anterior segment. The application of fluorescein allows for a better evaluation of the status of the corneal epithelium wetting of the ocular surface, and tension on the suture material. Tight sutures tend to cause pooling of fluorescein away from the graft host junction due to puckering of the wound. Loose interrupted sutures or loops of a running suture will protrude through the epithelium or prevent overlying epithelialization. Leakage of aqueous with and without gentle pressure on the globe can be visualized using a Seidel test.

The intraocular pressure may be measured in more regular corneas by applanation. Other methods such as using a pneumotonometry, a McKay-Marg tonometer, or Tonopen can provide more accurate information in more distorted corneas and in cases with intraoperative lateral tarsorrhaphies.[30] Elevations of intraocular pressure on the first postoperative day are more common in patients with preoperative glaucoma, combined keratoplasty and cataract surgery with lens implantation (triple procedures), aphakia, in cases requiring significant anterior segment reconstruction, and with extensive viscoelastic use especially with hyaluronate.[22,31,32] Early glaucoma is also associated with persistent or acquired peripheral anterior synechiae.[31] Early moderate elevations of intraocular pressure may be manifested by increased corneal epithelial edema, especially in the host rim of the cornea, and may cause the graft stroma to appear relatively compact. Higher pressures generally result in increased graft edema diffusely with delayed reepithelialization.

Treatment of early intraocular pressure elevations involve the use of topical beta blockers followed by carbonic anhydrase inhibitors if needed.[22,31] Topical miotics are generally avoided in the early postoperative period unless needed for other indications. Nonsteroidal antiinflammatory agents administered topically may also be useful. In more extreme pressure elevations, systemic osmotics can be given.

Most early postoperative glaucoma can be treated with rather simple measures. Attention must be given to the status of the anterior chamber and iris. Elevated intraocular pressure, with a narrowed anterior chamber due to pupillary block, can be relieved by mydriasis or laser iridotomy. A similar clinical presentation can also be seen with suprachoroidal hemorrhage with a forward shift of the iris diaphragm.

A surgical wound leak is usually accompanied by a shallowed anterior chamber, low intraocular pressure, and a positive Seidel test. Suture tract or small wound disparity leaks can usually be treated with pressure patching, collagen shields, or with a therapeutic soft contact lens. More significant leaks usually require suture adjustment or placement of new sutures. The application of tissue adhesive seems to be less effective in the presence of suture material. Anterior wound disparities have been treated successfully with long-term soft contact lens application.[33]

Once the status of the anterior segment has been assessed, topical and systemic treatment can be planned and the patient and family can be educated regarding appropriate medications. The type of treatment will vary depending on the nature of the procedure, any intraoperative complications, and the early postoperative status. Sticking to a fixed formula of early treatment will often lead to keratitis medicamentosa in more routine cases and under-treatment in higher risk cases or cases with complications.

Generally, topical steroid treatment is initiated with prednisolone acetate 1% or prednisolone sodium phosphate 1% drops.[34] These are administered at a minimum of four times daily and in severe inflammation, can be used up to every hour when the patient is awake. Dexamethasone sodium phosphate ointment may be administered at bedtime for a more sustained dosage during sleep. Ofloxacin or another fluoroquinolone antibiotic is given four times daily in routine cases until the graft epithelium is intact. When additional lubrication is necessary, preservative-free preparations are generally used due to the sensitive nature of the graft epithelium and the combined toxicity of multiple preservative–containing medications.

Nonspecific topical beta blockers should be used with caution due to their systemic effect, and their application should be followed immediately by punctal occlusion for a period of approximately 3 minutes. To avoid potential interactions, concomitant systemic steroids, carbonic anhydrase inhibitors, or antibiotic therapy should be initiated only with a thorough knowledge of the patient's medical history and other current systemic medications. Topical cycloplegia in the early postoperative period is probably underutilized, and may be a significant factor in relieving early postoperative pain due to ciliary spasm in the phakic patient or in cases with significant preoperative inflammation. Atropine sulfate 1%, scopolamine hydrobromide 0.25%, or homatropine hydrobromide 5% are usually administered twice daily, and cyclopentolate hydrochloride 1% may be administered up to four times daily. The patient should be instructed thoroughly in the proper administration of eye drops and ointments. A Fox shield is worn at night for at least the first week postoperatively and longer in high-risk individuals. Normal activities are encouraged, and physical exercise should be increased progressively as tolerated. Eye protection with glasses or wrap-around shields should be worn during increased activity in the early postoperative period. Safety glasses or goggles should be worn by postkeratoplasty patients in high-risk activities for the rest of their lives.

The treatment of an early persistent epithelial defect in a corneal transplant may be controversial. Traditionally, most keratoplasty patients wore pressure patches until the epithelium was intact. More recent data has demonstrated that the healing time of the defect is approximately the same if the patch is removed and just topical medications and lubricants are used. Although collagen shields may be useful immediately following surgery, they do not seem to be as effective in healing persistent epithelial defects in grafts.[35] Therapeutic soft contact lenses or disposable contact lenses may be used in cases where there is additional concern about the reepithelialization due to other external eye disease factors. Other treatment options to consider for persistent epithelial defects include reduction of potentially toxic topical medications, especially in patients with ocular surface disease, and lateral tarsorrhaphy for patients not responding to other treatments.

This author has found that even in grafts denuded entirely of epithelium at the time of surgery, once the epithelium has crossed the graft host junction and covered most of the suture material, the central epithelial defects tend to resolve just as quickly with topical lubrication without patching or contact lenses. Patients with epithelial defects should be reassessed regularly in the first days after surgery and therapy adjusted if there is significant delay or reversal of the spreading of the epithelium over the new graft. If therapeutic soft contact lenses are used, a flatter base curve lens usually does better due to the presence of conjunctival edema, which often leads to a tight lens syndrome with steeper base curve lenses. A new or unusual appearing epithelial defect occurring in the early postoperative period, which does not respond to conventional therapy, may be caused by herpes simplex keratitis.[36]

The corneal transplant patient and family should be instructed to notify the surgeon immediately with significant symptoms of pain, irritation, loss of vision, and ocular injection in the first week following surgery. Endophthalmitis following penetrating keratoplasty occurs at an incidence of approximately twice that found in cataract surgery. With early diagnosis and aggressive treatment, the overall visual outcome in these cases may be improved.[16,17,37,38]

Postoperative Care, 1 to 12 Weeks

One week to three months following surgery is the period of greatest change and highest risk for the corneal graft.[39,40] Care during this period should be directed towards prevention of rejection, infection, and cystoid macular edema along with early manipulation of corneal astigmatism. Identifying patients who are of higher risk for complications, and educating them to recognize the early signs and symptoms of problems, can greatly improve the outcome in penetrating keratoplasty.

The postoperative graft patient should be examined on a regular basis, particularly until the epithelium is intact over the graft. The new graft epithelium is extremely vulnerable to external influences especially during the first 3 months following reepithelialization. Topical antibiotics should generally be discontinued once the epithelium is intact. Continuing long-term topical antibiotic therapy selects out more resistant

> **Frequency of follow-up visits in routine cases**
>
> 1 day
> 1 week
> 2 weeks
> 1 month
> 2 months
> 3 months
> Then every 2 to 3 months for the first year

organisms, but does act significantly to prevent infection in the absence of other problems such as persistent epithelial defects, suture removal, exposure, or wound leaks.[41,42] The added toxicity of topical antibiotics, notably those such as the aminoglycosides, can be detrimental to the graft epithelium. Topical steroids may be continued or increased as needed for control of inflammation with an intact corneal epithelium.

The examination 1 week following the surgery is the time of greatest recognition of early endophthalmitis in penetrating keratoplasty. Endophthalmitis occurring early in penetrating keratoplasty is usually related to contaminated donor material, continuation of preexistent host disease, or a result of significant inoculation at the time of surgery.[37,43] Studies with cataract surgery have demonstrated that many patients will show positive anterior chamber cultures even after routine surgery. The goal of early antibiotic treatment in penetrating keratoplasty is to treat any possible inoculum. The majority of pathogens in early cases of endophthalmitis are gram-positive organisms that are often related to the normal flora of the eye. The early prophylaxis of endophthalmitis should be directed at this type of organism. In contrast, pathogens recovered from late cases of endophthalmitis associated with therapeutic contact lenses or eroded sutures, show a higher incidence of gram-negative organisms.

It may be difficult to distinguish between continuing postoperative inflammation or a rebound uveitis following surgery compared to an early endophthalmitis. The poor outcome of cases with endophthalmitis should prompt the corneal surgeon to be vigilant in these cases and to proceed with diagnostic and therapeutic measures aggressively in suspect cases.

With reestablishment of the corneal epithelium in the absence of other complications, the continuing follow-up care can be planned. Routine patients in the author's practice are seen at weekly intervals for the first 2 weeks following the surgery and then at monthly intervals over the next 3 months (box). Follow-up beyond that time is generally every 2 or 3 months depending on the suture technique or the type of visual rehabilitation. High-risk patients are generally seen twice as frequently.

At each examination, an interval history of symptoms should be obtained and any significant changes in systemic medications, systemic illnesses, or blood transfusions should be noted.[40] Visual acuities without correction, with a pinhole, and at least objective refraction are measured. Abnormalities in pupillary and motility evaluations and any significant external eye disease, such as blepharitis and lagophthalmos, should be identified.

The slit lamp examination in the postoperative patient includes an assessment of the corneal epithelium. The presence of any stromal vessels is significant especially if they enter the graft. The level of graft edema and folds is documented first by observation. Ultrasonic pachometry has been very helpful in following the progression of graft clearing, and corneal pachometry may be useful in identifying graft rejection as manifested by corneal thickening even before other signs of rejection are noted.[44] The endothelium is examined for the presence of any keratic precipitates, and the status of the endothelial cells may be assessed at the slit lamp by specular reflection. The anterior chamber reaction is graded separately for aqueous flare and any cellular components.

Careful attention must be paid in the postoperative period to identify any of the findings of graft rejection.[45] Epithelial rejection lines begin at the graft periphery and migrate towards the center of the graft with time. They are seen as hazy elevations in the epithelium and may stain with either fluorescein or rose bengal. These lines are usually seen in a relatively quiet or mildly inflamed eye. They are seen at a median of approximately 3 months following surgery and may occur in up to 15% of corneal transplants.

Although the epithelial rejection line may be a relatively self-limiting process heralding the replacement of the graft donor epithelium with host cells, in most cases, they precede other signs of endothelial rejection. This should alert the transplant surgeon to treat these patients more vigorously with steroids and to be more vigilant in the number and frequency of follow-up examinations.

Subepithelial infiltrates are often a component of graft rejection and are seen as gray-white infiltrates, approximately 0.2 to 0.5 millimeters in diameter, and are confined to the donor cornea. They are seen best with broad oblique slit lamp illumination or with scleral scatter. They have been reported in up to 15% of corneal transplants. Treatment with topical steroids results in resolution of the infiltrates. However, in larger or more dense infiltrates, a slight subepithelial scar or haze may persist even after successful treatment.

Signs of stromal rejection are seen as a haze or infiltrate spreading from the graft periphery towards the center of the donor cornea. These are associated with findings of endothelial rejection, and are frequently accompanied by stromal vascularization. The classic finding of endothelial rejection is a rather sharply demarcated line (Khodadoust line) that is seen as contiguous keratic precipitates. The Khodadoust line progresses across the endothelial surface, preceded on the advancing edge by endothelial edema and followed by endothelial findings of more diffuse keratic precipitates. Endothelial rejection results in the loss of endothelial function with stromal and epithelial edema. Accompanying signs to endothelial rejection include conjunctival hyperemia, ciliary flush, and varying degrees of anterior chamber reaction. Endothelial rejection often starts in quadrants involving deep neovascularization to the graft host junction or in areas of suture exposure or erosion. The risk factors predisposing to endothelial rejection include: young age at the time of corneal transplantation; history of previous anterior segment surgery; preoperative glaucoma; the number of quadrants of anterior synechiae present, quadrants of stromal vascularization; previous corneal transplants; the primary diagnosis of chemical burn; and blood group ABO incapability. Donor and preservation characteristics probably have no significant association with epithelial rejection.[2-5]

Epithelial downgrowth, occurring 1 to 12 weeks after penetrating keratoplasty, may also appear as an advancing line with signs of inflammation. The edge of the downgrowth is smooth or scalloped with a more refractile appearance and involves both donor and host cornea. Epithelial downgrowth progresses despite vigorous steroid therapy and ultimately has a poor prognosis.

Treatment of epithelial rejection and subepithelial infiltrates with topical steroids is usually quite successful. Treatment of endothelial rejection could also be initiated with topical steroids administered up to every hour when patient is awake and combined with one or more of the following additional modes of steroid administration: subconjunctival steroid injections, oral prednisone at approximately 1 milligram per kilogram per day, intravenous methylprednisolone 125 milligram to 500 milligram, and dexamethasone sodium phosphate ointment applied at night.[10,46] Concomitant cycloplegia may be necessary, and antiviral prophylaxis should be used in the treatment of endothelial rejection in patients with a previous history of herpes simplex keratitis. The transplant surgeon should also keep in mind any systemic disorders such as hypertension, diabetes, history of tuberculosis, or peptic ulcer disease, which could be affected significantly by systemic steroid administration. Ocular complications

Suggested tapering doses of topical steroids in routine cases*

Prednisolone acetate 1% or prednisolone sodium phosphate 1%

4 times a day for 3 weeks
3 times a day for 3 weeks
2 times a day for 3 weeks
Once a day for 3 weeks

Fluorometholone 0.1%

4 times a day for 3 weeks
3 times a day for 3 weeks
2 times a day for 3 weeks
Once a day for 3 weeks

* Topical steroids may be tapered sooner in phakic cases or with steroid-induced increases in intraocular pressure.

such as elevated intraocular pressure in steroid responders, cataract development in phakic individuals, and the epithelial toxicity in certain surface disorders that requires corneal transplantation should be considered when choosing the dose and type of administration of steroid therapy. Other agents such as systemic nonsteroidal antiinflammatory agents and systemic and topical cyclosporine have been used in cases with steroid complications or in combination with steroids in high-risk individuals.[47] Laser photocoagulation of stromal vessels has been successful in some cases to treat stromal neovascularization associated with graft rejection or in an attempt to prevent rejection and lipid deposition in affected individuals.[48,49]

In the absence of complications, topical steroids should be tapered during the first 3 months following penetrating keratoplasty. The box suggests a schedule of steroid tapering using two topical medications. Some surgeons find that patient compliance is better using clear topical medications rather than suspensions. Medications such as dexamethasone 0.1% drops or prednisolone sodium phosphate 1% may be used initially without significant loss of therapeutic effect. In cases requiring a slower steroid taper, medications including prednisolone acetate 0.125%, prednisone sodium phosphate 0.125%, fluorometholone acetate 0.1%, or fluoromethalone 0.25% are often substituted in the middle of steroid taper. In phakic individuals, the cataractogenic properties of topical steroids must be considered, and topical steroids should be tapered and discontinued as soon as possible. Although topical nonsteroidal anti-inflammatory drugs have been substituted successfully in the postcataract or refractive surgery patient, their role in routine treatment of the postkeratoplasty patient is not as defined.[50]

An assessment of intraocular pressure should be done on each postoperative visit. Electronic tonometry may be more successful and accurate in measuring pressures on irregular surfaces. With high corneal astigmatism postoperatively, applanation pressures can be best estimated by taking one measurement, rotating the prism 90 degrees to get a second measurement, and then using the average of the two measurements for estimation of the actual intraocular pressure.[30] Approximately 10% to 20% of patients on chronic topical steroid therapy will develop elevated intraocular pressure. This should be managed by steroid tapering, concomitant antiglaucoma therapy and assessment of any positive factors such as progressive peripheral anterior synechiae, intraocular bleeding, pupillary block, pigmentary dispersion, or inaccurate measurement. Fluorometholone 0.1% drops or nonsteroidal antiinflammatory drugs administered topically may be very beneficial in steroid tapering in affected individuals.[50] Laser trabeculoplasty may be an alternative to other more aggressive measures in managing persistent glaucoma in the postkeratoplasty patient.[51]

Once the graft has been stabilized with an intact epithelium, the surgeon can direct attention to the management of corneal astigmatism. Early manipulation of corneal astigmatism will depend greatly on the nature of the keratoplasty and the suturing method. Many claims have been made regarding the ultimate astigmatic result of certain suturing methods. The purpose of discussion in this chapter will be to encourage the surgeon to maximize control of the astigmatism with whatever method that has been selected.

The careful examination of the postkeratoplasty cornea by slit lamp examination may identify tight sutures that can cause a donut effect of the cornea with steepening around the suture and central flattening. In addition, epithelial and endothelial stress lines may be seen radiating from the tight sutures.[52] Conversely, loose suture material is associated with anterior wound gape and flattening immediately around the suture with relative central steepening. Methods to access the initial corneal astigmatism include refraction, retinoscopy, keratometry, corneoscopy, photokeratoscopy, and videokeratography. Any of these methods will often show very irregular corneal astigmatism on the early postkeratoplasty cornea (Figure 135-1).

The author recommends using whatever method or combination of methods necessary to feel comfortable about the nature of the astigmatism and effect of the suture material prior to any suture adjustment. For example handheld corneoscopy may be extremely helpful in identifying areas of tight suture when they are not obvious with standard keratometry or refraction. Certain features of any placido disc–based image system can be recognized in real time by corneoscopy. Tight sutures tend to compress the rings together. A D-pattern may be seen with relative flattening of the rings on one side of the area of tight sutures, and a bowing in of the rings may be seen in excessively tight sutures.[52,53] Videokeratography may be extremely helpful in identifying areas of tight or loose sutures when they are not obvious by other methods, in asymmetric astigmatism, and in cases when initial suture manipulation, indicated by other methods, did not produce the desired effect.[39,54]

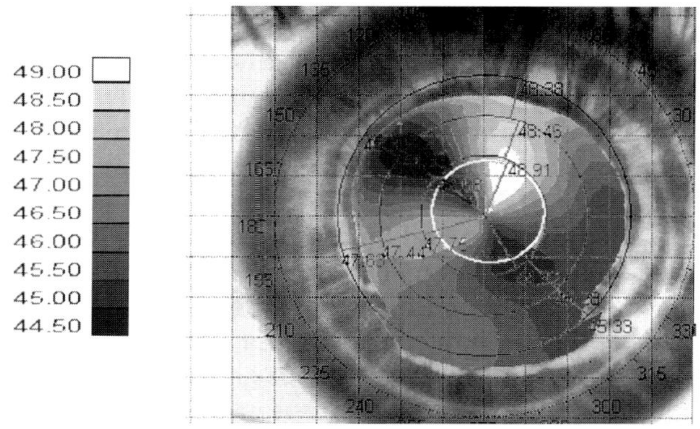

FIGURE 135-1 Irregular astigmatism postkeratoplasty as demonstrated by videokeratography. Four diopters of refractive astigmatism with steep axis at 49 degrees are present. Suture manipulation may reduce astigmatism by running suture rotation or selective interrupted suture removal. **See color plate 135-1.**

Four common types of suturing methods are used in penetrating keratoplasty: a single running suture technique, double running sutures, a combination of a running suture and interrupted sutures, and interrupted sutures only. Interrupted sutures tend to be used more in complicated grafts, especially those with preoperative neovascularization, large graft diameter, and in children. Early suture manipulation or removal may be applied to all of these techniques and may have early beneficial effects on visual rehabilitation.[55] Factors such as graft-host disparity, type of trephination employed, the placement of cardinal sutures, donor astigmatism, and presence of a scleral-fixated posterior chamber intraocular lens, etc. affect astigmatism following suture removal.[56] The ideal suturing system would be surgically fast and easy to perform, require the fewest number of suture manipulations postoperatively, result in a more stable cornea, and be associated with the fewest suture-related complications. Many surgeons, including the author, feel that the single-running suture technique, in selected cases, combined with early postoperative adjustment provides most of these benefits.[57-60]

Once the nature of the astigmatism has been identified and the plan made for adjustment, the procedure can generally be performed at a slit lamp in a cooperative adult patient. Topical anesthesia is in-

should be identified, and therapy altered if necessary. Many patients experience resolution of the macular edema with ongoing postkeratoplasty treatment independent of any specific treatment for cystoid macular edema. Other patients benefit by specific topical, local, or systemic treatment of cystoid macular edema. Topical steroids may be used particularly if there is associated anterior segment inflammation. Topical nonsteroidal antiinflammatory drops have been successful especially when used for longer periods of time in the treatment of cystoid macular edema.[50,63,64] Subtenons injections of deposteroid preparations may be used in cases without contraindications to their use. Systemic nonsteroidal agents and carbonic anhydrase inhibitors have been beneficial treatment for some individuals.[65] Pars plana vitrectomy has been used in cases of significant vitreous reaction or with anterior-posterior vitreous traction. Other causes of maculopathy, such as age-related maculopathy or light phototoxicity to the retina from the operating microscope, may be difficult to differentiate clinically from postoperative cystoid macular edema.

Care After 3 Months

Care after 3 months in routine cases focuses on the final visual rehabilitation of the patient, management of any long-term complications, and avoidance of iatrogenic problems. The ultimate refractive error in the transplant patient and how it is handled is the essential measure of "success" in corneal transplantation. A clear graft with ten diopters of irregular corneal astigmatism can hardly be judged "successful" from the patient's perspective.

In older published series, average postoperative astigmatism was in the 4 to 6 diopter range. Newer surgical methods and postoperative suture management have improved the initial refractive results but significant changes may still occur once sutures are removed.[66,67] The refractive status of the post-keratoplasty patient will challenge even the most experienced refractionist.[68] Multiple accurate refractions are necessary until the result is stable as the graft wound heals.

Some form of objective measurement of the corneal toricity is extremely helpful in beginning the refraction. Simple keratometry measurements and the qualitative appearance of the mires are useful in refraction because the visual axis or refractive portion of the graft is being assessed. Placing one half to two thirds of the measured total corneal astigmatism into the initial refraction with the plus cylinder in the steep axis, may expedite the subjective refinement.[68,69] Retinoscopy is often difficult due to the effects of the peripheral graft, especially with larger or irregular pupils and with intraocular lenses. Much less subjective cylinder correction may be accepted by the postkeratoplasty patient when compared to similar measured levels in naturally occurring astigmatism.[69] High levels of refractive cylindric correction should prompt reevaluation of the adequacy of suture manipulation. Videokeratography can be very useful in these cases, because both central and peripheral areas of the graft can be measured. Anisometropia, especially with high toricity, may require slab-off lens designs, separate distance and reading corrections, or may altogether preclude spectacle correction.[68]

Contact lens correction is generally indicated for convenience when the other eye requires contact lenses, in cases of high toricity and anisometropia, and in aphakia.[40,70] The presence of corneal sutures in these patients in the absence of other complications does not seem to alter the success rate of contact lens rehabilitation. Spherical gas-permeable hard contact lenses (GPHCL) may be successful even in visually rehabilitating patients with significant corneal toricity.[71,72]

A starting point for the initial GPHCL fit over a graft would be a base curve fit on the flattest keratometry reading and a contact lens diameter slightly larger than the donor corneal trephine size. Fitting programs are available on some videokeratography units and these may offer suggestions on initial values to be considered.[73] The final evaluation usually involves a trial fitting. The ideal lens should have adequate apical clearance on topical fluorescein evaluation, and good centration and movement. Centration may be difficult with high or irregular corneal astigmatism or a decentered graft, and larger diameter lenses with prism ballast or toric designs may be needed. Smaller lenses often show better centration within the suture line in cases with running sutures in place. Aspheric GPHCL designs and contact lenses incorporating a central GPHCL button surrounded by a soft contact lens skirt, have been used in cases with over 5 diopters of residual corneal toricity.[74,75] In cases in which contact lens wear does not show an improvement over best spectacle–corrected acuity or in cases with high levels of toricity precluding contact lens wear, surgical manipulation of the residual astigmatism should be considered. Methods such as repair of significant graft-host disparities, relaxing incisions with and without compression sutures, and corneal wedge resections could be selected depending on the nature and extent of the corneal toricity.

Soft contact lenses for visual rehabilitation following keratoplasty are generally used in aphakic children and adults, in anisometropic children, and in cases of low residual astigmatism, especially in nondominant eyes.[76] Higher oxygen permeability (K value) lenses with base curves flatter than the flattest K reading are generally used. The slit lamp evaluation should show at least 1 millimeter of lens movement with blinking and good centration. Since these lenses are often extended wear, the patients should be closely monitored for corneal neovascularization, graft rejection, and microbial keratitis.[77-79]

Corneal sensitivity may take years to return to normal in the corneal graft, and this may be a significant factor in the development and late recognition of microbial keratitis from contact lens wear or suture erosion.[78,80] The delayed return of corneal sensation may also explain why many postkeratoplasty patients may tolerate GPHCL fitting well, even in cases where these lenses were unsuccessful prekeratoplasty.

Significant iatrogenic complications may be induced by the chronic long-term administration of topical steroids in the post-keratoplasty patient. Steroids in combination with graft hypesthesia increases the risks of infectious crystalline keratopathy and other late graft infections often caused by very unusual pathogens.[42,78,81-85] Herpetic epithelial keratitis may be seen in long-term steroid use, even without a history of previous herpetic keratitis.[86] Glaucoma may be initiated or aggravated by long-term steroid use. The main risk factor for cataract development in the phakic postkeratoplasty patient seems to be age at the time of transplant, but the injudicious use of topical steroids may accelerate the process, which results in the risk of graft rejection at the time of cataract surgery.[87,88]

Topical steroids should be tapered and discontinued early, especially in low-risk phakic cases. If they are to be continued in aphakic, pseudophakic, or high-risk cases, the minimal effective dose should be prescribed and the potential for complications should be recognized. Effective long-term management of other risk factors such as keratoconjunctivitis sicca, chronic external eye disease, suture breakage or erosion, and contact lens wear is necessary.[89,90] Even following visual rehabilitation with glasses or contacts, postkeratoplasty patients should be followed regularly, usually every 2 or 3 months, while corneal sutures are in place. Patients with transsclerally-fixated IOLS, especially those without scleral flaps, have a long-term risk of proline suture exposure through the conjunctiva and possible endophthalmitis. Due to the permanent weakened nature of the keratoplasty wound, protective eyewear needs to be worn during high-risk activities. Since rejections have been described decades after keratoplasty and because of the higher risks of cataract development, glaucoma, and retinal detachment, regular comprehensive ocular examinations should be encouraged in the long-term care of the keratoplasty patient.

Postoperative Care in Infants and Children

A team approach combining the skills of the corneal surgeon, pediatric ophthalmologists, anesthesiologists, other hospital staff, and cooperative parents is necessary for successful postoperative care of the postkeratoplasty patient, especially under the age of 6. A clear graft combined with early visual rehabilitation and amblyopia therapy is necessary for visual and not just anatomical success.[91-94]

Children often have an intense inflammatory reaction in the anterior segment following keratoplasty. Treatment needs to be vigorous with cycloplegia, subconjunctival and often systemic steroids, in addition to frequent application of topical steroids in the early postoperative period. Perioperative antibiotic administration can be followed by topical fluoroquinolone drops given at least four times daily. Once pressure patching has been discontinued, a Fox shield should be used for protection along with hand mitts or arm restraints in uncooperative younger children and infants. This same group may need to be exposed to frequent examination under anesthesia (EUA) for monitoring of the early postoperative course, measurement of intraocular pressures, and suture manipulation or removal. A portable slit lamp or a handheld light and condensing lens are helpful in examining hospitalized infants and during EUA. Intraocular pressures should be measured often, particularly in patients with congenital anterior segment problems and in combined procedures.[91,92,94,95] Office slit lamp examination may be possible in children ages 4 and older. By the age of 7 or 8, sutures may often be removed with topical anesthesia at the slit lamp, especially if the child is comfortable with the environment and the surgeon.

Epithelial and stromal healing are very rapid in children resulting in early suture loosening, exposure, secondary vascularization, and subsequent rejection. Infants and young children may need to be examined every 2 days until the sutures are removed. Older children should be examined at least every week for the first few months or until suture removal. Nursing personnel and parents should be trained to recognize signs such as loss of graft clarity, ocular injection, mucus around sutures, and should report symptoms such as insomnia, frequent attempts at eye rubbing, eyelid closure, or photophobia in the nonverbal child. Tight sutures will often cheesewire through the very pliable host pediatric cornea. Exposed interrupted or running sutures should be removed promptly with appropriate antibiotic prophylaxis.[94]

Optical rehabilitation of the visually immature child must be done quickly and effectively to avoid irreversible amblyopia and strabismus. This is especially challenging in cases with significant anisometropia such as high postoperative myopia caused by very young donor tissue, high corneal toricity, and in cases of pediatric aphakia, especially if unilateral.[96-99]

Aphakic contact lenses may be placed at the time of surgery or within the first few days following surgery in infantile aphakia and should be monitored with frequent EUA. Corneoscopy, keratometry, and retinoscopy should be performed regularly to aid in the selection and use of optical devices for visual rehabilitation.[94,95] Occlusion therapy should be initiated as early as possible to treat and avoid further development of amblyopia. Care should be taken not to induce deprivation amblyopia of the fellow eye in younger children by excessive occlusion. Similarly, bilateral corneal disease should be treated with surgery on the fellow eye as soon as tolerated in infants. Although rapid visual rehabilitation is less critical in visually mature children and adolescents, these patients will still need frequent monitoring due to rapid healing and the propensity to develop inflammation, vascularization, and rejection. These patients should be examined at least monthly over the first year following keratoplasty. Since the cornea is more compliant in children, suture manipulation and incisional techniques for control of astigmatism usually have a more pronounced effect than with the adult cornea. Due to the difficulty in restricting activities and the higher risk of inadvertent trauma in children, adequate protective eyewear use should be encouraged.

Repeat penetrating keratoplasty in children carries a less optimistic prognosis for successful visual rehabilitation. Every attempt should be made to insure the success of first grafts by good patient and family education, close follow-up examinations, rapid suture removal, and the judicious use of topical steroids to control inflammation and reduce rejection episodes. Successful application of these measures may allow a lifetime of improved vision for the visually compromised child.[94]

REFERENCES

1. Council on Scientific Affairs: Report on the organ transplant panel: corneal transplantation, *JAMA* 259:719-722, 1988.
2. Vail A et al: Corneal graft survival and visual outcome. A multicenter study, *Ophthalmology* 101:120-127, 1994.
3. The Collaborative Corneal Transplantation Studies Research Group: The collaborative corneal transplantation studies, *Arch Ophthalmol* 110:1392-1403, 1992.
4. Maguire MG et al: Risk factors for corneal graft failure and rejection in the collaborative corneal transplantation studies, *Ophthalmology* 101:1536-1547, 1994.
5. Beekhuis WH: Current clinician's opinions on risk factors in corneal grafting. Results of a survey among surgeons in the eurotransplant area, *Cornea* 14(1):39-42, 1995.
6. Hyman L et al: Indications and techniques of penetrating keratoplasties, 1985-1988, *Cornea* 11(6):573-576, 1992.
7. Rapuano CJ et al: Indications for and outcomes of repeat penetrating keratoplasty, *Am J Ophthalmol* 109:689-695, 1990.
8. Kenyon KR, Starck T, Hersh PS: Penetrating keratoplasty and anterior segment reconstruction for severe ocular trauma, *Ophthalmology* 99(3):396-402, 1992.
9. The Collaborative Corneal Transplantation Studies Research Group: Design and methods of the collaborative transplantation studies, *Cornea* 12(2):93-103, 1993.
10. Rinne JR, Stulting RD: Current practices in the prevention and treatment of corneal graft rejection, *Cornea* 11(4):326-328, 1992.
11. Price FW, Whitson WE, Marks RG: Progression of visual acuity after penetrating keratoplasty, *Ophthalmology* 98:1177-1185, 1991.
12. Williams KA et al: Long-term outcome after corneal transplantation. Visual result and patient perception of success, *Ophthalmology* 98(5):651-657, 1991.
13. Bower KS, Kowalski RP, Gordon YJ: Which quinolone when combined with fortified Cefazolin would be best for the treatment of bacterial keratitis? *Ophthalmol Vis Sci* 34:1674, 1994.
14. Aquavella JV et al: Use of collagen shields as a surgical adjunct, *J Cataract Refract Surg* 14:492-495, 1988.
15. Ruffini JJ, Aquavella JV, Lo Cascio JA: Effect of collagen shields on corneal epithelialization following penetrating keratoplasty, *Ophthalmic Surg* 20(1):21-25, 1989.
16. Cameron JA et al: Endophthalmitis from contaminated donor corneas following penetrating keratoplasty, *Arch Ophthalmol* 109:54-59, 1991.
17. Kloess PM et al: Bacterial and fungal endophthalmitis after penetrating keratoplasty, *Am J Ophthalmol* 115:309-316, 1993.
18. Mounier M, Adenis JP, Denis F: Intraocular penetration of ciprofloxacin after infusion and oral administration, *Pathol Biol (Paris)* 36(5 Pt):724-727, 1988.
19. Fadi A et al: Intravitreal penetration of oral ciprofloxacin in humans, *Ophthalmology* 99:483, 1992.
20. Lesk MR et al: The penetration of oral ciprofloxacin into the aqueous humor, vitreous, and subretinal fluid of humans, *Am J Ophthalmol* 115:623, 1993.
21. Mounier M et al: Study of intraocular diffusion of ofloxacin in humans and rabbits, *Pathol Biol (Paris)* 40(5):529, 1992.
22. Chien AM et al: Glaucoma in the immediate postoperative period after penetrating keratoplasty, *Am J Ophthalmol* 115:711-714, 1993.
23. Geyer O, Rothkoff GO, Lazar M: Atropine in keratoplasty for keratoconus, *Cornea* 10(5):372-373, 1991.
24. Collin J, Robinet A, Malet F: Preventive treatment of herpetic keratitis with acyclovir tablets, *J Fr Ophtalmol* 16(1):6-9, 1993.
25. Barney NP, Foster CS: A prospective randomized trial of oral acyclovir after penetrating keratoplasty for herpes simplex keratitis, *Cornea* 13(3):232-236, 1994.
26. Donnefeld ED, Perry HD, Nelson DB: Cyanoacrylate temporary tarsorrhaphy in the management of corneal epithelial defects, *Ophthalmic Surg* 22:591-593, 1991.
27. Adams FFW, Kirkness CM, Lee JP: Botulinum toxin A induced protective ptosis, *Eye* 1:603-608, 1987.
28. Koenig SB, Harris GJ: Temporary suture tarsorrhaphy after penetrating keratoplasty, *Cornea* 10(2):121-122, 1991.
29. Reed JW, Joyner SJ, Knauer WJ III: Penetrating keratoplasty for herpes zoster keratopathy, *Am J Ophthalmol* 107:257-261, 1989.
30. Whitacre MM, Stein R: Sources of error with use of Goldmann-type tonometers, *Surv Ophthalmol* 38(1):1-29, 1993.
31. Foulks GN: Glaucoma associated with penetrating keratoplasty, *Ophthalmology* 94:871-874, 1987.
32. Kirkness CM, Ficker LA: Risk factors for the development of postkeratoplasty glaucoma, *Cornea* 11(5):427-432, 1992.

33. Mannis MJ, Zadnik K: Hydrophilic contact lenses for wound stabilization in keratoplasty, *CLAO J* 14(4):199-202, 1988.
34. Sousa FJ: The bioavailability and therapeutic effectiveness of prednisolone acetate vs prednisolone sodium phosphate: a 20 year review, *CLAO J* 17(4):282-284, 1991.
35. Groden LR, White W: Porcine collagen corneal shield treatment of persistent epithelial defects following penetrating keratoplasty, *CLAO J* 16(2):95, 1990.
36. Sundmacher R, Wolff M: Four years experience with triple procedures in herpes afflicted eyes, *Ger J Ophthalmol* 2(2):65, 1993.
37. Aiello LP, Javitt JC, Canner JK: National outcomes of penetrating keratoplasty, *Arch Ophthalmol* 111:509, 1993.
38. Guss RB et al: Endophthalmitis after penetrating keratoplasty, *Am J Ophthalmol* 95:651, 1983.
39. Khong AM et al: Computerized topographic analysis of the healing graft after penetrating keratoplasty for keratoconus, *Am J Ophthalmol* 115(2):209, 1993.
40. Smiddy WE et al: Visual correction following penetrating keratoplasty, *Arch Ophthalmol* 105:138, 1987.
41. Driebe WT, Stern GA: Microbial keratitis following corneal transplantation, *Cornea* 2(1):41, 1983.
42. Fong LP et al: Microbial keratitis complicating penetrating keratoplasty, *Ophthalmology* 95:1269, 1988.
43. Kloess PM et al: Bacterial and fungal endophthalmitis after penetrating keratoplasty, *Am J Ophthalmol* 115(4):548, 1993.
44. McDonnell PJ et al: Corneal thickness changes after high-risk penetrating keratoplasty, *Arch Ophthalmol* 111:155, 1993.
45. Alldredge OC, Krachmer JH: Clinical types of corneal transplant rejection: Their manifestations, frequency, preoperative correlates, and treatment, *Arch Ophthalmol* 99:599, 1981.
46. Hill JC, Ivey A: Corticosteroids in corneal graft rejection: double versus single pulse therapy, *Cornea* 13(5):383, 1994.
47. Belin MW et al: Topical cyclosporine in high-risk corneal transplants, *Ophthalmology* 96:1144, 1989.
48. Nirankari VS, Baer JC: Corneal argon laser photocoagulation for neovascularization in penetrating keratoplasty, *Ophthalmology* 93(10):1304, 1986.
49. Baer JC, Foster CS: Corneal laser photocoagulation for treatment of neovascularization, *Ophthalmology* 99:173, 1992.
50. Flach AJ: Cyclo-oxygenase inhibitors in ophthalmology, *Surv Ophthalmol* 36(4):259, 1992.
51. Van Meter WS et al: Laser trabeculoplasty for glaucoma in aphakic and pseudophakic eyes after penetrating keratoplasty, *Arch Ophthalmol* 106:185, 1988.
52. Rowsey JJ et al: Use of keratoscopy, slitlamp biomicroscopy, and retinoscopy in the management of astigmatism after penetrating keratoplasty, *Refractive Corneal Surgery* 7(1):33-41, 1991.
53. Harris DJ Jr, Waring Go III, Burk LL: Keratography as a guide to selective suture removal for the reduction of astigmatism after penetrating keratoplasty, *Ophthalmology* 96(11):1597, 1989.
54. Strelow S et al: Corneal topography for selective suture removal after penetrating keratoplasty, *Am J Ophthalmol* 112:657, 1991.
55. Linch Te et al: An adjustable double running suture technique for keratoplasty, *Am J Ophthalmol* 116(2):201, 1993.
56. Hardten DR et al: Clinical and anatomical study of the effect of transscleral fixation of posterior chamber lenses on early postkeratoplasty astigmatism, *Cornea* 12(4):282, 1993.
57. McNeill JI, Wessels IF: Adjustment of single continuous suture to control astigmatism after penetrating keratoplasty, *Refractive Corneal Surgery* 5:216-223, 1989.
58. Van Meter WS et al: Postkeratoplasty astigmatism control: single continuous suture adjustment versus selective interrupted suture removal, *Ophthalmology* 98:177, 1991.
59. Lin DT et al: An adjustable single running suture technique to reduce postkeratoplasty astigmatism. A preliminary report, *Ophthalmology* 97(7):934, 1990.
60. Filatov V, Steinert RF, Talamo JH: Postkeratoplasty astigmatism with single running suture or interrupted sutures, *Am J Ophthalmol* 115:715, 1993.
61. Burk LL, Waring Go III, Harris DJ Jr: Simultaneous and sequential selective suture removal to reduce astigmatism after penetrating keratoplasty, *Refractive Corneal Surgery* 6(3):179-187, 1990.
62. Flach AJ et al: Prophylaxis of aphakic cystoid macular edema without corticosteroids, *Ophthalmology* 97:1253, 1990.
63. Flach AJ et al: Improvement in visual acuity in chronic aphakic and pseudophakic cystoid macular edema after treatment with topical 0.5% ketorolac tromethamine, *Am J Ophthalmol* 112(5):514, 1991.
64. Solomon LD: Efficacy of topical flurbiprofen and indomethacin in preventing pseudophakic cystoid macular edema, *J Cataract Refract Surg* 21:73, 1995.
65. Cox SN, Hay E, Bird AC: Treatment of chronic macular edema with acetazolamide, *Arch Ophthalmol* 106:190, 1988.
66. Mader TH et al: Changes in keratometric astigmatism after suture removal more than one year after penetrating keratoplasty, *Ophthalmology* 100:119, 1993.
67. Mathers WD et al: Corneal steepening with final suture removal after penetrating keratoplasty, *Cornea* 10(3):221, 1991.
68. Mannis MJ, Zadnik K: Perspectives in refraction: refracting the corneal graft, *Surv Ophthalmol* 34(6):436, 1990.
69. Judge D et al: Refractive versus keratometric astigmatism postkeratoplasty, *Refractive Corneal Surgery* 6(3):174-178, 1990.
70. Smiddy WE et al: Keratoconus: contact lens or keratoplasty? *Ophthalmology* 95(4):487, 1988.
71. Mannis MJ, Zadnik K, Deutch D: Rigid contact lens wear in the corneal transplant patient, *CLAO J* 12(1):39, 1986.
72. Beekhuis WH et al: Contact lenses following keratoplasty, *CLAO J* 17(1):27, 1991.
73. Lopatynsky M et al: Corneal topography for rigid gas permeable lens fitting after penetrating keratoplasty, *CLAO J* 19(1):41, 1993.
74. Weiner BM, Nirankari VS: A new biaspheric contact lens for severe astigmatism following penetrating keratoplasty, *CLAO J* 18(2):81, 1992.
75. Binder PS, Kopecky L: Fitting the SoftPerm contact lens after keratoplasty, *CLAO J* 18(3):170, 1992.
76. Mannis MJ, Matsumoto ER: Extented-wear soft contact lenses after penetrating keratoplasty, *Arch Ophthalmol* 101:1225, 1983.
77. Fong LP et al: Microbial keratitis complicating penetrating keratoplasty, *Ophthalmology* 95(5):1269, 1988.
78. Harris DJ Jr et al: Late bacterial and fungal keratitis after corneal transplantation. Spectrum of pathogens, graft survival, and visual prognosis, *Ophthalmology* 95(10):1450, 1988.
79. Varley GA, Meisler DM: Complications of penetrating keratoplasty: graft infections, *Refractive Corneal Surgery* 7(1):62-66, 1991.
80. Tugal Tutkun I et al: Corneal sensitivity after penetrating keratoplasty, *Eur J Ophthalmol* 3(2):66, 1993.
81. Meisler DM et al: Infectious crystalline keratopathy, *Am J Ophthalmol* 97:337, 1984.
82. Reiss GR, Campbell RJ, Bourne WM: Afterimages: infectious crystalline keratopathy, *Surv Ophthalmol* 31(1):69, 1986.
83. Weisenthal RW et al: Postkeratoplasty crystalline depositis mimicking bacterial infectious crystalline keratopathy, *Am J Ophthalmol* 105(1):70, 1988.
84. Lubniewski AJ et al Posterior infectious crystalline keratopathy with staphylococcus epidermidis, *Ophthalmology* 97(11):1454, 1990.
85. Lam S, Meisler DM, Krachmer JH: Enterococcal infectious crystalline keratopathy, *Cornea* 12(3):273, 1993.

86. Mannis MJ et al: Herpes simplex dendritic keratitis after keratoplasty, *Am J Ophthalmol* 112(3):355, 1991.
87. Wood TO, Waltman SR, Kaurman HE: Steroid cataracts following penetrating keratoplasty, *Annals of Ophthalmology* 3:496, 1971.
88. Martin TP et al: Cataract formation and cataract extraction after penetrating keratoplasty, *Ophthalmology* 101:113, 1994.
89. Dana MR et al: Suture erosion after penetrating keratoplasty, *Cornea* 14(3):243, 1995.
90. Spigelman AV et al: Visual loss following suture removal postkeratoplasty, *Cornea* 7(3):214, 1988.
91. Cowden JW: Penetrating keratoplasty in infants and children, *Ophthalmology* 97(3):324, 1990.
92. Erlich CM, Rootman DS, Morin JD: Corneal transplantation in infants, children and young adults: experience of the Toronto hospital for sick children, *Can J Ophthalmol* 26(4):206, 1991.
93. Legeais JM, Jobin D, Pouliquen Y: Keratoplasty in children, analysis of 127 surgically treated eyes over 10 years, *J Fr Ophtalmol* 13(3):116, 1990.
94. Stulting RD et al: Penetrating keratoplasty in children, *Ophthalmology* 91(10):1222, 1984.
95. Parmley VC, Stonecipher KG, Rowsey JJ: Peters' anomaly: a review of 26 penetrating keratoplasties in infants, *Ophthalmic Surg* 24(1):31, 1993.
96. Gloor P, Keech RV, Krachmer JH: Factors associated with high postoperative myopia after penetrating keratoplasties in infants, *Ophthalmology* 99:775, 1992.
97. Baker JD: Visual rehabilitation of aphakic children. II. Contact lenses, *Surv Ophthalmol* 34(5):366, 1990.
98. Levin AV et al: Extended-wear contact lenses for the treatment of pediatric aphakia, *Ophthalmology* 95:1107, 1988.
99. Neumann D et al: The effectiveness of daily wear contact lenses for the correction of infantile aphakia, *Arch Ophthalmol* 111:927, 1993.

CHAPTER 136

BRADLEY H. SCHARF

Early Postoperative Complications

Modern microsurgical techniques and improved methods of eye banking and cornea preservation have resulted in a decreased incidence of early postoperative complications of penetrating keratoplasty. Occasionally however, one must manage complications including wound leaks and/or wound displacements, persistent epithelial defects, filamentary keratitis, suture complications, elevated intraocular pressure, severe intraocular inflammation, anterior synechia formation, pupillary block, choroidal detachment or hemorrhage, hyphema, fixed dilated pupil, infectious keratitis, endophthalmitis, and primary donor failure. In this chapter, we will discuss how these complications may be prevented, and if they should occur, how they may be managed. The proper diagnosis and management of complications in the critical early postoperative period may prevent early graft failure and improve long-term graft survival.

Wound Leaks and Wound Displacement

During the early postoperative period, low intraocular pressure and/or the presence of a shallow or flat anterior chamber suggests the possibility of a wound or suture tract leak. Pupillary block or choroidal detachment may also result in a shallow or flat anterior chamber but a coexistent wound leak must be ruled out. Seidel's test is useful for detecting an area of leakage. Even in the presence of a flat anterior chamber, the Seidel's test may be positive. The test is performed by placing concentrated fluorescein dye on the surface of the cornea. Under cobalt blue light, concentrated fluorescein appears black. The leakage of aqueous from the wound or a suture tract results in dilution of the fluorescein and a change in color from black to bright green.

If the anterior chamber is flat and a wound or suture tract leak is present, immediate surgical repair is indicated. The presence of iris prolapse associated with a wound leak also necessitates immediate surgical repair. Prolonged contact between the donor cornea and the iris, lens, or intraocular lens implant may result in extensive and irreversible endothelial cell damage.

If the anterior chamber remains formed in the presence of a wound or suture tract leak, a pressure patch may be used initially to achieve reapposition of the wound and to seal the wound or suture tract. An alternative is to use a soft bandage contact lens, which also may aid in reapposing the wound, tamponading the leak, and decreasing trauma from the lids on the wound. The use of topical or systemic aqueous suppressants may also facilitate sealing by decreasing aqueous flow through the leak. If a continuous suture is present, its rotation may facilitate wound leak closure.

A persistent wound or suture tract leak may lead to the development of a persistent fistula, peripheral anterior synechia, glaucoma, endophthalmitis, or epithelial ingrowth. If nonsurgical attempts fail to result in sealing of the leak after 24 to 48 hours, surgical repair is recommended. If leakage occurs along a single interrupted suture tract, removal of the suture may be considered. The wound must then be observed closely for the development of displacement or dehiscence. If the wound does not remain well apposed, the suture must be replaced.

If an interrupted suture breaks or loosens, it may result in an irregular, anterior displacement of the wound without an associated wound leak. If this appears to cause a high degree of astigmatism, a bandage contact lens may be used to reappose the wound. If the wound is not adequately reapposed, the suture should be replaced.

A wound dehiscence in the immediate postoperative period usually occurs secondary to technical problems such as a thin, necrotic recipient bed. Binder et al.[1] studied wound separations in 40 postkeratoplasty patients. Five patients developed immediate postoperative wound separations due to the condition of the recipient tissue. Six additional patients, who developed wound separations before suture removal, had severe glaucoma with intraocular pressure greater than 40 mm Hg. Therefore, the control of postoperative intraocular pressure may be important in preventing a postoperative wound dehiscence.

A full thickness wound dehiscence must be repaired surgically. If iris prolapse is present, avoid excision of

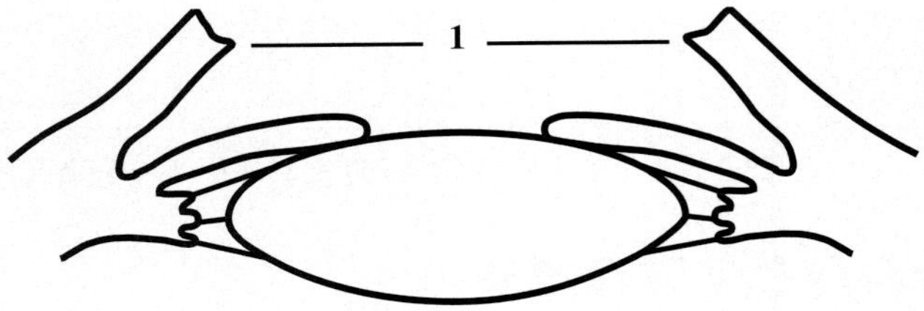

FIGURE 136-1 Host trephination with a thin posterior ledge *(1)* of rim tissue as a method to reduce wound leaks.

the iris since excision may result in significant glare problems. If the prolapsed tissue appears healthy, and the duration of prolapse is less than 24 hours, the tissue should be replaced with the use of a blunt spatula and viscoelastic agents. If the prolapsed tissue appears necrotic or macerated, or the duration of prolapse is greater than 24 hours, the tissue should be excised with microsurgical scissors held flush to the wound. To aid in the repositioning of prolapsed tissue, consider preoperative systemic osmotic agents to shrink the vitreous.

Although not approved by the Food and Drug Administration for ocular use, tissue adhesives have become a treatment option for corneal perforations since they were first described by Webster et al.[2] In a study of the use of tissue adhesive, Leahey et al.[3] reported its use in three patients for postkeratoplasty wound leaks. In two patients, the wounds sealed with good visual outcomes. The third patient ultimately required a repeat penetrating keratoplasty. The use of tissue adhesive is limited by the size of the perforation and the condition of the surrounding tissue. The future role of tissue adhesives and wound leaks remains to be defined.

The prevention of wound leaks begins with good wound construction. Good donor-recipient apposition, symmetric tissue distribution, and proper suture placement are all essential for the construction of a watertight wound.

Good donor-recipient apposition begins with the preparation of an adequate host-cornea rim. One technique to reduce wound leaks is to construct a posterior recipient ledge. During host trephination, the formation of a small (0.5 millimeter) posterior ledge of host cornea can greatly facilitate wound closure by providing a greater surface area for donor-recipient apposition (Figure 136-1). The presence of a posterior ledge takes on even greater significance when same-size donor and recipient trephination is planned. Without the presence of a posterior ledge, watertight wound closure of a same-size graft may be difficult and will mandate tight suturing.

To construct a posterior ledge, trephination should

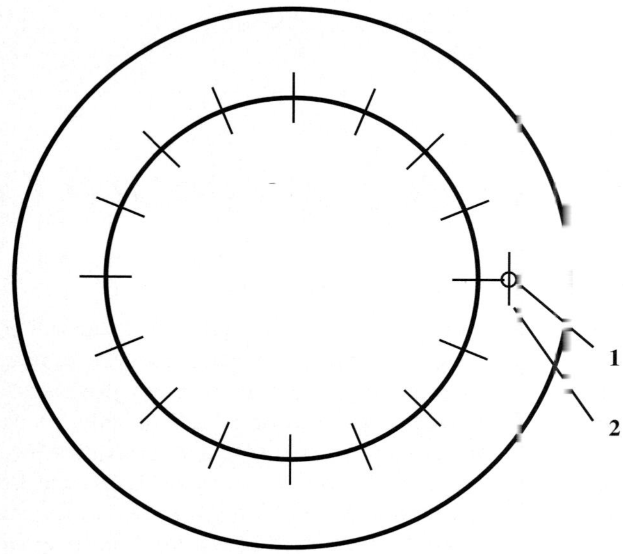

FIGURE 136-2 10-0 proline suture *(2)* sealing a suture track leak *(1)*.

be performed to a depth of approximately 90% of corneal thickness. The anterior chamber should then be entered from deep within the trephination groove at an angle with the cornea that results in the formation of the posterior ledge. Excision of the cornea is then completed with corneal scissors held at an angle; this will result in a symmetric continuation of the posterior ledge of rim tissue. After excision of the host cornea is completed, any areas of excess posterior ledge tissue should be carefully trimmed with small microsurgical scissors. It is essential that the posterior ledge be symmetric in order to minimize postoperative astigmatism. It is also important not to construct too thick of a posterior ledge since this will have the tendency to displace the graft anteriorly, especially after suture removal or relaxing incisions within the wound

When suturing begins, the proper placement of four cardinal sutures is essential. If distribution of the donor tissue is not symmetric, the cardinal sutures should be replaced until symmetric tissue distribution is achieved. To ensure good wound apposition, interrupted sutures must be radial and pass through the deep stroma of both the donor and recipient tissue. Full thickness suturing is not recommended, however, because the suture tracts are more likely to leak.

Once suturing is completed, the wound should be checked for the presence of leaks. Flourescein dye should be applied to the surface of the cornea, and light manual pressure should be applied to the globe. If a wound leak is noted, additional sutures should be placed. If a suture tract leak is noted, a 10-0 proline suture on a noncutting vascular needle may be placed perpendicular to the suture tract (Figure 136-2). This is especially important in pediatric keratoplasty because the cornea is less rigid and there is a greater tendency for leakage around suture tracts.

Persistent Epithelial Defects

During the early postoperative course of penetrating keratoplasty, reepithelialization and the maintenance of an intact epithelium is critical for postoperative wound healing, improved visual acuity, graft transparency, graft survival, and protection of the stroma against infection and melting. In patients with ocular surface disease secondary to dry eye, alkali burn, Stevens-Johnson syndrome, ocular cicatricial pemphigoid, neurotrophic keratopathy, and eyelid abnormalities, persistent epithelial defects may lead to graft failure. Aggressive management is necessary in these patients to facilitate epithelial healing and the maintenance of epithelial integrity.

If the graft recipient has a healthy ocular surface, reepithelialization is usually uneventful. However, even in those patients without surface disease, epithelial problems may develop. Twenty-seven percent of graft patients have developed a filamentary keratitis regardless of their preoperative diagnosis.[4] Grafts have also developed a whorl-like epithelial keratitis that has been related to toxicity and poor epithelial healing.[5]

Epithelial defects heal initially by the sliding of neighboring cells over the defect until it is closed. The cells move in an ameboid fashion with flattening of the infolded cell membranes that extend the cytoplasm. This is followed by mitosis that results in an increased epithelial thickness over the healed defect.[6] Once the defect is closed, any edema or leukocytic infiltration in the stroma usually disappears, restoring stromal transparency.[7]

The status of the donor epithelium depends upon several factors including donor medical history, death to preservation time, handling of the donor tissue, type of storage media, and donor cornea preservation time. The prevention of epithelial healing problems should begin before performing the penetrating keratoplasty. Patients suffering from severe keratoconjunctivitis sicca should undergo punctal occlusion before or at the the time of surgery. In addition, any patients with a significant loss of stem cells secondary to a chemical burn, a thermal burn, Stevens-Johnson syndrome, ocular cicatricial pemphigoid, or other ocular surface disease should be considered for an autologous transplant of limbal conjunctiva from the contralateral eye or a keratoepithelioplasty procedure before performing penetrating keratoplasty.[8,9] Any lid or lash abnormalities including trichiasis, ectropion, entropion, and lagophthalmos should be corrected before corneal surgery.

In penetrating keratoplasty for herpetic keratitis, the incidence of persistent epithelial defects ranges from 0%[10] to 44%.[11] Penetrating keratoplasty performed during active ocular inflammation or for corneal perforation secondary to herpetic eye disease has been significantly associated with epithelial healing problems. When possible, in eyes with a history of herpetic keratitis, penetrating keratoplasty should be performed at a time when inflammation is controlled. In a retrospective study of 76 penetrating keratoplasties and 9 lamellar keratoplasties for herpes simplex keratitis, an early persistent epithelial defect was experienced in 8% of penetrating keratoplasties and 44% of lamellar keratoplasties. All of the procedures that were performed during an active stage of herpetic disease developed a persistent epithelial defect.[12] A recent prospective study of 14 eyes in 13 patients who underwent penetrating keratoplasty for scarring secondary to herpes simplex keratitis showed that the long-term prophylactic use of oral acyclovir significantly decreased the recurrence of herpes simplex keratitis.[13] The use of perioperative oral acyclovir (800 to 1000 miligrams daily) may decrease the risk of persistent epithelial defects associated with active herpetic disease.

In the past, it was hypothesized that removal of the histocompatability antigen on the donor epithelial cells would decrease the incidence of allograft rejection. Based upon this hypothesis, removal of the donor epithelium became commonplace during penetrating keratoplasty. In 1988, Stulting et al.[14] showed that removal of the donor epithelium did not reduce the likelihood of allograft rejection or graft failure. Since that time, techniques to protect the donor epithelium have resulted in the decreased incidence of postoperative epithelial defects. When epithelial defects occur in the immediate postoperative period, they are usually due to sloughing of the donor epithelium or intraoperative surgical trauma to the epithelium. Meyer and Bobb[15] showed that in patients with bullous keratopathy treated with penetrating keratoplasty, the length of time required for postoperative epithelial healing was directly related to the amount of donor corneal epithelium that remained intact through the preservation and surgical periods. Therefore, careful handling of the epithelium is essential.

In patients in whom problems with epithelialization are anticipated, the use of a donor cornea with good epithelium is essential. The use of donor corneas with significant epithelial sloughing should be avoided. Additionally, as preservation time increases, the donor epithelium becomes less adherent. Therefore, donor tissue with the shortest preservation time as possible should be used in these cases. Intraoperatively, it is imperative to avoid trauma to the donor epithelium. Before harvesting the donor button, the surface of the Teflon cutting block should be carefully examined. This is usually done by running one's finger along the surface in order to detect any rough areas. When the donor cornea is placed on the block, the surface should be moist but not so moist as to cause slippage. Once the donor button is harvested, it should remain bathed in storage solution until its use.

During suturing of the donor button to the host rim tissue, it is important to keep the epithelium well lubricated and well protected. Dessication and excessive irrigation are both damaging to the corneal epithelium. Reed et al.[16] showed that using intraoperative sodium hyaluronate, as opposed to balanced saline solution, to hydrate the cornea and protect it from surgical trauma resulted in an improved corneal epithelial integrity 1 week postoperatively. The use of balanced saline solution alone may actually result in loosening of the epithelium. One disadvantage to using sodium hyaluronate, however, is that nylon suture may become sticky and difficult to handle.

Good graft apposition is also important for epithelialization since graft overide can cause problems with epithelial migration. An elevation of the graft at the graft-host junction or surface irregularities associated with sutures may result in abnormal tear-film distribution and epithelial healing problems.

The postoperative prevention and treatment of epithelial defects may include the use of a permanent or temporary tarsorrhaphy, pressure patching, a bandage soft contact lens, or a collagen shield. Using nonpreserved artificial tears and limiting medications toxic to the epithelium are also helpful. Once an epithelial defect is present, it must be treated aggressively. If the defect persists for greater than 1 week, it will heal more slowly. If it persists for greater than 3 weeks, the risks of stromal scarring and ulceration become significantly greater.

A permanent or temporary tarsorrhaphy at the time of keratoplasty or early in the postoperative period is the most powerful prophylactic and treatment modality available for epithelial defects. By decreasing the amount of exposed surface area, a tarsorrhaphy increases the effectiveness of the patient's own tears and any additional lubricants. When a postoperative epithelial defect is present, the tarsorrhaphy should be performed in a manner that results in maximal coverage of the defect. If the defect is located on the temporal cornea, a lateral tarsorrhaphy should be performed. If the defect is located on the nasal cornea, a medial tarsorrhaphy should be performed. Some cases may require the placement of both lateral and medial tarsorrhaphies. Koenig and Harris[17] described the use of a reversible central suture tarsorrhaphy to protect the eye in primary gaze. Temporary glue tarsorrhaphies have been described,[18] but they run the risk of the glue migrating onto the posterior aspect of the lids, thus adding to problems with epithelialization.

Since an extensive tarsorrhaphy often hinders examination of the globe, and when opened, may result in distortion of the lid margin, Adams et al.[19] described the use of botulinum A toxin to produce a protective ptosis. The toxin is injected into the levator muscle where it blocks the release of acetylcholine from the presynaptic nerve endings. The toxin was used in 15 patients. The time taken for full ptosis to develop was 30 hours to 10 days. Full ptosis lasted for 7 days to 2 weeks, and recovery took a maximum of 7 months (mean 8.1 weeks). Weakness of the superior rectus was observed in 12 of the 15 cases but in only two cases did the patient experience vertical diplopia when the lid began to open.

Pressure patching aids epithelialization by decreasing eyelid motion over the healing surface. A major disadvantage of pressure patching, however, is that the use of topical medication is limited. In addition, patching results in an environment that favors microorganism growth. In a study of pressure patching for postoperative epithelial defects 2 mm^2 or larger, Sugar et al.[20] found no significant difference in healing time between patched and unpatched eyes. The role of pressure patching has, therefore, been limited to short-term trials followed by the use of another treatment modality if pressure patching fails to result in improvement. Pressure patching may also be used on a part-time basis in combination with a tarsorrhaphy for the treatment of unresponsive epithelial defects.

Collagen shields and bandage soft contact lenses have also been used to prevent and treat postoperative epithelial defects. Collagen shields have been found to improve the healing of epithelial defects when used in the immediate postoperative period.[21,22] However, they have had limited success in the treatment of chronic epithelial defects.[21,22] In a prospective study, Ruffini et al.[21] found that the application of a 24-hour collagen shield at the conclusion of surgery resulted in less epithelial staining and smaller epithelial defects on the first postoperative day. On day 8, however, no significant difference in epithelial staining was noted. In a prospective study of 23 eyes, Groden and White[23] compared the effect of a 24-hour collagen shield versus a hydrophilic soft bandage contact lens for the treatment of persistent epithelial defects that failed to reepithelialize after 2 weeks. The use of a bandage contact lens was found to be significantly more effective than the use of a collagen shield.

The use of either a collagen shield or a bandage soft contact lens is not without risk. In a retrospective study of 47 patients requiring a therapeutic soft bandage contact lens in the early postoperative period, 23% developed corneal ulcers.[24] The only statistically significant risk factor for infection was the presence of a persistent epithelial defect. When bandage contact lenses are used, prophylactic coverage with a broad-spectrum topical antibiotic and close follow-up are recommended. The oxygen permeability of a collagen shield is greater than that of a bandage soft contact lens, and as degradation occurs, the oxygen permeability of a collagen shield continues to increase.[16] On this basis alone, the use of a collagen shield should be associated with less risk for infection than the use of a bandage soft contact lens. However, after insertion, the fit of a collagen shield may tighten, resulting in hypoxia and increased risk for infection and inflammation.

Postoperative medications should result in as little epithelial toxicity as possible. When antibiotics are used to treat an infection, the antibiotic most effective against the infectious agent should be used. However, when antibiotics are used prophylactically in the postoperative period, an antibiotic with minimal epithelial toxicity should be used. Pfister and Burstein[25] found that solutions containing neomycin, polymixin, gramicidin, thimerisol, and benzalkonium chloride caused desquamation of epithelial cells and loss of surface microvilli. Mackman et al.[5] described a characteristic "hurricane" shaped epithelial keratopathy in 15 cases of penetrating keratoplasty that was caused by the use of an antibiotic-steroid combination containing neomycin, polymixin, dexamethasone, and benzalkonium chloride. In six of the cases, the epitheliopathy was noted within the first 2 weeks of surgery. The keratitis took the form of a whorling spiral extending from the peripheral border of the graft inward. In three of the cases, the keratitis progressed to a large epithelial defect that required 1 to 3 weeks to heal once the medication was discontinued.

Topical corticosteroids inhibit corneal epithelial wound healing.[26,27] Therefore, in the presence of a persistent epithelial defect, the use of topical corticosteroids should be kept to a minimum. In routine cases, topical corticosteroids may be used only twice daily while the epithelial defect heals. In cases which remain resistant to healing, it may be necessary to temporarily discontinue the topical corticosteroids and prescribe oral corticosteroids to the patient.

The use of topical agents such as epidermal growth factor, eye-derived growth factor, and fibronectin for the enhancement of epithelial healing has had mixed reports of success.[28,29] Purified epidermal growth factor isolated from mice submaxillary glands was found to increase the corneal epithelium healing rates in rabbits with no sign of toxicity.[28] However, in a study of 35 patients, topically applied epidermal growth

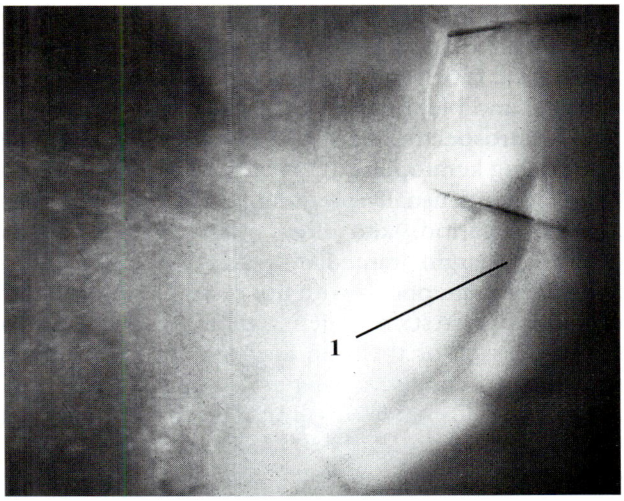

FIGURE 136-3 Active herpes keratitis resulting in a persistent epithelial defect *(1)*.

factor after penetrating keratoplasty was found to have no benefit on epithelial healing.[30] Fibronectin, a glycoprotein present at corneal wounds has had variably reported effects on epithelial wound healing in rabbits.[31,32] Autologous fibronectin has been used topically in 2 patients with trophic ulceration unresponsive to conventional therapy, and it resulted in complete epithelialization.[33] Additional clinical trials are required to determine the future use of these agents.

The possibility of active herpes virus infection must always be considered when an epithelial defect does not respond to treatment. Surgical incision of the trigeminal nerve has been shown to reactivate latent herpes simplex virus in humans.[34,35] Since a majority of the population carries herpes simplex virus in a latent phase, penetrating keratoplasty may lead to its reactivation even in patients with no clinical history of active disease.[36,37] Mannis et al.[38] described the development of late-appearing epithelial defects due to herpes simplex virus in penetrating keratoplasty patients who had no history of herpes simplex keratitis. The defect usually begins at the graft-host junction, and it may not resemble a typical herpetic epithelial keratitis (Figure 136-3). Viral culture or other diagnostic tools such as immunofluorescent staining may be helpful in evaluating unresponsive epithelial defects. If the defects are secondary to herpetic disease, then appropriate topical antiviral treatment is indicated.

Filamentary Keratitis

Filaments consist of abnormal collections of mucus and corneal epithelial cells on the corneal surface. The

Elevated Intraocular Pressure

The measurement of intraocular pressure in the early postoperative period is important. Because postoperative graft edema usually results in surface irregularity and pooling of fluorescein around sutures, pressure readings obtained by Goldmann applanation tonometry are inaccurate. The use of a pneumotonometer or an electronic tonometer is recommended.

The control of postoperative intraocular pressure is important because elevated pressure may result in endothelial cell damage. Bigar[45] reported decreased endothelial cell counts in 5 of 13 eyes following acute angle-closure attacks. Svedbergh[46] showed that elevated intraocular pressure could cause irreversible damage to monkey corneal endothelial cells in vitro. Charlin and Polack[47] found that an elevated intraocular pressure in rabbit eyes caused endothelial cell loss, distention of endothelial cell junctions, and graft edema.

The association between penetrating keratoplasty and postoperative glaucoma was first described by Irvine and Kaufman in 1969.[48] Elevated intraocular pressure (>25 mm Hg) in the immediate postoperative period in patients with aphakia or patients undergoing combined cornea and cataract procedures was reported as high as 60% to 90%.[48] Olson and Kaufman[49] found that 46% of eyes undergoing aphakic or combined penetrating keratoplasty had an intraocular pressure greater than 35 mm Hg during the first postoperative week. Goldberg et al.[50] found an early increase in intraocular pressure in 41% of patients undergoing combined penetrating keratoplasty procedures, in 38% of patients undergoing aphakic penetrating keratoplasty, and in only 3% of patients undergoing phakic penetrating keratoplasty.

Zimmerman et al.[51] postulated that in aphakic and combined penetrating keratoplasties, elevated intraocular pressure in the first postoperative week was related to trabecular meshwork collapse. Interruption of Descemet's membrane by the penetrating keratoplasty incision results in a loss of anterior support of the trabecular meshwork. In aphakia, absence of the lens results in a loss of the posterior support normally provided by the lens and zonules. This combined loss of both anterior and posterior support may result in collapse of the trabecular meshwork and decreased outflow.

Olson and Kaufman[52] developed a mathematical model to predict postoperative intraocular pressure. They showed that tight suturing, long suture bites, larger trephine sizes, a smaller recipient total corneal diameter, same size donor-host trephination, and increased recipient peripheral corneal thickness could all result in greater iridocorneal angle compression and elevated intraocular pressure. Zimmerman et al.[51] also showed a marked reduction of early postoperative intraocular pressure elevation in aphakic and combined penetrating keratoplasties when a 0.5 millimeter oversized versus same sized donor graft was used. Bourne et al.[53] showed that the use of an oversized donor button in aphakic penetrating keratoplasty resulted in a significantly lower mean intraocular pressure over the first 5 postoperative days when compared to the use of same size buttons. Some studies, however, found no difference in postoperative intraocular pressure in aphakic penetrating keratoplasty with oversize versus same size donors.[54,55] Therefore, variations in surgical technique may also play a role in postoperative intraocular pressure.

Other causes of elevated early postoperative intraocular pressure include retained viscoelastic, intraocular inflammation, anterior synechia causing angle closure, and pupillary block. Although it is common practice to use a viscoelastic agent to coat the intraocular structures and the host cornea rim tissue during graft suturing, as soon as the anterior chamber is able to maintain its depth, it should be filled with balanced saline solution. This helps to prevent the excessive use of viscoelastic agents and may help to prevent postoperative intraocular pressure elevations. Intraocular inflammation associated with elevated intraocular pressure should be treated aggressively with topical and/or systemic corticosteroids. The prevention and treatment of anterior synechia and pupillary block is discussed later.

If elevated postoperative intraocular pressure is expected, the use of a topical beta-blocker and/or an oral carbonic anhydrase inhibitor may be considered at the conclusion of surgery. These agents may be continued in the postoperative period if the intraocular pressure remains elevated. Topical apraclonidine 0.5% may also be used on a short-term basis. Attempts should be made to avoid the use of miotic agents because they may result in increased anterior segment inflammation. All topical medications should be used with caution because they may result in variable degrees of epitheliopathy. Systemic osmotic agents may be used on a short-term basis if other treatments fail to produce an adequate response.

If the intraocular pressure remains significantly elevated after all modalities of treatment have been attempted, the surgical wound may be manipulated at the slit lamp with a pair of tying forceps in an attempt to release viscoelastic or aqueous from the anterior chamber. This maneuver, however, should only be attempted in patients with an intact anterior hyaloid face.

The persistence of an elevated intraocular pressure refractory to medical treatment may require surgical intervention in the form of glaucoma filtration surgery, anterior chamber shunt implantation,[56,57] cyclocryotherapy, or laser cyclophotocoagulation.[58,59]

Postoperative Inflammation

Postoperative inflammation can usually be well controlled with topical corticosteroids. Occasionally, uncontrolled inflammation may lead to the formation of intraocular fibrin. This forms when a breakdown of the blood-aqueous barrier leads to the intraocular accumulation of fibrinogen, which is converted to fibrin by the enzymatic action of thrombin. The fibrin may serve as a scaffold for cellular proliferation and the formation of strands or membranes in the eye. This may lead to the development of pupillary block and glaucoma, or it may cause direct damage to the endothelial cells.

The initial treatment of fibrin in the anterior chamber should consist of intense topical corticosteroids on an hourly basis. Mydriatics should be used to prevent the development of posterior synechia and pupillary block. If the condition fails to improve, the use of periocular and/or systemic corticosteroids are recommended.

Tissue plasminogen activator (TPA) is a 70,000 dalton protein that has been approved by the Food and Drug Administration for the treatment of coronary thrombosis. Its mechanism of action is the conversion of plasminogen to plasmin. Plasmin then results in clot dissolution by fibrinolysis. TPA has been shown to be effective in the treatment of postvitrectomy fibrin formation.[60] A 25 microgram intraocular dose completely cleared intraocular fibrin membranes in three patients. In all patients, evidence of fibrinolysis was seen after 20 minutes. The time course for complete lysis varied from 30 minutes to 3 hours.

Intraocular TPA (25 micrograms) has been used successfully after penetrating keratoplasty for the treatment of postoperative fibrin formation[61] (Figures 136-7 and 136-8). Corneal endothelial perfusion studies have shown that this dose does not adversely affect corneal endothelial cell function. In addition, transmission and scanning electron microscopy failed to reveal any structural alterations in endothelial cells caused by the TPA.[62] Hemorrhage is an important risk factor associated with the intraocular use of TPA. Its use, therefore, should be limited to patients with extensive fibrin formation who have not responded to corticosteroid treatment. It would also be prudent to use as low a dose of TPA as possible. The use of as little as 6 to 10 micrograms in the anterior chamber has resulted in complete fibrinolysis postkeratoplasty.[63] Additional studies are needed to determine the optimal intraocular dose for anterior chamber use.

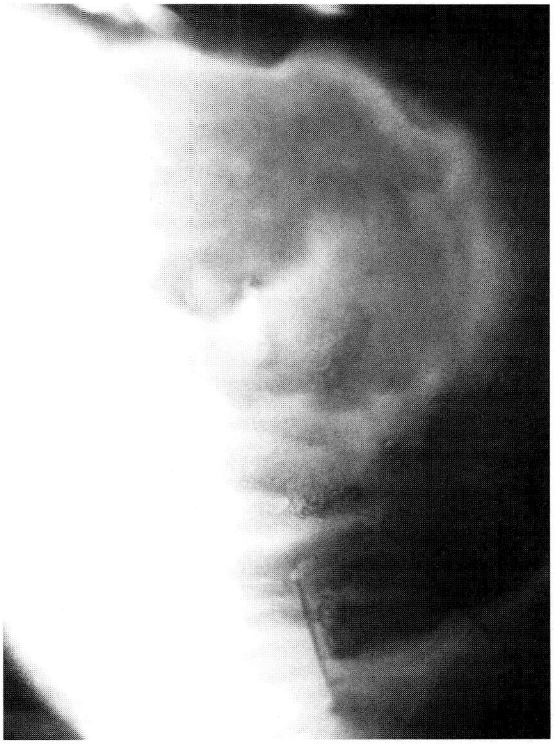

FIGURE 136-7 Severe postoperative inflammation.

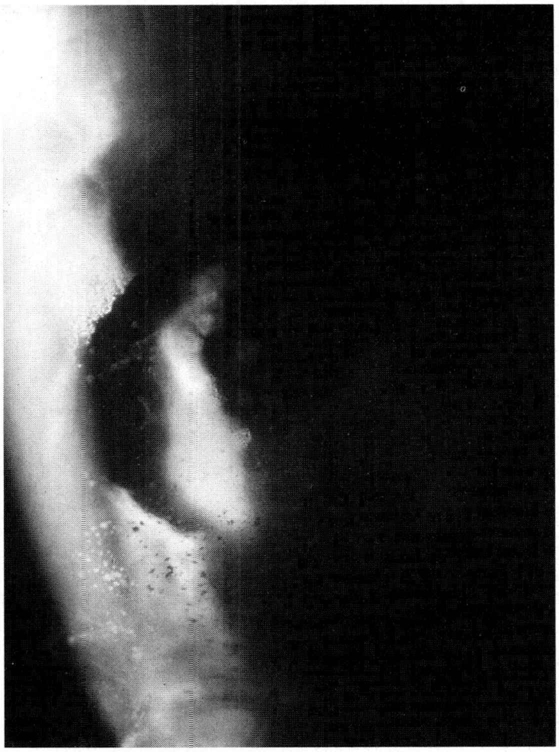

FIGURE 136-8 Post-TPA injection into the anterior chamber featuring same patient as in Figure 136-7.

Anterior Synechia Formation

The presence of anterior synechia is undesirable in the postkeratoplasty patient. The presence of anterior synechia may result in the development of a difficult to manage secondary angle-closure glaucoma, which may then cause damage to both the optic nerve and the corneal endothelial cells. In addition, the presence of anterior synechia increases the risk of graft failure.[64-66] Mechanical traction or persistent anterior segment inflammation secondary to the anterior synechia may also result in a progressive loss of endothelial cells.[66] Anterior synechia may also expose the corneal endothelium to blood vessels, which may increase the risk of graft rejection. In one study, 13 of 15 patients with anterior synechia and only 7 of 45 patients without anterior synechia had episodes of graft edema. Patients with anterior synechia also had a higher incidence of multiple episodes of graft edema.[66]

The risk of developing anterior synechia is increased in larger grafts. Aphakic and pseudophakic eyes also more commonly develop anterior synechia,[65] likely due to the loss of posterior support provided by the lens and zonules. The presence of a flaccid iris, either secondary to surgery or trauma, may also predispose to anterior synechia formation.

In order to prevent the formation of postoperative anterior synechia, it is important that the existing anterior synechia be released. Both blunt and sharp dissection should be used to perform a complete synechiolysis. A viscoelastic agent should then be injected into the anterior chamber angle before suturing the corneal graft to maintain the anterior chamber angle. Foulks et al[67] found that the use of an oversized donor was associated with a decreased incidence of anterior synechia formation and progressive angle closure. Performing a surgical iridoplasty during the penetrating keratoplasty procedure in order to produce a mechanically rigid iris diaphragm may also be useful in patients with flaccid irides.[68] In large grafts, the performance of one or more peripheral iridectomies may prevent angle closure. Good wound apposition and meticulous wound closure is essential to avoid iris incarceration in the wound during surgery or secondary to a postoperative wound leak.[69]

Mydriatics may be used postoperatively to prevent the formation of posterior synechiae, but wide dilation in the presence of a large graft may result in iris adhesion to the wound. Additionally, dilation in an eye with a posterior chamber intraocular lens increases the risk of synechia forming on the lens and developing iris capture. The use of atropine should be avoided in patients with keratoconus since it may result in permanent mydriasis.[70,71] The aggressive control of postoperative inflammation is also essential for the prevention of synechia formation.

Postoperatively, a small synechia may often be broken by movement of the iris with mydriatics or miotics. If the synechiae are small and not progressive, it is wise to leave them alone rather than risk more serious problems by entering the anterior chamber. However, the areas involved should be watched for the future development of rejection. If the synechiae are progressive, argon laser surgery to the basal iris at the advancing edge of the progressive angle closure has been suggested to halt progression. If anterior synechia close greater than 50% of the anterior chamber angle, surgical correction should be performed before permanent damage to the angle and trabecular meshwork occurs.

Pupillary Block

The presence of a flat or shallow anterior chamber and a securely closed wound, confirmed by Seidel's test, suggests the presence of pupillary block or a choroidal detachment. Pupillary block is usually associated with an elevated intraocular pressure but the condition can exist in normal or low pressure states. A choroidal detachment, on the other hand, is usually associated with a low intraocular pressure Posterior synechia or vitreous protruding through the pupil and peripheral iridectomy sites helps to confirm a diagnosis of pupillary block.

Medical management includes the repeated application of mydriatic and cycloplegic agents in a vigorous attempt to dilate the pupil. Topical beta-blockers, carbonic anhydrase inhibitors, and osmotic agents may be used to control intraocular pressure. If inflammation is present, additional topical and possibly systemic corticosteroids should be used.

Because prolonged shallowing of the anterior chamber may result in the formation of anterior synechia, a peripheral iridectomy should be performed if there is no response to medical treatment. Depending upon anterior chamber depth, this may be performed with a laser or surgically, possibly in conjunction with a pars plana vitrectomy. Performance of an iridectomy usually results in immediate resolution of the block with restoration of anterior chamber depth.

Choroidal Detachment and Choroidal Hemorrhage

Choroidal detachments are smooth, rounded elevations restricted by the vortex veins and the optic nerve.

They sometimes extend forward to the scleral spur resulting in an anterior displacement of the iris, shallowing of the anterior chamber, and secondary angle closure. They are usually diagnosed by direct or indirect ophthalmoscopy, but in cases where visualization is not possible, B-scan ultrasonography may be diagnostic.

Choroidal detachments in the early postoperative period are usually due to uveal effusion. Surgically-induced inflammation probably plays a role in causing hypotony and/or vascular permeability changes that result in the development of effusions.[72,73] Effusions that develop almost immediately after opening an eye are likely due to the sudden change in pressure gradient between the choroid and the suprachoroidal space. It is important to perform the Seidel's test to be certain that a wound leak is not causing the hypotony and the choroidal detachment. Once a choroidal or ciliochoroidal detachment occurs, it may result in decreased formation of aqueous and an increased outflow of aqueous through the uveoscleral route. This further perpetuates hypotony and the persistence of the choroidal detachment.

Postoperative choroidal detachments are usually self-limited. However, those that do not resolve and are associated with persistent hypotony and anterior displacement of the iris, may result in the development of anterior synechia, angle-closure glaucoma, pupillary block, and cystoid macular edema. If the anterior chamber angle is compromised for more than 48 to 72 hours and the choroidal detachment is persistent, surgical drainage of the suprachoroidal space with reformation of the anterior chamber is recommended.

Occasionally, a choroidal hemorrhage may occur in the early postoperative period. This usually appears as a sudden onset of pain and decreased vision. Risk factors include advanced age, atherosclerotic vascular disease, hypertension, and glaucoma.[74,75] In the postoperative period, patients should be warned against excessive straining, which may also play a role. Patients who experience a postoperative choroidal hemorrhage should be followed closely for resolution or possible drainage.

Hyphema

The postoperative occurrence of hyphema is uncommon after penetrating keratoplasty. Its incidence increases in cases where extensive synechiolysis, iridoplasty, or iridectomy have been performed. When it occurs, postoperative hemorrhage usually clears spontaneously without treatment. It may, however, be associated with an elevated intraocular pressure that should be treated aggressively. If topical beta-blockers alone are not adequate to control the intraocular pressure, topical apraclonidine and/or systemic carbonic anhydrase inhibitors should be used. Systemic osmotic agents may be required in instances of acute intraocular pressure elevation. A mydriatic agent is recommended to prevent the formation of posterior synechiae, and topical corticosteroids are recommended to control intraocular inflammation.

If the hemorrhage fails to clear spontaneously, the risk for the development of posterior synechia, peripheral anterior synechia, or corneal blood staining increases with time. The presence of uncontrollable elevated intraocular pressure or the prolonged persistence of intraocular hemorrhage may necessitate surgical intervention. Surgical methods may include (1) clot irrigation with trabeculectomy, (2) hyphema aspiration with vitrectomy instruments through a small limbal or clear corneal incision, (3) irrigation and aspiration of the hyphema through a small limbal or clear corneal incision, or (4) manual expression of the clot through a limbal incision.

Fixed Dilated Pupil

The development of a fixed, dilated pupil following penetrating keratoplasty for keratoconus has been observed as part of a syndrome associated with iris atrophy, scattered pigment granules over the lens capsule and corneal endothelium, and secondary glaucoma with posterior synechia.[70,71] In a study in 1977, 5.8% of eyes with keratoconus that underwent penetrating keratoplasty developed a fixed, dilated pupil in either a complete form or an incomplete form with recovery after 1 to 18 weeks.[71] The syndrome has also been reported in patients with Down syndrome and keratoconus who have not undergone penetrating keratoplasty.

Parasympatholytics including atropine and scopolamine hydrochloride (and to a lesser degree, adrenergic drugs including phenylephrine hydrochloride) have been associated with this syndrome. The syndrome has been explained by ischemic atrophy of the sphincter pupillae muscle secondary to iris strangulation associated with dilation. It remains unknown why this phenomenon occurs only in association with keratoconus. When dilation becomes necessary in patients with keratoconus, the use of mild, short-acting agents is recommended.[70]

Postoperative Infection

Bacterial or fungal keratitis in the early postoperative period may result from contamination of donor material, incomplete excision of an infected host cornea, or acquisition of microorganisms from the environment. Graft infection usually manifests within 24 to 48 hours with ciliary injection, graft edema, mucopurulent discharge, and occasionally an infiltrate in the graft or around a suture.

Risk factors associated with the development of postoperative infectious keratitis include persistent epithelial defects, contact lens usage, loose or broken sutures, corticosteroid therapy, and keratoconjunctivitis sicca. Corticosteroids and other immunosuppressive agents impair the host defenses and decrease inflammation, resulting in fewer symptoms and a more advanced presentation of the disease. Prevention of infection requires aggressive treatment and close follow-up of patients with persistent epithelial defects. Patients requiring the use of a soft bandage contact lens should be treated prophylactically with topical antibiotics and followed closely.

If a patient develops an early postoperative infectious keratitis, Gram stain and culture with sensitivities should be performed. The patient should be treated with broad-spectrum topical antibiotics until culture results are obtained. If a graft becomes extensively involved with infection, it should be replaced to prevent the development of endophthalmitis.

The incidence of endophthalmitis after penetrating keratoplasty ranges from 0.2% to 0.77%.[76-81] In one study, eyes receiving corneas with positive rim cultures had a 22-fold increased incidence of endophthalmitis.[76] In another study, there was a 12-fold increase. When endophthalmitis developed in a patient with a positive rim culture, the organism isolated from aqueous or vitreous aspirate was usually the same organism identified in the rim culture.[76,80,81] Donor rim cultures are important because they identify patients at increased risk of endophthalmitis, and they may enable more specific treatment if endophthalmitis develops. Patients with positive donor rim cultures should be followed closely in the early postoperative period.

Prior to treatment, 100% of postmortem eyes were culture positive.[82] Despite vigorous irrigation of donor tissue before enucleation and irrigation with antibiotics when placed in storage media, approximately 12% of donor corneoscleral rim tissue remained positive for aerobic or anaerobic bacteria or fungus.[83] Therefore, most bacteria and fungi are eliminated by residual antibiotics from the storage media, rinsing of the donor tissue during transplantation, postoperative antibiotics, or the host's immune system.[80] If the recipient is immunocompromised or if a high dose of corticosteroids is used postoperatively, there may be an increased risk of developing postoperative infection.

Chittum et al.[84] found a significantly higher incidence of contamination in donors who died of systemic infections. Therefore, careful screening must be done to prevent the use of eyes from donors with documented or suspected sepsis. In addition, donor corneas are more often culture positive when the donor has been on a respirator before enucleation.[85] The use of these eyes should be determined on an individual case basis, taking into account the length of time the donor had been on the respirator.

The use of antibiotics in storage media is standard. However, it has been shown that at the standard storage temperature of 4 degrees Celsius, antibiotics cannot reliably sterilize an inoculum of sensitive bacteria. The current recommendation is for donor tissue to be brought to room temperature for 1 hour immediately before using. Studies have shown that after 1 hour, the number of bacterial colonies cultured was decreased but not totally eliminated.[86] A marked reduction in bacterial concentration was not demonstrated until a warming time of 5 hours was reached.[87] Although periods of preoperative warming longer than 1 hour may result in a better antibacterial effect, the effect on donor cornea tissue is unknown. Future research may clarify this issue.

Primary Donor Failure

Primary donor failure results in irreversible edema of the corneal graft in the immediate postoperative period. It is a result of inadequate endothelial cell function due to unhealthy donor endothelium, inadequate tissue preservation, or surgical trauma. Edema usually develops within the first day or two after surgery and is unresponsive to steroids and hypertonic solutions. Hyposecretion of aqueous humor, which may occur after penetrating keratoplasty, may result in a thickened cornea due to a decreased supply of metabolites to the endothelium. Once a normal rate of aqueous production is restored, endothelial function improves, and the cornea begins to clear. In the presence of postoperative hypotension, it is important to give the ciliary body and the corneal endothelium time to resume their normal functions before diagnosing primary donor failure.[88]

A major goal of cornea preservation and cornea transplantation is to maintain as high a postoperative endothelial cell count as possible. The donor cornea should have at least 2000 endothelial cells/mm^2 for a good chance of long-term survival. Good technique is essential when removing the corneoscleral rim from the donor globe because poor technique can result in trauma to the endothelium secondary to contact with other ocular structures or secondary to marked corneal distortion. When this type of damage occurs, it is usually localized and may be overlooked by specular microscopy.[89] Therefore, all corneas should be examined preoperatively with a slit lamp for any areas of damage.

In phakic patients and in aphakic or pseudophakic patients with an intact vitreous face, preoperative hypotony has been associated with decreased endothelial cell loss.[64] This is likely related to the fact that increased vitreous pressure increases the chances of contact between the endothelium and other intraocular structures. It is therefore recommended that a Honan balloon, digital massage, or intravenous mannitol be used preoperatively in all patients with an intact vitreous face.

During suturing of the corneal graft, most of the damage to the endothelium occurs at the beginning when the borders of the graft can rub against the host corneal rim tissue. The use of a viscoelastic agent to coat the intraocular structures and the host cornea rim tissue has improved protection of the graft endothelium and eased surgical manipulation by stabilizing the graft.[90] Postoperative examination of 40 patients several months after penetrating keratoplasty showed that eyes in which sodium hyaluronate was used to protect the endothelium had an average endothelial cell count 42% greater than control patients in whom balanced saline solution was used.[91] During surgical manipulation, distortion of the donor tissue should be minimized, and it is imperative that no surgical instruments contact the endothelium.

Once a diagnosis of primary donor failure is made, regrafting may be performed as soon as the eye is no longer inflamed. Primary donor failure is relatively rare, and all cases should be investigated. Defective preservation media or intraocular fluids including irrigating solutions, viscoelastics, and intraocular medications should be suspected. The failed donor button should be evaluated, and the eye bank providing the tissue should be notified.

Conclusion

Proper postoperative care is critical for a successful penetrating keratoplasty. The anticipation of postoperative complications in high-risk patients is important, and preventative measures should be taken. When complications do occur, prompt and proper management is essential and will result in earlier visual rehabilitation and greater long-term graft survival.

REFERENCES

1. Binder PS et al: Keratoplasty wound separations, *Am J Ophthalmol* 80(1):109-115, 1975.
2. Webster RG Jr et al: The use of adhesive for the closure of corneal perforations. Report of two cases, *Arch Ophthalmol* 80:705-709, 1968.
3. Leahey AB, Gottsch JD, Stark WJ: Clinical experience with N-butyl cyanoacrylate (nexacryl) tissue adhesive, *Ophthalmology* 100 (2):173-180, 1993.
4. Rotkis WM, Chandler JW, Forstot SL: Filamentary keratitis following penetrating keratoplasty, *Ophthalmology* 89:946-949, 1982.
5. Mackman GS, Polack FM, Sydrys L: Hurricane keratitis in penetrating keratoplasty. *Cornea* 2(1):31-34, 1983.
6. Friedenwald JS, Buschke W: Mitotic and wound-healing activities of the corneal epithelium, *Arch Ophthalmol* 32:410-413, 1944.
7. Kuwabara T, Perkins DG, Cogan DG: Sliding of the epithelium in experimental corneal wounds, *Invest Ophthalmol Vis Sci* 15(1): 4-14, 1976.
8. Thoft RA: Conjunctival transplantation, *Arch Ophthalmol* 95: 1425-1427, 1977.
9. Thoft RA: Keratoepithelioplasty, *Am J Ophthalmol* 97:1-6, 1984.
10. Cobo LM et al: Prognosis and management of corneal transplantation for herpetic keratitis, *Arch Ophthalmol* 98:1755-1759, 1980.
11. Foster CS, Duncan J: Penetrating keratoplasty for herpes simplex keratitis, *Am J Ophthalmol* 92:336-343, 1981.
12. Gutow A et al: Corneal epithelial healing after keratoplasty for herpes simplex keratitis, *Cornea* 5(1):5-9, 1986.
13. Barney NP, Foster CS: A prospective randomized trial of oral acyclovir after penetrating keratoplasty for herpes simplex keratitis, *Cornea* 13(3):232-236, 1994.
14. Stulting RD et al: Effect of donor epithelium on corneal transplant survival, *Ophthalmology* 95(6):803-812, 1988.
15. Meyer RF, Bobb KC: Corneal epithelium in penetrating keratoplasty, *Am J Ophthalmol* 90:142-147, 1980.
16. Reed DE et al: Corneal epithelial healing after penetrating keratoplasty using topical healon versus balanced salt solution, *Ophthalmic Surg* 18(7):525-528, 1987.
17. Koenig SB, Harris GJ: Temporary suture tarsorrhaphy after penetrating keratoplasty, *Cornea* 10(2):121-122, 1991.
18. Donnenfeld ED, Perry HD, Nelson DB: Cyanoacrylate temporary tarsorrhaphy in the management of corneal epithelial defects, *Ophthalmic Surg* 22(10):591-593, 1991.
19. Adams GGW, Kirkness CM, Lee JP: Botulinum toxin A induced protective ptosis, *Eye* 1:603-608, 1987.
20. Sugar A, Meyer RF, Bahn CF: A randomized trial of pressure patching for epithelial defects after keratoplasty, *Am J Ophthalmol* 95:637-640, 1983.
21. Ruffini JJ, Aquavella JV, LoCascio JA: Effect of collagen shields on corneal epithelialization following penetrating keratoplasty, *Ophthalmic Surg* 20(1):21-25, 1989.
22. Poland DE, Kaufman HE: Clinical uses of collagen shields, *J Cataract Refract Surg* 14:489-491, 1988.
23. Groden LR, White W: Porcine collagen corneal shield treatment of persistent epithelial defects following penetrating keratoplasty, *CLAO J* 16(2):95-97, 1990.
24. Smith SG et al: Corneal ulcer-infiltrate associated with soft contact lens use following penetrating keratoplasty, *Cornea* 3:131-134, 1984.
25. Pfister RR, Burstein N: The effects of ophthalmic drugs: electron microscopic study, *Invest Ophthalmol Vis Sci* 15:246-259, 1976.
26. Gasset AR et al: Quantitative corticosteroid effect on corneal wound healing, *Arch Ophthalmol* 81:589-591, 1969.
27. Aquavella JV, Gasset AR, Dohlman CH: Corticosteroids in corneal wound healing, *Am J Ophthalmol* 58:621-626, 1964.
28. Ho PC et al: Kinetics of corneal epithelial regeneration and epidermal growth factor, *Invest Ophthalmol Vis Sci* 13(10):804-809, 1974.
29. Thompson P et al: The effect of an eye derived growth factor (EDFG) on corneal epithelial regeneration, *Exp Eye Res* 34:191-199, 1982.

30. Kandarakis AS, Page C, Kaufman HE: The effect of epidermal growth factor on epithelial healing after penetrating keratoplasty in human eyes, *Am J Ophthalmol* 98:411-415, 1984.
31. Nishida T et al: Fibronectin enhancement of corneal epithelial wound healing of rabbits in vivo, *Arch Ophthalmol* 102:455-456, 1984.
32. Newton C et al: Topical fibronectin and corneal epithelial wound healing in the rabbit, *Arch Ophthalmol* 106:1277-1279, 1988.
33. Nishida T et al: Fibronectin—a new therapy for corneal trophic ulcer, *Arch Ophthalmol* 101:1046-1048, 1983.
34. Pazin GJ, Ho M, Jannetta PJ: Reactivation of herpes simplex virus after decompression of the trigeminal nerve root, *J Infect Dis* 138:405, 1978.
35. Carton CA, Kilbourne ED: Activation of latent herpes simplex by trigeminal sensory-root section, *N Engl J Med* 246(5):172-176, 1952.
36. Salisbury JD et al: Herpesvirus infection of cornea allografts, *Ophthalmic Surg* 15:406-408, 1984.
37. Beyer CF et al: Oral acyclovir reduces the incidence of recurrent herpes simplex keratitis in rabbits after penetrating keratoplasty, *Arch Ophthalmol* 107:1200-1205, 1989.
38. Mannis MJ et al: Herpes simplex dendritic keratitis after keratoplasty, *Am J Ophthalmol* 111:480-484, 1991.
39. Thygeson P: Observation on filamentary keratitis, *Trans Sect Ophthalmol* 49-55, 1963.
40. Sugar A, Meyer RF: Giant papillary conjunctivitis after keratoplasty, *Am J Ophthalmol* 91:239, 1981.
41. Shahinian L Jr, Brown SI: Postoperative complications with protruding monofilament nylon sutures, *Am J Ophthalmol* 83:546, 1977.
42. Nirankari VS, Karesh JW, Richards RD: Complications of exposed monofilament sutures, *Am J Ophthalmol* 95:515, 1983.
43. Leahey AB et al: Suture abscesses after penetrating keratoplasty, *Cornea* 12(6):489-492, 1993.
44. Kaye DB: Epithelial response in penetrating keratoplasty, *Am J Ophthalmol* 89:381-387, 1980.
45. Bigar F: Specular microscopy of the endothelium. In Straub W, editor: *Developments in ophthalmology,* vol 6, Basel, 1982, Karger.
46. Svedbergh B: Effects of artificial intraocular pressure elevation on the endothelium in the vervet monkey, *Acta Ophthalmol (Copenh)* 53:839-855, 1975.
47. Charlin R, Polack FM: The effect of elevated intraocular pressure on the endothelium of corneal grafts, *Cornea* 1:241-249, 1982.
48. Irvine AR, Kaufman HE: Intraocular pressure following penetrating keratoplasty, *Am J Ophthalmol* 68(5):835-844, 1969.
49. Olson RJ, Kaufman HE: Prognostic factors of intraocular pressure after aphakic keratoplasty, *Am J Ophthalmol* 86:510-515, 1978.
50. Goldberg DB, Schanzlin DJ, Brown SI: Incidence of increased intraocular pressure after keratoplasty, *Am J Ophthalmol* 92:372-377, 1981.
51. Zimmerman TJ et al: Transplant size and elevated intraocular pressure postoperatively, *Arch Ophthalmol* 96:2231, 1978.
52. Olson RJ, Kaufman HE: A mathematical description of causative factors and prevention of elevated intraocular pressure after keratoplasty, *Invest Ophthalmol Vis Sci* 16:1085-1092, 1977.
53. Bourne WM, Davison JA, O'Fallon WM: The effects of oversize donor buttons on postoperative intraocular pressure and corneal curvature in aphakic penetrating keratoplasty, *Ophthalmology* 89(3):242-246, 1982.
54. Karesh JW, Nirankari VS: Factors associated with glaucoma after penetrating keratoplasty, *Am J Ophthalmol* 96:160-164, 1983.
55. Perl T, Charlton KH, Binder PS: Disparate diameter grafting: astigmatism, intraocular pressure, and visual acuity, *Ophthalmology* 88:774-781, 1981.
56. McDonnell PJ, Robin JB, Schanzlin DJ: Molteno implant for control of glaucoma in eyes after penetrating keratoplasty, *Ophthalmology* 95:364-369, 1988.
57. Minckler DS, Heuer DK, Hasty B: Clinical experience with the single-plate Molteno implant in complicated glaucomas, *Ophthalmology* 95:1181-1188, 1988.
58. Levy NS, Bonney NS: Transscleral YAG cyclocoagulation of the ciliary body for persistently high intraocular pressure following penetrating keratoplasty, *Cornea* 8:178-181, 1989.
59. Zaidman GW, Wandel T: Transscleral YAG laser photocoagulation for uncontrolled glaucoma in corneal patients, *Cornea* 7:112-114, 1988.
60. Williams GA et al: Treatment of postvitrectomy fibrin formation with intraocular tissue plasminogen activator, *Arch Ophthalmol* 106:1055, 1988.
61. Snyder RW, Sherman MD, Allinson RW: Intracameral tissue plasminogen activator for treatment of excessive fibrin response after penetrating keratoplasty, *Am J Ophthalmol* 109(4):483-484, 1990.
62. McDermott ML et al: Tissue plasminogen activator and the corneal endothelium, *Am J Ophthalmol* 108(1):91, 19[illegible].
63. Krachmer JH: Personal communication, 1995.
64. Bourne WM: Reduction of endothelial cell loss during phakic penetrating keratoplasty, *Am J Ophthalmol* 89:787-79[illegible], 1980.
65. Rowsey JJ, Gaylor JR: Intraocular lens disasters, peripheral anterior synechia, *Ophthalmology* 87(7):646-664, 198[illegible]
66. Tragakis MP, Brown SI: The significance of anterior synechiae after corneal transplantation, *Am J Ophthalmol* 74:532-533, 1972.
67. Foulks GN, Perry HD, Dohlman CH: Oversize corneal donor grafts in penetrating keratoplasty, *Ophthalmology* 86:490-494, 1979.
68. Cohen EJ, Kenyon KR, Dohlman CH: Iridoplasty for prevention of post-keratoplasty angle closure and glaucoma, *Ophthalmic Surg* 13(12):994-996, 1982.
69. Ainslie D: Recent advances in keratoplasty, *Br J Ophthalmol* 58:335, 1974.
70. Urrets-Zavalia A Jr: Fixed dilated pupil, iris atrophy and secondary glaucoma, a distinct clinical entity following keratoplasty in keratoconus, *Am J Ophthalmol* 56:257-265, 1963.
71. Gasset AR: Fixed dilated pupil following penetrating keratoplasty in keratoconus (Castroviejo syndrome), *Ann Ophthalmol* 9:623, 1977.
72. Bellows AR, Chylack LT Jr, Hutchinson BT: Choroidal detachment, *Ophthalmology* 88:1107, 1981.
73. Pederson JE: Discussion of: Bellows AR, Chylack LT Jr, Hutchinson BT: Choroidal detachment, *Ophthalmology* 88:1107, 1981.
74. Purcell JJ et al: Expulsive hemorrhage in penetrating keratoplasty, *Ophthalmology* 89(1):41-43, 1982.
75. Davison JA: Acute intraoperative suprachoroidal hemorrhage in extracapsular cataract surgery, *J Cataract Refract Surg* 12:606, 1986.
76. Leveille AS, McMullan FD, Cavanagh HD: Endophthalmitis following penetrating keratoplasty, *Ophthalmology* 9[illegible]:38-39, 1983.
77. Guss RB et al: Endophthalmitis after penetrating keratoplasty, *Am J Ophthalmol* 95:651-658, 1983.
78. Antonios SR et al: Contamination of donor cornea, post-penetrating keratoplasty endophthalmitis, *Cornea* 10(3):217-220, 1991.
79. Aiello LP, Javitt JC, Canner JK: National outcomes of penetrating keratoplasty—risks of endophthalmitis and retinal detachment, *Arch Ophthalmol* 111:509-513, 1993.
80. Kloess PM et al: Bacterial and fungal endophthalmitis after penetrating keratoplasty, *Am J Ophthalmol* 115:309-31[illegible], 1993.
81. Cameron JA et al: Endophthalmitis from contaminated donor

corneas following penetrating keratoplasty, *Arch Ophthalmol* 109:54-59, 1991.

82. Polack FM, Locatcher-Khorazo D, Gutierrez E: Bacteriologic study of 'donor' eyes: evaluation of antibacterial treatments prior to corneal grafting, *Arch Ophthalmol* 78:219-225, 1967.
83. Mascarella K, Cavanagh HD: Penetrating keratoplasty using McCarey-Kaufman preserved corneal tissue, *South Med J* 72: 1268-1271, 1979.
84. Chittum ME et al: Contamination of corneal tissue from infected donors, *Arch Ophthalmol* 103:802-804, 1985.
85. Karjalainen K, Vannas A: Bacterial contamination of donor corneas, *Ophthalmic Surg* 15:770-772, 1984.
86. Baum J, Barza M, Kane A: Efficacy of penicillin G, cefazolin, and gentamicin in M-K medium at 4 C, *Arch Ophthalmol* 96:1262-1264, 1978.
87. Baer JC, Nirankari VS, Glaros DS: Survival of *Streptococcus viridans* in gentamicin-supplemented McCarey-Kaufman medium, *Cornea* 8:131, 1989.
88. Berkowitz RA, Kyce SD, Kaufman HE: Aqueous hyposecretion after penetrating keratoplasty, *Ophthalmic Surg* 15:323-324, 1984.
89. Buxton JN et al: Donor failure after corneal transplantation surgery, *Cornea* 7:89-95, 1988.
90. Polack FM, Demong T, Santaella H: Sodium hyaluronate (Healon) in keratoplasty and IOL implantation, *Ophthalmology* 88:425-431, 1981.
91. Miller D, Stegman R: Use of Na-hyaluronate in corneal transplantation, *J Ocular Ther Surg* 1:28, 1981.

Additional Readings

Abrams GW et al: Management of postoperative suprachoroidal hemorrhage with continuous-infusion air pump, *Arch Ophthalmol* 104:1455, 1986.

Al-Hazzaa SAF, Tabbara KF: Bacterial keratitis after penetrating keratoplasty, *Ophthalmology* 95(11):1504-1508, 1988.

Baer JC, Nirankari VS, Glaros DS: Streptococcal endophthalmitis from contaminated donor corneas after keratoplasty—clinical and laboratory investigations, *Arch Ophthalmol* 106:517-520, 1988.

Bates AK et al: Microbial keratitis after penetrating keratoplasty, *Eye* 4:74-78, 1990.

Beyer CF et al: Herpes simplex dendritic keratitis after keratoplasty, *Am J Ophthalmol* 109:95, 1990.

Beyer CF et al: Herpes simplex virus and persistent epithelial defects after penetrating keratoplasty, *Am J Ophthalmol* 109(1):95-96, 1990.

Chien AM et al: Glaucoma in the immediate postoperative period after penetrating keratoplasty, *Am J Ophthalmol* 115:711-714, 1993.

Driebe WT Jr, Stern GA: Microbial keratitis following corneal transplantation, *Cornea* 2:41-45, 1983.

Escapini HE Jr, Olson RJ, Kaufman HE: Donor cornea contamination with McCarey-Kaufman medium preservation, *Am J Ophthalmol* 88:59, 1979.

Fong LP et al: Microbial keratitis complicating penetrating keratoplasty, *Ophthalmology* 95(9):1269-1275, 1988.

Foulks GN: Glaucoma associated with penetrating keratoplasty, *Ophthalmology* 94(7):871-874, 1987.

Heidemann DG et al: Oversized donor grafts in penetrating keratoplasty, *Arch Ophthalmol* 103:1807-1811, 1985.

Ingraham HJ, Donnenfeld ED, Perry HD: Massive suprachoroidal hemorrhage in penetrating keratoplasty, *Am J Ophthalmol* 108: 670-675, 1989.

Keates RH, Mishler KE, Riedinger KD: Bacterial contamination of donor eyes, *Am J Ophthalmol* 84(5):617, 1977.

Khodadoust AA, Franklin RM: Transfer of bacterial infection by donor cornea in penetrating keratoplasty, *Am J Ophthalmol* 87:130-132, 1979.

Kirkness CM, Ficker LA: Risk factors for the development of postkeratoplasty glaucoma, *Cornea* 11(5):427-432, 1992.

Kirkness CM, Moshegov C: Post-keratoplasty glaucoma, *Eye* (Suppl) 2:S19-26, 1988.

Lamensdorf M et al: Microbial keratitis after penetrating keratoplasty, *Ophthalmology* 89:124, 1982.

Olson R, Zimmerman TJ, Kaufman HE: Elevated intraocular pressure after aphakic keratoplasty: iatrogenic desease and prevention, *Ann Ophthalmol* 10:931-932, 1978.

Olson RJ: Aphakic keratoplasty, determining donor tissue size to avoid elevated intraocular pressure, *Arch Ophthalmol* 96:2274, 1978.

Pardos GJ, Gallagher MA: Microbial contamination of donor eyes, a retrospective study, *Arch Ophthalmol* 100:1611-1613, 1982.

Poole TG, Insler MS: Contamination of donor cornea by gentamicin-resistant organisms, *Am J Ophthalmol* 97:560-564, 1984.

Simmons RV et al: Elevated intraocular pressure following penetrating keratoplasty, *Trans Am Ophthalmol Soc* 87:79-91, 1990.

White JH: Fungal contamination of donor eyes, *Br J Ophthalmol* 53:30, 1969.

Wood TO, West C, Kaufman HE: Control of intraocular pressure in penetrating keratoplasty, *Am J Ophthalmol* 74:724, 1972.

Wysenbeek YS et al: The effect of sodium hyaluronate on the corneal epithelium, *Invest Ophthalmol Vis Sci* 29(2):194-199, 1988.

CHAPTER 137

CHARLES S. REING MARK G. SPEAKER

Postkeratoplasty Astigmatism

Advancements in microsurgical techniques, eye-banking, and the ability to detect and treat early graft rejection have led to very high success rates in achieving and maintaining optical clarity in corneal grafts. Success rates of 70% to 95% have been reported since the early 1970s.[1-3] However, visual acuity, binocular visual function, and patient satisfaction may be severely limited by postoperative astigmatism and anisometropia. Most studies document average postkeratoplasty astigmatism in the range of 4 to 5 diopters.[3-9] Numerous factors are theorized to contribute to the ultimate shape of the cornea. These can be divided into preoperative, operative, and postoperative considerations.

In the postoperative state, multiple factors influence the cylindrical component of the refraction. For example the tension of each interrupted suture acts as an independent vector on the central corneal curvature. Interrupted sutures act by causing local flattening and central steepening (Figure 137-1). The greater the number of independent forces acting on the cornea, the more complicated the corneal topography can be. Although the cylindrical spectacle prescription or the vector sum of forces acting on the cornea (Figure 137-2) adequately describes simple astigmatism, it is only a mathematical approximation if the corneal surface is more complex or irregular. Under these circumstances, irregular astigmatism may limit the best achievable spectacle corrected acuity. As will be discussed, the goal of postoperative corneal topography is not only to reduce the magnitude of the cylindrical refractive error, but also to decrease irregular astigmatism by eliminating unbalanced vector forces.

Reports concerning postkeratoplasty astigmatism must be interpreted with an understanding of the potential limitations of study data in this area. The causes of postkeratoplasty astigmatism are multifactorial (box). Variability introduced by the host and donor corneas and by operative and postoperative factors specific to a single surgeon or group, makes comparison of data from one surgeon to another difficult. Removal of sutures even 3 years after keratoplasty can result in substantial changes in corneal toricity so that sutures-in and sutures-out astigmatism are usually different. One must be careful to distinguish between the two when interpreting the data in these studies.

Furthermore, the technique used in the measurement and evaluation of astigmatism may affect reported results. Retinoscopy and or subjective refraction yields the total refraction of the eye, which includes lenticular astigmatism. Keratometry provides information regarding the central 3 millimeters of corneal curvature but does not describe irregular astigmatism well. Corneal topography provides the most useful and complete information regarding corneal shape. It is particularly helpful in identifying irregular or asymmetric astigmatism and localized abnormalities of corneal contour. In addition, corneal statistics such as simulated keratometry, and indices of surface regularity and asymmetry can be generated. However, because most currently available topography units generate data regarding corneal curvature from reflections of placido-discs off the corneal epithelium (Figure 137-3), focal areas of drying or defects in the corneal epithelium may degrade the image quality and can produce misleading information. Furthermore, fixation appears to be critical because a small decentration can result in significant distortion of the corneal map (Figure 137-4).

Preoperative Factors

Postoperative astigmatism may be analyzed with respect to the preoperative donor and recipient corneas, although neither can be readily controlled by the surgeon. Information regarding the average steepness or astigmatism of the donor is generally not available to the surgeon preoperatively. This information could theoretically be obtained from the donor patient's spectacles or family, or with preoperative computerized topography. However, because of technical and logistic factors, no studies to date have evaluated this relationship. Irregularities or defects in the corneal epithelium make using commonly available placido-ring corneal topography unfeasible, but nonplacido disc systems are currently under development that could make it possible to preoperatively evaluate the donor cornea in combination with an artificial anterior chamber in the future.

displacement.[23] For this reason, we avoid decentering the graft except when absolutely necessary. Typically, we make the donor the same size as the host (donor trephine 0.25 millimeters larger than the recipient when the donor is punched from the endothelial side) in all cases. The donor is oversized by 0.25 millimeter in cases in which iris abnormalities or severe inflammation may result in extensive angle closure, or in cases in which an anterior chamber intraocular lens (IOL) is to be implanted or left in place. IOL calculations need to be adjusted accordingly for the resultant steeper cornea.

Disparity between the shape of the donor and recipient corneas induces significant astigmatism. Tissue deficiency at the wound will decrease the chord length in that axis thereby steepening the cornea in that meridian. Conversely, the cornea is flattened in the meridian of tissue excess.[24,25] A 0.5 by 6.0 millimeter crescent shape block resection has been shown to induce 4 to 7 diopters of corneal steepening in the axis of the resected tissue in an animal model.[26] This concept forms the basis of the technique of wedge resection for correction of postkeratoplasty astigmatism that will be discussed later in this chapter. Similarly, misalignment between donor and recipient edges can change the chord length so that graft override and underride can produce flattening and steepening respectively. Alignment of the epithelial edges of the donor and host should be carefully monitored during suturing.

Several technical factors during surgery have been implicated in producing uneven, irregular, or oval trephination of the tissues. Small degrees of tilting of the trephine or decentration on the Teflon block will produce an oval cut. A tilt of 20 degrees results in approximately 0.5 millimeter of disparity between the major and minor axes.[27]

Presently, tissue is supplied to most surgeons in the form of a cornea with a scleral rim, and is cut from the endothelial surface. A vertically guided corneal punch system for the donor tissue should be used to create a trephination as close to perpendicular as possible. Newer punch systems, which maintain an artificial anterior chamber and allow the cutting of the donor tissue from the epithelial surface, may improve the match between host and donor edge profiles. The Krumeich guided trephine system uses the same disposable blade for trephination of the recipient and donor corneas after the intraocular pressure in the artificial chamber and the host eye are equalized. In a small prospective study, Belmont et al. found less keratometric astigmatism when this system was used compared with manual trephination.[28] For trephination of the host tissue, suction trephine systems such as the Hanna, Hessberg-Barron, or Krumeich are preferred because they stabilize the globe during trephination, ensuring that the cutting surface is held perpendicular to the cornea. However, a narrow palpebral fissure, filtration blebs, or irregularities of the conjunctiva may prevent adequate suction. In fact, suction trephines should be avoided when filtering blebs are present at the limbus because rupture of the bleb with postoperative hypotony may result.

A dull or damaged trephine or corneal block, poor punch technique, pressure on the globe from the lid speculum, bridle suture, fixation ring, or fixation forceps can adversely affect the trephination.[29] In addition, an abnormally elevated or low intraocular pressure may result in uneven or beveled trephination.[21] Distortion of the globe from the lid speculum also results in trephination of an oval opening in the host tissues and a mismatch in apposition of the recipient and donor corneas. Barraquer's wire speculum (the simplest of the many lid specula available), can induce 1 to 3 diopters of with-the-rule astigmatism keratometrically depending on the spring tension.[21] The McNeill-Goldmann ring combines scleral support rings with a blepharostat, but suturing of support rings to the globe may in itself induce in excess of 10 diopters of astigmatism.[27] Perhaps the ideal is direct eyelid sutures or Jaffe lid retractors.

In an attempt to reduce postkeratoplasty astigmatism, Troutman et al. performed two controlled studies evaluating the effect of selective positioning of the donor cornea in patients undergoing penetrating keratoplasty for keratoconus. In the study group, the corneal button was rotated before suturing until apparent sphericity was obtained using an intraoperative qualitative keratometer. This group was compared to another group in which the button was sutured in place with random orientation. In the earlier study, no statistical difference in astigmatism was found between the two groups after all sutures were removed.[30] But in the more recent study, the rotated group had significantly lower sutures-out astigmatism (2.27 diopters versus 4.64 diopters). The authors suggested increased experience with rotating the graft as a possible explanation for the different results.[31]

A device as simple as a handheld keratoscope or a surgical keratometer can be used intraoperatively to monitor astigmatism. These instruments are most useful in checking the tension of interrupted sutures or adjusting the running suture. It is important to have a deep, stable anterior chamber, and to have the plane of the patient's cornea perpendicular to the optical axis of the microscope. It is our impression that this technique reduces postoperative astigmatism and speeds visual rehabilitation. However, no controlled study to date has been performed to prove it. A new computerized nonplacido disc intraoperative topography system is

B

D

F

H

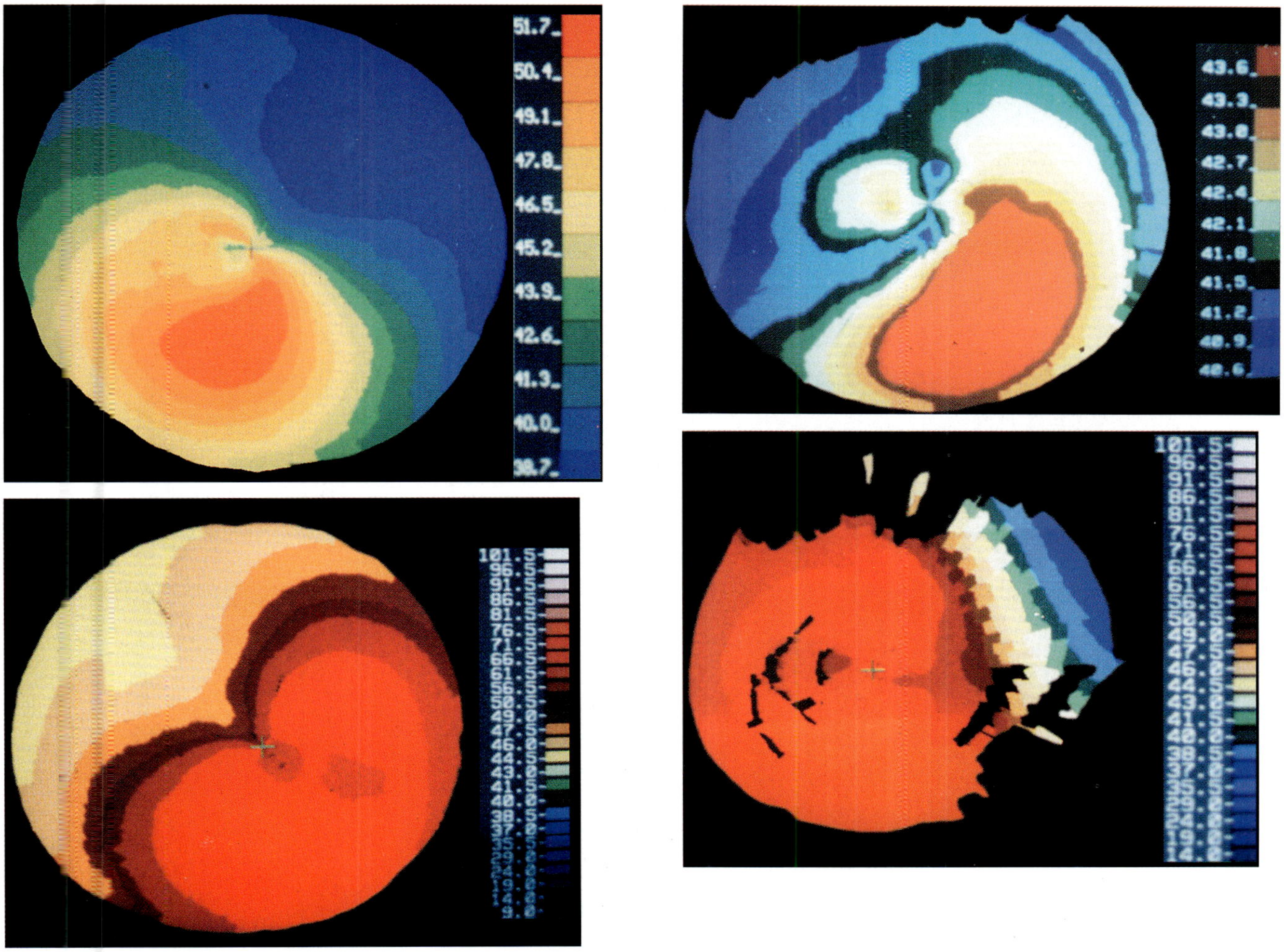

COLOR PLATE 91-10

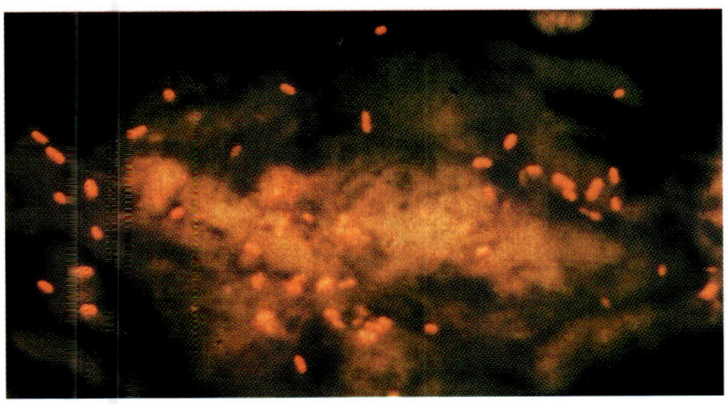

COLOR PLATE 94-29

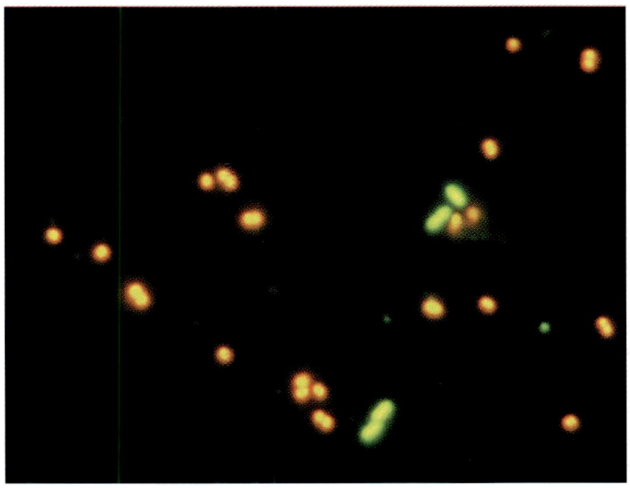

COLOR PLATE 94-30

A

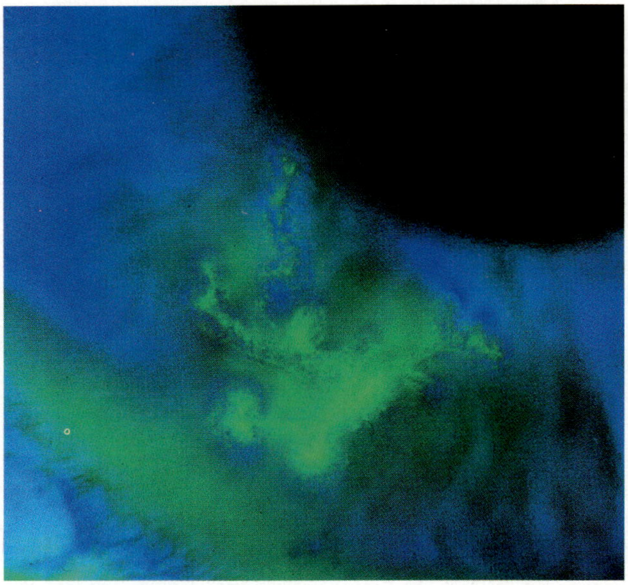

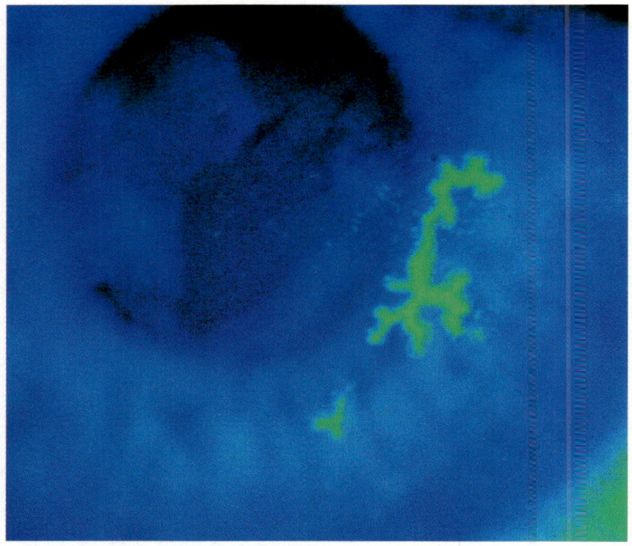

B

COLOR PLATE 95-5

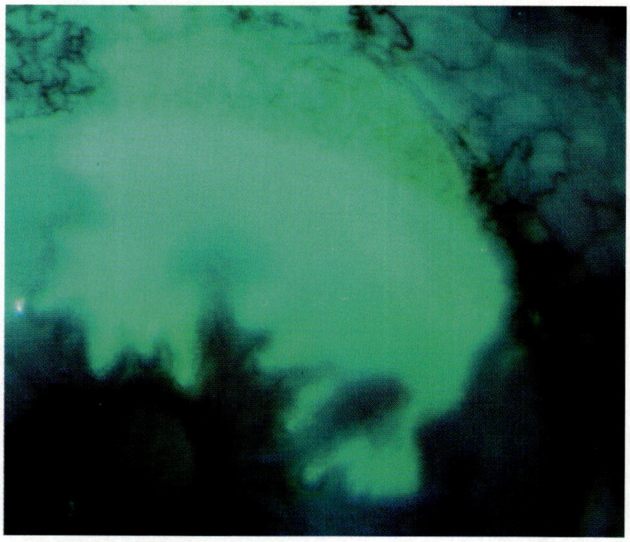

COLOR PLATE 95-7, B

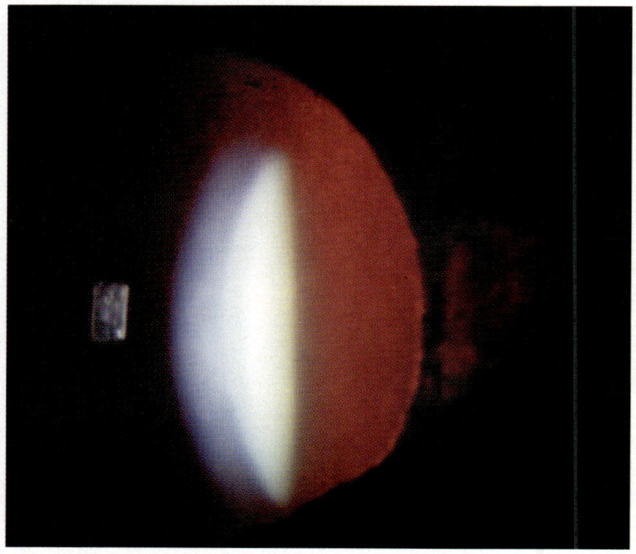

COLOR PLATE 95-26, B

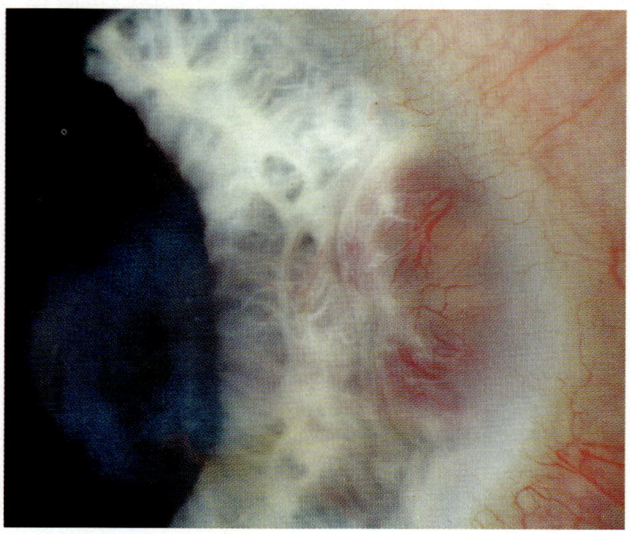

COLOR PLATE 95-27

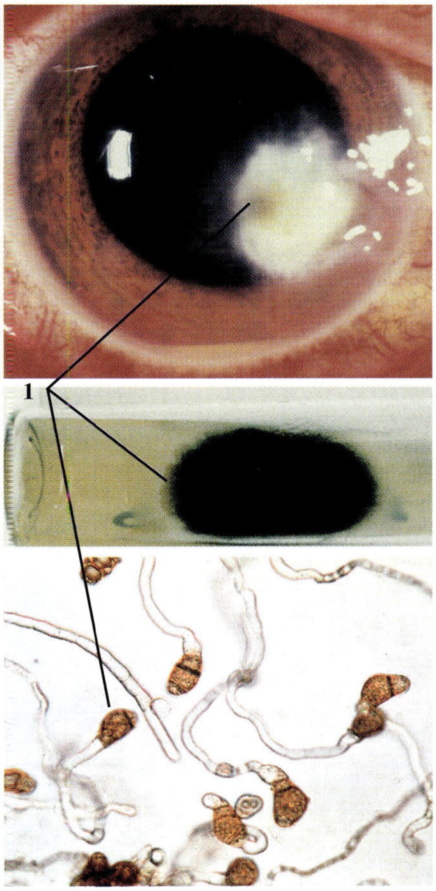

COLOR PLATE 98-6

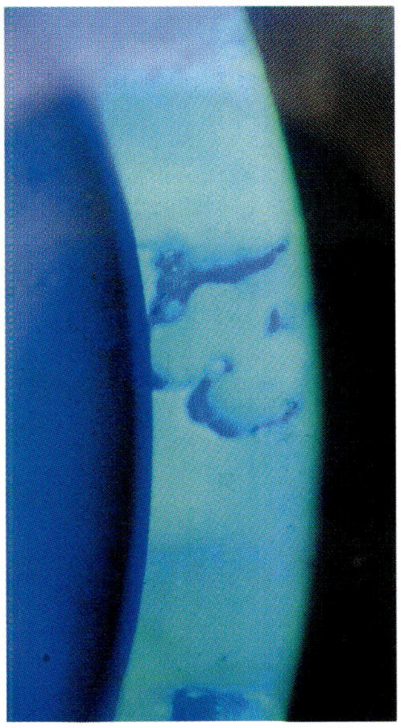

COLOR PLATE 102-3

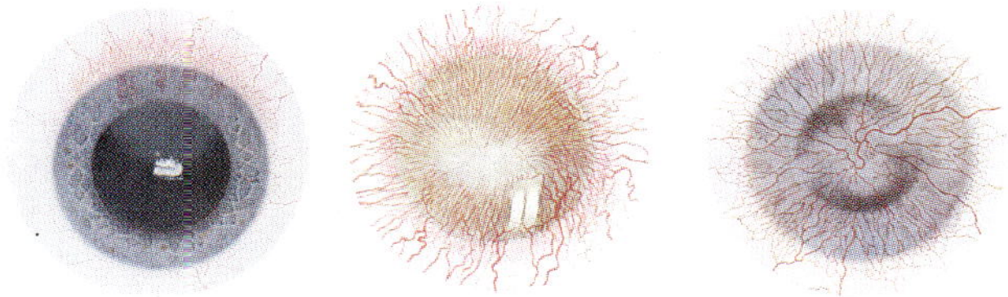

COLOR PLATE 100-7

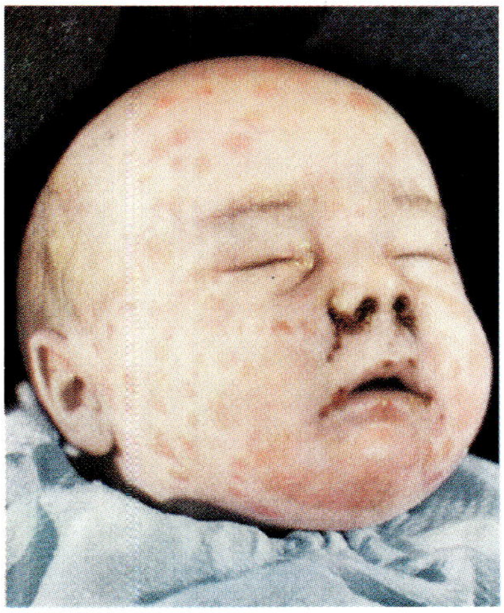

COLOR PLATE 100-31

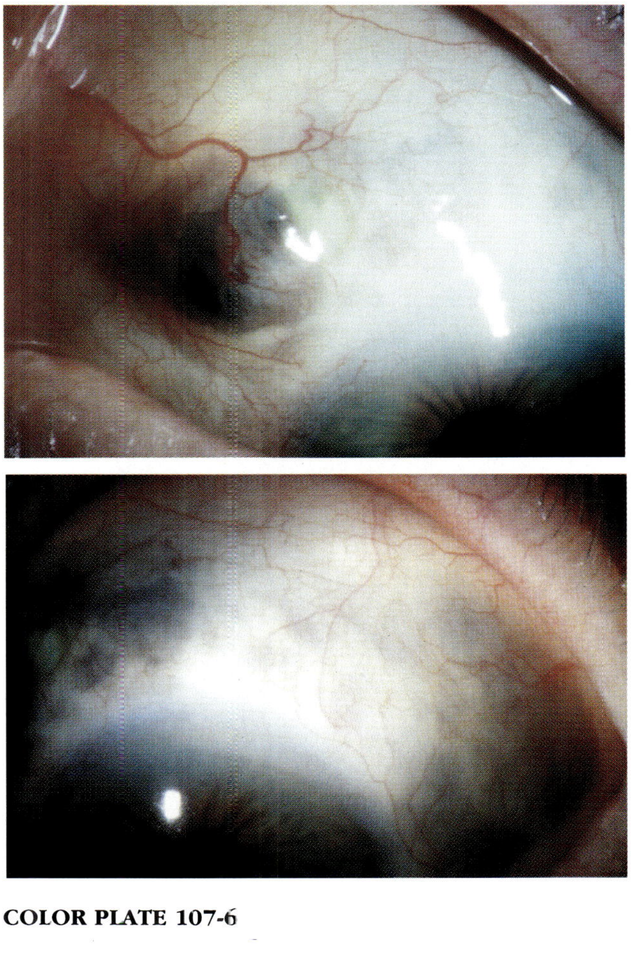

A

B

COLOR PLATE 107-6

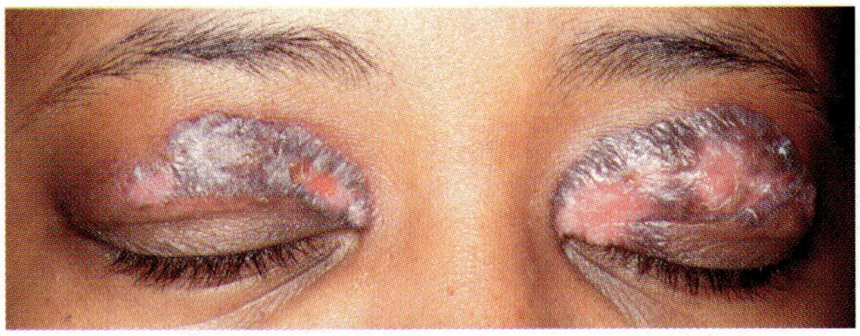

COLOR PLATE 108-2

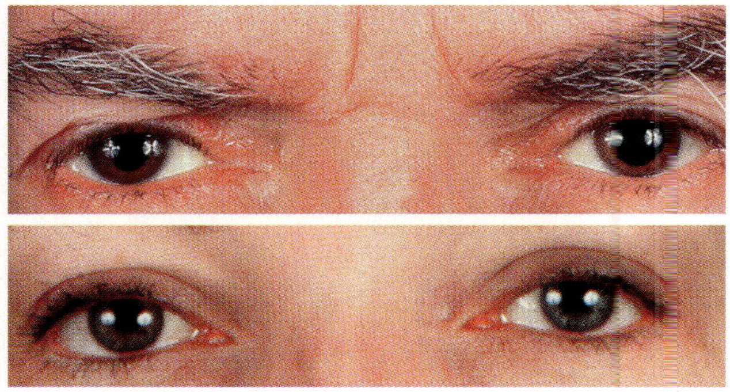

COLOR PLATE 125-1

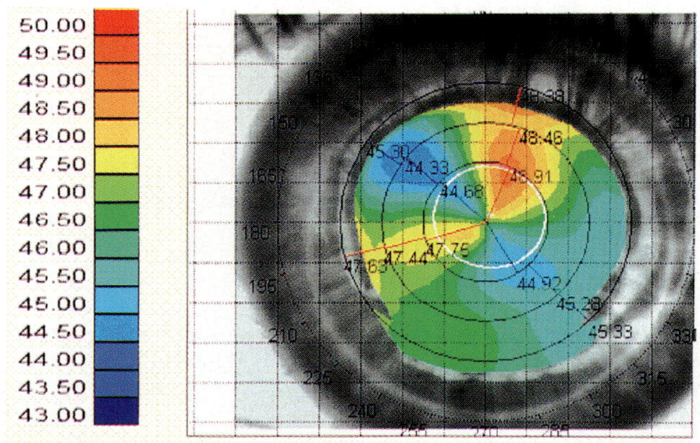

COLOR PLATE 135-1

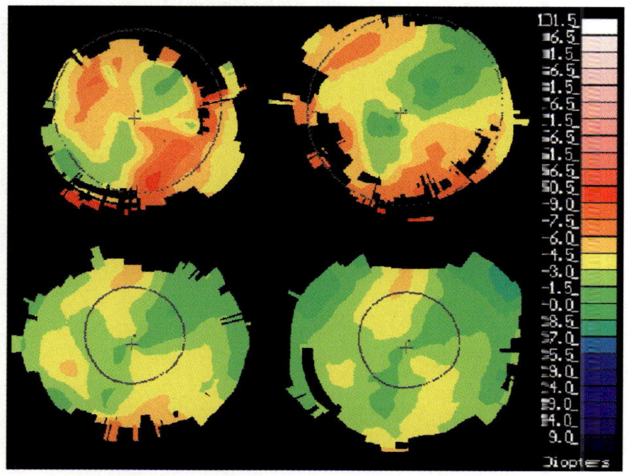

COLOR PLATE 137-5

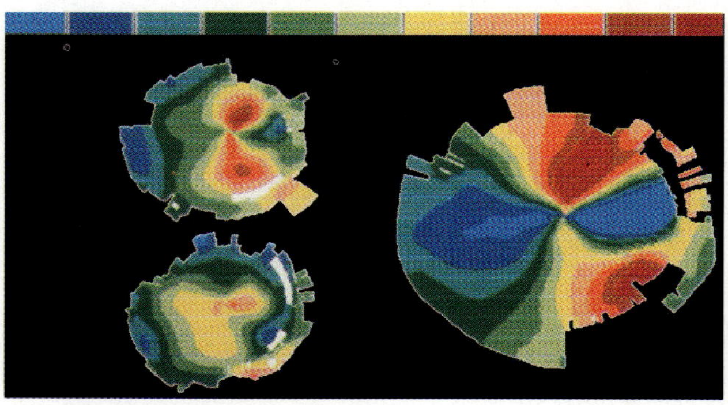

COLOR PLATE 137-6

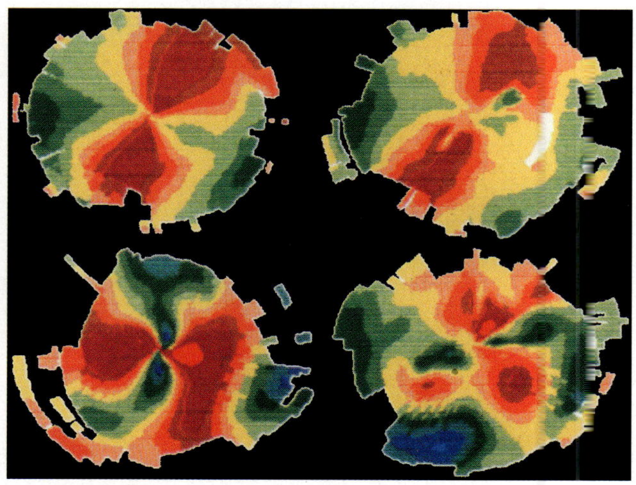

COLOR PLATE 137-7

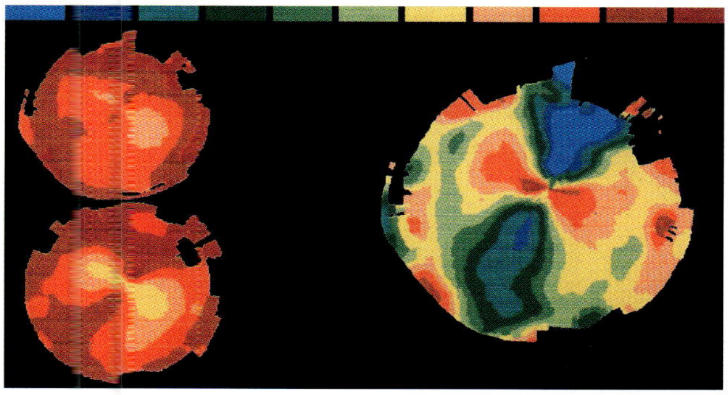

COLOR PLATE 137-10

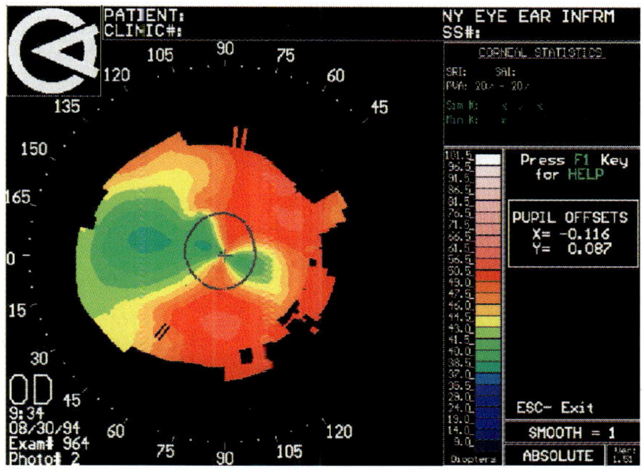

COLOR PLATE 137-11

A B C D

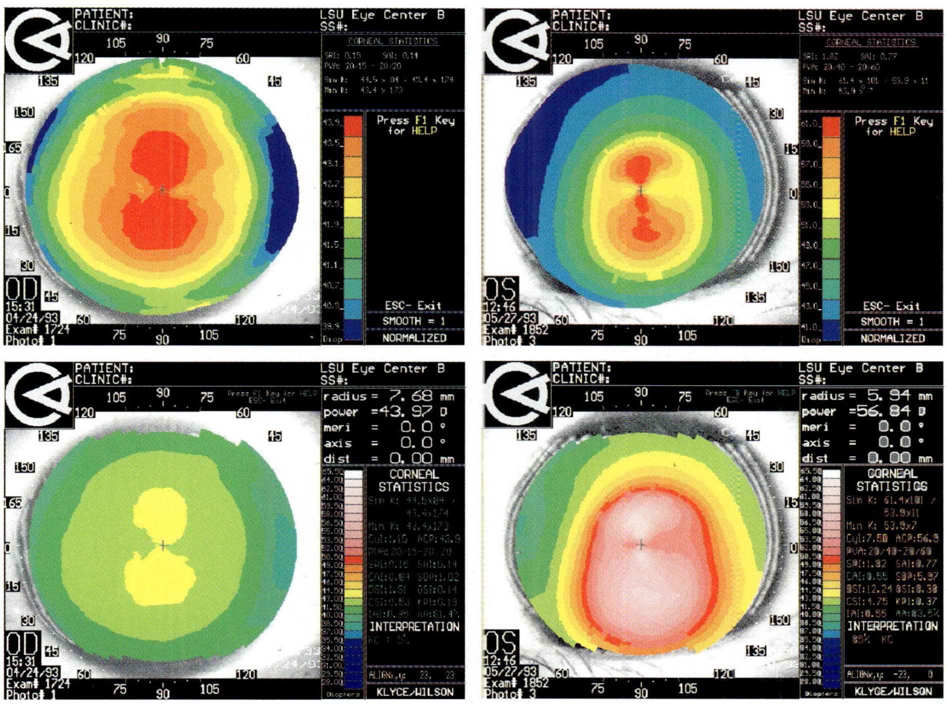

COLOR PLATE 165-1

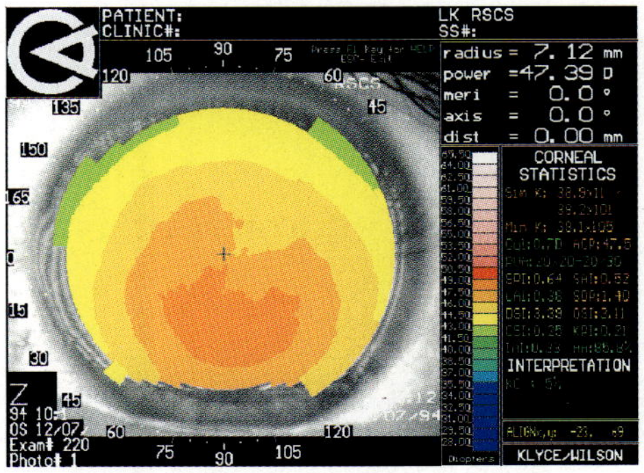

COLOR PLATE 165-2

A

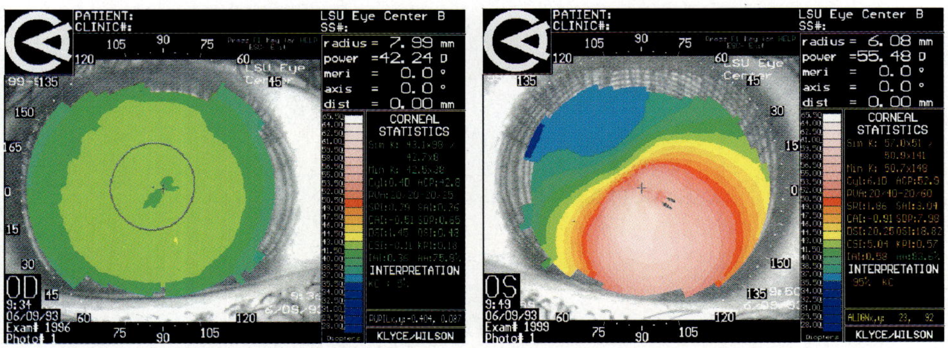

B

COLOR PLATE 165-3

A

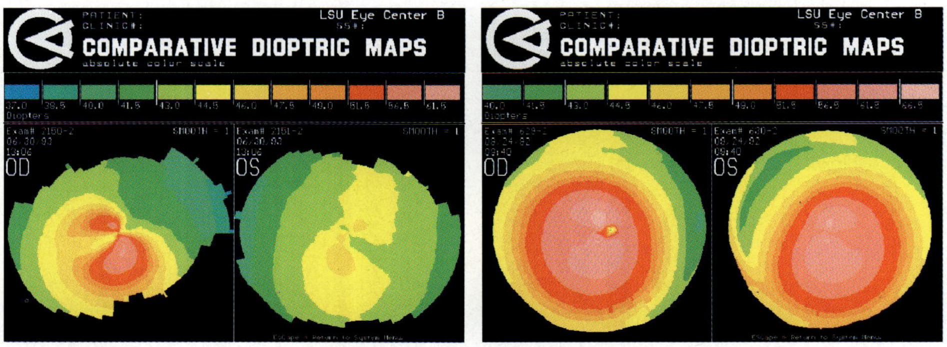

B

COLOR PLATE 165-4

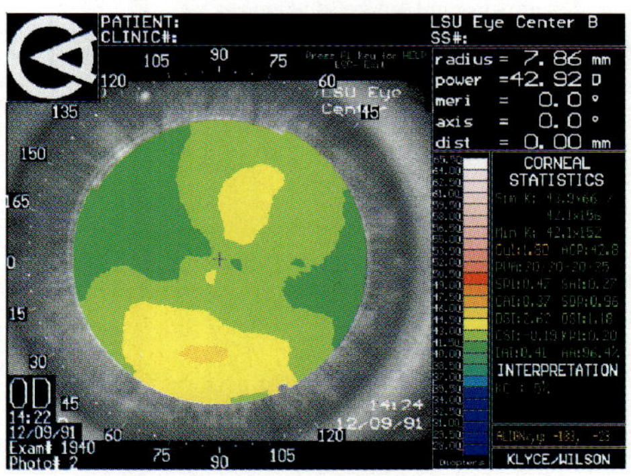

COLOR PLATE 165-5

A

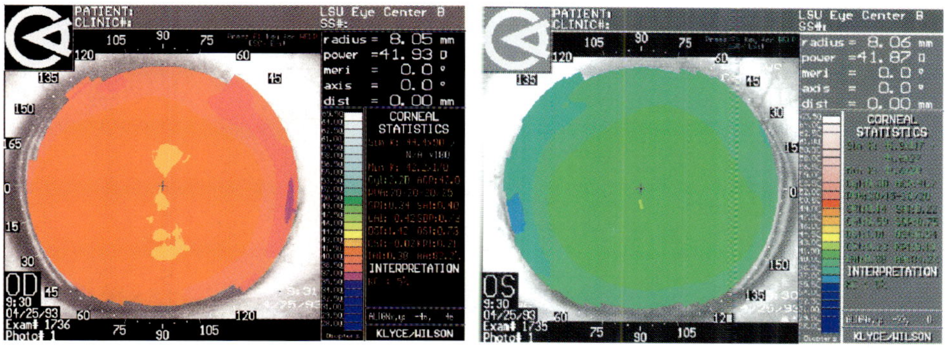

B

COLOR PLATE 165-6

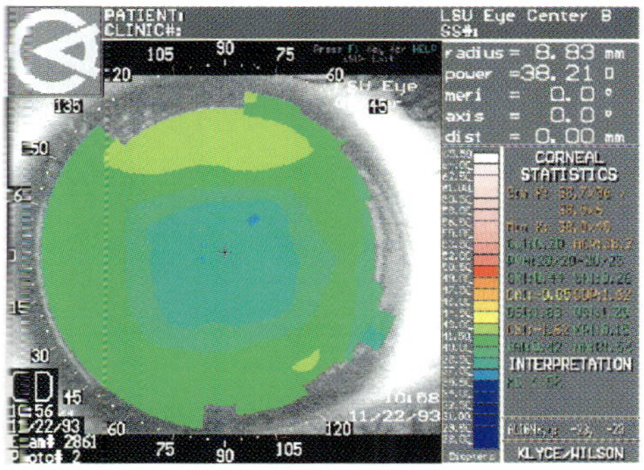

COLOR PLATE 165-8

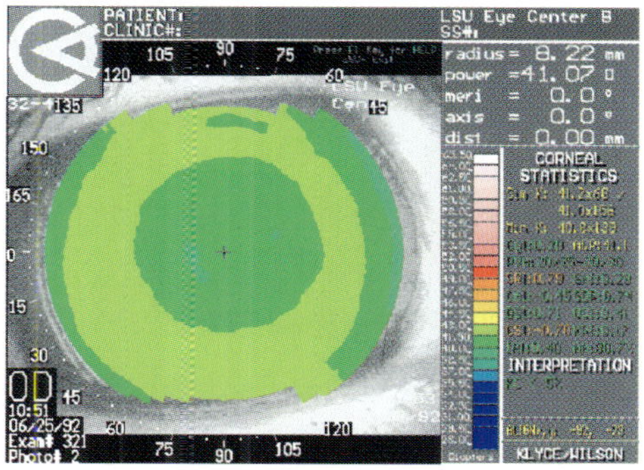

COLOR PLATE 165-9

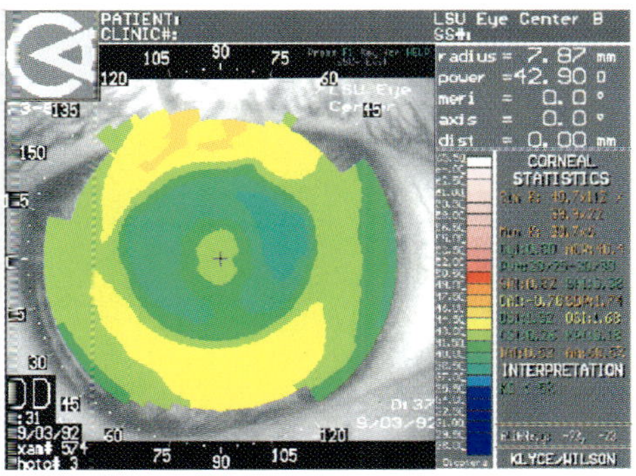

COLOR PLATE 165-10

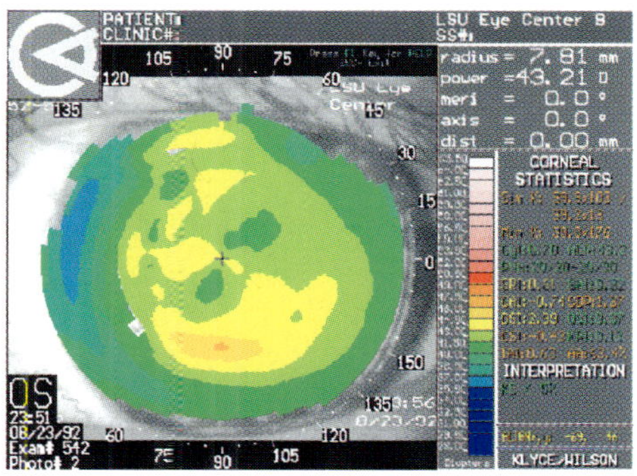

COLOR PLATE 165-11

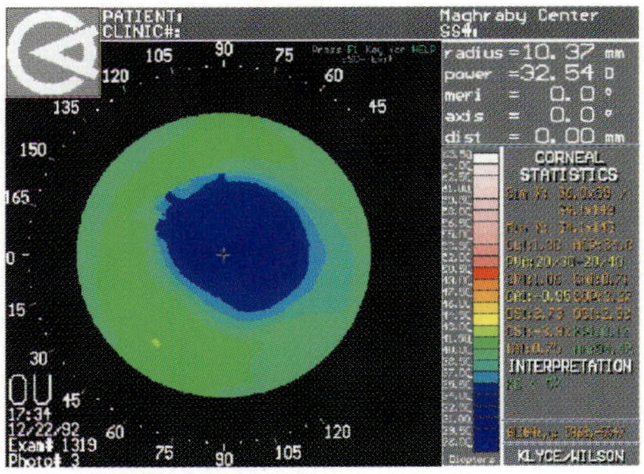

COLOR PLATE 165-12

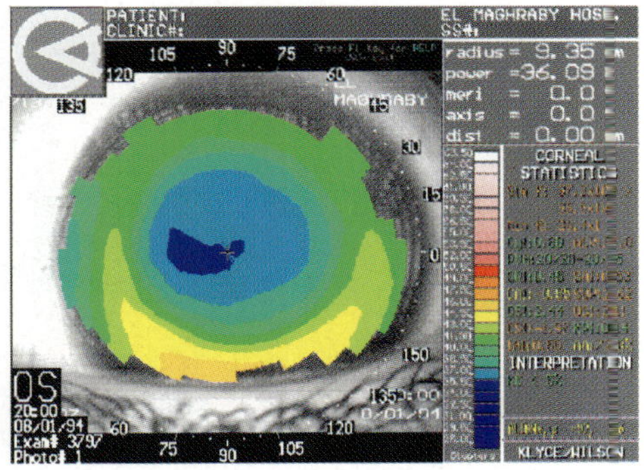

COLOR PLATE 165-13

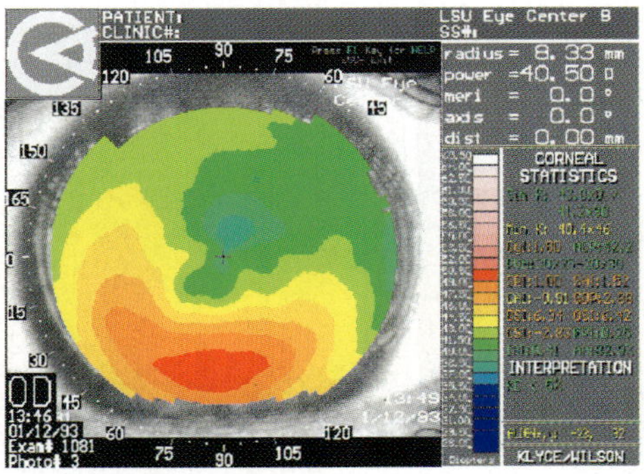

COLOR PLATE 165-14

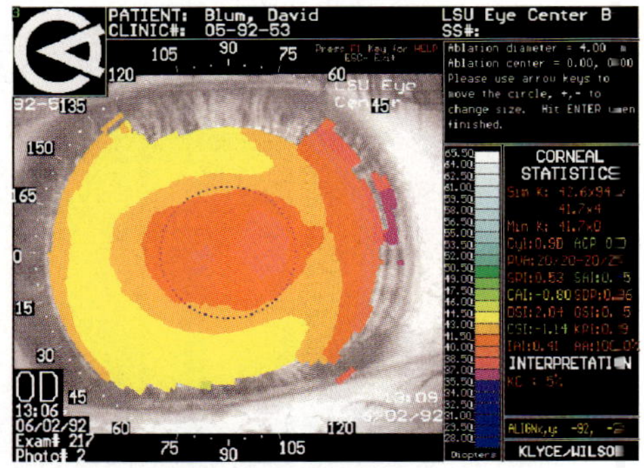

COLOR PLATE 165-15

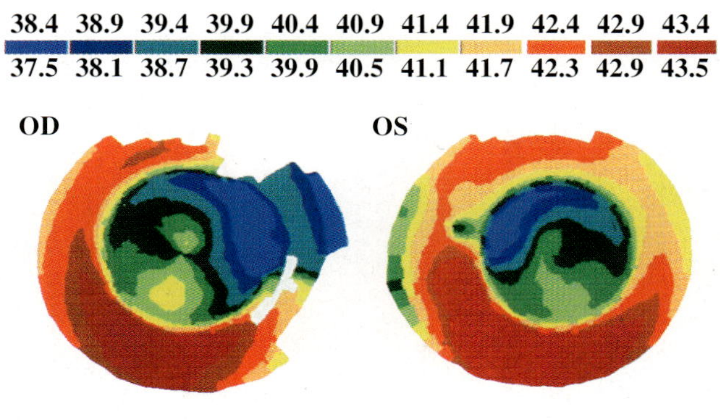

COLOR PLATE 172-14

currently under development that may provide more quantitative information during surgery despite donor surface irregularity or lack of epithelium.

Many surgeons advocate the use of a scleral support ring such as the McNeil-Goldmann ring described above or Flieringa's ring, a single metal ring, to provide support to the globe especially when performing aphakic keratoplasty. We are no longer routinely using such rings, since they may interfere with the use of newer vacuum trephines, and as mentioned previously, may in themselves induce distortion of the globe. If one is needed in special circumstances, it should be removed after placement of the cardinal sutures when the anterior chamber can be deepened and the corneal shape assessed with a qualitative keratometer.

Hardten et al. evaluated the effect of intraocular lens implantation at the time of keratoplasty on postkeratoplasty astigmatism. They found no predominant axis of astigmatism or relationship of the axis of astigmatism to the meridian of lens position in patients who had placement of an anterior chamber intraocular lens with flexible haptics.[32] For transclerally fixated posterior chamber intraocular lenses (TSPCL), the distance behind the limbus, at which the transcleral suture was placed, correlated with the orientation of early postoperative astigmatism. Patients with the TSPCL fixated 2 to 3 millimeters posterior to the limbus were more likely to have steepening in the same meridian as the haptics, whereas patients with the lens fixated within 0.75 millimeters of the limbus, presumably in the ciliary sulcus, were likely to have astigmatism oriented perpendicular to the meridian of the haptics. This relationship did not hold in the late postoperative period after suture removal.[33] Furthermore, the authors found in an eye bank model that the recipient bed was widened in the meridian of the haptics an average of 0.3 millimeters when a TSPCL was fixated in the ciliary sulcus (within 0.75 millimeters from the limbus). The recipient bed narrowed by an average of 0.2 millimeters when the lens was fixated 3 millimeter posterior to the limbus. This effect was probably due to the use of 13.5 to 14.0 millimeters diameter IOLs, which are too large for the ciliary sulcus. The average internal diameter of the eye at the ciliary sulcus has been measured to be 10.83 millimeters in the vertical and 11.17 millimeters in the horizontal direction.[34]

The numerous operative factors affecting the shape and regularity of the recipient bed and donor button mentioned above, as well as equal distribution of the corneal tissue during surgery, appear to be more critical than suture technique in determining the final astigmatism after all sutures have been removed. Unequal distribution of the donor tissue during placement of the cardinal sutures is as important as matching the shape of the donor and host during trephination. The distribution of the donor tissue should be scrupulously examined during placement of the four cardinal sutures. We check the tissue distribution during the second through fourth sutures by filling the anterior chamber with viscoelastic and passing the suture needle without pulling it out of the tissue. The donor tissue is then positioned in the recipient opening so that the epithelial edges of the donor and host are aligned as best as possible with support to the donor provided by the viscoelastic. The needle, which is still bridging the wound, is observed. Nonradiality indicates uneven tissue distribution. If necessary the needle is removed and passed again until radiality is achieved, at which point, the needle pass is completed and the suture tied.

Radial suture placement is of critical importance as described by Eisner.[35] As a guide, we mark the host cornea prior to trephination with a radial marker inked by a surgical marking pen. If an artificial anterior chamber is used in the trephination of the donor cornea, radial marks can also be made on the donor tissue.

Postoperative Factors

Careful intraoperative adjustment of suture tension and selective postoperative suture removal or adjustment in the postoperative period may decrease early astigmatism and promote earlier visual rehabilitation.[36-38] Beginning as early as 2 weeks after surgery, tight interrupted sutures can be identified using keratometry, keratoscopy, or corneal topography. But the topography of the donor cornea generally is not stable until 4 to 8 weeks after surgery (Figure 137-5). Corneal edema, epithelial irregularity, and fixation errors all may affect the topography image in the early postoperative period. For this reason, decisions concerning suture removal should be made only after stability has been confirmed with images obtained on two consecutive visits.

While topography provides the most useful information in directing suture removal, it does not correlate precisely with the amount of tension in the donor cornea. Therefore the amount of effect from removal of a single suture cannot be easily predicted. Removal of a tight interrupted suture typically results in an average of 2 to 3 diopters of flattening in the meridian of the suture, but may result in as much as a 10 diopter change (Figure 137-6). When vector analysis, which accounts for a shift in axis, is used, the reduction in astigmatism is approximately double this value.[39] Removal of one suture per postoperative visit allows more predictable adjustment and results in lower postoperative astigmatism when compared with mul-

CHAPTER 138

GARY N. FOULKS

Clinical Aspects of Corneal Allograft Rejection

Corneal transplantation is the most successful tissue transplantation procedure in humans. While much of the success in corneal grafting is due to improved surgical technique and better donor tissue management, the appreciation of the varied clinical manifestations and improved medical management of corneal allograft rejection have produced survival rates of up to 95% in some reported series of low-risk patients.[1,2] Yet of the 40,000 corneal transplants performed annually in the United States, corneal allograft rejection is still the leading cause of corneal graft failure.[3,4] Review of the reported prevalence of corneal graft rejection events compared to prevalence of corneal graft failure due to rejection over the past 25 years chronicles an improvement in our ability to manage allograft rejection (Figure 138-1) but also reveals that we do not sufficiently understand the process to control it completely.[1,5,6,7] The clinical challenge remains to recognize those patients who are at high risk of rejection, to communicate well with the patient the need for prompt recognition and therapy of rejection, to maintain a high level of suspicion for allograft rejection, to recognize the early and subtle signs of corneal allograft rejection, and to institute prompt and aggressive therapy. While future developments in immunosuppression and immunomodulation promise to mitigate the effects of corneal allograft rejection, our most effective strategy presently in corneal transplantation is to recognize allograft rejection early and treat it aggressively.

Historical Perspective

A brief historical review of our developing understanding of corneal graft rejection not only increases appreciation of the mechanism of corneal graft rejection but also identifies some of the important clinical principles that apply to recognition and therapy of rejection. Paufique, Sourdille, and Offret first described graft failure ("maladie du greffon") in 1948 as an opacification of the corneal graft occurring after an interval of clarity. They suggested that host sensitivity to the donor was the cause.[8] In laboratory studies of allograft rejection, Maumenee confirmed in 1951 that sensitization of the host to the donor was the underlying basis of this graft failure.[9] Maumenee's subsequent clinical observations in the 1960s characterized the clinical features of corneal allograft failure and emphasized the importance of the endothelium as relevant cells damaged by the immunologic assault.[10,11] Experimental studies in animals by Silverstein and Khodadoust in the late 1960s demonstrated the clinical and histopathologic events of corneal allograft rejection. These investigators observed that each layer of the cornea (epithelium, stroma, and endothelium) could induce host sensitization and undergo allograft rejection either individually or in concert.[12] Polack's laboratory studies extended these observations by experimentally determining the fate of the various layers of the transplanted cornea. Polack showed that donor epithelial cells are replaced rapidly by the host's epithelial cells and while susceptible to rejection when present, are not present for late immunologic assault. Conversely, stromal and endothelial tissues persist and are subject to subsequent immunologic attack.[13,14] With such supportive studies, it has been further asserted that allograft rejection was a form of delayed hypersensitivity. More recent studies, particularly by Streilein and associates, have raised the possibility that anterior chamber associated immune deviation (ACAID) phenomena contributes to graft survival and that allograft rejection represents a breakdown in the protection afforded the graft by ACAID.[15,16]

Recognition of Risk Factors

A number of clinical studies performed in the 1970s and 1980s by Casey in England,[17] Volker-Dieben in the Netherlands,[18] Arentsen in the United States,[1] Boisjoly in Canada,[19] and a large prospective collaborative study in the United States[20] characterized clinical

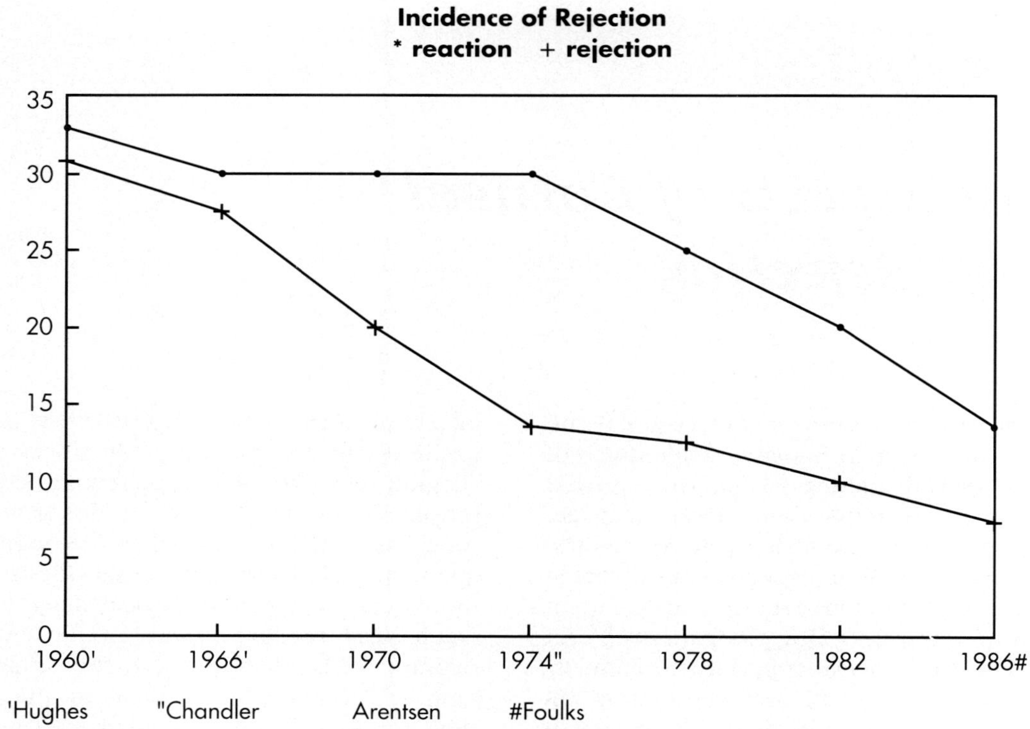

FIGURE 138-1 Progress in corneal graft survival. Comparison of prevalence of allograft reaction (*) versus rejection (+) in selected reported series over the past 30 years. The decline in graft failure despite prevalence of reaction episodes is apparent.[1,5,6,7]

aspects of corneal allograft rejection. These studies and others have identified certain patient characteristics as presenting increased risk for corneal allograft rejection. A young recipient age has been identified in two clinical series as carrying increased risk of rejection.[19,21] While data from two large transplant registries[22,23] do not demonstrate such a risk, statistically rigorous evaluation of the prospective data from the Collaborative Corneal Transplantation Studies (CCTS) confirms young recipient age (less than 40) as a strong risk factor for allograft rejection.[24]

A majority of published clinical studies have demonstrated the higher risk of rejection associated with vascularization of the host cornea either preoperatively[1,17,18] or postoperatively.[25] Typically there is an increasing risk associated with increasing degree of stromal vascularization. Based on such observations it is now generally accepted to consider any patient with greater than two quadrants of corneal stromal vascularization to be at high risk of graft rejection.[26] Additionally, it should be noted that at least one clinical study has shown that any vascularization of the recipient cornea to the graft margin confers a greater risk of rejection.[27]

The early clinical observation that large diameter corneal grafts were more susceptible to rejection was explained by the donor tissue proximity to the limbal vasculature.[28] Recently, more consideration has been given to the presence of immunocompetent cells in the recipient tissue. Investigations into the role of the Langerhans cells in corneal graft rejection performed by Gillette and Chandler postulate that the presence of Langerhans cells in the peripheral cornea could explain the increased risk of rejection when the donor-host junction extends further into the peripheral donor and recipient cornea.[29] The presence of such cells in the diseased central cornea might also increase the risk of allograft rejection in some high-risk disease states (e.g., chemical burn).[30] Interestingly, in at least two recent studies evaluating high-risk patients, graft rejection was greater for small diameter grafts suggesting that inflammatory disease or prior surgical intervention may alter the distribution of immunocompetent cells in the recipient corneas of high-risk patients.[24,31,32] Likewise, contact of the donor with the host vascular system through the presence of iris synechiae to the graft/host junction increases the risk of rejection.[1,23] Loose sutures in the graft, whether by induction of vascularization or stimulation of localized inflammation, also have been reported to increase the risk of rejection.[21]

One of the long recognized major risk factors for corneal allograft rejection is prior graft failure, particularly due to rejection.[33] With the more rigorous statistical analysis applied to recent prospective clinical trials in high-risk patients,[19,24] this risk factor has been further defined to reveal that in over 3 years of observation, the rate of failure due to rejection increases from 8% when there has been no prior graft, to 40% when there have been two or more previous grafts.[24] Interestingly, the same study demonstrated that any previous surgery (other than corneal grafting) also conferred an increased risk of graft failure.

The presence of pre-existing inflammation in the eye predisposes to corneal allograft rejection.[1,34] Corneal grafts performed in the presence of active inflammation are more likely to experience allograft rejection than those performed in noninflammed eyes,[35] and it is therefore preferable to control inflammation with corticosteroids or other antiinflammatory medication prior to transplantation when at all possible. The presence of immunocompetent cells in the host cornea (passenger cells) and the enhanced expression of antigens pertinent to subsequent allograft rejection (class II histocompatibility antigens, intercellular adhesion molecules) can be induced in the cornea as a consequence of prior inflammation or disease in the recipient cornea.[36,37] These histologic features have been associated with increased graft rejection, and infiltrating cell counts greater than 50 cells/mm^2 can be predictive of subsequent graft failure.[38]

When any of the previously identified risk factors are present, the surgeon should consider the patient at high risk for graft rejection, and the clinician should raise the level of suspicion for any inflammatory episode that occurs. Indeed, any inflammation in an eye with a prior corneal graft should be suspected of being graft rejection until proved otherwise.

Clinical Features of Corneal Allograft Rejection

Appreciation of the clinical features of corneal allograft rejection is critical to early recognition of rejection, and is the first step toward effective therapy. This is true for the patient as well as the clinician. The patient often is the first to notice that something is awry and therein is the need for clear, specific education of the patient about the symptoms of graft rejection. Communication with the patient should emphasize repeatedly that symptoms of redness of the eye, decreased vision, light sensitivity, or discomfort in the eye that lasts longer than a few hours requires evaluation to exclude an episode of graft rejection and that there is a need for a rapid start of therapy if treatment is to be successful. In a large group of high-risk patients who were followed very closely in the postoperative period, 70% of reactions were heralded

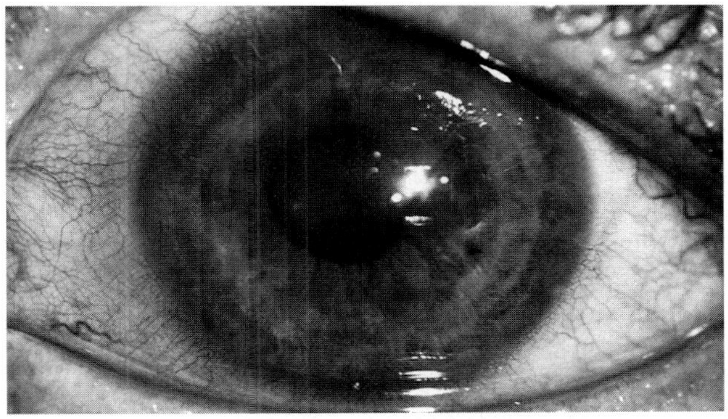

FIGURE 138-2 Physical signs of ciliary flush, conjunctival injection. Circumcorneal vascular injection can be an early sign of rejection reaction.

by patient symptoms, while 30% were identified by the clinician on the basis of physical signs at a routine follow-up visit. This recent evaluation of the reliability of patient symptoms as first identifier of allograft rejection showed poor sensitivity and specificity of symptoms as indicators of onset of graft rejection, despite a strong association of the symptoms of eye redness and decreased vision with rejection.[39] Nevertheless, when a patient experiences changes in visual performance or ocular symptoms, graft rejection must be excluded or treated.

Since allograft rejection is an immune mediated inflammatory process, it shares the traditional features of an inflammatory response: vascular dilation, vascular transudation, cellular infiltration, and tissue edema. These basic features are uniquely expressed in the eye, with vascular dilation occurring in both the conjunctival and uveal tissues with resultant conjunctival vascular engorgement and the circumcorneal vascular flush indicative of deeper vascular engorgement (Figure 138-2). Often circumcorneal (ciliary) flush is the earliest sign of rejection reaction and can occur before clinical appearance of cellular infiltrates in the cornea or the anterior chamber.

Anterior chamber flare indicates elevated levels of protein in the aqueous humor that has leaked from the uveal vasculature, and this can be a clinical sign of corneal allograft rejection. Obviously other forms of ocular inflammation also produce such anterior chamber flare, and thus it is a nonspecific sign of rejection. But if it occurs in an eye without previous history of inflammatory disease, it should be considered as evidence of rejection.

Cellular infiltration of the anterior segment of the eye during allograft rejection occurs in several patterns. Cellular infiltration of the cornea as discrete subepithelial infiltrates reminiscent of those seen in epidemic keratoconjunctivitis was first described by Krachmer and Alldredge in 1978.[40] These small (0.2 to

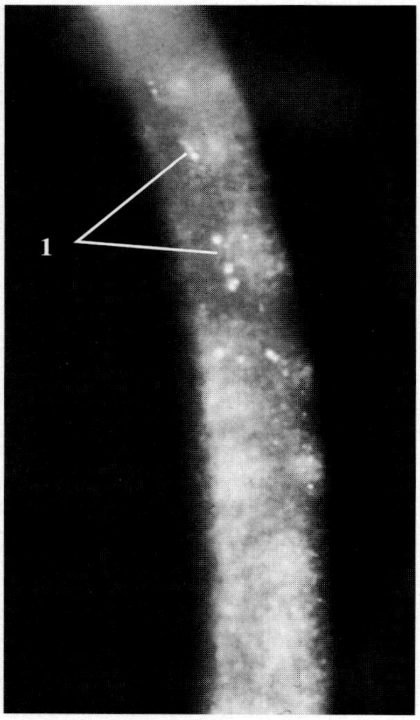

FIGURE 138-3 Subepithelial infiltrates. Scattered discrete, hazy subepithelial infiltrates 0.2 to 0.5 mm in size *(1)* confined to donor tissue can be seen in 10% to 15% of patients undergoing corneal allograft rejection.

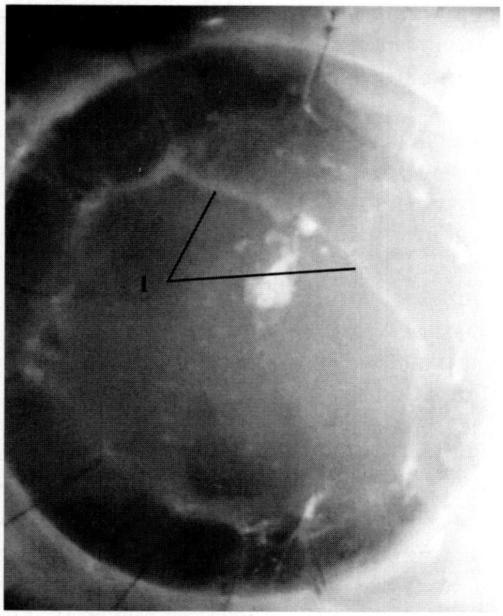

FIGURE 138-4 Epithelial rejection. Cellular infiltrates in the epithelium forming an advancing wave *(1)* across the corneal surface (epithelial rejection line).

0.5 mm), hazy infiltrates are usually scattered in the central cornea and occur exclusively in the donor tissue but not the peripheral recipient tissue (Figure 138-3). These lesions have been observed in 10% to 15% of cases of corneal graft rejection and can occur alone or

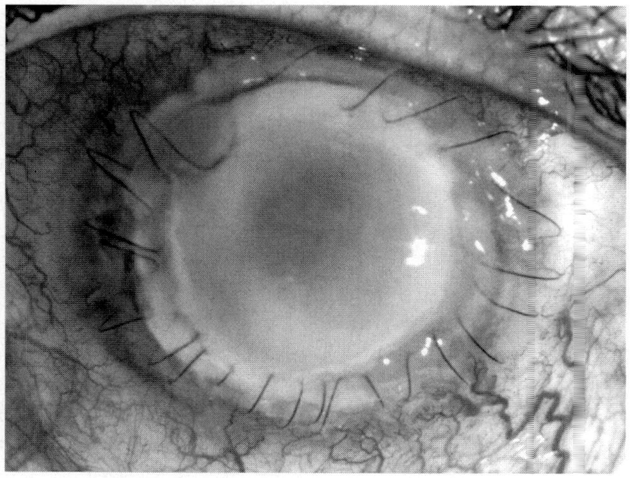

FIGURE 138-5 Stromal necrosis due to severe rejection of all corneal layers. Severe rejection reactions can result in infiltration of the cornea with resultant stromal necrosis.

in concert with signs of epithelial or endothelial rejection.[1,41] These lesions are an early sign of rejection and serve as a harbinger of more intense reaction, but they usually respond rapidly to topical steroid therapy and usually leave no residual infiltrate or scar.

An additional type of cellular infiltration is that of inflammatory cells invading the specific portion of the corneal graft that is being rejected: epithelium, stroma, or endothelium. Epithelial rejection (Figure 138-4) has been reported at a rate of 10% of those patients experiencing rejection, and it is usually seen earlier in the postoperative period (1 to 13 months) since gradual replacement of the epithelium obviates its rejection in patients with older grafts.[41] Isolated stromal rejection is not common but can be seen as stromal infiltrates and neovascularization. In very aggressive episodes of graft rejection the stroma can become necrotic during severe or prolonged bouts of rejection (Figure 138-5). Endothelial rejection is the most common of the three types, with reported rates of from 8% to 37% of cases undergoing rejection.[1,2,6,41] Endothelial keratic precipitates can occur as scattered lesions (Figure 138-6) or as a linearly oriented wave of leukocytes migrating from the peripheral cornea toward the center (Figures 138-7 and 138-8). Occasionally referred to as the Khodadoust line in recognition of one investigator who provided much insight into the mechanism of allograft rejection, this sign has been considered the hallmark of corneal allograft rejection, but it is not a *sine qua non* for rejection. Often there is associated edema of the stroma overlying the area that has been traversed by the advancing keratic precipitates. Inflammatory cells may also be apparent in the anterior chamber but are usually much less than would be expected given the number of keratic precipitates present.

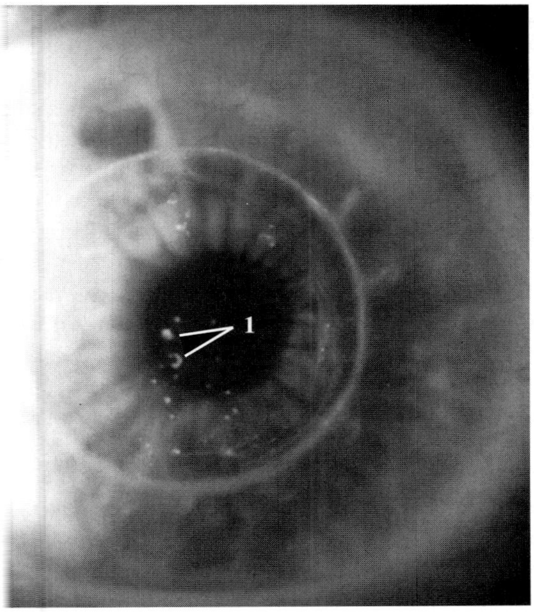

FIGURE 138-6 Endothelial keratic precipitates. Keratic precipitates *(1)* occurring on the donor tissue is a definitive sign of corneal allograft rejection affecting the endothelium.

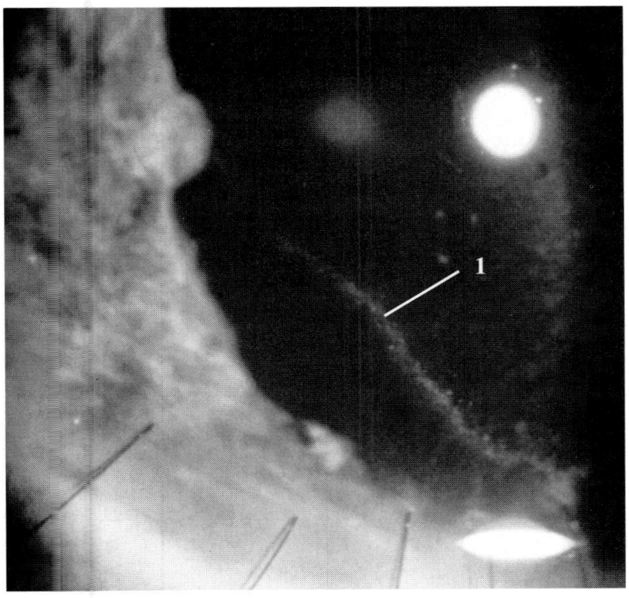

FIGURE 138-7 Endothelial line of keratic precipitates. Keratic precipitates *(1)* aligning themselves on the endothelial surface as the rejection reaction proceeds.

Edema of the graft can occur as a part of the inflammatory reaction, but more commonly as the result of the stress or damage to the corneal endothelium (Figure 138-8). Once the endothelium has been irreversibly damaged, the clearing of the stromal and epithelial edema is dependent upon migration of

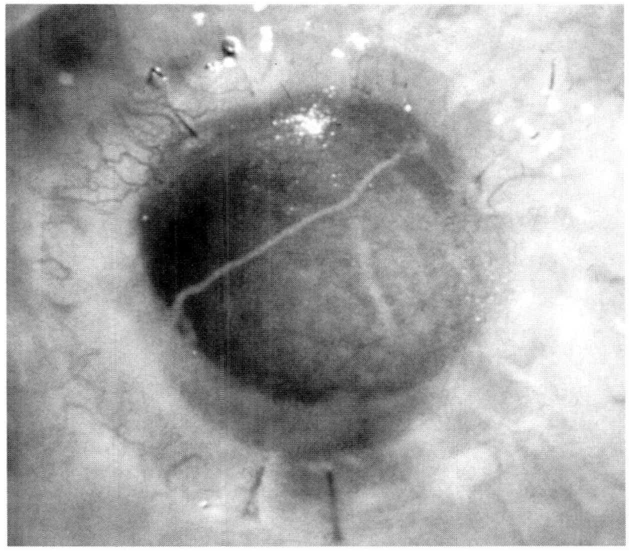

FIGURE 138-8 Endothelial rejection line. A wave of endothelial keratic precipitates marches across the endothelial surface leaving stromal edema in its wake. This represents the classic picture of a Khodadoust line.

adequate endothelial cells from the remaining endothelial cell population of the rest of the graft. Ultrasonic corneal pachymetry has been evaluated as a possible method for determining allograft rejection in a recent clinical trial. While an isolated increase in corneal thickness can be a sign of allograft rejection reaction in possibly 14.8% of patients, it is not a precise indicator, since only 49% of patients with other accepted signs of allograft rejection showed increased pachymetry.[42] Corneal thickness usually stabilizes by the third postoperative month, and if the corneal thickness is greater than 0.59 mm at the sixth postoperative month, there is a greater risk of ultimate graft failure.[42] Persistent edema, particularly if associated with continued inflammation, permits stromal neovascularization with subsequent opacification of the graft.

There are several unusual manifestations of corneal allograft rejection that deserve mention. While infrequent, elevated intraocular pressure can be a sign of rejection and on occasion can be an early manifestation of such an event.[43,44] This elevation of pressure may be due to engorgement or edema of the trabecular meshwork during the vascular dilation phase of rejection. It should also be remembered that elevated intraocular pressure can be a complication of the corticosteroid therapy necessary to treat the rejection episode.[45] Another unusual manifestation of corneal allograft rejection occurs particularly in young black males receiving corneal grafts in treatment of keratoconus who subsequently develop peripheral graft edema, epithelial ulceration, and inflammatory melting of the underlying stroma (author's observation) (Fig-

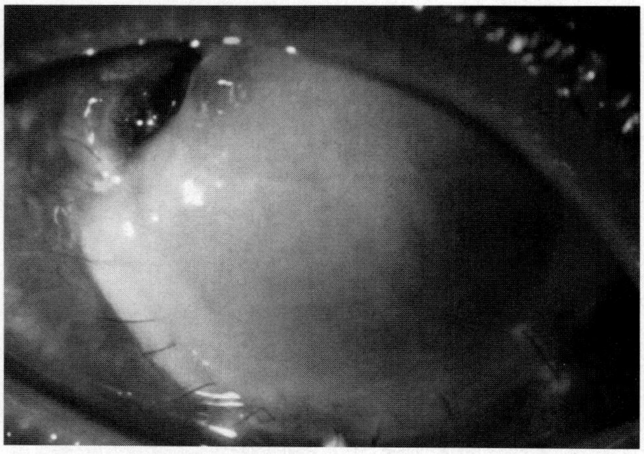

FIGURE 138-9 Peripheral corneal melt. An unusual pattern of corneal allograft rejection that is seen particularly in young black males receiving corneal grafts for treatment of keratoconus. The perilimbal intense inflammation is associated with peripheral graft lysis.

ure 138-9). This event usually presents with marked engorgement of segmental vessels near the limbus and can have a modest resemblance to the melting that occurs in Mooren's ulcer. The event is often followed by stromal vascularization in the area that was affected by the inflammation.

An additional unusual manifestation of corneal allograft rejection occurs more commonly in very young graft recipients. Acute epithelial defects of the corneal surface in conjunction with ocular inflammation may be the presenting sign of corneal allograft rejection in infants, and such events can spell demise of the graft.[45] Admittedly, infants and children with congenital corneal anomalies have a higher incidence of decreased corneal sensation and associated epithelial healing problems, but the sudden onset of an epithelial defect in a previously well-healed corneal graft must be considered suspect for allograft rejection as well.

In summary, any event or manifestation of inflammation occurring in a patient with a previous corneal graft must be considered a possible corneal allograft rejection. The specific characteristics of vascular engorgement and cellular infiltration that typify corneal graft rejection should be evaluated and once identified, should be promptly treated if the graft is to be saved.

Differential Diagnosis of Corneal Allograft Rejection

There are a number of clinical situations that challenge the clinician's ability to diagnose corneal allograft rejection, and it is valuable to review those situations and the differential features that would resolve the question. Certainly the most challenging situation is the patient who has had corneal transplantation in treatment of herpes simplex keratitis. The recurrent ocular inflammatory reaction present in herpes simplex keratouveitis is the most difficult condition to differentiate from corneal allograft rejection, and the therapeutic consequences are the most profound. Therapy for graft rejection with intense corticosteroids can aggravate the sequelae of herpetic keratouveitis; specific therapy against herpetic infection will not control allograft rejection, and the withholding of steroid medication can mean the demise of the graft. Unfortunately, the occurrence of corneal allograft rejection is a common event in patients grafted for herpes simplex, and repeated bouts of inflammation carry a more dismal prognosis for the graft.[46] There are a few features of herpetic keratouveitis that can help the clinician. Obviously the presence of a typical dendriform epithelial lesion serves as guide to the initial cause of the inflammatory episode. In the absence of epithelial lesions, an inflammatory episode in which the anterior chamber reaction is out of proportion to the endothelial reactions indicates greater likelihood of herpetic inflammation. Often, however, the only clue is the observation that the endothelial keratic precipitates in herpetic inflammation are not confined to the graft but involve as well the peripheral host endothelium. Unfortunately, we are presently lacking a clinical diagnostic test of sufficient rapidity and specificity to separate the inflammatory episodes of herpetic keratouveitis and corneal allograft rejection.

The recurring inflammation associated with herpes zoster ophthalmicus provides a further clinical situation that can confuse the clinician who is evaluating a corneal transplant for possible graft rejection. Here again, the anterior chamber reaction is often greater than expected for allograft rejection, and the diffuse location of keratic precipitates may be a useful clue, but most often topical or pulse systemic steroid therapy will be indicated because the exact diagnosis cannot be established, and the inflammation in any event warrants therapy.

An additional confounding clinical condition is that of epithelial downgrowth. When epithelial downgrowth presents as the classic linear wavefront of epithelium spreading from the periphery of the cornea at the site of previous penetration or perforation across the posterior surface of the corneal graft, there is usually little confusion as to the cause, and inflammation is often not a prominent part of the clinical presentation. When, however, epithelial downgrowth has provoked an inflammatory response, particularly in

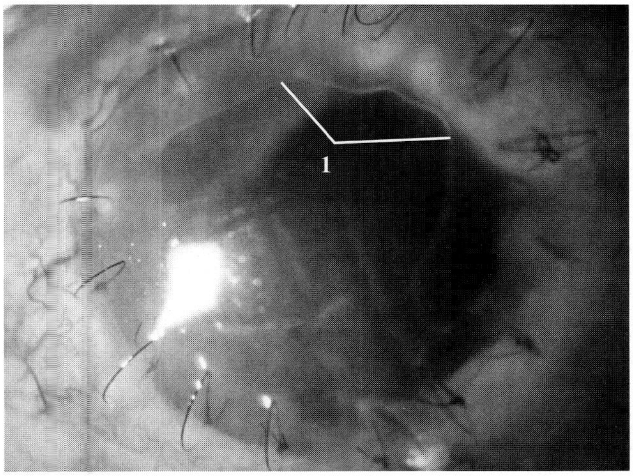

FIGURE 138-10 Epithelial downgrowth. The scalloped leading edge of epithelial downgrowth *(1)* advancing from the periphery towards the central cornea can be confused with an endothelial rejection line in some cases.

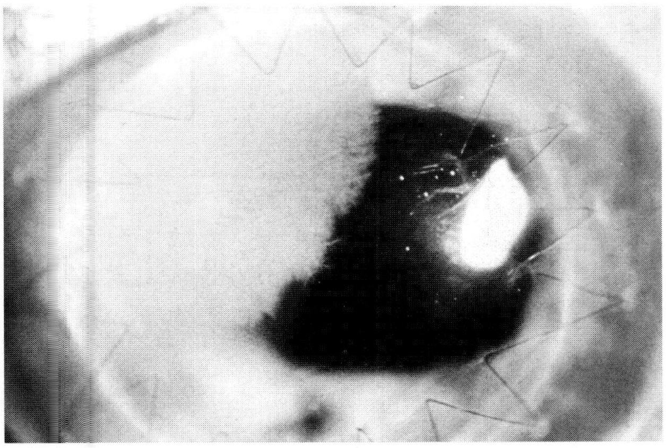

FIGURE 138-11 *Candida* keratitis masquerading as allograft rejection. The stromal infiltration of this *Candida parapsilosis* infection was initially misdiagnosed as allograft rejection yet transiently improved on topical steroid therapy.

the context of elevated intraocular pressure, the epithelial cells that can be free-floating in the anterior chamber may not be easily distinguished from inflammatory cells of allograft rejection. The presence of epithelial and stromal edema further confounds differentiation of the epithelial line from that of a Khodadoust rejection line (Figure 138-10). Steroid therapy usually will ultimately differentiate the conditions, since the epithelial downgrowth will not respond to steroid therapy. When epithelial downgrowth has involved the iris, it is possible to use low level application of the argon laser to document epithelium on the iris surface. If epithelium is present argon laser will result in blanching.

Finally, the unusual presentation of a low-grade corneal infection can masquerade as corneal allograft rejection. Figure 138-11 illustrates the corneal graft of a patient who underwent penetrating keratoplasty in treatment of aphakic bullous keratopathy and who subsequently developed late inflammation during soft contact lens wear. Based on the inflammation and corneal opacification in the absence of an epithelial defect, an initial diagnosis of allograft rejection was made, and treatment with topical steroids transiently improved the clarity of the graft and the inflammation. Only when repeated attempts to wean the steroid therapy resulted in recrudescence of inflammation and stromal opacity was referral made to the corneal specialist who identified *Candida parapsilosis* keratitis as the correct diagnosis. Obviously, it is the unusual and low virulence infection that can be so clinically confounding, but such infections can occur not only with fungal, but also with alpha-hemolytic streptococcus as seen in infectious crystalline keratopathy.

A further caution should be exercised when evaluating a corneal graft patient who has undergone previous cyclodestructive therapy to control glaucoma. Many of the patients who have undergone cyclocryotherapy and some of those treated with cyclophototherapy can manifest low grade aqueous flare as a chronic condition in the absence of active inflammation. It is advisable to establish whether chronic aqueous chamber flare is present once the inflammation from the acute treatment has subsided in order to minimize confusion with subsequent graft rejection.

Treatment of Corneal Allograft Rejection

Fortunately, most episodes of corneal allograft rejection reaction can be reversed if therapy is initiated early and aggressively. In a series of 587 corneal transplant patients reviewed at Duke University Eye Center in the 1980s, a frequency of rejection reaction of 29% resulted in frequency of graft failure of only 10% when the patient was treated promptly with aggressive local corticosteroid therapy. Interestingly, while the frequency of reaction was higher in the high-risk group of patients (55%) as compared to the frequency in the low-risk group of patients (18%), the frequency of failure due to rejection was 20% for the high-risk and 6% for the low-risk patients, thus demonstrating reversibility of rejection reaction in 66% of cases in both groups. This observation further emphasizes the need for prompt and aggressive therapy in all corneal transplant patients experiencing graft rejection regardless of their high or low risk predisposition.

Corticosteroid therapy by topical, periocular, or systemic administration is the treatment of choice for acute corneal allograft rejection reaction. A recent survey of the membership of the Castroviejo Cornea Society indicated that while wide variability exists in the preferred current practice for prevention and treatment of corneal allograft rejection among corneal specialists, topical preparations were favored over subconjunctival or systemic preparations with 1% prednisolone acetate being the most popular topical preparation.[47] Eighty five percent of surgeons responding to the survey stated that they modified their routine postoperative regimen for those patients identified as being at high risk of rejection by the risk factors discussed previously. The results of the CCTS clinical trial suggest that the use of higher frequency postoperative topical steroids, close follow-up of the patient, and the aggressive treatment of suspected or diagnosed rejection reaction (including the use of hourly topical prednisolone acetate for mild reactions plus intravenous methylprednisolone pulse therapy [3 to 5 mg/kg IV push] followed by 5 days of oral prednisone [1 mg/kg/day] for severe reactions) results in graft survival rates that obviate the need for histocompatibility matching of donors with recipients.[32] A prospective study by Hill and associates suggests that intravenous methylprednisolone (500 mg) in a single dose is more effective and better tolerated than daily oral prednisone (60 to 80 mg) when combined with topical therapy[48] in treatment of corneal allograft rejection. Repetition of the treatment within 48 hours did not significantly improve outcome.[49]

Immunosuppression by long-term corticosteroid therapy is associated with unacceptable ocular and systemic side effects. The newer immunosuppressive agents such as cyclosporin and tacrolimus (FK506) have improved corneal graft survival when used systemically,[50,51] but there are possible systemic side effects produced by both agents, including impaired renal and hepatic function.[52] It is wise to monitor systemic cyclosporin therapy with a fellow physician experienced in the use of systemic immunosuppressive drugs since therapy is often prolonged and periodic evaluation of hematologic, renal, and hepatic function is necessary. Studies by Hill and associates suggest that graft survival with systemic cyclosporin therapy is better with longer term (more than 1 year) rather than shorter term (6 month) therapy.[50] While evidence is increasing as to effectiveness of topically administered cyclosporin in the prevention of graft rejection,[53,54] at least one ointment-based formulation of 2% cyclosporin was not demonstrably better than intensive topical steroid therapy with close follow-up in prophylaxis of allograft rejection.[55] The possible benefit of topical cyclosporin to allow steroid sparing to avoid the ocular complications of steroid treatment (particularly steroid-induced glaucoma) remains a valuable potential of the newer cyclosporin formulations. Additional immunosuppressive agents are continuously being developed and evaluated. Additional agents may provide future benefit in treating graft reaction if side effects and toxicity can be controlled.[56]

The therapy of corneal allograft rejection by biologic methods also shows some promise. Ippoliti has successfully reversed acute allograft rejection by the intracameral administration of anti-T lymphocyte monoclonal antibodies.[57] Monoclonal antibody therapy directed at other relevant portions of the molecules involved in the immune response (CD4+ cells, ICAM-1, IL-2) also offers promise in the attempt to mitigate graft rejection[58,59] but the laboratory experimental data has not been extended as yet to clinical trials.

Prevention of Corneal Allograft Rejection

A variety of strategies to prevent corneal allograft rejection have been explored. The most extensive clinical trials have evaluated the role of histocompatibility matching of donor and recipient to prevent graft rejection. Early studies from Great Britain[17] and the Netherlands[18] suggest that histocompatibility matching can improve graft survival, particularly in high-risk patients in these homogeneous populations. The Canadian experience also demonstrates improved survival using histocompatibility matching.[60] An early prospective clinical trial in the United States suggested a benefit from histocompatibility matching in high-risk patients,[61] but a larger multicenter collaborative trial using higher dose corticosteroid therapy postoperatively was unable to demonstrate any improvement by histocompatibility matching. However, a trend toward reduced graft rejection was noted in recipients receiving ABH blood type antigen-compatible donor tissue.[32] This is an aspect of donor-recipient matching that will require further study and validation, however.

Manipulation of antigen expression in the donor tissue has been an area of research for the past 10 years. Depletion of immune-competent Class II positive-Langerhans cells from the donor cornea tissue has been demonstrated to be achievable by exposure of the tissue to hyperbaric oxygen and ultraviolet light.[62] No clinical trials have been done to corroborate clinical effectiveness, however.

Management Strategy

Given the present options for managing corneal allograft rejection, a management strategy can be proposed. Identification of high-risk patients and recognition of the clinical risk factors predisposing to allograft rejection should be done before transplantation. There should be clear and frequent communication with the patient to describe the symptoms of allograft rejection and to emphasize the importance of prompt evaluation and therapy. The clinician should maintain a high level of suspicion for allograft rejection and remember the unusual as well as the traditional signs of graft rejection so that early recognition of a graft rejection episode can be made. Finally, prompt and aggressive therapy with frequent topical applications of corticosteroids supplemented in severe reactions with pulse intravenous steroid therapy and possible oral systemic steroid therapy should be initiated and monitored until the acute reaction is controlled.

REFERENCES

1. Arentsen JJ: Corneal transplant allograft rejection: possible predisposing factors, *Trans Amer Ophthalmol Soc* 81:361-402, 1983.
2. Polack FM: Clinical and pathological aspects of the corneal graft reaction, *Trans Amer Acad Ophthalmol* 77:418-431, 1973.
3. Khodadoust AA: The allograft rejection reaction: the leading cause of late failure of clinical corneal grafts. In Corneal graft failure ciba symposium Elsevier, Amsterdam, 1973, p 151-167.
4. Eye Bank Association of America Annual Report 1993.
5. Hughes WF: The treatment of corneal dystrophies by keratoplasty, *Am J Ophthalmol* 50:1100-1105, 1960.
6. Chandler JW, Kaufman HE: Graft reactions after keratoplasty for keratoconus, *Am J Ophthalmol* 77:543-547, 1974.
7. Foulks: unpublished data, 1988.
8. Paufique L, Sourdille P, Offret G: *Les Greffes del la Cornee,* Paris, 1948, Masson et Cie.
9. Maumenee AE: The influence of donor-recipient sensitization on corneal grafts, *Am J Ophthalmol* 34:142-152, 1951.
10. Maumenee AE: Clinical aspects of the corneal homograft reaction, *Invest Ophthalmol Vis Sci* 1:244-252, 1962.
11. Maumenee AE: Clinical patterns of corneal graft failure, Corneal graft failure ciba symposium, Elsevier, Amsterdam, 1973, p 5-15.
12. Khodadoust AA, Silverstein AM: Transplantation and rejection of individual cell layers of the cornea, *Invest Ophthalmol Vis Sci* 8:180-195, 1969.
13. Polack FM: Clinical and pathological aspects of the corneal graft reaction, *Trans Amer Acad Ophthalmol* 77:418-431, 1973.
14. Polack FM: *Corneal transplantation,* New York, 1977, Grune and Stratton.
15. Sonoda Y, Streilein JW: Orthotopic corneal transplantation in mice—evidence that the immunogenetic rules of rejection do not apply, *Transplantation* 54:694-704, 1992.
16. Sonoda Y, Strelein JW: Impaired cell-mediated immunity in mice bearing healthy orthotopic corneal allografts, *J Immunol* 150: 1727-1734, 1993.
17. Batchelor JR et al: HLA matching and corneal grafting, *Lancet* 1:551-554, 1976.
18. Volker-Dieben HJ, D'Amaro J, Kok-van Alphen CC: Hierarchy of prognostic factors for corneal allograft survival, *Aust N Z J Ophthalmol* 15:11-20, 1987.
19. Boisjoly HM: Effect of factors unrelated to tissue matching on corneal transplant endothelial rejection, *Am J Ophthalmol* 107:647-654, 1989.
20. Maguire MG et al: Risk factors for corneal graft failure and rejection in the collaborative corneal transplantation studies, *Cornea* 14:43-48, 1993.
21. Musch DC, Meyer RF: Risk of endothelial rejection after bilateral penetrating keratoplasty, *Ophthalmology* 96:1139-1143, 1989.
22. Volker-Dieben HJ, D'Amaro J, Kok-van Alphen CC: Hierarchy of prognostic factors for corneal allograft survival, *Aust N Z J Ophthalmol* 14:11-18, 1987.
23. Williams KA et al: The Australian Graft Registry: 1990-1992 report, *Aust N Z J Ophthalmol* 21:1-48, 1993.
24. Maguire MG et al Risk factors for corneal graft failure and rejection in the Collaborative Corneal Transplantation Studies, *Ophthalmology* 101:1536-1547, 1994.
25. Paque J Poirier RH: Corneal allograft reaction and its relationship to suture site neovascularization, *Ophthalmic Surg* 8:71-74, 1977.
26. The Collaborative Corneal Transplantation Research Group: design and methods of the collaborative corneal transplantation studies, *Cornea* 12:93-103, 1993.
27. Foulks GN et al: Presensitization to HLA antigens in low risk keratoplasty patients, *Invest Ophthalmol Vis Sci* (supp): 1987, p. 227.
28. Cherry PMH et al: An analysis of corneal transplantation. I. Graft clarity, *Ann Ophthalmol* 11:461-469, 1979.
29. Gillette TE, Chandler JW, Greiner JV: Langerhans cells of the ocular surface, *Ophthalmology* 89:700-710, 1982.
30. Ross J et al: The differential effects of donor versus host Langerhans cells in the rejection of MHC-matched corneal allografts, *Transplantation* 52:857-861, 1991.
31. Sanfilippo F et al: Reduced graft rejection with good HLA-A and HLA-B matching in high risk corneal transplantation, *N Eng J Med* 315:29-35, 1986.
32. Collaborative Corneal Transplantation Studies Research Group: Effectiveness of histocompatibility matching in high risk corneal transplantation, *Arch Ophthalmol* 110:1392-1403, 1992.
33. Khodadoust AA, Abizadeh A: The fate of corneal regrafts after previous rejection reactions. In Silverstein AM, O'Connor GR, editors: *Immunology and immunopathology of the eye,* New York, 1979, Masson Publishing.
34. Polack FM: The effect of ocular inflammation on corneal grafts, *Am J Ophthalmol* 60:259-269, 1965.
35. Williams KA et al: Factors predictive of corneal graft survival, *Ophthalmology* 99:403-414, 1992.
36. Williams KA, Ash JK, Coster DJ: Histocompatibility antigens and passenger cell content of normal and diseased human cornea, *Transplantation* 39:265-269, 1985.
37. Elner VM et al: Intercellular adhesion molecule-1 (ICAM) in human corneal endothelium, *Am J Pathol* 138:525-531, 1991.
38. Williams KA et al: Leukocytes in the graft bed associated with corneal graft failure, *Ophthalmology* 96:38-44, 1989.
39. Kamp MT et al: Patient-reported symptoms associated with graft reactions in high-risk patients in the Collaborative Corneal Transplantation Studies, *Cornea* 14:43-48, 1995.
40. Krachmer JH, Alldredge OC: Subepithelial infiltrates: a probable sign of corneal transplant rejection, *Arch Ophthalmol* 96:2234-2237, 1978.
41. Alldredge OC, Krachmer JH: Clinical types of corneal transplant rejection: their manifestations, frequency, preoperative correlates and treatment, *Arch Ophthalmol* 99:599-604, 1981.
42. McDonnell PJ et al: Corneal thickness changes after high-risk

literature reveals that 55% of endophthalmitis after keratoplasty is due to gram-positive organisms (66% Streptococci and 34% Staphylococci). Gram-negative organisms are implicated in 19% of reported cases, which include *Pseudomonas aeruginosa*, *Klebsiella* species, *Serratia*, *Citrobacter*, and *Flavobacterium*. Fungi account for 21% of reported cases, the most common organisms being *Candida albicans* (46%) and *Torulopsis glabrata* (23%). Individual cases of *Cryptococcus neoformans*, *Cephalosporium*, *Aspergillus flavus*, and *Aspergillus fumigatus* are also documented.[42-45] Data regarding information on the causative pathogen were not specified in five percent of cases. These overall percentages may not reflect the experience of the general population because cases of unusual organisms are more likely to be reported, and under-reporting of common pathogens may also occur.

CLINICAL APPROACH

Subjectively, the patient with endophthalmitis may complain of pain beyond the normal level of discomfort after keratoplasty. Clinical signs of endophthalmitis include marked inflammation with or without hypopyon, and a diminished or poor red reflex. Additional findings such as corneal wound dehiscence may also be present. The integrity of the transplant wound must be assessed, preferably with a Seidel's test. Careful documentation of all findings should be made in the medical record.

B-scan ultrasonography should be performed, since it typically reveals vitreous debris, which supports the diagnosis of endophthalmitis. B-scan photographs should be part of the permanent, carefully documented medical record.

After informed consent is obtained, the patient should be taken emergently for aspiration of aqueous humor as well as vitreous sampling. Diagnostic vitrectomy or vitreous aspiration should be performed in addition to aqueous sampling, since vitreous cultures may be positive in the absence of microbial growth in the aqueous specimen.[46] The technical aspects of vitrectomy are reviewed elsewhere.[47]

After specimens have been obtained from both aqueous and vitreous, they should be plated directly onto blood, chocolate, and Saboraud's agar, as well as innoculated into tubes of thioglycolate broth and brain-heart infusion broth. The specimens should also be plated directly onto glass slides for stat Gram stain and Giemsa stain. One should consider reviewing these stain results personally to minimize the chance of laboratory error.

THERAPEUTIC APPROACH

Several routes of antibiotic administration should be used to combat endophthalmitis. Intraocular injection

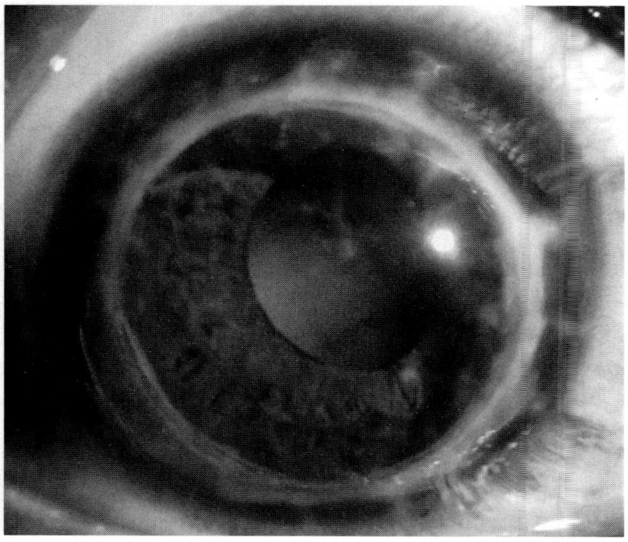

FIGURE 139-12 Same patient as in Figure 139-11 after graft exchange, vitrectomy, and injection of intraocular antibiotics. Vision was restored to 20/80.

of vancomycin 1mg in 0.1 cc and ceftazidime 2.25 mg in 0.1 cc should be carried out after a diagnostic or therapeutic vitrectomy has been performed.[47] If the intraoperative Gram stain or Giemsa stain reveals fungal elements or if the clinical suspicion for fungal endophthalmitis is very high, intravitreal injection of amphotericin B 0.005 mg in 0.1 cc should be performed.

Fortified broad-spectrum topical antibiotics should be administered with an intensive dosing regimen of at least every hour around the clock. Topical cycloplegics are also useful in cases of severe inflammation. Subconjunctival antibiotics at the time of aqueous aspiration and vitrectomy should also be given as an adjunct to therapy. Some clinicians feel intravenous antibiotics such as vancomycin and ceftazidime are important in the management of endophthalmitis. Antibiotic therapy should be tailored to the clinical response and with guidance from the results of cultures and sensitivities. If the use of systemic amphotericin B is required, the clinician should consider obtaining the services of an infectious disease consultant who is familiar with antifungal therapy and its complications.

Several authors recommend the replacement of the corneal button at the time of diagnostic aqueous aspiration and vitrectomy in cases of early postoperative endophthalmitis since the donor cornea is presumed to be contaminated (Figure 139-12).[38,45] However, it may not be possible to obtain corneal tissue emergently, and the treatment of endophthalmitis should not be delayed while waiting for tissue.

The complete management of endophthalmitis is beyond the scope of this chapter. The reader is referred to several excellent sources on the management of endophthalmitis.[46-48] Results of the Endophthalmitis Vitrectomy Study should further elucidate effective management strategies.[48a]

OUTCOMES

In a survey of the literature, only 3% of all eyes with endophthalmitis after penetrating keratoplasty had a visual acuity of 20/40 or better. Acuities of 20/50 to 20/200 were achieved in 19% of cases. An additional 19% of eyes had acuities ranging from 20/300 to hand motions. Fourteen percent retained light perception, whereas 9% lost light perception. Fourteen percent of cases resulted in phthisis, 7% in evisceration, and 15% in enucleation.

Recurrence of Herpetic Keratitis after Keratoplasty

Herpes simplex keratitis is a relatively infrequent indication for penetrating keratoplasty.[49] The incidence of recurrence of herpetic disease after modern PKP ranges from 6% to 38%.[50-53] Manifestations of recurrent disease include dendritic ulceration within the graft (Figure 139-13), geographic ulceration, and herpetic stromal infiltration of the graft.[51] Subsequent graft edema, vascularization, scarring, or perforation may result. Corneal transplant patients without a history of herpetic keratitis may also present with persistant epithelial defects at the graft host interface, which are culture-positive for Herpes simplex I and respond to topical antiviral medication.[54] In one series of penetrating keratoplasties for herpetic keratitis, 32% of eyes with graft rejection experienced a recurrence of epithelial herpetic disease, whereas only 6% of non-inflammed grafts had such a recurrence.[52] In this series, no antiviral coverage was used in the postoperative period while these patients were receiving topical corticosteroids. Sixty-four percent of grafts remained clear at 2 years and 62% remained clear at 5 years.[52]

The risk of recurrent viral infection may be increased by the application of topical corticosteroids without the concomitant use of antiviral, since steroids enhance viral replication. Antiviral coverage should be used prophylactically during the treatment of graft rejection when frequent topical corticosteroids are used.[53] There is no clear consensus as to whether topical antiviral coverage should be used during the routine postoperative period.[52,53] In one series of penetrating keratoplasties for herpetic keratitis, the incidence of recurrent herpetic disease during a rejection episode was decreased from 34% to 1% by employing a topical antiviral prophylactically.[53] The surgeon should consider a prolonged maintenance regimen of oral acyclovir in any patient undergoing corneal transplantation for active or inactive herpetic keratitis. Oral acyclovir is effective in the treatment of herpetic epithelial disease[55-57] and may decrease the incidence of herpetic recurrence within the graft.[58,59] Recurrent epithelial disease should be treated with gentle debridement, topical antiviral therapy, and the withdrawal of corticosteroids.

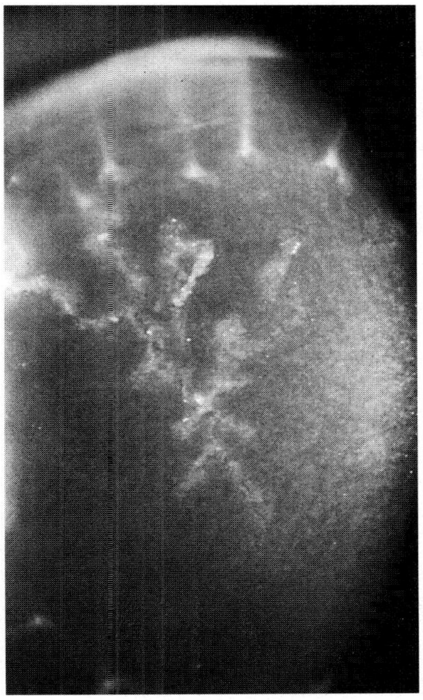

FIGURE 139-13 Recurrence of herpes simplex keratitis in a graft as manifested by a dentritic ulcer.

Transmission of Unusual Infections

RABIES

Person-to-person transmission of the rabies virus by corneal transplantation was reported in 1979.[60] A 39-year-old forester-rancher died from a rapidly progressive illness characterized by ophthalmoplegia, facial diplegia, flaccid quadriparesis, and areflexia. The right cornea was transplanted into a 37-year-old woman with keratoconus. Four weeks postoperatively, she complained of an ipsilateral retroorbital headache, which progressed to hemifacial numbness, ataxia, areflexia, and quadriparesis. The patient died 50 days after keratoplasty. Autopsy results showed meningoencephalitis and the presence of rabies virus in the cornea, optic nerve, temporal lobe, and brainstem. Rabies virus was then demonstrated in the donor's eyes, confirming the transmission by corneal transplantation. Additional cases of rabies transmission by corneal transplantation have been reported.[60a,b] Eye banks currently exclude donors with infectious neurologic disease or in cases of neurologic diseases of unestablished diagnosis.

CREUTZFELDT-JAKOB DISEASE

The transmission of Creutzfeldt-Jakob disease by corneal transplantation was first documented in 1974 after a donor cornea was obtained from a man later found to have "spongy" change and astrocytosis of the gray matter at autopsy.[61] Transplantation was performed in a 55-year-old woman with Fuchs' dystrophy before the availability of donor autopsy results. She presented with signs of ataxia 18 months after keratoplasty and died after 8 months of neurologic deterioration. Recipient autopsy revealed signs consistent with Creutzfeldt-Jakob disease. Creutzfeldt-Jakob disease is due to a "slow virus" that causes a fatal spongiform encephalopathy. Experimental studies by Manuelidis and associates have duplicated the transmission of Creutzfeldt-Jakob disease by corneal transplantation in guinea pigs.[62]

HEPATITIS B VIRUS

A possible case of hepatitis B transmission by corneal transplantation led to the recommendation that donors be screened for hepatitis B virus (Eye Bank Association of America Medical Standards, 1986).[62a] The virus has been documented in the tears of patients who are serum-positive for hepatitis B surface antigen (HBsAg).[63] Emulsified corneal tissue and washings of intact globes obtained from infected donors also tested positive for HBsAg.[64]

HUMAN IMMUNODEFICIENCY VIRUS

There are no documented cases implicating corneal transplantation in the transmission of the human immunodeficiency virus (HIV). However, the virus has been isolated in the tears of patients with AIDS[65,66] and in corneal tissue from a seropositive donor[67] as well as from donors with overt AIDS.[68] Corneal tissue from cadavers has been transplanted before knowing that the donors were positive for HIV. None of the recipients have seroconverted.[69] Serologic testing is currently performed on all donors.

REFERENCES

1. Bates AK et al: Microbial keratitis after penetrating keratoplasty, *Eye* 4:74-78, 1990.
2. Tuberville AW, Wood TO: Corneal ulcers in corneal transplants, *Curr Eye Res* 1:479-485, 1981.
3. Lamensdorf M et al: Microbial keratitis after penetrating keratoplasty, *Ophthalmology* 89(suppl):124, 1982.
4. Harris DJ et al: Late bacterial and fungal keratitis after corneal transplantation: spectrum of pathogens, graft survival, and visual prognosis, *Ophthalmology* 95:1450-1457, 1988.
5. Gandhi SS, Lamberts DW, Perry HD: Donor to host transmission of disease via corneal transplantation, *Surv Ophthalmol* 25:306-311, 1981.
6. Driebe WT, Stern GA: Microbial keratitis following corneal transplantation, *Cornea* 2:41-45, 1983.
7. Smith SG et al: Corneal ulcer-infiltrate associated with soft contact lens use following penetrating keratoplasty, *Cornea* 3:131-134, 1984.
8. Fong LP et al: Microbial keratitis complicating penetrating keratoplasty, *Ophthalmology* 95:1269-1275, 1988.
9. Confino J, Brown SI: Bacterial endophthalmitis associated with exposed monofilament sutures following corneal transplantation, *Am J Ophthalmol* 99:111-113, 1985.
10. Paglen PG, Webster RG, Abbott RL: The advantages of interrupted sutures and a therapeutic lens in keratoplasty, *Ophthalmic Surg* 12:95-97, 1981.
11. Waring GO, Laibson PR: A systematic method of drawing corneal pathologic conditions, *Arch Ophthalmol* 95 1540-1542, 1977.
12. Abbott RL, Kremer PA, Abrams MA: Bacterial corneal ulcers. In Tasman, W, Jaeger E, editors: *Duanes' clinical ophthalmology,* Philadelphia, 1994, JB Lippincott.
13. Leahey AB et al: Suture abscesses after penetrating keratoplasty, *Cornea* 12(6):489-492, 1993.
14. Gorovoy MS et al: Intrastromal noninflammatory bacterial colonization of a corneal graft, *Arch Ophthalmol* 101 1749-1752.
15. Stern GA: Infectious crystalline keratopathy, *Int Ophthalmol Clin* 33:1-7, 1993.
16. Meisler DM et al: Infectious crystalline keratopathy *Am J Ophthalmol* 97:337-343, 1984.
17. Kincaid MC, Fouraker BD, Schanzlin DJ: Infectious crystalline keratopathy after relaxing incisions, *Am J Ophthalmol* 1[illegible]:374-375, 1991.
18. Kintner JC et al: Infectious crystalline keratopathy associated with topical anesthetic abuse, *Cornea* 9:77-80, 1990.
19. Davis RM et al: *Acanthamoeba* keratitis and infectious crystalline keratopathy, *Arch Ophthalmol* 105:1524-1527, 1987.
20. Brooks SB et al: Crystalline keratopathy and epikeratophakia, *Am J Ophthalmol* 113:337-339, 1992.
21. McDonnell JM et al: Infectious crystalline keratopathy with ring opacity, *Cornea* 11:479-483, 1992.
22. Matoba AY et al: Infectious crystalline keratopathy due to *Streptococcus pneumoniae:* possible association with serotype, *Ophthalmology* 101:1000-1004, 1994.
23. Zabel RW et al: Infectious crystalline keratopathy, *Can J Ophthalmol* 23:311-314, 1988
24. Weisenthal RW et al: Postkeratoplasty crystalline deposits mimicking bacterial infectious crystalline keratopathy, *Am J Ophthalmol* 105:70-74, 1988.
25. Ormerod LD et al: Infectious crystalline keratopathy: role of nutritionally variant streptococci and other bacterial factors, *Ophthalmology* 98:159-169, 1991.
26. Hunts JH et al: Infectious crystalline keratopathy: the role of bacterial exopolysaccharide, *Arch Ophthalmol* 111:523-530, 1993.
27. Wilhelmus KR, Robinson NM: Infectious crystalline keratopathy caused by *Candida albicans, Am J Ophthalmol* 112:32[illegible]-325, 1991.
28. Eiferman RA, Ogden LL, Snyder J: Anaerobic peptostreptococcal keratitis, *Am J Ophthalmol* 100:335-336, 1985.
29. Groden LR, Pascucci SE, Brinser JH: *Haemophilus aphrophilus* as a cause of crystalline keratopathy, *Am J Ophthalmol* 1[illegible]4:89-90, 1987.
30. Hu FR: Infectious crystalline keratopathy caused by *Mycobacte-*

rium fortuitum and *pseudomonas aeruginosa*, *Am J Ophthalmol* 109:738-739, 1990.

31. Lam S, Meisler DM, Krachmer JH: Enterococcal infectious crystalline keratopathy, *Cornea* 12:273-276, 1993.
32. Hwang DG: Lamellar flap corneal biopsy, *Ophthalmic Surg* 24: 512-515, 1993.
33. Pardos GJ, Gallagher MA: Microbial contamination of donor eyes: a retrospective study, *Arch Ophthalmol* 100:1611-1613, 1982.
34. Leveille AS, McMullan FD, Cavanagh HD: Endophthalmitis following penetrating keratoplasty, *Ophthalmology* 90:38-39, 1983.
35. Guss RB et al: Endophthalmitis after penetrating keratoplasty, *Am J Ophthalmol* 95:651-658, 1983.
36. Aiello LP, Javitt JC, Canner JK: National outcomes of penetrating keratoplasty: risks of endophthalmitis and retinal detachment, *Arch Ophthalmol* 111:509-513, 1993.
37. Antonios SR et al: Contamination of donor cornea: postpenetrating keratoplasty endophthalmitis, *Cornea* 10:217-220, 1991.
38. Kloess PM et al: Bacterial and fungal endophthalmitis after penetrating keratoplasty, *Am J Ophthalmol* 115:309-316, 1993.
39. Speaker MG et al: Role of external bacterial flora in the pathogenesis of acute postoperative endophthalmitis, *Ophthalmology* 98:639-650, 1991.
40. Menikoff JA et al: A case-control study of risk factors for postoperative endophthalmitis, *Ophthalmology* 98:1761-1768, 1991.
41. Forstot SL, Abel R, Binder PS: Bacterial endophthalmitis following suture removal after penetrating keratoplasty, *Am J Ophthalmol* 80:509-512, 1975.
42. Beyt BE, Waltman SR: Cryptococcal endophthalmitis after corneal transplantation, *N Engl J Med* 298:825, 1978.
43. Rao GN, Aquavella JV: Cephalosporium endophthalmitis following penetrating keratoplasty, *Ophthalmic Surg* 10:34, 1979.
44. Cameron JA et al: Endophthalmitis from contaminated donor corneas following penetrating keratoplasty, *Arch Ophthalmol* 109:54-59, 1991.
45. Boucher P et al: Endophthalmie a *Aspergillus fumigatus* secondaire a une keratoplastie transfixiante, *J Mycol Med* 2:99-102, 1992.
46. Forster RK, Abbott RL, Gelender H: Management of infectious endophthalmitis, *Ophthalmology* 87:313-319, 1980.
47. Kremer PA, Abbott RL: Management of endophthalmitis, *Ophthalmol Clin N Am* 7:39-50, 1994.
48. Stern GA, Engel HM, Driebe WT: The treatment of postoperative endophthalmitis: results of differing approaches to treatment, *Ophthalmology* 96:62-67, 1989.

48a. Results of the endophthalmitis vitrectomy study: a randomized trial of immediate vitrectom and of intravenous antibiotics for the treatment of postoperative bacterial endophtalmitis, *Arch Ophthalmol* 113:1479-1496, 1995.

49. Cohen EJ, Laibson PR, Arentsen JJ: Corneal transplantation for herpes simplex keratitis, *Am J Ophthalmol* 95:645-650, 1983.
50. Foster CS, Duncan J: Penetrating keratoplasty for herpes simplex keratitis, *Am J Ophthalmol* 92:336-343, 1981.
51. Pfister RR, Richards JSF, Dohlman CH: Recurrence of herpetic keratitis in corneal grafts, *Am J Ophthalmol* 73:192-196, 1972.
52. Cobo LM et al: Prognosis and management of corneal transplantation for herpetic keratitis, *Arch Ophthalmol* 98:1755-1759, 1980.
53. Ficker LA et al: The changing management and improved prognosis for corneal grafting in herpes simplex keratitis, *Ophthalmology* 96:1587-1596, 1989.
54. Mannis MJ et al: Herpes simplex dendritic keratitis after keratoplasty, *Am J Ophthalmol* 111:480-484, 1991.
55. Collum LMT, Akhtar J, McGettrick P: Oral acyclovir in herpetic keratitis, *Trans Ophthalmol Soc UK* 104:629-632, 1985.
56. Schwab IR: Oral acyclovir in the management of herpes simplex ocular infections, *Ophthalmology* 95:423-430, 1988.
57. Hung SO et al: Oral acyclovir in the management of dendritic herpetic corneal ulceration, *Br J Ophthalmol* 68:398-400, 1984.
58. Beyer CF et al: Oral acyclovir reduces the incidence of recurrent herpes simplex keratitis in rabbits after penetrating keratoplasty, *Arch Ophthalmol* 107:1200-1205, 1989.
59. Barney NP, Foster CS: A prospective randomized trial of oral acyclovir after penetrating keratoplasty for herpes simplex keratitis, *Cornea* 13:232-236, 1994.
60. Houff SA et al: Human-to-human transmission of rabies virus by corneal transplant, *N Engl J Med* 300:603-604, 1979.

60a. Centers for Disease Control: Human-to-human transmission of rabies via corneal transplant-France, *MMWR* 29:25-26, 1980.

60b. Centers for Disease Control: Human-to-human transmission of rabies via corneal transplant-Thailand, MMWR 30:473-475, 1981.

61. Duffy P et al: Possible person-to-person transmission of Creutzfeldt-Jakob disease, *N Engl J Med* 290:692, 1974.
62. Manuelidis EE et al: Experimental Creutzfeldt-Jakob disease transmitted via the eye with infected cornea, *New Engl J Med* 296:1334-1336, 1977.

62a. Hoff et al: Unpublished data presented at the 1988 AAO annual meeting.

63. Darrell RW, Ginette BJ: Hepatitis B surface antigen in human tears, *Arch Ophthalmol* 96:674-676, 1978.
64. Raber IM, Friedman HM: Hepatitis B surface antigen in corneal donors, *Am J Ophthalmol* 104:255-258, 1987.
65. Fujikawa LS et al: Isolation of human T-cell leukemia/lymphotropic virus type III (HTLV-III) from the tears of a patient with acquired immunodeficiency syndrome, *Lancet* 2:529, 1985.
66. Fujikawa LS et al: HTLV-III in the tears of AIDS patients, *Ophthalmology* 93 1479-1481, 1986.
67. Salahuddin SZ et al: Isolation of human T-cell leukemia/lymphotropic virus type III from the cornea, *Am J Ophthalmol* 101:149-152, 1986
68. Doro S et al: Confirmation of HTLV-III virus in cornea, *Am J Ophthalmol* 102:390-391, 1986.
69. Pepose JS et al: Serologic markers after the transplantation of corneas from donors infected with human immunodeficiency virus, *Am J Ophthalmol* 103:798-801, 1987.

CHAPTER 140

STEPHEN Y. LEE CHRISTOPHER J. RAPUANO

Retrocorneal Membranes

Evaluation of membranes on the posterior surface of the cornea has intrigued ophthalmologists for many generations. Although rare, the specter of epithelial ingrowth and its devastating consequences has been a foremost concern. Fortunately, not all membranes on the posterior surface of the cornea represent epithelial ingrowth. Fibrous ingrowth and varieties of inflammatory and degenerative processes may also produce membranous opacities behind the cornea. This chapter will focus on epithelial and fibrous ingrowth but will also include discussions of other clinical entities that may be entertained in the evaluation of membranes on the posterior surface of the cornea. The terminology has been inconsistent in prior literature, but in this chapter, retrocorneal membrane, as the name suggests, will encompass all membranes on the posterior surface of the cornea.

Epithelial Ingrowth

HISTORY

The earliest description of the epithelialization of the anterior chamber is given by Collins and Cross in 1892 who described two cases of epithelial implantation cyst after cataract extraction and confirmed histologically the presence of epithelium in the anterior chamber.[1] Guaita linked epithelialization of the anterior chamber to postoperative hypotony, and Meller confirmed the entrance of epithelium through an incompletely healed wound, suggesting the theory of progressive epithelialization of the anterior chamber derived from the epithelium of the ocular surface.[2,3] Salus presented the first biomicroscopic description of epithelial ingrowth, and attempts at experimental reproduction of the disease added greatly to the understanding of its pathogenesis.[4,5,6,7] Therapeutically, Calhoun presented 20 patients with epithelial ingrowth and concluded that x-ray therapy may be the only hope for these eyes and that surgery may exacerbate the condition.[8] Maumenee, however, emphasized the importance of confirming the diagnosis with biopsy and suggested that if most of the epithelium could be removed from the eye, surgical intervention may be curative.[9] Since then, more refined histopathologic studies and better diagnostic techniques have prompted earlier diagnosis and better prognosis.

INCIDENCE AND ETIOLOGY

Studies on the clinical incidence of epithelial ingrowth must be viewed with caution, since determining the diagnosis is difficult and the certainty of pathologic diagnosis necessarily underestimates the incidence. Nevertheless, estimates from prior clinical studies allow an appreciation of the scope of the problem.

Virtually all types of traumatic and surgical perforations of the globe have been implicated. Terry estimated that 0.6% of all traumatic and surgical perforations result in epithelial ingrowth based on 28 diagnostic laboratory specimens out of 45,000 cases between 1900 and 1939.[10] Cataract extraction remains the most frequent cause of epithelial ingrowth.[11] Older studies have reported incidences of up to 1.1%, but newer studies report lower incidences of 0.2,%, 0.06%, and 0%.[12,13,14,15] Previous authors have reported a greater incidence of epithelial ingrowth with intracapsular versus extracapsular techniques of cataract removal and fornix-based versus limbus-based conjunctival peritomy, but current microsurgical techniques probably render such distinctions moot.[16,17] Nevertheless, the bleak prognosis of epithelial ingrowth is demonstrated by studies that report incidences of epithelial ingrowth in enucleations after cataract extractions of 7.2% to 45.7%.[14,18,19]

Penetrating keratoplasty appears to have a lower incidence of epithelial ingrowth than cataract surgery, but an incidence of up to 0.27% has been reported.[20] Numerous other surgical procedures have also resulted in epithelial ingrowth. Glaucoma surgeries, pterygium excision, discission of posterior capsule, and even a transcorneal (McCannel) suture have reportedly caused epithelial ingrowth.[11,21,22,23] Regardless, two facts appear certain: epithelial ingrowth is rare, and its incidence is decreasing.

PATHOGENESIS

Despite identification of risk factors that promote epithelial ingrowth, a cohesive understanding of its pathogenesis is still elusive. The source of the invading epithelium appears to be surface conjunctival and/or corneal epithelium. Careful sectioning of enucleated specimens occasionally reveals a continuity between the surface epithelium and the epithelial ingrowth into the anterior chamber through a fistulous tract. In addition, goblet cells are occasionally found, suggesting conjunctival epithelium. However, in some cases of epithelial ingrowth that occur after penetrating keratoplasty, goblet cells are absent, suggesting that corneal epithelium may be the source.[24]

Regardless of the source of epithelium, an entry site into the anterior chamber is a necessary, although insufficient, requisite. Most eyes affected with epithelial ingrowth, if not all, display a delayed closure or dehiscence of the surgical wound, often with a fistula or inadvertent bleb and incarceration of tissue in the surgical margin. However, mere access to the anterior chamber is insufficient to develop epithelial ingrowth. Free conjunctiva, cornea, or cilia implanted into the anterior chamber typically degenerate or form cysts on rare occasions. Drastic measures are required to sustain epithelial ingrowth in experimental models such as keeping a wick of conjunctival tissue within the surgical margin of a hypotonous, inflamed eye, or the use of a carcinogen such as methylcholanthrene.[6,25] Indeed, even a fibrin plug in a surgical wound margin is sufficient to prevent an epithelial invasion.[26] Therefore, other factors must be present concurrently.

Modern science has focused attention on cell-cell interactions and growth factors that may promote epithelial proliferation. Contact inhibition by healthy corneal endothelium may inhibit the advance of epithelium, and its absence may promote it.[27,28,29] In addition, the presence of a smooth surface (for example, lens capsule or a fibrin-laden surface) may facilitate the movement of the invading epithelium.[30,31] Also, the loss of the blood-aqueous barrier in hypotonous, inflamed eyes may provide growth factors required for the proliferating epithelium.[32,33] As suggested above, normal uninflamed aqueous may be able to sustain an epithelium but may not be able to support its proliferation. In any case, better animal models may elucidate specific cellular interactions required for the production of this rare but devastating disease and allow a better understanding of its pathogenesis and perhaps provide a more specific avenue of intervention.[34,35,36]

DIAGNOSIS

The clinical diagnosis of epithelial ingrowth rests on heightened suspicion as well as the recognition of clinical signs. Surgery may have been difficult or complicated with poor wound construction or tissue incarceration. Previous authors have felt that deep placement of silk sutures, aphakia, or fornix-based conjunctival peritomy predispose to epithelial ingrowth.[16,17] However, modern surgical techniques such as the biplanar incision, separate corneoscleral and conjunctival closure with better visualization, and finer suture materials probably mitigate many of these risk factors.

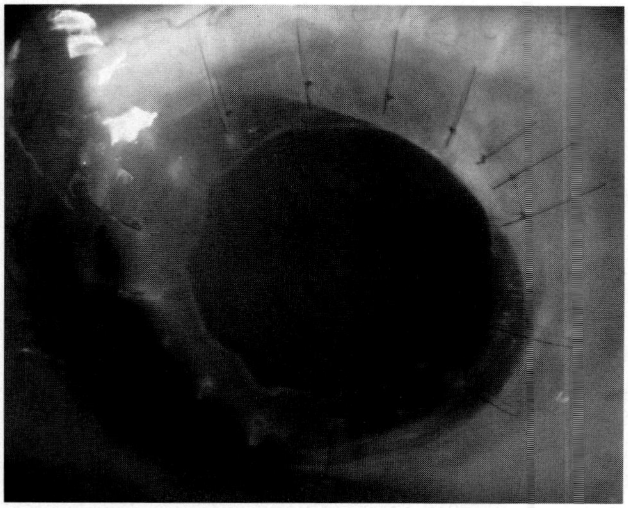

FIGURE 140-1 Epithelial ingrowth 3 months after a repeat penetrating keratoplasty. The previous failed graft revealed epithelial ingrowth on histologic examination. It commonly invades the periphery in a 360 degree fashion before moving centrally after a penetrating keratoplasty.

Patients present with recognizable clinical findings as early as 4 days and as late as 10 years after surgery.[3,37] They complain of nonspecific symptoms such as a dull aching pain, photophobia, and blurred vision.[17] Clinical examination reveals a hypotonous, normal, or elevated intraocular pressure, and the incision site may contain incarcerated tissue, a conjunctival bleb, or a fistula. Most remarkably, a faint gray line with scalloped, rolled edges may be visible on the posterior surface of the cornea and/or iris and represent the leading edge of the epithelial invasion[38] (Figure 140-1). This leading edge can be stable over months to years or rapidly progressive over days to weeks (Figure 140-2). Band keratopathy may be present with vascularization of deep corneal stroma, although the epithelial membrane itself is avascular.[14,38] The anterior chamber reaction is variable. Epithelial cells can be seen in the anterior chamber and are typically larger than white blood cells. The pupil may be distorted with ectropion uveae, and the fine iris architecture may be blurred by the overlying epithelial membrane.[38]

Two percent fluorescein Seidel testing may reveal a leaking wound, and gonioscopy often reveals incarcerated iris, lens cortex, capsule, or vitreous.[21] Some authors have advocated a sector iridectomy biopsy

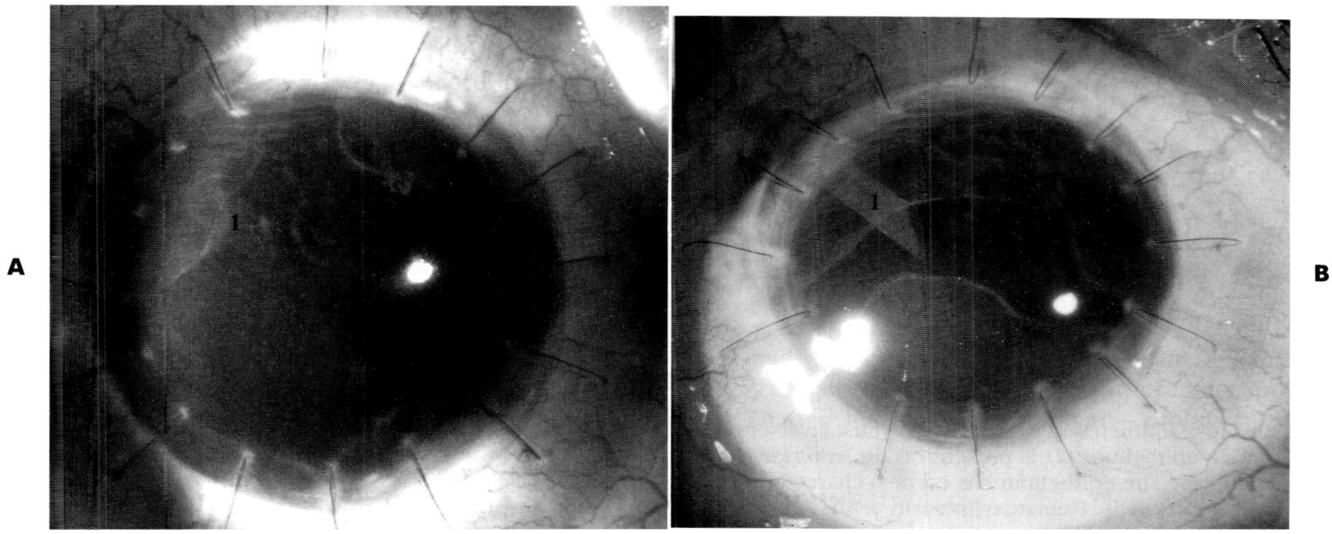

FIGURE 140-2 **A,** Epithelial ingrowth 2 years after a third penetrating keratoplasty. The shunt from previous glaucoma surgery *(1)* is less visable than in **B. B,** Three weeks later, the same eye demonstrated rapid central advancement of the epithelial ingrowth. This rapid progression is much more common with epithelial than fibrous ingrowth. The shunt from glaucoma surgery is more visable *(1)*.

specimen or curretting of the posterior surface of the cornea for definitive diagnosis.[39,40] However, argon laser photocoagulation and specular microscopy are often sufficient for diagnosis when combined with the clinical picture.[41] The argon laser settings of 0.1 to 0.2 sec, 100 to 500 micron spot size, and 100 to 500 mW are used to outline the extent of epithelial invasion over the iris. The involved areas turn white when the laser energy is applied as opposed to an inapparent burn to the normal iris (Figure 140-3). The specular microscope can also confirm the diagnosis if the leading edge of the epithelium can be visualized by focusing just posterior to the endothelium.[42] Thus, the diagnosis of epithelial ingrowth requires clinical suspicion with careful examination and confirmation with specular microscopy or argon laser photocoagulation.

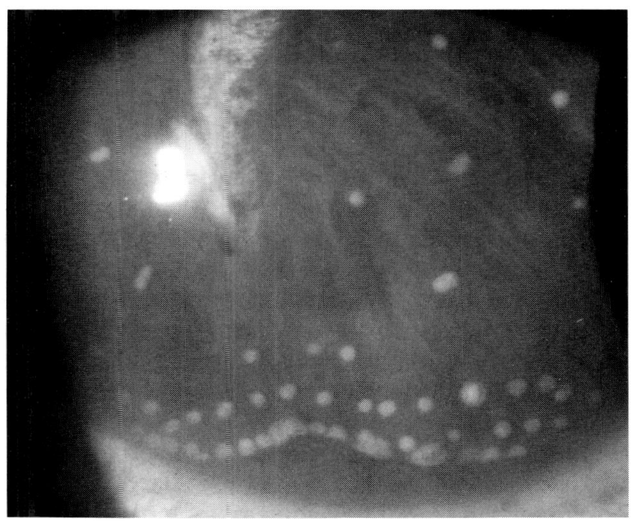

FIGURE 140-3 Epithelial ingrowth 18 months after microsurgical repair of a corneal laceration. The diagnosis was confirmed with argon laser treatment (0.1 sec, 100 mW, 100-500 micron spot size) to the involved (blanched) and uninvolved (normal) iris. The laser spots straddle the line of involvement inferiorly, delineating the extent of the epithelial membrane.

PATHOLOGY

Nonkeratinized stratified squamous epithelium on the posterior surface of the cornea or over the iris is diagnostic for epithelial ingrowth[43] (Figure 140-4). The multilayered epithelium is avascular and thicker over the uvea suggesting that the nutrition is provided by the aqueous and the uvea.[44] Careful sectioning occasionally reveals a continuity with the surface epithelium through a fistulous tract, and goblet cells may be present, suggestive of conjunctival epithelium.[38] The epithelium can create a "false angle" over the trabecular meshwork, accounting for frequent glaucoma, and can continue over the iris, ciliary body, and even retina.[45] The contraction of such a membrane may cause ectropion uveae.

Electron microscopy reveals numerous surface microvilli, wide intercellular borders, and prominent tonofilaments at the leading edge of the membrane, consistent with active migration of epithelium.[46] Goblet cells can be seen with electron microscopy, suggesting a conjunctival source of the epithelium. However, epithelial ingrowth after penetrating keratoplasty typi-

Table 140-1. Epithelial versus fibrous ingrowth

	Epithelial ingrowth	Fibrous ingrowth
Cellular source	Corneal or conjunctival epithelium	Subepithelial connective tissue, corneal stromal fibroblasts, others
Clinical signs	Fistula or bleb often present scalloped, thickened edge; nonvascular	Frayed, irregular edge may be vascular
Adjunctive tests	Argon laser photocoagulation; specular microscopy	None
Course	Usually rapidly progressive	Usually slowly progressive or stable

poorly apposed wound and chronic inflammation or hemorrhage certainly favor its production.

DIAGNOSIS

Like epithelial ingrowth, the diagnosis of fibrous ingrowth rests on high clinical suspicion and careful examination (Table 140-1). Preoperative and operative risk factors are similar to those for epithelial ingrowth. Difficult surgery complicated by vitreous loss or tissue incarceration in wound margins with hypotony or endothelial damage favor fibrous proliferation. Peripheral anterior synechiae, postoperative inflammation, or hyphema may also be risk factors.[65] Finally, one series reported that tube-shunt glaucoma surgery may favor development of diffuse fibrous ingrowth.[66]

Symptoms are nonspecific, and patients are usually not uncomfortable. Examination, however, often reveals a translucent membrane on the posterior surface of the cornea near the wound. The edges may be frayed or irregular, and unlike epithelial ingrowth, the stroma of the membrane may be vascular.[17] Stripped Descemet's membrane or vitreous touch to endothelium or wound may be evident. The overlying cornea is often edematous. Variable amounts of intraocular inflammation are present.

Prognosis of patients with fibrous ingrowth is quite variable. The invasion of the fibrous membrane is frequently limited with few functional sequelae. Occasionally, fibrous proliferation can be exuberant with growth over the angle structures into the posterior chamber of the globe. Subsequent inflammation and contraction of the membrane may lead to retinal detachment, cystoid macular edema, or phthisis bulbi.[17] Glaucoma is frequent but less aggressive than with epithelial ingrowth. The angle structures may be obliterated by the proliferating fibrous membrane, or progressive peripheral anterior synechiae may develop secondary to prolonged inflammation or shallow anterior chamber. Rarely, hemolytic glaucoma may result from repeated hemorrhage from friable and inflamed tissues.[57]

Despite careful examination, many cases of fibrous ingrowth are recognized only after pathologic examination (Figure 140-5). Laboratory findings mirror the clinical observations. Fibrous ingrowth from limbal incisions display poorly apposed wounds with intervening fibrocellular proliferative tissue and occasionally incarcerated iris, lens capsule or fragments, or vitreous. The surrounding sclera and cornea are often quite inflamed with deep vascularization. Fibrous ingrowth after penetrating keratoplasty may reveal breaks in Descemet's membrane with fibrocellular proliferation through the break suggesting a corneal stromal source of the fibrous ingrowth. The surrounding endothelium appears irregular with occasional pigmentation, attenuation, or metaplasia.[17]

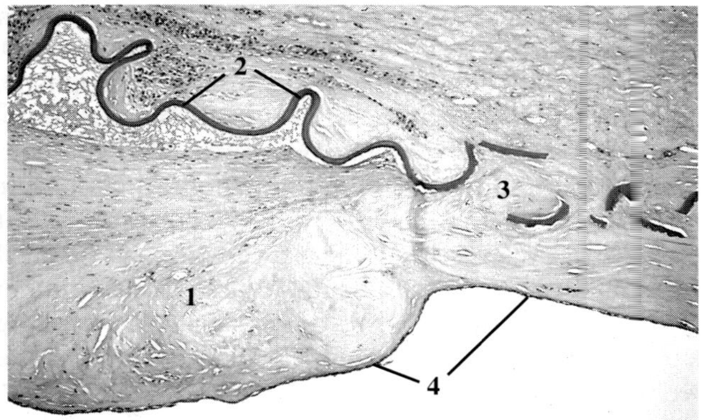

FIGURE 140-5 Fibrous ingrowth. A mass of dense fibrous connective tissue rests *(1)* on the posterior surface of Descemet's membrane *(2)*, which is sinuously folded. The fibrosis communicates with the corneal stroma via breaks in Descemet's membrane at the site of a surgical wound *(3)*. Vitreous loss occurred during surgery. A thin layer of epithelial ingrowth *(4)* is seen posterior on the surface of the fibrous ingrowth. Periodic acid-Schiff ×25. (Courtesy of Ralph C. Eagle, Jr., MD.)

Unfortunately, unlike epithelial ingrowth there are no adjunctive tests for confirming the diagnosis before pathologic examination. Nevertheless, the clinical behavior of fibrous ingrowth is characteristically less malignant than epithelial ingrowth and typically allows serial examination of patients to confirm the clinical suspicions.

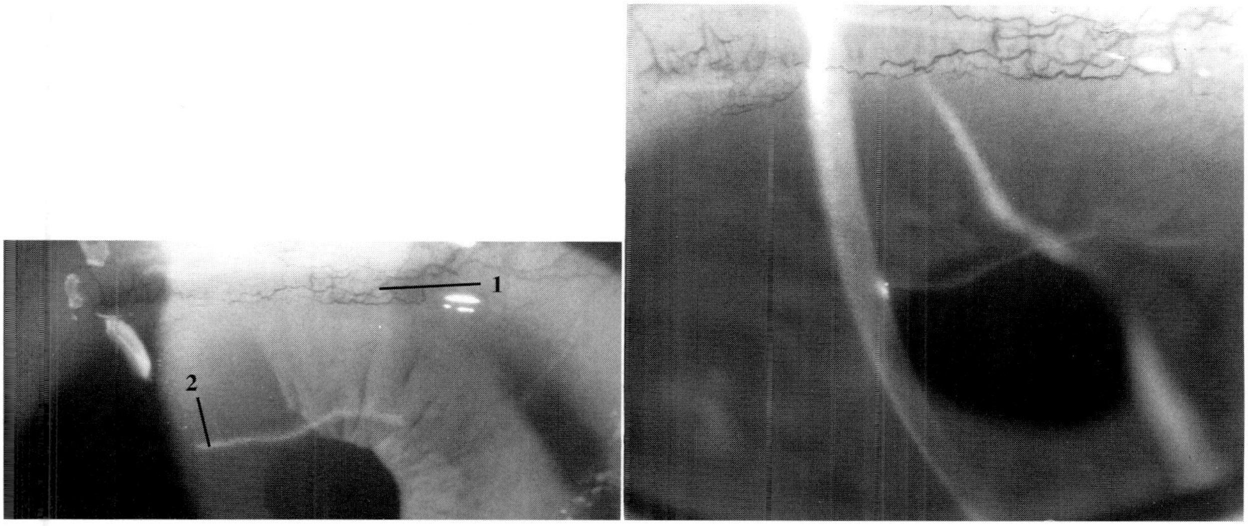

FIGURE 140-6 **A,** An extremely bevelled sutureless cataract incision can mimic the edge of a retrocorneal membrane. This patient was 3 months status postcataract surgery. Vascularization at the scleral wound *(1)* and a white line *(2)* at the entrance into the anterior chamber through the cornea are seen. **B,** Slit view of the same eye. Clues to distinguish this line from epithelial or fibrous ingrowth include history, observation of the lamellar corneal incision just superior to the endothelial line, and that the line begins and ends in the midperipheral cornea. A true retrocorneal membrane would demonstrate medial and lateral sides.

TREATMENT

Fortunately, fibrous ingrowth is not as aggressive as epithelial ingrowth. Often medical management of inflammation, glaucoma, or corneal edema is sufficient, and the fibrous proliferation matures into a quiescent scar and can even fade considerably. Nevertheless, uncontrolled proliferations do occur. Steroids have not been effective, and radiation therapy remains a poor theoretical possibility.[67]

With current technology, surgical intervention can be attempted. Unlike epithelial ingrowth, removal of all proliferating tissue is not required, and management of the sequelae of fibrous proliferation may be sufficient. Trabeculectomy or cyclodestructive procedures for glaucoma, repeat penetrating keratoplasty for failed corneal transplants, and vitrectomy for posterior segment proliferation are a few of the potential interventions.

Differential Diagnosis

Not all membranous opacities behind the cornea represent epithelial or fibrous ingrowth. Occasionally transient postoperative changes can appear suspicious. Beveled corneal incisions, especially those associated with phacoemulsification, can appear cloudy from stromal hydration, and the leading edge can become thickened and white from retraction of Descemet's membrane, simulating the thickened edge of epithelial ingrowth[59] (Figure 140-6). Peripheral corneal edema from persistent vitreocorneal touch or operative endothelial trauma or detached Descemet's membrane can also provide a whitish opacity near the operative incision.[68]

Penetrating incision is not needed for other sources of retrocorneal membrane. The endothelium itself can undergo fibrous metaplasia and produce a cloudy membrane on the posterior surface of the cornea. Trauma, inflammation, infection, and other stimuli can cause endothelial damage, and the regenerating endothelium can produce excessive amounts of Descemet's membrane. Notably, alkaline injury, HSV keratitis, corneal freezing, and anterior chamber inflammation have been reported to produce a fibrous membrane created by the regenerating endothelium through intact Descemet's membrane.[62,69,70,71] Finally, a pigmented membrane can appear on the posterior surface of the cornea as a result of proliferation of iris stromal melanocytes from trauma or surgery.[72]

Conclusion

The evaluation and management of membranes on the posterior surface of the cornea offer a special challenge to ophthalmologists. The urgency of the diagnosis and treatment of epithelial ingrowth must be tempered with the consideration of the more benign forms of retrocorneal membrane previously discussed. Clearly, accurate history, including operative details and postoperative course, and thorough examination are critical, but careful follow-up may be equally important. It is hoped that a clearer understanding of the pathogenesis of the myriads of retrocorneal membranes may allow a more selective and definitive therapy in the future.

REFERENCES

1. Collins ET, Cross FR: Two cases of epithelial implantation cyst in the anterior chamber after extraction of cataract, *Trans Ophthal Soc UK* 12:175, 1892.
2. Guaita M: Proliferation de l'endothelium corneen sur l'iris et le champ pupillaire apres l'extraction de la cataracte, *Arch D'opht* 13:507, 1893.
3. Meller J: Ueber Epitheleinsenkung and Cystenbildung im Auge, *Arch F Ophth* 52:436, 1901.
4. Salus R: Geheilte Epithelaus-Kleidung der Vorderkammer, *Klin Monatsbl Augenheilkd* 78:368, 1927.
5. Gunderson T: Results of autotransplantation of cornea into the anterior chamber: Their significance regarding corneal nutrition, *Trans Am Ophthalmol Soc* 36:207, 1938.
6. Cogan DG: Experimental implants of conjunctiva into the anterior chamber. II. *Am J Ophthalmol* 39:165, 1955.
7. Patz A, Wulff L, Rogers S: Experimental production of epithelial invasion of the anterior chamber, *Am J Ophthalmol* 47:815, 1959.
8. Calhoun FP Jr: The clinical recognition and treatment of epithelialization of the anterior chamber following cataract extraction, *Trans Am Ophthalmol Soc* 47:498-553, 1949.
9. Maumenee AE, Shannon CR: Epithelial invasion of the anterior chamber, *Am J Ophthalmol* 41:929, 1956.
10. Terry TL, Chisolm JF Jr, Schonberg AL: Studies on surface epithelium invasion of the anterior segment of the eye, *Am J Ophthalmol* 22:1083, 1939.
11. Weiner MJ, Trentacoste J, Pon DM et al: Epithelial downgrowth: a 30-year clinicopathological review, *Br J Ophthalmol* 73:6, 1989.
12. Theobald GD, Haas JS: Epithelial invasion of the anterior chamber following cataract extraction, *Trans Am Acad Ophthalmol Otol* 52:470, 1948.
13. Otradovec J, Zicha Z: Epithelial invasion into the anterior chamber after cataract extraction, *Cesk Oftalmol* 16:131, 1960.
14. Bernardino VB, Kim JC, Smith TR: Epithelialization of the anterior chamber after cataract extraction, *Arch Ophthalmol* 82:742-750, 1969.
15. Merenmies L, Tarkhanen A: Causes of enucleation following cataract surgery, *Acta Ophthalmol* 55:347, 1977.
16. Blodi FC: Failures of cataract extractions and their pathologic explanation, *J Iowa Med Soc* 44:514-516, 1954.
17. Smith P et al: Epithelial, fibrous, and endothelial proliferation. In *The Glaucomas.* Ritch R, Shields MB, Krupin T, editors: St Louis, 1989, Mosby—Year Book.
18. Schulze RR, Duke JR: Causes of enucleation following cataract extraction, *Arch Ophthalmol* 73:74, 1965.
19. Dunnington JH: Ocular wound healing with particular reference to the cataract incision, *Arch Ophthalmol* 56:639, 1956.
20. Sugar A, Meyer RF, Hood I: Epithelial downgrowth following penetrating keratoplasty in the aphake, *Arch Ophthalmol* 95: 464, 1977.
21. Theobald GD, Haas JS: Epithelial invasion of the anterior chamber following cataract extraction, *Ophthalmology* 52:470, 1948.
22. Zavala EY, Binder PS: The pathologic findings of epithelial ingrowth, *Arch Ophthalmol* 98:2007, 1980.
23. Abbott RI, Spencer WH: Epithelialization of the anterior chamber after transcorneal (McCannel) suture, *Arch Ophthalmol* 96:482, 1978.
24. Yamaguchi T, Polack FM, Valenti J: Electron microscopy study of epithelial downgrowth after penetrating keratoplasty, *Br J Ophthalmol* 65:374, 1981.
25. Perera CA: Epithelium in the anterior chamber of the eye after operation and injury, *Ophthalmology* 42:142, 1937.
26. Christensen L: Epithelialization of the anterior chamber. In Transactions of the New Orleans Academy of Ophthalmology: *Symposium on Cataracts,* St Louis, 1965, Mosby—Year Book.
27. Sidrys LA, Demong T: Epithelial downgrowth after penetrating keratoplasty, *Can J Ophthalmol* 17:29, 1982.
28. Davanger M, Olsen EG: Experimental epithelial ingrowth. Epithelial/endothelial interaction through a corneal perforation, studied in organ culture, *Acta Ophthalmol* 63:443, 1985.
29. Cameron JD, Flaxman BA, Yanoff M: *In vitro* studies of corneal wound healing: epithelial-endothelial interactions, *Invest Ophthalmol* 13:575, 1974.
30. Bruner WE, Green WR, Stark WJ: A case of epithelial ingrowth primarily involving the lens capsule, *Ophthalmic Surg* 17:483-485, 1986.
31. Matsumoto S: Contribution to the study of epithelial movement: the corneal epithelium of the frog in tissue culture, *J Exp Zool* 26:545, 1918.
32. Puck A, Tso MO, Yue B: Cellular deposits on intraocular lenses, *Acta Ophthalmol* (suppl) (Copenh) 170:54, 1985.
33. Smith DR, Somerville GM, Shew M: An experimental model of epithelialization of the anterior chamber, *Can J Ophthalmol* 2:158, 1967.
34. Burris TE, Rowsey JJ, Nordquist RE: Model of epithelial downgrowth. II. Scanning and transmission electron microscopy of corneal epithelialization, *Cornea* 3:141-151, 1984.
35. Burris TE, Rowsey JJ, Nordquist RE: Model of epithelial downgrowth. III. Scanning and transmission electron microscopy of iris epithelialization, *Cornea* 4:249-255, 1985.
36. Zagorski Z, Michelson G, Naumann GOH: Experimental autologous inverse keratoplasty – epithelial, stromal, and endothelial interactions, *Graefe's Arch Clin Exp Ophthalmol* 228:55-57, 1990.
37. Papolczy F: Partielle Epithelauskleidung der vorder Kammer nach graefescher Strextraktion, *Klin Monatsbl Augenheilkd* 84:266, 1930.
38. Sullivan GL: Treatment of epithelialization of the anterior chamber following cataract extraction, *Trans Ophthalmol Soc UK* 87:835, 1968.
39. Dixon WS, Speakman JS: Epithelial downgrowth following cataract surgery, *Arch Ophthalmol* 84:303, 1970.
40. Calhoun FP: An aid to the clinical diagnosis of epithelial downgrowth into the anterior chamber following cataract extraction, *Am J Ophthalmol* 61:1055, 1966.
41. Stark WJ et al: Surgical management of epithelial ingrowth, *Am J Ophthalmol* 85:772, 1978.
42. Smith RE, Parrett C: Specular microscopy of epithelial downgrowth, *Arch Ophthalmol* 96:1222, 1978.
43. Spencer WH, Font RL, Green WR et al: *Ophthalmic pathology: an atlas and textbook,* ed 3, Philadelphia, 1985, WB Saunders.
44. Lytle RA, Simmons RJ: Epithelial and fibrous proliferation. In Jakobiec A, Albert D, editors: *Principles and practice of ophthalmology,* Philadelphia, 1994, WB Saunders.

45. Vannas S: Epithelial downgrowth into the anterior chamber and deep into the eye, *Arch Ophthalmol* 35:190, 1957.
46. Iwamoto T, Srinivasan BD, DeVoe AG: Electron microscopy of epithelial downgrowth, *Ann Ophthalmol* 9:1095, 1977.
47. Epstein DL: Epithelialization of the anterior chamber. In Epstein DL, editor: *Chandler and Grant's glaucoma,* ed 3, Philadelphia, 1986, Lea & Febiger.
48. Layden WE, Torczynski E, Font RL: Mucogenic glaucoma and goblet cell cyst of the anterior chamber, *Arch Ophthalmol* 96:2259, 1978.
49. Loane ME, Weinreb RN: Glaucoma secondary to epithelial downgrowth and 5-fluorouracil, *Ophthalmic Surg* 21:704, 1990.
50. Lazarus S: Epitheliosis of the anterior chamber of the eye following cataract operation, *Orv Hetil* 76:776, 1932.
51. Pincus MH: Epithelial invasion of anterior chamber following cataract extraction: effect of radiation therapy, *Arch Ophthalmol* 43:509, 1950.
52. Vail D: Epithelial downgrowth into the anterior chamber following cataract extraction arrested by radium treatment, *Trans Am Ophthalmol Soc* 56:606, 1958.
53. Maumenee AE, Paton D, Morse PH et al: Review of 40 histologically proven cases of epithelial downgrowth following cataract extraction and suggested surgical management, *Am J Ophthalmol* 69:598, 1970.
54. Brown SI: Results of excision of advanced epithelial downgrowth, *Ophthalmology* 86:321-328, 1979.
55. Henderson T: A histological study of the normal healing of wounds after cataract extraction, *Ophthalmology Review* 26: 27, 1907.
56. Swan KC: Fibroblastic ingrowth following cataract extraction, *Arch Ophthalmol* 89:445, 1973.
57. Allen JC: Epithelial and stromal ingrowths, *Am J Ophthalmol* 65:179-182, 1968.
58. Waring GO, Laibson PR, Rodrigues M: Clinical and pathological alteration of Descemet's membrane: with emphasis on endothelial metaplasia, *Surv Ophthalmol* 18:325, 1974.
59. McDonnell PJ, de la Cruz ZC, Green WR: Vitreous incarceration complicating cataract surgery, *Ophthalmology* 93:247, 1986.
60. Silbert AM, Baum JL: Origin of the retrocorneal membrane in the rabbit, *Arch Ophthalmol* 97:1141, 1979.
61. Matsuda H, Smelser GK: Endothelial cells in alkali-burned corneas. Ultrastructural alterations, *Arch Ophthalmol* 89:402, 1973.
62. Polack FM, Kanai A: Electron microscopic studies of graft endothelium in corneal graft rejection, *Am J Ophthalmol* 73:711, 1972.
63. Leigh AG: Complications of corneal grafting, *Int Ophthalmol Clin* 2:776, 1962.
64. Bushmich DG, Stepanik J: Clinical and morphologic investigation of retrocorneal membranes after keratoplasty, *Oftalmol Zh* 4:223, 1963.
65. Bloomfield SE, Jakobiec FA, Iwamoto F: Fibrous ingrowth with retrocorneal membrane, *Ophthalmology* 88:459-465, 1981.
66. Kremer I, Rapuano CJ, Cohen EJ et al: Retrocorneal fibrous membranes in failed corneal grafts, *Am J Ophthalmol* 115:478-483, 1993.
67. Friedman AH, Hendkind P: Corneal stroma overgrowth after cataract extraction, *Br J Ophthalmol* 54:528, 1970.
68. Snip RC, Kenyon ER, Green WR: Retrocorneal fibrous membrane in the vitreous touch syndrome, *Am J Ophthalmol* 79:233, 1975.
69. Townsend WM, Kaufman HE: Pathogenesis of glaucoma and endothelial changes in herpetic keratouveitis in rabbits, *Am J Ophthalmol* 71:904-910, 1971.
70. Michels RG, Kenyon KR, Maumenee AE: Retrocorneal fibrous membrane, *Invest Ophthalmol* 11:822-831, 1972.
71. Maumenee AE: Treatment of epithelial downgrowth and intraocular fistula following cataract extraction, *Trans Am Ophthalmol Soc* 62:153, 1964.
72. Snip RC et al: Posterior corneal pigmentation and fibrous proliferation by iris melanocytes, *Arch Ophthalmol* 99:1232-1238, 1981.

CHAPTER 141

DAVID GEORGE O'DAY

Glaucoma after Penetrating Keratoplasty

Perhaps the most devastating complication after penetrating keratoplasty is the development of intractable glaucoma. Although corneal allograft rejection, astigmatism, and cystoid macular edema are common clinical problems complicating keratoplasty, none have such irreversible consequences for vision. Postkeratoplasty glaucoma is a significant clinical problem because of its frequency of occurrence, difficulty in recognition and monitoring, and complexity of management. It is often refractory to medical therapy, and surgical alternatives may lead to complications detrimental to the graft. If the glaucoma remains uncontrolled, irreversible visual loss occurs from progressive optic nerve damage, and graft clarity may be compromised from endothelial cell damage.[1]

Advances in the methods used to measure intraocular pressure in abnormal corneas have led to increased awareness and recognition of postkeratoplasty glaucoma.[2] In the last 25 years since the problem was first emphasized, understanding of the mechanisms and risk factors has increased, thus influencing prevention and management.

Postkeratoplasty glaucoma is defined as an elevated intraocular pressure greater than 21 mm Hg after penetrating keratoplasty, with or without associated visual field loss or optic nerve changes, necessitating the addition of medications to reduce the intraocular pressure. This definition is limited invariably by an inability to evaluate progressive optic nerve cupping clinically and by the unreliability of visual field testing after keratoplasty. Although these structural and functional changes undoubtedly occur, they are not easily documented because of changes in astigmatism and varying degrees of graft edema after surgery. These problems are also compounded in aphakic eyes. Postkeratoplasty glaucoma is thus one of the most difficult of the glaucomas to monitor.

Incidence

Improvements in technology, microsurgical techniques, and eye banking have led to greater functional success rates after keratoplasty. Yet for many years, little was known about changes in intraocular pressure occurring after keratoplasty, because there was no accurate technique for measuring it. Schiotz readings are inaccurate after keratoplasty.[3] Goldmann applanation is difficult in recently grafted eyes because of surface irregularity and fluorescein pooling around corneal sutures, and it may not be reliable in edematous corneas. With the development of the electronic applanation tonometer in the 1960s,[4,5] the ability to accurately monitor intraocular pressure after keratoplasty was realized. Using the Mackay-Marg electronic applanation tonometer, Irvine and Kaufman[2] in 1969 noted an alarming incidence of elevated intraocular pressure in the early postkeratoplasty period. They reported that during the first postoperative week, intraocular pressure higher than 25 mm Hg occurred in 37% of phakic eyes, 88% of aphakic eyes, and 100% of eyes undergoing combined cataract extraction with penetrating keratoplasty. The average maximum intraocular pressure during the first week was 24 mm Hg in phakic eyes, 40 mm Hg in aphakic eyes, and 50 mm Hg in eyes undergoing combined procedures. Although this study called attention to an early rise in intraocular pressure after keratoplasty in a majority of aphakic patients, little was known about the true incidence of persistent glaucoma after keratoplasty. This incidence was subsequently shown to vary with the study population by defined risk factors.

Further studies on the long-term course of intraocular pressure after penetrating keratoplasty were forthcoming. Wood et al.[6] reported an incidence of intraocular pressure greater than 25 mm Hg the morning after surgery in 15% of 423 aphakic eyes; in most patients, the pressure returned to normal after 1 to 2 weeks. However, persistent glaucoma developed in some and was more common in the groups with preoperative glaucoma. Thoft et al.[7] noted an incidence of postkeratoplasty glaucoma lasting at least 2 months in 11% of 153 consecutive patients studied after keratoplasty. However, patients with preexisting glaucoma, adherent leukomas, corneal perforations, and early postoperative pressure rise were excluded. Additionally, intraocular pressures were measured by Goldmann applanation. Olson and Kaufman[8] retrospectively reviewed the course of patients after aphakic keratoplasty or combined cataract extraction with

trabeculectomy for postkeratoplasty glaucoma. Gilvarry et al.[40] reported results of 35 consecutive trabeculectomies performed after penetrating keratoplasty for uncontrolled glaucoma with a mean follow-up of 3 years. Using survival analysis, the risk that the filtration surgery would not control intraocular pressure was 50% at 2 years. Further surgery to control intraocular pressure was required in 49% of patients. Few serious complications were encountered, and graft survival was 80% at 2 years in this series. Ficker et al.[41] reporting results of 29 eyes that underwent trabeculectomy after penetrating keratoplasty, found a 62% probability of graft survival at 4 years after surgery. Insler et al.[42] reported that 71% of seven eyes undergoing combined penetrating keratoplasty and trabeculectomy had successful control of intraocular pressure. Only one graft failed, but follow-up was limited in this study. Kirkness et al.[43] compared combined penetrating keratoplasty and trabeculectomy in 26 eyes versus trabeculectomy followed by penetrating keratoplasty in 22 eyes. Using survival analysis, there was an equal probability of maintenance of normal intraocular pressure with additional medications (approximately 50% in each group), but graft survival probabilities were 70% at 5 years in the combined group and 50% in the group with sequential surgery. These data point towards partial success with trabeculectomy in controlling intraocular pressure in postkeratoplasty eyes. There may be an advantage of combined surgery with regard to ultimate graft survival. If one considers the nature of eyes at risk, it is clear that many have extensive anterior segment abnormalities that lower the success rate of filtration surgery. The use of fibrinolytic agents with trabeculectomy in these cases may increase the rate of successful intraocular pressure control in postkeratoplasty glaucoma.

Cyclodestructive procedures provide an alternative to further intraocular surgery in eyes with uncontrolled glaucoma after keratoplasty. Cyclocryotherapy has been regarded as the procedure of choice in the past for the treatment of postkeratoplasty glaucoma unresponsive to medical therapy. West et al.[44] reported results on nine eyes that underwent cyclocryotherapy before penetrating keratoplasty. After grafting, intraocular pressure remained controlled in 78% of eyes. One eye required three treatments before control was achieved. In 14 additional eyes receiving cyclocryotherapy after keratoplasty, control of intraocular pressure was achieved in five eyes with one procedure, in six eyes with two procedures, and in one eye with four procedures. Reported complications included uveitis (23 eyes), phthisis (three eyes), cystoid macular edema (three eyes), retinal detachment (one eye), and choroidal detachment (one eye). Graft failure occurred in 3 of 23 eyes (13%). Thoft et al.[7] reported that intraocular pressure was reduced to less than 21 mm Hg in 12 of 15 eyes after one to three applications of cyclocryotherapy 180 degrees around the limbus in postkeratoplasty eyes. However, two eyes became phthisical. Binder et al.[45] treated 36 eyes with 360 degrees cyclocryotherapy for postkeratoplasty glaucoma. Although intraocular pressure was >40 mm Hg in all eyes before cyclocryotherapy, 30 eyes were controlled with one treatment, five eyes with two treatments and one eye with three treatments. Eighteen percent of grafts failed during the follow-up period, and 14% of eyes developed complications including phthisis (one eye), vitreous hemorrhage (two eyes), cystoid macular edema (one eye), and graft failure (two eyes) after cyclocryotherapy. Kirkness et al.[43] reported long-term results of cyclocryotherapy for postkeratoplasty glaucoma, with none of 13 patients maintaining both a clear graft and controlled intraocular pressure. Despite these complications, the use of cyclocryotherapy continues to be viewed favorably by some as a preferred treatment for postkeratoplasty glaucoma. However, its unpredictability, high failure rate, and incidence of severe complications in up to 25% of patients have led others to recommend it only in patients with poor visual potential.[46]

Transscleral Nd:YAG cyclophotocoagulation has been used through either contact or noncontact methods and has supplanted cyclocryotherapy as the cyclodestructive procedure of choice for refractory glaucomas in most centers. It is more predictable and less painful than cyclocryotherapy, with less incidence of significant complications. This procedure has been used to treat postkeratoplasty glaucoma with some success. Zaidman and Wandel[47] initially reported successful control of intraocular pressure with transscleral Nd:YAG cyclophotocoagulation in a patient after penetrating keratoplasty with anterior vitrectomy and intraocular lens removal complicated by hyphema, vitreous hemorrhage, and increased intraocular pressure.

Levy and Bonney[48] reported results of nine postkeratoplasty eyes treated with transscleral Nd:YAG cyclophotocoagulation using 7 to 10 Joules to 360 degrees of the limbus. Preoperative intraocular pressures were between 30 and 56 mm Hg. All eyes achieved intraocular pressures of less than 21 mm Hg, with a mean decrease of 75% from the preoperative intraocular pressure. However, two eyes (22%) became hypotonous. Other complications included severe fibrinous iritis, loss of light perception, pupillary block, hyphema, and graft failure. Levy and Bonney[48] recommended limiting initial total energy to less than 256 Joules to avoid hypotony.

Cohen et al.[49] reported results of Nd:YAG cyclophotocoagulation in 28 postkeratoplasty eyes with uncontrolled glaucoma with a median follow-up of 18 months. Using a mean pulse energy of 4.13 Joules, 30 to 50 applications were given for 180 degrees (29%) or 360 degrees (71%). Control of intraocular pressure was achieved in 64% at 3 months, 74% at 6 months, 67% at 1 year, and in 73% of eyes at 2 years, although multiple treatments (two to five) were required in 46% of eyes. At the 3-month postoperative interval, the 360 degree treatments were effective in 65%, whereas the 180 degree treatments were effective in 14% of eyes. Complications encountered included hypotony (two eyes), pain, iritis, and hyphema. Phthisis did not develop in any eye. Of 14 grafts that were clear before cyclophotocoagulation, 46% failed after the first procedure. These authors recommend transscleral Nd: YAG cyclophotocoagulation as the procedure of choice for postkeratoplasty glaucoma refractory to medical therapy.

Wheatcroft et al.[50] confirmed the efficacy of transscleral Nd:YAG cyclophotocoagulation in treating refractory postkeratoplasty glaucoma. Using a mean 4.2 Joules applied initially to 180 degrees of the limbus in most eyes, control of intraocular pressure was achieved in 9 of 13 eyes (69%), with a mean follow-up of 20 months. Of these, 23% were controlled with one treatment, 23% with two treatments, and 8% each with three, five, or six treatments of cyclophotocoagulation. Graft failure occurred in 23% of eyes after surgery. Two eyes (15%) became hypotonous after multiple treatments. No eye became phthisical. Because of these results, these authors recommended initial therapy with 180 degrees of Nd:YAG cyclophotocoagulation.

Hardten et al.[51] addressed the question of whether initially 180 or 360 degree treatments should be used, stating that control of intraocular pressure can be achieved ultimately with both strategies. However, more patients are controlled initially with fewer complications using 360 degree cyclophotocoagulation. They subsequently reported successful control of intraocular pressure in 13 of 19 eyes (68%) with uncontrolled glaucoma after keratoplasty using Nd: YAG cyclophotocoagulation.[52] Graft clarity was later lost in 14% of eyes. No patient developed persistent hypotony, and postoperative inflammation and pain were minimal.

Results of these studies indicate that successful control of intraocular pressure is possible in a majority of eyes with this procedure. However, the effect of Nd:YAG cyclophotocoagulation on ultimate graft clarity has not been well studied. It is not known whether postoperative inflammation and other complications accompanying cyclophotocoagulation are inherently more deleterious to the graft than other surgical modalities available to treat postkeratoplasty glaucoma.

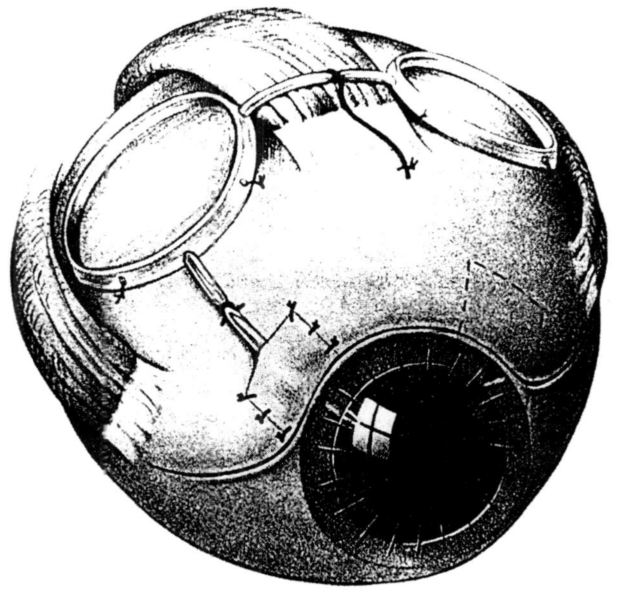

FIGURE 141-2 Double-plate Molteno implant for postkeratoplasty glaucoma. The anterior chamber tube exits at the limbus and is buried under a scleral graft anteriorly. Tube ligatures are present to avoid early postoperative hypotony. (From Beebe WE et al: *Ophthalmology* 97:1414-1422, 1990.)

Aqueous drainage devices have been used successfully for the treatment of refractory glaucomas after penetrating keratoplasty. Modern-day implants are translimbal-equatorial shunts that channel aqueous from the anterior chamber through a long tube to an episcleral, equatorial, bleb-promoting device or plate. The surface area of the fibrous cocoon that develops over this device is a key factor in promoting postoperative aqueous drainage and control of intraocular pressure. Commercially available aqueous shunts include devices described by Molteno,[53] Schocket et al.,[54] Krupin et al.,[55] Joseph et al.,[56] and Smith et al.,[57] Of these, the Molteno implant is the most frequently used and widely available (Figure 141-2). These devices are advantageous in previously operated eyes with conjunctival scarring, or in eyes with total synechial angle closure in which filtration procedures are difficult or have previously failed.

Recently, successful control of postkeratoplasty glaucoma with aqueous shunts has been reported. Kirkness[58] initially reported favorable results with the use of a Schocket-type implant (an inverted 220 silicone band) in a one- or two-stage procedure in 11 patients with postkeratoplasty glaucoma. Kirkness et al.[59] reported results of 20 aphakic patients followed prospectively for a mean of 26 months after using a two-stage Schocket-type implant to control postkeratoplasty glaucoma. All eyes had previously undergone surgery for glaucoma before tube insertion. Control of intraocular pressure was attained in 80% of eyes. Graft failure occurred in 31% of eyes. Using survival analysis, the probability of maintenance of a clear graft with control of intraocular pressure was 68% 4 years after surgery. Complications included severe uveitis, delayed suprachoroidal hemorrhage, tube blockage, and graft rejection.

Subsequent reports by McDonnell et al.,[60] Beebe et al.,[61] O'Day et al.,[62] and Sherwood et al.,[63] using either Molteno or Schocket implants in separate series, have confirmed control of intraocular pressure in 71%, 86%, 93%, and 96% of eyes, respectively. However, the incidence of graft rejection and failure was high in these series. McDonnell et al.[60] reported that corneal allograft rejection occurred in 7 of 16 eyes (44%) and was irreversible in five eyes (31%) after Molteno implantation. Beebe et al[61] reported that graft rejection occurred in 12 of 35 eyes (34%) and was irreversible in nine eyes (26%). Nonimmunologic graft failure occurred in an additional nine eyes (26%). Using strict criteria for graft rejection, O'Day et al.[62] reported that immunologic rejection occurred in 10 of 44 eyes (23%) and was irreversible in four eyes (9%). The most frequent cause of graft loss in this study was nonimmunologic failure, which occurred in 13 eyes (30%). Using Kaplan-Meier analysis, graft survival was 33% at 2 years.

Kirkness[58] postulated that the risk of graft rejection may be increased after aqueous shunt surgery because the drainage tubing may provide an additional limb for the efferent arc of the immune response by allowing retrograde passage of inflammatory cells into the anterior chamber. The findings in the study by O'Day,[62] however, that nonimmunologic graft failure occurred most frequently, indicate that other factors that affect endothelial viability play a role. Considering the results of repeated grafts, eventually 71% to 81% of eyes maintained clear grafts in these series. Other complications occurred frequently, including choroidal detachment, retinal detachment, cystoid macular edema, hypotony, tube occlusion and exposure, vitreous hemorrhage, and malignant glaucoma. Most of these complications did not affect ultimate control of intraocular pressure. Similar complication frequencies are reported in the literature after the use of aqueous shunts for complicated glaucomas.[63-68] These studies indicate that aqueous shunts offer a viable alternative for the control of glaucoma after keratoplasty. The increased rates of graft loss may reflect the high-risk nature of these eyes or an as yet unidentified risk factor specific to equatorial shunting of aqueous humor. Finally, graft failure after aqueous shunting may not preclude repeat keratoplasty. As long as the glaucoma is successfully controlled, visual rehabilitation is possible.

Summary

Postkeratoplasty glaucoma is one of the most difficult complications of corneal transplantation to manage. Knowledge of risk factors allows for increased vigilance and aggressive management of elevated intraocular pressure both before and after keratoplasty. Although prevention is difficult, attention to surgical detail can minimize the incidence of significant iridocorneal angle distortion and collapse. When preventive measures fail, logical, stepwise medical management can control intraocular pressure in a majority of cases. When surgical therapy becomes necessary, however, individualized selection of an appropriate intervention is necessary to control the intraocular pressure and ultimately salvage vision in many severely compromised eyes. Corneal graft failure may occur in a significant number of these eyes after any further surgical procedure, especially those associated with anterior segment inflammation or complications detrimental to endothelial viability. Therefore surgical control of intraocular pressure before penetrating keratoplasty is advised in all high-risk cases and in those where control of intraocular pressure is inadequate.

REFERENCES

1. Charlin R, Polack FM: The effect of elevated intraocular pressure on the endothelium of corneal grafts, *Cornea* 1:241-249, 1982.
2. Irvine RA, Kaufman HE: Intraocular pressure following penetrating keratoplasty, *Am J Ophthalmol* 68:835-844, 1969.
3. Kaufman HE et al: Measurement and control of intraocular pressure in corneal disease, *Int Ophthalmol Clin* 10:387-401, 1970.
4. Mackay RS, Marg E: Fast, automatic electronic tonometers based on an exact theory, *Acta Ophthalmol (Copenh)* 37:495-507, 1959.
5. Moses R, Marg E, Oechsli R: Evaluation of the basic validity and clinical usefulness of the Mackay-Marg tonometer, *Invest Ophthalmol* 1:78-85, 1962.
6. Wood TO, West C, Kaufman HE: Control of intraocular pressure in penetrating keratoplasty, *Am J Ophthalmol* 74:724-728, 1972.
7. Thoft RA, Gordon JM, Dohlman CH: Glaucoma following keratoplasty, *Trans Am Acad Ophthalmol Otolaryngol* 78:352-364, 1974.
8. Olson RJ, Kaufman HE: Prognostic factors of intraocular pressure after aphakic keratoplasty, *Am J Ophthalmol* 86:510-515, 1978.
9. Robinson CH: Indications, complications and prognosis for repeat penetrating keratoplasty, *Ophthalmic Surg* 10:27-34, 1979.
10. Polack FM: Keratoplasty in aphakic eyes with corneal edema: results in 100 cases with 10-year follow-up, *Ophthalmic Surg* 11:701-707, 1980.
11. Goldberg DB, Schanzlin DJ, Brown SI: Incidence of increased intraocular pressure after keratoplasty, *Am J Ophthalmol* 92:372-377, 1981.
12. Karesh JW, Nirankari VS: Factors associated with glaucoma after penetrating keratoplasty, *Am J Ophthalmol* 96:160-164, 1983.
13. Foulks GN: Glaucoma associated with penetrating keratoplasty, *Ophthalmology* 94:871-874, 1987.
14. Simmons RB et al: Elevated intraocular pressure following

penetrating keratoplasty, *Trans Am Ophthalmol Soc* 87:79-91, 1989.

15. Kirkness CM, Ficker LA: Risk factors for the development of postkeratoplasty glaucoma, *Cornea* 11:427-432, 1992.
16. Sekhar GC et al: Post-penetrating keratoplasty glaucoma, *Indian J Ophthalmol* 41:181-184, 1993.
17. Chien AM et al: Glaucoma in the immediate postoperative period after penetrating keratoplasty, *Am J Ophthalmol* 115:711-714, 1993.
18. Olson RJ, Kaufman HE: Intraocular pressure and corneal thickness after penetrating keratoplasty, *Am J Ophthalmol* 85:97-100, 1978.
19. Rootman DS et al: Accuracy and precision of the Tono-Pen in measuring intraocular pressure after keratoplasty and epikeratophakia and in scarred corneas, *Arch Ophthalmol* 106: 1697-1700, 1988.
20. Svedburgh B: Effects of artificial intraocular pressure elevation on the corneal endothelium in the vervet monkey, *Acta Ophthalmol (Copenh)* 53:839-855, 1975.
21. Bigar F, Witmer R: Corneal endothelial changes in primary acute angle-closure glaucoma, *Ophthalmology* 89:596-599, 1982.
22. Vannas A, Setala K, Ruusuvaara P: Endothelial cells in capsular glaucoma, *Acta Ophthalmol (Copenh)* 55:951-958, 1977.
23. Williams KA et al: Factors predictive of corneal graft survival, *Ophthalmology* 99:403-414, 1992.
24. Zimmerman TJ et al: The effect of suture depth on outflow facility in penetrating keratoplasty, *Arch Ophthalmol* 96:505-506 1978.
25. Zimmerman TJ et al: Intraocular pressure after aphakic penetrating keratoplasty "through-and-through" suturing, *Ophthalmic Surg* 10:49-52,
26. Olson RJ, Kaufman HE: A mathematical description of causative factors and prevention of elevated intraocular pressure after keratoplasty, *Invest Ophthalmol Vis Sci* 16:1085-1092, 1977.
27. Olson RJ: Aphakic keratoplasty. Determining donor tissue size to avoid elevated intraocular pressure, *Arch Ophthalmol* 96:2274-2276, 1978.
28. Zimmerman TJ et al: Transplant size and elevated intraocular pressure postkeratoplasty, *Arch Ophthalmol* 96:2231-2233, 1978.
29. Perl T, Charlton KH, Binder PS: Disparate diameter grafting. Astigmatism, intraocular pressure, and visual acuity, *Ophthalmology* 88:774-781, 1981.
30. Foulks GN, Perry HD, Dohlman CH: Oversize corneal donor grafts in penetrating keratoplasty, *Ophthalmology* 86:490-494, 1979.
31. Heideman DG et al: Oversized donor grafts in penetrating keratoplasty. A randomized trial, *Arch Ophthalmol* 103:1807-1811, 1985.
32. Olson RJ: Variation in corneal graft size related to trephine technique, *Arch Ophthalmol* 97:1323-1325, 1979.
33. Bourne WM, Davison JA, O'Fallon WM: The effects of oversize donor buttons on postoperative intraocular pressure and corneal curvature in aphakic penetrating keratoplasty, *Ophthalmology* 89:242-246, 1982.
34. Burke S, Sugar J, Farber MD: Comparison of the effects of two viscoelastic agents, Healon and Viscoat, on postoperative intraocular pressure after penetrating keratoplasty, *Ophthalmic Surg* 21:821-826, 1990.
35. Lass JH, Pavan-Langston D: Timolol therapy in secondary angle-closure glaucoma post penetrating keratoplasty, *Ophthalmology* 86:51-59, 1979.
36. Olson RJ, Kaufman HE, Zimmerman TJ: Effects of Timolol and Daranide on elevated intraocular pressure after aphakic keratoplasty, *Ann Ophthalmol* 11:1833-1836, 1979.
37. Cohen EJ, Kenyon KR, Dohlman CH: Iridoplasty for prevention of post-keratoplasty angle closure and glaucoma, *Ophthlamic Surg* 13 994-996, 1982.
38. Van Meter WS et al: Laser trabeculoplasty for glaucoma in aphakic and pseudophakic eyes after penetrating keratoplasty, *Arch Ophthalmol* 106:185-188, 1988.
39. Casey TA, Gibbs D: Complications in corneal grafting, *Trans Ophthalmol Soc UK* 92:517-530, 1972.
40. Gilvarry AME et al: The management of post-keratoplasty glaucoma by trabeculectomy, *Eye* 3:713-718, 1989.
41. Ficker LA et al: Intraocular surgery following penetrating keratoplasty: the risks and advantages, *Eye* 4:693-697, 1990.
42. Insler MS et al: Penetrating keratoplasty with trabeculectomy, *Am J Ophthalmol* 100:593-595, 1985.
43. Kirkness CM et al: Co-existent corneal disease and glaucoma managed by either drainage surgery and subsequent keratoplasty or combined drainage surgery and penetrating keratoplasty, *Br J Ophthalmol* 76:146-152, 1992.
44. West CE, Wood TO, Kaufman HE: Cyclocryotherapy for glaucoma pre- or postpenetrating keratoplasty, *Am J Ophthalmol* 76:485-489, 1973.
45. Binder PS, Abel R, Kaufman HE: Cyclocryotherapy for glaucoma after penetrating keratoplasty, *Am J Ophthalmol* 79:489-492, 1975.
46. Krupin T, Mitchell KB, Becker B: Cyclocryotherapy in neovascular glaucoma, *Am J Ophthalmol* 86:24-26, 1978.
47. Zaidman GW, Wandel T: Transscleral YAG laser photocoagulation for uncontrolled glaucoma in corneal patients, *Cornea* 7:112-114, 1988.
48. Levy NS, Bonney RC: Transscleral YAG cyclophotocoagulation of the ciliary body for persistently high intraocular pressure following penetrating keratoplasty, *Cornea* 8:178-181, 1989.
49. Cohen EJ et al: Neodymium: YAG laser transscleral cyclophotocoagulation for glaucoma after penetrating keratoplasty, *Ophthalmic Surg* 20:713-716, 1989.
50. Wheatcroft S et al: Treatment of glaucoma following penetrating keratoplasty with transscleral YAG cyclophotocoagulation, *Int Ophthalmol* 16:397-400, 1992.
51. Hardten DR, Brown JD: Transscleral Neodymium:YAG cyclophotocoagulation: comparison of 180-degree and 360-degree initial treatments, *Ophthalmic Surg* 24:181-184, 1993.
52. Hardten DR, Brown JD, Holland EJ: Results of Neodymium: YAG laser transscleral cyclophotocoagulation for postkeratoplasty glaucoma, *Glaucoma* 2:241-245, 1993.
53. Molteno ACB: New implant for glaucoma clinical trial, *Br J Ophthalmol* 53:606-615, 1969.
54. Schocket SS, Lakhanpal V, Richards BD: Anterior chamber tube shunt to an encircling band in the treatment of neovascular glaucoma, *Ophthalmology* 89:1188-1194, 1982.
55. Krupin T et al: A long Krupin-Denver valve implant attached to a 180 scleral explant for glaucoma surgery, *Ophthalmology* 95:1174-1180, 1988.
56. Joseph NJ et al: A one piece drainage system for glaucoma surgery, *Trans Ophthalmol Soc UK* 105:657-664, 1986.
57. Smith S et al: Early clinical experience with a Baerveldt 350-mm^2 glaucoma implant and associated extraocular muscle imbalance, *Ophthalmology* 100:914-918, 1993.
58. Kirkness CM: Penetrating keratoplasty, glaucoma, and silicone drainage tubing, *Dev Ophthalmol* 14:161-165, 1987.
59. Kirkness CM, Ling Y, Rice NC: The use of silicone drainage tubing to control post-keratoplasty glaucoma, *Eye* 2:583-590, 1988.
60. McDonnell PJ et al: Molteno implantation for control of glaucoma in eyes after penetrating keratoplasty, *Ophthalmology* 95:364-369, 1988.
61. Beebe WE et al: The use of Molteno implant and anterior tube shunt to encircling band for the treatment of glaucoma in keratoplasty patients, *Ophthalmology* 97:1414-1422, 1990.

62. O'Day DG et al: Graft survival and intraocular pressure control after Molteno implantation for post-keratoplasty glaucoma, *Invest Ophthalmol Vis Sci* 34 (suppl):1273, 1992.
63. Sherwood MB, Smith MF, Driebe WT: Drainage tube implants in the treatment of glaucoma following penetrating keratoplasty, *Ophthalmic Surg* 24:185-189, 1993.
64. Melamed S et al: Postoperative complications after Molteno implant surgery, *Am J Ophthalmol* 111:319-322, 1991.
65. Lotufo DG: Postoperative complications and visual loss following Molteno implantation, *Ophthalmic Surg* 22:650-656, 1991.
66. Lloyd MA et al: Clinical experience with the single-plate Molteno implant in complicated glaucomas. Update of a pilot study, *Ophthalmology* 99:679-687, 1992.
67. Wilson RP et al: Aqueous shunts. Molteno versus Schocket, *Ophthalmology* 99:672-678, 1992.
68. Smith MF, Sherwood MB, McGoray SP: Comparison of the double-plate Molteno drainage implant with the Schocket procedure, *Arch Ophthalmol* 110:1246-1250, 1992.

SECTION FOUR Complicated Penetrating Keratoplasty

CHAPTER 142

PETER GLOOR

Pediatric Penetrating Keratoplasty

In 1958, an article entitled "Corneal Grafting" contained the following dictum: "A perforating keratoplasty should never be attempted in any child who is under sixteen years of age."[1] Because of advances in surgical technique and postoperative care, a clear transplant can now often be attained in an infant or a child. Therefore penetrating keratoplasty is no longer contraindicated in pediatric patients. In fact, prompt penetrating keratoplasty may be the necessary first step in averting irreversible loss of visual function to amblyopia. The visual results of pediatric penetrating keratoplasty, however, are often disappointing. Many special difficulties encountered in the management of an infant or a child requiring corneal transplantation conspire to make these patients among the most challenging for the corneal surgeon.

Many aspects of an infant's or a child's preoperative, intraoperative, and postoperative care differ from those of an adult undergoing a corneal transplantation. The child and the child's parents are generally more fearful and anxious when they present for preoperative evaluation. The difficulty in assessing the visual function of an infant or a young child, a child's inability to cooperate with the eye examination, and the great variability in outcome all make the physician's decision regarding surgery more difficult.

In the operating room, the corneal surgeon encounters other difficulties unique to pediatric penetrating keratoplasties. In infants, the cornea and anterior segment are smaller, and the cornea is often thinner and more pliable, requiring more exacting surgical technique. Compared to an adult eye, the eye of a young keratoplasty patient is much more likely to have scleral collapse and alarming posterior pressure. The iris of infants and children seems to have a greater tendency to adhere to the posterior corneal surface and the wound. Many young patients with congenital or traumatic corneal disease have significant anterior segment abnormalities, which may be difficult to anticipate but must be addressed during surgery. In children requiring vitrectomy, the vitreous is more tenacious, which makes its safe, rapid removal more difficult.

Compared to adults, infants and children appear to be more prone to a severe inflammatory response during the early postoperative period and are more likely to have endothelial graft rejection or graft failure. The corneal wound heals more rapidly in infants and children, increasing the risks that sutures will erode, vascularize, and become infected. Therefore all sutures must be removed early, making selective suture removal to minimize transplant astigmatism impossible.

Postoperatively, infants and young children are unable to cooperate with examinations. Therefore the examination must be either suboptimal or performed with the patient under restraint, under sedation, or under anesthesia. Infants and children cannot effectively communicate that they have visual loss, pain, or other symptoms that require evaluation. Therefore compared to adults, they require more frequent examinations. Infants and children are dependent on their parents to report problems, instill medications, provide other treatment, and transport them to and from eye appointments. Children are more likely than adults to rub or otherwise traumatize their eyes. Refraction must be accomplished by retinoscopy, which may be difficult if there is irregular astigmatism or the graft is not completely clean.

The greatest difference between the management of pediatric and adult corneal transplantation patients is that infants and young children with a visually significant corneal opacity develop deprivation amblyopia. The specter of amblyopia affects the decision to proceed with surgery, the timing of the surgery, and almost every aspect of postoperative care. In fact, the fundamental goal of pediatric penetrating keratoplasty and all the postoperative care is to reverse or limit the effects of amblyopia. The duration of time the eye is capable of perceiving a clear, well-focused image and the effectiveness of the amblyopia therapy during a patient's first years of life establish the eye's visual potential for the rest of the patient's life. The surgery itself should be viewed, by physician and parents alike, as the first in a long series of interventions designed to treat amblyopia.

This chapter describes treatment of the uncommon cases of pediatric corneal disease encountered in economically developed nations that are privileged to have plentiful food, adequate sanitation, and modern medical facilities. It should be noted, however, that childhood corneal blindness is perhaps 100 times more prevalent in some developing regions, particularly Africa.[2] Pediatric penetrating keratoplasty is performed in some developing nations.[3,4] However, the surgery is currently not feasible on any large scale in underdeveloped nations; in these countries, preventive measures currently hold the only hope for reducing the worldwide prevalence of corneal blindness.

Review of the Literature

About 30 years ago, reports of success with pediatric penetrating keratoplasty began to appear in the literature.[5-7] Until recently, these reports generally included the percentage of grafts that remained clear during follow-up periods that ranged from months to years. Visual outcome was often not reported. Factors associated with a clear graft were reported without statistical analysis.[8-13] In the last 10 years, the use of increasingly sophisticated statistical analysis, including survival analysis and multivariate analysis, has provided more useful information.[13-15] Identifying the factors associated with graft survival and good visual outcome help define the indications for pediatric penetrating keratoplasty and point the way to improving the outcome when the surgery is performed. In general, the work reviewed here has appeared in the English-language, peer reviewed literature over the last 20 years, with emphasis on larger series that used statistical analyses. Most series included patients who were under 12 to 18 years of age when they underwent penetrating keratoplasty.

INDICATIONS

Among 348 eyes described in six series of pediatric penetrating keratoplasties, 55% of the eyes had congenital opacities and 45% had acquired opacities.[9,10,12-15] Among the eyes with congenital opacities, 54% had Peters' anomaly, 15% had congenital glaucoma, 12% had congenital hereditary endothelial dystrophy, 6% had posterior polymorphous dystrophy, 4% had sclerocornea, 1% had a dermoid, and 8% had other disorders. Among the acquired opacities, the diagnoses were globe lacerations, 43%; infectious keratitis, 32%; keratoconus, 18%; nonpenetrating trauma, 6%; and other disorders, 1%.

Of 220 patients undergoing pediatric penetrating keratoplasty, 63% of patients had a unilateral opacity.[9,14,15] Bilateral disease was seen in 63% of patients with congenital opacities, but only 10% of patients with acquired opacities.[9,14] Of the patients with bilateral corneal disorders, only 49% underwent bilateral surgery.[9,14,15] The earliest postconception, successful corneal transplantation described was performed for a large corneal perforation on a 34-week postconception, 1 lb infant.[16]

GRAFT SURVIVAL

In the studies reviewed, a graft was generally considered to have failed when it became cloudy and was no longer compatible with good visual function. In most cases, failure resulted from edema, often secondary to endothelial graft rejection or presumed rejection. Other causes of failure were glaucoma, phthisis, or stromal scarring from a persistent epithelial defect or corneal infection. In Figure 142-1, the survival curves from two large series of pediatric penetrating keratoplasties have been combined.[14,15] The curves represent a total of 228 eyes from five medical centers. Repeat keratoplasties were not included. The failure rates for all pediatric first keratoplasties in these studies were 26% at 1 year and 36% at 2 years. There were few additional failures after the second postoperative year.

The graft failure rates for pediatric keratoplasty are greater than that reported for adults. For instance the failure rate at 1 year after surgery is about 7% for adults.[17-19] There are several possibilities for the difference in the failure rates. The surgery on young patients is technically more difficult. Younger recipient age has been associated with an increased rejection rate,[20,21] and the eyes of infants and children can mount a severe inflammatory reaction.[15,22] Because infants and young children cannot effectively communicate pain and decreased vision, treatment of rejection or other complications is often delayed. Two reports indicate that as few as 10% of pediatric graft rejections are reversible.[10,12]

The causes of pediatric penetrating keratoplasty failure are not well defined, and reports are contradictory. In the two large series, the causes of failure among failed grafts were distributed as follows: transplantation rejection, 11% to 50%; glaucoma, 0 to 14%; corneal ulcer or infection, 10% to 25%; phthisis, 5% to

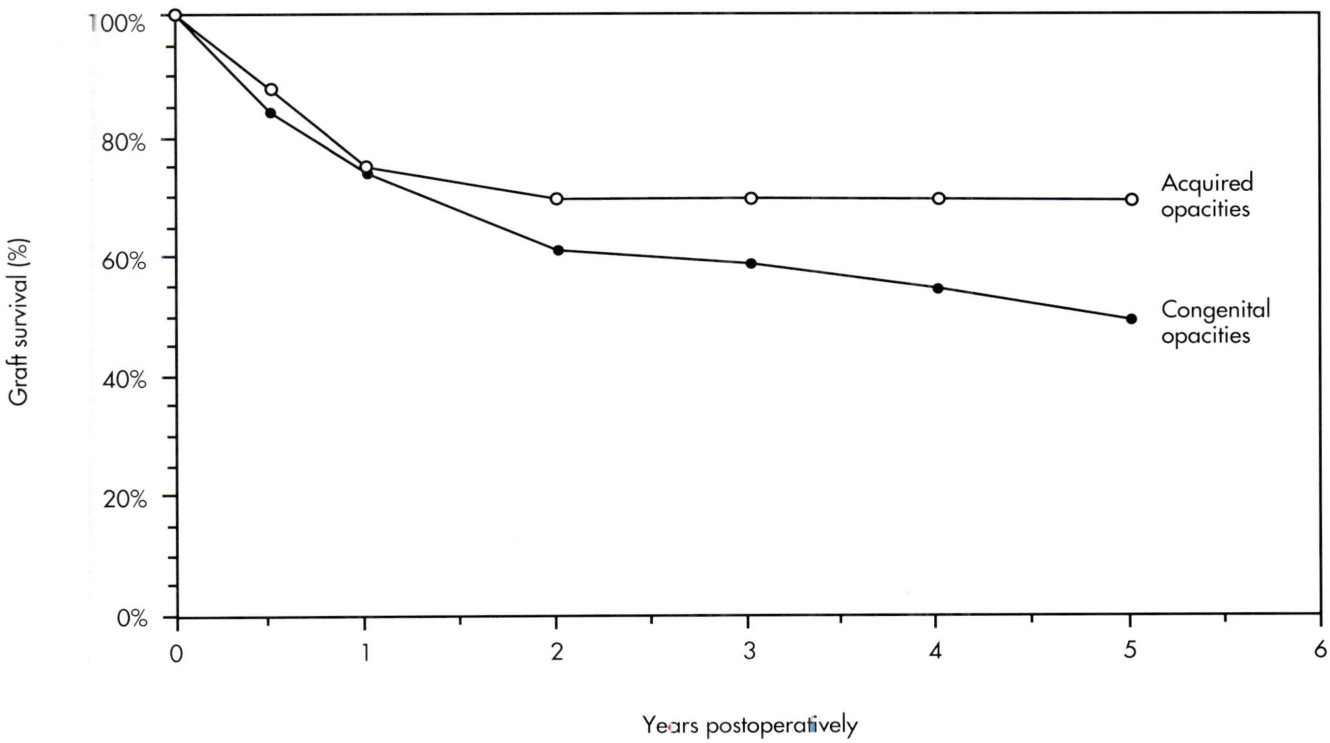

FIGURE 142-1 Survival curves for pediatric penetrating keratoplasties using data combined from five eye centers.[14,15] The plot shows the percentage of grafts remaining clear at different follow-up periods. Repeat penetrating keratoplasties were not included. The number of grafts (N) performed for a congenital opacity and followed for 6 months was 100, but only 39 of these grafts had 3 year follow-up. The N for acquired opacities was 89 at 6 months and 24 at 3 years.

8%; retrocorneal membrane, 4% to 8%; endophthalmitis, 0 to 3%; and unknown, 0 to 47%.[14,15] The difference in the rates of rejection as a cause of failure is probably due to differing definitions of rejection. The study reporting only an 11% rejection rate among failures defined a rejection more narrowly.[14] Because the same study noted that many pediatric grafts fail with gradual loss of clarity, the cause of almost half of the failures in this study was "unknown."

Factors statistically associated with pediatric penetrating keratoplasty failure are tear or surface abnormalities,[14] prior persistent epithelial defect,[14] corneal ulceration,[15] deep or superficial corneal vascularization at the time of surgery,[14] persistent postoperative inflammation,[15] pupillary membranes,[14] lensectomy and vitrectomy,[14,15] and repeat keratoplasty.[14,15] In one study, vascularization was associated with rejection, but not with failure in general.[15] Among pediatric keratoplasties, congenital opacities,[14,15] and younger age at the time of the first transplantation[14] tended to be associated with greater rates of graft failure; but these associations did not reach statistical significance. Even when the results from the two studies were combined, the rates of graft failure among congenital and acquired opacities were not significantly different (Figure 142-1; $P=0.3$).

Vascularization has been associated with graft failure and rejection in adults,[18-21,23] as well as the pediatric population, presumably because vascularization increases the access of the immune system to the graft.[19-21] Pupillary membranes may be associated with retrocorneal membranes, which could explain their association with pediatric graft failure.

Lensectomy and vitrectomy were also associated with greater rates of pediatric penetrating keratoplasty failure. In adults, aphakic eyes have increased rates of graft failure compared to phakic or pseudophakic eyes.[18] One possible explanation is that vitreous touch damages the endothelium,[24] but this complication should be unusual with modern anterior vitrectomy techniques. Anterior vitrectomy during keratoplasty has been associated with diffuse retrocorneal fibrous membrane formation in failed grafts.[25] Perhaps formation of retrocorneal membranes explains why many grafts fail by gradual loss of clarity.[14]

Even though children are generally considered to have a resilient corneal epithelium, many pediatric graft failures were thought due to or associated with

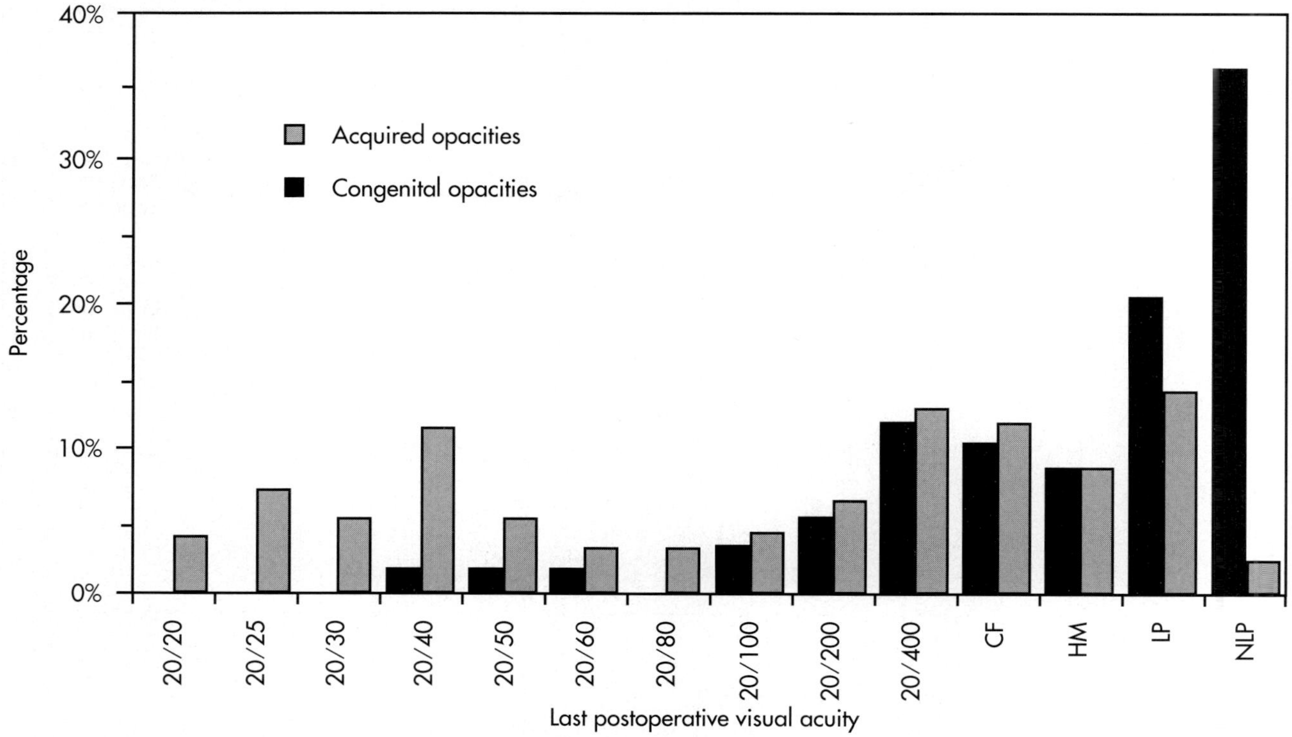

FIGURE 142-2 The distribution of the most recent postoperative visual acuities from five series of pediatric penetrating keratoplasties in which individual visual acuities were reported separately for eyes with acquired and dense congenital opacities.[9-11,13,14,22] A total of 59 eyes that had a dense congenital corneal opacity and 94 eyes that had an acquired corneal opacity are represented.

epithelial disease or ulceration. Early suture erosion, uneven wounds, and the use of frequent topical medications may contribute to these surface problems. As in adults,[18,21,23] repeat keratoplasty has also been associated with graft failure in children. It is unclear whether this failure is a true effect of multiple keratoplasties or whether eyes that require repeat keratoplasty are by their nature more prone to graft failure.

Recipient gender, recipient race, graft size, the length of time sutures were left in place, and "social support" factors were not found to be associated with graft failure.[15] A shorter time of donor death to transplantation appeared to be associated with longer graft survival, although this association was not statistically significant.[14] Donor age, donor endothelial cell count, time of donor death to enucleation, and time of donor death to storage in media were not associated with graft failure.[14]

VISUAL OUTCOME

The distribution of the most recent postoperative visual acuities from the five large series of pediatric penetrating keratoplasties that reported individual visual acuities separately for eyes with acquired and congenital opacities is shown in Figure 142-2.[9-11,13,14,22] The median visual acuity after all pediatric penetrating keratoplasties was count fingers. The median visual acuity after pediatric penetrating keratoplasties for acquired opacities was 20/200, but for congenital opacities it was light perception.[9-11,13,14,22]

These results for congenital opacities are probably worse than expected and certainly worse than the results of congenital cataract surgery.[26] Among 178 eyes receiving a cataract extraction for a unilateral congenital cataract in the first year of life, 41% of eyes achieved a visual acuity of 20/100 or better and 16% achieved 20/40 or better.[27] Among 84 eyes receiving a penetrating keratoplasty for a dense congenital corneal opacity, only 8% achieved a visual acuity of 20/100 or better and 2% achieved 20/40 or better.[9-11,13,14,22]

Possible explanations for the poor visual outcome after pediatric penetrating keratoplasty are frequent graft failures; optical distortion from the graft; irreversible, untreated, or ineffectively treated amblyopia; and the other pathology frequently found in eyes requiring pediatric penetrating keratoplasty. In one large study, the children with congenital opacities were an average of 2.5 years old at the time of first penetrating keratoplasty, so many had deep amblyopia at the time of surgery.[14] In a second study, however, a statistically significant association between the age at surgery and visual outcome could not be demonstrated among patients with congenital opacities. On the other hand, only 62% of grafted eyes in this second study received optical correction, and 69% of patients with unilateral disease who were less than 8 years old received amblyopia therapy.[15]

Younger age at the onset of the opacity has been associated with a poor visual outcome in one large series.[14] When the results from several series[9-11,13,14,22] were combined (Figure 142-2), congenital opacities had a significantly worse visual outcome than acquired opacities ($P = 0.0001$). In a recent large series of grafts in children up to 12 years of age, however, multivariate analysis showed that age of onset of the opacity was not an independent predictor of visual outcome,[15] perhaps because many of the eyes with congenital opacities had "posterior segment abnormalities," which were independently associated with poor visual outcome.

Other factors associated with poor visual outcome were preoperative corneal edema,[14] preoperative glaucoma,[14] preoperative anterior synechiae,[14] preoperative and postoperative aphakia,[14] vitrectomy,[14,15] posterior segment abnormalities,[15] no optical correction,[15] no amblyopia therapy,[15] and bilateral corneal disease.[15]

Although the visual outcome reported in the literature is disappointing, the postoperative visual acuity is often better than the preoperative visual acuity, which is frequently poor. Preoperative and postoperative visual acuities are generally available only for acquired corneal diseases in older children. In two large pediatric series, 64% to 70% of such eyes had an improved visual acuity after transplantation surgery.[14,15]

COMPLICATIONS

Amblyopia and strabismus are often listed among the common complications of pediatric penetrating keratoplasty, but reporting is too inconsistent to summarize. Rates of significant but less common complications have generally been reported as a percentage of eyes in the series, but some are a percentage of grafts performed in the series. The reported complication rates are expulsive choroidal hemorrhage, 2% to 3%[10,12,13]; inadvertent lens loss, 1% to 2%[10,15]; wound leak or dehiscence, 2% to 10%[10,12,13,15,28]; corneal ulcer and/or infection, 4% to 9%[12,13,15,28]; endophthalmitis, 2%[12-14]; new onset glaucoma, 5% to 9%[13,15]; cataract, 2% to 7%[10,13,15]; retinal detachment, 3% to 5%[13,15]; and phthisis, 4% to 13%.[9,10,12,14] Of 94 eyes undergoing penetrating keratoplasties for an acquired opacity, 2% had a final visual acuity of no light perception. Of 59 eyes undergoing penetrating keratoplasties for a dense congenital opacity, 36% had a final visual acuity of no light perception.[9-11,13,14,22]

FUTURE STUDIES

There are two major challenges for those investigating strategies for improving the outcome of pediatric penetrating keratoplasty. The first is to determine ways to improve graft survival. The second is to improve amblyopia therapy. Prospective, multicenter trials allow for the use of advanced statistical analysis and are most likely to yield valid results that can be applied to improving outcome.

In one large study, the cause of nearly half the graft failures was unknown.[14] A study of the histology of failed pediatric grafts would help determine the cause of such failures. In a study of high-risk grafts in adults, defined as grafts in a recipient with two or more quadrants of corneal vascularization and/or a history of previous graft rejection, ABO blood group compatibility, but not HLA compatibility, was associated with a statistically significant reduction in graft failure and graft failure caused by rejection.[29] The study was limited to patients 10 or more years old. Although infant grafts are high risk, it is unclear whether the high failure rate is due to rejection, and it is unknown whether ABO compatibility would benefit pediatric penetrating keratoplasty patients.

Topical cyclosporin A has been used to treat anterior segment inflammatory diseases[30] and for corneal transplantation rejection prophylaxis.[31,32] Its safety and efficacy in pediatric penetrating keratoplasty patients should be studied. The development of treatments to inhibit or reverse corneal vascularization would also benefit pediatric keratoplasty patients. Glaucoma management in pediatric penetrating keratoplasty patients should be investigated, as many of these patients have glaucoma. High pressure, hypotony, and other complications of glaucoma treatment all threaten graft survival and visual outcome. Additionally, work is needed to determine whether simple strategies, such as increased emphasis on parental examination of the graft or more frequent thorough examinations, can improve graft survival in infants and children.

The optimum treatment for amblyopia in pediatric penetrating keratoplasty patients has not been defined. In the analogous situation of congenital cataracts, early surgery, early optical correction, and good compliance with aggressive amblyopia therapy have been associated with excellent visual outcomes, even in patients with unilateral cataracts.[26,27,33] A recent study appears to confirm some of these results in pediatric penetrating keratoplasties.[15]

Two large studies have divided pediatric keratoplasty patients into congenital, acquired traumatic, and

7. What will be the cost to the family in terms of anxiety, disruption of home life, loss of time to attend to the other needs of this child and the needs of other dependents, loss of income, and cost of medical care? In a large series of grafts from several centers, pediatric penetrating keratoplasty patients required an average of 40 visits over a mean follow-up of 5 years. The average distance they traveled was about 100 miles per visit.[15] The cost of medical care for the eye depicted in Figure 142-3 has been $32,000 over 4 years. The deleterious effects on the family of undertaking the corneal transplantation vary among families. The patient's parents are in the best position to gauge the impact, providing the surgeon has given them a realistic description of the treatment.
8. Are there any other treatments that have a better chance of improving this patient's visual function or have less risk and cost? Many acquired opacities and some congenital opacities involve only a portion of the cornea. In these cases, alternative treatments may offer better or equal visual outcome with fewer risks and costs.

Consideration of these questions will help the corneal surgeon decide whether it is in the overall best interest of the child to offer no treatment, alternative treatment, offer transplantation; recommend transplantation; or urge transplantation. Although no set of guidelines can be applied to every patient, the following strategies are reasonable based on the currently available outcome data and the recommendations of experienced corneal surgeons.

Alternatives to penetrating keratoplasty

Given the risks and costs of pediatric penetrating keratoplasty, virtually any alternative with a better or equal chance of success of improving vision and limiting amblyopia should be attempted rather than embarking on treatment with penetrating keratoplasty. Central corneal lacerations, in particular, diminish visual function less than one would expect. In a study of 26 eyes with corneal lacerations in children and adults, a contact lens could be fitted in all but one patient; 54% of the 24 verbal patients achieved a visual acuity of 20/30 or better, and 92% achieved 20/60 or better. Many of these patients had been referred for corneal transplantation.[47] The eye depicted in Figure 142-4 has visual acuity of 20/30 with a spectacle correction and 20/20 with a rigid contact lens.

If the entire cornea in front of the pupil is opacified, a contact lens will not improve vision. If a portion of the peripheral cornea is clear, however, a rotational autokeratoplasty[48] or peripheral optical iridectomy[49-51]

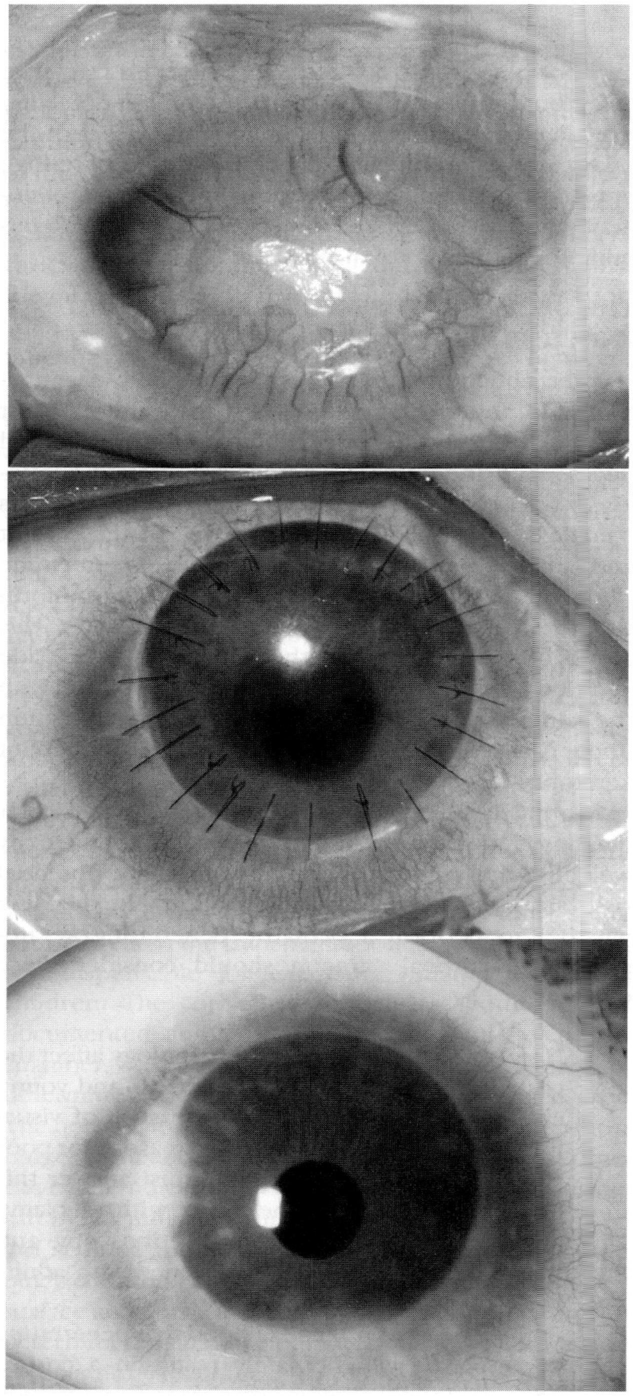

A

B

C

FIGURE 142-3 **A,** The preoperative appearance of the right eye of an infant with a unilateral congenital corneal opacity. The patient underwent penetrating keratoplasty with lysis of iridocorneal adhesions at 1 month of age. **B,** The appearance of the same eye, immediately before suture removal 4 weeks after surgery. Two months later the patient had a reversible endothelial graft rejection. Two years later graft astigmatism had increased from 2 to 14 diopters. Unsuccessful relaxing incisions with compression sutures were followed by a successful wedge resection temporally. **C,** Four years after the penetrating keratoplasty, the graft is clear with 6 diopters of astigmatism. The eye is otherwise normal. The parents have not been compliant with the occlusion therapy prescribed by the patient's pediatric ophthalmologist. The best corrected visual acuity is 20/400 because of amblyopia.

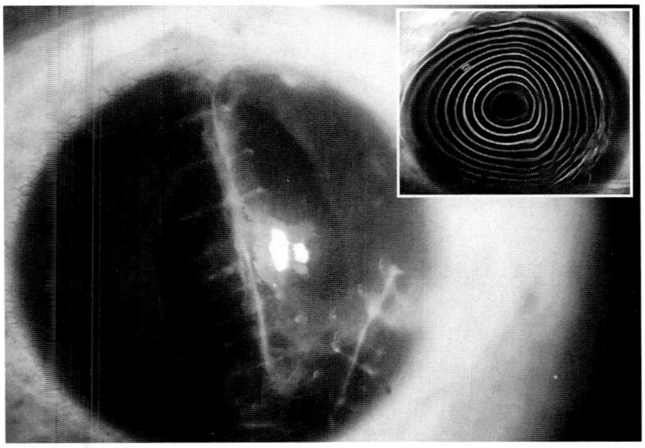

FIGURE 142-4 An example of an eye that has excellent visual acuity despite a large central scar from a laceration. Visual acuity is 20/30 with a spectacle correction and 20/20 with a rigid contact lens. Keratoscopy of the same eye shows moderate irregular astigmatism (inset).

may provide better vision with less risk and cost than corneal transplantation. Superficial keratectomy or lamellar keratoplasty should be considered if the endothelium is functioning and the opacity is superficial (see Chapter 149).[12] Mild edema can be treated with hypertonic drops. A very high or low intraocular pressure, an anterior chamber foreign body,[52] or even a loose crystalline lens may be a reversible cause of corneal edema and should be treated before making a decision about corneal transplantation. In summary, given the current pediatric transplantation outcome data, any alternative that seems likely to provide vision better than perhaps 20/400 in an infant or better than perhaps 20/100 in a young child should be recommended rather than the transplantation. Treatment should be coupled with amblyopia therapy when appropriate.

Bilateral opacities

In most cases, bilateral dense corneal opacities in an infant or a child who is young enough to develop significant amblyopia and has some visual potential, require the surgeon to urge the parents to consent to corneal transplantation. Both corneas should probably be transplanted promptly.[22,53] Because these patients may require multiple surgeries, it is quite possible that one eye will be lost because of a complication. Therefore it is probably unwise to "save" an eye with a dense opacity for future surgery, because the eye will develop a dense and possibly irreversible amblyopia.[22] (There are little data about visual potential of adult eyes with untreated, dense, congenital opacities. There is, however, a report of a 16-year-old patient with bilateral, dense sclerocornea since birth who attained visual acuity of 20/400 as a result of penetrating keratoplasty.[54]) Furthermore, if one graft fails, while waiting to repeat the transplantation, the vision in the other eye will minimize the effect on the child's early development and education.[22] The transplantation of both corneas in bilateral disease is usually not indicated if one eye has a mild opacity, consistent with ambulatory vision, or if the child is no longer in the amblyogenic age range.

Unilateral opacities

The decision to perform a corneal transplant for a unilateral dense opacity in an infant or a child less than 7 or 8 years old is difficult. Some surgeons consider the situation a relative contraindication to penetrating keratoplasty.[12] Because these patients are in the amblyogenic age range, transplantation surgery may be the only option to improve the visual potential of the eye. However, if the visual outcome of transplantation is to count fingers, the median from the literature,[9-11,13,14,22] and the other eye is normal, the child may gain little from the surgery unless the normal eye is lost to injury or disease. The risk of a vision-threatening injury is low,[55,56] but the risk of visual loss to disorders such as glaucoma and age-related macular degeneration accumulates over the patient's lifetime. In the Framingham Eye Study, 4% of the study population had a visual acuity of 20/200 or worse in at least one eye because of an apparently untreatable condition. Among those over 75 years of age, this value increased to 10%, although three-fourths of these people had a visual acuity greater than 20/60 in their better eye.[55] Consequently, the benefit to the patient of a "spare" eye with ambulatory vision may outweigh the risks and costs of a corneal transplantation in the majority of such cases. Therefore, it is reasonable to offer surgery for a unilateral dense opacity, but to support the parents' decision if, after appropriate counseling, they decide against surgery.

If a moderate unilateral opacity is consistent with visual acuity of perhaps 20/400 to count fingers in an infant or perhaps 20/100 to 20/200 in a child up to the age of 8 years, it seems reasonable either to offer corneal transplantation or to recommend against it, depending partly on whether the eye has other pathology that may limit vision or threaten graft survival. If a mild unilateral opacity is consistent with better than 20/400 vision in an infant or better than 20/100 in a child, or if other pathology will almost certainly limit visual prognosis, it is probably best to recommend against transplantation surgery.

Older children

In children beyond the amblyogenic age range who have good vision in one eye, it is probably best to defer corneal transplantation or repeat corneal transplantation in the other eye as long as doing so does not put it at significant risk of losing visual potential. In these older children, amblyopia is no longer one of these risks, so transplantation can be delayed until the patient can better participate in his or her care, has a better chance of success, has greater visual needs, and has less chance of injury. Athletic teenagers often prefer poor vision in one eye to having their activities restricted after surgery. If the eye that sees well has had surgery or has a significant chance of becoming unstable for some other reason, the case against performing a transplantation of the poor-seeing eye is even stronger. Once the risk of amblyopia has passed, it is prudent to "save" such a poor-seeing eye in case the abnormal better-seeing eye is lost. Surgical results are likely to improve substantially as the decades go by, and the goal in such a patient is to retain good vision in at least one eye for a lifetime, which may span 80 or more years.

COUNSELING THE PARENTS AND INFORMED CONSENT

The corneal surgeon should remember that the family is likely to be upset and anxious and may have misconceptions about transplantation surgery. Many pediatric penetrating keratoplasties are performed on newborn infants with isolated, sporadic, eye anomalies. Because these patients should be referred promptly to a corneal surgeon, the family often has had little time to adjust to the threat to their child's vision and perhaps an obvious abnormal appearance. Because the parents' knowledge of transplantation surgery is probably based on popular coverage of organ transplantation, they may feel corneal transplantation surgery is a desperate measure and likely to fail with dire results. On the other hand, the parents may hold the false hope that simply replacing the cloudy cornea with a clear one will make their child's eye completely normal.

Counseling of the parents should include a discussion of the findings and the diagnosis or possible diagnoses. A model of the eye and photos of a corneal transplantation (Figure 142-3) are helpful to show them the cornea, its refractive function, the portion of the cornea that is transplanted, the other parts of the eye, and their functions. The surgeon should indicate the cause of the disorder, if it is known, and refer the patient for systemic evaluation and the parents for genetic counseling if appropriate. Many parents of children with congenital disorders may silently fear that they are responsible for the disorder. The parents should be explicitly assured that they are in no way responsible for the disorder whenever there is no evidence to the contrary. The ophthalmologist should also address the parents' concerns about the appearance of the eyes. Ophthalmologists tend to view this concern as secondary to concerns about visual function, but the parents may not.

The parents must be thoroughly counseled, so they can make an informed decision about surgery and begin their participation in the care of their child's eye condition. The corneal surgeon can use loose lenses and a trial frame to demonstrate different levels of vision to the parents. (Providing a person has normal vision, is not a latent hyperope or over-minused, does not squint, and is looking in the distance, these spherical lenses over his or her distance correction produce vision as follows: +1.50 = 20/100; +2.50 = 20/200; +3.50 = 20/400; +10.00 = count fingers at 3 feet; +30.00 = hand motion at 3 feet.)

The following is an example of one approach to providing the realistic information to parents as they take part in the decision to operate. In this example, a newborn has a moderately dense, left, unilateral, corneal opacity and no other ocular abnormalities. Because the rest of the eye is normal, the predictions made about outcome are somewhat more optimistic than indicated previously.

By my examination I estimate that the vision in the left eye is like this (occlude the right eye and cover the left with both a +10.00 and +20.00 sphere). If we go ahead with a corneal transplantation and all the other care required afterward, then about half the time we could gain vision only this good even when wearing the best glasses (remove the +20.00 sphere, leaving the +10.00 sphere). There is some chance it could be better but also some chance it could be worse. However, the right eye is normal and will almost certainly see this well (remove the occluder from the right eye) whether or not we decide to do surgery of the left eye. The vision from the left eye after the surgery may not be very useful because the right eye is normal, but would be very useful if something unexpected happened to the good eye, like an injury (occlude the right eye for a moment again). That is what the surgery might gain for your child.

Now let us talk about risks and difficulties involved in doing a corneal transplantation. There is perhaps a 1 in 10 chance that the eye could end up completely blind and look more abnormal than it does now. There is a good chance that the corneal transplantation will become cloudy and need replacement once or twice during childhood and several times during adulthood. Other types of eye surgery might be needed. During the first years of your child's life, you may need to put in drops every day, patch the other eye every day, and come in for about 25 visits in the first year. Especially early on, patching the other eye might cause your child to cry or withdraw because initially the left eye will be lazy. Unless you are willing to go through all this, performing the transplantation is not worthwhile.

You should know two other things. If you decide to proceed with transplantation surgery, the sooner it is done the better. The vision that can be gained from the surgery probably starts to decline if the surgery is delayed a few months. After a few years, there will be very little chance of improving the vision because the eye will become what is often called a lazy eye. Finally, you should know that if you decide against the surgery, or if the surgery is done, fails, and is not repeated, things can be done to improve the appearance of the eye.

This information is complicated, and the parents' decision is a difficult one. Some of the information will need to be repeated, and the parents will have many questions. Giving them written information and the opportunity to phone or return with questions is helpful. The patient should be given age-appropriate information about the condition and treatment.

If the surgeon and parents decide against surgery for a unilateral opacity, three other issues should be discussed. First, less aggressive alternative treatments should be considered. Even though they may offer less potential for visual improvement, their risks and cost are much lower. For instance, occlusion therapy may keep a 20/100 translucent cornea from resulting in 20/400 amblyopia. Second, options to reduce the abnormal appearance should be discussed and revisited as the child grows up. Finally, the ophthalmologist should counsel the parents about the importance of guarding the visual function of the eyes, particularly if one is normal. Full-time safety glasses, goggles when engaging in sports and other hazardous activities, and examinations at least once a year should be recommended. The importance of these precautions should be reinforced as the child matures.

PREPARING FOR THE TRANSPLANTATION SURGERY

The pediatric penetrating keratoplasty literature is limited but shows no statistically significant association between visual outcome and the time from the onset of the opacity to surgery for congenital[14,15] and acquired opacities.[14] The literature on congenital cataracts is more extensive and perhaps could be applied to congenital corneal opacities. A recent review of the literature uncovered 178 patients with congenital and presumed congenital unilateral cataracts who underwent surgery before 1 year of age.[27] Of the 123 patients undergoing surgery in the first 4 months of life, 52% attained vision of 20/100 or better and 22% attained 20/40 or better. Of the 55 undergoing surgery after the first 4 months of life, only 16% attained a visual acuity of 20/100 or better, and only 2% attained 20/40 or better. Although there appears to be no firm data, the feeling among anesthesiologists is that general anesthesia has fewer risks after the first month of life.[57] Therefore for a congenital corneal opacity, surgery at about 5 weeks of life is probably optimal. For a patient needing bilateral transplantations, the second transplantation surgery should be performed optimally 1 to 2 weeks after the first. Some surgeons advocate performing surgery on both eyes simultaneously.[58]

Before surgery, any lid or adenexal anomalies that might threaten the health of the graft should be repaired. In a patient with glaucoma, it is important to bring the pressure into the normal range before attempting transplantation surgery if at all possible. Very high pressures, hypotony, and glaucoma procedures performed after the transplantation are all threats to graft clarity. If the patient has posterior segment anomalies, such as retinal detachment, a retinal surgeon should be involved in developing a surgical plan. The child's pediatrician should be asked to "clear" the patient for anesthesia and make recommendations for perioperative care.[59] Because Peters' anomaly has been associated with heart anomalies, it has been recommended that all these patients be evaluated for these anomalies.[60] This evaluation should be performed before surgery.

THE DONOR TISSUE

The surgeon should alert the eye bank about the tissue requirements as soon as he or she is prepared to perform the surgery. As in all transplantations, a careful donor history, examination of the donor eye, and blood work on the donor serum are necessary to reduce the risks of transmission of infection and primary graft failure. Because transplantations in infants and children have a high failure rate, and because each failure deepens the child's amblyopia, an effort should be made to transplant tissue with the greatest possible density of viable endothelial cells. If excellent tissue is not available when the patient is ready for surgery, the benefits of using excellent tissue must be weighed against the risk of deepening the amblyopia by waiting.

Endothelial cell barrier function declines with increasing storage time.[61] In a large pediatric series, donor age,[14,15] donor cell count,[15] and time from death to storage media[14] did not affect graft survival. Decreased time from donor death to transplantation was associated with increased graft survival, but the relationship was not statistically significant.[14] The donor epithelium is more likely to remain intact with shorter storage times.[62] Despite the absence of data to support these recommendations,[63,64] for pediatric keratoplasties, it seems prudent to use tissue in which the time from cardiovascular collapse to storage in media was short (perhaps, less than 8 hours with at least half this time under refrigeration) and the time the tissue is in storage media was short (perhaps optimally, less than 5 days in Optisol). Ideally, the endothelial cell count should be about 3,000 or more cells/mm^2.

Donor age is generally inversely proportional to the cell count,[63,65] and increased donor age is an independent risk factor for increased endothelial cell loss over the first postoperative year.[66,67] Therefore, a cornea from a young donor should be used. It has been reported, however, that use of tissue from donors less than 3 years of age can result in a very steep graft in adult recipients.[68-70] Use of tissue from donors less than 2 years old in infant recipients can also result in a graft curvature of over 60 diopters, particularly if the graft is 0.5 mm or more oversized.[71] The resulting high myopia complicates amblyopia therapy. Therefore, tissue from healthy donors from 4 to perhaps 30 years of age should be used for pediatric penetrating keratoplasties on phakic eyes. In a penetrating keratoplasty of an eye of a monocular aphake, there may be some advantage to using infant tissue to produce a steep graft and reduce anisometropia. This practice has been advocated in aphakic adults[68,69] and children[13] requiring penetrating keratoplasty. However, very young donor tissue is more difficult to manipulate during surgery,[12,22,69] and the refractive result may be unpredictable.

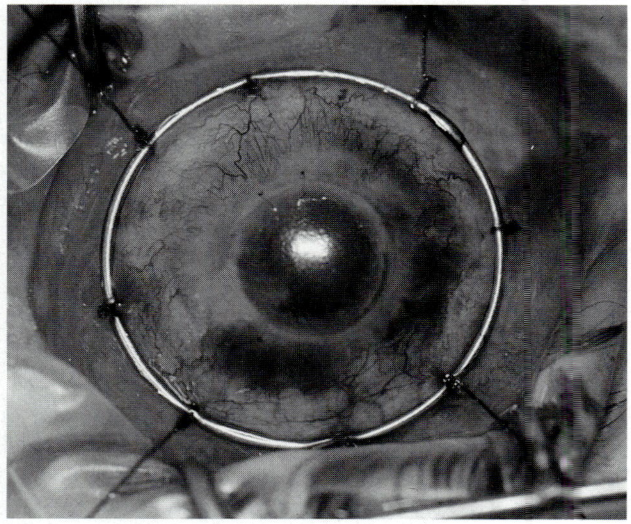

FIGURE 142-5 A repeat penetrating keratoplasty in a 4-year-old who was born with bilateral, idiopathic, dense, corneal opacities and congenital glaucoma. A lateral canthotomy has been performed to improve exposure and reduce posterior pressure. A Flieringa ring was fastened to the episclera with eight sutures. Four of these sutures were left long enough to be fastened to the drapes to further support the eye.

Surgical Management

BEFORE THE INCISION

Pediatric penetrating keratoplasties are performed with an operating microscope, with the patient under general anesthesia. The surgery in infants and children is marked, more than anything else, by scleral collapse and alarming posterior pressure.[9,10,22,53] Particularly in infants, lens expulsion often seems imminent. However, a review of 161 keratoplasties found only one episode of inadvertent lens loss.[15] Nonetheless, posterior pressure that requires the use of the graft to push the lens and iris posteriorly may result in the loss of endothelial cells[72]; therefore steps should be taken to minimize and prepare for posterior pressure.

Every available maneuver to reduce posterior pressure should be used. It is desirable to have an anesthesiologist experienced in pediatric anesthesia. The anesthesiologist should also be informed that if the patient "bucks" while the cornea is off, it could be catastrophic for the eye; therefore, the patient must be deeply anesthetized and paralyzed until the end of the case. Paralysis with a nondepolarizing muscle relaxant monitored with a peripheral nerve stimulator eliminates the risk of movement[73,74] and contraction of the extraocular muscles.[22,73] The anesthesiologist should be asked to hyperventilate the patient, which reduces intraocular pressure.[75] Positioning the patient with the head slightly higher than the feet probably also decreases posterior pressure.

Digital massage reduces posterior pressure and endothelial cell loss during penetrating keratoplasty.[21,72] Alternatively, a Honan balloon should be applied at 30 mm Hg for 5 or more minutes. Experimental evidence suggests that these maneuvers reduce vitreous volume, as well as lower intraocular pressure.[76,77] Care should be taken to ensure the speculum, surgeon, and assistant do not apply pressure to the globe. A lateral canthotomy is helpful in improving exposure in infants and may reduce posterior pressure. A Flieringa ring should be used in every pediatric penetrating keratoplasty. It should be fastened to the episclera with six to eight sutures. Four sutures should be left long so that they can be fastened to the drapes to gently support the eye (Figure 142-5). Some surgeons recommend a double scleral ring[10] with attached blepharostat secured with up to 16 sutures.[22,53] However, a poorly fitting double ring may increase posterior pressure.[72]

Mannitol reduces vitreous volume as well as intraocular pressure[78] and thus reduces posterior pressure. Because it causes systemic fluid shifts that can lead to hemodynamic instability, it should be used with care. Mannitol is of little benefit in a patient who has already had an anterior vitrectomy and may be of little benefit in older children, who generally have less posterior pressure. The dose of 20% mannitol is 0.5 to 1.5 g/kg by slow intravenous infusion. To reduce the possibility of hemodynamic instability, each 0.5 g/kg should be given over a period no less than 20 to 30 minutes.[78,79] The peak action is about 45 minutes after administration.[78]

The scrub nurse should have a lens loop available so that an assistant can quickly use it to gently place pressure on the iris and lens if loss of the lens seems imminent. The nurse should also have an "emergency suture" (8-0 nylon or silk on a cutting needle) loaded and immediately available if the posterior pressure is so great that 10-0 nylon would break during placement of the cardinal sutures. Some surgeons recommend use of preplaced bridging sutures to hold the graft in place in the face of severe posterior pressure.[13,80] Finally, the surgeon should be sure that the donor button is punched and all instruments that may needed are nearby and in working order before entering the anterior chamber.

Preoperative miotic or mydriatic drops can be used depending on the procedure. If the lens is known to be clear, miotics will help protect the lens, especially in the setting of posterior pressure. Topical miotic drops can be used preoperatively, or an intraocular miotic can be injected into the anterior chamber as soon as it is entered. If the eye has a visually significant cataract and the surgeon plans an "open sky" lensectomy, mydriatics can be used preoperatively. If the status of the lens is unknown, it is probably best to use no agent preoperatively and then apply an intraocular miotic to the iris if cataract extraction is unnecessary. If the lens has a marked opacity, the pupil can be dilated with the epinephrine in the irrigating solution or mechanically.

A final examination immediately preoperatively may aid the surgeon in making a final surgical plan and may eliminate the need for a separate preoperative examination under anesthesia. A portable slit lamp and possibly pachymetry will help the surgeon avoid trephining through particularly thin areas, which would make secure wound closure more difficult. If prior intraocular pressure measurements, funduscopic examination, or ultrasound examination were not optimal, or if there is reason to suspect interim change, these measurements and examinations should be repeated immediately preoperatively under anesthesia.

Three series of pediatric penetrating keratoplasties report a rate of endophthalmitis of about 2%,[12-14] about 20 times that reported for adults[81] and infants undergoing other intraocular procedures.[82] Because of the inability of infants and small children to communicate pain and the limitations of postoperative examinations, any reasonable precaution that may reduce the risk of postoperative endophthalmitis should be taken. Preoperative topical antibiotics appear to reduce the risk of postoperative endophthalmitis,[81] and preoperative antibiotics combined with preoperative irrigation of the ocular surface with dilute povidone-iodine reduces ocular surface bacterial counts better than either of these treatments alone.[83] The patient's head should be carefully positioned so that it is stable and the limbus is parallel to the floor. The contralateral eye should be taped closed. If it has had a transplant, it should be protected with a metal shield before the patient is draped.

PENETRATING KERATOPLASTY

In infants, the cornea and anterior segment are smaller, and the cornea is often thinner and more pliable, making the surgery technically more difficult. Because an infant cornea is smaller, and because of the marked posterior pressure, most surgeons perform a smaller transplantation in infants than in adults. In a study of 161 pediatric transplantations from four centers, the mean recipient trephine size was 7.1 mm.[15] Children often have larger pupils, so a small graft may be less than optimal optically.

Another potential disadvantage of performing a small graft is that a lower total number of endothelial cells are transplanted. For instance, reducing the donor diameter from 8.0 to 6.0 mm reduces the number of endothelial cells transplanted by 44%. This reduction becomes important if the recipient rim has a low density of viable endothelial cells. For instance, if a 6.0 mm graft with 3,000 viable endothelial cells/mm^2 is placed into a 12 mm cornea devoid of endothelial cells, and the transplanted cells distribute themselves evenly on the cornea, the final density will be 750 cells/mm^2. This may, in part, explain the observation that many pediatric grafts fail by gradual loss of clarity without signs of inflammation.[14] On the other hand, if the density and function of the recipient rim endothelium are normal, a small graft may improve the likelihood that the recipient endothelium will repopulate and clear the graft if irreversible endothelial rejection occurs. Therefore, an estimate of the recipient rim's endothelial cell density should be an important determinate of the size of the graft.

Infants and children are more active postoperatively and are probably more likely than adults to stress the wound with crying, rubbing, and injury. Because of these factors, the posterior pressure, and the thin recipient tissue, it is important to use a donor trephine 0.5 mm or more larger than the recipient trephine (0.5 mm oversized) to facilitate secure closure of the eye. In a study of 161 pediatric transplantations from four centers, the grafts were an average of 0.5 mm oversized.[15] The more a graft is oversized, the steeper its final curvature.[84] By geometry alone, and not accounting for the variables of wound healing, this effect is greater in smaller grafts.[71] As in adults, the recipient bed is formed by bevelling in the corneal scissors after trephining two-thirds or three-fourths the thickness of the cornea. This technique will create a posterior lip to help form an aqueous-tight wound. In a case where the entire recipient cornea is too thin or soft to hold sutures, a total corneal or corneal-scleral graft can be performed (Figure 142-6).[85] An alternative in this situation is to perform a large lamellar keratoplasty followed by a smaller penetrating keratoplasty.[86]

Because the graft is often needed to push the lens and iris back, copious viscoelastic agent should be placed on the lens-iris diaphragm before bringing the graft to the wound to limit endothelial trauma.[22,87] The increased fibrin production in infants and young children, combined with posterior pressure, can produce iris adhesions to the wound. These adhesions can often be avoided by placing viscoelastic in the anterior chamber as soon as the eye is opened, before the anterior chamber collapses.[13] If adhesions form, they can be lysed by placing viscoelastic in the anterior chamber after the wound is closed, entering a distant portion of the wound with a vitreous sweep, and sweeping the adherent iris out of the wound. It is sometimes difficult to verify through the operating microscope that there are no adhesions to the wound. Using the slit beam of a portable slit lamp while the infant or child is still under anesthesia aids in the visualization of any iris adhesion to the wound. Blood clot can be manually removed from the anterior chamber, and tissue plasminogen activator (25 μg) can be used to lyse a fibrin clot intraoperatively.[22,87]

Wound closure is accomplished with three-fourths depth 10-0 nylon sutures, as in adult penetrating keratoplasties. Because the sutures cannot be removed selectively in very young patients, equal distribution of the donor tissue in the recipient bed is probably important to minimize graft astigmatism. If there is severe posterior pressure and preplaced sutures have not been placed, a few 8-0 sutures can be used to secure the graft to the recipient bed inferiorly before opening the superior half of the wound. Most corneal surgeons close pediatric penetrating keratoplasty wounds exclusively with interrupted sutures.[12,13,15] Eighty-four percent of 161 pediatric grafts performed at four centers were closed with interrupted sutures only.[15] Some surgeons advocate a running closure providing there is no asymmetric vascularization.[11,22,53] However, interrupted sutures are preferred because they reduce the chance that a broken suture will result in wound dehiscence. They also allow for staged removal if some sutures begin to erode before the wound is sufficiently healed to allow removal of all sutures. One study reports that 15% of 40 transplantations performed

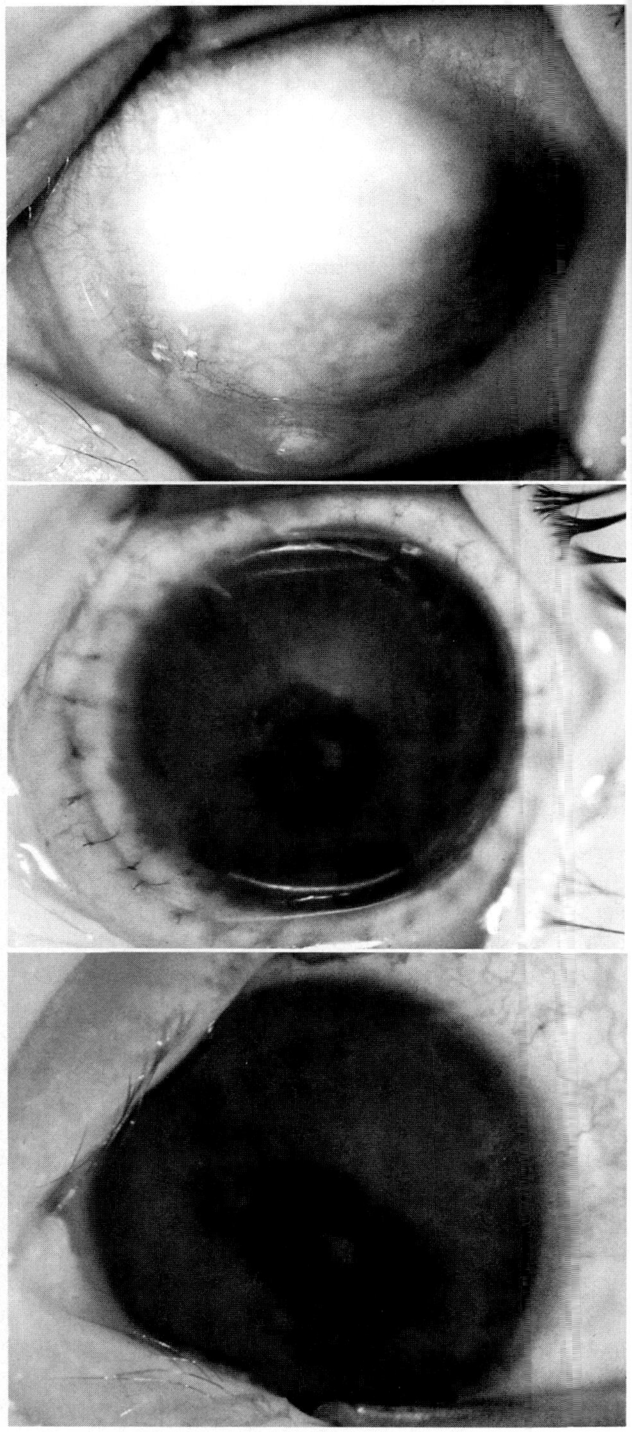

A

B

C

FIGURE 142-6 **A,** A congenital opacity in a 1-month-old infant. From limbus to limbus, the opacity consisted of loose connective tissue, which would not have held sutures. Therefore a total corneal transplantation was performed. **B,** The same eye 1 month postoperatively, immediately before suture removal. A 12 mm trephine had been used to form the recipient bed, and 13 mm trephine had been used to punch the corneal-scleral donor tissue. **C** Six months later the graft remains clear, the anterior chamber is deep, and the surgical wound has healed without a visible scar. The intraocular pressure had remained between 12 and 20 mm Hg.

for congenital opacities were complicated by wound dehiscence.[13] Because of the risk of postoperative trauma, a generous number of sutures, perhaps 20 to 24 for a 7.0 mm transplantation, should be placed in infants and children. All suture knots should be buried to reduce the risk of ocular surface complications.

CONCOMITANT IRIS PROCEDURES

Other procedures may be necessary at the time of penetrating keratoplasty. Because pediatric penetrating keratoplasties may be associated with posterior synechiae and persistent intraocular inflammation, a peripheral iridectomy could be indicated in every pediatric keratoplasty. However, the risks of bleeding and the difficulty of safely placing a peripheral iridectomy in a phakic eye with posterior pressure outweigh the benefits of the procedure in most cases. A peripheral iridectomy should be performed as prophylaxis against a sequestered pupil if the eye is inflamed or already has significant posterior synechiae at the time of surgery. A peripheral iridectomy is also indicated if a lensectomy with vitrectomy is being performed. Despite an anterior vitrectomy, blockade of the pupil with vitreous is possible.

Anterior synechiae have been associated with graft failure.[21,88] Therefore synechiolysis should be performed when possible during pediatric penetrating keratoplasties. If there is high posterior pressure, "open sky" synechiolysis may not be possible. If the view is sufficient, lysis can be most easily accomplished with a vitreous sweep after making a 1 mm incision at the base of the trephine groove and injecting viscoelastic into the anterior chamber. In many cases, however, visualization will not be sufficient before removing the cornea, and synechiolysis can be accomplished only after suturing the graft into place.[22] However, blunt dissection with a vitreous sweep through the wound after forming the anterior chamber with viscoelastic may be ineffective or result in a hyphema. Furthermore, synechiae tend to re-form, especially if there has been bleeding; therefore the benefits of lysis may outweigh its risks in some cases. In an aphakic eye, with a sector iridectomy creating a smaller pupil with 10-0 prolene suture on a noncutting needle (Ethicon BV100-4) will tighten the iris diaphragm and may prevent re-formation of synechiae.[89]

LENSECTOMY AND ANTERIOR VITRECTOMY

Twenty-seven percent of eyes in a large pediatric penetrating keratoplasty series underwent lensectomy and vitrectomy at the time of their first transplantation.[15] Some surgeons recommend against such combined procedures.[12] If it can be determined before or during surgery that the patient has a dense cataract, then it can be removed during the keratoplasty. The lens must also be removed if is adherent to the cornea in Peters' type II anomaly. However, the decision to remove a lens with only a mild or moderate opacity during pediatric penetrating keratoplasty should be made judiciously. Lensectomy and vitrectomy are statistically significant risk factors for graft failure[14,15] and poor visual outcome.[14] If the resulting aphakia is unilateral, amblyopia therapy will be more difficult. Furthermore, evaluation of a lens opacity may be impossible preoperatively and difficult intraoperatively. Finally, some congenital lens opacities do not progress.[26] Therefore, if it is not absolutely evident that a lens opacity will significantly reduce vision, it is probably best to leave the lens in place and reevaluate the opacity after the transplantation wound is healed. Even though a subsequent lensectomy with anterior vitrectomy can be performed in a controlled fashion with a vitrectomy instrument and infusion port,[26,90] the graft will loosen some endothelial cells. However, this outcome is preferable to removing a lens that need not have been removed.

If lensectomy is performed at the time of penetrating keratoplasty, it is generally performed "open sky," as in adults. After anterior capsulotomy and expression or aspiration of the nucleus, the cortical material is removed. Removal will be difficult in the face of posterior pressure. An irrigation-aspiration device or anterior vitrectomy instrument with its cutting action turned off can be used for cortical aspiration. The one part per million concentration of epinephrine in the balanced salt solution, which is generally used in adults, appears to be well tolerated by infants.[73,91]

As virtually every pediatric posterior capsule will opacify,[26] a partial posterior capsulotomy and anterior vitrectomy should be performed in infants and perhaps children. Even though older children might cooperate for a Nd:YAG capsulotomy, in the absence of a posterior chamber lens, Nd:YAG capsulotomy usually results in vitreous prolapse into the anterior chamber.[92] This prolapse can cause pupillary block or vitreous-endothelial touch, which will threaten the graft.[24,25] The posterior capsulotomy and anterior vitrectomy are performed with an automated vitrector with a cut rate of about 300 to 400 cycles/minute and maximum suction setting of about 180 mmHg. The vitrector should be used to create a circular hole of about 7 mm diameter in the posterior capsule. The capsulotomy should be this large, as the capsular remnants can contract and opacify postoperatively to block the visual axis, especially in infants. If the capsulotomy is circular, it will not tear and would provide support if a posterior chamber lens is implanted later. Care should be taken to remove enough vitreous so that none can prolapse into the anterior chamber to cause pupillary block or threaten the graft.

Some surgeons recommend implanting a posterior chamber lens, particularly in children with isolated, unilateral cataracts.[26,34-36] In a large study of adults, which used multivariate analysis, aphakic eyes were nearly twice as likely to develop graft failure as were pseudophakic eyes.[18] The alternative for visual rehabilitation is a contact lens or use of a aphakic spectacle when the other eye is being patched. The series of 161 pediatric penetrating keratoplasties from four centers reports only one lens implantation; therefore data about the effect of a posterior chamber lens on pediatric penetrating keratoplasty outcome are sparse. The posterior chamber lens has only about a 25-year follow-up, and these pediatric patients may very well have life spans of three times that period. The Food and Drug Administration considers the implantation of intraocular lenses into patients less than 18 years of age as investigational.[93] It is difficult to calculate the power of the lens in an infant because the final corneal curvature and final axial length are difficult to predict. Placement of an intraocular lens in infants with a normal cornea is associated with high complication rates, including a 10% rate of corneal edema, an 8% rate of dislocated lenses, and a 15% rate of "iris complications."[35] Finally, eyes requiring pediatric penetrating keratoplasty often have preexisting anomalies or injuries and often require multiple procedures. Therefore, it seems prudent to avoid introducing the additional variable of an artificial lens into these eyes.

CONCOMITANT RETINAL SURGERY

If the eye requires pars plana vitrectomy for retinal detachment, use of an intraoperative keratoprosthesis for the retinal surgery affords the retinal surgeon a better view than through a new transplant. After the retinal surgeon completes the retinal reattachment, the keratoprosthesis is replaced with the transplantation tissue. In this way the transplantation tissue is protected from the surgical trauma of the vitrectomy. The Landers wide field temporary keratoprosthesis (Ocular Instruments; and the Eckhardt temporary keratoprosthesis[94] (Dutch Ophthalmic, USA) are two currently available models.

AFTER WOUND CLOSURE

After the transplantation is completed, subconjunctival injections of antibiotics and steroids are generally given. There is evidence that subconjunctival antibiotics reduce the risk of postoperative endophthalmitis.[81,95] It is reasonable to give subconjunctival gentamicin and vancomycin for broad coverage. Although the amount of subconjunctival antibiotics that are absorbed systemically is unknown, it is wise to limit the subconjunctival injections to no more than the intravenous doses for the infant's weight (2.5 mg/kg for gentamicin and 10 mg/kg for vancomycin). Some surgeons advocate the use of prophylactic intravenous antibiotics in pediatric penetrating keratoplasties[12]; 0.5 ml 10 mg/ml dexamethasone is also generally given subconjunctivally.

It may be useful to perform a postoperative examination while the child is still under anesthesia. A portable slit lamp is useful to confirm that there are no iris adhesions to the wound and can be used to provide a blue light to perform a Seidel test of the wound. The new transplantation may afford the surgeon the first view of the retina with an indirect ophthalmoscope. An axial eye length can be determined to help in later estimating an aphakic eye's refractive error. The intraocular pressure should be normal for an accurate measurement.

Before applying a pressure patch and metal shield, a single drop of 0.5% atropine in healthy full-term infants or 1% atropine in children should be applied. When seeing the family after surgery, it is wise to remind them of the guarded prognosis for vision and that the transplantation is only the first step in the visual rehabilitation of the eye.

Postoperative Care

IMMEDIATE POSTOPERATIVE PERIOD

Pediatric penetrating keratoplasty patients are generally admitted to the hospital for 1 or 2 days. Infants and children with cardiac or respiratory diseases, in particular, require careful postoperative monitoring, and the recommendations of the patient's pediatrician and anesthesiologist should be sought. Infants born at less than 37 week's gestation are at increased risk for postoperative apnea, periodic breathing, and bradycardia until they reach 60 weeks of postconception age. It is also thought that full-term healthy infants are at risk for these serious complications during their first month of life. Therefore, both groups should be hospitalized and placed on apnea and electrocardiogram monitoring for at least the first day after general anesthesia. If apnea occurs, the patient may need to be monitored for several days.[57,96]

A pediatrician should be asked to provide orders for sedation and an antiemetic if they are needed to obtain a careful examination of the eye or limit stress to the wound for the first postoperative days. Droperidol substantially reduces the incidence of postoperative vomiting.[73,97,98] The patient may be discharged on the first or second postoperative day if the vital signs are normal, oral intake is normal, and the eye is doing well.

EARLY POSTOPERATIVE CARE

The goals of the examinations and interventions in the first weeks after surgery are to make certain the wound is secure and watertight, monitor and promote epithelialization of the graft if there is an epithelial defect, monitor and promote the decline in postoperative inflammation, monitor and control intraocular pressure, rule out or treat endophthalmitis and other postoperative complications, and begin amblyopia therapy. Infants and young children are unable to communicate effectively that they have pain, visual loss, or other symptoms that may indicate a complication. Therefore they require frequent early postoperative examinations.

The first postoperative examination should be within 24 hours after surgery. A reasonable schedule of routine postoperative examinations includes examinations on the first, second, fourth, seventh, tenth, and fourteenth postoperative days. Some surgeons examine these patients every day or two during the first 2 to 3 weeks.[11,22] Thereafter, a reasonable schedule is roughly weekly for the rest of the first postoperative month. Additional examinations are also required if the parents seem unlikely to recognize problems or if there is delayed resolution of an epithelial defect, unusual postoperative inflammation, increased intraocular pressure, or other complications.

The parents should be given careful verbal and written instructions to phone if any signs of complication appear. These signs include increased redness, light sensitivity, refusal to open the eye, eye rubbing, lid swelling, discharge, loss of graft clarity, a spot on the cornea, change in the shape of the pupil, evidence of decreased vision, or any other change. The parents can be given a penlight and asked to examine the eye every day while instilling drops.

At each early postoperative visit, the visual acuity and alignment of the eyes should be evaluated. Before attempting to examine the eye more closely, which may precipitate a struggle and cause lid swelling or red eyes, the eye should be examined from a distance for obvious signs of inflammation. Signs of inflammation should decline steadily with each visit during the first few postoperative weeks.

A slit lamp examination should be performed at every visit to the corneal surgeon. Pneumotonometry and indirect ophthalmoscopy should be attempted at every visit during the first few postoperative weeks and thereafter perhaps every second or third visit. During the first few postoperative visits, a clearing graft and irregular epithelium may preclude a clear view of the retina. In this case, B-scan ultrasonography can be used to rule out vitreous infiltrate and retinal detachment.

EARLY POSTOPERATIVE COMPLICATIONS

If the eye is unusually inflamed, endophthalmitis should be suspected. If it has a hypopyon, vitreous haze, or retinal infiltrates, endophthalmitis is likely and prompt treatment by a vitreoretinal specialist is mandatory. If there is marked inflammation without infection, consideration should be given to a short course of systemic steroids. Tissue plasminogen activator (25 μg)[87] can be injected into the anterior chamber to lyse a fibrin clot postoperatively, although this would require return to the operating room.

If the anterior chamber is shallow or the intraocular pressure is low, a Seidel test should be performed with a portable slit lamp. If a leak is discovered, the child can be followed daily. If the leak does not stop in a day or so, the anterior chamber flattens, or iris becomes adherent to the wound, the child should be brought back to the operating room for repair of the wound and removal of any iris from the wound.

If the graft has an epithelial defect, it must be monitored for signs of corneal infection, and topical antibiotics should be used at least until the defect is healed. Persistent defects in adult keratoplasty patients have been associated with stromal opacification, poor wound healing, ulceration, infection, and vascularization.[21] In one pediatric series, tear and surface abnormalities, as well as prior persistent epithelial defects, were associated with graft failure. Fifteen percent of failed grafts were thought to result from a sterile ulcer.[14] Any underlying cause of the epithelial defect should be treated. For instance, topical medications should be limited, and punctal occlusion should be performed for a dry eye. If pressure patching fails, a tarsorrhaphy[99] appears to be the most effective treatment for a persistent defect.[62] Because of the risk of amblyopia, temporary[100] or lateral tarsorrhaphy is preferred in infants and children.

Bacterial keratitis was reported in 5% of eyes in a large pediatric series.[14] Management of an infected ulcer is the same as for adults, removal of any eroded sutures, scraping for microbiologic studies, and fortified topical antibiotics (see Chapter 94).

POSTOPERATIVE MEDICATIONS

Five percent of eyes in a large series of pediatric penetrating keratoplasties had intraocular inflammation longer than 6 weeks after the operation. Because infants and children can have an exaggerated inflammatory response postoperatively, it seems reasonable to use more topical steroids than in adult keratoplasty patients. Ointments are less likely to be cried out than drops but interfere with vision. Therefore, one reasonable regimen is to alternate a topical antibiotic-steroid ointment combination four times a day with 1% prednisolone or 0.1% dexamethasone drops four times a day for the first 2 postoperative weeks. The alcohol and acetate forms of these drugs penetrate the anterior chamber better than the phosphate forms when the corneal epithelium is intact.[101] After 2 weeks, the ointment can be discontinued and the drops continued. Some surgeons recommend steroid drops every hour for the first 1 or 2 days after surgery.[22,102]

A long-acting topical cycloplegic, generally atropine, should also be given during the first 2 preoperative weeks. Anticholinergics dilate the pupil to reduce synechiae formation, reduce ciliary spasm, and reduce abnormal iris vascular permeability.[103] Posterior synechiae formation was reported as a complication in 5% of a large series of pediatric penetrating keratoplasties.[15] All topical anticholinergics can be absorbed systemically to produce systemic toxicity including tachycardia, flushing, dry mouth and skin, fever, urinary retention, intestinal hypomotility, hallucinations, and somnolence.[103,104] There have been several reports of death from ophthalmic atropine in children.[105] Because of their body weight, children and infants are more prone to these effects; thus the lowest effective dose should be used. In the first year of life, atropine, 0.25%, one drop a day or every other day may be adequate. In older children atropine, 0.5% a day, may be adequate.[104] If these doses are not effective, higher doses may be needed, particularly in children with dark irides. Parents should be warned to apply only one drop. Because atropine is active if taken orally, parents should also be told to keep the bottle out of reach of children.[37]

EXAMINATION OF PEDIATRIC PATIENTS

A close examination is critical to the postoperative care of pediatric penetrating keratoplasty patients, but requires patience and some special techniques. Children over age of 4 years will often allow themselves to be examined at the slit lamp or in a parent's lap with a portable slit lamp. Allowing a young child to play with different parts of the instrument and turn on the different color lights often helps enlist his or her cooperation. Showing a child that the pneumotonometer "tickles" when touched to the finger, cheek, and forehead often helps a child cooperate with tonometry. A mechanical toy, used as a fixation device at the end of the examination lane, will often cajole a reluctant young patient.

Children less than 3 or 4 years of age usually need to be restrained or sedated for an adequate examination. Some surgeons believe that examination with the patient under anesthesia is required for an adequate examination of the graft in young children,[22] but the mean number of examinations with the patient under anesthesia for first grafts was 3.2 in a large series.[15] Examinations with the patient under anesthesia or sedation have some risks, should be performed with the patient with an empty stomach, require that the patient awakens before leaving, and are generally time consuming. Sedation is sometimes ineffective, and a pediatrician, as well as equipment for resuscitation, should be nearby in case of a complication. Guidelines for sedation from the American Academy of Pediatrics call for informed consent, considerable documentation, and continuous monitoring of oxygen saturation and heart rate.[106] An examination with the patient under anesthesia has a total cost of about $2,500. Therefore restraining the child seems preferable for routine, careful examinations. The parents generally consent to a restrained examination if they are informed of its importance, the difficulties of sedation, and that the child's discomfort is minimal.

The child who requires a restrained examination should be held flat on an examination table. Infants less than 6 months of age can be held effectively by a single assistant. A Velcro fastening papoose board (Regular size; Olympic Medical Corporation;) will restrain an older infant or a young child sufficiently to allow a thorough examination. If a cycloplegic refraction or dilated fundus examination is required, the drops are given in advance, and the restrained examination is timed, so that it is performed only once during the visit. If a restrained examination is inadequate, sedation of a healthy child or full-term infant more than 1 month of age can usually be achieved safely with chloral hydrate (75 to 100 mg/kg, up to a maximum of 3.0 g).[107] Examination with the patient under anesthesia should probably be reserved for suture removal or when sedation in the office is deemed ineffective or unsafe.

A portable slit lamp allows the evaluation of the stability of the wound, eroded sutures, epithelial defects, graft clarity and thickness, keratic precipitates, anterior chamber depth, and lens clarity. It generally does not allow detection of anterior chamber cell. A pneumotonometer or other nonapplanation technique is best for measurement of intraocular pressure while the corneal surface is irregular. Often a pacifier will quiet a restrained infant sufficiently to obtain an accurate pressure.

OPTICAL CORRECTION AND AMBLYOPIA THERAPY

Without effective optical correction and amblyopia therapy, a pediatric penetrating keratoplasty may be useless. The duration of time the eye is capable of perceiving a clear, well-focused image and the effectiveness of the amblyopia therapy during a patient's first years of life establish the eye's visual potential for the rest of his or her life. The younger the patient, the deeper the amblyopia will become if the eye has a structural or refractive abnormality that limits vision. However, amblyopia is more easily reversed in younger patients if it is treated promptly and appropriately.[108] Therefore, after surgery reverses the structural abnormality, refraction and amblyopia therapy should be started as soon as possible. In pediatric penetrating keratoplasty patients, the evaluation of vision, correction of refractive error, and amblyopia therapy are

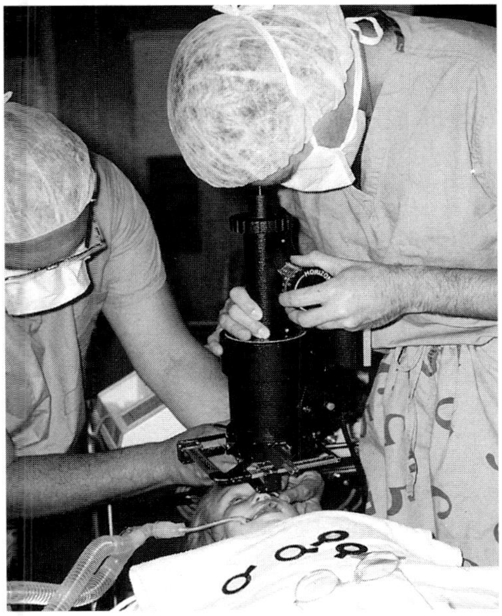

FIGURE 142-7 The head of a keratometer can be removed from its base to perform keratometry during an examination under anesthesia.

difficult; therefore, care of these patients should be shared with a pediatric ophthalmologist.

Correction of refractive error is a vital part of amblyopia therapy. At about 2 postoperative weeks, the epithelium has generally healed and the graft has cleared sufficiently to perform cycloplegic retinoscopy. Retinoscopy may be difficult, and the refraction will change as the wound heals and sutures are removed; but a correction of any moderate or large refractive error should be prescribed at this time, even if it is not exact. The refraction should be repeated every 3 to 6 weeks until the sutures have been out for several months. Thereafter, the refraction should be repeated several times a year.

All cycloplegic drops can have systemic side effects.[103] One percent cyclopentolate has been associated with abdominal distention, leading to death in two premature infants.[109] Premature infants should be given one drop of 0.2% cyclopentolate with 1% phenylephrine. Dilation and cycloplegia in full-term infants less than 4 months of age should be achieved with one drop of 0.5% cyclopentolate. Older children can receive one drop of 1% cyclopentolate. The peak cycloplegic effect is about 40 minutes after instillation. Preceding the cyclopentolate drop with a proparacaine drop increases absorption.[37]

The retinoscopic reflex in a pediatric penetrating keratoplasty patient is often irregular and may be difficult to interpret.[110] Using a bright halogen retinoscope and a short working distance[110] is helpful. If the refractive error cannot be determined in the office, an examination with the patient under anesthesia may be justified. In this case, keratometry, keratoscopy, direct ophthalmoscopy, and axial eye length measurements can help confirm the results of retinoscopy. Keratometry will determine corneal power and astigmatism. (The head of a Bausch and Lomb keratometer can be removed for use on a supine patient as shown in Figure 142-7 by removing a stop screw and turning the focus knob fully counterclockwise.) The spectacle astigmatism is generally about two thirds of the corneal astigmatism.[110]

If an examiner uses his or her distance correction and uses the weakest minus lens or strongest plus lens of a direct ophthalmoscope to focus on the retina of a cyclopleged eye, an estimate of the eye's spherical distance correction can be read off the ophthalmoscope's focusing dial.[111] In a phakic patient with unilateral cornea disease, bilateral keratometry, bilateral axial lengths, and cycloplegic refraction of the normal eye can also be used to confirm the retinoscopy of the transplant eye (assuming the crystalline lens in each eye has the same power).

Refraction of an aphakic eye can be confirmed if the axial eye length is known. The following formula is an approximation for an aphakic eye and assumes a keratometry measurement of 45 diopters and a vertex distance of 10 mm:

$$\text{Distance spectacle power} = 63.7 - (2.28 \times \text{axial eye length in mm}).^{*}$$

The results from this formula can be modified by keratometry measurements. For an aphakic eye, an infant is generally prescribed a near correction, that is, +1.00 to +2.50 sphere over the distance correction.[26,33,90] At 1.5 to 3 years of age, the aphakic child should be put in a bifocal, with the top of the segment at the inferior border of the pupil.[33,92]

Contact lenses are sometimes useful in the visual rehabilitation of pediatric keratoplasty patients. In a large multicenter study, 35% of eyes receiving an optical correction were fitted with a contact lens.[15] A gas-permeable rigid lens or a thick, aphakic soft lens will mask irregular astigmatism.[112] Silicone lenses (Silsoft, Bausch and Lomb,) offer the highest oxygen permeability of all lenses and are often well tolerated in aphakic infants with normal corneas.[113] A monocular aphake or monocular high myope requires a contact lens to develop some fusion.[26,92] The goal of fusion may be unrealistic, and spectacle correction is a

*This formula is an approximation for aphakic eyes with axial eye lengths 16 to 24 mm, keratometry of 45 diopters, and a vertex distance of 10 mm. It is based on the general formula: $P = (1.33/L) - K)^{-1} + V)^{-1}$, where P is the distance spectacle correction (D), K is the keratometry reading (D), L is the axial eye length (m), and V is the vertex distance (m).

practical alternative.[92] The risks of contact lenses include endothelial loss, corneal ulceration, and corneal vascularization,[115] which are each associated with pediatric graft failure.[14] Fitting a contact lens may also delay refractive error correction if the fitting is difficult, or the parents have difficulty applying the lens. Because of the added risk of infection, a contact lens should probably not be used in pediatric penetrating keratoplasty patients before all sutures are removed. Some advocate the use of extended-wear contact lenses in pediatric penetrating keratoplasties.[53] However, these lenses should probably be avoided, as they are associated with an increased risk of ulceration, even when fit to a normal cornea.[115,116]

Because selective suture removal is not possible in young transplantation patients, they may have high astigmatism. If the astigmatism is deemed to interfere with amblyopia therapy, relaxing incisions, with or without compression sutures, a wedge resection, and other wound revisions can be performed, as in adults[117] (see Figure 142-3 and Chapter 137).

Virtually all infants and young children who have undergone penetrating keratoplasty have some amblyopia because of visual deprivation before the surgery, graft astigmatism, anisometropia, or some combination of these. There are many published approaches to amblyopia therapy.[33,108,114] The following approach is widely accepted and has been effective in the analogous setting after extraction of a unilateral congenital cataract.[33]

If the contralateral eye is normal in an infant or a young child, occlusion therapy should be started as soon as the graft has partially cleared, and correction of any significant refractive error is being worn. Optimally, this should be no later than 2 postoperative weeks. There is concern that a normal eye is more prone to amblyopia if occluded during the first months of life, and it is difficult to monitor vision during this period. Therefore occlusion during the first 6 months of life is usually limited to one fourth to three fourths of the infant's waking hours.[33,108] If the child is older than 6 months old, full-time occlusion therapy should be started.[33]

The vision in both eyes is monitored carefully to check for improvement of the amblyopic eye or worsening of the normal eye. In preverbal children older than 6 months of age, vision is measured by evaluating the fixation pattern or preferential looking tests.[108,114] One-year-olds have their vision assessed weekly, two-year-olds are examined every 2 weeks, three-year-olds are examined every 3 weeks; those older than 4 years of age are examined every 4 weeks.[33,108,114] If the occluded eye becomes amblyopic, occlusion therapy is discontinued, and occlusion of the contralateral eye is sometimes necessary.[108,114]

If the amblyopic eye has not improved after three examination intervals of full-time occlusion, it is assumed that an abnormality other than amblyopia limits the eye's visual potential. If this occurs or if vision becomes equal in the two eyes, part-time occlusion is instituted, usually until the patient is out of the amblyogenic age range, at about age 8 years. If the vision worsens during part-time occlusion because of worsening amblyopia, another course of full-time occlusion should be prescribed.[33,114] In the setting of pediatric keratoplasty, it is often difficult to determine whether worsening vision is due to subtle graft opacity, irregular astigmatism, amblyopia, or some combination of these.

If the patient has required bilateral penetrating keratoplasties, he or she may still have amblyopia. For example, an eye that has a mild clouding that does not justify repeat transplantation, has some uncorrected irregular astigmatism, or has had a graft failure that required repeat transplant may develop amblyopia. If amblyopia is suspected, it should be treated as outlined previously after doing everything reasonable to correct the structural and refractive abnormalities.

Parents are critical to the success of occlusion therapy. Enforcing occlusion therapy is naturally very difficult for parents if their infant or child withdraws, cries, or removes the patch whenever it is applied. They need to be instructed about the importance of the amblyopia therapy and how to administer it properly.

WOUND INTEGRITY AND SUTURE REMOVAL

The transplant wound heals rapidly in children and infants; however, infants and children rub their eyes, are prone to trauma, and otherwise challenge the integrity of the wound. The wound should be protected in a way that minimizes interference with visual function and amblyopia therapy. A metal shield with multiple perforations or a clear plastic shield[58] can be fastened over the eye with the tape on the side so that there is minimal obstruction to vision. For infants, the tabs on the shield can be bent over to make a smaller shield. If repeated taping is leading to breakdown of the skin, stoma adhesive can be placed on the cheek and forehead and the tape applied to it. Occasionally, a child will persist in removing the shield to rub the eye. Arm restraints can then be used for a short period until the eye is more comfortable, and the child stops rubbing.

Two weeks postoperatively, the shield can be replaced with a pair of polycarbonate glasses during waking hours. If the child reaches under the new glasses, the metal shield should be reinstituted for a few weeks until the glasses are attempted again. It is prudent to continue using the metal shield while the child sleeps for the first 3 postoperative months.

As the wound heals, sutures will erode. Sutures erode as early as 2 weeks postoperatively in infants.[10,12,53] These eroded sutures can lead to eye rubbing, vascularization, epithelial defects, and corneal infection.[22] The goal is to remove the sutures before erosion and its complications can occur but after there is any significant chance of wound dehiscence.

Typically, all sutures can be removed safely according to the following schedule. During the first year of life, sutures are removed at 5 weeks after surgery, in 1-year-olds at 6 to 7 postoperative weeks, in 2- and 3-year-olds at 8 to 10 postoperative weeks, in 4- to 6-year-olds at 3 to 4 postoperative months, and in 7- to 10-year-olds at 5 to 6 months postoperatively. Patients 10 to 20 years of age often require removal of all sutures because of rapid erosion by the sixth to eighth postoperative month. These periods should be somewhat longer if more topical steroids than usual were used or if the child is particularly prone to injury or eye rubbing. When all remaining sutures need to be removed in a child too young to allow removal at the slit lamp, suture removal is probably best accomplished in the operating room. An examination with the patient under anesthesia is performed at that time.

Some sutures may erode ahead of this schedule. For instance, vascularized portions of the wound will heal more rapidly, so the sutures will erode first in these areas. Young patients cannot report the foreign body sensation that adults generally feel when a suture erodes. Therefore, until all sutures are removed, infants and very young children probably require weekly examination. Older children who are approaching the expected time of suture removal should also be examined weekly. Parents should be instructed to report new eye rubbing, new squinting, new discharge or mucous, and any white spot or irregularity on the cornea. Any eroded suture should be removed as soon as it is recognized. Sutures that are inducing vascularization should also be removed promptly. If a few sutures need to be removed in an infant or a young child before the surgeon thinks it is safe to remove all remaining sutures, they can often be removed by restraining an infant or sedating a healthy older child in the office. If many sutures suddenly erode around the entire graft, this is a sign that the removal of all sutures is overdue.

Some children older than 6 years of age will allow suture removal at the slit lamp, particularly if a fixation device is used, so that selective suture removal can begin about 12 weeks after surgery to attempt to modulate wound healing and reduce astigmatism. Keratometry or keratoscopy is used to determine which meridian is steep and so requires suture removal (see Chapter 137). Nevertheless, little may be gained, as all sutures will probably need to be removed by 4 to 6 months postoperatively in children 6 to 10 years of age.

As the child grows older, the patient and parents should be reminded that both eyes, including one that is normal, must be protected from injury for the rest of the child's life. Polycarbonate glasses should be worn during all waking hours, and goggles are needed for sports or any other activity that might put either eye at risk.

PREVENTION AND TREATMENT OF REJECTION

Infants and young children are unable to effectively communicate that they have visual loss, probably the best early sign of graft rejection. Survival analysis from two large recent studies shows that of pediatric grafts that have failed by 3 years after surgery, 30% to 70% failed in the first 6 months, and 65% to 85% failed in the first year (Figure 142-1).[13-15] Therefore, examinations should be especially frequent in the first year after surgery. If the eye is progressing well, and all sutures have been removed, a reasonable schedule for careful examination of the penetrating keratoplasty is every 2 to 3 weeks during the first postoperative year, every month during the second postoperative year, and every 2 months thereafter. Some surgeons advocate examinations every 1 to 2 weeks for the first postoperative year.[22,53] The pediatric ophthalmologist may require more frequent examinations to monitor the amblyopia therapy. Social service personnel may be able provide services to help the family adhere to the rigorous examination schedule.

Parents should share in the responsibility for monitoring the health of the transplant. They should be frequently reminded that rejection can occur even many years after the transplant and that only prompt treatment can reverse the rejection. Parents should be given written instructions to phone immediately for redness, signs of discomfort, decreased graft clarity, and signs of decreased vision. They can perform a penlight examination daily. Parents of older children should be given a near card and asked to check the vision daily, one eye at a time. If parents are following this regimen reliably, examinations of older children can be somewhat less frequent than indicated earlier. Nursing personnel can play an important role in instructing the family.

Because infants and children have a higher rate of graft rejection and are more likely to present late during the course of a rejection, it is wise to use prophylactic topical steroids more frequently and for a longer time than typical for adult transplantation patients. A reasonable regimen is to use topical steroids eight times a day for the first 2 weeks, then 1% prednisolone drops four times a day until 6 weeks postoperatively, then three times a day for 6 weeks, then twice a day for 6 weeks, and then once or twice a

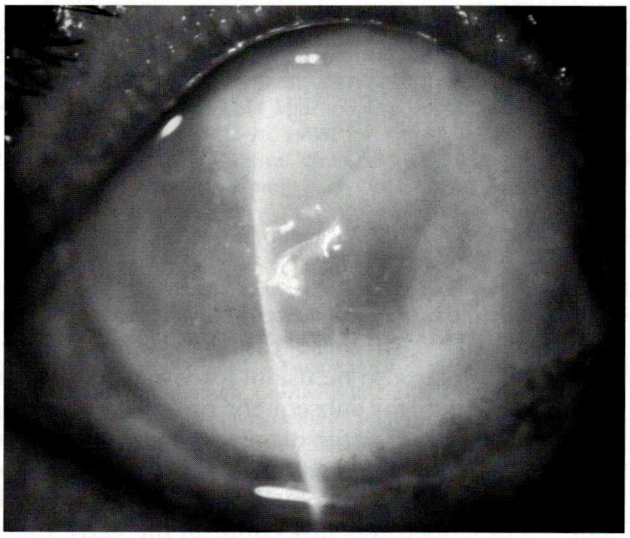

FIGURE 144-1 Severe bacterial corneal ulcer caused by a gram-negative bacillus, dysgonic fermenter, type 2 (DF 2).

anterior chamber is entered with a super blade, and the host cornea is excised using corneal scissors. Synechiae may be broken using a viscoelastic agent, Wescott scissors, or dissection with an iris spatula. An anterior vitrectomy using an automated vitrector is usually required in aphakic eyes. Extracapsular cataract extraction (usually without intraocular lens implantation) is performed if a cataract is present. In noninfected cases, an intraocular lens may be implanted. The donor cornea is sutured to the recipient using 16 or more interrupted 9-0 or 10-0 nylon sutures. The recessed conjunctiva is reattached to the limbus by bipolar cautery or sutures. At the conclusion of the operation, sub-Tenon injections of gentamicin sulfate, 100 mg, and methylprednisolone, 80 mg, are given in most cases.

Total penetrating keratoplasty or sclerokeratoplasty with the use of a corneal scleral graft to replace large areas of excised diseased corneal and scleral tissue and to restore structural integrity was first described by Castroviejo in 1951.[19] Barraquer[20] and Taylor and Stern[21] further developed this type of reconstructive keratoplasty. The technique, as modified by Cobo et al.,[22] consists of a 14 mm or larger corneal scleral graft. A 360 degree, 50% depth lamellar dissection of the donor sclera is carried into clear cornea just anterior to the trabecular meshwork before entering the anterior chamber with a sharp blade. Vannas scissors are used to complete the internal corneal incision 1 to 2mm anterior to the angle. The diseased corneal scleral host tissue is removed in a similar fashion. Four equally spaced 10-0 Prolene double armed sutures are placed through the internal corneal lip in a mattress fashion, passed through the donor cornea and tied, and the knots are buried. The scleral incision is closed using

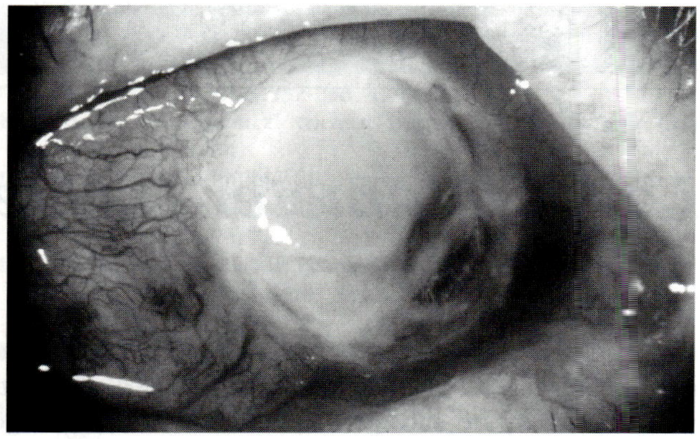

FIGURE 144-2 Perforation caused by chronic recurrent rheumatoid melting in transplanted cornea.

interrupted 10-0 nylon sutures and covered with conjunctiva.

The Malbran procedure is used in advanced keratoconus and consists of making a partial-thickness large diameter trephination of the host of 9.5 mm or greater in diameter. The dissection is carried down to just above Descemet's membrane and is extended in a lamellar plane using blunt dissection with excision of the overlying cornea. The large donor corneal button is fashioned from the donor globe after increasing the intraocular pressure in the donor eye by injection of air or saline through the optic nerve. A donor cornea with the scleral rim may also be used by placing it in a fixation device such as an artificial anterior chamber permitting the dissection of the lamellar graft. The donor cornea should be oversized by only 0.5 mm in order to flatten the cornea. Same-sized donor-recipient grafts are difficult to suture without wound gape and may result in increased intraocular pressure because of partial angle closure.

Postoperative Management

Postoperatively, all eyes are treated with topical antibiotics. Prednisolone acetate or prednisolone sodium phosphate 1% four times a day is used once the corneal epithelium is intact. A cycloplegic agent and more frequent use of steroid drops are indicated in inflamed eyes. After 2 weeks, the topical antibiotic drops are usually tapered, and the steroid drops are maintained at four times a day. Intraocular pressure is measured using a Tono-Pen or similar device. Increasing corneal thickness indicating endothelial cell dysfunction and corneal edema may be the first sign of an impending graft rejection/reaction. If present, appropriate antirejection medications must be used to maintain graft clarity. Postoperative keratometry read-

A B C

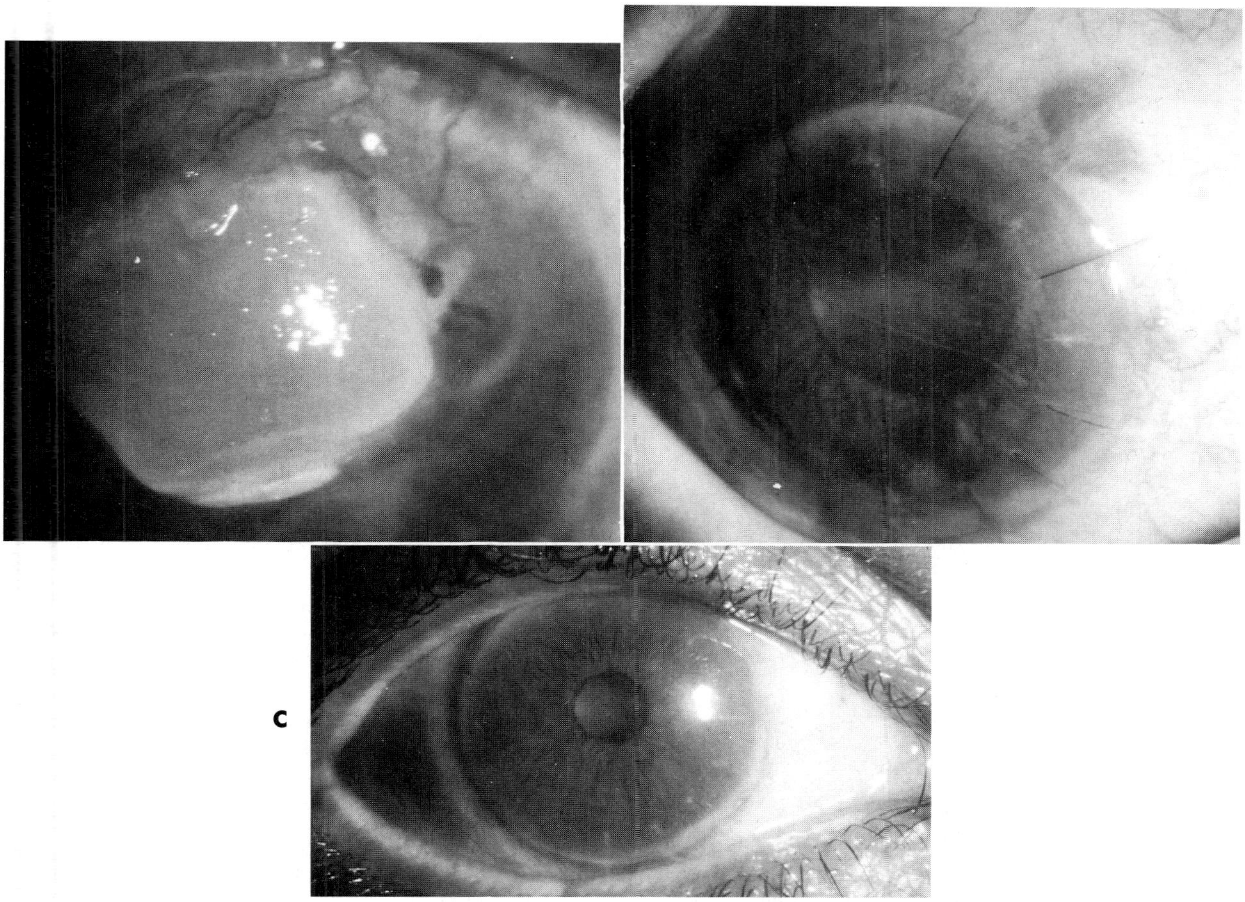

FIGURE 144-3 **A,** Severe Mooren's ulcer of 18 month's duration with 360 degrees of peripheral thinning and central deepithelialized island of stroma. Mooren's ulcer 4 months later with descemetocele. (See Fig. 144-3.) **B,** One month postoperative oversized (11.0/10.0mm) deep lamellar keratoplasty for Mooren's ulcer. **C,** Six month postoperative oversized deep lamellar graft for Moorens ulcer.

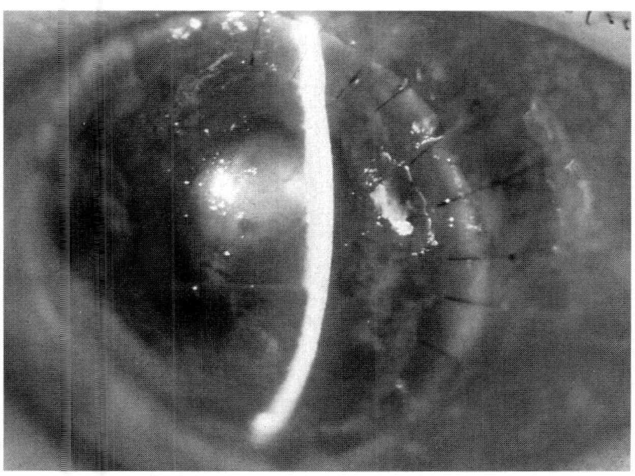

FIGURE 144-4 10.0 mm penetrating keratoplasty for total *Pseudomonas* corneal ulcer 1 day after surgery with hyphema.

ings and visual acuity are measured with a +10.00 diopter sphere in aphakes, correction from manifest refraction, or a pinhole. All exposed sutures are removed once the wound has healed. Buried sutures may be left in place if they are not causing excessive astigmatism.

Topical or systemic therapy for subsequent or coexisting elevated intraocular pressure, rejection reaction, graft melting and microbial infections is used as appropriate. Surgical intervention for nonhealing epithelial defects, graft melting or uncontrolled intraocular pressure is often necessary and may require tube implantation, trabeculectomy, or a laser cyclodestructive procedure.

Complications

Large diameter grafts are associated with many complications because of the nature of the primary

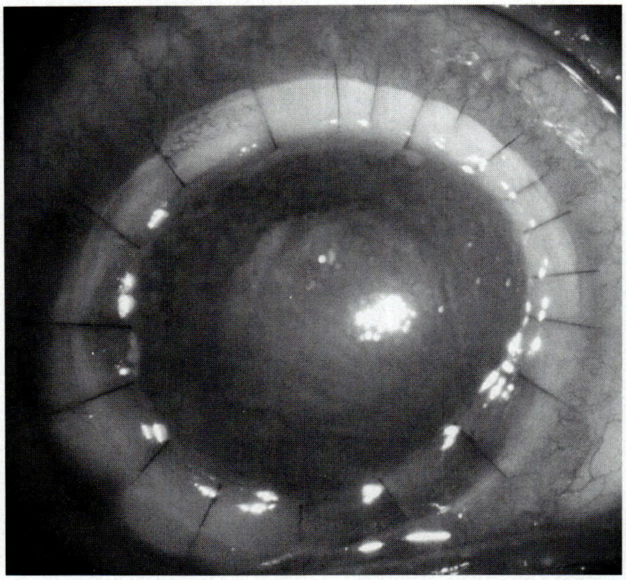

FIGURE 144-5 A 10.0 mm corneal transplant with rim of sclera 1 month postoperatively.

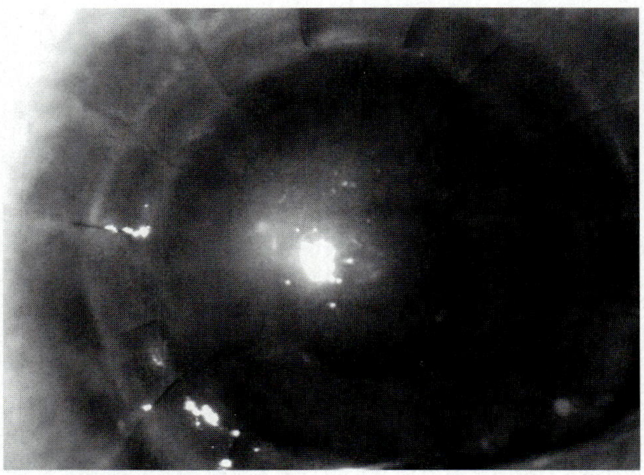

FIGURE 144-6 Large diameter lamellar keratoplasty for keratoconus.

problem and the complexity of the procedure. Graft failure caused by rejection is a frequent complication of large diameter keratoplasty despite intensive steroid use.[18,23] Conditions that predispose the graft to failure are its proximity to the limbal vessels and effector cells, the presence of antigen-bearing Langerhans cells in the donor tissue, inflammation, regraft associated sensitization and synechia formation.[24] Total keratoplasty except in cases of autografting as reported by Maumenee,[25] are at high risk for allograft rejection.

A "hyperacute" graft rejection with a dense, white, sterile ring infiltrate can occur in some cases where multiple penetrating keratoplasties have been performed, necessitating a repeat large diameter keratoplasty with intensive steroid and antirejection medications, such as the use of cyclosporine A topically or systemically (Figures 144-8 and 144-9).

The most frequent complication other than rejection in a large diameter keratoplasty is the recurrence of the original disease in the new large diameter graft. This usually means recurrent melting with descemetocele formation. A repeat, large diameter keratoplasty may be required if such a condition recurs. A nearly complete tarsorrhaphy may be necessary to prevent repeat melting. Bacterial corneal reinfection may occur in the graft in infected cases (Figure 144-10).

The ophtholmologist should be prepared for this probability by culturing the excised tissue for purposes of microbial indentification and sensitivity determination.

Persistent epithelial defects must be prevented or managed successfully by using a tarsorrhaphy or the graft will fail (Figures 144-11 and 144-12).

Large diameter therapeutic sclerokeratoplasty of 12 mm or greater performed to salvage an eye in cases of severe infectious keratitis or Mooren's ulcer may fail because of intractable glaucoma from the peripheral anterior synechiae and angle closure.[26,27] Trabeculectomy, a cyclodestructive procedure, or tube shunt implant may be necessary to adequately control intraocular pressure. Cobo et al.[22] report successful management of the intraocular pressure using angle-support sutures in 14 mm sclerokeratoplasty cases.

Placement of a smaller diameter penetrating keratoplasty for visual purposes within the rejected large diameter graft may result in visual improvement in some cases.[27] Ticho and Ben Sira[18] reported functional visual improvement in 14 cases of total therapeutic keratoplasty performed as eye saving operations in Africa. Kirkness et al.[28] reported 17 grafts of 10 mm or more in diameter in 16 eyes of 15 patients with a 1-year survival probability of 46%. Thirteen of these eyes had clear grafts, although multiple grafts were required in a number of cases and the follow-up was relatively short.

I have performed 14 penetrating keratoplasties on 10 patients using a 9.5 mm or larger diameter graft.[27] Five large diameter grafts were performed for perforation or impending perforation of large descemetoceles caused by bacterial ulceration and sclerokeratitis three for herpes simplex virus keratouveitis, four grafts for severe keratoconjunctivitis sicca with ulceration, and one each for alkaline burn and Mooren's ulcer. The average duration of graft clarity was 67.2 days, ranging from 14 days to 6 months. Best corrected visual acuity ranged from light perception to 20/40 vision. Two patients had recurrent ulcerations, each requiring a

A 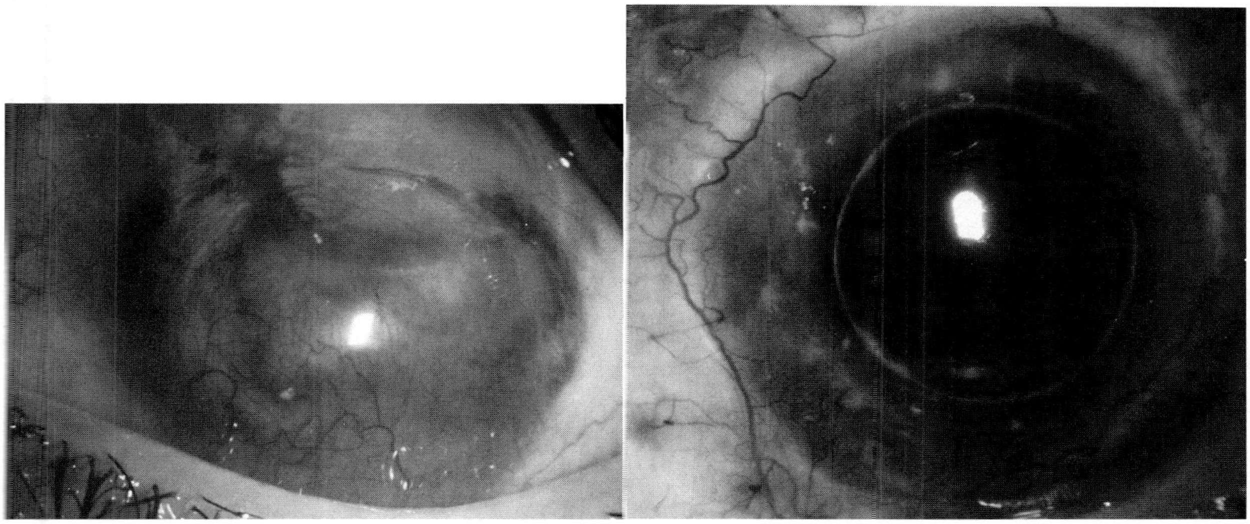 B

FIGURE 144-7 **A,** Extensive corneal thinning and scarring caused by trauma. **B,** Clear central graft in oversized lamellar graft 8 months later.

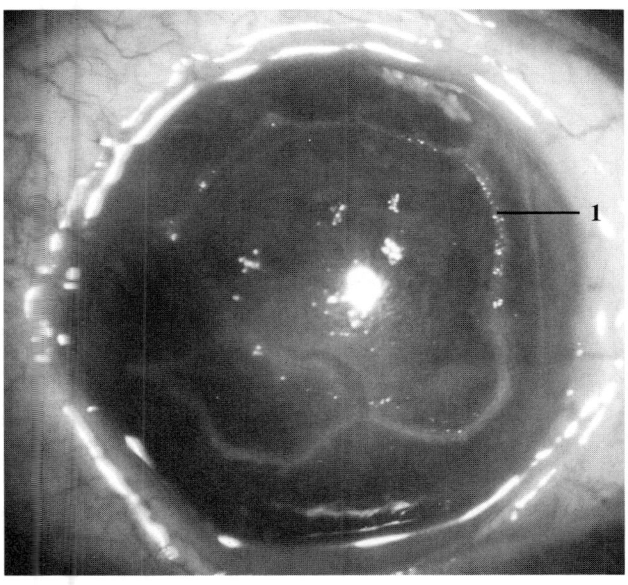

FIGURE 144-8 Three-month post operative 12. mm graft with epithelial rejection line (*1*) The transplant was performed for a perforated *Pseudomonas* corneal ulcer with endophthalmitis.

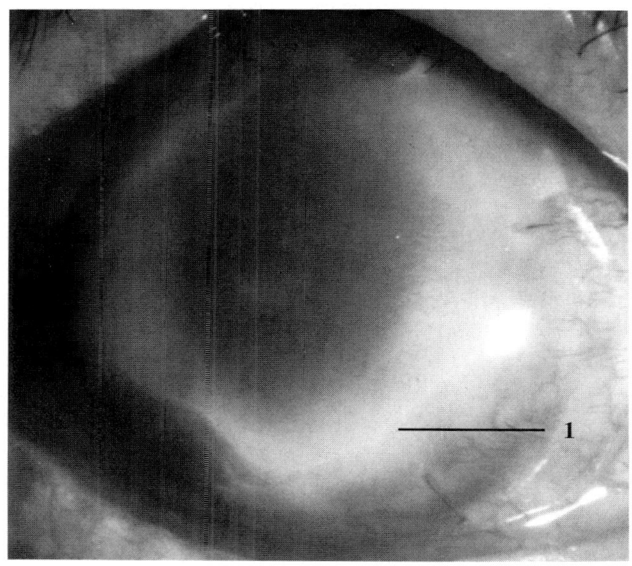

FIGURE 144-9 Immune ring (*1*) in 11.0 mm graft with hyperacute rejection reaction.

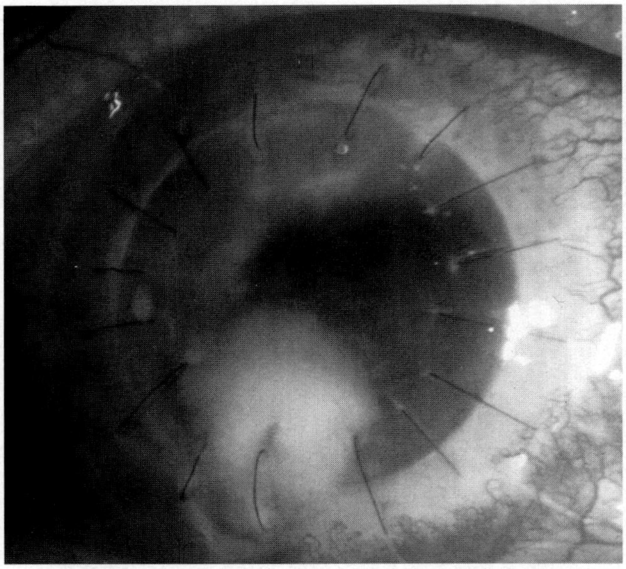

FIGURE 144-10 Suture abscess in 7.25 mm central graft placed in 10.0 mm transplantation for bacterial corneal ulcer.

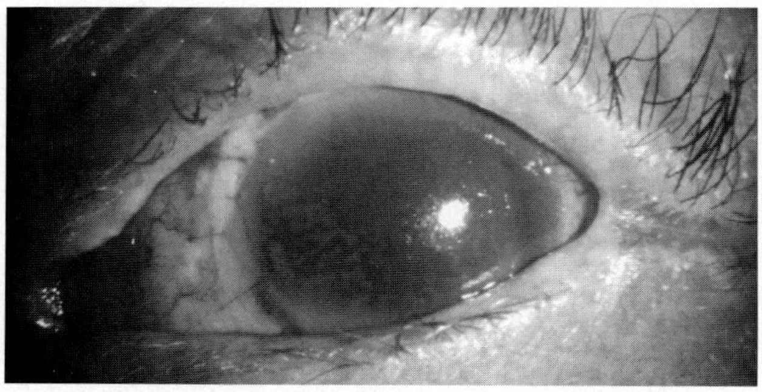

FIGURE 144-11 11.0 mm large diameter graft in dry eye patient showing lateral tarsorrhaphy.

large diameter regraft. The average period of clarity in these repeat grafts was 26 days. A small graft placed inside the failed large graft remained clear for at least 1 year in 50% of the 6 eyes operated for visual restoration.

Complications in this series of cases included graft rejection (13 eyes); recurrent disease (5 eyes) including recurrent Mooren's ulcer (3 eyes), and herpetic sclero-keratitis (2 eyes); secondary infection (4 eyes), bacterial ulcers (3 eyes) and endophthalmitis (1 eye); glaucoma (8 eyes), 2 requiring cyclocryotherapy and 2 requiring trabeculectomy and one retinal detachment. Two eyes eventually required enucleation. More than 50 ocular surgical procedures were performed on the 10 eyes, with a range of 3 to 10 procedures per eye.[27] The economic impact of such extensive and multiple surgical procedures to salvage the eye when only 30% will have any useful vision may be questionable.

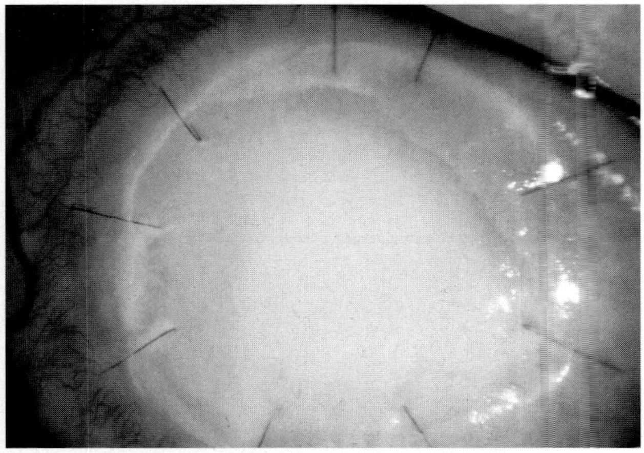

FIGURE 144-12 Large diameter graft. Failure caused by persistent epithelial defect.

However, if the patient's only eye is involved, these heroic measures are usually indicated. It thus becomes necessary to consider the cost and potential benefit for the patient's well-being before proceeding with such a procedure, which may require multiple operations and little visual improvement.

Large diameter penetrating keratoplasty is an eye-saving procedure, that, if successful in eliminating the disease process, may eventually allow some visual restoration. Many of these grafts are rejected because of the large diameter or intraocular inflammation. However, a subsequent, smaller diameter repeat keratoplasty may result in improved vision in some cases. In most circumstances, the only alternative to a large diameter therapeutic penetrating keratoplasty is enucleation.

REFERENCES

1. Malik SRK, Singh G: Therapeutic keratoplasty in *Pseudomonas pyocyaneus* corneal ulcers, *Br J Ophthalmol* 55:326-330, 1971.
2. Du NZ et al: Therapeutic keratoplasty in the management of purulent corneal ulceration: report of 100 cases, *JNJ Ophthalmol* 23:412-420, 1979.
3. Forster RK, Rebell G: Therapeutic surgery in failures of medical treatment for fungal keratitis, *Br J Ophthalmol* 59:366-371, 1975.
4. Singh G, Malik SRK, Bhatnagar PK: Therapeutic value of keratoplasty in keratomycosis, *Arch Ophthalmol* 92:48-50, 1974.
5. Hirst LW et al: Non-traumatic mycotic keratitis, *Eye* 6:391-395, 1992.
6. Panda A, Vajpayee RB, Kumar TS: Critical evaluation of therapeutic keratoplasty in cases of keratomycosis, *Annals Ophthalmol* October 23:373-376, 1991.
7. Guildford J et al: Large therapeutic penetrating keratoplasty in microbial keratitis, *Invest Ophthalmol Vis Sci* 29:6, 1988.
8. Qiu XZ: Large grafts for penetrating keratoplasty: clinical analysis of 48 cases, *Chung Hua Yen Ko Tsa Chih 22:81-84, 1986.*
9. Raizman MB, dela Maza MS, Foster CS: Surgical therapy of progressive peripheral ulcerative keratitis., *American Academy of Ophthalmology Meeting, Las Vegas, Nevada, October 1988.*
10. Bialasiewicz AA, Naumann GOH: Tectonic keratoplasty for

corneal perforations in Sjogren's syndrome: 12 years follow up, *American Academy of Ophthalmology Meeting, Las Vegas, Nevada, October 1988.*

11. Foster RK: The role of excisional keratoplasty in microrbital keratitis. In Cavanagh HD, editor: The cornea transactions of the world congress on the cornea III, New York, 1988, Raven Press.
12. Casey TA, Mayer DJ: *Corneal grafting principles and practices,* Philadelphia, 1984, WB Saunders.
13. Varley GA,Macsai MS, Krachmer JH: The results of penetrating keratoplasty for pellucid marginal corneal degeneration, *Am J Ophthalmol* 110:149-152, 1990.
14. Cameron JA: Keratoglobus, *Cornea* 12:124-130, 1993.
15. Speaker MG, Arentsen JJ, Laibson PR: Long-term survival of large diameter penetrating keratoplasties for kerotoconus and pellucid marginal degeneration, *Acta Ophthalmol Suppl (Copenh)* 192:17-19, 1989.
16. Malbran E: Lamellar keratoplasty in keratoconus. In King, Mezique, editors: *The cornea, world congress,* Washington, 1965, Butterworths.
17. Malbran E, Stefani C: Lamellar keratoplasty in corneal ectasias, *Ophthalmologica* 164:50-58, 1972.
18. Ticho V, Ben Sira I: Total keratoplasty, *Arch Ophthalmol.* 90:104-106, 1973.
19. Castroviejo R: Total penetrating keratoplasty: a preliminary report, *Am J Ophthalmol* 34:1697-1706, 1951.
20. Barraquer J: Total penetrating keratoplasty, *Proc R Soc Med* 54:1116-1118, 1961.
21. Taylor DM, Stern AL: Reconstructive keratoplasty in the management of conditions leading to corneal destruction, *Ophthalmology* 87(9):892-904, 1980.
22. Cobo M, Ortiz JR, Safran SG: Sclerokeratoplasty with maintenance of the angle, *Am J Ophthalmol* 113(5):533-537, 1992.
23. Boisjoly HM et al: Effect of factors unrelated to tissue matching on corneal transplant endothelial rejection, *Am J Ophthalmol* 107:647-654, 1989.
24. Arentsen JJ: Corneal transplant allograft reaction: possible predisposing factors, *Trans Am Ophthalmol Soc* 181:361-401, 1983.
25. Maumenee AE: Penetrating autokeratoplasty of the entire cornea, *Am J Ophthalmol* 47:125-133, 1959.
26. Cowden JW, Kaufman HE, Polack FM: The prognosis of keratoplasty after previous graft failures, *Am J Ophthalmol* 78:523-525, 1974.
27. Cowden JW, Copeland RA, Schneider MS: Large diameter therapeutic penetrating keratoplasties, *Refract Corneal Surg* 5:244-248, 1989.
28. Kirkness CM, Ficker LA, Rice NSC, Steele A: Large corneal grafts can be successful, *Eye* 3:48-55, 1989.

CHAPTER 145

H. KAZ SOONG

Penetrating Keratoplasty in Ocular Surface Disease

The functional dynamics of corneal and conjunctival epithelia are closely interdependent, mutually forming a physiologic and anatomic continuum. Ocular surface disease is a generic term referring to disorders affecting both the corneal surface and conjunctiva.[1] Etiologies are manifold and include the six "I's": immunologic, infectious, inflammatory, injury-related, iatrogenic, and idiopathic. Examples include pemphigoid, Stevens-Johnson syndrome, graft-versus-host disease, atopy, herpes zoster ophthalmicus, trachoma, rosacea, blepharitis and other eyelid disorders (lagophthalmos, ectropion, entropion, and trichiasis), chemical and thermal burns, medicamentosa, radiation keratoconjunctivitis, dry eyes, and aniridic keratopathy. Moreover, secondary ocular surface scarring, dryness, and keratinization may result from various primary ocular surface pathology, further aggravating the original situation in a vicious, cyclical fashion. There is a common tendency of ocular surface disorders in general to cause tear deficiency states and corneal surface breakdown. This, in turn, promotes corneal vascularization and scarring, reduction of visual acuity, compromise of antimicrobial protective mechanisms, and weakening of corneal structural integrity. Uncontrolled ocular surface disorders therefore are deleterious to the overall survival of a corneal graft.

Penetrating keratoplasty is adversely affected by concomitant ocular surface disease. In the presence of surface disorders, the normal, orderly transdifferentiation of conjunctival epithelium to corneal epithelium is disrupted, corneal epithelial healing is retarded, and the vision may be compromised by corneal surface irregularities.[2-7] Nonstem cell conjunctival epithelium may cover the cornea (conjunctivalization), resulting in poor optical clarity. Chronic inflammation and irritation may promote vascularization and melting of the donor cornea, resulting not only in decreased vision, but also in an increased likelihood of immune graft rejection and corneal scarring. Damaged ocular surface defense mechanisms may increase the probability of infectious keratitis after corneal transplantation.

Ideally, ocular surface problems should be treated aggressively before performing penetrating keratoplasty to improve the chances of survival of the donor graft. Postoperatively, any lingering or recurrent surface problems should be addressed immediately. As a rule, the decision to perform penetrating keratoplasty on an eye with significant ocular surface disease should be one of restraint and conservatism. Only when all other treatment modalities are exhausted should one proceed with penetrating keratoplasty.

Preoperative History and Examination: Special Concerns

In the penetrating keratoplasty patient who has overt or occult ocular surface disease, certain historical information may raise a red cautionary flag.[1] Chronic or recurrent conjunctival inflammation may signify atopy or mucous membrane cicatricial diseases, such as pemphigoid and Stevens-Johnson syndrome.[4,8] A history of previous chemical burns, no matter how minor, should alert the surgeon to pay particular heed to the eyelid anatomy and function, tear dynamics of the eye, and the presence of chronic ocular surface inflammation.[9-14] Congenital aniridia is often associated with chronic ocular surface problems with mild inflammation, characterized by low Schirmer tests, Bitot's spots, and irregular corneal epithelium with underlying stromal vascularization and scarring.[15] A patient who has undergone radiation treatment to the head region or one who has undergone bone marrow transplantation should be examined closely for signs of radiation keratoconjunctivitis or graft-versus-host disease (Figure 145-1).[16,17] Patients from regions where trachoma is endemic should be evaluated closely for bulbar and palpebral conjunctival scarring, corneal pannus, and dryness.[18] Individuals with collagen vascular diseases or women who are postmenopausal (involutional or preinvolutional) should be evaluated

A

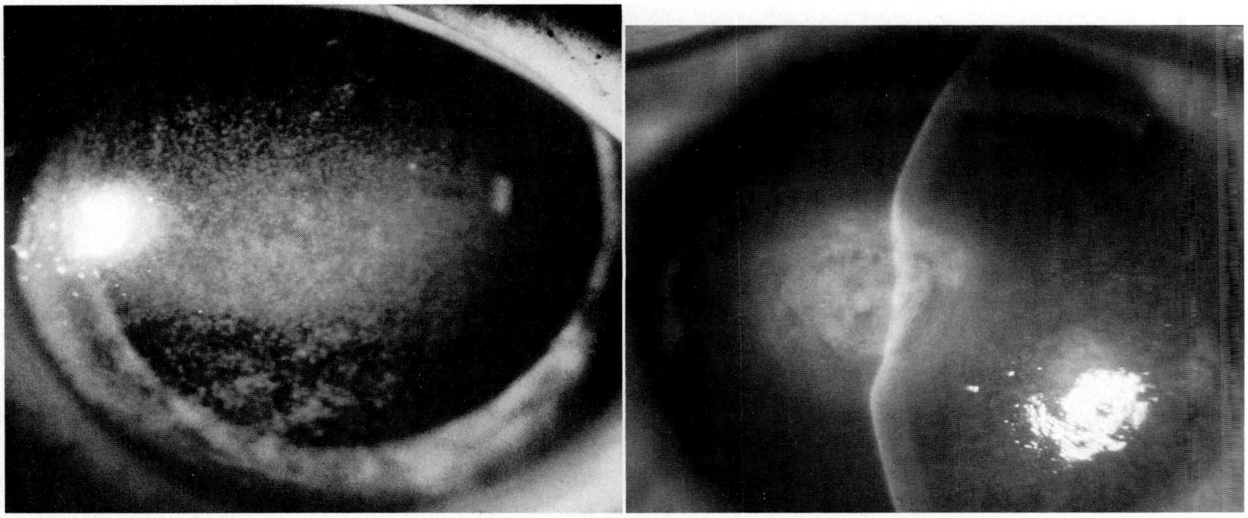

B

FIGURE 145-1 The cornea in graft-versus-host disease. **A**, Punctate fluorescein staining of cornea caused by dryness from conjunctival scarring and exposure keratopathy from eyelid scarring with secondary lagophthalmos. **B**, Corneal epithelial defect with early stromal necrosis.

for primary aqueous tear deficiency syndromes.[19] A careful medication history indicating types of medication, as well as their dosages, may unravel the existence of drug-induced ocular surface problems.[20]

The condition of the patient's skin may help in the correlative diagnosis of acne rosacea, psoriasis, or an antecedent history of herpes zoster ophthalmicus.[21-24] In advanced cases, the diagnosis could be quite obvious from dermatopathologic features such as rhinophyma, psoriatic scaling, and dermatomal skin scarring (Figure 145-2).

The condition of the eyelids may also provide vital clues for the diagnosis of existing ocular surface disease. Cicatrization of the palpebral conjunctiva from pemphigoid,[4,5] Stevens-Johnson syndrome,[25,26] radiation keratoconjunctivitis,[16] graft-versus-host disease,[17] severe infectious conjunctivitis,[27] conjunctival neoplastic processes, and certain topical medications (e.g., antiviral and antiglaucoma agents)[27-29] may result in entropion, trichiasis, lagophthalmos, retroplacement of the meibomian gland orifices, and keratinization of the inside surface of the eyelids.[30] Eyelid margin findings, such as collarette formation, crusting, madarosis, thickening, telangiectasis, lipid soap formation, and glandular inspissation may be associated with blepharitis and acne rosacea.[22,31] Chemical or thermal burns, as well as skin tumors, xeroderma pigmentosum (Figure 145-3), lacerations, and radiation dermatitis, often spare the conjunctival side of the eyelids, but preferentially damage the eyelid skin and the margins.[30] These conditions tend to cause eyelid retraction on the skin side, resulting in ectropion and lagophthalmos with corneal exposure. Scarring from herpes zoster ophthalmicus is associated not only with ocular surface damage from eyelid retraction, entropion, ectropion, and trichiasis, but may also be associated with neurotrophic keratopathy, dry eye syndromes and primary corneal scarring. A papillary reaction present on the tarsal conjunctiva may signify an underlying allergic etiology, such as vernal conjunctivitis and giant papillary conjunctivitis.[32-34] The latter may result from contact lenses[35,36] or exposed nylon suture ends.[37]

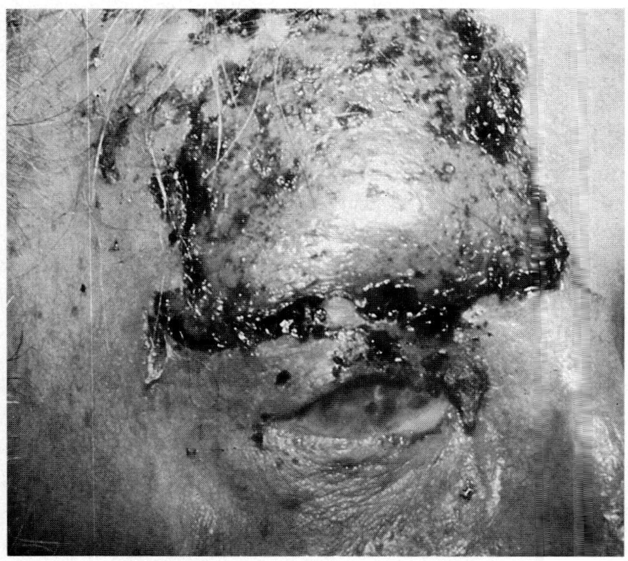

FIGURE 145-2 Herpes zoster ophthalmicus (acute stage) with corneal surface breakdown and edema.

Abnormalities in the tear dynamics may be based on dysfunction of the aqueous, surfactant (mucin), and/or

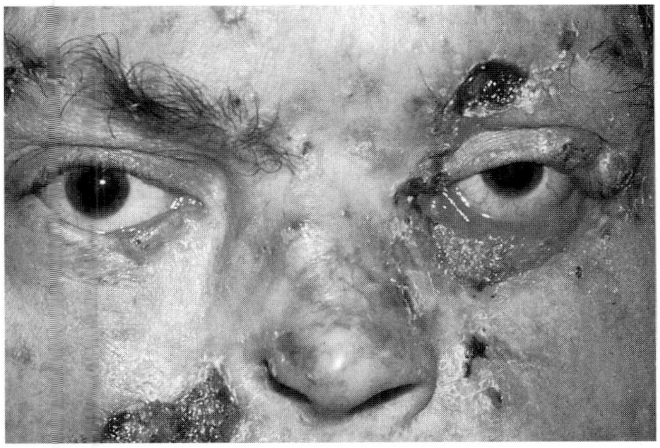

FIGURE 145-3 Eyelid skin scarring from xeroderma pigmentosum, resulting in lagophthalmos and ectropion of left eye.

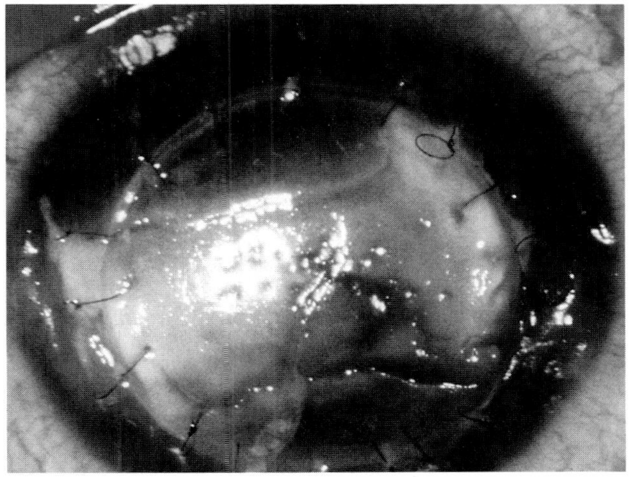

FIGURE 145-4 Persistent epithelial defect (stained with fluorescein) in corneal graft from exposure keratopathy.

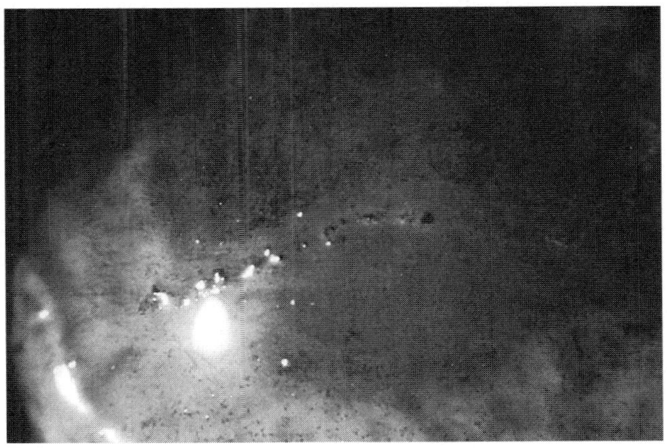

FIGURE 145-5 Medicamentosa keratopathy showing typical diffuse punctate staining of cornea with fluorescein.

lipid moieties of the tear film. Alternatively, they may result from insufficiencies of the blink mechanism. Localized corneal surface drying resulting from an interruption in tear film spreading from limbal masses may result in dellen formation.[38] The Schirmer test,[19,39] tear film meniscus height,[39] tear breakup time,[40] lysozyme test,[41] fluorescein dilution test,[42] and tear osmolality measurements[42,43] may aid in the diagnosis of dry eye. Tear meniscus debris, filaments, and mucous strands are also sometimes associated with dry eye disease.[19] Primary or secondary damage to the conjunctival goblet (mucin-producing) cells may be associated with ocular surface keratin plaques[42] and rose bengal punctate staining[42] and may be diagnosed definitively by impression cytologic examination.[44] Dryness and improper eyelid blink or closure (Figure 145-4) may cause the corneal graft to undergo vascularization, scarring, infection, melting, perforation, and recurrent or persistent epithelial breakdown or ectasia. All these complications increase the chances of eventual graft failure.

With most ocular surface disorders, the cornea may show evidence of punctate epithelial staining, pannus formation, previous thinning, and scarring. Rose Bengal staining of the cornea (and conjunctiva) is of particular value in the assessment of surface epithelial damage.[45] The location and distribution of all these findings on the cornea may not only be crucial for determining the etiology of the ocular surface problem, but also may aid in deciding on the appropriate preoperative treatment strategies before corneal transplantation. For instance, the presence of such findings on the inferior cornea may often suggest blepharitis, exposure, and dry eye, whereas the presence of similar findings on the superior cornea may often suggest trachoma, contact lens intolerance, and superior limbic keratoconjunctivitis. Diffuse punctate staining, coupled with a suspicious medication history, may suggest topical drug toxicity (Figure 145-5).[20] If possible, any persistent corneal epithelial defect should be allowed to heal completely before penetrating keratoplasty is performed. A persistent epithelial defect often signifies that the corneal dynamics have not yet stabilized and that residual surface inflammation may still persist. There are, of course, occasional clinical circumstances that require exigent corneal transplantation, even in the presence of corneal surface defects and active stromal melting. Such corneal grafts tend to be unstable and are often fraught with postoperative healing problems.

Persistent epithelial defects may be inflammatory or noninflammatory in origin.[46] In inflammatory conditions, polymorphonuclear leukocytes or their products are capable of inhibiting corneal epithelial healing.[46] Furthermore, the chronic use of topical corticosteroids

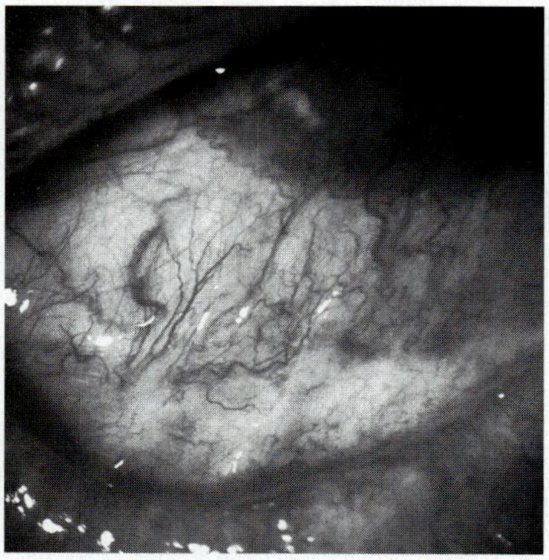

FIGURE 145-6 Inferior symblepharon formation with blunting of the cul-de-sac in ocular cicatricial pemphigoid.

in the presence of such persistent epithelial defects may be associated with problems such as stromal melting, delay of epithelial healing, infection, glaucoma, and cataract formation (see Prekeratoplasty Therapeutic Management). Persistent epithelial defects associated with dry eyes, exposure, trichiasis, and neurotrophic states, on the other hand, generally do not show a significant underlying inflammatory component. These are probably secondary to abnormal wetting, damaged substrata, and mechanical irritation.

Because the anatomy and function of the corneal epithelium is so intimately related to the conjunctival surface, corneal findings are often associated with conjunctival abnormalities. The bulbar and cul-de-sac conjunctiva may show evidence of scarring (subepithelial fibrosis, cul-de-sac blunting, and symblepharon formation) as a result of any severe inflammation (Figure 145-6), such as pemphigoid, Stevens-Johnson syndrome, chemical and thermal burns, neoplasms, infections, xerophthalmia caused by vitamin A deficiency,[47] atopy, previous eye surgery, and radiation. Late changes after chronic conjunctival insult may show extreme clinical pathology such as severe goblet cell attrition, ankyloblepharon formation, and keratinization.[48] In essence, these changes convert the normal secretory conjunctival epithelium into skinlike, nonsecretory epithelium. The conjunctival goblet cells, which normally produce the mucin secretions necessary for the spreading of the aqueous tear film over the hydrophobic corneal epithelial surface, are gradually annihilated.[2,48-50] Concurrent blunting of the cul-de-sac may compromise eyelid closure and contact lens insertion.

The preoperative therapy should be guided to a certain extent by the reduction of conjunctival, episcleral, and scleral erythema. The eye should have little or no inflammatory activity before corneal transplantation. Failure to reduce inflammation adequately before surgery may increase the chances of postoperative corneal surface breakdown, corneal melting, graft rejection or failure, and vascularization. For instance, penetrating keratoplasty in a patient with pemphigoid and active disease-related conjunctival inflammation may have disastrous consequences, resulting in graft failure and rapidly progressive anterior segment destruction. Unfortunately for advanced ocular cicatricial pemphigoid, the prognosis for penetrating keratoplasty is bleak even if the disease is quiescent, especially with severe conjunctival scarring, keratinization, corneal vascularization, and eyelid abnormalities. However, good control of the inflammation associated with pemphigoid before surgery with immunosuppression may improve the chances of success by preventing stimulation of pemphigoid inflammatory activity by surgical trauma.[51] At the other extreme, preoperative ischemia of the conjunctival vasculature, especially at the limbus, may also portend poor epithelial healing of the corneal graft, resulting in attenuated graft survival. Limbal ischemia is commonly encountered after severe chemical or thermal burns,[52,53] and occasionally during active herpes simplex involvement of the limbus and conjunctiva.[54] Although the exact mechanism of vascular ischemia remains unknown in the case of herpetic disease, it may possibly be due to either direct tissue invasion by the virus or to immune-mediated vascular inflammation.

In addition to the ocular surface examination, the importance of a meticulous examination of the deeper, internal structures of the eye to rule out corneal endothelial disease, glaucoma, intraocular inflammation, and macular disease cannot be stressed more emphatically. A conservative, careful, and considerate decision to operate only on stable, quiescent eyes will avert many postoperative disappointments, difficulties, and disasters.

Prekeratoplasty Therapeutic Management

MEDICAL

Several nonsurgical therapeutic modalities that can improve graft survival are available before performing penetrating keratoplasty. Topical and systemic corticosteroids are important mainstays of reducing ocular inflammation before surgery. In the presence of active corneal melting, however, it is preferable to use systemic medication to reduce the possibility of local corticosteroid-mediated enhancement of the collagenolytic process. Moreover, systemic corticosteroids are beneficial in treating underlying systemic inflammatory disease. Topical progestational steroids, such as medroxyprogesterone (Provera) 1% three times a day, may help manage inflammation, with minimal inhibition of wound repair and minimal enhancement of the collagenolytic process.[55] Topical or systemic cyclosporine A may have some efficacy in reducing the immune process in atopic keratoconjunctivitis,[56] severe keratoconjunctivitis sicca,[57] corneal melting,[58] and perhaps also in graft-versus-host disease.[59,60]

Cromolyn[61] and lodoxamide,[62] both mast cell stabilizers, may be used to reduce inflammatory activity in ocular allergy. Topical antihistamines (including the newer H-1 antihistamines) and human IgE pentapeptide are also helpful in reducing atopic activity.[63] Oral, nonsedating antihistamines, such as loratadine (Claritin), astemizole (Hismanal), and terfenadine (Seldane) may be beneficial in the control of chronic allergic or atopic keratoconjunctivitis. Topical nonsteroidal anti-inflammatory agents may help reduce the ocular surface inflammatory response in atopic and nonatopic states,[64] without many of the side effects associated with corticosteroids. Topical fibronectin, vitamin A derivatives, and epidermal growth factor may have beneficial effects in the therapy of persistent corneal epithelial defects; however, clinical studies have at best shown equivocal, if not conflicting, results. Fibronectin (as well as laminin) is thought to be a key element in mediating cell-to-substratum adhesion and cell migration.[65,66] Topical fibronectin eyedrops have demonstrated efficacy in accelerating corneal epithelial healing in persistent epithelial defects associated with several conditions, including herpes simplex keratitis, cataract surgery, and trophic keratitis.[65-67] On the other hand, fibronectin was not effective in the treatment of epithelial defects after corneal alkali injury[68] and in dry eye conditions.[69] Furthermore, exogenous fibronectin by itself did not enhance epithelial wound closure rates in an in vitro study using spatula-scraped corneal epithelial defects, nor did it enhance the concomitant effects of epidermal growth factor.[70]

Topical tretinoin (all-trans-retinoic acid), a vitamin A analog, may show some efficacy in the treatment of various dry eye disorders[71] by reversing squamous metaplasia and goblet cell loss. However, such beneficial effects were seen mostly in dry eyes associated with conjunctival scarring disorders, such as ocular cicatricial pemphigoid, Stevens-Johnson syndrome, and radiation keratoconjunctivitis. The benefits were insignificant in primary keratoconjunctivitis sicca.[72] Topical retinoids also enhanced corneal epithelial wound closure rates in experimental rabbit investigations.[73]

Growth factors have been shown to accelerate epithelial healing by increasing cellular mitosis.[74-78] Although primarily mitogenic agents, growth factors also stimulate production of extracellular matrix components to enhance cell-to-substratum adhesion.[74] Whether growth factors enhance cellular migration and spreading is unclear.[74,79]

Moisturizing and lubricating the ocular surface with artificial tears and ointment may be extremely beneficial in patients with dry eyes, ocular surface scarring, exposure keratopathy, and neurotrophic keratopathy. Preservatives in these ocular moisturizing and lubricating products, however, may be irritative, producing adverse effects on the ocular surface of these patients.[20] Therefore, it may be advantageous to use preservative-free products, especially if the agents are used frequently.

Oral tetracyline[80] and lid scrubs with detergent (either dilute "baby shampoo" or commercial eyelid scrub packs) aid in the control of blepharitis and other eyelid oil gland problems, such as ocular rosacea.[81] Interestingly, tetracycline may also have some anti-collagenolytic effects.[82] Based on studies of systemic metronidazole (Flagyl) for facial acne rosacea, the efficacy of topical metronidazole is now being investigated for the treatment of rosacea blepharoconjunctivitis.

SURGICAL MANAGEMENT

Eyes with ocular surface problems may often require conjunctival, corneal, or eyelid surgery to optimize graft survival. Transplantation of conjunctiva or limbal stem cells may vastly improve the orderly transdifferentiation of surface epithelia and therefore, may significantly improve the chances of graft success.[83-87] If the contralateral eye has healthy, undamaged conjunctiva, a conjunctival limbal autograft may be transferred to the diseased eye with minimum risk to the donor eye. Alternatively, if both eyes have surface disease or damage, conjunctival allografts from another individual (preferably with good HLA-genetic matching) may be used.[88,89] Such allografts carry a significant risk of immunologic rejection, manifested by cellular destruction and sloughing of the conjunctival graft. Oral cyclosporin is necessary in the immediate postoperative period to reduce the rejection risk of the transplanted conjunctival limbal autografts. A starting daily oral dose of 5 mg/kg body weight is recommended. After 3 months, the dose should be reduced to 3 mg/kg.

Keratoepithelioplasty is a surgical procedure similar to conjunctival grafting, with the major difference being the use of allogenic corneal epithelium to block conjunctival invasion of the corneal surface.[90,91] Incorporation of limbal epithelial cells with the donor corneal epithelial tissue will also provide a source of stem cells.

Laser photocoagulation of corneal neovascularization may provide a more stable corneal surface, both from an immunologic and humoral standpoint. Photocoagulation may be performed by focal laser treatment of vessels or by concomitant use of photosensitizing dyes or photoporhyrins.[92-96] The yellow laser or blue-green argon laser may be used for this purpose. Use of a focusing contact lens (e.g. Abraham lens) enhances the treatment efficiency. A relatively small spot size of 50 to 100 μm diameter allows focal treatment with minimal adjacent stromal heating. This is applied at a power level of 200 to 300 mW at a duration of 50 to 100 ms. The additional use of photosensitization allows the use of lower power levels to achieve closure of vessels.

Eyelid surgical procedures may include (1) punctal occlusion for dry eye patients; (2) tarsorraphy for exposure, neurotrophic keratopathy, and other recurrent corneal surface breakdown conditions; (3) ectropion/entropion corrective surgery; (4) trichiasis surgery (cryotherapy versus incisional surgery); and (5) reconstructive surgery to improve eyelid closure. Preferably, these procedures should be performed before penetrating keratoplasty. However, if surface problems recur after keratoplasty, these procedures may need to be repeated.

DONOR SELECTION

There are no specific recommendations for donor corneal tissue for eyes with surface disease. As a minimum criterion, the donor cornea should have a healthy epithelial substrate and preferably no significant epithelial breakdown. Furthermore, the allograft tissue should be as fresh as possible. These criteria are not absolute, however, since no published studies have yet supported these recommendations.

Special Considerations for Corneal Surgery and Its Postoperative Management

In eyes with significant ocular surface disease, it is best not to rely exclusively on continuous (running) sutures for closure of the keratoplasty. Unpredictable postoperative vascularization, uneven healing rates, and thinning of the corneal graft may necessitate premature cutting and removal of the sutures. It is safer to use interrupted sutures, either exclusively or in combination with continuous sutures. Because of an increased tendency of corneal sutures in vascularized corneas to loosen prematurely as a result of corneal fibroblast contraction, it may be prudent to tie all corneal sutures tighter in vascularized corneas than for nonvascularized corneas. Loose or vascularized sutures should be removed to reduce the chances of microbial infection or immune rejection from the invading vessels. Bandage contact lenses and collagen lenses may also be inserted at the time of surgery to protect the corneal surface. Partial tarsorrhaphy is a useful and much underused procedure that may be performed easily in conjunction with the penetrating keratoplasty if one expects an unstable corneal surface after keratoplasty.

Aggressive surface lubrication and wetting with nonpreserved artificial tears, ointments, or viscoelastic (sodium hyaluronate) may be necessary to protect the graft after surgery. High-dose systemic and/or topical corticosteroids may be required in the immediate postoperative period. The tapering process should proceed under close observation and caution. The patient should be followed closely for evidence of surface breakdown, persistent epithelial defects, corneal melting, inflammation, infection, vascularization, and immune rejection.

The patient with ocular surface disease represents a special challenge for the corneal surgeon and requires presurgical planning and alternatives in intraoperative techniques to maximize chances for graft success.

REFERENCES

1. Thoft RA: Conjunctival transplantation, *Arch Ophthalmol* 95:1425, 1977.
2. Tseng SCG et al: Topical retinoid treatment for various dry-eye disorders, *Ophthalmology* 92:717, 1985.
3. Kinoshita S et al: Goblet cell density in ocular surface disease: a better indicator than tear mucin, *Arch Ophthalmol* 101:1284, 1983.
4. Foster CS: Cicatricial pemphigoid, *Trans Am Ophthalmol Soc* 84:527, 1986.
5. Mondino BJ, Brown SI: Ocular cicatricial pemphigoid, *Ophthalmology* 88:95, 1981.
6. Shapiro MS, Friend J, Thoft RA: Corneal re-epithelialization from the conjunctiva, *Invest Ophthalmol Vis Sci* 21:135, 1981.
7. Thoft RA, Friend J: Biochemical transformation of regenerating ocular surface epithelium, *Invest Ophthalmol Vis Sci* 16:14, 1977.
8. Mondino BJ, et al: The acute manifestations of ocular cicatricial pemphigoid: diagnosis and treatment, *Ophthalmology* 86:543, 1979.
9. Pavilack M, Chang P, Soong H: Corneal alkali burns. In Schachat AP et al, editors: *Current practice in ophthalmology*, St Louis, 1992, Mosby.
10. Brown SI, Bloomfield SE, Pearce DB: A followup report on transplantation of the alkali-burned cornea, *Am J Ophthalmol* 77:538, 1974.
11. Brown SI, Tragakis MP, Pearce DB: Corneal transplantation for severe alkali burns, *Trans Am Acad Ophthalmol Otolaryngol* 76:1266, 1972.
12. Casey TA, Mayer DJ: Grafting in chemical burns. In Casey TA, Mayer DJ, editors: *Corneal grafting: principles and practice*, Philadelphia, 1984, WB Saunders.
13. Thoft RA: Chemical and thermal injury, *Int Ophthalmol Clin* 19:243, 1979.

14. Belin ME, Krachmer JH: Chemical burns of the cornea. In Easty DL, Smolin G, editors: *External eye disease,* London, 1985, Butterworths.
15. Mackman G, Brightbill FS, Optiz JM: Corneal changes in aniridia, *Am J Ophthalmol* 87:497, 1979.
16. Parrish CM, Chandler JW: Corneal trauma. In Kaufman HE, Barron BA, McDonald MB, Waltman SR, editors: *The cornea,* New York, 1988, Churchill Livingstone.
17. Franklin RM et al: Ocular manifestations of graft-vs-host disease, *Ophthalmology* 90:4, 1983.
18. Whitcher JP: Chlamydial diseases. In Smolin G, Thoft RA, editors: *Cornea,* vol 2, Boston, 1987, Little, Brown.
19. Holly FJ, Lemp MA: Tear physiology and dry eyes, *Surv Ophthalmol* 22:69, 1977.
20. Pfister RR, Burstein N: The effects of ophthalmic drugs, vehicles, and preservatives on corneal epithelium: a scanning electron microscope study, *Invest Ophthalmol Vis Sci* 15:246, 1976.
21. Moschella SL, Pillsbury DM, Hurley HJ, editors: *Dermatology,* vol 1, Philadelphia, 1975, WB Saunders.
22. Jenkins MS et al: Ocular rosacea, *Am J Ophthalmol* 88:618, 1979.
23. Liesegang T: Corneal complications from herpes zoster ophthalmicus, *Ophthalmology* 92:316, 1985.
24. Liesegang T: The varicella zoster virus: systemic and ocular features, *J Am Acad Dermatol* 11:165, 1984.
25. Chan LS et al: Ocular cicatricial pemphigoid occurring as a sequela of Stevens-Johnson syndrome, *JAMA* 266:1543, 1991.
26. Howard GM: The Stevens-Johnson syndrome: ocular prognosis and treatment, *Am J Ophthalmol* 55:893, 1963.
27. Wright P: Cicatrizing conjunctivitis, *Trans Ophthalmol Soc UK* 105:1, 1986.
28. Patten JT, Cavanaugh HD, Allansmith MR: Induced ocular pseudopemphigoid, *Am J Ophthalmol* 83:443, 1977.
29. Hirst LW et al: Drug-induced cicatrizing conjunctivitis simulating ocular pemphigoid, *Cornea* 1:121, 1982.
30. Wolfley DE: Surgical management of eyelid abnormalities. In Kaufman HE, McDonald MB, Barron BA, Waltman SR, editors: *The cornea,* New York, 1988, Churchill Livingstone.
31. Smolin G, Tabbara K, Whitcher J: Lids. In Smolin G, Tabbara K, Whitcher J, editors: *Infectious diseases of the eye,* Baltimore, 1984, Williams & Wilkins.
32. Smolin G, O'Connor GR: *Ocular immunology,* Philadelphia, 1981, Lea & Febiger.
33. Jay JL: Clinical features and diagnostis of adult atopic keratoconjunctivitis and the effect of treatment with sodium cromglycate, *Br J Ophthalmol* 65:335, 1981.
34. Gormaz A, Essers C: Vernal keratoconjunctivitis and keratoconus, *Am J Ophthalmol* 96:555, 1984.
35. Henriquez AS, Kenyon KR, Allansmith MR: Mast cell ultrastructure. Comparison in contact lens-associated giant papillary conjunctivitis and vernal conjunctivitis, *Arch Ophthalmol* 99: 1266, 1981.
36. Stenson S: Focal giant papillary conjunctivitis from retained contact lenses, *Ann Ophthalmol* 14:881, 1982.
37. Sugar A, Meyer RF: Giant papillary conjunctivitis after keratoplasty, *Am J Ophthalmol* 91:239, 1981.
38. Baum JL, Mishima S, Boruchoff SA: On the nature of dellen, *Arch Ophthalmol* 79:657, 1968.
39. Lamberts DW, Foster CS, Perry HD: Schirmer test after topical anesthesia and the tear meniscus height in normal eyes, *Arch Ophthamol* 97:1082, 1979.
40. Lemp MA, Hamill J: Factors affecting tear film breakup in normals, *Arch Ophthalmol* 89:103, 1973.
41. Avisar R et al: Lysozyme content of tears in patients with Sjögren's syndrome and rheumatoid arthritis, *Am J Ophthalmol* 87:148, 1979.
42. Lamberts DW: Dry eyes. In Smolin G, Thoft RA, editors: *Cornea,* vol 2, Boston, 1987, Little, Brown.
43. Gilbard JP, Farris RL, Santamaria J II: Osmolarity of tear microvolumes in keratoconjunctivitis sicca, *Arch Ophthalmol* 96:677, 1978.
44. Nelson JD: Ocular surface impressions using cellulose acetate filter material. Ocular pemphigoid, *Surv Ophthalmol* 27:76, 1982.
45. Farris RL et al: Diagnostic tests in keratoconjunctivitis sicca, *CLAO J* 9:23, 1983.
46. Wagoner MD et al: Polymorphonuclear neutrophils delay corneal epithelial wound healing in vitro, *Invest Ophthalmol Vis Sci* 25:1217, 1984.
47. Vitamin A deficiency and xerophthalmia, WHO Technical Report, No 590, 1976.
48. Sporn MB, Roberts AB: Role of retinoids in differentiation and carcinogenesis, *Cancer Res* 43:3034, 1983.
49. Tseng SCG: Staging of conjunctival squamous metaplasia by impression cytology, *Ophthalmology* 92:728, 1985.
50. Maumenee AE: Keratinization of the conjunctiva, *Trans Am Ophthalmol Soc* 77:133, 1979.
51. De la Maza MS, Tauber J, Foster CS: Cataract surgery in ocular cicatricial pemphigoid, *Ophthalmology* 95:481, 1988.
52. Hughes WF: Alkali burns of the eye. 1 Review of the literature and summary of present knowledge, *Arch Ophthalmol* 35:423, 1946.
53. Hughes WF: Alkali burns of the eye. 2: clinical and pathological course, *Arch Ophthalmol* 36:189, 1946.
54. Brown DC et al: Recurrent herpes simplex conjunctivitis, *Arch Ophthalmol* 79:733, 1968.
55. Newsome DA, Gross J: Prevention by medroxyprogesterone of perforation in the alkali-burned rabbit cornea: Inhibition of collagenolytic activity, *Invest Ophthalmol Vis Sci* 16:21, 1977.
56. Ben Ezra D et al: Cyclosporine eye drops for the treatment of severe vernal keratoconjunctivitis, *Am J Ophthalmol* 101:278, 1986.
57. Ben Ezra D, Matamoros N, Cohen E: Treatment of severe keratoconjunctivitis with cyclosporin A eyedrops, *Transplant Proc* 20 (Suppl 2) 644, 1988.
58. Kruit PJ, Van Balen AThM, Stilma JS: Cyclosporin A treatment in two cases of corneal peripheral melting syndrome, *Doc Ophthalmol* 59:33, 1985.
59. Culbertson WW, Tseng SCG: Personal communication, July 1995.
60. Nussenblatt RB, Palestine AG: Cyclosporine: immunology, pharmacology and therapeutic uses, *Surv Ophthalmol* 31:159, 1986.
61. Sorkin EM, Ward A: Ocular sodium cromoglycate: an overview of its therapeutic efficacy in allergic eye disease, *Drugs* 31:131, 1986.
62. Collum LMT: A three-month clinical evaluation of topical lodoxamide tromethamine for the control of allergic conjunctivitis, *26th International Congress Ophthalmology Abstracts* SP-177, 1990.
63. Rodriguez RD et al: Recent advances in the therapy of ocular allergy. In Sugar A, Soong HK, editors: *Ophthalmology clinics of North America,* Philadelphia, 1990, WB Saunders.
64. Abelson MB et al: Topical arachidonic acid: a model for screening anti-inflammatory agents, *J Ocul Pharmacol* 3:63, 1987.
65. Nishida T et al: Fibronectin promotes epithelial migration of cultured rabbit cornea in situ, *J Cell Biol* 97:1653, 1983.
66. Nishida T et al: Fibronectin, *Arch Ophthalmol* 101:1046, 1983.
67. Nishida T et al: Spontaneous persistent epithelial defects after cataract surgery, *Cornea* 6:32, 1987.
68. Fujikawa LS et al: Fibronectin in healing rabbit corneal wounds, *Lab Invest* 45:120, 1981.

A

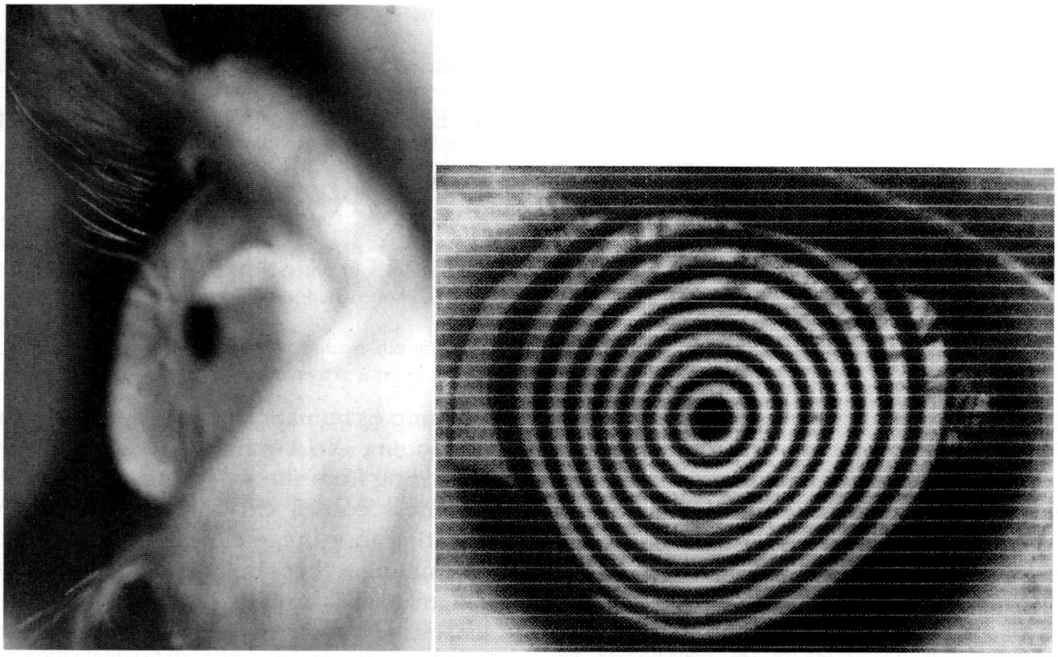

B

FIGURE 146-1 **A,** Pellucid marginal degeneration (PMCD) with normal cornea protruding above abnormal thin cornea. **B,** Corneal topography of PMCD showing vertical inferior steepening and central flattening.

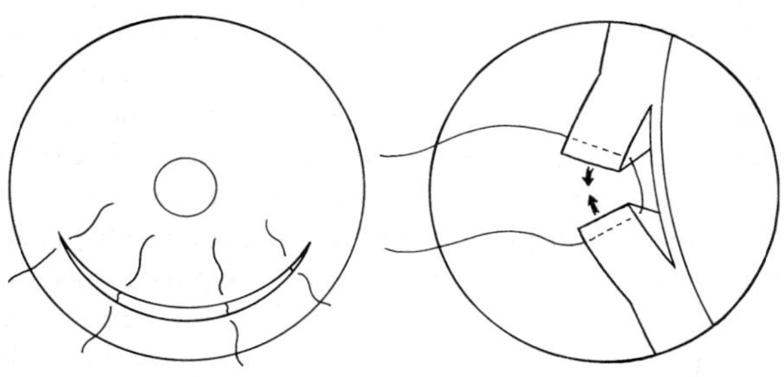

FIGURE 146-2 Corneal resection for PMCD. Sutures reappose normal-thickness stroma to normal-thickness stroma after crescent has been resected. (From Cameron JA: *Am J Ophthalmol* 113:296, 1992.)

full-thickness stroma on both sides (Figure 146-2). In a study by Cameron,[19] four of five eyes obtained 20/40 or better visual acuity with minimum follow-up of 27 months.[19] Although inferior peripheral corneal vascularization occurred in all patients, the use of donor tissue and subsequent rejection episodes are avoided. However this technique is technically more difficult and may be complicated by postoperative astigmatism.

Another method used to correct PMCD is epikeratoplasty using a 12 mm graft as described by Fronterre and Portesani.[22] Tectonic correction of the irregular astigmatism occurred in all cases to varying degrees, allowing either spectacle or contact lens wear. Total keratoplasty has also been used to correct peripheral thinning disorders. However, success has been marginal because of high rejection rates.[23-25]

Full-thickness wedge resection has also been described,[20,26] but is technically difficult, especially in phakic patients. An inferior lamellar wedge resection of the abnormal cornea will also cause corneal flattening, but is difficult to quantitiate and can lead to high postoperative astigmatism.

Our preferred technique is an inferior perpendicular incision parallel to the limbus down to Descemet's membrane. The affected tissue is undermined with a Martinez corneal dissector, and the redundant tissue is resected analogous to a facelift. The edges can be difficult to appose and may require multiple interrupted 10-0 nylon sutures with four throws or alternatively 9-0 silk (Figure 146-3). Occasionally, a paracentesis is necessary to allow reapproximation. Intraoperative keratometry is often helpful to determine the proper amount of resection and suture tension.

TERRIEN'S MARGINAL DEGENERATION

Terrien's marginal degeneration is a rare peripheral corneal thinning disorder that may take decades to progress to perforation or visually significant amounts of irregular astigmatism. More common among men in their fourth decade, the earliest changes typically occur near the superior limbus and consist of opacification and superficial neovascularization. In more advanced cases, stromal thinning and a limbal gutter with

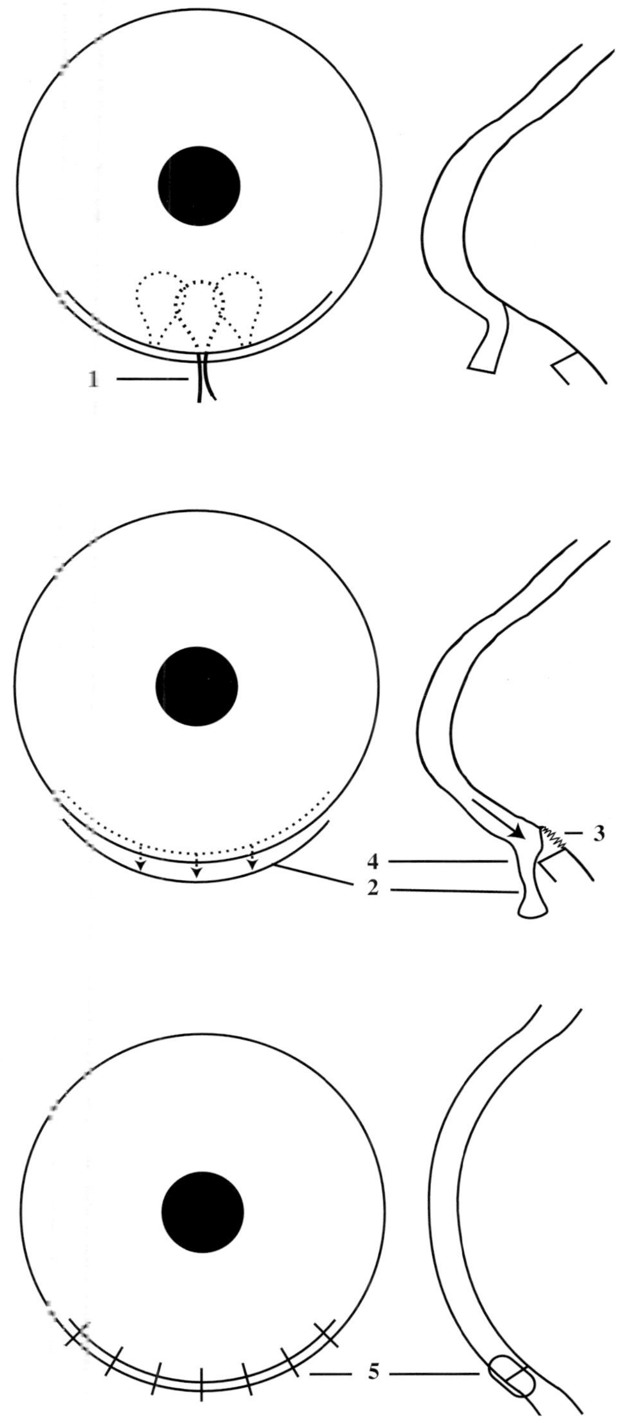

FIGURE 146-3 "Face lift" maneuver for PMCD. A Martinez lamellar dissection knife *(1)* is used to perform a pre-Descemet's dissection. Undermined corneal tissue is pulled down *(2)*, wrinkling Descemet's membrane *(3)*. The excess tissue is resected where it overhangs the incision wound *(4)*. Interrupted sutures *(5)* close the wound.

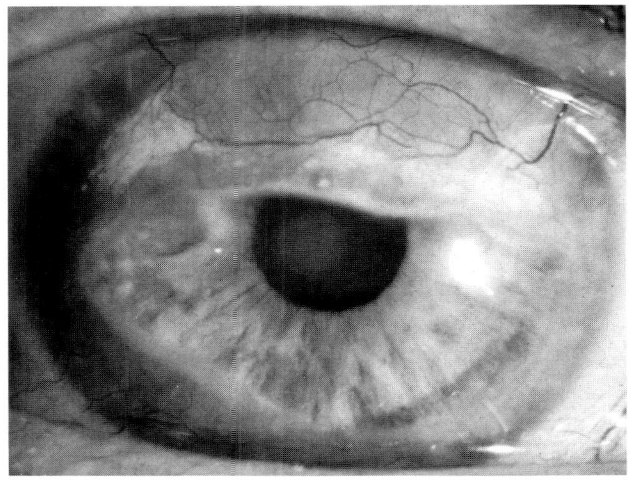

FIGURE 146-4 Terrien's marginal degeneration having 360 degrees of involvement with a large superior ectasia.

progressive ectasia may occur, causing against-the-rule astigmatism[27-28] (Figure 146-4).

Surgical correction for Terrien's degeneration is indicated for progressive thinning with imminent perforation or for severely reduced visual acuity caused by excessive astigmatism. Historically, improvement of astigmatism was accomplished through use of cautery and trichloroacetic acid.[29,30] More recently, scleral autotransplantation and lamellar keratoplasty have been used to treat this disorder.[31-33] The use of corneoscleral lamellar grafts in four eyes reported by Pettit[34] yielded satisfactory results and demonstrated long-term stability (Figure 146-5).

Full-thickness peripheral grafting has been reported by several authors for Terrien's marginal degeneration.[35-37] Brown et al.[37] noted the technical difficulties associated with a full-thickness freehand annular corneal graft and its astigmatic unpredictability.

Anderson[38] described another technique used to repair perforations caused by Terrien's marginal degeneration using a limbus-based lamellar scleral flap covered by a fornix-based conjunctival flap.

Dissection of the ectatic area down to Descemet's membrane with subsequent approximation of full-thickness stroma to full-thickness stroma was described by Caldwell et al.[39] with good results at 30 months follow-up (Figure 146-6). Another technique, described by Hahn and Kim,[40] is the two-step annular lamellar keratoplasty for severe 360 degree marginal degeneration. Annular lamellar grafts were performed 180 degrees at a time in an effort to avoid extensive donor and host surgical manipulation.

Our preferred technique is to use a corneal/scleral horseshoe graft to repair the defect. A caliper is used to determine the proper length and width of the resec-

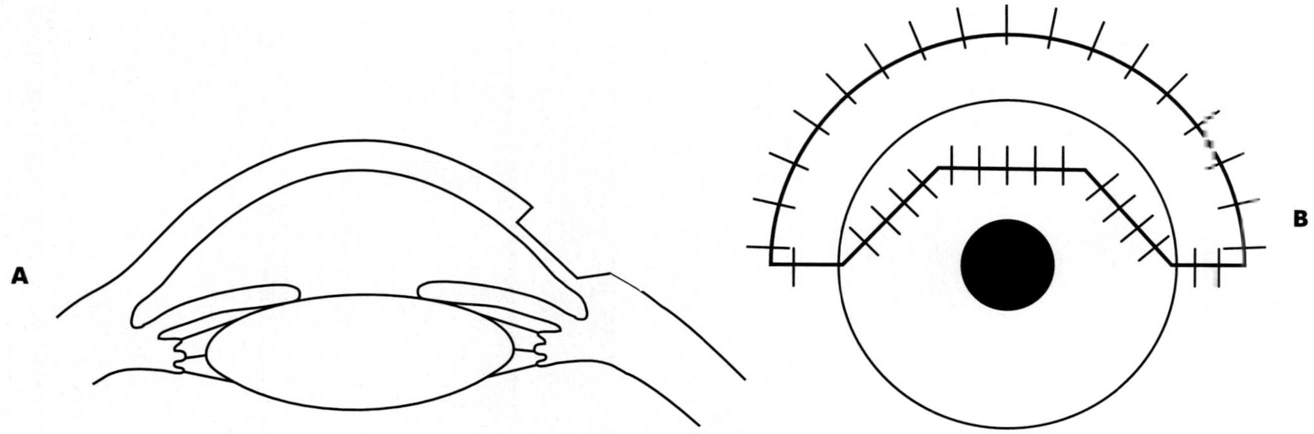

FIGURE 146-5 Diagrams of recipient bed preparation for corneoscleral lamellar graft. (Modified from Pettit TH: *Refrac Corneal Surg* 7:28, 1991.)

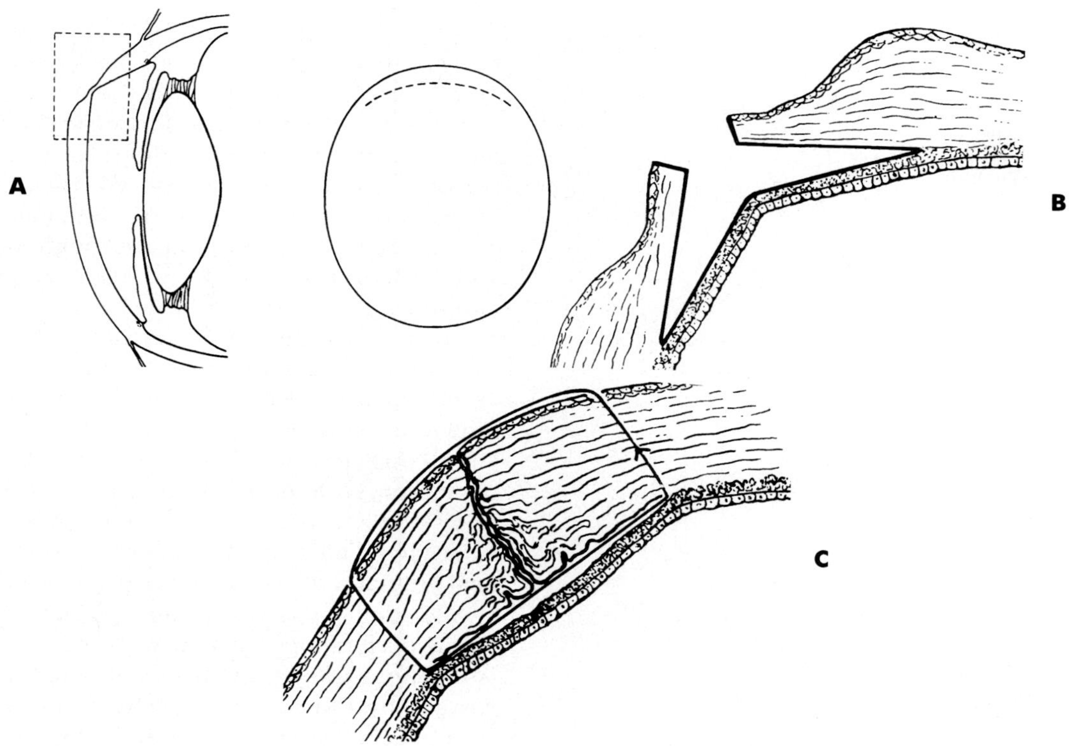

FIGURE 146-6 Dissection, resection, and approximation of corneal tissue for Terrien's marginal degeneration. **A,** Area of ectasia with resultant increased vertical diameter and flattened meridian. **B,** The area and extent of the incision at the level of Descemet's membrane. **C,** Completed suturing of dissected ectatic area. (Modified from Caldwell DR et al: *Am J Ophthalmol* 97:332, 1984.)

tion. The greater curve is outlined on the sclera with a 12 to 13 mm trephine and the lesser curve is marked on the cornea with an 8 mm trephine. Tipping the trephine results in a partial-thickness incision, which is easily completed with corneal scissors or a knife. A congruent graft is harvested from the peripheral rim of donor tissue using the same technique (Figure 146-7). In our experience, clear cornea or preserved sclera are unsatisfactory because of differing thickness and consistency. Annular, crescentric, and semicircular grafts are difficult to fashion and are technically demanding.

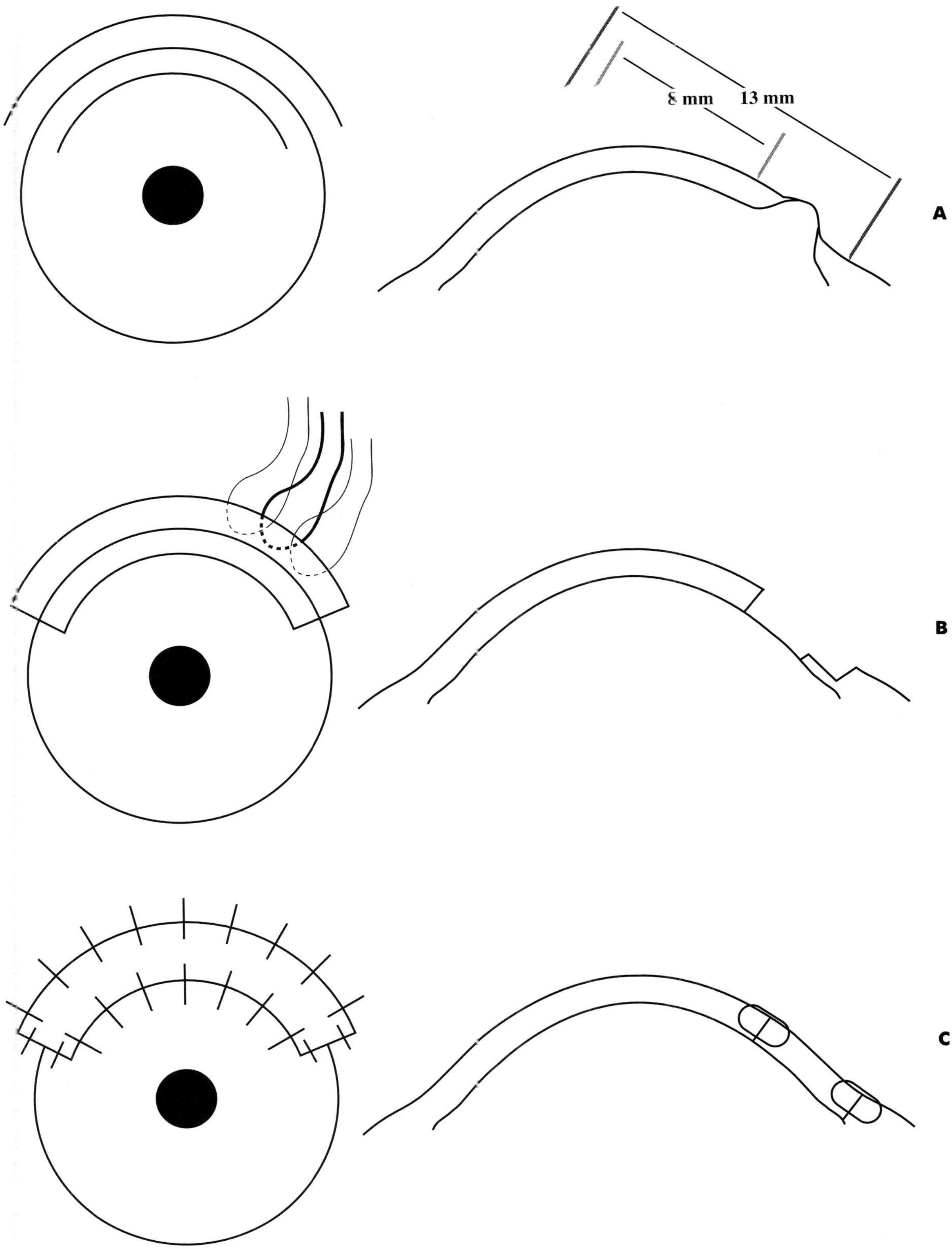

FIGURE 146-7 Method using two trephines to delineate a horseshoe graft on both donor and recipient. **A,** A greater curve is begun with a 13 mm trephine and a lesser curve with an 8 mm trephine. **B,** A lamellar bed is then dissected. Tissue is harvested from a similar location from a donor eye. **C,** The scleral portion of the wound is sutured with 8-0 vicryl while the corneal portion is sutured with 10-0 nylon.

Surgery for Peripheral Corneal Ulceration

When medical therapy fails, a variety of surgical techniques are in the ophthalmologist's armamentarium to treat peripheral corneal disease. These include lid modification, conjunctival surgery, and corneal procedures.

EYELID SURGERY

Nonhealing epithelial defects of any etiology may predispose to corneal infection and melting. If concomitant dry eye is present, it should be treated aggressively with punctal occlusion and supplemental wetting agents.

Tarsorrhaphy is a vastly underused technique for a wide variety of corneal diseases. Baum[41] described rapid healing of persistent epithelial defects following temporary tarsorrhaphy after failure with prolonged patching. Increased oxygenation and tear flow proximity were the proposed mechanisms for improvement, although other factors are probably involved. Lateral tarsorrhaphy has also been advocated in nonhealing sterile corneal ulcers.[42]

Apposition of the lids can be achieved by Frost suture, tarsal pillar,[43] intermarginal adhesion, or cyanoacrylate glue. Patients with seventh or fifth cranial nerve denervation and those with lid contour abnormalities may also benefit from tarsorrhaphy.[44] The tarsorraphy should be maintained until the cornea heals and should be combined with punctal occlusion if the eye is dry.

CONJUNCTIVAL SURGERY

Partial or total *conjunctival flaps* are useful for patients with corneal disease unresponsive to or intolerant of bandage soft contact lenses (with or without tissue adhesive), as well as for those who respond poorly to tarsorrhaphy. Debilitated patients and others may benefit from this procedure, which often allows a future sight-restoring penetrating keratoplasty.

Eyes with severe corneal thinning and poor visual potential may also be candidates for conjunctival flaps.[45,46] Before the introduction of antibiotics, conjunctival flap surgery was frequently used and was greatly improved after Gunderson advocated dissection of Tenon's capsule from the conjunctival sling.[47,48] Conjunctival flaps are of questionable value in cases of imminent perforation in which tectonic support is necessary or as a sole procedure once perforation has occurred.

In the past, peripheral corneal ulcerations were managed using the *"blow-out" patch* technique. A large piece of Tenon's capsule (obtained from the fornix) was sutured over a perforation. Dohlman et al.[49] later described the use of transparent silicone rubber to overlay a lamellar plug in corneal perforations. Penetrating keratoplasty would be performed at a later time when the inflammation had subsided; however, others described complications of this technique including ulceration of the patch, dehiscence of the graft with "cheese wiring," and persistent defects.[50]

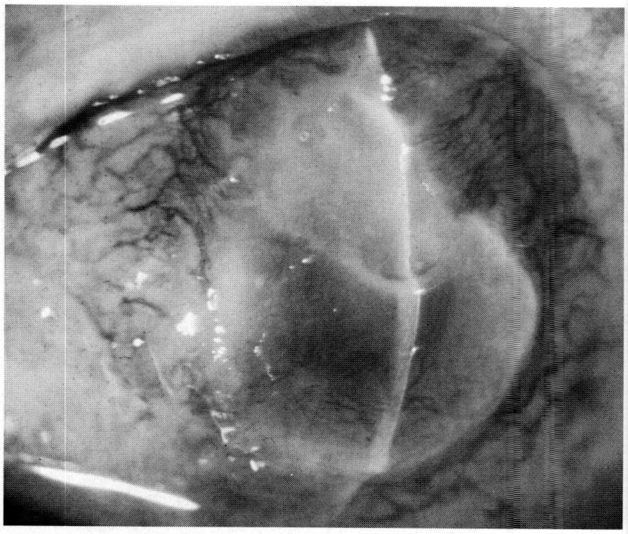

FIGURE 146-8 Mooren's ulcer with corneal destruction and overhanging edge.

Limbal conjunctival resection is indicated in cases of noninfected peripheral thinning disorders associated with Mooren's ulcer, rheumatoid arthritis, Wegener's granulomatosis, and Sjögren's syndrome.[51,52] Presumably, this technique removes the source of collagenase as described by Eiferman et al.[53] The resection should extend 3 to 4 mm posteriorly and well beyond the affected area.[7,42] Concomitant use of cytotoxic agents (e.g., cyclophosphamide) as described by Foster,[7] has shown improved rates of arrest of the thinning process.

Mooren's ulcer exemplifies a peripheral ulcerative disorder for which conjunctival resection is the first step. First described in 1849, its cause remains obscure and it is often resistant to medical-surgical therapies.[54] The disease affects the peripheral cornea as an undermining sterile ulcer spreading circumlimbally or centripetally[55] (Figure 146-8). Evidence that this is an immunologically mediated disease is suggested by some authors,[56,57] and medical treatment is directed toward reversing a type III immune complex disorder by immunosuppression.[7]

Surgical correction for Mooren's typically begins with conjunctival resection as previously described.[7,58]

A 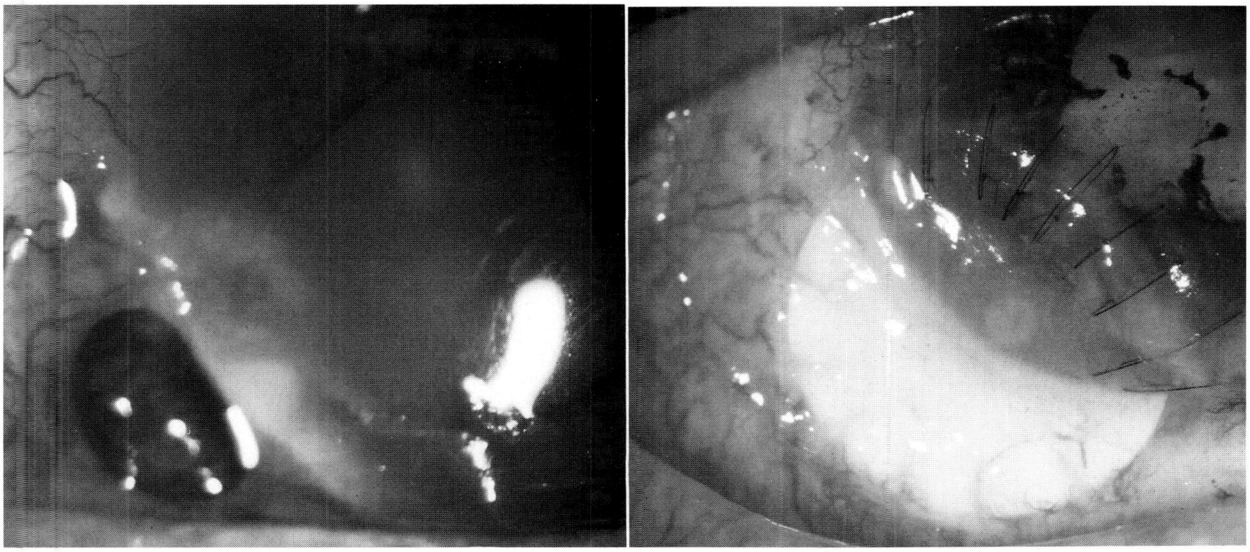 B

FIGURE 146-9 **A,** Peripheral ulcerative keratitis with perforation in a patient with rheumatoid arthritis. **B,** Corneal/scleral graft for the perforation. The donor was trephined eccentrically to match the limbal involvement.

If perforation has occurred, tectonic support using tissue adhesives may obviate the need for patch graft or conjunctival flap. Extensive ulceration may be treated with a lamellar graft, which may temporarily provide tectonic support for a future penetrating graft. Recurrence of the disease in the graft is well documented, and immunosuppression before treatment is necessary.[7,59] In unrelenting cases, removal of the remaining clear cornea may be the only way to control the disease. Lamellar or penetrating grafts can then be attempted.[60]

CORNEAL SURGERY

If a peripheral corneal graft is necessary, it is technically easier to place full-thickness donor tissue into a lamellar bed than to perform a penetrating keratoplasty. The donor tissue must be cut eccentrically using the limbus as a reference; this technique ensures proper peripheral thickness and orientation, especially if the graft includes the sclera (Figure 146-9). However, if a circular graft impinges on the visual axis it will produce objectionable irregular astigmatism.

A combination of lamellar donor graft and tissue adhesive has also been described.[61] Penetrating keratoplasty performed during active inflammation and infection is often unsuccessful, and a patch graft (with or without adhesive) can provide a temporizing or permanent solution.[62]

TISSUE ADHESIVE

The application of tissue adhesive is a useful modality for both imminent and actual corneal perforations. Early formulations of the cyanoacrylates were first used for ocular purposes in 1963, but were noted to produce moderate corneal haze and inflammatory reactions.[63,64] Glue was used initially to bond alloplastic materials to the cornea in the case of severe chemical burns.[65]

Current formulations of tissue adhesive have significantly improved tissue compatibility (especially n-butyl-2-cyanoacrylate), although none have been approved by the Food and Drug Administration. Glue has multiple beneficial effects. It provides tectonic support and antibacterial action. It physically excludes the collagenases present in polymorphonuclear leukocytes both in the tears and in the stroma, which are believed to be responsible for keratolysis.[66-69] Healing occurs under the adhesive by fibroblast formation and occasional vascular ingrowth.

Techniques of application are varied. We prefer to deliver the cyanoacrylate to the dried cornea through a small-bore needle and then draw it across the defect by capillary action with a cellulose sponge. It rapidly polymerizes without excessive accumulation and permits easy application of a bandage lens. Perforations less than 1.5 mm are easily plugged by using this technique. In addition, tissue adhesives are an excellent temporizing measure before definitive surgical correction is undertaken.[70]

ALTERNATIVE SURGICAL APPROACHES

Deep peripheral defects occasionally can be treated with cryotherapy. An iceball is placed at the limbus and allowed to encompass the ulcer. A triple freeze-thaw cycle causes fibroblast formation and neovas-

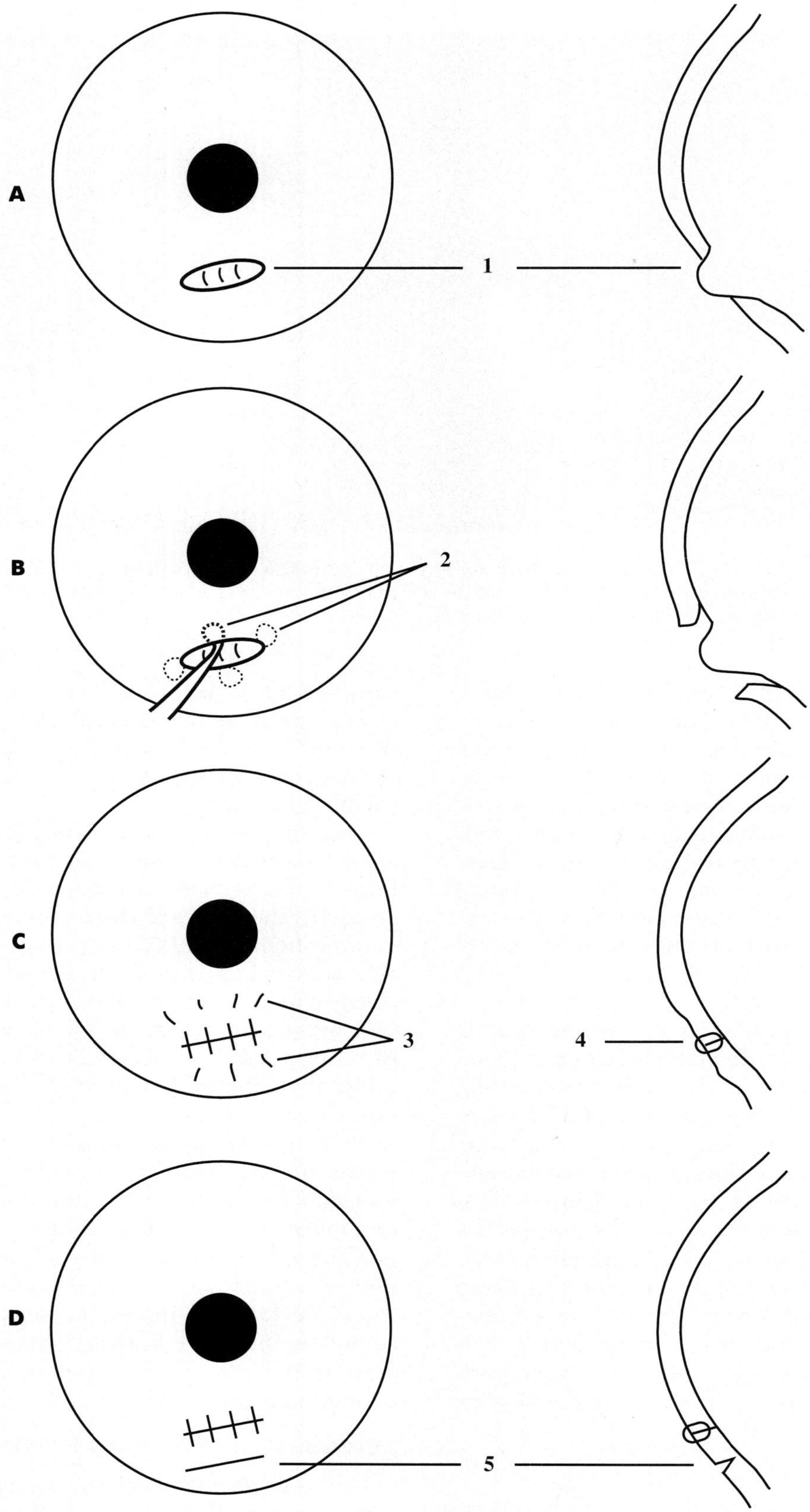

FIGURE 146-10 **A,** Large oval descemetocele *(1).* **B,** A lamellar dissector is used to undermine surrounding tissue *(2)* so that it can slide toward sutured wound. **C,** Closing the wound results in stress on surrounding tissue *(3)* and localized corneal flattening *(4).* **D,** A relaxing incision *(5)* relieves the stress and flattening.

cularization and may avoid the need for invasive surgery.

If a nonsighted eye or an eye with a poor prognosis presents with a large descemetocele, it can be oversewn by undermining the edges. This maneuver is facilitated by a deep relaxing incision parallel to the defect, which allows corneal tissue to slide toward the affected area (Figure 146-10).

Periosteal grafting from the anterior tibial plateau has been used to patch both sclera and peripheral corneal ulcers recalcitrant to other treatments.[50,71] The strength, avascularity, and lack of immune reaction make this tissue favorable for corneal tectonic support. The graft is easily harvested with a Freer elevator, placed under the conjunctiva, and anchored to the limbus, using either absorbable or nylon sutures.

REFERENCES

1. Grayson M: Marginal furrows: a characteristic corneal lesion of rheumatoid arthritis, *Arch Ophthalmol* 79:563, 1968.
2. Gold DH, Henkind P: Ocular findings in systemic lupus erythematosus, *Br J Ophthalmol* 56:800, 1972.
3. Spaeth GL: Corneal staining in systemic lupus erythematosus, *N Engl J Med* 276:1168, 1967.
4. Halmay O, Ludwig K: Bilateral band-shaped deep keratitis and iridocyclitis in systemic lupus erythematosus, *Br J Ophthalmol* 48:558, 1964.
5. Berman MB, Davidson P, Dohlman CH: Characterization of collagenolytic activity in the cornea, *Exp Eye Res* 11:255, 1971.
6. Wise GN: Ocular periarteritis nodosa, *Arch Ophthalmol* 48:1, 1952.
7. Foster CS: Conjunctiva, cornea, and sclera. In Albert D, Jakobiec F, editors: *Principles & practice of ophthalmology,* Philadelphia, 1994, WB Saunders.
8. Fauci AS, Wolff SM: Wegener's granulomatosis: studies in 18 patients and review of the literature, *Medicine* 52:535, 1973.
9. Bullen CL et al: Ocular complications of Wegener's granulomatosis, *Ophthalmology* 90:270, 1983.
10. Krachmer JH: Pellucid marginal corneal degeneration, *Arch Ophthalmol* 96:1217, 1978.
11. Zucchini G: Su di un caso di degenerazione marginale della cornea-varieta inferiore pellucida-studio clinico ed istologico, *Ann Ottalmol Clin Ocul* 88:47, 1962.
12. Parker DL, McDonnell PJ, Barraquer J, Green WR: Pellucid marginal corneal degeneration, *Cornea* 5:115, 1986.
13. Carter JB, Jones DB, Wilhelmus KR: Acute hydrops in pellucid marginal corneal degeneration, *Am J Ophthalmol* 107:167, 1989
14. Rodrigues MM et al: Pellucid marginal corneal degeneration: clinicopathologic study of two cases, *Exp Eye Res* 33:277, 1981.
15. Pouliquen Y et al: Acute corneal edema in pellucid marginal degeneration or acute marginal keratoconus, *Cornea* 6:169, 1987.
16. Speaker MG, Arentsen JJ, Laibson PR: Long-term survival of larger diameter penetrating keratoplasties for keratoconus and pellucid marginal degeneration, *Acta Ophthalmol Suppl (Copenh)* 192:17, 1989.
17. Varley GA, Macsai MS, Krachmer JH: The results of penetrating keratoplasty for pellucid marginal corneal degeneration, *Am J Ophthalmol* 110:149, 1990.
18. Schanzlin DJ, Sarno EM, Robin JB: Crescentic lamellar keratoplasty for pellucid marginal degeneration, *Am J Ophthalmol* 96:253, 1983.
19. Cameron JA: Results of lamellar crescentic resection for pellucid marginal corneal degeneration, *Am J Ophthalmol* 113:296, 1992.
20. Barraquer F: Results of the crescent resection in keratotorus, *Dev Ophthalmol* 5:49, 1981.
21. Duran JA, Rodriguez-Ares MT, Torres D: Crescentic resection for the treatment of pellucid corneal marginal degeneration, *Ophthalmic Surg* 22:153, 1991.
22. Fronterre A, Portesani GP: Epikeratoplasty for pellucid marginal corneal degeneration, *Cornea* 10:450, 1991.
23. Mohammadi H, Morton RL, Wetterholm D: Total keratoplasty in peripheral corneal degeneration, *Ophthalmic Surg* 13:400, 1982.
24. Ticho U, Ben-Sira I: Total keratoplasty, *Arch Ophthalmol* 90:104, 1973.
25. Barraguer J: Total penetrating keratoplasty, *Proc R Soc Med* 54:1116, 1961.
26. Dubroff S: Pellucid marginal corneal degeneration. Report on corrective surgery, *J Cataract Refract Surg* 15:89, 1989.
27. Richards WW: Marginal degeneration of the cornea with perforation, *Arch Ophthalmol* 70:72, 1963.
28. Terrien F. La dystrophie marginale ectatizue de la cornee, *Arch Ophtalmol (Paris)* 38:523, 1921.
29. Gifford RS: Marginal dystrophy of cornea: furrow keratitis, *Am J Ophthalmol* 8:16, 1925.
30. Admantidades B: Un cas d'ectasie circonscite de la cornee, *Arch Ophtalmol (Paris)* 30:46, 1910.
31. Hinken MV: Marginal degenerations of the cornea, *Arch Ophthalmol* 72:29, 1964.
32. Leigh AG: *Corneal transplantation,* Oxford, 1966, Blackwell Scientific Publications.
33. Christensen L: Corneoscleroplasty with scalpel, *Trans Pac Coast Otoophthalmol Soc Annu Meet* 45:323, 1964.
34. Pettit TH: Corneoscleral freehand lamellar keratoplasty in Terrien's marginal degeneration of the cornea-long term results, *Refract Corneal Surg* 7:28, 1991.
35. Binder PS, Zavala FY, Stainer GA: Noninfectious peripheral corneal ulceration: Mooren's ulcer or Terrien's marginal degeneration, *Ann Ophthalmol* 14:425, 1982.
36. Legrand J, Hervouet F: Ectasie marginale de la cornee (maladie de Terrien) keratoplastie-etude anatomopathologique, *Ann Ocul (Paris)* 186:7, 1953.
37. Brown AC, Rao GN, Aquavella JV: Peripheral corneal grafts in Terrien's marginal degeneration, *Ophthalmic Surg* 14:931, 1983.
38. Anderson FG: Repair of marginal furrow perforation, *Ophthalmic Surg* 8:25, 1977.
39. Caldwell DR et al: Primary surgical repair of severe peripheral marginal ectasia in Terrien's marginal degeneration, *Am J Ophthalmol* 97:332, 1984.
40. Hahn TW, Kim JH: Two step annular tectonic lamellar keratoplasty in severe Terrien's marginal degeneration, *Ophthalmic Surg* 24:831, 1993.
41. Baum J: The advantages of partial patching or tarsorrhaphy over complete eyelid closure, *Am J Ophthalmol* 103:339, 1987.
42. Donzis PB, Mondino BJ: Management of noninfectious corneal ulcers, *Surv Ophthalmol* 32:94, 1987.
43. Tanenbaum M et al: The tarsal pillar technique for narrowing and maintenance of the interpalpebral fissure, *Ophthalmic Surg* 23:418, 1992.
44. Grayson M: *Diseases of the cornea,* St Louis, 1983, Mosby.
45. Paton D, Milauskas AT: Indications, surgical technique, and results of thin conjunctival flaps on the cornea: a review of 122 consecutive cases, *Int Ophthalmol Clin* 10:329, 1970.
46. Insler MS, Pechous B: Conjunctival flaps revisited, *Ophthalmic Surg* 10:329, 1970.

47. DeSchweinitz GE: *Diseases of the eye,* Philadelphia, 1924, WB Saunders.
48. Gunderson T: Conjunctival flaps in the treatment of corneal disease with reference to a new technique of application, *Arch Ophthalmol* 60:880, 1958.
49. Dohlman CH, Boruchoff SA, Sullivan GL: A technique for the repair of perforated corneal ulcers, *Arch Ophthalmol* 77:519, 1967.
50. Portnoy SL, Insler MS, Kaufman HE: Surgical management of corneal ulceration and perforation, *Surv Ophthalmol* 34:1, 1989.
51. Wilson FM, Grayson M, Ellis FD: Treatment of peripheral corneal ulcers by limbal conjunctivectomy, *Br J Ophthalmol* 60:713, 1976.
52. Bloomfield SE et al: Bilateral necrotizing scleritis with marginal corneal ulceration after cataract surgery in a patient with vasculitis, *Br J Ophthalmol* 64:170, 1980.
53. Eiferman RA, Yankeelov J, Carothers D: Peripheral rheumatoid ulceration and evidence for conjunctival collagenase production, *Am J Ophthalmol* 87:703, 1979.
54. Bowman W: Case 12, p. 112 in the parts concerned in the operations of the eye (1849), cited by Nettleship, E.: Chronic serpiginous ulcer of the cornea (Mooren's ulcer), *Trans Ophthalmol Soc UK* 22:103, 1902.
55. Wood TO, Kaufman HE: Mooren's ulcer, *Am J Ophthalmol* 71:417, 1971.
56. Foster CS et al: The immunopathology of Mooren's ulcer, *Am J Ophthalmol* 88:149, 1979.
57. Berkowitz PJ et al: Presence of circulating immune complexes in patients with peripheral corneal disease, *Arch Ophthalmol* 101:242, 1983.
58. Brown SI, Mondino BJ: Therapy of Mooren's ulcer, *Am J Ophthalmol* 98:1, 1984.
59. King JH: Destructive marginal ulceration. A saga of surgical therapy, *Trans Am Ophthalmol Soc* 63:311, 1965.
60. Martin HF, Stark WJ, Maumenee AC: Treatment of Mooren's and Mooren's-like ulcer by lamellar keratectomy, *Ophthalmic Surg* 181:564, 1987.
61. Hyndiuk RA, Hull DS, Kinyoun JL: Free tissue patch and cyanoacrylate in corneal perforations, *Ophthalmic Surg* 5:50, 1947.
62. Nobe JR et al: Results of penetrating keratoplasty for the treatment of corneal perforations, *Arch Ophthalmol* 108:939, 1990.
63. Straatsma BR et al: Experimental studies employing adhesive compounds in ophthalmic surgery, *Trans Am Ophthalmol Otolaryngol* 57:320, 1963.
64. Bloomfield S, Barnert A, Kanter P: The use of Eastman 910 monomer as an adhesive in ocular surgery. I. Biologica effects on ocular tissues, *Am J Ophthalmol* 55:742, 1963
65. Wagoner MD, Kenyon KR: Chemical injuries. In Shingleton BJ, Hersh PS, Kenyon KR, editors: *Eye Trauma,* St Louis, 1991, Mosby.
66. Hirst LW, Smiddy WE, Stark WJ: Corneal perforations: changing methods of treatment, 1960-1980, *Ophthalmology* 89:630, 1982.
67. Eiferman RA, Snyder J: Antimicrobial properties of cyanoacrylate adhesives, *Invest Ophthalmol Vis Sci (Suppl)* 22:2 198[illegible].
68. Snip RC, Kenyon KR: Acute inflammatory cells in melting human corneas, *Invest Ophthalmol Vis Sci (Suppl)* 17:252 1978.
69. Fogle JA, Kenyon KR, Foster C: Tissue adhesive arrests stromal melting in human cornea, *Am J Ophthalmol* 89:795, 1980.
70. Refojo MF et al: Evaluation of adhesives for corneal surgery, *Arch Ophthalmol* 80:645, 1968.
71. Koenig SB, Kaufman HE: The treatment of necrotizing scleritis with an autogenous periosteal graft, *Ophthalmic Surg* 14:1029, 1983.

CHAPTER 147

ROGER H.S. LANGSTON

Penetrating Keratoplasty in Herpes Simplex Disease

Performing penetrating keratoplasty in eyes that have been damaged by herpes simplex disease is challenging. Even in the best of circumstances, one can anticipate unpredictable episodes of recurrent epithelial, stromal, or uveitic herpetic disease; epithelial healing problems; and graft rejections. Surgery may be required in severely inflamed eyes with complicating anterior segment problems such as glaucoma and cataract. Treatment modalities are often in conflict. Topical corticosteroids tend to exacerbate dendritic keratitis and stromal melting. Topical antivirals tend to contribute to epithelial healing problems. Nonetheless, the results of surgery for this difficult problem continue to improve as we understand more of the pathophysiology and refine our surgical, perioperative, and postoperative management efforts.

Indications

Indications for corneal transplantation in herpetic keratitis may be, singly or severally, improvement in vision, restoration of the structural integrity of the eye, arrest of the disease process, and rehabilitation of the patient.

With respect to restoration of vision, it is worth noting that most patients who require a transplantation for herpetic disease have a normal fellow eye. Bilateral herpetic keratitis is unusual.[1] Consider also that the average amount of astigmatism after keratoplasty is approximately 4 diopters, that the astigmatism may be oblique, and that penetrating keratoplasty tends to induce myopia. Thus even if the patient has a clear graft after surgery, a contact lens may be required to achieve balanced binocular vision. This information should be included in the patient's preoperative counseling.

Reports in the literature about the prognosis for a clear graft and the potential for good vision vary substantially. At 2 years or more after surgery, it may be as low as 15% or as high as 90%, depending mainly on the disease activity at the time of surgery.[2] Visual outcome is usually less satisfactory than the chance for clear graft. Ficker et al.,[3] in reviewing recent experience at Moorefields Eye Hospital, noted a best corrected vision of 20/40 or better in only 71% of patients who had clear grafts. Causes for the discrepancy included cataract, glaucoma, amblyopia, retinal detachment, traumatic expulsive hemorrhage, and macular degeneration, in order of decreasing frequency.

Surgery to maintain the structural integrity of the eye is usually required because of perforation or impending perforation of a corneal ulcer with stromal melting, often exacerbated by the use of topical corticosteroids. Although the chance of success, as measured by clear vision, is low under these circumstances, the chance of maintaining or restoring the structural integrity of the eye is excellent.[2] Some surgeons have suggested managing perforations with glue or lamellar patch grafts and then performing a penetrating keratoplasty for vision at a later date.[2,4] In one report, 11 of 13 grafts remained clear when the initial treatment of a perforation had been cyanoacrylate tissue adhesive or a lamellar patch, followed with a penetrating keratoplasty for vision, in comparison to only one of six in which the initial perforation had been repaired by a penetrating keratoplasty.[2]

Herpetic disciform, interstitial, and neurotrophic keratitis tend to be both persistent and recurrent and often are associated with uveitis, cataract formation and secondary glaucoma. Hence, on occasion surgery is undertaken to limit the secondary anterior segment damage caused by the chronic inflammation and also to limit the socioeconomic consequences of chronic illness. To be sure, herpetic eye disease is recurrent, primarily because the virus is repeatedly shed from the trigeminal ganglion. It is also clear that the results of surgery are better in an eye without active disease. Nonetheless, a smoldering keratouveitis may be treated by a penetrating keratoplasty once it is clear that vision will not be restored without it, and it is also established that letting the disease "burn out" is not satisfactory for the patient. Studies have shown that with vigorous use of topical corticosteroids before and after surgery and concomitant coverage with topical

the eye to be operated on. It should include a review of others' records on the patient, if available, to look for evidence of concomitant disease including cataract, glaucoma, pressure rises associated with steroid use or maculopathy. In addition, other conditions that might affect the outcome such as AIDS, atopy, rosacea, and tear deficiency should be looked for. Evidence of blepharitis should be sought and treated when found. The tendency for herpetic patients to have recurrent and persistent epithelial defects may make them more likely to have secondary bacterial infections from blepharitis and other sources.[13] In one series the incidence of bacterial infection complicating recurrent epithelial disease was 10%.[3]

Preoperative examination should address the same issues and should include an accurate measurement of the intraocular pressure, and gonioscopy, if possible, to assess the status of the angle.

It may be interesting to check corneal sensation preoperatively, although in herpes simplex disease, as opposed to herpes zoster, it is unusual for the anesthesia to be so profound as to influence outcome. In any case, grafts in patients with herpes simplex disease appear to remain anesthetic for years.[14]

Preoperative keratometric readings will probably be irregular, but may show a flat cornea if scarring is extensive. This finding may influence surgical technique, as discussed later. Temporary placement of a hard contact lens may facilitate preoperative assessment of visual potential, because in many cases an irregular corneal surface, rather than stromal scarring, is the major cause of the patient's visual loss.

As mentioned previously, the preoperative evaluation should include an assessment and a frank discussion of the patient's ability to participate in postoperative care. Because of this issue in children and because studies show that in unilateral surgery the major determinant of outcome with regard to amblyopia is the age of the patient when vision was lost (not the age at the time of surgery),[15] it may be sensible to postpone surgery until adulthood. This approach avoids the technical problems of pediatric keratoplasty. Further, the pediatric cornea remodels much more rapidly than that of the adult. In some cases, in which the major vision loss was due to an irregular cornea surface, vision may improve spontaneously as the cornea smooths. When pediatric keratoplasty is required, careful preoperative counseling of the family and continued support postoperatively are usually necessary because the infant or child often will not spontaneously report problems.

Donor Tissue Requirements

Uveitis, glaucoma, and recurrent graft rejection episodes—all of which damage the corneal endothelium—are common after penetrating keratoplasty for herpetic keratitis. This finding argues for selecting younger donor tissue with a high endothelial cell density. Although there are no studies to support this need, Cobo et al.[8] noted a greater incidence of early graft failure in herpetic patients who had active inflammation at the time of surgery. They postulated that this outcome might be due to the technical difficulties of the surgery in an inflamed or perforated eye, coupled with the damage from the anterior segment inflammation.

Persistent epithelial defects are also common after penetrating keratoplasty for herpetic keratitis. Although retrospective studies do not show a difference in the incidence of persistent epithelial defects between donor corneas with intact epithelium and those in which it was removed at the time of surgery,[2] many surgeons prefer to use tissue with intact epithelium and without exposure damage in herpetic cases. Tissue with a short death-to-preservation time may have some advantage in this regard.

Because grafting for herpes is often performed in high-risk patients, there has been interest in assessing the value of tissue matching. Volker-Dieben et al. reviewed their experience in 288 penetrating keratoplasties for herpetic keratitis, 110 of which were human leukocyte antigen (HLA) matched. They found a 2-year survival rate of 74% for matched grafts, compared to 59% for unmatched grafts.[16] However, the results of the Collaborative Corneal Transplantation Studies[17] in the United States did not support the value of tissue matching.

Preoperative Medications

A broad-spectrum prophylactic antibiotic regimen, like that used for cataract surgery, is probably wise. Mydriatic drops should be given if the patient is undergoing concomitant cataract surgery. If the patient is not, miotics may be given to protect the lens or hyaloid face, but should be withheld in very inflamed eyes. In severely inflamed eyes, pretreatment with topical corticosteroids, as often as every hour, is helpful. Systemic corticosteroids may also be of value. It is important to minimize the inflammation in order to limit damage to the graft and to the rest of the anterior segment. The use of diamox or osmotic agents is generally unnecessary before penetrating keratoplasty.

A B

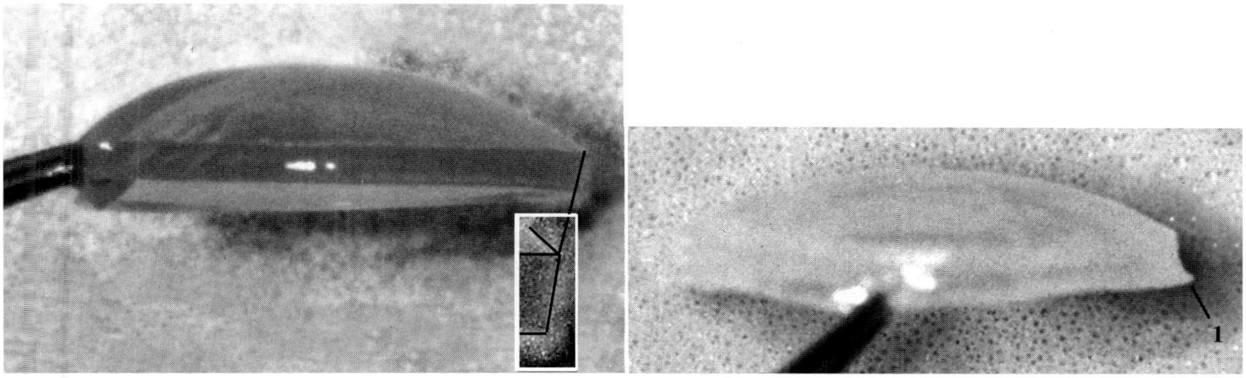

FIGURE 147-2 **A,** A donor button punched from the endothelial side has a narrower diameter posteriorly (*inset*). **B,** In contrast a host button obtained by full-thickness trephination with a vacuum trephine has a larger diameter posteriorly *(1)*. This mismatch leads to a posterior wound disparity, which induces myopia and astigmatism. Consequently, full-thickness trephination with a vacuum trephine should be avoided.

Anesthesia

Local anesthesia, using a combination of lidocaine and bupivacaine, achieves excellent results in penetrating keratoplasty in an intact globe under elective conditions. General anesthesia is more appropriate in a perforated globe.

Some sort of pressure reducer, such as the Honan balloon, may have value in penetrating keratoplasty. Bourne[13] has shown that preoperative hypotony induced by intermittent digital massage results in less endothelial cell loss in phakic keratoplasties.

Surgical Technique

Because no recent studies have compared surgical techniques in grafting for herpes simplex, the following discussion is my preference based on 25 years of experience.

A Flieringa, or other scleral support ring, is unnecessary except in younger patients who are or will become aphakic. It seems wise to limit the surgical trauma in herpetic patients.

The donor button should be cut before the host button. If it is punched from the endothelial side it should be 0.1 to 0.2 mm larger than the host button and, perhaps, 0.5 mm larger if the host cornea has been severely flattened by scarring. Heavily scarred corneal tissue does not swell as much as normal tissue. Under these circumstances using a larger donor button or fashioning a large bevel on the host tissue helps avoid wound leaks and dehiscences.

If the host cornea is heavily vascularized, it may be useful to make several small incisions through the corneal vessels at the limbus to allow bleeding and clotting to occur there, rather than in the trephine wound where it can obscure the surgeon's view or bleed into the vitreous and delay visual rehabilitation.

The host button must be large enough, usually 7.0 to 9.0 mm, to encompass the pathology and provide an optically satisfactory result. Clinical studies evaluating the effect of graft size on rejection and graft failure are contradictory. Animal studies show that grafts that approach the limbus have a higher risk of rejection.[19] The graft should be centered as much as possible to minimize astigmatism in the visual axis. If a vacuum trephine is used, viscoelastic may be necessary to improve fixation on a scarred cornea. Trephination is ordinarily carried through the anterior one third of the host cornea and excision completed with scissors, because full-thickness trephination with a vacuum trephine tends to lead to a disparity in shape between the host and donor, with a posterior dehiscence that results in increased astigmatism and myopia (Figure 147-2). The host button should be kept in saline until the donor button is in place, because occasionally some misadventure will preclude the use of the donor button.

In a perforated eye, the intraocular pressure must be raised before trephination is undertaken. If the perforation is small, placing viscoelastic in the anterior chamber through a paracentesis incision may suffice. Otherwise cyanoacrylate adhesive or a patch graft may be necessary to close the perforation before trephination (Figure 147-3). Under these circumstances, patch grafts can be fashioned from the rim of donor tissue, unused or preserved donor tissue, the patient's sclera, or even soft contact lens material.

In general, viscoelastics are useful as space maintainers in the anterior chamber. In inflamed eyes, they

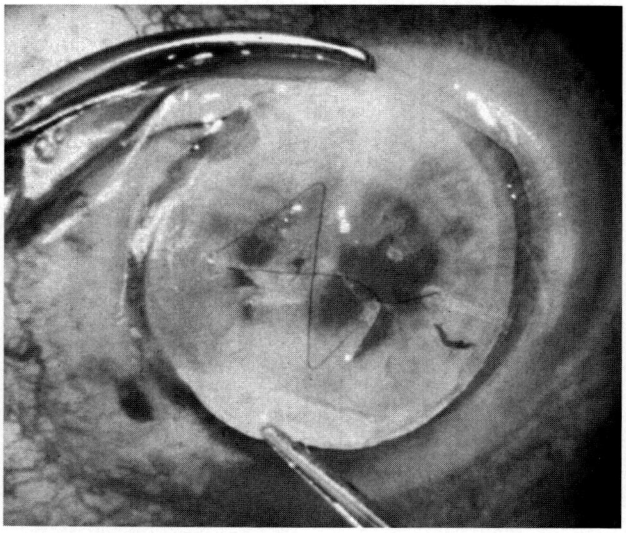

FIGURE 147-3 A small patch graft can be used to close a large perforation temporarily to facilitate trephination of the host cornea.

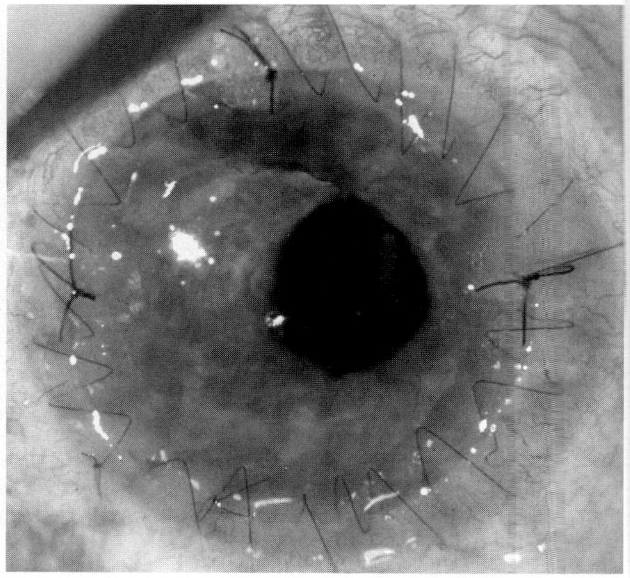

FIGURE 147-4 Stabilization of the iris diaphragm by suturing iris defects may prevent formation of synechiae and postoperative angle-closure glaucoma.

are especially useful to keep iris tissue from adhering to the cornea and to limit bleeding and exudation of fibrin from the iris. Most of the viscoelastic should be replaced with saline solution at the end of surgery to avoid extreme pressure rises. However, some can generally be left in the angle if necessary to prevent synechia formation. Inflamed iris tissue tends to form synechiae to the keratoplasty wound. This can lead to a progressive postoperative "zippering" shut of the angle over time. Because of this phenomenon, there may be value in performing a simple iris repair with prolene sutures on a vascular needle if the iris is floppy and unstable (Figure 147-4). Anterior synechiae are also associated with an increased risk of graft rejection.[20]

Concomitant anterior segment surgery can be performed as needed. In noninflamed eyes, there appears to be no difference in graft survival rate when penetrating keratoplasties are compared with penetrating keratoplasties combined with cataract surgery.[21] Because of the tendency of herpetic patients to have recurrent inflammation, capsule fixated intraocular lenses should be used during cataract surgery rather than sulcus or iris fixated lenses.

In an inflamed eye, it may be preferable to limit surgical manipulation and perform cataract surgery later. On the other hand, removal of the cataractous lens may deepen the anterior chamber and reduce the risk of postoperative glaucoma. Graft failure is more likely when combined surgery is performed in inflamed eyes.[3] Intracapsular cataract extraction, especially combined with vitrectomy, has a much worse prognosis than extracapsular extraction.[3]

Vitrectomy should be performed when vitreous appears in the anterior chamber, as vitreoendothelial contact is clearly associated with an increased risk of graft decompensation. Vitreous in the anterior chamber also predisposes to anterior synechiae and glaucoma.[20]

Monofilament nylon sutures are appropriate. Although a running suture can be placed more quickly and often requires less care after surgery than do interrupted sutures, there is a tendency for the corneal wound to heal asymmetrically in vascularized or scarred corneas. The suture often loosens in the healed area. Because loose sutures tend to be associated with inflammation, recurrence of keratitis, and rejection,[3] they should be removed when encountered. Removal is difficult with a running suture that must be adjusted to remove the slack or cut and retied, which often leads to excessive astigmatism. Consequently, interrupted sutures are preferable. Sutures must not be too tight, as they can bunch the tissue at the wound margin and lead to a flat cornea centrally (Figure 147-5), predisposing to epithelial defects in the graft. Knots should be buried to minimize inflammation.

Because of the tendency for epithelial healing problems in herpetic eyes, particular attention should be paid to keeping the donor epithelium from drying or being otherwise traumatized during the surgery.

At the end of the case, prophylactic antibiotics are given along with topical corticosteroids. In cases of severe inflammation, use of systemic steroids may be warranted. Depot corticosteroids should never be injected in patients with herpes simplex disease because

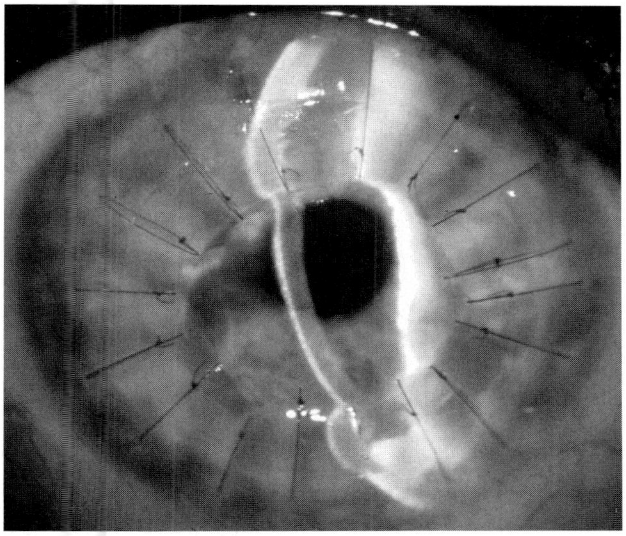

FIGURE 147-5 Excessively tight sutures should be avoided as they can predispose to corneal wetting problems and persistent epithelial defects.

they cannot be removed if there is a recurrence of dendritic keratitis. Corticosteroid dosage is arbitrarily titrated against inflammatory activity. Usually the initial dose is prednisolone 1% or dexamethasone 0.1% drops given four times a day or hourly while awake and tapering to once or twice a day for approximately 1 month. The use of nonsteroid antiinflammatory drugs, topically or systemically, have not been effective in controlling anterior segment inflammation in herpetic patients.

The prophylactic use of antiviral agents following keratoplasty is controversial, whether used in general or as "coverage" of topical corticosteroids. Clinical and animal studies show that topical corticosteroids tend to make dendritic keratitis worse and may increase the risk of recurrence, although this finding has not been demonstrated in operated eyes. The effect has been shown to be ameliorated by the concomitant use of antiviral agents.[22,23] On the other hand, animal studies have demonstrated that antiviral drugs applied to healing epithelium can produce histologic and biomicroscopic evidence of damage,[6,24] even though they did not retard the rate of epithelial healing.[25] Clinically, epithelial healing problems seem to be more common in eyes in which prophylactic antiviral medication is regularly used. Two studies from the Massachusetts Eye and Ear Infirmary, in which antiviral medications were used prophylactically whenever topical corticosteroids were used after penetrating keratoplasty, showed that persistent epithelial defects developed in 25% to 44% of cases.[2,5] In comparison, epithelial defects were uncommon in two studies from Moorefields Eye Hospital in which topical corticosteroids were not used prophylactically or were used only to cover high-dose topical corticosteroid treatment of rejection episodes.[3,8]

Comparison of these studies suggests that topical antiviral prophylaxis, when topical corticosteroids are used, is helpful in reducing the rate of recurrence of dendritic keratitis postkeratoplasty. In the groups treated with routine antiviral prophylaxis, the recurrence rate varied between 6% after, on average, 4 years and 15% after 2 years[2,5]; in the group with no antiviral prophylaxis, the recurrence rate was 38% after 10 years.[3] In the groups in which antiviral prophylaxis was used only to cover high-dose topical corticosteroids, the incidence of epithelial keratitis varied between 15% after 4 years and 18% after 2 years.[3,8] Further, the use of antivirals along with corticosteroids in the treatment of graft rejection episodes reduced the incidence of dendritic keratitis at that time from 39% to 1%.[3]

A study from the University of Michigan also showed decreased recurrence rates with topical antiviral prophylaxis. After 3 years the recurrence rate was 21% in the group with prophylaxis and 32% in the group without prophylaxis.[21] In this study, an increased risk of graft failure, usually from rejection, was noted in eyes that sustained recurrence of herpetic keratitis, especially if it occurred during the first postoperative year. Others have made similar observations.[2,3,6,8]

If topical antiviral medication is used prophylactically, it may be advantageous to use vidarabine ointment rather than to idoxuridine; animal studies suggest that vidarabine is less toxic to the epithelium.[25] Trifluorothymidine is also less toxic than idoxuridine.

Data about the usefulness of oral acyclovir are accumulating. A prospective, randomized study from the Massachusetts Eye and Ear Infirmary showed no recurrences of herpetic keratitis in 13 patients (14 eyes) treated with oral acyclovir prophylactically after keratoplasty over a mean follow-up period of 16 months.[26] The recurrence rate in patients who did not receive acyclovir was 44% (four of nine eyes) over a mean follow-up of 20 months. In this study the percentage of grafts that experienced a rejection episode did not differ between groups, but the rate of graft failure was 56% in patients without prophylaxis compared to 14% in those on oral acyclovir. The treated patients received 800 to 1000 mg of acyclovir a day as an initial dose and were tapered to an average of 600 mg a day over 12 to 15 months. Acyclovir is expensive, but this small and unmasked study suggests the need for further work to establish dose-response curves over time.

Sutures should be removed as the wound heals, and should certainly be removed when they loosen. In some cases vascularization may be stimulated by the sutures.[27] When this occurs the surgeon must decide

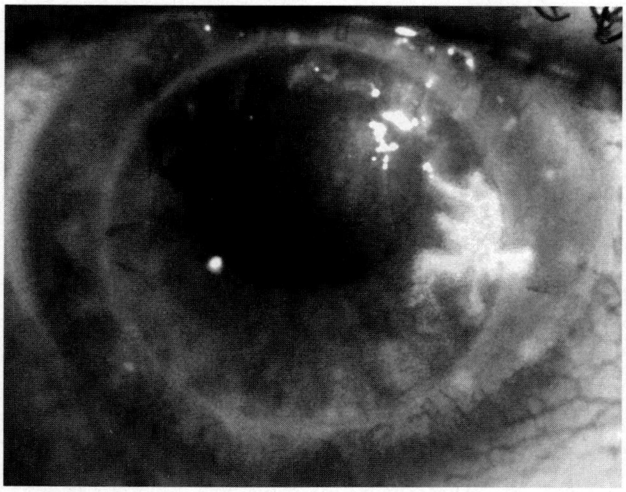

FIGURE 147-6 Recurrence of "dendritic" keratitis in a graft may be atypical in shape and commonly occurs at the graft margin.

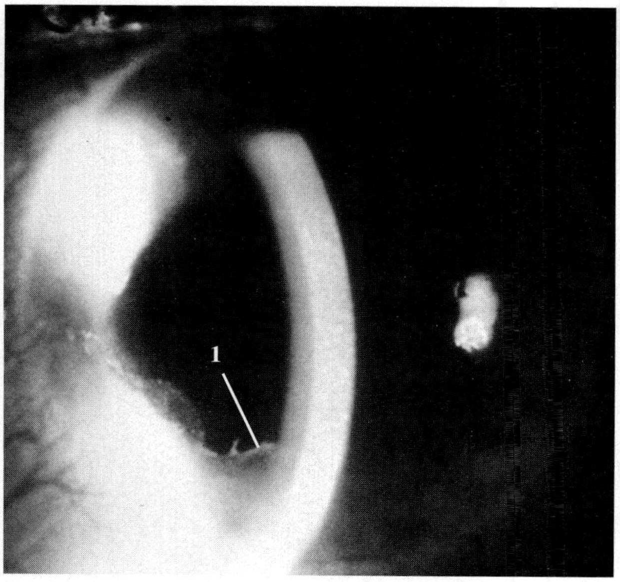

FIGURE 147-7 Epithelial rejection *(1)* is not associated with graft edema.

whether the wound is adequately healed for suture removal. Signs suggesting adequate healing include scarring or vascularization in the wound and lack of edema in the adjacent tissues. Argon laser has also been suggested as an alternative way to manage intracorneal neovascularization.[28,29] Deep stromal vascularization is more likely to be associated with rejection than is superficial.[5,30]

Complications

Recurrence of infectious epithelial keratitis is common, as indicated previously, particularly in eyes that were grafted when they were inflamed. In one series the incidence of recurrence was 75%.[4] Although most recurrences are seen in the first postoperative year,[21] they can occur at any time. The recurrence may take the classic dendritic form or it may be more ovoid. The ovoid form can often be distinguished from other causes of epithelial loss by its margin, which tends to appear thickened and vesicular as in dendritic keratitis. Recurrences commonly occur at the edge of the graft (Figure 147-6). Dendritic keratitis may also occur after keratoplasty performed for nonherpetic disease.[31] The management of dendritic keratitis in a graft is the same as it is in a nontransplanted cornea. Because of the tendency of these grafts to develop persistent epithelial defects, however, idoxuridine should be avoided because of its toxicity. If the patient is taking topical corticosteroids at the time of recurrence, these should be stopped or rapidly tapered, as they clearly exacerbate the dendritic keratitis.[23]

Although herpetic recurrence usually does not lead to immediate loss of graft clarity, it is significantly associated with graft failure. In one study of 40 grafts that failed, 20% failed because of rejection associated with herpetic recurrence, and 10% failed because of herpetic recurrence without rejection.[21]

Corneal graft rejection takes four forms: epithelial rejection, subepithelial infiltrates, stromal rejection, and endothelial rejection. Stromal rejection is rare.[32] Epithelial graft rejections take the form of a raised epithelial rejection line (Figure 147-7), which stains with fluorescein or rose bengal. The patient is usually asymptomatic if there are no other manifestations of the rejection. It can be confused with recurrent herpetic disease when initially seen, but does not lead to epithelial loss.

If these grafts are untreated, an epithelial rejection line moves across the cornea in about 1 week as the host epithelium replaces the damaged donor epithelium. Subepithelial infiltrates (Figure 147-8), as first described by Krachmer and Alldredge,[33] look similar to those caused by adenovirus. They are white, ovoid, approximately 0.2 to 1.0 mm in diameter, appear to be in or immediately below Bowman's layer, and are generally scattered randomly, although they may on occasion be confluent. They are best seen with diffuse direct illumination and may be overlooked if only a narrow slit beam is used for illumination. The patient rarely notices a change in vision or other symptoms. Neither epithelial rejection nor subepithelial infiltrates cause graft failure. Hence they do not require treatment per se. However, they do indicate that the host is sensitized to the donor tissue and that endothelial rejection may be impending.[30,33] Consequently, many

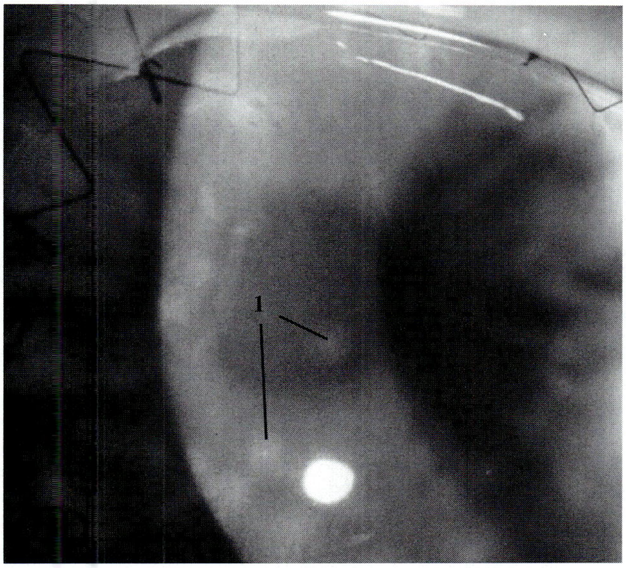

FIGURE 147-8 Subepithelial infiltrates (SEIs) *(1)* may be harbingers of an endothelial rejection episode.

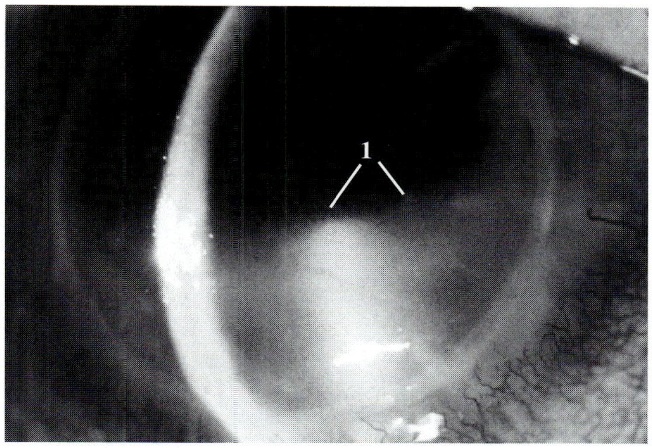

FIGURE 147-9 Endothelial rejection with segmental graft edema and a Khodadoust line *(1)*.

surgeons ordinarily treat them with some topical steroid routine, such as prednisolone 1% four times a day for a week, and then taper. Because of the previously outlined issues with the use of topical corticosteroids in patients with herpes simplex disease, corticosteroids must be used sparingly and judiciously, with close observation of the graft.

Endothelial rejection may present with the classic Khodadoust rejection line (Figure 147-9), which marches across the cornea over several days or may be diffuse with stromal edema and associated with a varying amount of keratic precipitates scattered over the graft endothelium (Figure 147-10, *A*). Endothelial rejections are treatable, and the results are better if treatment is initiated early.[30] Consequently, patients should be forewarned of the symptoms of a rejection episode, and when symptoms are seen, vigorous therapy should be instituted. There are no studies to validate one treatment regimen over another. Most surgeons use topical prednisolone 1% or dexamethasone 0.1% drops hourly while the patient is awake as initial therapy, with a tapering dose after approximately 1 week. Some also use dexamethasone 0.05% ointment at bedtime, and others recommend 2 mg of subconjunctival dexamethasone or oral corticosteroids as part of the initial treatment.[34] As indicated earlier, some surgeons feel strongly about "covering" the topical corticosteroids with prophylactic antiviral medication when treating graft rejections.[3] I prescribe trifluorothymidine drops four times a day for any patient who is using topical corticosteroids more frequently than four times a day.

The chance of reversing a rejection episode with clearing of the graft edema depends on the severity of the rejection, the amount of time treatment is delayed, and perhaps other risk factors.[30] All episodes should be treated promptly and vigorously, because even severely edematous grafts with bullous edema may recover with appropriate treatment (Figure 147-10).

A graft that is edematous from endothelial dysfunction caused by herpetic keratouveitis or progressive endothelial failure may be indistinguishable from one that is edematous because of rejection. Treatment should initially be instituted for rejection and then modified as needed. Herpes simplex can cause linear endotheliitis with a line of keratic precipitates, which is similar in appearance to an endothelial rejection episode.[35] Therefore many clinicians recommend treating patients with oral acyclovir, 200 mg five times a day, if there is iritis and an endothelial rejection line or diffuse keratic precipitates. This protocol has been used for the multicenter clinical trials in high-risk keratoplasty.

Occasionally, a graft rejection episode or its treatment will lead to a serious rise in intraocular pressure.[36] This complication should be treated with β-blockers and carbonic anhydrase inhibitors while the corticosteroid drops are continued.

Because of the possibility of exacerbating recurrent epithelial disease, it is probably unwise to keep patients with a history of herpetic keratitis on long-term prophylactic topical corticosteroids as is often the protocol in routine keratoplasty.

Cyclosporin A has the potential for decreasing the chance of graft rejection without the liabilities of corticosteroids. It suppresses antigenic sensitization and the resulting proliferation of immunocompetent T cells. In animal studies, both local and systemic administration have been shown to reduce the incidence of graft rejection. In a study with a follow-up of

A 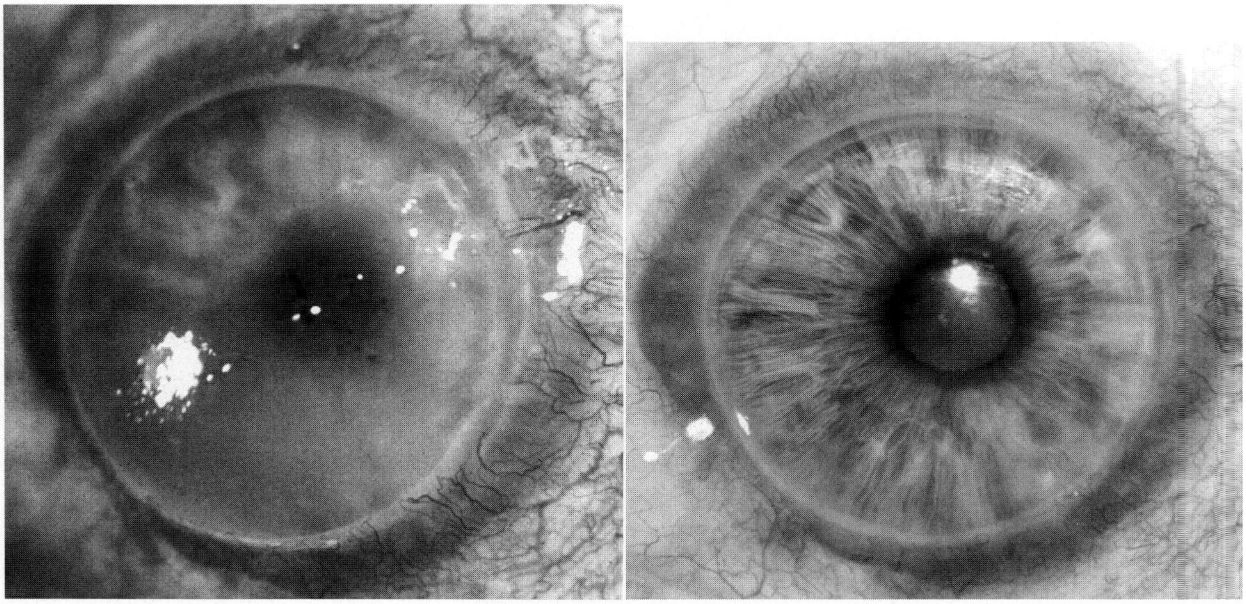 B

FIGURE 147-10 **A** and **B,** All episodes of endothelial rejection should be treated vigorously with topical corticoste- roids as even a grossly edematous cornea may clear.

14 to 82 months (mean 53), Hill[37] found that in high-risk, vascularized patients, a 12-month course of oral cyclosporin A was necessary to maximize the effect in reducing irreversible graft rejections. In a control group, 62% of the grafts were irreversibly rejected. Where cyclosporin A was used for 4 to 6 months, the rate dropped to 31% and when used for 12 months, it dropped to 9%.

Persistent epithelial defects are a serious problem in grafts for herpes simplex disease. The reported incidence varies widely. In two series from Boston, the incidence was 33% and 44%.[2,5] On the other hand, a large series from Ann Arbor showed an incidence of only 5%.[21] The difference may be due in part to the fact that both series from Boston contained a substantial number of eyes grafted while actively inflamed, compared to only 3% of eyes in the Ann Arbor series.

Persistent epithelial defects are commonly associated with lid abnormalities and lagophthalmos, tear film deficiencies, inflammation, and poor wound apposition. These issues should be addressed before or during surgery. Although one study showed that patching does not influence the rate of epithelial healing after penetrating keratoplasty,[38] some surgeons routinely patch or use a bandage lens after surgery until any epithelial defects are healed. If a bandage lens is used, prophylactic antibiotics should be considered because there is an increased risk of bacterial infection under these circumstances.[39] Nonpreserved tear substitutes and lubricants and ointments can be used frequently if needed. Eliminating or reducing the dose of toxic medications such as antiviral agents or aminoglycosides is important.[25,46] Corticosteroids may be beneficial by reducing inflammation, which has been shown to inhibit epithelial healing.[41] Epidermal growth factor does not appear to be useful[42] and may even exacerbate herpetic stromal keratitis.[43] Fibronectin may have potential by facilitating epithelial adhesion,[44,45] but it is not generally available.

A nonhealing epithelial defect in a graft may not be a persistent epithelial defect or trophic or metaherpetic ulcer, but in fact an infectious herpetic ulcer. This possibility should always be considered because infectious herpetic defects in grafts are often atypical in appearance.[31] Characteristically, the epithelium at the edge of a persistent defect has either a thin wispy appearance or a thick rolled edge (Figure 147-11). Ultimately, the diagnosis of a persistent defect is made over time, but an early diagnosis allows initiation of prompt treatment. Early treatment often leads to healing in a few days, whereas a defect that has persisted for a week or more may take months to heal, with increased risk of stromal ulceration, opacification, vascularization, and infection.[46] Consequently, the healing process of any epithelial defect in a herpetic patient should be closely monitored.

Glaucoma is a common problem after keratoplasty in herpes simplex, in part because of the need for prolonged corticosteroid use and in part because of the tendency toward chronic inflammation. Progressive angle closure resulting from synechia formation may also occur. Iridoplasty at the time of surgery may be

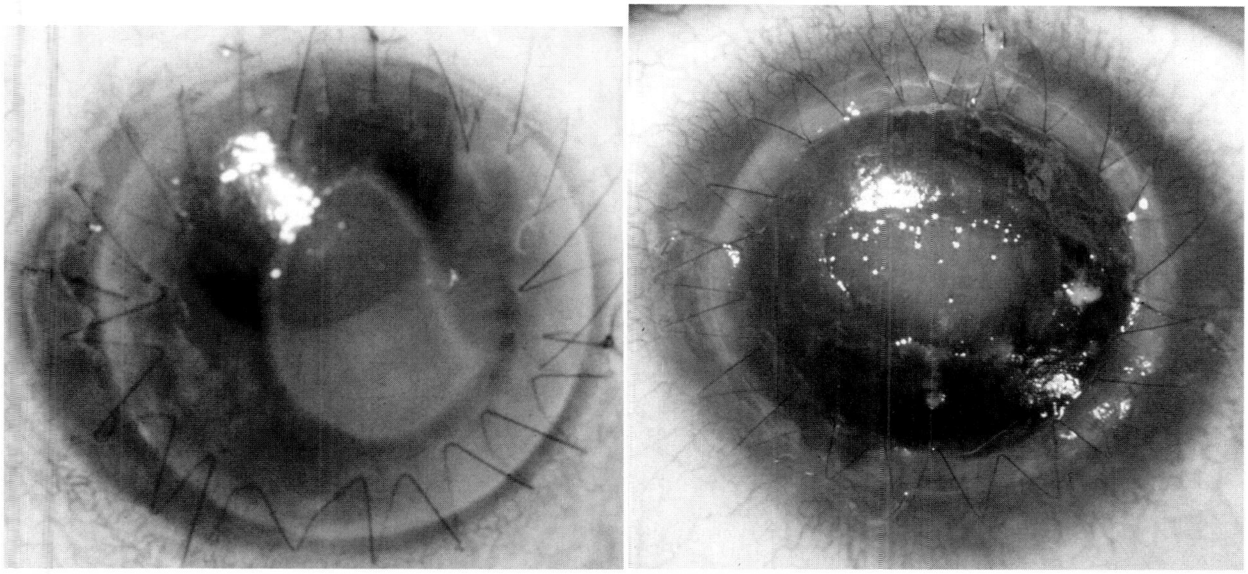

FIGURE 147-11 **A,** Persistent epithelial defects often have thick gray edges. **B,** Alternately, the margin may have a wispy appearance. In either case they tend to be ovoid.

helpful to prevent this devastating problem.[47] Viscoelastics are also useful, as mentioned earlier.[48]

Although animal studies have shown that elevated intraocular pressure can lead to endothelial damage in corneal transplantations,[49] it is not clear what level or duration of pressure rise causes damage in humans. Because failed grafts can be replaced but damaged optic nerves cannot, the critical issue in keratoplasty patients must be the optic nerve damage. In herpetic disease β-blockers and carbonic anhydrase inhibitors may have an advantage over miotics because of the tendency of the latter to exacerbate inflammation. If medical therapy fails, there are no good options for treatment because cycloablations, filters with or without antimetabolites, and setons all tend to lead to graft damage.[20,50,51] Rapuano et al.[52] found graft failure rates of 31% when setons were placed before keratoplasty, 29% when placed at the time of keratoplasty, and 44% when placed after keratoplasty, with a follow-up time of approximately 30 months.

Wound dehiscence is a largely, but not entirely, preventable complication of keratoplasty. It may be more common in grafts performed for herpes simplex disease because of the thinning and scarring of the donor tissue and the tendency to epithelial and stromal healing problems. Although antiviral and corticosteroid medications have been shown to retard stromal healing in animal studies,[25,53] they do not clinically cause healing problems in keratoplasty incisions. If sutures are placed deep, they are unlikely to erode before the wound is adequately healed. If interrupted sutures are used, as is appropriate in keratoplasty for herpes simplex infection, they can be removed at intervals, allowing observation of the wound response to suture removal before the decision is made to remove more. Occasionally, however, inflammation, vascularization, or a persistent epithelial defect will lead to premature loosening of the suture, requiring its removal. If repair of a dehiscence is needed, the wound should be opened down to Descemet's membrane before resuturing to ensure adequate apposition. If the wound has been separated for some time, any epithelium that has migrated into it should be removed before resuturing. Late wound dehiscences, long after suture removal, may occur with blunt trauma. The keratoplasty incision probably never regains the strength of a normal cornea.[54]

Keratoplasties performed for herpetic disease are particularly likely to develop secondary infections because of the high incidence of epithelial healing problems and the need for antiinflammatory agents.[13,55,56] Thus prophylactic antibiotics should be considered whenever a break in the epithelium occurs.

I have treated infectious crystalline keratopathy (Figure 147-12) in four eyes grafted for herpes simplex disease and in one other nongrafted eye with herpes simplex disease. This infection can occur even while the patient is receiving broad-spectrum antibiotics because it is extremely treatment resistant despite in vitro antibiotic sensitivity of the usual microbial cause, *Streptococcus viridans.*[57,58]

Overall, the chance of graft failure occurring from one of these complications is approximately 30% during the first 4 postoperative years in most se-

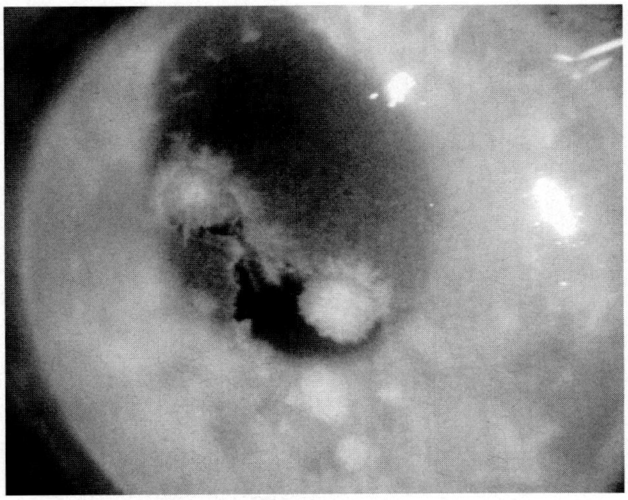

FIGURE 147-12 Infectious crystalline keratopathy is associated both with penetrating keratoplasty and herpes simplex disease.

ries.[3,11,21] It is much more likely that the graft will fail in inflamed or perforated eyes, regrafts, and in eyes in which additional anterior segment surgery is combined with keratoplasty.[2,3,8] Nonetheless, anticipation of and prophylactic measures against herpetic recurrence, epithelial healing problems, and rejection episodes, as indicated earlier, pay substantial dividends.

REFERENCES

1. Liesegang TJ: Epidemiology of ocular herpes simplex: natural history in Rochester, Minn, 1950 through 1982, *Arch Ophthalmol* 107:1160-1165, 1989.
2. Foster CS, Dunkin J: Penetrating keratoplasty for herpes simplex keratitis, *Am J Ophthalmol* 92:336-343, 1981.
3. Ficker L et al: The changing management and improved prognosis for corneal grafting in herpes simplex keratitis, *Ophthalmology* 96:1587-1596, 1989.
4. Polack FM, Kaufman HE: Penetrating keratoplasty in herpes simplex keratitis, *Am J Ophthalmol* 73:908-913, 1972.
5. Langston RHS, Pavan-Langston D, Dohlman CH: Penetrating keratoplasty for herpetic keratitis—prognostic and therapeutic determinants, *Trans Am Acad Ophthalmol Otolaryngol* 79:577-583, 1975.
6. Rice NSC, Jones BR: Problems of corneal grafting in herpetic keratitis. In Jones BR, editor: *Corneal graft failure. Ciba Foundation Symposium 16,* Amsterdam, 1973, Elsevier.
7. Moore TE, Aronson SB: The corneal graft: a multiple variable analysis of penetrating keratoplasty, *Am J Ophthalmol* 72:205-298, 1971.
8. Cobo LM et al: Prognosis and management of corneal transplantation for herpetic keratitis, *Arch Ophthalmol* 98:1755-1759, 1980.
9. Cohen EJ, Laibson PR, Arentsen JJ: Corneal transplantation for herpes simplex keratitis, *Am J Ophthalmol* 95:645-650, 1983.
10. Fine M, Cignetti FE: Penetrating keratoplasty in herpes simplex keratitis, *Arch Ophthalmol* 95:613-616, 1977.
11. Epstein RJ et al: Penetrating keratoplasty for herpes simplex keratitis and keratoconus: allograft rejection and survival, *Ophthalmology* 94:935-944, 1987.
12. Ficker LA et al: Long term prognosis for corneal grafting in herpes simplex keratitis, *Eye* 2:400-408, 1988.
13. Dohlman CH, Zucker BB: Long-term treatment with idoxuridine and steroids, *Arch Ophthalmol* 74:172-174, 1965.
14. Mathers WD, Jester JV, Lemp MA: Return of human corneal sensitivity after penetrating keratoplasty, *Arch Ophthalmol* 106:210-211, 1988.
15. Frey T, Friendly D, Wyatt D: Re-evaluation of monocular cataracts in children, *Am J Ophthalmol* 761:381-388, 1973.
16. Völker-Dieben HJ et al: The effect of prospective HLA-A and B matching in 288 penetrating keratoplasties for herpes simplex keratitis, *Acta Ophthalmol (Copenh)* 62:513-523, 1984.
17. The CCTS Research Group: The Collaborative Corneal Transplantation Studies (CCTS). Effectiveness of histocompatibility matching in high-risk corneal transplantation, *Arch Ophthalmol* 110:1392-1403, 1992.
18. Bourne WM: Reduction of endothelial cell loss during phakic penetrating keratoplasty, *Am J Ophthalmol* 89:787-790, 1980.
19. Grönemeyer V, Pülhorn G, Muller-Rucholtz W: Histocompatibility and allogenic corneal grafting between inbred strains of rats, *Mod Probl Ophthalmol* 16:161-166, 1976.
20. Tragakis MP, Brown SI: The significance of anterior synechiae after corneal transplantation, *Am J Ophthalmol* 74:532-533, 1972.
21. Moyes AL et al: Antiviral therapy after penetrating keratoplasty for herpes simplex keratitis, *Arch Ophthalmol* 112:601-607, 1994.
22. Patterson A, Jones BR: The management of ocular herpes, *Trans Ophthalmol Soc UK* 87:537-579, 1967.
23. Kaufman HE, Maloney ED: IDU and hydrocortisone in experimental herpes simplex keratitis, *Arch Ophthalmol* 68:396-398, 1962.
24. Foster CS, Pavan-Langston D: Corneal wound healing and antiviral medication, *Arch Ophthalmol* 95:2062-2067, 1977.
25. Langston RHS, Pavan-Langston D, Dohlman CH: Antiviral medication and corneal wound healing, *Arch Ophthalmol* 92:509-513, 1974.
26. Barney NP, Foster CS: A prospective randomized trial of oral acyclovir after penetrating keratoplasty for herpes simplex keratitis, *Cornea* 13:232-236, 1994.
27. Paque J, Poiner RH: Corneal allograft reacton and its relationship to suture site neovascularization, *Ophthalmic Surg* 8:71-74, 1977.
28. Narankari VS, Baer JC: Corneal argon laser photocoagulation for neovascularization in penetrating keratoplasty, *Ophthalmology* 93:1304-1309, 1986.
29. Corrent GC et al: Promotion of graft survival by photothrombotic occlusion of corneal neovascularization, *Arch Ophthalmol* 107:1501-1506, 1989.
30. Alldredge OC, Krachmer JH: Clinical types of corneal transplant rejection. Their manifestations, frequency, pre-operative correlates and treatment, *Arch Ophthalmol* 99:599-604, 1981
31. Mannis MJ et al: Herpes simplex dendritic keratitis after keratoplasty, *Am J Ophthalmol* 111:480-484, 1991.
32. Stark WJ: Transplantation immunology of penetrating keratoplasty, *Trans Am Ophthalmol Soc* 78:1079-1117, 1980.
33. Krachmer JH, Alldredge OC: Subepithelial infiltrates. A probable sign of corneal transplant rejection, *Arch Ophthalmol* 96:2234-2237, 1978.
34. Chandler JW: Immunologic considerations in corneal transplantation. In Kaufman HE, Barron BA, McDonald MB, Waltman SR, editors: *The cornea,* New York, 1988, Churchill Livingstone.
35. Olsen TW, Hardten DR, Meiusi RS, Holland EJ: Linear endotheliitis, *Am J Ophthalmol* 117:468-474, 1994.
36. Polack FM: Graft rejection and glaucoma, *Am J Ophthalmol* 101:294-297, 1986.

37. Hill JC: Systemic cyclosporine in high-risk keratoplasty. Short-view long-term therapy, *Ophthalmology* 101:128-133, 1994.
38. Sugar A, Meyer RF, Bahn CF: A randomized trial of pressure patching for epithelial defects after keratoplasty, *Am J Ophthalmol* 95:637-640, 1983.
39. Smith SG et al: Corneal ulcer-infiltrate associated with soft contact lens use following penetrating keratoplasty, *Cornea* 3:131-134, 1984.
40. Stern GA et al: Effect of topical antibiotic solutions on corneal epithelial wound healing, *Arch Ophthalmol* 101:644-647, 1983.
41. Wagoner et al: Polymorpho-nuclear neutrophils delay corneal wound healing in vitro, *Invest Ophthalmol Vis Sci* 25:1217-1220, 1984.
42. Kandarakis AS, Paye C, Kaufman HE: The effect of epidermal growth factor on epithelial healing after penetrating keratoplasty in human eyes, *Am J Ophthalmol* 98:411-415, 1984.
43. Romano A et al: Aggravation of herpetic stromal keratitis after murine epidermal growth factor topical application, *Cornea* 13:167-172, 1994.
44. Nishida T et al: Fibronectin. A new therapy for corneal trophic ulcer, *Arch Ophthalmol* 101:1046-1048, 1988.
45. Phan TM et al: Topical fibronectin in the treatment of persistent epithelial defects and trophic ulcers, *Am J Ophthalmol* 104:494-501, 1987.
46. Dohlman CH: The function of the corneal epithelium in health and disease, *Invest Ophthalmol* 10:383-407, 1971.
47. Cohen EJ, Kenyon KR, Dohlman CH: Iridoplasty for prevention of post-keratoplasty angle closure and glaucoma, *Ophthalmic Surg* 13:994-996, 1982.
48. Polack FM, Demong T, Santaelle H: Sodium hyaluronate (Healon) in keratoplasty and IOL implanation, *Ophthalmology* 88:425-431, 1981.
49. Charlin R, Polack FM: The effect of elevated intraocular pressure on the endothelium of corneal grafts, *Cornea* 1:241-249, 1982.
50. Binder PS, Abel R, Kaufman HE: Cyclocryotherapy for glaucoma after penetrating keratoplasty, *Am J Ophthalmol* 79:489-492, 1975.
51. Minckler DS, Heuer DK, Hasty B: Clinical experience with the single-plate Molteno implant in complicated glaucomas, *Ophthalmology* 95:1181-1188, 1988.
52. Rapuano CJ et al: Results of alloplastic tube shunt procedures before, during and after penetrating keratoplasty, *Cornea* 14:26-32, 1995.
53. Aquavella JV, Gasset AF, Dohlman CH: Corticosteroids in corneal wound healing, *Am J Ophthalmol* 58:621-626, 1964.
54. Farley MK, Petit TH: Traumatic wound dehiscence after penetrating keratoplasty, *Am J Ophthalmol* 104:44-49, 1987.
55. Fong LP et al: Microbial keratitis complicating penetrating keratoplasty, *Ophthalmology* 95:1269-1275, 1988.
56. Harris DJ et al: Late bacterial and fungal infections after corneal transplantation, *Ophthalmology* 95:1450-1457, 1988.
57. Meisler DM et al: Infectious crystalline keratopathy, *Ophthalmology* 97:337-343, 1984.
58. Langston RHS: Infectious crystalline keratopathy. In Fraunfelder FT, Roy FH, Meyer SM, editors: *Current ocular therapy* 3, New York, 1990, WB Saunders.

PART IX

THERAPEUTIC AND RECONSTRUCTIVE PROCEDURES

CHAPTER 148

MARC A. HONIG CHRISTOPHER J. RAPUANO

Management of Corneal Perforations

Corneal perforations can result from a variety of disorders and can lead to devastating visual sequelae. Descemetoceles and perforations are ophthalmic emergencies that require immediate recognition and intervention. The primary causes include infection, inflammation, and trauma. However, other conditions such as exposure and neurotrophic keratopathy, xerosis, and corneal degenerations can also cause ulceration and perforation (box). Conditions leading to descemetocele and perforation are briefly outlined here. The workup and treatment of these disorders are discussed at length elsewhere in the textbook.

Management should be directed toward prevention of corneal perforation, because once a perforation has occurred, visual outcome is often disappointing. Recognition of the conditions leading to perforation and management of the perforated cornea are discussed. Treatment of traumatic perforations are not discussed in depth here because this topic is covered in great detail in other chapters.

Etiology

The most common cause of corneal perforation is infection, either bacterial, fungal, or viral. Infection accounts for between 24% and 55% of all perforations,[1-6] with bacterial infections being most common.[2] A frequent predisposing factor leading to these and other types of perforations is early breakdown of the corneal epithelium. Once this barrier is compromised, the pathogen gains easy access to the stroma, inciting an inflammatory response in the host. Damage results from a combination of direct microbial invasion, and more importantly, through host chemotaxis of leukocytes causing collagenases to be released and corneal ulceration to occur. Viral keratitis, namely herpes simplex (HSV) and herpes zoster (HZV) may lead to corneal perforation secondary to recurrent active ulcerative keratitis, persistent epithelial defects, and neurotrophic keratopathy. Fungal infections are less common and often progress more slowly than other forms of infectious ulcerative keratitis, but nonetheless may lead to corneal perforation.

Inflammatory conditions such as collagen vascular disease, acne rosacea, Wegener's granulomatosis, and Mooren's (idiopathic) ulcer can also cause peripheral, and occasionally central, ulcerative keratitis and subsequent perforation. The use of topical corticosteroids may exacerbate or initiate a stromal melt in the presence of one of these disorders, but perforation can also occur spontaneously.[7,8]

Trauma, either chemical, thermal, surgical, or penetrating, is also a common cause of corneal perforation. Chemical injuries, alkali burns in particular, may cause devastating corneal damage, initially by direct tissue destruction and later by induction of stromal melting and necrosis because of the elaboration of collagenases.[9] Thermal injury normally causes superficial corneal damage but may, in rare instances, cause perforation because of extreme heat or associated mechanical injury.[10] Corneal ulceration and perforation have also been reported after cataract extraction, both with and without intraocular lens implantation.[11,12]

Xerosis and exposure keratopathy are also causes of corneal perforation. Xerosis may be idiopathic; related to collagen vascular disease (Sjögren's syndrome); or secondary to Stevens-Johnson syndrome, ocular cicatricial pemphigoid, or vitamin A deficiency. Exposure may result from seventh nerve palsy, thyroid ophthalmopathy, involutional ectropion, or other chronic cicatrizing eyelid disorders.

Neurotrophic keratopathy is most commonly encountered after a viral infection, typically HSV and HZV, as well as secondary to tumor, trauma, or surgery (e.g., penetrating keratoplasty, cataract extraction). The lack of corneal sensation leads to chronic epithelial breakdown with slow healing. This persistent epitheliopathy makes the cornea susceptible to a sterile melting process or infectious keratitis and potential perforation.

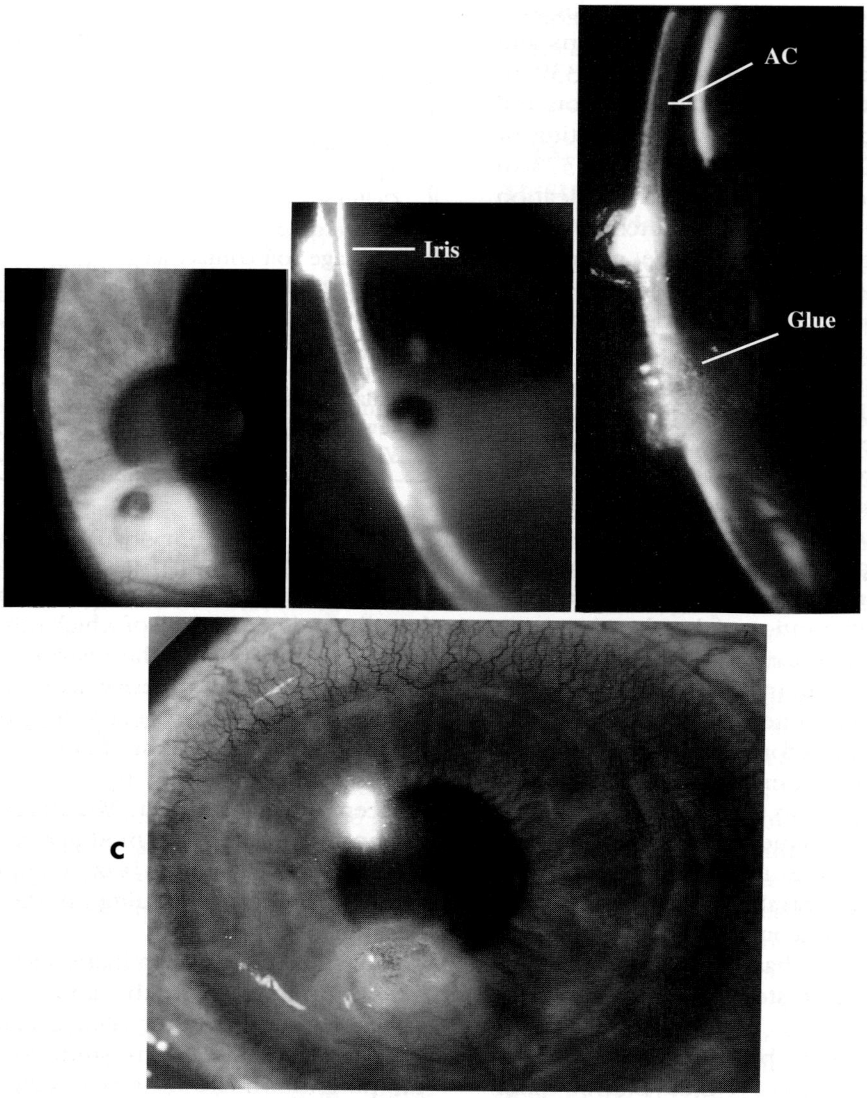

FIGURE 148-4 **A,** Small midperipheral full-thickness perforated corneal ulcer in a patient with acne rosacea keratitis. **B,** Slit lamp view demonstrates a flat anterior chamber. **C,** Perforation treated with cyanoacrylate tissue adhesive and a bandage soft contact lens. **D,** Slit lamp view one hour after placement of tissue glue demonstrating reformation of the anterior chamber (*AC*).

remains it can be trimmed. A small ring of any sterile ophthalmic ointment (e.g., erythromycin) is placed approximately 1 to 2 mm from the broken edge of the applicator (Figure 148-5, *A*). When a small amount of glue is required for small perforations, the ointment is placed closer to the tip, and vice versa for larger perforations.

Attention is then redirected to the operating microscope. Several drops of topical anesthetic are placed in the affected and unaffected eyes, and a Barraquer eyelid speculum is gently inserted. The perforation site is inspected and debridement of any loose or necrotic material is performed. In addition, it is extremely important to debride 1 to 2 mm of epithelium surrounding the ulcer with a cellulose spear or forceps, because glue does not adhere well to epithelium. Any lens material, vitreous, or foreign matter present should be removed. After debridement, the perforation site should be dried thoroughly with successively applied cellulose spears (Figure 148-5, *B*). If the wound is not completely dry, the likelihood of a satisfactory adhesion is greatly diminished. If the perforation site is actively leaking aqueous, several cellulose spears may be necessary to dry the area completely. In certain situations, if not contraindicated, the anterior chamber may be gently massaged

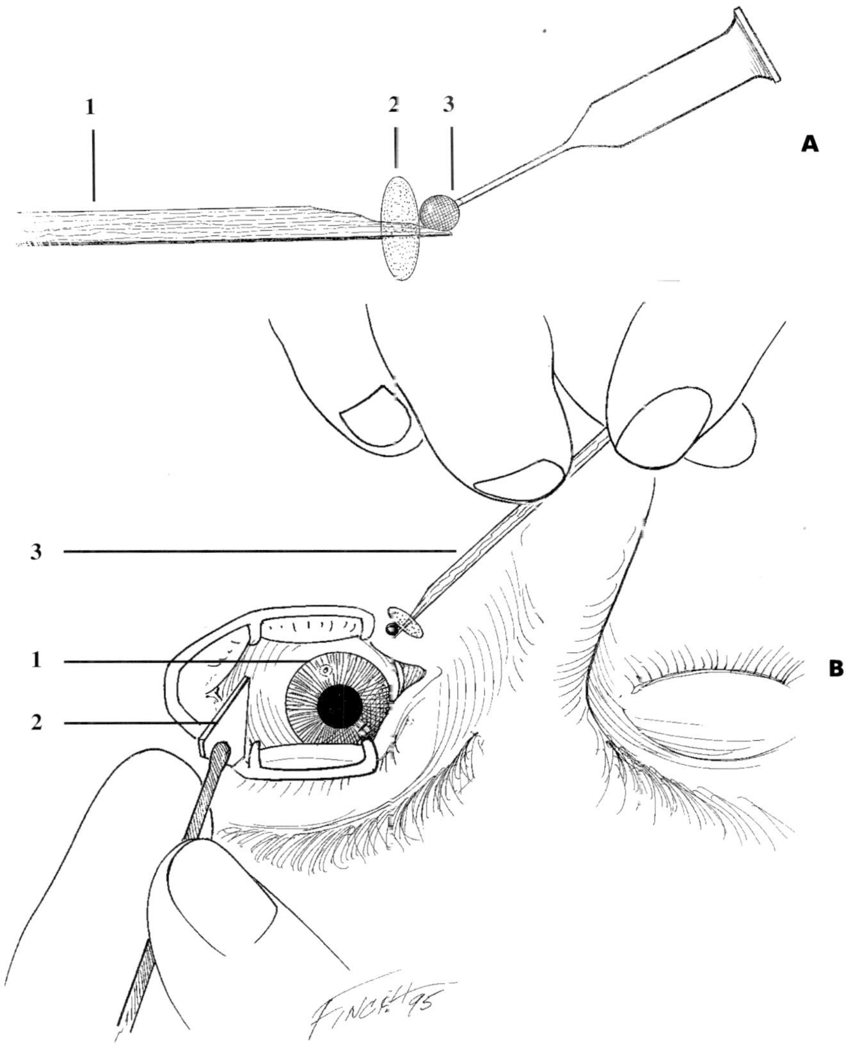

FIGURE 148-5 Technique for application of cyanoacrylate tissue adhesive. **A,** Sterile wooden applicator *(1)* with a broken, tapered, smooth end and a ring of ophthalmic ointment *(2)* placed approximately 1 mm from the edge. A small drop of tissue adhesive *(3)* is placed on the end of the applicator; the amount is limited by the ointment. The placement of the ring of ointment can be modified to control the amount of tissue adhesive that will be delivered to the wound. **B,** The patient is lying in a supine position under the operating microscope with the eyelid speculum in place. The perforation site *(1)* and the surrounding 1 to 2 mm have been debrided of epithelium and necrotic debris. The surgeon has a cellulose spear *(2)* in one hand and the wooden applicator with the tissue adhesive *(3)* in the other. *Continued.*

to express some aqueous so that with successive attempts at drying, aqueous does not immediately leak into the area to be glued.[30]

If the anterior chamber is totally flat and iris or lens is directly beneath the perforation, a small amount of viscoelastic or air may be injected in an attempt to avoid incarceration of the tissue into the glue or additional damage to underlying structures.[31] This step is difficult to achieve, especially with a flat chamber, and is not always necessary. Incarceration of tissue into the adhesive is often unavoidable and is not deemed a significant detriment to the ultimate success of the procedure.

One small drop of tissue adhesive is then carefully applied to the prepared end of the wooden applicator (Figure 148-5, *A*). With the glue in one hand and a cellulose spear in the other, the area to be glued is quickly dried with the tip of the spear, and the glue is then immediately applied (Figure 148-5, *C*). This maneuver is accomplished by gently touching the tip with the glue directly to the perforation site and then removing it quickly. The cellulose spear should not be

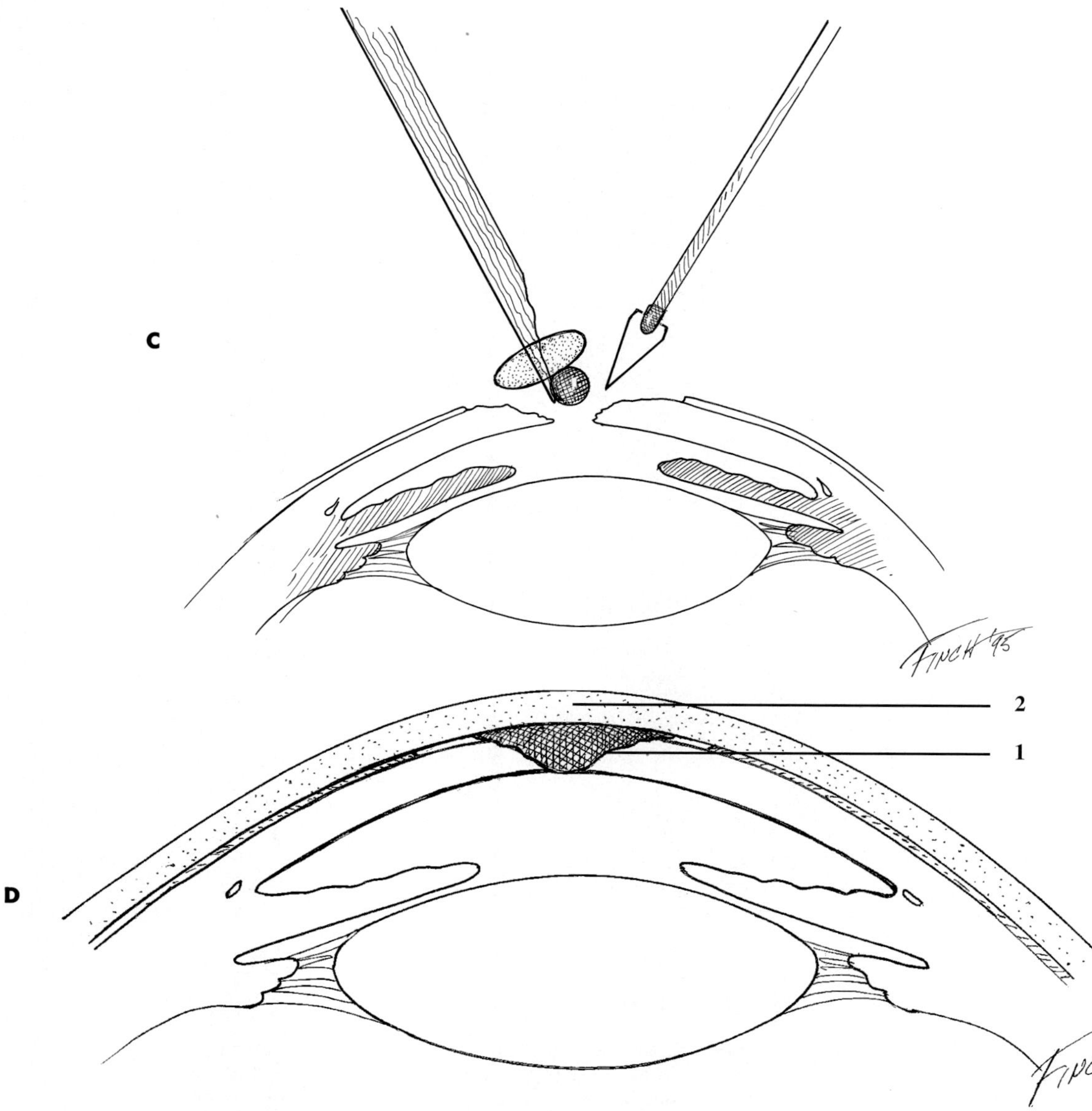

FIGURE 148-5, cont'd. **C,** The perforation site is dried with successively applied cellulose spears just before the application of the tissue adhesive. As the glue is applied to the wound, the cellulose spear and applicator are quickly removed. **D,** After successful application of tissue adhesive *(1),* the perforation site is sealed. A bandage soft contact lens *(2)* is in place and the anterior chamber is reforming.

applied near the glued area until the adhesive has totally dried because it will stick to the glue. The glue will solidify completely within several minutes. The polymerization process can be expedited by applying a few drops of fluid (e.g., proparacaine or preservative-free artificial tears) to the surface. The goal is to fill the ulcerated area with a minimal amount of glue. The ideal amount is just enough to secure it to the surrounding cornea without creating a large ring or mound of glue. Too much glue or excessive anterior protrusion of glue, which may cause discomfort even with a bandage contact lens, is undesirable.

If the entire defect is not covered or a small leak remains, additional applications of tissue adhesive to the existing plug or to an adjacent area may be necessary. If the wound is still leaking and the existing plug is unsatisfactory, the glue can be removed by gently rotating it at the corneal surface and then lifting it away from the cornea. Gluing may be reattempted, but repeated application and removal of glue may create or enlarge the defect.

After the adhesive solidifies, the area should be dried carefully with a cellulose spear and reinspected for an aqueous leak. If too generous an amount of glue has been applied, any excess glue that may have become adherent to adjacent normal epithelialized cornea can be removed carefully with a jeweler's forceps. However, this maneuver risks dislodging the entire plug. One additional recheck of the glued area is recommended before a bandage soft contact lens is applied. We use a loose fitting, flat, low power, low water content disposable extended wear soft contact lens such as a Seequence II, base curve 9.0 mm (Bausch and Lomb, Rochester, NY). If this particular lens is not available, any low water content extended wear soft contact lens with the flattest (i.e., highest) base curve can be used. Unlike soft contact lenses used for other purposes, these lenses will not move significantly with blinking after gluing and may have large folds with "edge off" because of surface irregularities caused by the tissue adhesive.

After placement of the bandage contact lens, the eyelid speculum is gently removed from the eye. Depending on the clinical setting, one may see reformation of the anterior chamber before completion of the entire procedure (Figure 148-5, *D*). The patient should be reexamined several minutes later to check for formation of the anterior chamber and for possible dislodging of the glue or contact lens. If the glue and contact lens remain in place at the initial examination after the procedure, the patient should be rechecked 30 to 60 minutes later and once again within the next 24 hours.

Small linear or curvilinear perforations may be sealed using a modification of the method described. First, glue is applied centrally, with subsequent applications adjacent to the previous glue until the entire defect is covered. There are several alternative techniques for application of the tissue adhesive. All attempt to provide a controlled method for placement of the minimum amount of glue necessary to close the perforation site. Several other methods are described briefly. This list is by no means exhaustive, and each practitioner may adopt his or her own modifications based on personal experience.

Ophthalmic ointment may be applied to the flat end of a wooden applicator with a drop of adhesive placed on the layer of ointment. The glue is then directly applied to the perforation site and quickly removed. Alternatively, a polyethylene disk (2 to 4 mm in diameter) can be attached by ointment to the flat end of a wooden applicator with glue applied to the disk.[30,32,33] Both the glue and disk are then directly applied to the defect with mild pressure. Fluid may be applied to the area to expedite polymerization. The applicator is then removed, with the disk in place. The disk may be removed gently with forceps or simply left in place. This method has the advantage of creating a smoother surface than with other techniques. However, a contact lens is still necessary for comfort. Similar variations include a circular piece of a dry collagen shield, plastic surgical drape, or collagen minishield (Bio Cor, Bausch and Lomb, Clearwater, FL) in lieu of a polyethylene disk.[26] By applying gentle pressure during application, this method allows both adhesive and disk to be applied to the depth of the defect because the disk is flexible. These methods may be particularly helpful in descemetoceles in which the surface to be glued has a convex anterior surface. The advantage of a collagen shield is that it dissolves within 24 hours, leaving a relatively smooth anterior surface to the tissue adhesive plug.

The tip of the plastic handle from a cellulose spear (either flat or cut at an angle), a metal spatula,[34] or the needle from a tuberculin syringe[3,24] can be used as an applicator. Because the latter two applicators are made of metal, polymerization of adhesive to the metallic surface may be a problem. A fine-gauge capillary tube provides an effective way to control the amount of glue placed on the eye. Unfortunately, these tubes are no longer commonly available in the United States. An angled polyethylene pipette used in dentistry called the "Squeez-ett" (Ellman Manufacturing, Hewlett, NY) has been described as a superior method for application of tissue adhesive.[27]

In larger perforations, a half-thickness corneal or scleral patch[35] or collagen shield can be fashioned and fit into the debrided bed of the perforation or descemetocele. This patch is then sealed in place with tissue adhesive, using any of the aforementioned applicators. This technique has the advantage of being able to seal relatively large perforations, limiting the chance that adhesive will enter the anterior chamber (Figure 148-6).

Postoperative management

All patients should be placed on aqueous suppressants consisting of either a topical β-blocker (e.g., timolol 0.5% twice a day) and/or an oral carbonic anhydrase inhibitor (e.g., acetazolamide 500 mg sequel twice a day or methazolamide 50 mg three times a day) if medically tolerable. This regimen decreases the pressure head against the perforation. If the ulcer is thought to be noninfectious, prophylactic broad-spectrum topical antibiotics such as trimethoprim/polymyxin B, ofloxacin, or ciprofloxacin should be used three to four times a day. A protective shield or glasses should be placed on the eye at all times. Preservative-free artificial tears can be added four to eight times a day to provide additional lubrication and prevent the contact lens from becoming dehydrated and tight. Severely dry eyes may require punctal occlusion in the acute setting or at a later time when the eye is more stable.

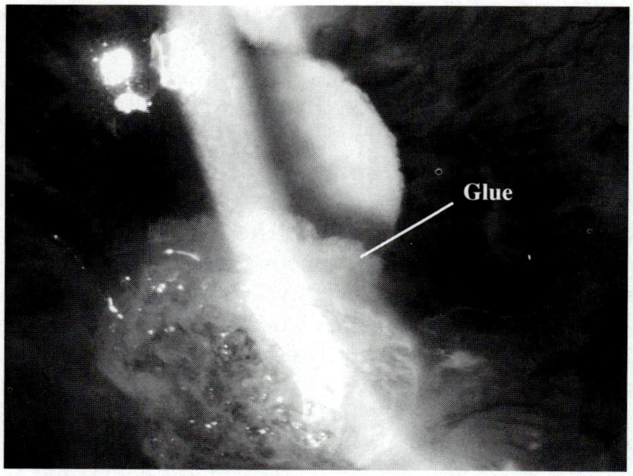

FIGURE 148-6 Cyanoacrylate tissue adhesive placed in a 3 mm perforation. Note the "barbell" shape of the glue with a large portion in the anterior chamber (Glue). In large perforations, this problem can be avoided by placing a small piece of collagen shield or corneal tissue in the base of the perforation before gluing to prevent the glue from entering the anterior chamber.

The need for hospital admission and the use of intravenous antibiotics in the case of a sterile perforation is controversial. Even in noninfectious perforations, we still prefer to admit the patients and initiate intravenous antibiotics (e.g., cefazolin and gentamicin) at standard systemic doses for at least 72 hours. If the patient is not admitted, outpatient antibiotic treatment with oral ciprofloxacin, 500 mg twice a day, seems most reasonable because of ciprofloxacin's excellent ocular penetration. It is also important to check the status of the fellow eye carefully and to add lubrication in this eye, if clinically indicated.

Infected corneal perforations are always admitted and, if a bacterial infection is suspected, the patient is started on fortified topical antibiotics (e.g., cefazolin, 50 mg/ml, or vancomycin, 25 mg/ml, and tobramycin, 14 mg/ml, every 1 to 2 hours). These medications can be tapered appropriately over the next several days, depending on the clinical response and culture and sensitivity results. Antiviral or antifungal therapy should be instituted if a herpetic or fungal etiology is suspected. One must carefully balance the need for frequent topical medications against the desire to manipulate the eye as little as possible. Prophylactic intravenous antibiotics are administered for at least 3 days. The position of the glue and contact lens are evaluated daily until discharge and then again in 3 to 5 days. If the glue and contact lens remain in place, the patient may be discharged after the full 72-hour course of intravenous antibiotics. Patients must be made aware that if they notice a sudden change in vision, pain, discharge, photophobia, tearing, or appearance of the eye, immediate follow-up examination is necessary.

If the glue becomes dislodged, the situation must be reevaluated. If the remaining defect can be reglued, this procedure should be attempted as needed. In some situations, several reapplications may be necessary before a stable adhesion is obtained. Any contact lens that has become dislodged should be replaced as soon as possible. If the glue repeatedly dislodges or if the resultant perforation is too large to repair with tissue adhesive, other modalities (e.g., penetrating keratoplasty or patch graft) must be considered.

Ideally, the glue should remain in place for weeks to months while stromal healing and vascularization occur beneath it to stabilize the cornea. The contact lens should remain in place for as long as the glue is present to maximize patient comfort. We typically replace the bandage contact lens every 2 to 3 months, or more frequently if necessary. Contact lens replacement must be performed with extreme care so as not to dislodge the glue. We use an eyelid speculum to prevent accidental eyelid closure and disturbance of the glue. Prophylactic topical antibiotics (e.g., trimethoprim/polymyxin B) should be continued during contact lens use. The appropriate time for removal of the glue is controversial. As a rule, we tend to leave the glue in place until it loosens excessively or becomes totally dislodged. If the stroma appears healed, the glue can theoretically be removed after several months. However, the risk of perforation still exists. Tissue adhesive has remained on the eye for up to 660 days before spontaneously sloughing, with subsequent perforation 30 days later from recurrent stromal thinning.[24]

Management after glue has been removed and stromal healing has occurred is also variable. Peripheral lesions not affecting the visual axis or other lesions in eyes with limited visual potential can be managed conservatively. Years after the gluing, one may see only a faint stromal scar, with little other evidence of previous perforation. In other cases, dense fibrosis, with or without uvea incorporated into the scar, and vascularization may persist. If visual rehabilitation is desired, elective penetrating keratoplasty and/or anterior segment reconstruction can be attempted 6 to 12 months later.

Complications

Although tissue adhesives are well tolerated by the eye, several complications have been reported. These include cataract formation[8,35] (thought to be due to direct contact of glue with the lens), corneal infiltration[3,24] (infectious and noninfectious), glaucoma,[3] giant papillary conjunctivitis,[36] retinal toxicity,[37] granulomatous keratitis,[38] and symblepharon formation.[24] It is often difficult, however, to determine whether the

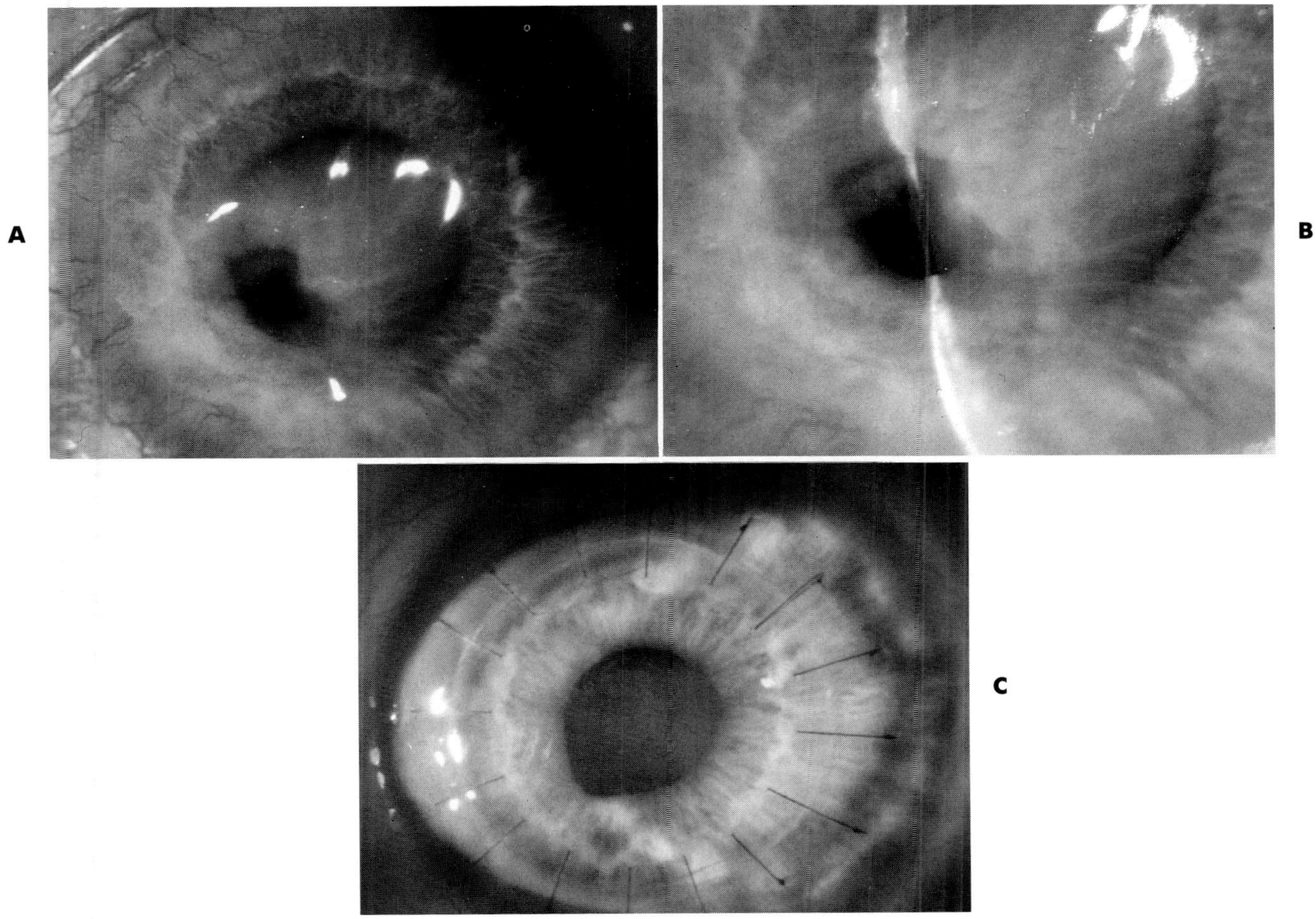

FIGURE 148-7 **A,** Large perforated corneal ulcer in a patient with chronic HSV keratitis. **B,** Slit lamp view demonstrating the large size of the full-thickness perforation. **C,** This patient was treated with an emergent penetrating keratoplasty.

complication was due to the use of tissue adhesive or the original perforation.

PENETRATING KERATOPLASTY

Larger perforations not amenable to repair using tissue adhesive or tissue adhesive failures are often treated with penetrating keratoplasty (Figure 148-7). The timing of surgery is quite variable. If tissue adhesive has been applied and the integrity of the eye restored, keratoplasty can be deferred for days to months, depending on the stability of the clinical situation.

Patients with acute perforations that require surgical repair by keratoplasty should be admitted to the hospital, given intravenous antibiotics (e.g., cefazolin, gentamicin, or ceftazidime), and not permitted to receive food or drink by mouth until the repair can be performed. If an infection is suspected, the appropriate topical and systemic antibiotics, antivirals, or antifungals should be administered. Some advocate medical therapy for at least 24 hours before attempting any surgical intervention.[4] In some situations, gentle B-scan ultrasonography can be invaluable in detecting the presence of hemorrhagic choroidal detachments. If detachments are present, one should obtain the advice of a vitreoretinal surgeon and seriously consider waiting several days before attempting keratoplasty and/or drainage of the choroidal effusions because of the increased risk for expulsive hemorrhage.

The use of general anesthesia, with the anesthesiologist well aware that the globe is open, is usually preferred. A Barraquer eyelid speculum is then inserted, making sure that no external pressure is placed on the globe. In situations in which the anterior chamber is flat or the eye is soft, attaching a Flieringa ring is quite difficult, and this step may be omitted. The recipient trephine size is generally determined by the size and location of the existing perforation. The smallest trephine capable of incorporating the perforation site and any infected or ulcerated border is generally chosen. Trephine sizes usually vary between 6.0 and 11.0 mm,[20,39] with 7.5 to 8.0 mm being optimal. The donor is generally oversized by 0.50 mm. Viscoelastic is occasionally helpful in reinflating the anterior chamber before trephination and also in maintaining tissue planes.

The method of trephination in the recipient is quite variable. In general, trephination is difficult to achieve in a soft eye. The standard handheld trephine without a guard may be used, taking great care to avoid causing protrusion of ocular contents through the perforation site. Some surgeons prefer to mark the superficial cornea with the trephine and deepen the mark freehand with a blade. The cornea is entered through the deepened trephination mark. If the perforation is not due to infection, curved corneal scissors can be introduced through the perforation and a free hand excision of the recipient cornea can be performed. In any case, extreme care must be taken to avoid cutting iris or lens. An alternative method involves the use of a suction trephine system such as the Hessburg-Baron trephine. In this way pressure is exerted outward by the suction apparatus, avoiding direct pressure on the open globe. Once the trephine is secured on the cornea by suction, trephination is accomplished by simply rotating the blade of the trephine.

Others have advocated the temporary use of tissue adhesive with or without scleral or corneal patches to restore the anterior chamber minutes before trephination.[40] In this way traditional trephination can then be accomplished in a safer, more effective manner. In our opinion, most lesions amenable to such patches and adhesive would benefit from reformation and observation followed by keratoplasty days to weeks later rather than on an emergent basis. In addition, perforations large and severe enough to require keratoplasty are unlikely to reform temporarily with adhesive and/or patch; however this technique is occasionally useful.

The recipient cornea is removed with curved corneal scissors. This step can be more difficult than usual because corneal opacification may hinder the surgeon's view. Care must be taken to avoid cutting uvea, lens, or intraocular lens, which may be displaced anteriorly. If vitreous is adherent to the cornea, it should be cut with Wescott or deWecker scissors before removal of the button. Once the recipient button is removed, the anterior chamber should be inspected for peripheral anterior synechiae, posterior synechiae, and cataract. In most situations, cataract removal is left for a subsequent procedure because the risk of expulsive hemorrhage, vitreous loss, endophthalmitis, and sequestered organisms may be higher at the time of the initial procedure. Posterior and anterior synechiae should be gently lysed and one or multiple peripheral iridectomies performed. The anterior chamber is then irrigated to remove any necrotic or inflammatory debris. A small amount of viscoelastic should be placed in the angle and over the iris and pupil.

The donor cornea is then placed onto the eye and secured with at least 16 interrupted 10-0 nylon sutures. The anterior chamber should be reinflated with balanced salt solution and the periphery swept with the tip of the cannula or cyclodialysis spatula to avoid peripheral anterior synechia formation. The wound is then checked for any possible leaks. Subconjunctival injections of antibiotics (e.g., cefazolin, 100 mg/0.5 ml, or vancomycin, 25 mg/0.5 ml, and gentamicin, 20 mg/0.5 ml) can be given in the inferior cul-de-sac. One may wish to withhold a depot injection of steroid, which might typically be administered (e.g., betamethasone sodium phosphate/betamethasone acetate, [Celestone] 3 mg/0.5 ml), if an infection is present and particularly in fungal and severe bacterial infections.

Postoperative care can be most challenging. The need for intensive topical steroids to reduce inflammation and the chance of graft rejection must be weighed against the reduced host immunity it may create or the sterile corneal melt it might incite or exacerbate. Nonetheless, topical corticosteroids (e.g., prednisolone acetate 1%) are typically given four times a day, except in fungal infections. Topical fortified antibiotics are used with a similar frequency if persistent bacterial infection is suspected. Antifungals and antivirals may also be used if necessary. A broad-spectrum commercial strength antibiotic such as trimethoprim/polymyxin B may be used three to four times a day in noninfected cases or when the infection is thought to be eradicated. Intravenous antibiotics should be continued for at least 72 hours and then discontinued when the patient is discharged. Oral steroids should be considered only if the patient develops an intensive inflammatory response or frank graft rejection. Some emergent grafts will be allowed to fail intentionally with future thoughts of a regraft when conditions are more conducive to graft survival. This is particularly true in some fungal infections in which topical and subconjunctival steroids should be withheld, with the understanding that the graft is likely to fail. Intraocular pressure should be monitored carefully, and antiglaucoma medications including β-blockers, apraclonidine, and carbonic anhydrase inhibitors, should be prescribed as needed.

Once the acute postoperative period is over, long-term care is similar as that for uncomplicated penetrating keratoplasty. Corticosteroids should be tapered gradually; and visual rehabilitation using spectacles, contact lenses, or selective suture removal may be attempted in the future.

A 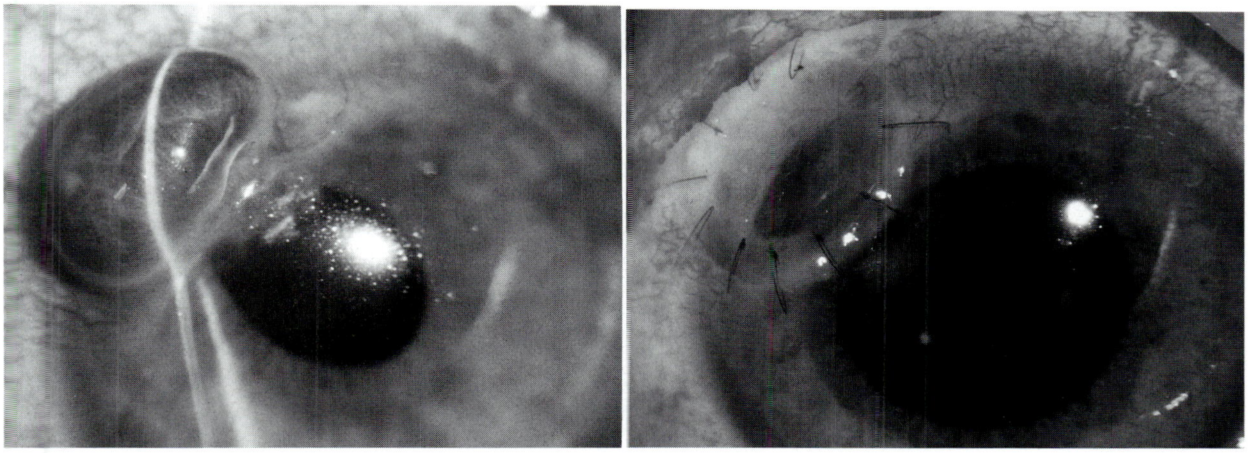 B

FIGURE 148-8 **A,** Large but peripheral area of iris prolapse covered with an intact epithelium and Descemet's membrane. It was not leaking and the anterior chamber was formed. **B,** It was treated with a patch graft, which involved full-thickness corneal dissection centrally and partial-thickness scleral dissection peripherally. A full-thickness corneal button was placed.

PATCH GRAFT

Patch grafts may be used to temporarily or permanently repair both peripheral or central descemetoceles and perforations. Such a graft is usually performed in lesions that are too large to use tissue adhesive but small enough to obviate the need for a full-sized penetrating keratoplasty (usually 5 mm or less) (Figure 148-8, *A*). It is important to ensure that the patch graft and its sutures will not interfere with the visual axis (Figure 148-8, *B*). If the lesion is small but a patch graft would interfere with vision, a full-sized penetrating keratoplasty is often preferable. A lamellar patch graft may be quite effective in reinforcing an area of thinned and necrotic stroma with descemetocele formation or to treat a chronic, nonhealing stromal ulceration. Alternatively, a full-thickness patch graft may be technically easier to perform and more effective if uveal tissue is permanently incorporated into the perforation site.

The preoperative preparation for a patch graft is identical to that described for penetrating keratoplasty. A Barraquer eyelid speculum is placed in the eye, but the Flieringa ring is usually omitted. Viscoelastic substance can be injected, preferably through a paracentesis site, but it can be instilled directly through the perforation site if paracentesis is difficult because of a flat anterior chamber. The ulcerated or thinned area is outlined with a small trephine for central and midperipheral circular ulcers (Figure 148-9, *A*). A sharp blade is used to deepen the trephination and ensure adequate and uniform depth (Figure 148-9, *B*). Peripheral ulcers may require conjunctival peritomy and scleral dissection if the lesion extends to the limbus or into sclera. Crescentic or irregular configurations are outlined on one side, typically the corneal side, using a standard circular trephine, while the scleral side is cut free hand with a blade. In some instances, a free hand incision may be necessary for the entire graft, after the cornea is marked on the surface.

A lamellar dissection is then performed within the margins of the trephined areas (Figure 148-9, *C*). Care must be taken to remove all the necrotic tissue and to achieve a proper depth (at least one-half normal thickness) for the lamellar dissection. A smooth recipient bed to the level of deep cornea or even Descemet's membrane should be created. A same size or slightly larger diameter lamellar donor button is then prepared from a donor globe or cornea in the usual fashion. The donor patch is then secured in position with multiple interrupted 10-0 nylon sutures. Sutures placed on the side of the graft closest to the visual axis can be made intentionally shorter to further reduce the possibility that vision will be affected. When dealing with irregular or noncircular patches, it is sometimes easier to suture one margin of the donor into place, trim the other margins of the button to ensure a good fit, and then suture the remaining margins of the patch.

A similar procedure using deep lamellar trephination and a full-thickness donor patch graft can also be performed with good results. In this procedure the chamber is entered with a sharp blade, and the recipient cornea is removed with curved corneal scissors. Great care should be taken to avoid damaging lens or iris. Any uveal tissue should be gently teased away from the excised cornea or simply cut away with scissors if it is too firmly adherent. If a large iridectomy remains after this maneuver, a pupilloplasty can be performed with a 10-0 polypropylene suture on a

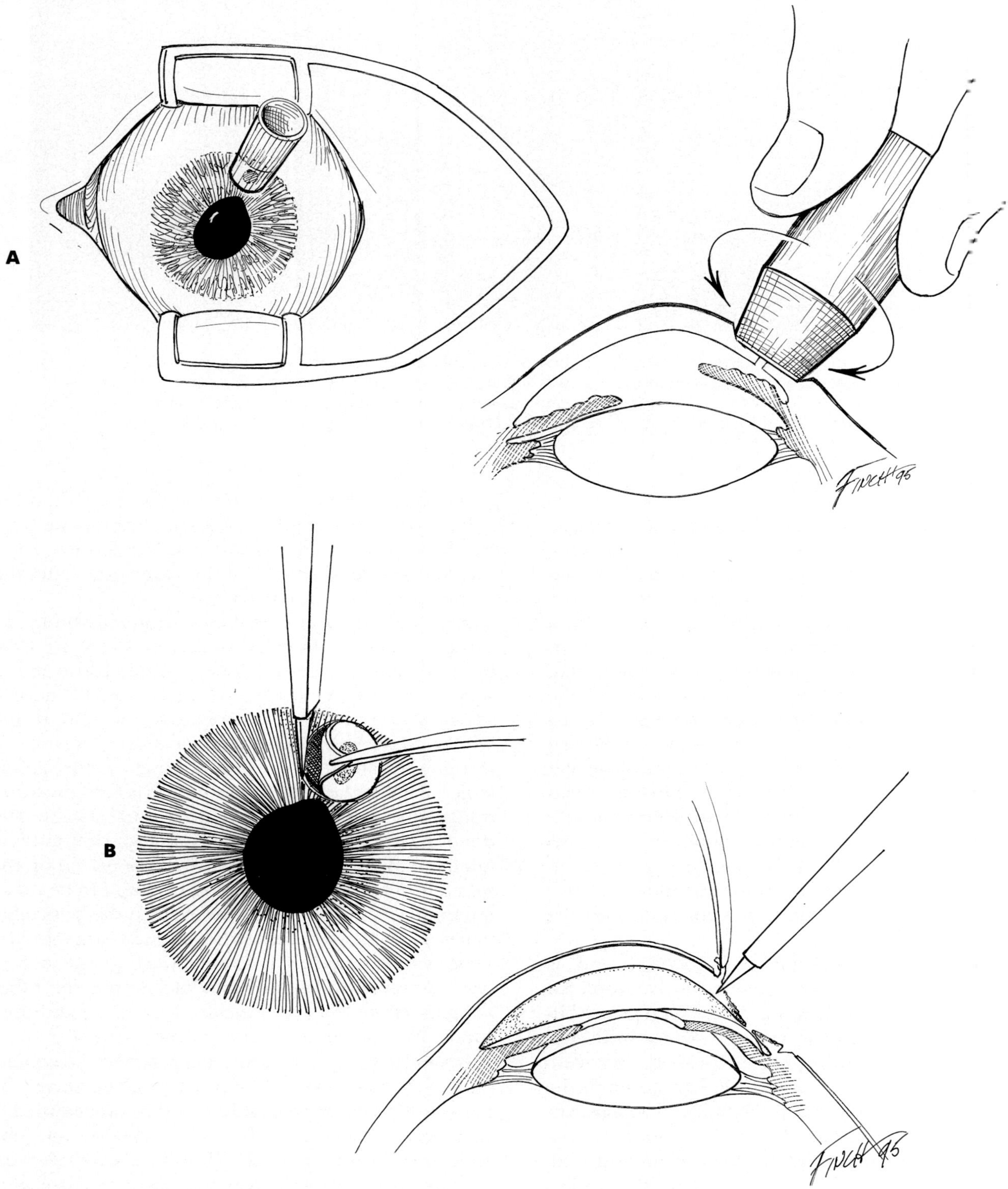

FIGURE 148-9 Repair of a corneal perforation with a patch graft, demonstrated by front and profile drawings. **A,** The perforated area is outlined with a small trephine and a partial-thickness trephination is performed. **B,** A sharp blade is used to deepen the trephination mark and ensure adequate and uniform depth. *Continued.*

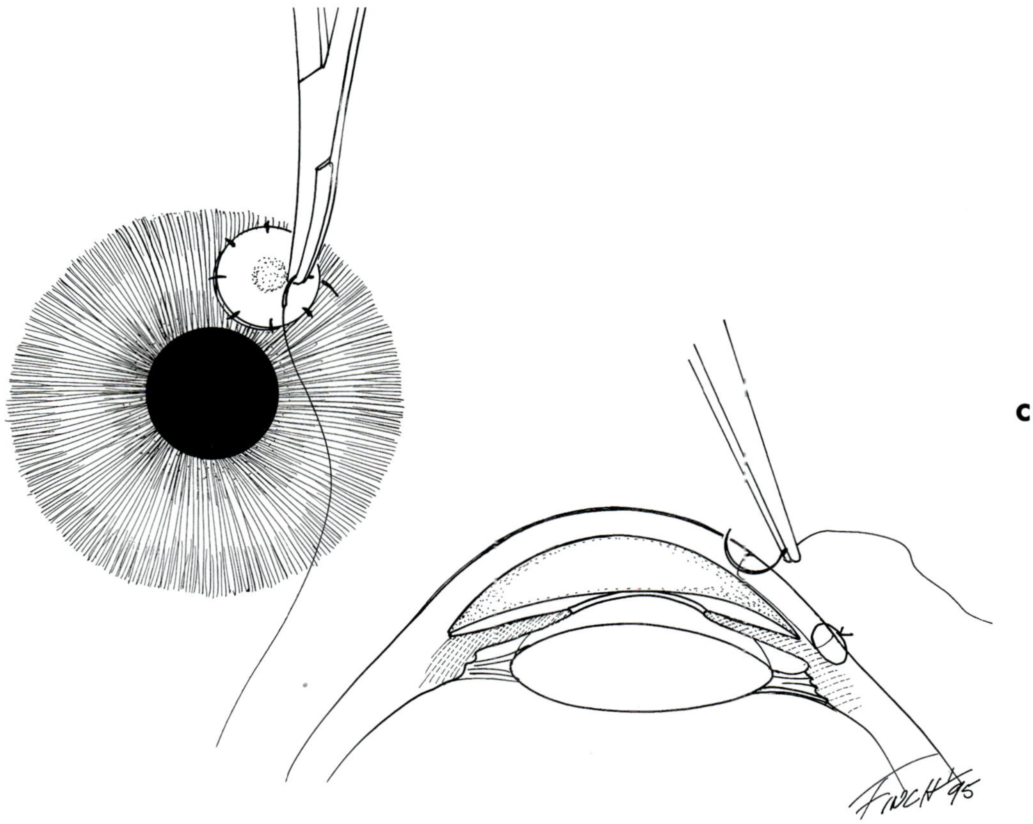

FIGURE 148-9, cont'd. **C,** Lamellar dissection is performed within the margins of the trephined areas. All necrotic tissue should be removed creating a smooth recipient bed to the level of deep cornea or even Descemet's membrane. The donor button is secured in place with multiple interrupted 10-0 nylon sutures.

vascular needle. Appositional 10-0 nylon sutures are used to secure the donor in place. The anterior chamber should be reinflated with balanced salt solution and the wound checked to assure watertightness. The principles of postoperative management are similar to that for full-sized penetrating keratoplasty. Because these grafts are often located outside the visual axis, however, permanent graft clarity is not as essential for good postoperative vision as it is for full-sized penetrating keratoplasty.

CONSERVATIVE MANAGEMENT

Selected cases not amenable to repair with tissue adhesive because of size, configuration, or degree of suppuration or in patients who are poor surgical candidates, may be treated by conservative methods. Descemetoceles and perforations in debilitated and combative patients can be treated with aggressive antibiotics and/or lubricants. In some cases, the perforation may self-seal because of tissue edema, fibrin, or uvea plugging the wound or because of spontaneous reepithelialization. Cases have been described in patients with small peripheral perforations and conditions that heal notoriously poorly (e.g., rheumatoid arthritis, Stevens-Johnson syndrome) where simply dilating the pupil has caused iris to plug the hole.[41] In these instances, the epithelium usually covers the perforation within 1 week, and new blood vessels invade the area to heal the stroma shortly thereafter. Conservative management should always remain an option of last resort, however, because the chance of a good visual outcome is generally poor.

Other less conventional methods to treat perforations have been described in the literature with variable results. These options are usually reserved for situations in which the preceding methods have already failed or when appropriate donor tissue is not readily available. Autologous donor tissue from the fellow blind, amblyopic, or even normal eye can be used to perform a lamellar patch graft.[42] Temporary lamellar and penetrating grafts have been described using Gore-Tex (expanded polytetrafluoroethylene, W.L. Gore Inc., Flagstaff, AZ) to keep the anterior chamber formed until a time that penetrating keratoplasty could be performed.[43] In general the material was well tolerated and eventually removed within 2 months of the original procedure.

Prevention of Corneal Perforation

Corneal ulcers that threaten perforation must be identified and treated aggressively. Once perforation has occurred, the management options and visual prognosis are greatly affected. The underlying condition will direct the treatment modality. The general principle is to promote reepithelialization and stromal repair. Some infected ulcers recalcitrant to conventional medical therapy may benefit more from the use of a conjunctival flap, whereas those caused by exposure or decreased sensation may best be treated with punctal occlusion, tarsorrhaphy, or bandage contact lens. Medications such as topical corticosteroids, which can initiate a sterile melt or exacerbate an existing infection, should be discontinued as soon as stromal thinning or impending perforation is recognized. Many other medications or their preservatives can be toxic to the cornea and may also require tapering or discontinuation. Treatment options may overlap in some conditions.

BANDAGE SOFT CONTACT LENS

Certain noninfectious and postinfectious surface healing problems can be helped with the use of bandage contact lenses. Because chronic, nonhealing epithelial defects are prone to ulceration, the use of a contact lens to promote reepithelialization may be of great benefit in some patients. If ulceration has already progressed to descemetocele formation, placement of a contact lens can protect Descemet's membrane and add additional tectonic support until reepithelialization and stromal repair can occur.[44] As with contact lens use after application of tissue adhesive, it is important to use a loose-fitting extended wear contact lens with prophylactic topical antibiotic coverage. Careful follow-up is imperative because of the high risk for infection. Patients must be informed that immediate ophthalmic care is needed if there is increased pain, redness, or discharge. Certain situations are particularly poorly suited for bandage lens use such as ocular cicatricial pemphigoid, severe dry eye, and active infection.

CONJUNCTIVAL FLAP

Conjunctival flaps are useful in the treatment of persistent corneal ulceration and descemetocele, primarily in eyes with poor visual potential. They are contraindicated after a perforation has occurred because persistence of the leak can occur under the flap, causing the flap to fail. A thin, total conjunctival flap such as that described by Gunderson[45] and others[4] is recommended for larger, more central ulcerations, whereas a partial conjunctival flap may be more appropriate in smaller, more peripheral lesions. The techniques for performing a Gunderson conjunctival flap are described in detail elsewhere in the textbook. Similarly, partial conjunctival flaps can be dissected easily and rotated to cover peripheral lesions and secured in place with interrupted 10-0 nylon or 9-0 polyglactin 910 (Vicryl) sutures after the edges and the base of the ulcer have been debrided of epithelium and necrotic material. Conjunctival flaps can work well in certain chronic infectious situations (e.g., herpes simplex or fungal ulcers) where recruitment of a vascular supply to the ulcer aids in the host defenses against the microorganism and also in stromal repair. It can also be used to successfully close chronic, nonhealing epithelial defects that have persisted because of lack of corneal sensation. Because the visual and cosmetic results of a conjunctival flap are poor, other therapeutic options should be considered first.

TARSORRHAPHY

Tarsorrhaphy, like a bandage contact lens punctal occlusion, and aggressive lubrication, is an effective modality in the treatment of chronic corneal ulcerations and in the prevention of perforations. It can be useful in the treatment of small descemetoceles because it provides a smooth surface (tarsal conjunctiva) to protect Descemet's membrane and promote reepithelialization. It has been reported as a possible treatment for very small peripheral perforations[46]; however, it is not a procedure of choice in this setting.

Tarsorrhaphy can be particularly effective in cases of exposure, xerosis, and neurotrophic keratopathy but can be used in numerous other clinical settings. It can be used alone or in conjunction with other techniques both before and after perforation such as tissue adhesive, penetrating keratoplasty, and patch grafting. Tarsorrhaphy can be temporary or "permanent." Temporary tarsorrhaphy, in which the eyelids are closed for several weeks, is indicated for short-term problems (e.g., healing an epithelial defect in a patient with rheumatoid arthritis). "Permanent" tarsorrhaphy, in which the eyelid margins are dissected and sutured together, is performed for more long-standing conditions (e.g., a nonhealing epithelial defect from a neurotrophic cornea). Although they are described as "permanent," these tarsorrhaphies may be taken down months to years later if desired. Unfortunately despite the effectiveness of these tarsorrhaphies, some patients are often disappointed with the cosmetic result.

MISCELLANEOUS

Other methods used to prevent corneal perforation include simple pressure patching, aggressive lubrication, and punctal occlusion in an effort to facilitate reepithelialization. Patching is contraindicated in potentially infectious situations and has other disadvantages such as removing the patient's ability to note any subsequent changes in visual acuity or appearance of the eye.

Conclusions

One of the major goals in managing corneal ulcers must be prevention of descemetocele formation and perforation. Regardless of the cause, any ulcer in which perforation is imminent, or in which a frank perforation exists, must be treated as a true ophthalmic emergency. If perforation has occurred, attempts to restore the structural integrity of the eye as soon as possible using tissue adhesives, penetrating keratoplasty, or a patch graft must be undertaken. The use of tissue adhesives is the simplest, quickest, and safest method of sealing small perforations in the acute setting until a more definitive repair can be performed. Long-term visual rehabilitation can be attempted later, using anterior segment reconstruction and corneal grafting, if the eye still has good potential vision.

REFERENCES

1. Arentsen JJ, Laibson PR, Cohen EJ: Management of corneal descemetoceles and perforations, *Ophthalmic Surg* 16:29-33, 1985.
2. Hirst LW, Smiddy WE, Stark WJ: Corneal perforations: changing methods of treatment, 1960-1980, *Ophthalmology* 89:630-635, 1982.
3. Weiss JL et al: The use of tissue adhesive in corneal perforations, *Ophthalmology* 90:610-615, 1983.
4. Portnoy SL, Insler MS, Kaufman HE: Surgical management of corneal ulceration and perforation, *Surv Ophthalmol* 34:47-58, 1989.
5. Kenyon KR: Corneal perforations: discussion, *Ophthalmology* 89:634-635, 1982.
6. Saini JS, Sharma A, Grewal SPS: Chronic corneal perforations, *Ophthalmic Surg* 23:399-402, 1992.
7. Krachmer JH, Laibson PR: Corneal thinning and perforation in Sjogren's syndrome, *Am J Ophthalmol* 78:917-920, 1974.
8. Gudas PP et al: Corneal perforations in Sjögren syndrome, *Arch Ophthalmol* 90:470-472, 1973.
9. Pfister RR: The effect of chemical injury on the ocular surface, *Ophthalmology* 90:601-609, 1983.
10. Vajpayee RB et al: Contact thermal burns of the cornea, *Can J Ophthalmol* 26:215-218, 1991.
11. Gelender H: Descemetocele after intraocular lens implantation, *Arch Ophthalmol* 100:72-76, 1982.
12. Insler MS, Boutros G, Boulware DW: Corneal ulceration following cataract surgery in patients with rheumatoid arthritis, *Am Intraocular Implant Soc J* 11:594-597, 1985.
13. Krachmer JH, Feder RS, Belin MW: Keratoconus and related noninflammatory corneal thinning disorders, *Surv Ophthalmol* 28:293-322, 1984.
14. Musco PS, Aquavella JV: Cornea fistula, *Ophthalmic Surg* 18: 574-575, 1987.
15. Lahoud S et al: Keratoconus with spontaneous perforation of the cornea, *Can J Ophthalmol* 22:230-233, 1987.
16. Duke-Elder S, Leigh AG: *System of ophthalmology: diseases of the outer eye*, part 2, vol VIII, St Louis, 1965, Mosby.
17. Goosey JD, Mosteller MW, Kaufman HE: Radiating folds in Descemet's membrane as a sign of impending corneal perforation, *Am J Ophthalmol* 98:625-626, 1984.
18. Webster RG Jr et al: The use of adhesive for the closure of corneal perforations, *Arch Ophthalmol* 80:705-709, 1968.
19. Hirst LW, Smiddy WE, DeJuan E: Tissue adhesive therapy for corneal perforations, *Aust J Ophthalmol* 11:113-118, 1983.
20. Nobe JR et al: Results of penetrating keratoplasty for the treatment of corneal perforations, *Arch Ophthalmol* 108:939-941, 1990.
21. Dohlman CH, Boruchoff SA, Sullivan GL: A technique for the repair of perforated corneal ulcers, *Arch Ophthalmol* 77: 519-525, 1967.
22. Tragakis MP, Rosen J, Brown SI: Transplantation of the perforated cornea, *Am J Ophthalmol* 78:518-522, 1974.
23. Eiferman RA, Snyder JW: Antibacterial effect of cyanoacrylate glue, *Arch Ophthalmol* 101:958-960, 1983.
24. Leahey AB, Gottsch JD, Stark WJ: Clinical experience with n-butyl cyanoacrylate (Nexacryl) tissue adhesive, *Ophthalmology* 100: 173-180, 1993.
25. Refojo MF: Current status of biomaterials in ophthalmology, *Surv Ophthalmol* 26:257-265, 1982.
26. Erdey RA et al: Techniques for application of tissue adhesive for corneal perforations, *Ophthalmic Surg* 22:352-354, 1991.
27. Wessels IF, McNeill JI: Applicator for cyanoacrylate tissue adhesive, *Ophthalmic Surg* 80:211-214, 1989.
28. Refojo MF, Dohlman CH, Koliopoulos J: Adhesives in ophthalmology: a review, *Surv Ophthalmol* 15:217-236, 1971.
29. Lagoutte FM, Gauthier L, Comte PRM: A fibrin sealant for perforated and preperforated corneal ulcers, *Br J Ophthalmol* 73:757-761, 1989.
30. Lin DTC, Webster RG, Abbott RL: Repair of corneal lacerations and perforations, *Int Ophthalmol Clin* 28:69-75, 1988.
31. Hirst LW, DeJuan E: Sodium hyaluronate and tissue adhesive in treating corneal perforations, *Ophthalmology* 89:1250-1253, 1982.
32. Refojo MF et al: Evaluation of adhesives for corneal surgery, *Arch Ophthalmol* 80:645-656, 1968.
33. Boruchoff SA, Donshik PC: Medical and surgical management of corneal thinnings and perforations, *Int Ophthalmol Clin* 15: 111-123, 1975.
34. Hirst LW, Stark WJ, Jensen AD: Tissue adhesives: new perspectives in corneal perforations, *Ophthalmic Surg* 10:58-64, 1979.
35. Hyndiuk RA, Hull DS, Kinyoun JL: Free tissue patch and cyanoacrylate in corneal perforations, *Ophthalmic Surg* 5:50-55, 1974.
36. Carlson AN, Wilhelmus KR: Giant papillary conjunctivitis associated with cyanoacrylate glue, *Am J Ophthalmol* 104:437-438, 1987.
37. Hida T et al: Retinal toxicity of cyanoacrylate tissue adhesive in the rabbit, *Retina* 8:148-153, 1988.
38. Ferry AP, Barnert AH: Granulomatous keratitis resulting from use of cyanoacrylate adhesive for closure of perforated corneal ulcer, *Am J Ophthalmol* 72:538-541, 1971.
39. Patten JT, Cavanagh HD, Pavan-Langston D: Penetrating keratoplasty in acute herpetic corneal perforations, *Ann Ophthalmol* 8: 287-294, 1976.
40. Mizuno K, Hayasaka S: Penetrating keratoplasty with use of

adhesives and scleral strip in acute corneal perforations, *Ophthalmic Surg* 13:475-477, 1982.
41. Brown SI: The treatment of corneal perforations, *Trans Pa Acad Ophthalmol Otolaryngol* 28:118-120, 1975.
42. Lam S et al: Lamellar corneal autograft for corneal perforation, *Ophthalmic Surg* 22:716-717, 1991.
43. Legeais JM et al: Surgical management of corneal perforation with expanded polytetrafluoroethylene (Gore-Tex), *Ophthalmic Surg* 22:213-217, 1991.
44. Leibowitz HM, Berrospi AR: Initial treatment of descemetocele with hydrophilic contact lenses, *Ann Ophthalmol* 7:1161 1166, 1975.
45. Gundersen T: Conjunctival flaps in the treatment of corneal disease with reference to a new technique of application *Arch Ophthalmol* 60:880-888, 1958.
46. Pakarinen M, Tervo T, Tarkkanen A: Tarsorrhaphy in the treatment of persistent corneal lesions, *Acta Ophthalmol (Copenh)* 65 (Suppl 182): 69-73, 1987.

CHAPTER 149

WILLIAM H. BENSON JOHN D. GOOSEY

Lamellar Keratoplasty

Lamellar keratoplasty consists of placing a partial-thickness donor corneal graft within a recipient corneal bed that is prepared with a lamellar dissection of abnormal corneal tissue. Lamellar keratoplasty can be performed for either optical or tectonic purposes. Optical lamellar keratoplasty can be performed for any corneal disorder that causes reduced corneal clarity or surface irregularity over the visual axis, resulting in significant visual impairment but sparing Descemet's membrane. Tectonic lamellar keratoplasty is usually performed to restore the normal peripheral corneal thickness that has been abnormally thinned because of any of various disease processes.

The criteria for lamellar keratoplasty include a reasonably healthy recipient ocular surface, adequate endothelial cell function, a corneal opacity that spares Descemet's membrane, or a grossly distorted corneal surface that precludes contact lens fit. The ideal patient population includes young active patients, one-eyed patients, and patients with a history of poor compliance.

Clinical Indications for Lamellar Keratoplasty

Clinical indications for optical lamellar keratoplasty include keratoconus or other corneal ectasias, corneal stromal dystrophies and degenerations that involve the visual axis and that spare Descemet's membrane, corneal leukomas from nonperforating trauma or resolved infectious keratitis (Figures 149-1 and 149-2), surgically induced abnormalities from refractive keratotomy or keratomileusis such as irregular astigmatism and autoimmune or neurotrophic corneal melting. Tectonic lamellar keratoplasty may be used for the surgical rehabilitation of corneal thinning disorders such as Terrien's marginal degeneration, Mooren's ulcer, any peripheral ulcerative process of an immunologic etiology, or restoration of the normal anatomic thickness after the surgical excision of tissue from the corneal surface, such as a dermoid, pterygium, or neoplasm.

Lamellar Versus Penetrating Keratoplasty

Three variables that require consideration for choosing the best method of keratoplasty with regard to underlying corneal disease and centration are optical, tectonic, and biological. Penetrating keratoplasty is the most common surgical procedure used for patients that require optical keratoplasty because it offers excellent visual results. Lamellar keratoplasty has become less popular because it is technically more difficult to perform than penetrating keratoplasty. Although lamellar keratoplasty has become less popular for the treatment of disorders that require optical keratoplasty, it has several advantages over penetrating keratoplasty. It is an extraocular procedure that offers intraoperative safety, especially for single-eyed patients and those that experienced a poor surgical result with penetrating keratoplasty in the other eye. In most cases, there are fewer intraoperative and postoperative complications than with penetrating keratoplasty, and the risks of intraocular surgery are avoided. Lamellar grafts have superior wound strength and can be considered for young and physically active patients. They can also be considered for patients with poor access or a history of poor compliance to ophthalmic care.

The use of lamellar keratoplasty can achieve the goals of both optical and tectonic rehabilitation. Patients with pellucid marginal corneal degeneration or keratoconus and eccentric corneal thinning may exhibit a large amount of astigmatism and visual impairment and both spectacle and contact lens intolerance. A large, eccentric lamellar graft can be used to reduce astigmatism and improve vision as well as to provide structural support to the thinned peripheral cornea. In these patients, lamellar keratoplasty can accomplish both optical and tectonic purposes (Figure 149-3).

Many patients with advanced keratoconus that will eventually require keratoplasty are young and physically active. Inadequate vision from anterior stromal scarring over the visual axis or contact lens intolerance resulting from corneal surface irregularities are the two

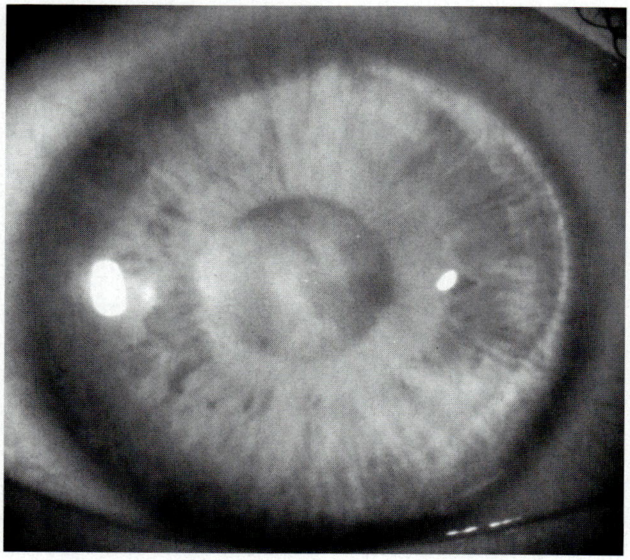

FIGURE 149-1 Corneal stromal scar from previous *Pseudomonas* corneal ulcer.

indications for surgical intervention in keratoconus patients. It is often difficult to decide which surgical procedure is optimal for an individual patient who requires visual rehabilitation. Because many patients have anterior stromal scarring over the visual axis, visual rehabilitation requires removal of the corneal scar with either penetrating keratoplasty or lamellar keratoplasty.

Penetrating keratoplasty can yield superior visual results to lamellar keratoplasty for patients with keratoconus.[1-3] However, penetrating keratoplasty has a greater likelihood for loss of graft clarity than lamellar keratoplasty as a result of allograft reaction episodes or intraoperative complications.[4,5] Numerous studies compiled by Wilhelmus[6] reported an 18% mean weighted incidence of allograft reaction episodes following penetrating keratoplasty for keratoconus. Although most allograft reactions can be treated successfully without a loss of graft clarity, long-term studies of penetrating keratoplasty report that 7% to 10% of grafts ultimately fail, with endothelial cell rejection being the most common reason for allograft failure. Lamellar keratoplasty, however, eliminates this undesirable biological outcome because the endothelial cell layer that is subject to rejection from inflammatory mediators is not transplanted with lamellar grafts.

Lamellar keratoplasty has several other advantages over penetrating keratoplasty. Lamellar grafts can replace large and eccentrically displaced areas of corneal surface irregularity and thinning without the risk for immune reactions to the endothelium, which carry an increased incidence among eccentric penetrating grafts adjacent to the limbus. There is a less rigid requirement for the quality of donor tissue because the age of the donor and the endothelial cell integrity is not important. Corneal tissue that would otherwise be rejected for penetrating keratoplasty may be used for lamellar keratoplasty. Patients in areas where tissue availability is limited as a result of increasing demand, stricter donor screening requirements, or a paucity of donor corneal tissue should be considered for lamellar grafting.

The advantages of lamellar keratoplasty have been affirmed in several studies.[7-13] Visual acuities achieved in those studies, however, were inferior by approximately one line of Snellen visual acuity to those published in comparable reports for penetrating keratoplasty. Visual acuity achieved after lamellar keratoplasty can be limited by four potential problems: (1) irregular and uneven dissection of donor corneal tissue, (2) particulate debris trapped in the lamellar interface, (3) irregular and uneven dissection of the recipient bed, and (4) mechanical folds in the posterior layer over the visual axis induced from flattening of this layer with donor corneal tissue. Mechanical folds are usually encountered in cases of advanced keratoconus, which comprise the most difficult population of patients that require a keratoplasty for visual rehabilitation because of the irregular and abnormal posterior corneal curvatures that are present at the time of surgery. Patients who require keratoplasty for corneal stromal dystrophies, degenerations, or stromal leukomas usually exhibit a normal posterior corneal curvature preoperatively and do not encounter this problem.

Preoperative Evaluation

Preoperative evaluation for those undergoing lamellar keratoplasty should include careful screening for the presence of any preexisting ocular surface diseases that could impair epithelialization of the donor graft or reduce postoperative graft clarity if the disease recurs. External diseases that either contraindicate keratoplasty or categorize it as a high risk for failure include previous herpes simplex keratitis, herpes zoster ophthalmicus, chemical or radiation injuries, Stevens-Johnson syndrome, ocular cicatricial pemphigoid, aniridia, neurotrophic keratopathy, lagophthalmos with exposure keratopathy, severe keratoconjunctivitis sicca, and severe type III or type IV hypersensitivity disease such as staphylococcal toxin hypersensitivity or phlyctenulosis. However, it is not always possible to avoid keratoplasty in these patients. If a high risk keratoplasty is performed, aggressive measures should be taken postoperatively to treat the underlying ocular surface disease and to promote epithelialization of the donor

A

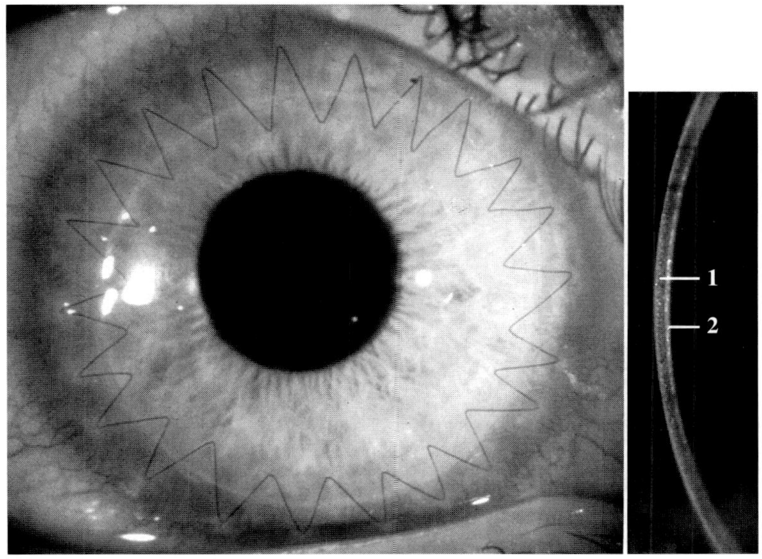

B

FIGURE 149-2 Deep optical lamellar keratoplasty performed for visual rehabilitation. **A,** Diffuse view. **B,** Slit view shows donor *(1)* and host *(2)* corneal tissue.

A

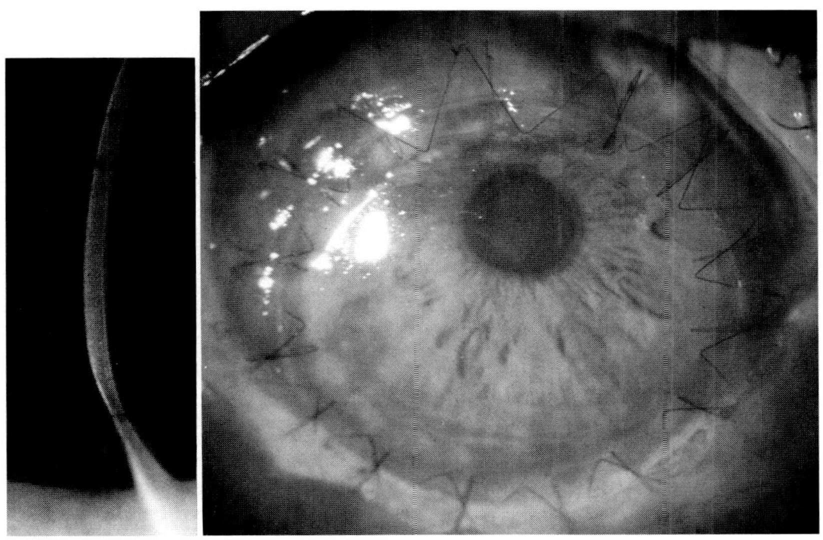

B

FIGURE 149-3 Surgery for pellucid marginal degeneration. **A,** Typical eccentric crescentric thinning of the inferior cornea in a patient with pellucid marginal corneal degeneration. **B,** A large, eccentric lamellar keratoplasty was performed for both optical and tectonic purposes.

graft. For example, in some instances a temporary tarsorrhaphy may be necessary to encourage epithelialization of the donor graft, and oral corticosteroids may be necessary to reduce inflammation when topical steroids cannot be administered.

Other preoperative considerations should include evaluation of Descemet's membrane and a determination of host endothelial cell integrity. Poor endothelial cell function or previous breaks in Descemet's membrane are contraindications for inlay lamellar keratoplasty. Patients with marginal endothelial cell function may not exhibit a sufficient reserve capacity to deturgesce the donor graft, which could delay or prevent epithelialization. A split in Descemet's membrane caused by previous trauma or corneal hydrops will remain a point of poor tissue strength that could separate again at the time of deep lamellar dissection. Although small tears in Descemet's membrane at the time of deep keratectomy can be managed with careful measures, these potential problems should be avoided

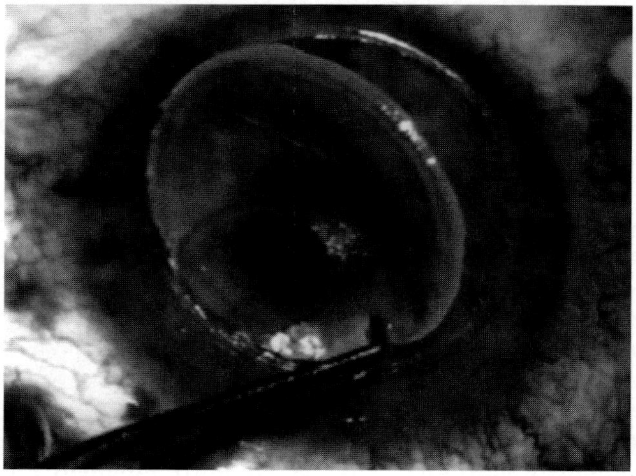

FIGURE 149-8 Fresh-frozen cryolathed tissue eliminates the technical difficulty of preparing donor tissue and provides a uniform posterior donor surface.

posterior donor surface (Figure 149-8). Donor lamellar tissue is commercially available as fresh tissue (Cryo-Optics, Houston, TX) that is frozen and lathed to a specified thickness and diameter. The tissue is stored in corneal storage media for up to 96 hours before surgery. We find that a plano donor graft with a thickness of 0.38 mm and a diameter of 9.2 mm apposes the recipient wound well within an 8.5 mm diameter circular keratotomy incision. Expanded use of the excimer laser may suggest a potential role for this instrument in the processing of fresh donor corneal tissue. As with cryolathed corneal tissue, this method provides a corneal lenticule with a smoother surface than that of a hand-cut lenticule.[23]

The presence of lint and talc in the operative field has the potential to create opacities in the graft interface. This complication can be minimized by using talc-free gloves and cellulose sponges. The recipient bed is then irrigated and wiped with a cellulose sponge to remove any debris from the surfaces and avoid entrapment of foreign material in the interface between the graft and the underlying recipient cornea. The donor graft is sutured into the host keratectomy bed with 16 interrupted 10-0 nylon sutures on adjustable knots. Each suture knot is tied with three single throws. The first two single throws are tied as an adjustable slip knot that can be tightened and loosened to a desired tension (Figure 149-9). After the corneal graft is secured with 16 interrupted sutures and tied with slip knots, the sutures can be adjusted to obtain a spherical surface over the visual axis as determined by qualitative keratometry (Figure 149-10). After the adjustment of suture tension, the slip knots are secured with a third single throw to create a square knot over each slip knot.

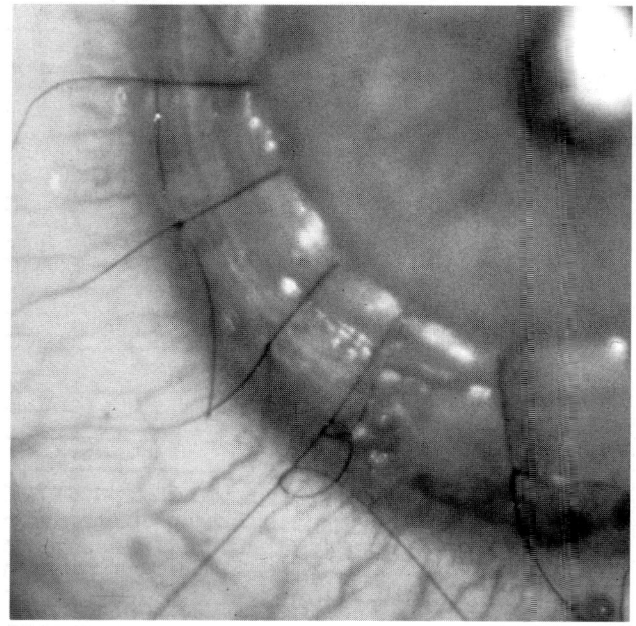

FIGURE 149-9 Slip knot tied to allow adjustment of suture tension.

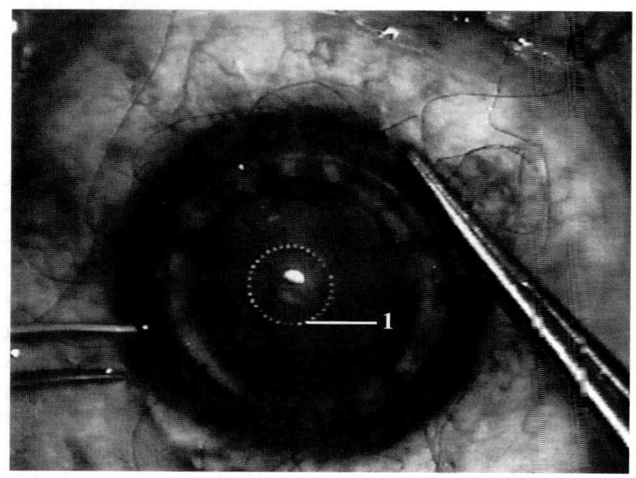

FIGURE 149-10 Intraoperative qualitative keratometry (1) used as a guide to selectively adjust suture tension at the time of wound closure to obtain a spherical surface over the visual axis.

Postoperatively, all patients are pressure-patched until the graft has epithelialized, a process that takes an average of 3 to 5 days. Suture removal is performed selectively to control astigmatism induced by the forces of wound healing. All sutures can be removed between 6 and 9 months after surgery.

For patients with advanced keratoconus who undergo deep lamellar keratoplasty, mechanically induced folds in the posterior layer are an inevitable consequence of donor tissue compression that produces uneven flattening of the posterior recipient bed.

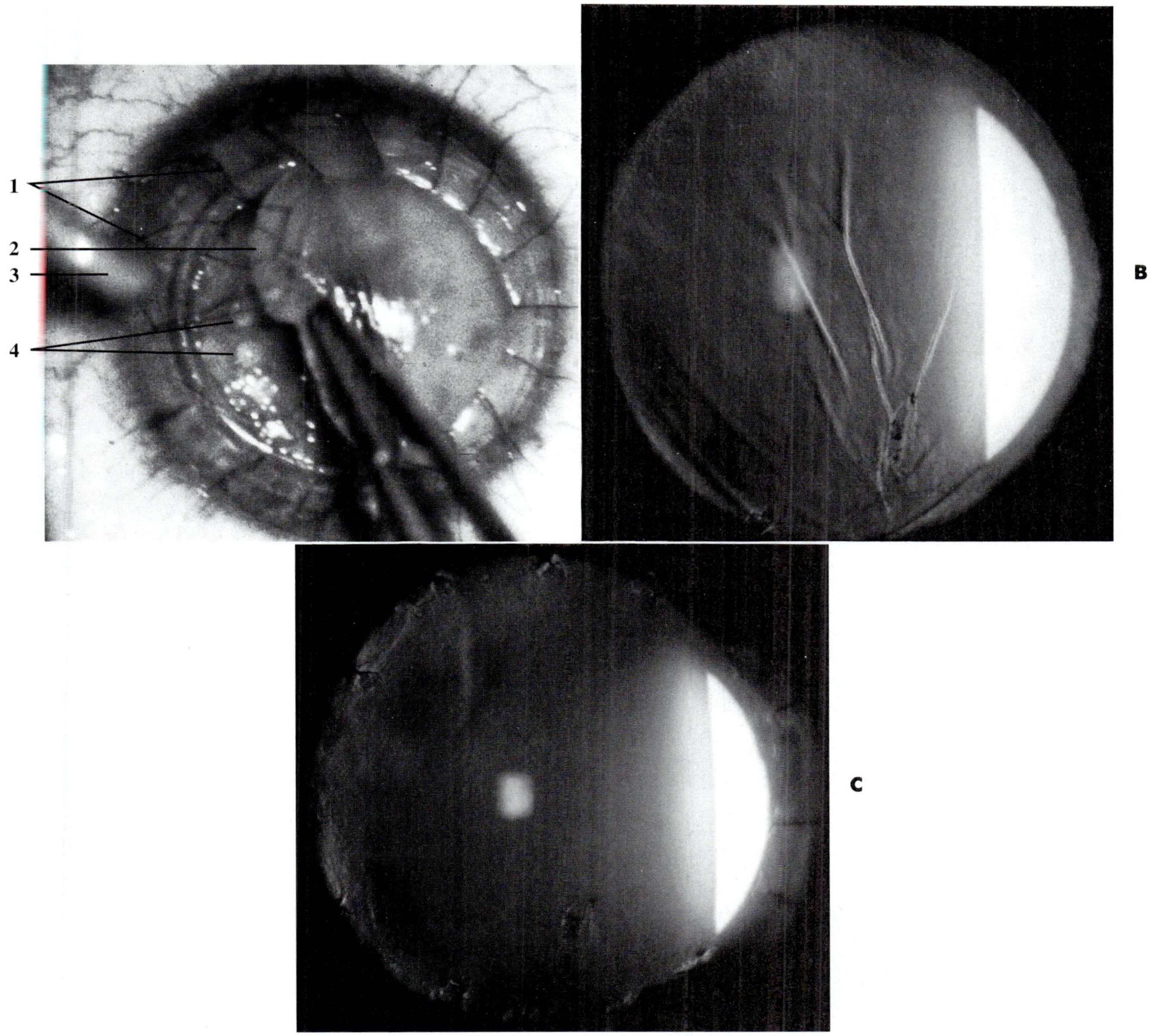

FIGURE 149-11 **A,** Slip knots *(1)* are loosened, the donor tissue *(2)* is lifted,and a diathermy instrument *(3)* is used to apply heat to the peripheral host bed *(4),* resulting in shrinkage of the tissue, thus ironing out the folds. **B,** Application of diathermy to the peripheral recipient bed caused the tissue to gather up by stretching. **C,** Smoothing of the posterior surface over the visual axis with resolution of the mechanical folds occurs after application of diathermy.

The persistence and extent of these folds are related to the age of the patient and usually disappear more rapidly for those less than 30 years of age. A method of reducing mechanical folds over the visual axis involves thermokeratoplasty to "shrink" the posterior layer. The application of diathermy to the peripheral aspects of the flattened, corrugated posterior recipient bed reduces the presence of folds. After diathermy, the peripheral tissue gathers or draws up, with resultant smoothing of the surface over the visual axis (Figure 149-11). These technical modifications of the procedure such as the use of cryolathed corneal donor tissue, wound closure with adjustable sutures, and the application of diathermy to the posterior recipient layer for those patients with keratoconus can improve the visual results with optical lamellar keratoplasty from those of previously described methods.[12]

Tectonic inlay lamellar keratoplasty consists of

A

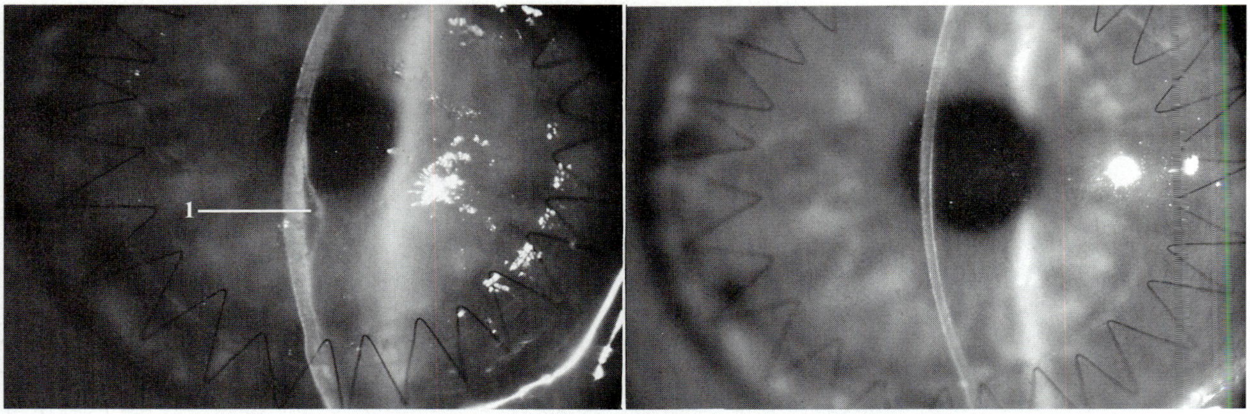

B

FIGURE 149-12 **A,** Postoperative interface separation *(1)* of the graft and posterior corneal layer following perforation of Descemet's membrane during deep lamellar keratoplasty. **B,** Spontaneous apposition of graft and posterior corneal layer 1 week postoperatively.

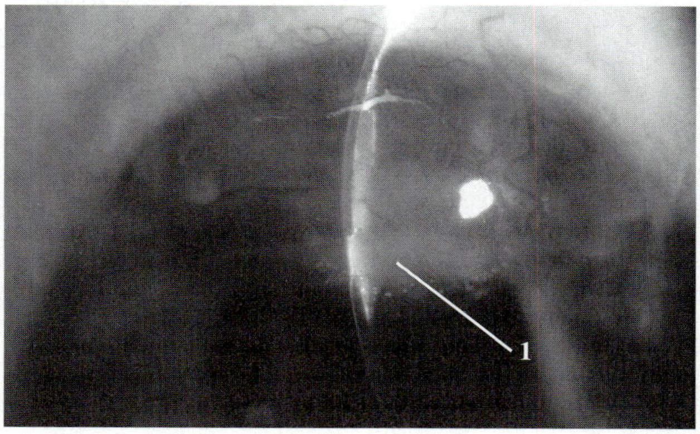

FIGURE 149-13 Interface epithelial inclusion cyst *(1)* following tectonic lamellar keratoplasty for Terrien's marginal degeneration.

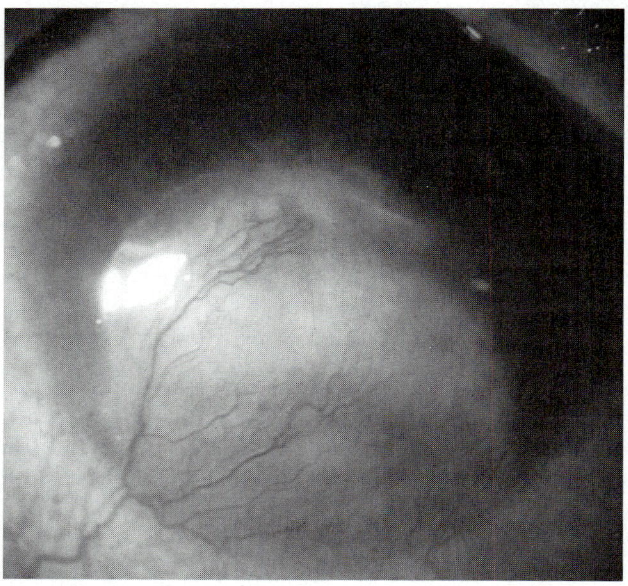

FIGURE 149-14 Corneal pannus with underlying stromal scarring and thinning following corneal ulceration from erythema multiforme (Stevens-Johnson syndrome).

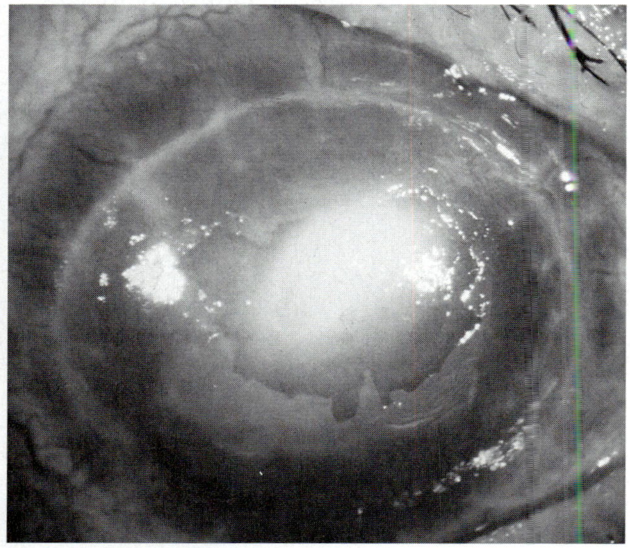

FIGURE 149-15 Lamellar graft with persistent epithelial defect and stromal infiltrate caused by preexisting ocular surface disease from Stevens-Johnson syndrome.

making keratotomy incisions in healthy corneal tissue beyond the abnormal corneal tissue to include removal of all diseased tissue. This technique provides healthy tissue at the keratotomy edge to obtain adequate wound apposition and tissue healing between the graft and host. The keratotomy incisions can be made with an unguarded blade by scratching down or with a guarded diamond knife set to the desired depth. If the abnormal tissue is adjacent to the limbus, a trephine can be used, with more pressure applied to the corneal side by tilting the trephine to avoid excising healthy scleral tissue beyond the limbus. After the incisional keratotomy, the abnormal corneal tissue is removed by the same cut-and-peel technique as described for optical lamellar keratectomy.

Preparation of donor material requires methodical

A B

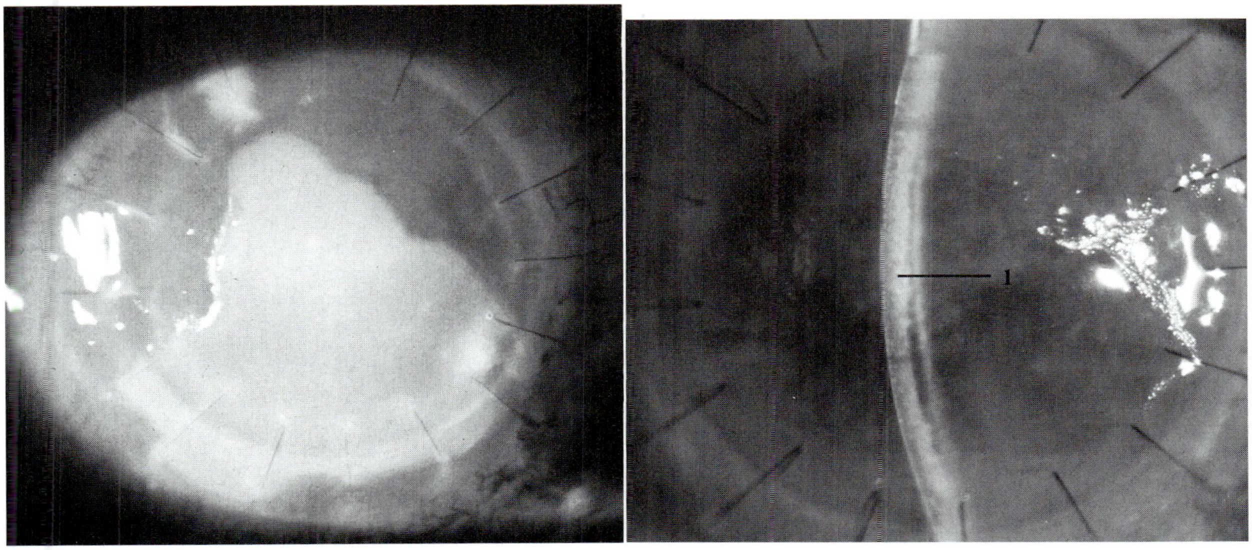

FIGURE 149-16 Lamellar graft with persistent epithelial defect caused by underlying stromal edema and endothelial decompensation sustained during a chemical blast injury preoperatively. **A,** Diffuse view showing defect. **B,** Slit view showing cornea edema (*1*).

whole globe dissection to obtain both the desired thickness and size. A guarded diamond blade can be used to make the keratotomy incision in the donor tissue to achieve the desired thickness. A blunt spatula can then be used to separate the overlying corneal tissue along the plane of dissection determined by the keratotomy incision. The keratectomy bed is often irregularly shaped. The donor tissue must be cut freehand with Vannas scissors to match the shape of the keratectomy bed. The graft is best fit into the keratectomy bed by suturing each wound edge into place after it is cut to the necessary size to fit the keratectomy bed. This approach allows the best fit and avoids errors in undersizing the graft.

Complications of Lamellar Keratoplasty

Perforation of Descemet's membrane is the most important intraoperative complication for lamellar keratoplasty (Figure 149-12). It can occur during the keratotomy incision or at the time of deep lamellar dissection. If perforation occurs with trephination, it is best managed with wound closure of the keratotomy incision at the time of its occurrence. The surgery should be postponed for at least 1 month until Descemet's membrane has healed. If perforation occurs during the keratectomy, the anterior chamber should be reformed with air using an air syringe and cannula through a paracentesis. The keratectomy can be completed with careful sharp dissection over an anterior chamber that maintains reformation with air. Reforming the anterior chamber with viscoelastic material can enlarge the tear in Descemet's membrane and should be avoided. Reapposition of the posterior corneal layer to the graft is best accomplished by introducing air into the anterior chamber through a paracentesis. More than 50% air fill of the anterior chamber should be avoided to prevent a significant rise in the intraocular pressure postoperatively.

Postoperative complications that can lead to loss of graft clarity include interface opacification caused by epithelial or vascular tissue, delayed epithelialization of the graft, and sterile corneal melting.[24-26] Epithelial proliferation along the graft-host interface can occur if epithelial tissue is incarcerated in the keratotomy wound before closure (Figure 149-13). Prolonged surgery with exposure and drying of the ocular surface correlates to the degree of arrested epithelialization. This delayed epithelialization of the graft surface may result from damage to the limbal conjunctival stem cells, which are the source of corneal epithelium for the graft. Persistent epithelial defects can stimulate the ingrowth of blood vessels along the graft interface or encourage the development of corneal melting, particularly in high-risk patients with preexisting ocular surface disease (Figures 149-14 and 149-15). Poor endothelial cell function with impaired deturgescence of the corneal stroma can delay epithelialization of the graft surface (Figure 149-16). Significant visual impairment from loss of graft clarity may require penetrating keratoplasty to accomplish functional visual rehabilitation.

REFERENCES

1. Anseth A: Keratoplasty for keratoconus: a report of fifty operated eyes, *Acta Ophthalmol (Copenh)* 45:684, 1967.
2. Boruchoff SA, Jenson AD, Dohlman CH: Comparison of suturing techniques in keratoplasty for keratoconus, *Ann Ophthalmol* 7:433-436, 1975.
3. Keates HR, Falkenstein S: Keratoplasty in keratoconus, *Am J Ophthalmol* 74:442-444, 1972.
4. Paglen PG et al: The prognosis for keratoplasty in keratoconus, *Ophthalmology* 89:651-654, 1982.
5. Epstein RJ et al: Penetrating keratoplasty for herpes simplex keratitis and keratoconus. Allograft rejection and survival, *Ophthalmology* 94:935-942, 1987.
6. Wilhelmus KR: (In Discussion) Epstein RJ et al: A penetrating keratoplasty for herpes simplex keratitis and keratoconus. Allograft rejection and survival, *Ophthalmology* 94:943-944, 1987.
7. Wood TO: Lamellar transplants in keratoconus, *Am J Ophthalmol* 83:543-545, 1977.
8. Richard JM, Paton D, Gassett AR: A comparison of penetrating keratoplasty and lamellar keratoplasty in the surgical management of keratoconus, *Am J Ophthalmol* 86:807-811, 1978.
9. Gassett AR: Lamellar keratoplasty in the treatment of keratoconus: Conectomy, *Ophthalmic Surg* 10:26-33, 1979.
10. Malbran E, Stefani C: Lamellar keratoplasty in corneal ectasias, *Ophthalmologica* 164:50-58, 1972.
11. Malbran E, Stefani C: Lamellar keratoplasty in corneal ectasias, *Ophthalmologica* 164:59-70, 1972.
12. Benson WH, Goosey CB, Prager TC, Goosey JP: Visual improvement as a function of time after lamellar keratoplasty for keratoconus, *Am J Ophthalmol* 116:207-211, 1993.
13. Vancea PP, Schwartzenberg T: Lamellar keratoplasty in keratoconus, *Graefes Arch Clin Exp Ophthalmol* 212:55-64, 1979.
14. Ehrlich ML et al: Techniques of lamellar keratoplasty, *Int Ophthalmol Clin* 28:24-29, 1988.
15. The cornea and sclera. In Fine BS, Yanoff M, editors: *Ocular histology*, Hagerstown, 163-192, 1979. Harper & Row.
16. Polack FM: Lamellar keratoplasty: Malbran's "peeling off" technique, *Arch Ophthalmol* 86:293-295, 1971.
17. Price FW Jr: Air lamellar keratoplasty, *Refract Corneal Surg* 5:240-243, 1989.
18. Hanna KD et al: Lamellar keratoplasty with the Barraquer microkeratome, *Refract Corneal Surg* 7:177-181, 1991.
19. Haimovici R, Culbertson WW: Optical lamellar keratoplasty using the Barraquer microkeratome, *Refract Corneal Surg* 7:42-45, 1991.
20. Barraquer JL: Lamellar keratoplasty (special techniques), *Ann Ophthalmol* 4:437-469, 1972.
21. Hamilton W, Wood TO: Inlay lamellar keratoplasty. In Kaufman HE et al, editors: *The cornea,* New York, 1988, Churchill Livingstone.
22. Kaufman HE, McDonald MB, Barron BA, Wilson SE: Inlay lamellar keratoplasty. In Wright KW et al, editors: *Corneal and refractive surgery,* Philadelphia, 1992, JB Lippincott.
23. Gabay S, Slomovic A, Jares T: Excimer laser-processed donor corneal lenticules for lamellar keratoplasty, *Am J Ophthalmol* 107:47-51, 1989.
24. Yee RD, Pettit TH: Corneal intrastromal cyst following lamellar keratoplasty, *Ann Ophthalmol* 7:644-646, 1975.
25. Pettit TH: Corneoscleral freehand lamellar keratoplasty in Terrien's marginal degeneration of the cornea long-term results, *Refract Corneal Surg* 7:28-32, 1991.
26. Bessant DA, Dart JK: Lamellar keratoplasty in the management of inflammatory ulceration and perforation, *Eye* 8(Pt 1):22-28, 1994.

CHAPTER 150

ERIC D. DONNENFELD   ANASTASIOS JOHN KANELLOPOULOS

Therapeutic Keratoplasty

Therapeutic keratoplasty is a surgical procedure whose primary purpose is to (1) restore the structural integrity of the eye (tectonic keratoplasty) or (2) resolve an infectious/inflammatory keratitis that is refractory to conventional medical therapy. Often, both these indications are present. Therapeutic keratoplasties are generally emergent or semiemergent procedures in which the survival of the globe is in jeopardy. Whereas visual restoration is the primary goal of an optical penetrating keratoplasty, in therapeutic keratoplasty, acute visual rehabilitation is of secondary importance. Visual rehabilitation, if necessary, can always be accomplished later under more controlled circumstances.

Indications for Therapeutic Keratoplasty

Despite recent advances in the medical management of infectious keratitis, a subgroup of bacteria, fungi, parasites, and viruses do not respond to antimicrobial therapy.[1-7] Therapeutic keratoplasty is indicated when inflammatory or infectious corneal disease is progressing despite maximum medical therapy and the integrity of the globe is compromised. Medical therapy should be continued or altered, if necessary, until there is no reasonable expectation that the infection or inflammation can be controlled or until there is a significant risk of corneal perforation or scleral extension. Corneal perforation dramatically increases the risk of endophthalmitis, and infectious scleritis should be avoided because of the severe morbidity of this disease.[8-11] Noninvasive surgical treatment, such as conjunctival flaps and tarsorrhaphies, can be attempted if indicated.

A therapeutic keratoplasty offers a surgical debridement of an infectious process. The goal of therapeutic keratoplasty is to remove completely the infectious inoculum or to decrease the organisms in the cornea to a level at which exogenous antiinfective/antiinflammatory agents and the patients' endogenous host defense mechanisms can be effective.[12] Robin et al[13] reviewed 497 corneal buttons and noted that penetrating keratoplasty was performed for active bacterial ulcerative keratitis in 7% of these patients and for viral keratitis in 6% of patients.[13] Killingsworth et al[12] reviewed 80 consecutive therapeutic keratoplasties performed in Gainesville, Florida, over a 9-year period. Twenty-six therapeutic keratoplasties were performed for bacterial infections, 15 for fungal infections, 11 for active herpetic keratitis, 4 for persistent epithelial defects following herpes simplex keratitis, 12 for dry eyes, 10 for nonherpetic persistent epithelial defects, and 2 for *Acanthamoeba* keratitis.

When an acute ulceration threatens perforation, the patient should receive systemic and topical therapy to reduce the likelihood of intraocular involvement. Subconjunctival antibiotics do not appear to offer a significant advantage over aggressive topical therapy.[14,15] Once an acute infectious corneal perforation has occurred, topical antimicrobials should be continued, but the physician and patient should be aware of the risk of intraocular toxicity.[16-18]

An attempt to seal the perforation with cyanoacrylate adhesives can be considered.[19,20] After the integrity of the anterior chamber has been reestablished, topical antimicrobial treatment can be reinstituted safely without the risk of intraocular toxicity. Sealing the perforation with cyanoacrylate may often be definitive management, but if the perforation progresses to require therapeutic keratoplasty, the patient will have been temporized with additional antimicrobials and the ulceration, it is hoped, will have been sterilized. When cyanoacrylate is applied, the patient must be monitored closely because bacterial infections can progress beneath the cyanoacrylate glue.[21]

THERAPEUTIC KERATOPLASTY FOR BACTERIAL INFECTIONS

Certain bacteria, notably *Pseudomonas aeruginosa,*[22] can infect the cornea and progress to corneal perforation over 24 to 48 hours. These bacteria may produce collagenase, which results in rapid corneal thinning. Most bacterial infections, when managed expediently, respond to therapy, but because of delay in seeking or obtaining medical treatment, they may progress rapidly to corneal perforation.[23,24] Bacterial keratitis has been treated with both lamellar and

A 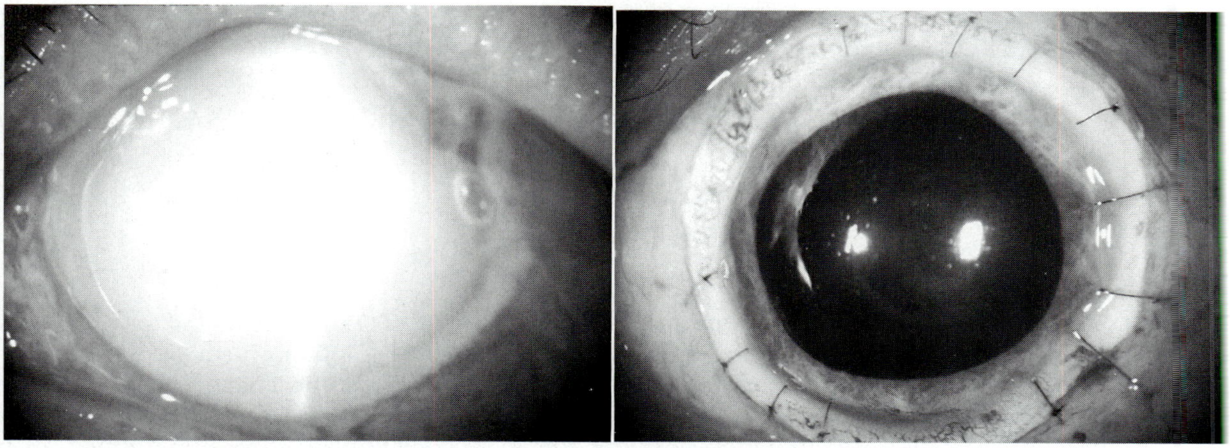 B

FIGURE 150-1 **A,** *Pseudomonas aeruginosa* corneal ulcer with perforation. **B,** A 12 mm therapeutic corneal transplantation. (Courtesy George Stern, MD.)

penetrating keratoplasty in an attempt to reduce the infectious organism count in the cornea when medical treatment has not been successful. Lamellar and penetrating grafts have also been used to prevent and/or treat perforation. Malik and Singh[3] in 1971 managed 36 *Pseudomonas* ulcers with lamellar and penetrating grafts. All eight of the lamellar grafts became reinfected, and one eye was enucleated. Only four of the 28 penetrating therapeutic grafts became reinfected. The authors conclude that penetrating grafts are more efficient in treating active infection than lamellar grafts. Hill[1] in 1986 presented 23 patients with deep, indolent ulceration and/or descemetoceles that were treated with therapeutic keratoplasty. Early surgery did not jeopardize the final outcome of the keratoplasty. The period of morbidity was shorter, and more rapid visual rehabilitation occurred with early keratoplasty, possibly secondary to the fact that corneal neovascularization was prevented by earlier surgical management. Removal of the infected cornea may necessitate a larger than customary keratoplasty to debride the infected tissue. Cowden et al[25] described 14 patients who underwent penetrating keratoplasty with 9.5 mm or larger diameter grafts (Figure 150-1). Five of these patients had bacterial keratitis. The authors concluded that larger diameter penetrating keratoplasties can salvage an eye that may have otherwise been lost and achieve reasonable visual rehabilitation. Although visual prognosis is best when the surgery is performed in a sterilized, minimally inflamed eye, perforation or threatened perforation with uncontrolled progression of disease and/or a necrotic stroma all mandate early intervention. Lam and Cooper[26] in 1989 presented 13 cases treated with therapeutic keratoplasty for bacterial suppurative keratitis, with satisfactory long-term optical results.

A separate subgroup of bacterial keratitis that may require therapeutic keratoplasty are bacterial infections unresponsive to conventional medical therapy. These infections are generally opportunistic and indolent, but continue to progress despite aggressive treatment. This subgroup includes crystalline keratoplasty (most commonly caused by α-hemolytic streptococcus,[12,27] but can be seen with a variety of bacteria, as well as *Candida*. These infections are most commonly seen after corneal surgery and progress relentlessly until a therapeutic keratoplasty is performed.

THERAPEUTIC KERATOPLASTY FOR FUNGAL KERATITIS

The introduction of topical antifungal agents has reduced the need for therapeutic penetrating keratoplasty for fungal keratitis and has also improved the prognosis and visual outcome of patients with medically uncontrolled fungal ulcers. Forster and Rebell[28] reviewed 61 eyes with corneal fungal infections, 13 of which were considered treatment failures. Nine of the 13 treatment failures underwent therapeutic keratoplasty. Five of these nine patients achieved a visual acuity of 20/70 or better. In all nine cases that underwent penetrating keratoplasty, the fungal disease process was halted by therapeutic keratoplasty.[28] Polack et al[29] had reviewed 30 patients with keratomycosis. Of the 22 treated surgically, penetrating keratoplasty was far superior to lamellar keratoplasty. Pathologic examination revealed fungal elements that appeared to penetrate Descemet's membrane, causing a high recurrence rate in lamellar keratoplasty grafts. Forster[30] observed that 17 of 29 corneas infected by fungi remained culture-positive at the time of keratoplasty, and 26 of the eyes had viable hyphal elements on pathology (Figure 150-2). Killingsworth et al[12] obtained a 100% cure rate in 15 fungal ulcers treated with therapeutic keratoplasty. Postoperatively fungal

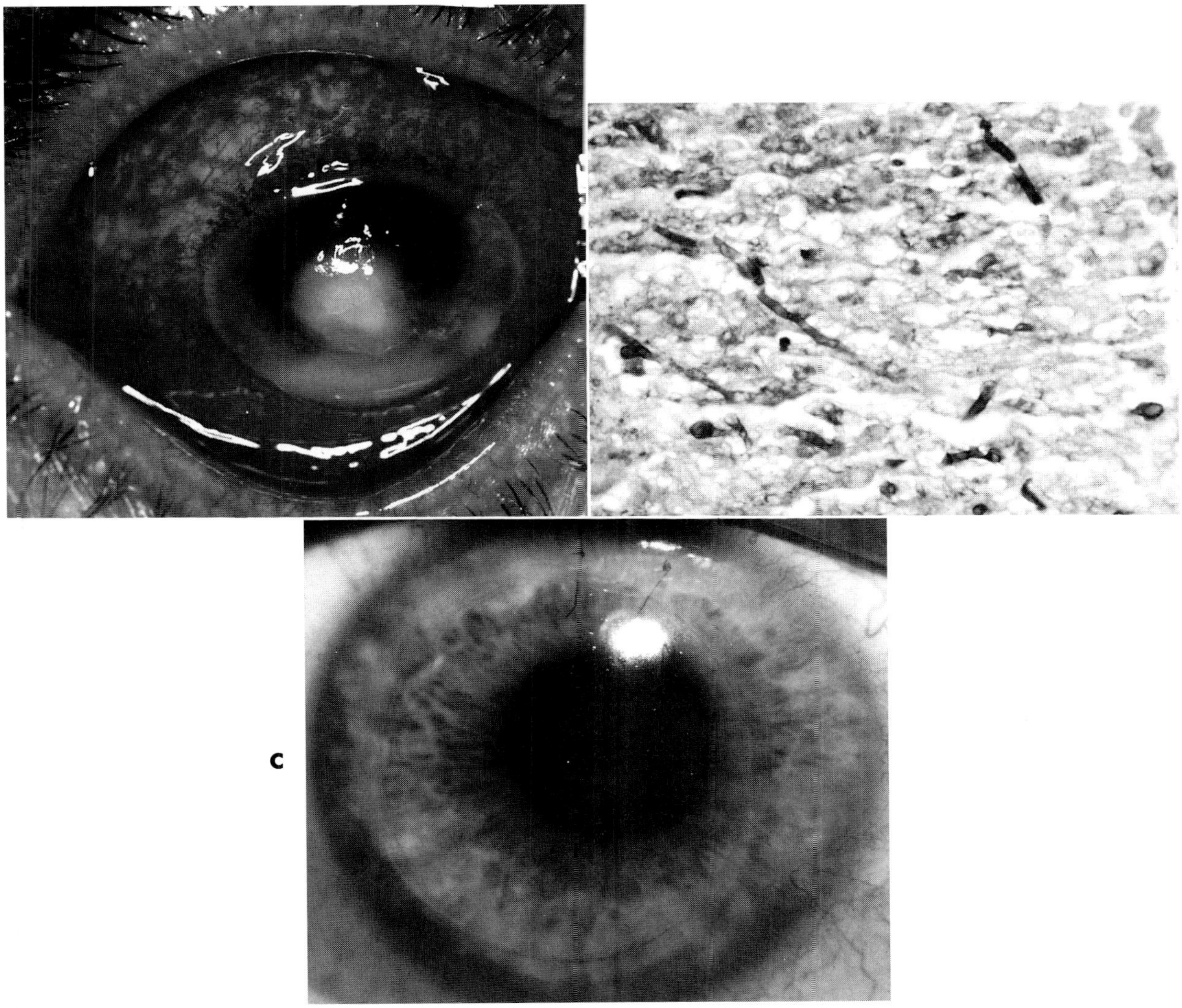

FIGURE 150-2 **A,** *Fusarium* corneal ulceration with hypopyon progressing despite 10 days of aggressive antifungal therapy. **B,** Hyphal elements visible on pathology of corneal button. Cornea was culture-positive. **C,** Therapeutic keratoplasty 1 year after surgery for *fusarium* keratitis.

infection may infiltrate the grafted tissue (Figure 150-3).

THERAPEUTIC KERATOPLASTY FOR *ACANTHAMOEBA* KERATITIS

The respective roles of medical and surgical intervention in *Acanthamoeba* keratitis are controversial. Some patients diagnosed early have been successfully treated with medication alone.[31] Early penetrating keratoplasty has been advocated to remove the bulk of infection and reduce the risk of intractable scleral contamination.[32] In a report by Ficker et al,[33] graft survival for *Acanthamoeba* keratitis was poor, with a more than 50% incidence of recurrence in the graft. Cullen et al[34] reported on seven patients. They concluded that early diagnosis helps with successful medical treatment, but penetrating keratoplasty continues to have a central role in the management of cases that are advanced or unresponsive to medical therapy. Cryotherapy of the host cornea has also been suggested in conjunction with penetrating keratoplasty for cases unresponsive to medical treatment.[35] The acute management of these active cases is to sterilize the infection as rapidly as possible and to delay surgical management until the patient receives adequate antiamebic treatment.

THERAPEUTIC KERATOPLASTY FOR HERPETIC KERATITIS

Herpes simplex viral disease of the cornea often requires surgical intervention. Most commonly intervention is indicated for significant residual corneal

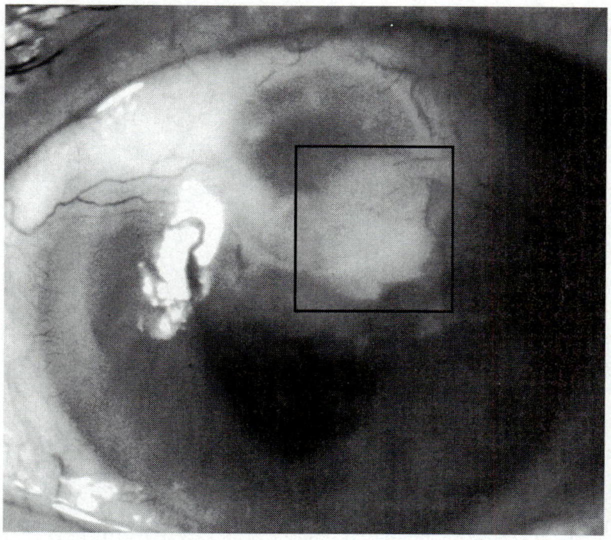

FIGURE 150-3 Recurrent fungal ulceration in therapeutic keratoplasty *(box)*.

scarring and is performed under quiescent, controlled circumstances. Recently, adjunctive medical management has made possible successful penetrating keratoplasty in the active stromal stage of herpes simplex keratitis. Therapeutic keratoplasty can be indicated for significant ulceration and/or perforation, or to remove viral antigenic material responsible for repeated immune inflammatory episodes (Figure 150-4). As noted by Langston et al,[36] success of the keratoplasty depends on the degree of inflammation, the presence of neovascularization, use of fine (10-0 nylon) sutures, and the use of high doses of topical steroids in the immediate postoperative period.

Recently, adjunctive use of oral acyclovir has been shown to improve prognosis (Figure 150-5).[37] Topical antiviral prophylaxis in the immediate postoperative period and during allograft rejection episodes while topical corticosteroids are used may prevent recurrent herpetic disease.[38] Ficker et al[39] found that the combination of prophylactic antivirals and corticosteroids increased the success rate in inflamed eyes undergoing therapeutic keratoplasty for herpes simplex keratitis to a rate comparable to that of quiescent eyes. The use of interrupted sutures, prompt removal of loose sutures, and the previously noted antivirals and topical steroid treatment combination reduced the recurrence rate of herpes simplex virus to 15%.

Killingsworth et al[12] divided 15 patients who required therapeutic penetrating keratoplasty for herpes simplex keratitis into two groups. The first group included patients with severe stromal keratitis who did not respond to medical treatment and patients who progressed to perforation. The second group consisted of patients who developed corneal perforation secondary to persistent epithelial defects with little or no active stromal inflammation. Only 4 of the 11 patients in the first group achieved clear grafts, whereas all four patients in the second group had successful grafts.

The prognosis for therapeutic keratoplasty in herpes zoster keratitis is generally worse than for herpes simplex keratitis. Patients with herpetic corneal disease commonly have neurotrophic corneas. However, the anesthesia tends to be more severe for herpes zoster than for herpes simplex. One of the most important prognostic variables for herpes zoster therapeutic keratoplasty is the level of corneal sensation. Therapeutic keratoplasty in patients with herpes zoster keratitis perforations often requires adjunctive therapy, such as conjunctival flaps or tarsorrhaphy.

THERAPEUTIC KERATOPLASTY FOR PERSISTENT EPITHELIAL DEFECTS

An additional subgroup that may require therapeutic keratoplasty is severe external disease resulting in a persistent epithelial defect that progresses to stromal loss. Killingsworth et al[12] found 26 of 80 patients (3[illegible]%) in their series had therapeutic keratoplasty for a persistent epithelial defect. This subgroup may often be secondarily infected. The underlying disease process may be extremely varied, but all have in common the inability to maintain a normal ocular surface and tear film. This category can be divided into three subclasses: neurotrophic disease, exposure keratitis, and dry eye.

Neurotrophic corneal perforation may be due to systemic disease, trigeminal nerve dysfunction, or localized to the eye. Systemic diseases include Riley-Day syndrome[40] (familial dysautonomia) and Wilson's disease (hepatolenticular degeneration).[41] Trigeminal nerve dysfunction produces corneal tissue damage by a poorly understood mechanism. The pathogenesis may be related to neurologically controlled mediators of the epithelium.[42] Trigeminal dysfunction may occur in 15% to 18% of patients following trigeminal ganglionectomies or inadvertent surgical trauma.[43] Additional nonsurgical causes of trigeminal dysfunction include cerebral vascular accidents, multiple sclerosis, tumors, and aneurysms. The most common cause of neurotrophic corneal disease is the herpes virus family.[44] The development of neurotrophic keratitis following herpes zoster ophthalmicus may be particularly debilitating.[45] Corneal anesthesia leading to perforation has been described following *Acanthamoeba* keratitis,[33,46-48] anesthetic abuse,[49] and penetrating keratoplasty.[50,51] Corneal perforation may be particularly devastating, as the patient is often unaware of the severity of the disease process because of the lack of pain.

Exposure keratitis may predispose to corneal perforation and the need for a therapeutic keratoplasty. In

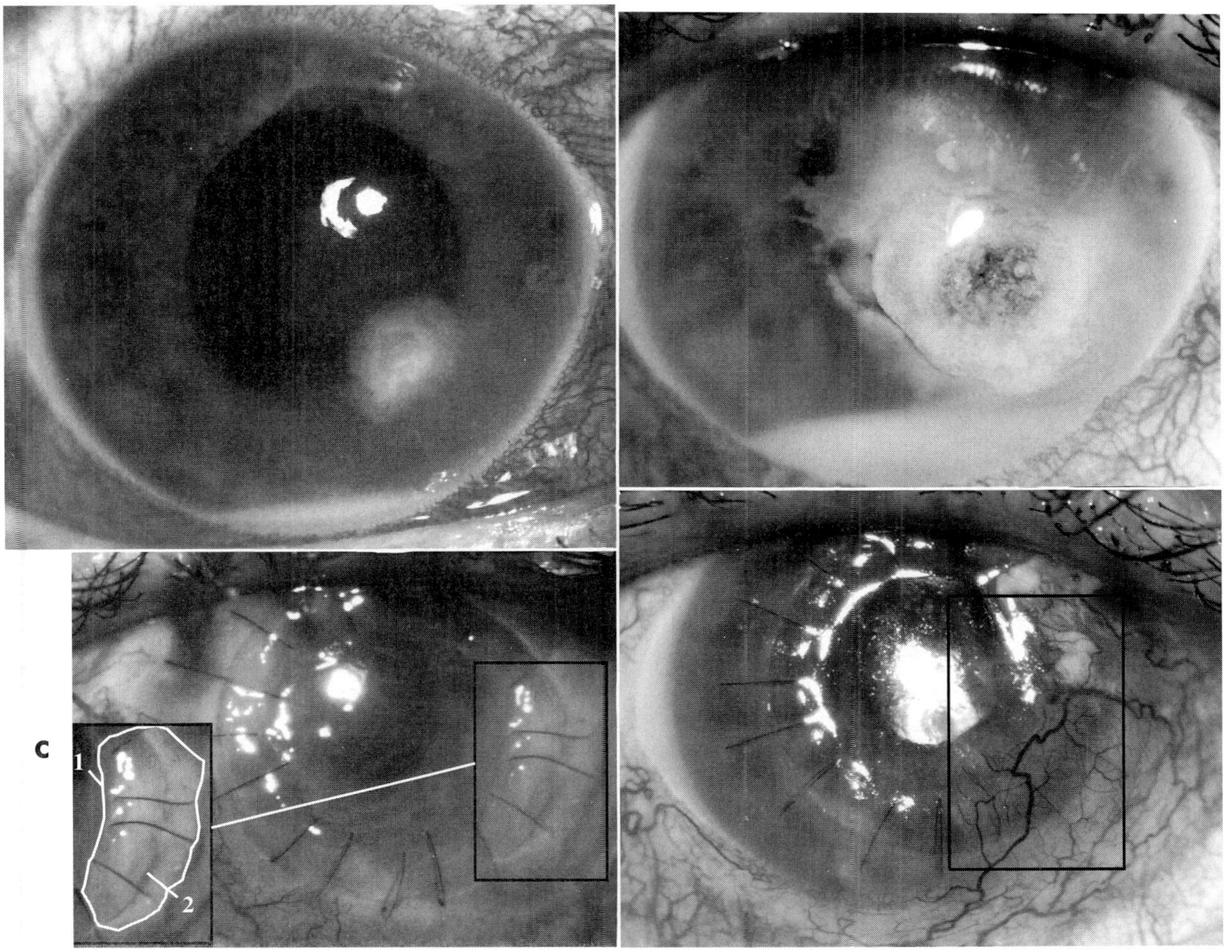

FIGURE 150-4 **A**, Herpes simplex stromal keratitis with corneal thinning. **B**, Progression of herpes simplex stromal keratitis requiring cyanoacrylate occlusion of corneal perforation. **C**, Therapeutic keratoplasty for acute herpes simplex keratitis. Note persistent epithelial defect *(1)* and corneal thinning *(2)* in donor cornea. **D**, Advancement conjunctival flap stabilizes corneal thinning in therapeutic keratoplasty *(box)*.

exposure keratitis, the common finding is breakdown of the epithelium and the loss of corneal integrity. Exposure keratitis can occur because of a variety of lid abnormalities, including facial nerve paralysis,[52] Parkinson's disease, entropion, ectropion, lid notching, and lid imbrication syndrome.[53] The combination of fifth and seventh nerve dysfunction can be particularly dangerous (Figure 150-6).[54]

Severe dry eye may also predispose to corneal perforation and therapeutic keratoplasty.[55] The dry eye may affect the mucin, aqueous, or goblet cell component in the tear film, or any combination of these.[56] Severe dry eye may be associated with systemic conditions[57] such as collagen vascular disease, ocular cicatricial pemphigoid,[58] rosacea, Riley-Day syndrome,[40] or Stevens-Johnson syndrome.[59,60] Localized causes of severe dry eye include radiation[61] and chemical injuries.[62] When a therapeutic keratoplasty is required and the patient has neurotrophic disease, exposure keratitis, or severe dry eye, attention must be paid to the underlying condition.

Presurgical Evaluation

Once the decision has been made to perform a therapeutic keratoplasty, a thorough presurgical examination should be performed. The visual axis is often opacified, precluding a comprehensive vitreoretinal examination. Regardless, a dilated funduscopic examination should be attempted, if at all possible. When an adequate view of the retina is not possible and the integrity of the globe is not compromised by a large corneal perforation, a B-scan ultrasound should be attempted. In addition to evaluating the retina, the B-scan ultrasonography can assess the vitreous for the

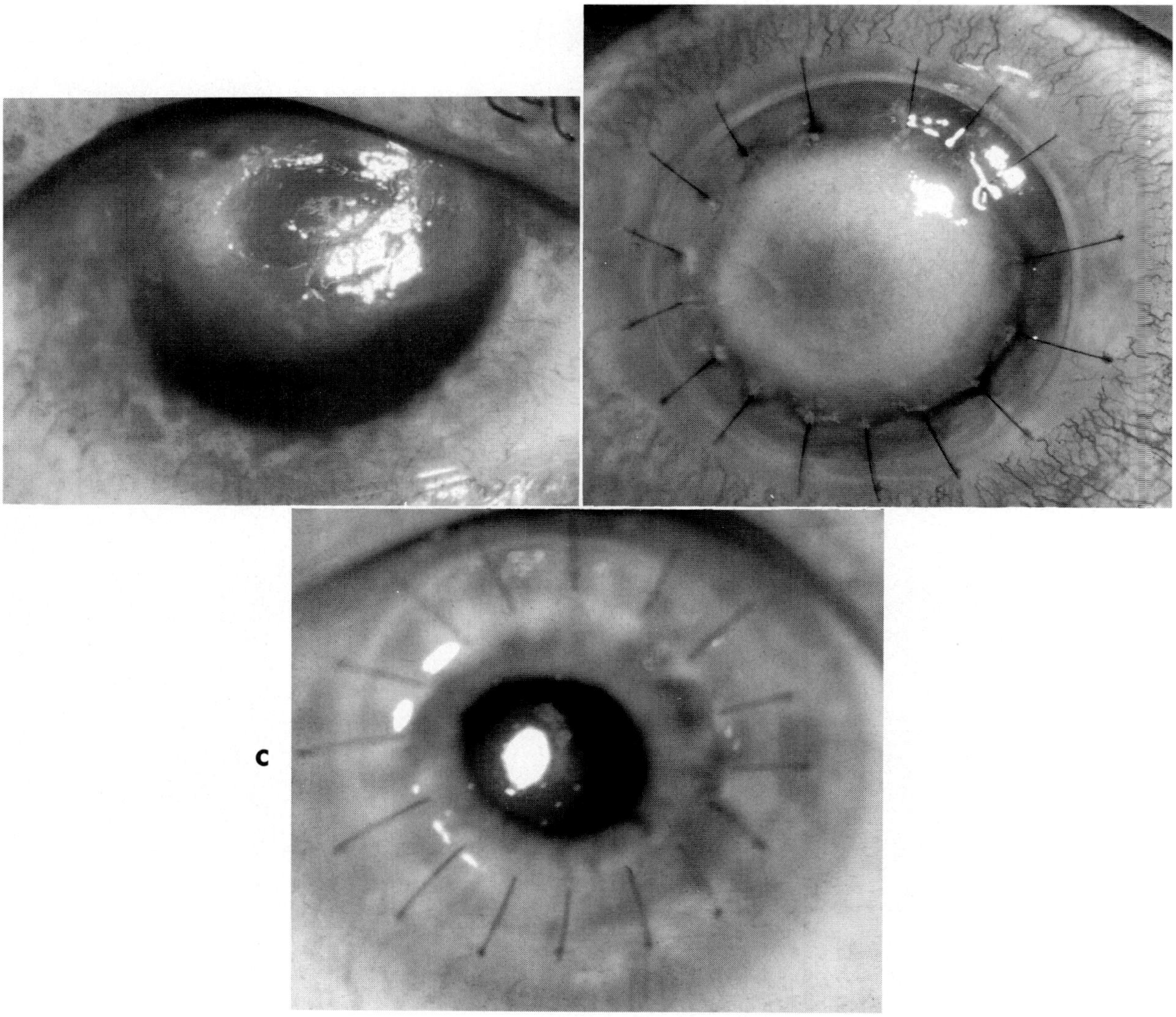

A B C

FIGURE 150-5 **A,** Herpes simplex stromal keratitis before perforation. **B,** Recurrent herpes simplex stromal keratitis 2 weeks after therapeutic keratoplasty. **C,** Repeat therapeutic keratoplasty, clear after 4 months of oral acyclovir.

possibility of endophthalmitis. Any time therapeutic keratoplasty is performed for infectious keratitis, the surgeon should be aware of the possibility of a concomitant endophthalmitis.[63] Increased risk for endophthalmitis at the time of therapeutic keratoplasty includes patients with fungal disease, corneal perforation, and patients who have undergone previous cataract extraction. Removal of the crystalline lens creates loss of a barrier to the vitreous.[64] Patients who have had previous intracapsular cataract extraction with vitreous in the anterior chamber may be at greater risk for endophthalmitis than patients who have had previous extracapsular cataract extraction with an intact posterior capsule.

Before surgery, intraocular pressure should be evaluated in eyes without a perforation. Adequate pressure control is essential.[65] In patients with markedly elevated intraocular pressure or in patients with a corneal perforation in which the lens-iris diaphragm has moved forward, we frequently give intravenous mannitol to control intraocular pressure and to reduce the vitreous volume. The decreased vitreous volume assists in anterior chamber reconstruction by allowing the lens-iris diaphragm to move posteriorly. In eyes with a crystalline lens or posterior chamber intraocular lens, and in patients with iris incarcerated in a wound, we give pilocarpine, 2%, 1 hour before surgery in an attempt to constrict the pupil, protect the lens, and maintain a posterior lens-iris diaphragm.

Although the majority of optical penetrating keratoplasties are performed with the patient under local anesthesia, many therapeutic keratoplasties are per-

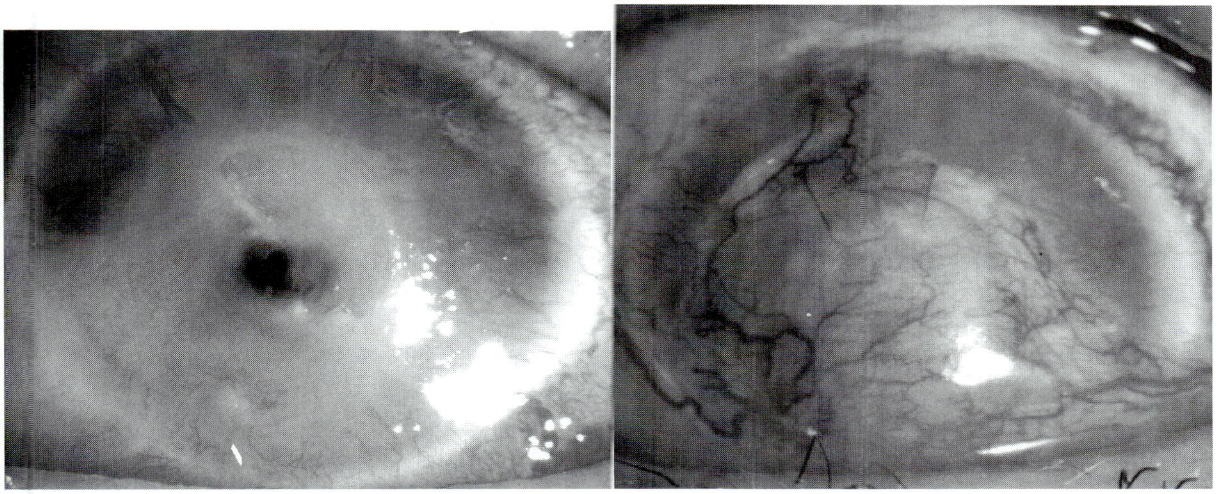

A B

FIGURE 150-6 **A,** Corneal perforation secondary to severe neurotrophic and neuroparalytic disease. **B,** Therapeutic keratoplasty with Gunderson conjunctival flap to prevent repeat corneal melting. Patient achieved a visual acuity of 20/80.

formed with the patient under general anesthesia, particularly when a corneal perforation is present. For this reason, we suggest a presurgical general medical evaluation. When a corneal perforation is present, the anesthesiologist should be informed because the use of depolarizing anesthetic agents in these patients is controversial.[66,67]

Antimicrobial Therapy

Before therapeutic keratoplasty for infectious keratitis, the patient should be treated with topical and systemic therapy directed toward the offending microbe. This treatment applies to bacterial, fungal, herpetic, and parasitic infections. Regardless of the infectious etiology, we always recommend topical antibiotic therapy to prevent bacterial superinfection. In sterile corneal necrosis with corneal perforation, the preoperative antibiotic prophylaxis should be broad-spectrum and nontoxic to help promote reepithelialization. In addition, we prefer an antibiotic that penetrates well into the cornea, aqueous, and vitreous to achieve levels above the MIC_{90} of most pathogenic bacteria.[68] We currently use topical ofloxacin hourly in conjunction with systemic ofloxacin, 400 mg orally, every 12 hours before admission. After the patient is hospitalized, we often place the him or her on intravenous vancomycin and tobramycin.

Donor Material

Exclusion criteria for therapeutic keratoplasties are similar to those for optical penetrating keratoplasties. Most eye banks will respond to an emergent request, and will either find a local donor or import a donor cornea from another eye bank. Under emergent circumstances, the donor cornea may not be of the same quality as it is for an optical penetrating keratoplasty. (Older donor corneas that have decreased endothelial cell counts or have been in storage media too long to be used for therapeutic keratoplasty.) When fresh tissue is not available, cryopreserved or glycerine-preserved corneal tissue or even sclera can be acceptable.[69-71] The surgeon should have a reasonable expectation of the size of keratoplasty before entering the operating room. In many operating rooms, small trephines less than 7.0 mm and trephines larger than 8.5 mm may not be readily available. It is the surgeon's responsibility to make certain these devices are available if there is any expectation that they are going to be needed. When the therapeutic keratoplasty is to be small and off of the visual axis, the donor cornea quality is not as important as it is when the visual axis is involved. Central therapeutic keratoplasties often become optical penetrating keratoplasties, and the availability of good donor tissue in these cases is even more important.

Surgical Technique

At the time of therapeutic keratoplasty, the size of the graft should be carefully determined by placing the appropriate trephine over the cornea and creating an indentation in the epithelium. The goal of surgery is to excise all necrotic or infected tissue during the trephination. If possible, a 1 mm rim of healthy corneal tissue should also be removed to leave a stable, noninfected recipient bed. We routinely suture a Flieringa ring in place to provide scleral support. Once the size of the recipient bed has been determined, the donor cornea can be trephined and is usually 0.25 to 0.5 mm larger than the host trephine. The donor trephination is the same as for optical penetrating keratoplasty.

During trephination of the recipient bed, care should be taken not to place pressure on the globe, which could lead to extrusion of the intraocular contents or an expulsive choroidal hemorrhage. Avoidance of pressure is particularly important in therapeutic keratoplasty for corneal perforation. A self-retaining lid speculum or lid sutures are helpful to prevent pressure on the globe. The host trephination in a therapeutic keratoplasty for corneal perforation can be difficult because of loss of scleral rigidity with decreased intraocular pressure. When cyanoacrylate adhesive has not successfully sealed a corneal perforation before therapeutic keratoplasty, it can often be attempted during the operation. A limbal or peripheral corneal stab incision can be made to sweep iris with a cyclodialysis spatula from the perforation under viscoelastic protection. When there is vitreous in the perforation, an anterior vitrectomy can often be performed through the limbal incision. If cyanoacrylate adhesive can be applied preoperatively or intraoperatively, the anterior chamber can be re-formed with viscoelastic, and the host trephination can be performed under a more controlled environment.

The corneal trephination should be centered over the infection or perforation to leave the maximal, noninfected tissue between the ulceration and the recipient bed. The one exception is the case of a small perforation or infection, in which decentering the therapeutic keratoplasty would provide a better optical result. Occasionally, the therapeutic transplantation is located near the limbus. This possibility occurs most frequently with limbal wound infections after cataract surgery, infections after pterygium surgery with adjunctive mitomycin or irradiation, and peripheral inflammatory disorders such as Mooren's ulceration. Small therapeutic grafts can be performed in a normal fashion with a corneal trephine straddling the limbus. With larger, eccentric therapeutic keratoplasties, however, a round trephine will not adequately excise the affected tissue. In these severe cases, a freehand graft is often required. The therapeutic patch graft can be excised with a corneal trephine and then approximated into the corneal defect by serially excising tissue from the donor cornea until it fits into the appropriate corneal scleral defect. Trephining a cornea in an eye with a flat anterior chamber or markedly decreased intraocular pressure can be challenging. Care should be taken to avoid pressure on the eye if a perforation is present. We recommend using an extremely sharp trephine and applying a minimal amount of pressure to the globe. Suction trephines, such as a Hessburg-Barron trephine,[72] can be advantageous. We have had success with a motorized trephine.

Rarely, an undiagnosed infectious keratitis patient will be brought to the operating room for a therapeutic keratoplasty. In a review by Cohen et al,[73] two cases of *Acanthamoeba* keratitis were found on retrospective pathologic evaluation. At the time of keratoplasty, suppurative areas of the specimen should be aggressively cultured on multiple media. In addition to chocolate agar, blood agar, Sabouraud's agar, and thioglycollate, we frequently culture specimens on Löwenstein-Jensen, brain-heart infusion, and blood agar with an *Escherichia coli* overlay, as indicated by the clinical findings. In cases of undiagnosed infectious keratitis, we also perform multiple scrapings and send a portion of the specimen for frozen section pathologic evaluation. Establishing the diagnosis in the operating room allows us to alter intraoperative therapy, including the use of intravitreal antimicrobial injections, if we are suspicious of a concomitant endophthalmitis. Establishing a diagnosis also allows the surgeon to modify the subconjunctival injections, soak a collagen shield in an appropriate medication, and initiate directed postoperative therapy.

Lamellar keratoplasty should be avoided for infectious therapeutic grafts, as there is increased risk of the infection spreading into the deeper tissue, particularly in cases of fungal ulcerative keratitis.[30] Fungi appear to have a tropism for Descemet's membrane. When the deeper cornea is viable, however, we recommend an 80% depth trephination with approximately 1 mm of beveling of the incision to create a deep lip of tissue, which provides support for the therapeutic keratoplasty and decreases the risk of postoperative wound leaks. Suturing technique in any inflamed or infectious keratitis should almost always be interrupted. The sutures should be approximately 75% corneal depth and should not be full-thickness, as this increases the risk for a conduit of infectious organisms from the cornea into the anterior chamber. The interrupted sutures should be placed radially and farther into the recipient bed than for a noninflamed optical penetrating keratoplasty. We use an increased number of sutures, but try to maintain only moderate suture tension. The goal of the longer interrupted sutures with moderate tension is to avoid "cheese-wiring" of the sutures through a potentially necrotic host bed. The interrupted sutures also allow early suture removal for excessive sectoral inflammation, vascularization, or recurrent infection.

At the time of keratoplasty, we recommend performing the minimal intraocular surgery necessary. When possible, the crystalline lens should be left in place, as it provides a barrier against vitreous seeding and infectious endophthalmitis.[64] The anterior chamber should be irrigated aggressively with balanced salt solution, and the iris should be inspected for infectious foci. Any iris lesions should be excised and cultured. When infection of the vitreous is suspected, particularly in aphakic eyes, the vitreous should be cultured. When the organism is known, intravitreal injections of an appropriate antimicrobial are indicated. When the organism is in question, broad-spectrum intravitreal injections are indicated. We currently use intravitreal vancomycin (1 mg in 0.1 ml) and ceftazadime (2.5 mg in 0.1 ml) for suspected bacterial endophthalmitis.

At the time of the operation, any predisposing factors that have contributed to the need for a therapeutic keratoplasty should be addressed. As previously mentioned, many patients who require a therapeutic keratoplasty have underlying external disease, which has been a significant part of their disease process. After a therapeutic keratoplasty, the donor cornea is more anesthetic than it was preoperatively,[51] and the tear film is significantly altered. Failure to address the predisposing external disease problem, in conjunction with the changes induced by the surgery, often leads to severe postoperative complications, including persistent epithelial defect, sterile corneal melts, infectious keratitis, would leaks, and corneal neovascularization. All lid abnormalities should be corrected. Patients with mild dry eyes should have punctal occlusion. Patients with moderate to severe dry eye should undergo tarsorrhaphy. Patients with severe dry eyes or anesthetic corneas, in which postoperative wound healing is jeopardized, should either have large tarsorrhaphies or should be offered a conjunctival flap at the time of therapeutic keratoplasty. A conjunctival flap is often a definitive procedure, which is further indicated if the eye has limited visual prognosis. A conjunctival flap is never indicated if there is active infection or perforation.

Postoperative Management of Therapeutic Penetrating Keratoplasty

The postoperative management of a therapeutic keratoplasty is often as challenging as the operation. Several basic principles should be followed:

1. Eradicate all remnants of infection and prevent reinfection. The therapeutic keratoplasty often provides a surgical excision of an infection. When there is a reasonsable doubt, however, antiinfectious therapy should be maintained until the corneal epithelium has healed. Duration of treatment depends on the severity of the infection and the causative organism. In general, the more opportunistic infections, such as *Acanthamoeba* and fungi, are the most resistant to therapy and require the longest postoperative antimicrobial treatment to prevent reinfection. This treatment may be required for several months.
2. Promote reepithelialization of the cornea and wound healing. Avoid prolonged overtreatment of the cornea with toxic medications, such as fortified antibiotics, amphotericin B, and antivirals.[74] Systemic acyclovir appears to offer the efficacy of topical antivirals without the risk of keratitis medicamentosa. We routinely maintain patients with a therapeutic keratoplasty for herpes simplex keratitis on acyclovir 400 mg twice a day for 6 months after surgery.[37] When treating epitheliopathy in therapeutic keratoplasties postoperatively, nonpreserved tears and lubricants are often useful. When these agents are ineffective, a cyanoacrylate temporary tarsorrhaphy can often resolve a persistent epithelial defect.[75] Milder medications should be substituted for toxic antibiotics when indicated. Therapeutic keratoplasty has been used for removal of dense antibiotic precipitates caused by prolonged use of topical antimicrobials.[74]
3. Control inflammation with corticosteroids. The use of topical corticosteroids after a therapeutic keratoplasty for an infectious organism is controversial. Most bacterial corneal infections are responsive to antibiotics. Therefore the concomitant use of corticosteroids is justified in an inflamed eye. In a therapeutic keratoplasty for herpetic keratitis, the corticosteroids can be given without significant risk, as long as the patient is managed with topical or oral antiviral therapy. There is controversy regarding the use of corticosteroids after therapeutic keratoplasty involves infections that do not respond readily to treatment, such as fungal or *Acanthamoeba* corneal ulceration. When there is any sign of active fungal or *Acanthamoeba* infection after a therapeutic keratoplasty, corticosteroids should be avoided.[18,76] When the eye has been treated extensively and a wide surgical debridement has been performed, however, corticosteroids are indicated and can be used safely.[12,77] For severe inflammation, the use of systemic corticosteroids should be considered.
4. Intraocular pressure control. Postoperatively, the patient's intraocular pressure should be followed carefully. Glaucoma is seen in approximately 50% of optical penetrating keratoplasties. After therapeutic keratoplasty, the patient may develop anterior synechiae, iritis, and trabeculitis, which may further contribute to an elevated intraocular pres-

tarsorrhaphy in the management of corneal epithelial defects, *Ophthalmic Surg* 22:591-593, 1991.

76. Moore MB, McCulley JP: *Acanthamoeba* keratitis associated with contact lenses. Six consecutive cases of successful management, *Br J Ophthalmol* 73:271, 1989.

77. Stern GA, Buttrosski H: Use of corticosteroids in combination with antimicrobial drugs in the treatment of infectious corneal disease, *Ophthalmology* 98:847-853, 1991.

78. Sanders N: Penetrating keratoplasty in treatment of fungus keratitis, *Am J Ophthalmol* 70:24-30, 1970.

CHAPTER 151

CLAES H. DOHLMAN

Keratoprosthesis

For patients with severe corneal opacity, transplantation using human cornea has been increasingly successful since the beginning of this century. Still, the prognosis for standard keratoplasty remains very poor in the category of patients with past or ongoing chronic inflammation such as end-stage Stevens-Johnson syndrome, pemphigoid, advanced dry eyes for other reasons, or severe chemical burns. Beyond this group there is a larger group of patients with repeated graft failures in whom the outlook for another transplant, while not hopeless, is still not good. For these patients with complicated corneal blindness, a keratoprosthesis seems like an obvious and logical alternative. The idea has attracted a number of clinical investigators spanning two centuries. However, despite considerable effort, their techniques have not become well accepted. The surgery has been complicated, and, more importantly, the short- and long-term complication rate has been discouraging. The approach has often been labeled biologically unsound and dangerous. Its present disrepute is exemplified by the fact that in 1992 only about 15 keratoprosthesis operations were attempted in the United States, as compared with more than 42,000 corneal transplants done during the same period. In the last few years, however, attention has shifted from concerns about prosthesis design and materials to the accompanying biologic problems and their solutions. As a result of this change of focus, there is now reason for cautious optimism regarding the prognosis for future keratoprosthesis surgery.

History

The concept of trying to restore vision to eyes with severely opaque corneas by implanting a piece of transparent material appeared early in the ophthalmologic literature. As early as 1789 the noted French surgeon Pellier de Quengsy suggested that a leukomatous cornea be replaced by a lens of glass in a silver ring.[1] It seemed that he never put his idea to the test. Much later, in 1855, Nussbaum initiated animal experiments and published the first human trial using a quartz crystal implant.[2] Over the next 50 years these early efforts were continued by Heusser,[3] von Hippel,[4] Dimmer,[5] and Salzer.[6] Only a few patients in total were subjected to these primitive keratoprostheses. They all failed, most of them within weeks or months. Characteristically, a retroprosthesis membrane formed quickly and, combined with necrosis of the tissue surrounding the device, caused it to extrude. Leak and infection followed.

During the first half of the twentieth century, keratoprostheses received little attention. In 1930 Verhoeff[7] reported the use in one patient of a quartz button that had to be removed shortly afterward. Filatov[8] in 1935 implanted a penetrating glass device into the leukomatous cornea of a patient and covered it with a double conjunctival flap. After 6 months the flap had thinned sufficiently to give the patient a vision of 1/200. More detailed information of the attempts at keratoprostheses before the mid-century has been reported in the reviews by Day,[9] Cardona,[10] and Lund.[11]

After 1950 keratoprosthesis research gained momentum. New inert plastics such as polymethylmethacrylate (PMMA) became available and Stone,[12] Cardona,[10] and others tested various prosthesis designs in rabbits. Bolder human applications followed as a number of ophthalmologists throughout the world tried to develop keratoprosthesis surgery into a standard procedure. Often initial enthusiasm turned into dismay after a few months or years when severe complications developed; the dropout rate among these surgeons was high. Some, however, persevered in using their favorite design and technique and have compiled fairly large series over many years. Thus Cardona and DeVoe,[13] Strampelli,[14] Lund,[15] Dohlman,[16,17] Casey,[18] Donn,[19] Buxton,[20] Choyce,[21] Puchkowskaya,[22] Girard,[23] Moroz,[24] Temprano,[25] Falcinelli,[26] Pintucci,[27] Marchi,[28] Legais,[29] Lacombe,[30] Worst,[31] Polack,[32] Aquavella,[33] Waring,[34] Berthelsen,[35] Singh,[36] Mohan,[37] Yakimenko,[38] Caldwell,[39] and others have reported their experience in a combined total of about 3000 cases—still a very small number compared to standard keratoplasty worldwide. Many genuine contributions regarding technique and follow-up have gradually emerged, but the literature has been somewhat difficult to interpret. Reporting of visual acuity, for instance, has usually been in the form of a

A 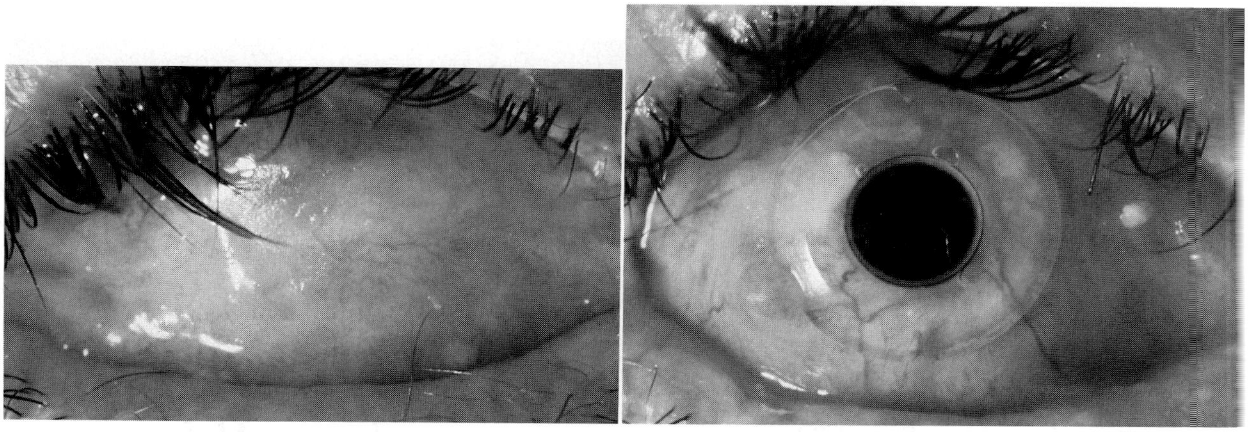 B

FIGURE 151-3 Chemical burn, before **(A)** and 2 years after **(B)** keratoprosthesis (type I). Vision 20/20.

A 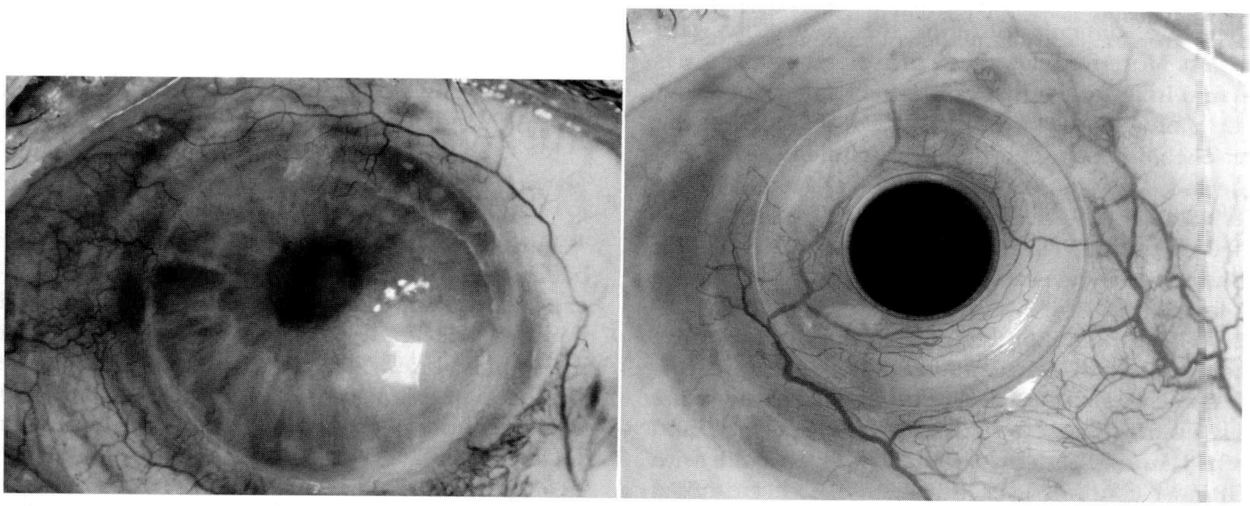 B

FIGURE 151-4 **A,** Graft failures in lattice dystrophy. **B,** Fifteen months after keratoprosthesis. Vision 20/20.

Prognostic categories in keratoprosthesis

Prognosis is best in the top group, then in falling order, with the last category the worst.

1. Noninflammatory conditions such as graft failure in edema, dystrophies, etc.
2. Graft failure after herpes simplex keratitis, zoster, infectious ulcer, etc.
3. Pemphigoid
4. Chemical burns
5. Stevens-Johnson syndrome

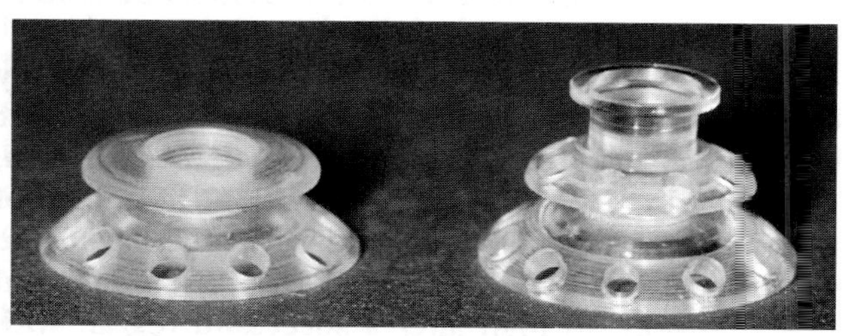

FIGURE 151-5 The two keratoprosthesis designs used by the author. Type I for wet eyes at left. Type II (through-the-lid) for very dry eyes, at right.

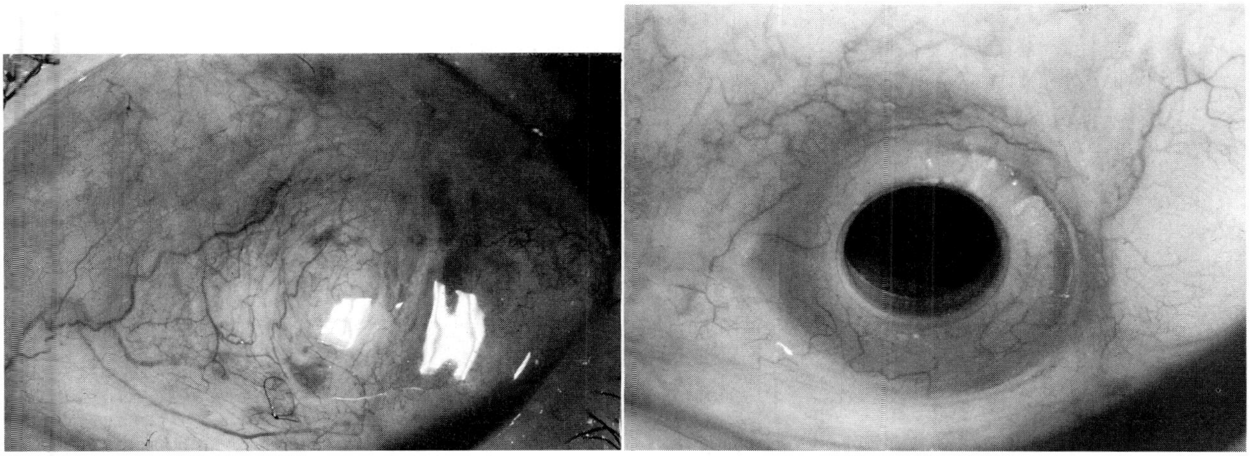

FIGURE 151-6 **A,** Keratoprosthesis (type I) temporarily covered with a total conjunctival flap, to be opened after about 2 months. **B,** Appearance 1 year later.

Development of the technique of insertion of the keratoprosthesis has been dictated by two obvious needs. One has been the simplification of the procedure and the elimination of need for nonocular support tissue. The goal has been a one-stage operation of such simplicity and brevity that even the occasional surgeon can readily become comfortable with it. Simplicity is one of the prerequisites for keratoprostheses becoming truly beneficial on a larger scale.

The other goal for the surgical procedure has been to incorporate measures that diminish future complications. Thus the inserted prosthesis is temporarily covered with a total conjunctival flap or with lid skin, a maneuver that has been found to reduce postoperative necrosis of the tissue surrounding the device.[16,17] The threat of devastating postoperative glaucoma often necessitates the simultaneous implantation of a drainage shunt.[45] If present, the lens is removed using extracapsular technique, if possible. Occasionally the iris is removed as well. Examples of my present technique using the two types of keratoprosthesis are shown in Figures 151-6 and 151-7.

Postoperatively it has become obvious that large doses of corticosteroids are needed, especially in cases of present or past severe inflammation of the eye (Stevens-Johnson syndrome, pemphigoid, chemical burns, etc). Topical, systemic, or, in particular, peribulbar routes are routinely used. Typically, 25 mg of dexamethasone is given by peribulbar injection through the lower lid at the end of surgery. At the end of 1 week, 20 mg of triamcinolone is administered in the same way, to be repeated every 2 weeks until the conjunctiva or lid skin is opened, usually after 2 months. Injections may have to be repeated later if postoperative uveitis is still present. In some inflammatory cases, systemically administered steroids may have to be added, starting with 30 to 75 mg of prednisone per day, to be tapered over the period of 1 or 2 months.

Perioperatively, antibiotics must be administered generously, and some prophylactic antibiotics may be advisable on a permanent basis. At particular risk are the Stevens-Johnson syndrome patients who might be vulnerable to infection because of the chronic skin pathogenic flora.

After the opening of the tissue covering the prosthesis, anticollagenase medication is applied topically for months or years. Presently, 1% medroxyprogesterone, which reduces collagenase synthesis, and 1% tetracycline, a potent direct enzyme inhibitor, are routinely used for this purpose.[17] The efficacy of these agents in reducing tissue necrosis has not been established in humans but has been well documented in experimental animals.

Complications

As has already been emphasized, complications after keratoprosthesis are frequent, often severe, and sometimes occur precipitously long after surgery. The patient is therefore never safe and requires frequent follow-up. Problems must be dealt with promptly by surgical revision, laser treatment, steroid injection, antibiotics, glaucoma medications, etc. If not handled properly, vision can easily become irreversibly damaged. Such involvement is demanding and can become very expensive. Therefore, keratoprosthesis surgery in its present state is unfortunately not possible in many

A

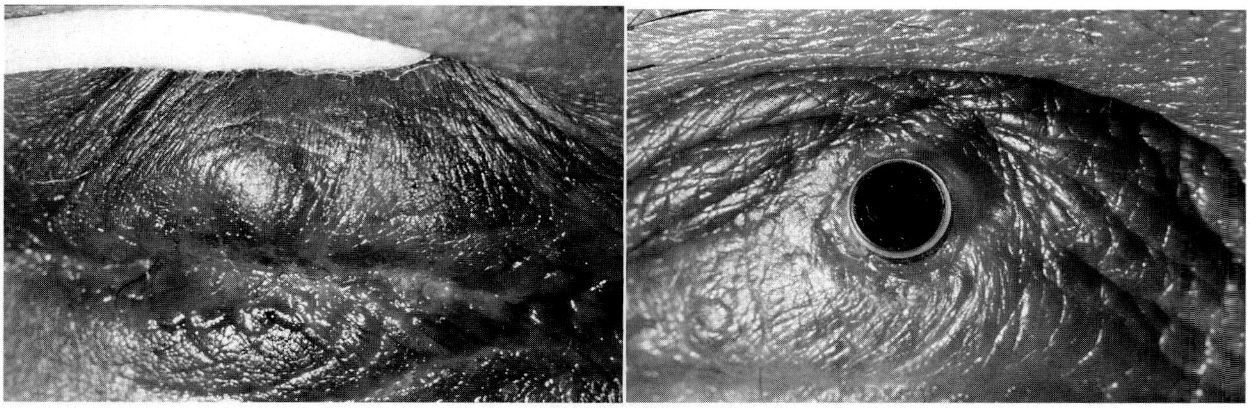

B

FIGURE 151-7 **A,** Keratoprosthesis (type II) in Stevens-Johnson syndrome, temporarily covered with lid skin. **B,** Appearance after 18 months. Vision 20/25.

Most important complications after keratoprosthesis surgery

- I. Necrosis of tissue around the keratoprosthesis (which if unchecked can lead to leak, infection, extrusion)
  - a. Melt in the wet eye (type I device)—now a minor problem
  - b. Skin retraction in the dry eye (type II device)—still a problem
  - c. Epithelial downgrowth—rare
- II. Postoperative uveitis—can lead to the following:
  - a. Keratoprosthesis membrane—now rare
  - b. Lens capsule opacification
  - c. Vitreous opacities, membranes
  - d. Retinal detachment
  - e. Macular edema, epiretinal membrane, etc.
- III. Glaucoma—especially in Stevens-Johnson syndrome, pemphigoid, chemical burns
- IV. Infection—postoperative endophthalmitis or later from skin retraction

countries where corneal blindness is very prevalent but where medical manpower is in short supply. Particularly frustrating for the surgeon is the situation in which an initially successful outcome reverses gradually to functional loss of the eye despite maximal attention and proactive treatment. An exasperated senior European keratoprosthesis surgeon recently stated that he had given up on the procedure because his long-term (many years) success, despite intense effort, has been in the range of 5%. However, there is now reason to be considerably more optimistic.

The most feared complications after keratoprosthesis implantation are listed in the box. The leading concern has, in the past, been necrosis of the tissue holding the device. Therefore, much of the attention of innovators in the field has been to find the ultimate design that prevents extrusion. It is questionable whether a particular design, even with holes or pores for tissue ingrowth, will be the final answer, since the dissolution of supporting tissue is probably an enzymatic process related to the degree of inflammation. In particular, collagenases derived from polymorphonuclear leukocytes must be suspected of playing a key role in this process. Drying damage to the skin wound in the through-the-lid prosthesis can also aggravate the tissue breakdown.

Skin retraction away from the plastic stem is still a considerable problem and, if allowed to proceed too far, can lead to disastrous perforation and infection. The retraction can usually be repaired in an early stage by shifting the surrounding lid skin using sutures. These repeated revisions make through-the-lid technique less manageable and more time consuming than the standard technique in the wet eye. In the very dry eye with extensive symblephara, however, the through-the-lid approach is the only feasible approach.

In the eye with adequate tears, deep fornices and an intact blink function, the standard collar button device (type I), temporarily covered with a total conjunctival flap, now runs little risk of exposure or extrusion from corneal necrosis. The combination of temporary flap coverage and subsequent treatment with enzyme-suppressing medication has made this complication rare. In only two out of 20 type I cases has early repair been indicated. The anterior plate of the prosthesis makes such revision easy. A thin slice of (frozen) corneal tissue with a central 3.0 mm trephine hole and a radial cut can be slipped under the plate with the aid of viscoelastics and sutured. There has been no need to repeat such repair in the two cases mentioned. In general, it can be stated that the once feared necrosis and extrusion has become much less common.[45]

Acute or chronic uveitis is the most frequent and severe complication after keratoprosthesis surgery and is the cause of most of the ultimate failures. In the short run, it can cause a retroprosthetic membrane or vitreous traction bands that later can result in retinal detachment. It can also lead to severe glaucoma or aggravate a preexisting pressure problem. In the long run, cystoid macular edema, epiretinal membrane or other hard-to-define macular dysfunction can follow. Therefore, monitoring the degree of postoperative uveitis is very important—but not easy. Visibility is obscured by the tissue coverage for 4 to 8 weeks. Even after baring the prosthesis, the presence of a few cells in the aqueous can be hard to detect because of the internal reflections of the slit lamp beam along the prosthesis stem. Still, every effort should be made to evaluate the anterior chamber and vitreous by slit lamp and ultrasound on an ongoing basis, since prophylaxis and treatment can be quite successful.

Control of postoperative uveitis has recently improved radically with the introduction of the high-dose steroid regimens, as mentioned earlier. In my own experience, retroprosthetic membrane and vitreous organization have become much rarer than in earlier cases. These steroid doses are not completely without risk, however. Systemic complications are theoretically possible. Repeated peribulbar injections through the altered lid anatomy may eventually result in an accident with ocular penetration. Wound healing is most likely delayed, and pressure rises certainly can occur if a glaucoma shunt is not in place. The benefits have nonetheless been striking, and they usually outweigh the risks. The incidence of retroprosthetic membrane as well as residual uveitis have been drastically reduced without any obvious steroid complications.[45]

A retroprosthetic membrane, once formed, is usually accessible to opening by YAG laser. The back plate of the prosthesis has a laser ridge that will keep the membrane away from the stem; it is nonetheless advisable to keep laser energy below 2.0 mJ to decrease the risk of causing heat cracks in the adjacent plastic. A heavier membrane may become dangerously vascularized and may require surgical opening with a Ziegler knife or similar instrument.

Glaucoma is a frequent occurrence after keratoprosthesis and is the most common direct cause of eventual blindness. In my own series, glaucoma is already present preoperatively in one third of patients, and has increased to two thirds postoperatively (unless a shunt has been implanted). One must assume that the pressure elevation is caused by the uveitis although outflow obstruction at the level of the ocular surface may contribute as well. Intraocular pressure is hard both to monitor and to treat. Tonometers are useless in this setting, and digital palpation of the globe, with

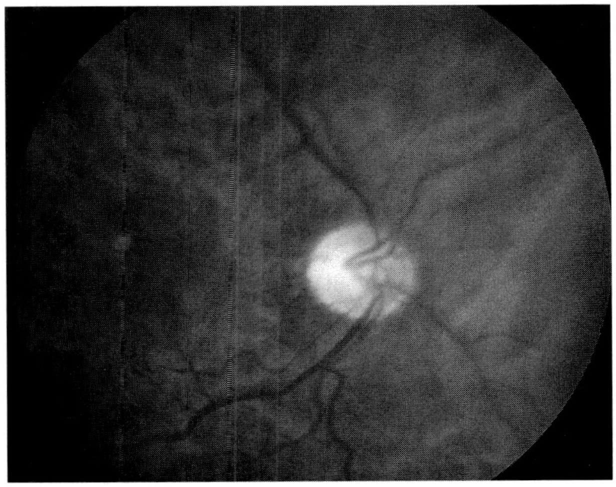

FIGURE 151-8 The central fundus can be easily inspected and photographed through the uncomplicated keratoprosthesis.

all its uncertainties, is the only available method. Disk appearance and field are usually easy to monitor and must be examined frequently (Figure 151-8). Treatment is also limited because only carbonic anhydrase inhibitors can be relied on. Topical medication may have some penetration in the wet eye, but is probably useless in the through-the-lid prosthesis. Because of the frequency of glaucoma and the limits of diagnosis and treatment, it has become clear that many of these eyes require a glaucoma shunt implanted together with the prosthesis. We have used the Ahmed valve shunt primarily, with adequate pressure control.[45]

Retinal detachment is fortunately not a common complication. It is presumably caused by traction from inflammatory membranes stimulated by postoperative uveitis or by surgical trauma. Repeated postoperative ultrasound (B-scan) examinations are advisable, since the peripheral retina cannot be observed with ophthalmoscopy.

Infection is uncommon but devastating if it occurs. Endophthalmitis immediately after surgery is a rare occurrence. Most cases come from the through-the-lid keratoprostheses where skin retraction has led to exposure, necrosis, and perforation. Many candidates for keratoprosthesis and shunt surgery, especially Stevens-Johnson syndrome patients, are carriers of pathogenic microorganisms, including *Candida* and need vigorous prophylactic antibiotic treatment during and after surgery.

Conclusions

The importance of keratoprosthesis design and material has been overemphasized in the past. It is unlikely that a future device will be designed so that all postoperative complications are eliminated. My preference is to use a double-plated (collar button) PMMA device for stability, wide visual field, and ease of tissue repair, if needed. Two models are available, one for the wet, normally blinking eye and the other for the very dry eye (through-the-lid).

Simplicity of surgery is important, and this can be reasonably achieved at the present time. Postoperative follow-up is still very time consuming and expensive, however, and revisions are often needed.

Postoperative necrosis of tissue around the prosthesis, resulting in leak, extrusion, or infection, has fortunately become less common, as long as the device has been covered with conjunctiva or lid skin for 1 to 2 months postoperatively, followed by collagenase-reducing agents given topically. Skin retraction around the prosthesis nub in the through-the-lid arrangement is still a problem, however.

Uveitis is the most destructive long-term postoperative complication but has been markedly reduced with a high dose regimen of corticosteroids. Retroprosthetic membrane and vitreous organization is now much less frequent, as are retinal detachment and infection.

Glaucoma is very frequently present in patients requiring a keratoprosthesis. Simultaneous implantation of a valve shunt seems to be effective in normalizing the pressure on a short-term basis, but long-term experience with this arrangement is lacking.

The indications for keratoprosthesis are imprecise at this time and depend on the interest and time commitment of the surgeon. Conditions with chronic inflammation, such as Stevens-Johnson syndrome, pemphigoid, and severe chemical burn, while in most desperate need of a well-functioning keratoprosthesis, are also at the greatest risk for hazardous complications. Noninflammatory conditions such as graft failure in bullous keratopathy in the elderly have a surprisingly good outcome.

A worldwide effort has improved the prognosis for keratoprosthesis substantially, and it is to be expected that the number of successful procedures will increase in the decade ahead. This work was sponsored by the Al-Rashed Foundation, Kuwait.

REFERENCES

1. Pellier de Quengsy G: *Precis au cours d'operations sur la chirurgie des yeux,* Paris, 1789, Didot.
2. Nussbaum N: Cornea Artificialis, ein Substitut für die Transplantatio Cornea, *Deutsche Klinik* 34:367, 1853.
3. Heusser J: Die Einheilung einer Cornea artificialis, *Oesterr Ztschr Pract Med* 26:424, 1860.
4. von Hippel A: Eine neue Methode der Hornhauttransplantation, *Arch Ophthalmol* 34:108, 1888.
5. Dimmer F: Zwei Fälle von Celluoidplatten der Hornhaut, *Klin Monatsbl Augenh* 29:104, 1891.
6. Salzer F: *Über den künstlichen Hornhautersatz,* Wiesbaden, 1898.
7. Verhoeff FH: Cited in Cardona H: Keratoprosthes , *Am J Ophthalmol* 54:284, 1962.
8. Filatov VP: Alloplastik bei vollständig "hoffnungslosen" Leukomen, *Sov Viest Opht* 9:400, 1936.
9. Day R: Artificial corneal implants, *Trans Am Ophthalmol Soc* 55:455, 1957.
10. Cardona H: Keratoprosthesis, *Am J Ophthalmol* 54:284, 1962.
11. Lund O-E: Die Keratoprosthese, *Berichte Deutsche Ophthalmologische Gesellschaft,* Munich, 1977, Bergmann.
12. Stone W Jr, Herbert E: Experimental study of plastic material and replacement for the cornea: preliminary report, *Am J Ophthalmol* 36:168, 1953.
13. Cardona H, DeVoe AG: Prosthokeratoplasty, *Trans Am Acad Ophthalmol Otolaryngol* 83:271, 1977.
14. Strampelli B: Osteo-odonto-keratoprosthesis, *Ann Ottalmol Clin Ocul* 89:1039, 1963.
15. Lund OE: Keratoprosthesis: 25 years experience, *Refract Corneal Surg* 9:186, 1993.
16. Dohlman CH, Schneider HA, Doane MG: Prosthokeratoplasty, *Am J Ophthalmol* 77:694, 1974.
17. Dohlman CH, Doane MG: Some factors influencing outcome after keratoprosthesis surgery, *Cornea* 13:214, 1994.
18. Casey TA: Osteo-odontokeratoprosthesis and chondrokeratoprosthesis, *Proc R Soc Med* 63:313, 1970.
19. Donn A: Aphakic bullous keratopathy treated with prosthokeratoplasty, *Arch Ophthalmol* 94:270, 1976.
20. Buxton JN: Keratoprosthesis: personal experiences, *Trans Am Acad Ophthalmol Otolaryngol* 83:268, 1977.
21. Choyce DP: Evolution of choice two-piece multistage perforating keratoprosthesis technique in 135 eyes (1967-1980). In Trevor-Roper editor: *VIth Congress of European Society of Ophthalmology,* New York, 1981, Grune & Stratton.
22. Puchkovskaia NA: Keratoprosthesis as a method of restoring vision in the sequelae of severe corneal lesions (Russian; English abstract), *Oftamol Zh* 3:132, 1985.
23. Girard LJ: Keratoprosthesis, *Cornea* 2:207, 1983.
24. Moroz ZI: Artificial cornea. In Fyodorov SN, editor: *Microsurgery of the eye, main aspects,* Moscow, 1987, Mir.
25. Temprano J: Keratoprosthesis with tibial autograft, *Refract Corneal Surg* 9:192, 1993.
26. Falcinelli G et al.: osteo-odonto-keratoprosthesis up to date. *Acta XXV Concilium Ophthalmologicum,* Milano, 1987, Kugler and Chedini.
27. Pintucci S, Pintucci F: Kératoprothèse avec un nouveau support haptique à la colonisation tissulaire pour oeil sec, *Ophthalmologie* 2:157, 1988.
28. Marchi V et al.: Osteo-odonto-keratoprosthesis, *Cornea* 13:125, 1994.
29. Legeais JM et al.: Keratoprosthesis with biocolonizable microporous fluorocarbon haptic: two-year study on 24 patients, *Arch Ophthalmol* 113:757-763, 1995.
30. Lacombe E: Keratoprosthesis by retrocorneal fixation: results in 30 eyes over 3 years, *Refract Corneal Surg* 9:199, 1993.
31. Worst JGF: Twenty-three years of keratoprosthesis research: present state of art, *Refract Corneal Surg* 9:188, 1993.
32. Polack F: Clinical results with a ceramic keratoprosthesis, *Cornea* 2:185, 1983.
33. Aquavella JA et al.: Keratoprosthesis. Results, complications and management, *Ophthalmology* 89:655, 1982.
34. Kozarsky AM, Knight SH, Waring, GO: Clinical results with a ceramic keratoprosthesis placed through the eyelid, *Ophthalmology* 94:904, 1987.
35. Sletteberg O, Hovding G, Bertelsen T: Keratoprosthesis. II.

Results obtained after implantation of 27 dismountable two-piece prostheses, *Acta Ophthalmol* 68:375, 1990.

36. Singh IR: Central and paracentral perforating keratoprostheses – an experience of 200 cases, *Refract Corneal Surg* 9:191, 1993.
37. Mohan M, Panda A: Artificial cornea. In Cavanagh HD, editor: *The cornea. transactions of the World Congress on the Cornea,* vol 3, New York, 1988, Raven.
38. Yakimenko S: Results of a PMMA/Titanium keratoprosthesis in 502 eyes, *Refract Corneal Surg* 9:197, 1993.
39. Caldwell DR: Personal communication.
40. Barber JC, Feaster F, Priour D: The acceptance of a vitreous carbon alloplastic material, Proplast, in the rabbit eye, *Invest Ophthalmol Vis Sci* 19:182, 1980.
41. Trinkaus-Randall V et al.: Development of a biopolymeric keratoprosthesis material, *Invest Ophthalmol Vis Sci* 29:393, 1988.
42. Kirkham SM, Dangel ME: Keratoprosthesis: improved biocompatibility through design and surface modification, *Ophthalmic Surg* 22:455, 1991.
43. Kain HL: The silicon-carbon keratoprosthesis: design and implant procedure (abstract), *Invest Ophthalmol Vis Sci* 33:992, 1992.
44. DeVore DP et al: Evaluation of collagen-based corneal grafts in the rabbit model, *Refract Corneal Surg* 9:208, 1993.
45. Dohlman CH, Netland PA, Fung WC: Unpublished data.

CHAPTER 152

LARRY F. RICH

Corneal Surgery for Ocular Surface Disease

Ocular surface disease is a broad category comprising many disorders. Any process that interrupts the structure or function of the surface of the eye could be included. Abnormalities of the lid margins, conjunctiva, and cornea must also be included, since the epithelial and subepithelial surfaces of these structures influence the integrity of the ocular surface. Infectious processes, by tradition, have been excluded from this category.

The box lists most of the entities falling within the definition of ocular surface disease, although it could be argued that several others should be included. The causes and characteristics of these conditions have been described elsewhere in this book, and a discussion of etiology is outside the scope of this chapter. However, research efforts aimed at identifying the causes of these diseases have uncovered a number of useful therapeutic approaches. Many treatment modalities were discovered fortuitously, while others were deduced from studies of histopathologic changes commonly found in patients with these disorders.

Treatment Options

MEDICAL APPROACHES

Nonsurgical therapy of ocular surface diseases are generally regarded as being more conservative than surgical approaches. The use of lubricants, drugs, or devices such as contact lenses is considered less invasive than the mechanical alteration of tissues. Except in cases where surgical treatments are clearly more effective than medical options, the physician should first consider using the less invasive treatment.

SURGICAL APPROACHES

There are many surgical approaches for treating ocular surface diseases (see box), but these are rarely used alone. Chemicals, drugs, or radiation often supplement surgery. Although numerous surgical techniques have been suggested for the eyelids, conjunctiva, or cornea, this discussion will be limited to those procedures directly applicable to the cornea, namely, anterior stromal puncture, epithelial debridement, superficial keratectomy, heat and chemical cautery, and phototherapeutic keratectomy. Transposition or transplantation of the conjunctiva and other methods of managing corneal stem cell disease, such as keratoepithelioplasty, have been discussed in separate chapters.

Corneal Surgery for Ocular Surface Disease

Defective adhesion of the corneal epithelium has been recognized by ophthalmologists for over 100 years.[1,2] Early observers noted that the corneal epithelium was loosely attached to underlying stroma in the recurrent erosion syndrome.[3,4] With the advent of biomicroscopy, clinicians were able to describe irregularities of the epithelial surface, including dots and lines at the level of Bowman's membrane.[5,6] Numerous treatments were attempted, but it was not until histopathologic correlation could be obtained with light and electron microscopy that a rationale for a particular treatment modality could be supported. For example, hypertonic ointment was advocated for recurrent erosions as early as 1914 after Szily described corneal epithelial edema in patients with recurrent erosions.[3,7] Numerous case reports and anecdotal evidence have been cited to support the use of hypertonic agents, but no satisfactory experimental data have established the superiority of these agents over bland ointments alone in the treatment of recurrent erosions or corneal dystrophies because of epithelial adhesion deficiencies.[8,9] Therefore, the most effective therapies are those in which the underlying etiologic deficiency can be identified histopathologically and logical therapy developed that is aimed at its correction.

In recurrent corneal erosion there is absence or discontinuity of the basement membrane in the corneal epithelium.[10,11] In epithelial basement membrane dystrophies, incomplete basement membrane complexes, such as hemidesmosomes, are associated with epithelial cells misdirected into cysts or folds, the deposition of amorphous granular substance in the subepithelial area, and subsequent nonadherence of the epithelium to the underlying structures.[12-15] In both erosion syndromes and dystrophies of the corneal

Ocular surface diseases

Aniridia
Bank keratopathy
Contact lens–induced keratopathy
Dystrophies
  Lattice
  Reis-Bückler's
  Salzmann's nodular
Persistent epithelial defects
Pterygium
Recurrent erosions
Superficial punctate keratitis
Superior limbic keratitis
Trauma
  Chemical
  Radiation
  Thermal
Vortex keratopathy

Surgical modalities for the treatment of ocular surface disease

Anterior stromal puncture
Cautery
  Chemical
  Heat
Conjunctival flap
Conjunctival transplant
  Autologous
  Homologous
Epithelial debridement
  Local excision
  Wide excision
Keratoepithelioplasty
Keratoplasty
Phototherapeutic keratectomy
Superficial keratectomy (sub-Bowman's, intrastromal)
Tarsorrhaphy

epithelial basement membrane, therefore, "the critical factor [. . .] is the incomplete formation and maintenance of basement membrane complexes, the basic effectors of adhesion."[16] The aim of treatment should be to establish secure, tight adhesion of epithelial cells to the underlying structures and ultimately the formation of a smooth corneal surface.

Of the treatment modalities listed in the box, five are aimed at altering the adherence of the epithelium to the underlying cornea: anterior stromal puncture (ASP), epithelial debridement, superficial keratectomy, cauterization, and phototherapeutic keratectomy (PTK). The remaining—keratoepithelioplasty, conjunctival transplant and flaps, tarsorrhaphy, and keratoplasty—either reconstruct or replace altered structures that reestablish the ocular surface.

CAUTERIZATION

Chemical cauterization

Early in this century, chemical cauterization of the epithelium was favored in the treatment of recurrent corneal erosions.[17,18] Chemicals frequently used included fresh chlorine water, iodine, or trichloroacetic acid.[8,19,20] With this technique the cauterizing solution is applied with a cotton-tipped applicator to the affected area of the cornea after topical anesthetic has been instilled. The corneal epithelium may be removed before cauterization. The applicator tip is rolled over the area several times, often beyond the area of visible epithelial disturbance.[19] More recently, the use of chemical cauterization has been questioned, because chemical cauterization may induce additional damage to the compromised basement membrane of these patients.[21]

Heat cauterization

Heat cauterization for recurrent corneal erosion was introduced by T.O. Wood.[22] After a topical anesthetic is instilled, the surgeon presses a fine, pointed microdiathermy needle onto the corneal surface. A short duration (0.05 seconds) radiofrequency current is activated, and the needle is then removed. Multiple applications are applied up to the limits of the erosion. Immediately after the treatments are applied the surrounding epithelium is white, and permanent superficial stromal scars are produced.[22] Patients usually become asymptomatic within a few weeks of treatment, and retreatments are occasionally required. Histopathologic analysis of animal eyes subjected to microdiathermy in this fashion revealed, however, that basement membrane reformation was not complete as long as 1 month after treatment.[23]

SUPERFICIAL KERATECTOMY

Superficial keratectomy is a vague term because the precise level of keratectomy is not specified. The most superficial keratectomy is removal of the epithelium. Procedures that advocate removal of basement membrane or invade no deeper than Bowman's membrane are distinctly different from dissections into anterior stroma. Thus, it is best to consider each of these therapeutic approaches separately.

Epithelial debridement

Debridement of the epithelium without cautery was advocated for the treatment of recurrent erosions as early as 1889.[24] It continued to be an accepted

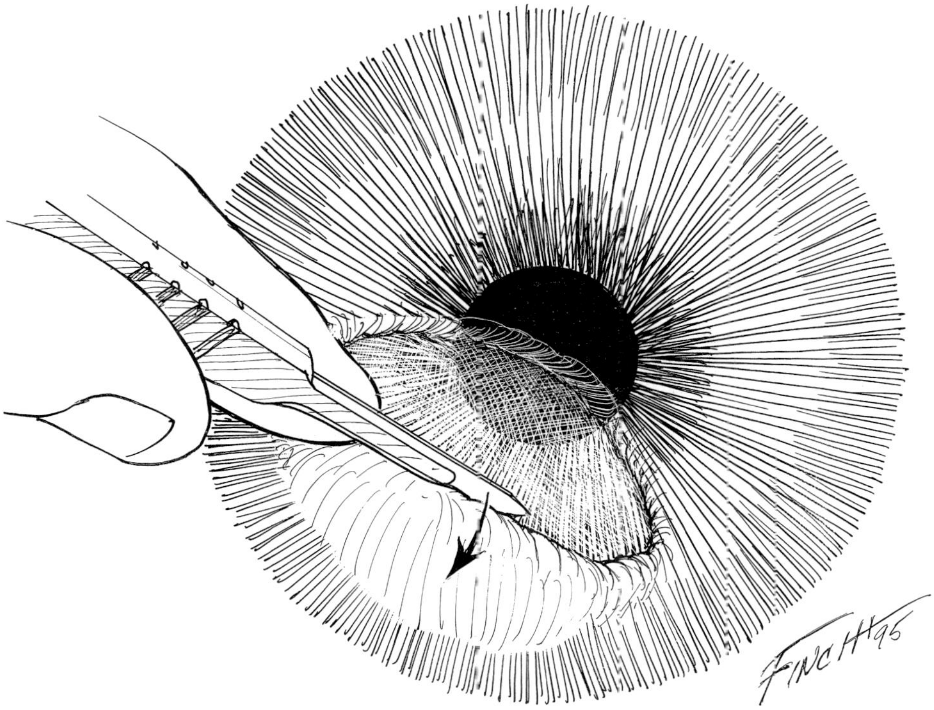

FIGURE 152-1 Technique of epithelial debridement using a scalpel.

treatment, and the technique was embellished over the succeeding decades.[25] Kaufman advocated vigorous curettage for irregularities of Bowman's membrane but cautioned against disturbing the basement membrane in recurrent erosion syndromes.[21,26] Cogan et al advocated removing the epithelium in a single sheet whenever the symptoms of microcystic dystrophy of the cornea warranted surgical intervention.[13]

Khodadoust et al described a series of experiments using electron microscopy to compare the healing characteristics of rabbit corneas that had the epithelium removed by simple scraping versus anterior stromal keratectomy, in which the basement membrane was also removed.[27] Following simple scraping, epithelial adhesion was nearly normal after approximately 1 week, perhaps because the basal epithelial cells were broken in the process, leaving basement membrane and adherence complexes intact.[27] In contrast, the reformation of adhesion complexes took up to 6 weeks when an anterior stromal keratectomy was the method of epithelial removal.[27]

In a clinical report by Brown and Bron, local epithelial debridement did not prevent the recurrence of corneal erosions.[28] Furthermore, although debridement combined with either chemical cautery or vigorous scarification of Bowman's seemed to reduce the tendency toward recurrence, permanent scarring resulted.[28] Thus their findings appeared to be in conflict with the work of Khodadoust et al.[27]

Thoft and Friend hypothesized that the regeneration and maintenance of the corneal epithelium was a multidimensional process depending heavily on those cells closest to the limbus.[29] This outer zone contains "stem cells," which act as the source of new cells for epithelial regeneration.[29,30] After deepithelialization and subsequent healing, these cells appear to be more firmly attached than those that are central.[27]

Buxton advocated total superficial epithelial keratectomy (to the limbus) for the treatment of epithelial basement membrane dystrophy.[31] With this technique, he described a high degree of success in preventing recurrence of both the signs and symptoms of the dystrophic process.[32] Buxton et al believed that total removal of the epithelium in this manner permitted reepithelialization of the cornea with a completely new layer of cells, which reestablished normal basement membrane and adhesion complexes.[31,32] Subsequent studies suggested that removal of the perilimbal corneal stem cells may be harmful or delay reepithelialization.[33]

When both efficacy and cost are considered, removal of the epithelium with a scalpel (Figure 152-1) leaving the perilimbal stem cells intact (Figure 152-2), is perhaps the best treatment currently available for epithelial basement membrane dystrophies. The use of topical diclofenac sodium with or without a soft bandage contact lens relieves much of the postoperative pain.[34] This approach takes advantage of the knowledge

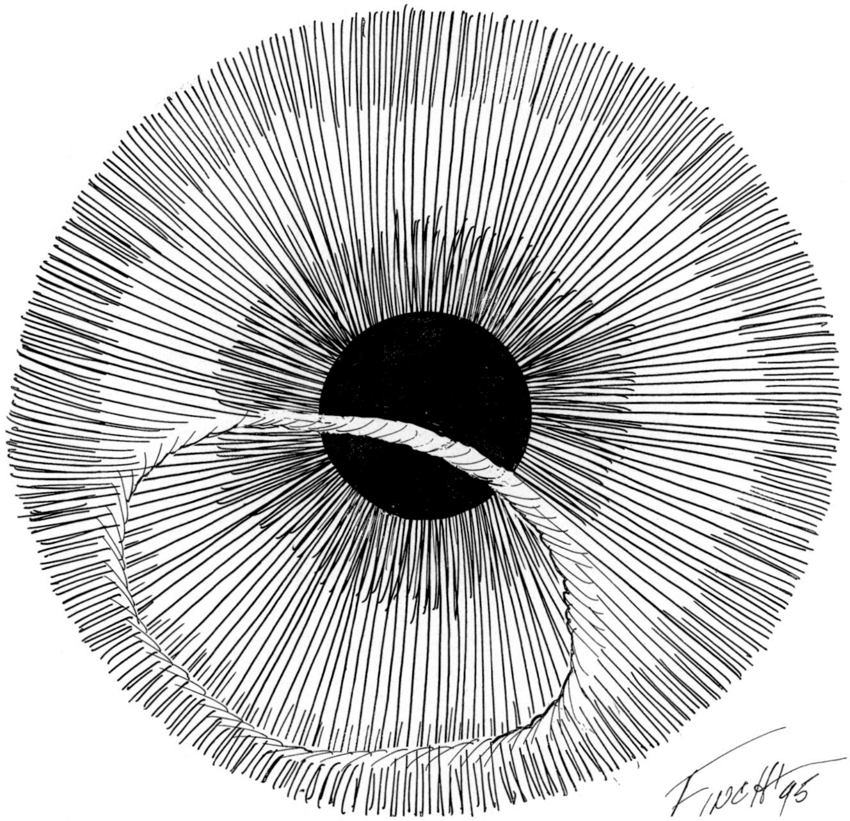

FIGURE 152-2 Completion of epithelial debridement to within 0.5 to 1.0 mm of the limbus, sparing epithelial stem cells.

gained from histopathologic studies and is aimed at correcting the basement membrane redundancy and associated misdirection of the epithelium common to the epithelial basement membrane dystrophies.

Anterior stromal keratectomy

When the ocular surface is irregular because of disturbances beneath the epithelium or its basement membrane, anterior keratectomy may become necessary. In the traditional manner this is performed mechanically by hand dissection; more recently, excimer laser phototherapeutic keratectomy has become available (see later discussion). Sub-Bowman's dissection removes not only the epithelium but also its basement membrane. Although the regenerated epithelium attempts to remodel the surface to form a smooth contour, the adhesion of the new cells is slow and they must be protected with a soft contact lens or ocular lubricants long after the defect has reepthelialized.[27,35]

ANTERIOR STROMAL PUNCTURE

Based on the clinical observation that recurrent erosions were usually seen after superficial trauma but rarely after lacerations into the stroma or when foreign bodies were present, McLean described a technique of intentionally breaching Bowman's membrane with a needle in an attempt to form a more secure adhesion of the epithelium.[36]

McLean suggests using a 20-gauge disposable hypodermic needle to make multiple micropunctures through the epithelium and Bowman's membrane into anterior stroma (Figure 152-3). He advocates the use of a disposable hypodermic needle because no special equipment is necessary other than that which is commonly found in an ophthalmologist's office. The treatment can be performed at the slit lamp. The needle is held perpendicular to the cornea, and multiple puncture wounds are made into the anterior third of the stroma. The lesions are placed 0.5 to 1.0 mm apart, and the cornea is intentionally indented during penetration (Figure 152-3). An attempt is made to avoid the visual axis, but the entire area of loose epithelium is treated, which is most easily identified by the negative staining produced after fluorescein instillation (Figure 152-4). The treatment marks are made 1 mm beyond the area of negative staining and frequently encompass one third to one half of the total corneal surface.[36] Not uncommonly, 40 or 50 micro-

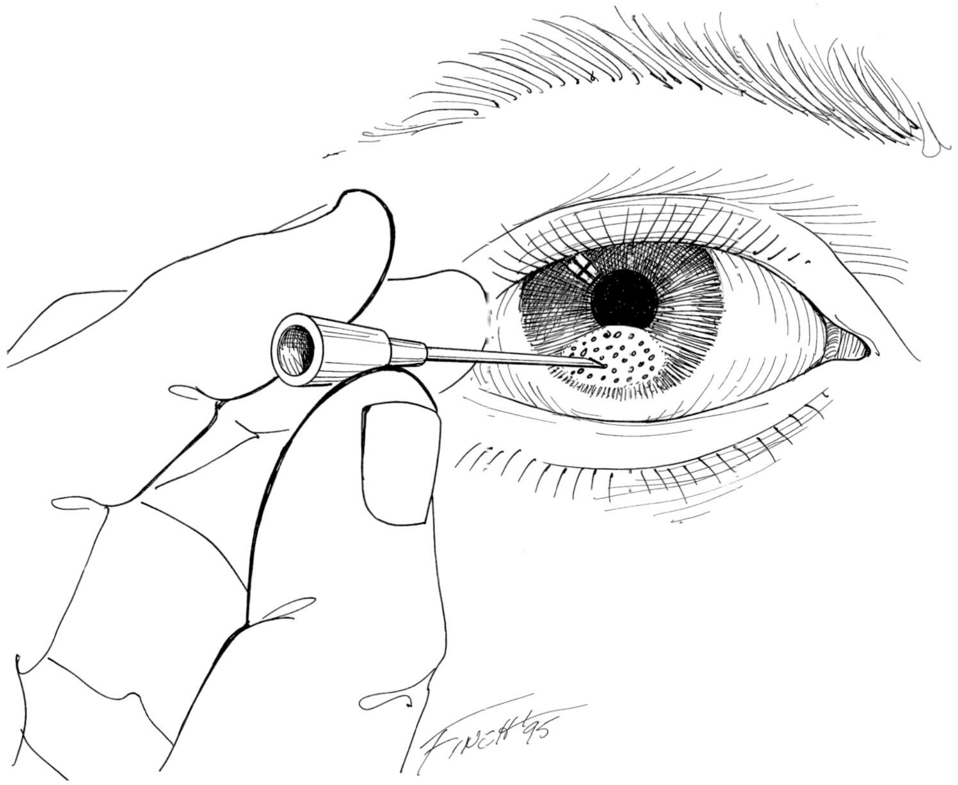

FIGURE 152-3 Technique of anterior stromal puncture.

punctures are necessary (Figure 152-5). Subsequent experience has shown that placing these wounds in the visual axis produces minimal impact on visual acuity.[37]

Since penetration through Bowman's membrane into anterior stroma is all that is required to obtain the beneficial effect, a needle designed specifically for anterior stromal puncture can be used, limiting penetration and minimizing inadvertent entry into the anterior chamber[38] (Figure 152-6). Scarring appears to be less significant, and postoperative discomfort is minimized with the use of this needle.[38]

After anterior stromal puncture, the operated eye can be treated with a bandage soft lens or an antibiotic ointment and a pressure patch. After 2 to 4 days, patching is discontinued and ocular lubricants, such as a bland ointment, are initiated. The scars become sharply defined and then fade over a period of weeks to months.

Histopathologic evaluation of corneas subjected to anterior stromal puncture reveals that basement membrane reproduction occurs more rapidly than when microdiathermy is used.[23] The enhancement of epithelial reattachment is ostensibly caused by the protection of extracellular matrix proteins such as fibronectin, type IV collagen, and laminin in corneas treated with anterior stromal puncture.[39]

In a high percentage of cases, freedom from recurrence is obtained after a single anterior stromal puncture session. If repeat treatment is needed, it usually results in permanent prevention of recurrences.[35,36,38,40]

Anterior stromal puncture has also been performed with the Nd:YAG laser.[41] Compared to needle puncture, laser treatment produces less stromal scarring.[42] However, the depth of the Nd:YAG treatment applications was less predictable and Descemet's membrane can be violated.[37,42] Furthermore, the use of a laser instead of an inexpensive disposable needle negates one of the advantages of anterior stromal puncture because costs are increased significantly.

PHOTOTHERAPEUTIC KERATECTOMY

The value of treating corneal pathology with the excimer laser is becoming increasingly obvious. Excimer ablation can be used to remove Salzmann's nodules, band keratopathy, anterior corneal dystrophies, recurrent erosions, and superficial stromal scars.[43-61] These reports illustrate that excimer laser phototherapeutic keratectomy (PTK) is a viable procedure for the treatment of certain pathologic corneal conditions, but to date, none demonstrates that excimer laser PTK is superior to existing treat-

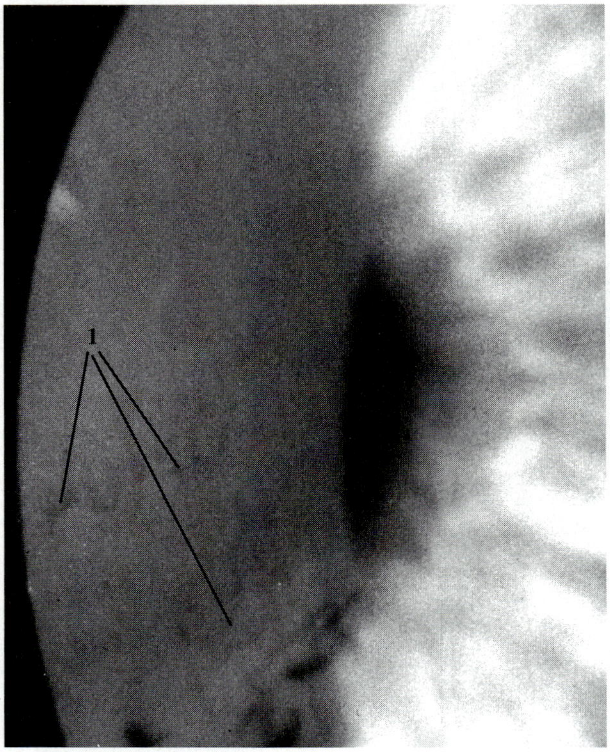

FIGURE 152-4 Area of recurrent erosion identified by negative fluorescein staining *(1)*.

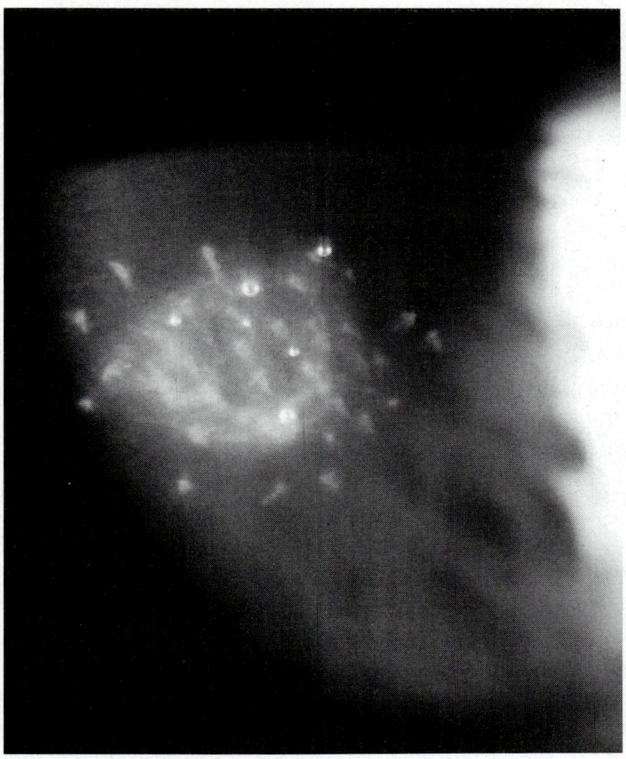

FIGURE 152-5 Cornea immediately after anterior stromal puncture.

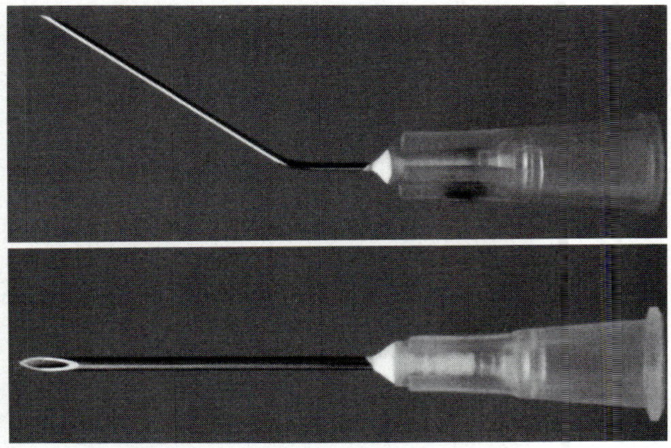

FIGURE 152-6 Two types of anterior stromal puncture needles. *Bottom,* 20-gauge disposable hypodermic needle. *Top,* 27-gauge needle specifically designed for anterior stromal puncture.

ment modalities with regard to safety, efficacy, and cost.*

There are drawbacks to the use of the excimer laser for therapeutic reasons. A shift of the patient's refractive error toward the hyperopic direction occurs in a significant number of cases.[44,46,51-53,57,62] Since the excimer laser irradiates the cornea uniformly, without regard to the height or depth of a lesion, the preexisting surface irregularity is translated into the ablation bed. Therefore masking fluids, which fill in low spots and minimize variations of corneal height, are required when treating surface disorders.[63] Occasionally, scars are resistant to excimer PTK.[64] Efficacy and cost savings are most demonstrable when treating superficial corneal dystrophies, such as Reis-Bucklers, crystalline keratopathy, or the stromal dystrophies, which would otherwise require keratoplasty.[50-52,56,57,64] Phototherapeutic keratectomy for corneal erosions may be helpful in cases wherein the visual axis is involved but the increased cost, pain, and healing time, when compared with anterior stromal puncture, makes PTK less attractive than it is in the treatment of other ocular surface diseases.

The increased cost of using an expensive laser must be justified before its use can be expanded onto a large scale. Until such time, excimer laser PTK must remain an investigational supplement to existing treatments.

Conclusions

Contemporary ophthalmologists are fortunate to have multiple options for the treatment of ocular surface disease. New surgical concepts are conceived as

*References 32, 36, 38, 40, 60, 62.

histopathologic correlations expand our understanding of the causes of these disorders. At the present time, anterior stromal puncture is the most effective, cost-containing treatment for recurrent corneal erosions. Epithelial debridement to within 0.5 to 1.0 mm of the limbus, followed by topical diclofenac sodium and a bandage soft contact lens for pain control, is the most logical treatment for epithelial basement membrane dystrophies. Phototherapeutic keratectomy with the excimer laser holds a great deal of promise for the treatment of nodular dystrophy, anterior stromal dystrophies, and superficial corneal scars, but future studies must determine its relative value in the treatment of each pathologic condition.

REFERENCES

1. Hansen E: Om den intermitterende keratitis visicularis neuralgica af traumatisk oprindelse, *Hospitals-Tidende* 51:201-203, 1872.
2. Arlt von F: Ueber die verletzungen des auges in gerichtsärztlicher beziehung, *Wien Med Woch* 23:447-449, 1874.
3. Szily A: Ueber disjunction des hornhautepithels, *Albrecht Von Graefes Arch Ophthalmol* 51:486-531, 1900.
4. Peters A: Über traumatische hornhauterkrandungen und ihre beziehungen zum herpes corneae, *Albrecht von Graefes Arch Ophthalmol* 57:93-137, 1904.
5. Vogt A: Weitre ergebnisse der spaltlampenmikroskopie des vorderen bulbusabschnittes, *Albrecht von Graefes Arch Ophthalmol* 106:63-113, 1921.
6. Vogt A: *Lehrbuch und Atlas der Spaltlampenmikroskopie Des Lebenden Auges,* Berlin, 1930, Verlag Von Julius Springer.
7. Schreiber L: Die behandlung der rezidivierenden hornhauterosionen mit Scharlachsalbe, *Albrecht von Graefes Arch Ophthalmol* 87:174-184, 1914.
8. Chandler P: Recurrent erosion of the cornea, *Am J Ophthalmol* 28:355-363, 1945.
9. Leibowitz H: *Corneal disorders, clinical diagnosis and management,* Philadelphia, 1984, Saunders.
10. Goldman J, Dohlman C, Kravitt B: The basement membrane of the human cornea in recurrent epithelial erosion syndrome, *Trans Am Acad Ophthalmol Otolaryngol* 73:471-481, 1969.
11. Tripathi R, Bron A: Ultrastructural study of non-traumatic recurrent corneal erosion, *Br J Ophthalmol* 56:73-85, 1972.
12. Brodrick J, Dark A, Peace G: Fingerprint dystrophy of the cornea, *Arch Ophthalmol* 92:483-489, 1974.
13. Cogan D et al: Microcystic dystrophy of the cornea, *Arch Ophthalmol* 92:470-474, 1974.
14. Rodriques M et al: Disorders of the corneal epithelium, *Arch Ophthalmol* 92:475-482, 1974.
15. Tripathi R, Bron A: Cystic disorders of the corneal epithelium. II. Pathogenesis, *Br J Ophthalmol* 57:376-390, 1973.
16. Fogle J et al: Defective epithelial adhesion in anterior corneal dystrophies, *Am J Ophthalmol* 79:925-940, 1975.
17. Franke E: Ueger erkrankungen des epithels der hornhaut, *Klin Monatsbl Augenheilk* 44:508-533, 1906.
18. Verhoeff F: Neuropathic keratitis and some allied conditions with special reference to treatment, *J Am Med Assoc* 53:191-198, 1909.
19. Gundersen T: Herpes corneae with special reference to its treatment with strong solution of iodine, *Arch Ophthalmol* 15:225-249, 1936.
20. Thygeson P: Observation on recurrent erosion of the cornea, *Am J Ophthalmol* 47:48-52, 1959.
21. Kaufman H: Epithelial erosion syndrome: metaherpetic keratitis, *Am J Ophthalmol* 57 983-987, 1964.
22. Wood T: Recurrent erosion, *Trans Am Ophthalmol Soc* 82:850-898, 1984.
23. Judge D et al: Anterior stromal micropuncture electron microscopic changes in the rabbit cornea, *Cornea* 92:152-160, 1990.
24. Bronner A: On some cases of traumatic keratalgia, *Trans Ophthalmol Soc UK* 9:89-94, 1889.
25. Guerry D: Observations on Cogan's microcystic dystrophy of the corneal epithelium, *Trans Am Ophthalmol Soc* 63:320-334, 1965.
26. Kaufman H, Clower J: Irregularities of Bowman's membrane, *Am J Ophthalmol* 61:227-230, 1966.
27. Khodadoust A et al: Adhesion of regenerating corneal epithelium, *Am J Ophthalmol* 65:339-348, 1968.
28. Brown N, Bron A: Recurrent erosion of the cornea, *Br J Ophthalmol* 60:84-96, 1976.
29. Thoft R, Friend J: The X,Y,Z hypothesis of corneal epithelial maintenance, *Invest Ophthalmol Vis Sci* 24:1442-1443, 1983.
30. Schermer A, Galvin S, Sun T: Differentiation-related expression of a major 64K corneal keratin in vivo and in culture suggests limbal location of corneal epithelial stem cells, *J Cell Biol* 103:49-62, 1986.
31. Buxton J, Fox M: Superficial epithelial keratectomy in the treatment of epithelial basement membrane dystrophy, *Arch Ophthalmol* 101:392-395, 1983.
32. Buxton J, Constad W: Superficial epithelial keratectomy in the treatment of epithelial basement membrane dystrophy, *Ann Ophthalmol* 19:92-96, 1987.
33. Huang A, Tseng S: Corneal epithelial wound healing in the absence of limbal epithelium, *Invest Ophthalmol Vis Sci* 32:96-105, 1991.
34. Eiferman R, Hoffman R, Sher N: Topical diclofenac reduces pain following photorefractive keratectomy, *Arch Ophthalmol* 111: 1022, 1993.
35. Laibson P: Recurrent erosion. In Fraunfelder FT, Roy FH, editors: *Current ocular therapy,* ed 4, Philadelphia, 1994, Saunders.
36. McLean E, MacRae S, Rich L: Recurrent erosion: treatment by anterior stromal puncture, *Ophthalmology* 93:784-788, 1986.
37. McLean E: Update on stromal puncture technique, *Ophthalmology* 97:1245, 1990.
38. Rubinfeld R et al: Anterior stromal puncture for recurrent erosion: further experience and new instrumentation, *Ophthalmic Surg* 21:318-326, 1990.
39. Hsu J et al: Anterior stromal puncture. Immunohistochemical studies in human corneas, *Arch Ophthalmol* 111:1057-1063, 1993.
40. Reinhard T, Sundmacher R, Strunck-Kortenbusch B: Hornhautschelung bei rezidivierenden hornhauterosionen, *Ophthalmologie* 90:694-697, 1993.
41. Geggel H: Successful treatment of recurrent corneal erosion with Nd:YAG anterior stromal puncture, *Am J Ophthalmol* 110:404-407, 1990.
42. Geggel H, Maza C: Anterior stromal puncture with the Nd:YAG laser, *Invest Ophthalmol Vis Sci* 31:1555-1559, 1990.
43. Steinert R, Puliafito C: Excimer laser phototherapeutic keratectomy for a corneal nodule, *Refract Corneal Surg* 6:352, 1990.
44. Sher N et al: Clinical use of the 193 nm excimer laser in the treatment of corneal scars, *Arch Ophthalmol* 109:491-498, 1991.
45. Wu W, Stark W, Green W: Corneal wound healing after 193 nm excimer laser keratectomy, *Arch Ophthalmol* 109:1426-1432, 1991.
46. Stark W et al: Clinical follow-up of 193-nm ArF excimer laser photokeratectomy, *Ophthalmology* 99:805-812, 1992.
47. McDonnell P, Seiler T: Phototherapeutic keratectomy with

excimer laser for Reis-Bückler's corneal dystrophy, *Refract Corneal Surg* 8:306-310, 1992.
48. Fagerholm P et al: Phototherapeutic keratectomy: long term results in 166 eyes, *Refract Corneal Surg Suppl* 9:76-80, 1993.
49. Thompson V, Durrie D, Cavanaugh T: Philosophy and technique for excimer laser phototherapeutic keratectomy, *Refract Corneal Surg Suppl* 9:81-85, 1993.
50. Förster W et al: Phototherapeutic keratectomy in corneal diseases, *Refract Corneal Surg Suppl* 9:85-90, 1993.
51. Hersh P et al: Phototherapeutic keratectomy: strategies and results in 12 eyes, *Refract Corneal Surg Suppl* 9:90-95, 1993.
52. Lawless M, Cohen P, Rogers C: Phototherapeutic keratectomy for Reis-Bücklers dystrophy, *Refract Corneal Surg Suppl* 9:96-98, 1993.
53. Hahn T, Sah W, Kim J: Phototherapeutic keratectomy in nine eyes with superficial corneal diseases, *Refract Corneal Surg Suppl* 9:115-118, 1993.
54. John M et al: Excimer laser photoablation of primary familial amyloidosis of the cornea, *Refract Corneal Surg Suppl* 9:138-141, 1993.
55. Rapuano C, Laibson P: Excimer laser phototherapeutic keratectomy, *CLAO* 19:235-240, 1993.
56. O'Brart D, et al: Treatment of band keratopathy by excimer laser phototherapeutic keratectomy: surgical techniques and long term follow up, *Br J Ophthalmol* 77:702-708, 1993.
57. Rogers C, Cohen P, Lawless M: Phototherapeutic keratectomy for Reis-Bückler's corneal dystrophy, *Aust NZ J Ophthalmol* 21:247-250, 1993.
58. Örndahl M, et al: Treatment of corneal dystrophies with excimer laser, *Acta Ophthalmol* 72:235-240, 1994.
59. Poirier L et al: Resultats de la photokeratectomie therapeutique par laser excimer. A propos de 12 cas, *J Fran D'Ophtalmologie* 17:262-270, 1994.
60. Dausch D et al: Phototherapeutic keratectomy in recurrent corneal epithelial erosion, *Refract Corneal Surg Suppl* 9:419-424, 1993.
61. John M et al: Excimer laser phototherapeutic keratectomy for treatment of recurrent corneal erosion, *J Corneal Refract Surg* 20:179-181, 1994.
62. Fountain T et al: Reassembly of corneal epithelial adhesion structures after excimer laser keratectomy in humans, *Arch Ophthalmol* 112:967-972, 1994.
63. Kornmehl E, Steinert R, Puliafito C: A comparative study of masking fluids for excimer laser phototherapeutic keratectomy, *Arch Ophthalmol* 109:860-863, 1991.
64. McDonnell J, Tseng S: Corneal epithelial wound healing in the absence of limbal epithelium, *Invest Ophthalmol Vis Sci* 32:96-105, 1991.

CHAPTER 153

MICHAEL R. GRIMMETT EDWARD J. HOLLAND

Management of Pterygium

The term *pterygium* is derived from the Greek combining form *pteron* meaning "wing." Clinically, a pterygium appears as a fleshy, vascular mass that occurs in the interpalpebral fissure. The typical pterygium is triangular and is made up of a cap, head, and body. The cap, or gray zone, is an arcuate, gray-white, subepithelial, corneal opacity that is at the leading edge of the pterygium (Figure 153-1). With chronicity, abnormal tear pooling in advance of the cap leads to the deposition of a corneal epithelial iron line (Stocker's line).[1] The head of the pterygium is an elevated white mass that forms a firm adhesion to the globe. The body of the pterygium is a fleshy fibrovascular mass that is demarcated from normal conjunctiva superiorly and inferiorly by sharp folds. Vital staining reveals selective rose bengal uptake on the surface of pterygia in approximately half the cases.[2] Although simultaneous nasal and temporal pterygia can occur, pterygia are more frequently located nasally rather than temporally.[3] Isolated temporal pterygia are considered an uncommon occurrence.[4] Bilateral ocular involvement occurs in approximately one third of patients with pterygia.[3,4] Active pterygia are characterized by marked vascular engorgement and progressive growth. Some pterygia will become quiescent with resolution of the vascular injection and flattening of the pterygium mass. The ultimate reasons for variable growth characteristics of pterygia are largely unknown.

In advanced cases, the pterygium encroaches onto the cornea and may cause visual loss secondary to (1) loss of corneal transparency within the visual axis or (2) irregular corneal astigmatism (localized flattening). Regarding the latter phenomenon, a recent study disclosed that the induced irregular corneal astigmatism results largely from pooling of tears in advance of the pterygium apex.[5] In select cases, however mechanical forces may predominate, leading to tractional corneal flattening.[6] Additional evidence suggests that both spatial contrast sensitivity and glare disability are worsened in patients with pterygia even when the Snellen visual acuity is minimally affected.[7]

Symptomatically, patients may experience foreign body sensation, burning, tearing, and blurred vision. Most of these symptoms are related to active inflammation of the pterygium. In some patients with advanced pterygia, ocular motility may be restricted, leading to diplopia in certain fields of gaze. Detrimental cosmetic effects caused by large pterygia are common.

Prevalence

Epidemiologic surveys indicate that the prevalence rates of pterygia vary, depending on the exact population under scrutiny. Overall, prevalence rates range from 0.7% to 31% in various populations around the world.[3,4,8-11] Prevalence rates for pterygia in the United States are reported to range from 2% in the northern states to 7% in the southern states.[8] As a general rule, prevalence rates for pterygia increase with age, although a decline in prevalence rates has been reported for patients over 60 to 70 years of age.[3,8] Reasons cited for this decline include a lack of self-reporting by the elderly and the regression of pterygia with senescence.[3] Furthermore, certain studies report an equal occurrence of pterygia in males or females,[3] while others report a male predominance.[8,9] It is possible that the reported differences in prevalence rates for men and women reflect different exposure rates to environmental risk factors. Additionally, prevalence rates for pterygia have been found to vary according to race. A population study in West Malaysia found that pterygia were more likely in those of Chinese descent as compared to those of Malaysian or Indian descent.[10] Other authors have similarly reported racial differences in prevalence rates.[4,12]

surgical techniques used, the proportion of secondary recurrent pterygia treated, the postoperative medical regimens prescribed, the age and location of the populations studied, the length of the follow-up periods, and the specific definition of a recurrence used by a given author.[49]

Complications from conjunctival autografting are infrequent and not generally sight threatening. Before performing an autograft, the interested reader is referred to an excellent review of postoperative problem prevention and management for conjunctival autografts that was published by Starck et al in 1991.[50] Minor problems such as conjunctival graft edema, corneoscleral dellen, and epithelial inclusion cysts are encountered infrequently. Less common problems include corneal astigmatism, hematomas, Tenon's granuloma, retraction and/or necrosis of the graft, and extraocular muscular disinsertion. For optimal surgical results, Starck et al[50] emphasize careful dissection of Tenon's tissue from the conjunctival graft and recipient bed, minimal manipulation of tissues, and accurate orientation of the graft. Allan et al[49] concur with the low complication rate of conjunctival autografting while reporting one Tenon's granuloma, one conjunctival inclusion cyst, and three wound dehiscences after 93 procedures performed. All complications in Allan's[49] series were corrected with minor surgical revision without recurrences. Vrabec et al[51] reported two cases of subconjunctival fibrosis at the harvest site causing extraocular muscle restriction with concomitant diplopia in one patient. Suggestions for management of this fibrosis included early frequent topical corticosteroids and/or possible primary closure of the harvest site conjunctiva at the time of the original surgery.

The specific procedure for conjunctival autografting has been previously published by Kenyon et al.[36] With only a few variations from Kenyon's[36] original report, what follows will be a description of the general procedural technique for conjunctival autografting (Figure 153-2). After the excision of the pterygium as described previously in this chapter, the size of the scleral defect created is measured with Castroviejo calipers. The globe is then rotated downward using the stay sutures to expose the superior bulbar conjunctiva. The dimensions of the intended conjunctival graft (adjacent to the limbus) are marked with a gentian violet marking pen based on the previous measurements of the recipient bed. The gentian violet marks not only aid in the excision of an appropriately sized donor graft but are invaluable in preventing inadvertent upside-down orientation of the graft in the recipient bed. Adamis et al[35] note that free grafts as large as 15 mm by 15 mm can be prepared and used without difficulty. Balanced salt solution is then injected subconjunctivally outside of the gentian violet marks to elevate the conjunctiva to aid in the conjunctival dissection. Blunt Wescott scissors are used to incise the conjunctiva outside the gentian violet marks along the posterior border of the graft. The conjunctiva is then undermined using blunt dissection with care taken to not include underlying Tenon's capsule in the final graft. The lateral edges of the donor graft are incised outside of the gentian violet marks as the dissection is carried forward. It is important to note that the graft is purposely excised outside of the gentian violet marks so that these marks can be used for later orientation. (In the final graft, the limbus is the edge without any marks.) The donor conjunctival graft should be as thin as possible so that postoperative healing will occur with less shrinkage. It is also important that the limbal conjunctiva is incised last after the entire graft has been dissected forward to the limbus. This assures that the graft will not retract and become difficult to handle. The tissues are not allowed to dry during the procedure and are moistened with frequent applications of balanced salt solution. Handling of the donor conjunctival tissue only occurs with nontoothed forceps (e.g., a McGregor conjunctival forcep) so as to avoid a buttonhole in the conjunctiva. At this point the graft is repositioned into the recipient bed, with adjustment of the traction sutures as necessary. The graft is oriented with the unmarked limbal donor edge adjacent to the limbus in the recipient bed and the gentian violet marks on the exposed surface of the conjunctiva. Adamis et al[35] advocate securing the graft with approximately eight 8-0 vicryl sutures; we routinely secure the graft to the recipient conjunctival edge and underlying episclera with numerous 10-0 nylon sutures (buried knots) to avoid a postoperative graft dehiscence. The majority of these sutures usually extrude on their own by 1 month postoperatively, while the rest usually epithelialize and remain buried. Because of the use of permanent sutures, patient discomfort is usually not a problem. The occasional exposed stitch can be removed after adequate conjunctival healing in the early postoperative period. The donor harvest site is left to epithelialize on its own, which usually occurs in the first several days postoperatively. Kenyon et al[36] advocate postoperative steroid and antibiotic ointments. We typically use a steroid/antibiotic drop six times a day during the first 1 or 2 weeks and switch to a steroid drop alone after that time. Drops are titrated according to the degree of inflammation and may be continued for 4 to 8 weeks, depending on the clinical circumstance (Figure 153-3).

The primary disadvantage of the conjunctival autograft technique is the prolonged operative time required when compared to other bare sclera or primary closure techniques. Additionally, an operating

A B C D

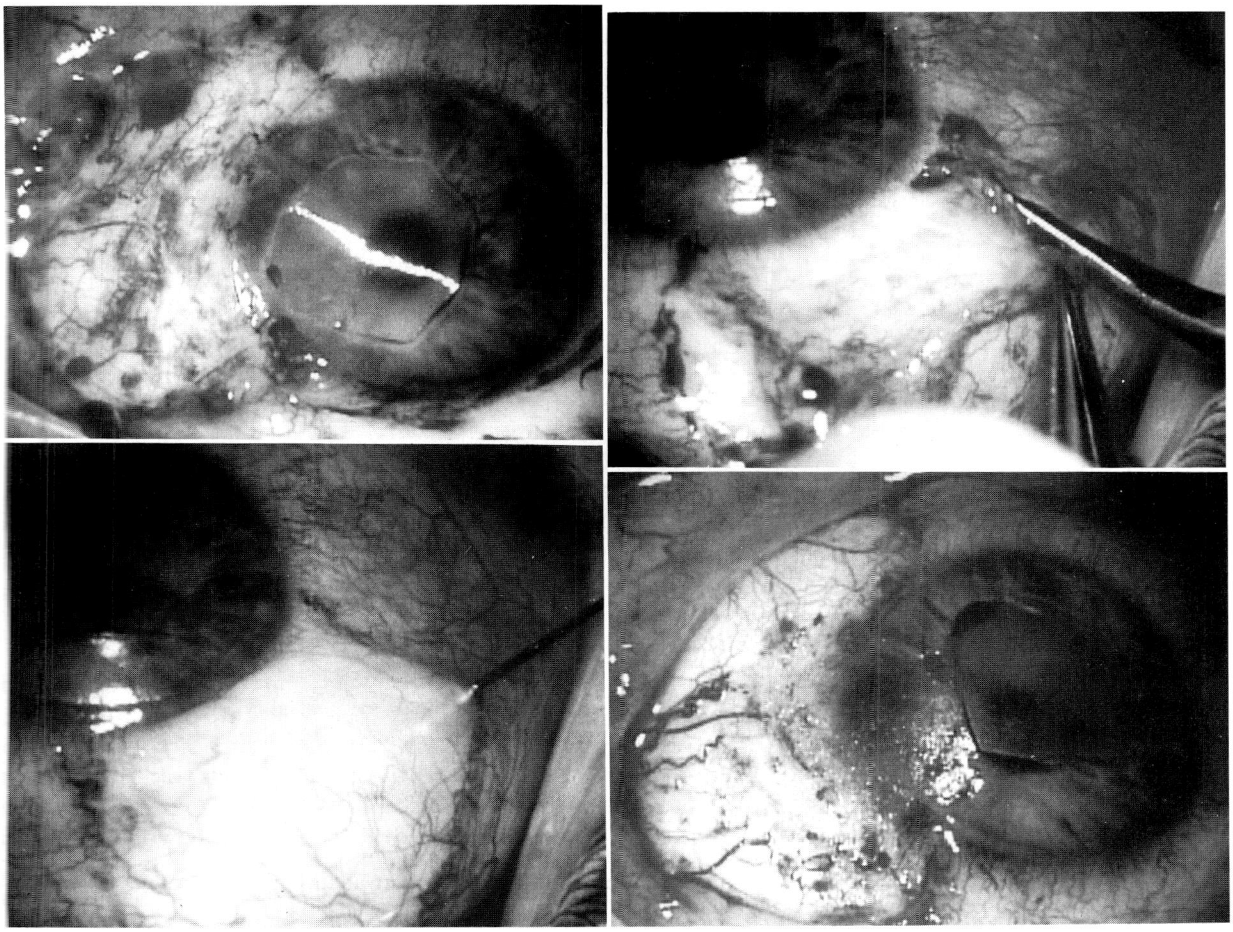

FIGURE 153-2 Conjunctival autograft. **A,** Conjunctival defect present immediately after excision of pterygium. The central corneal polygonal material protects the fundus from light toxicity. **B,** Harvesting of conjunctival autograft tissue from the superotemporal quadrant. Gentian violet demarcates the margins of the autograft. Balanced salt solution is injected subconjunctivally. **C,** Excision of the conjunctival autograft starts with the posterior border of the graft followed by each lateral border. The limbal border is removed last. Note that the incision is made outside of the gentian violet mark to retain the marks on the graft. These marks assist the surgeon in orientating the graft. **D,** Conjunctival autograft is secured over bare sclera with interrupted 10-0 nylon sutures.

microscope is required for optimum results, which can be a problem for ophthalmologists in developing countries.[52] However, these disadvantages are outweighed by the lack of sight-threatening complications and the relatively low recurrence rates after conjunctival autografts.

Lamellar keratoplasty and penetrating keratoplasty

If significant corneal thinning is present as a consequence of previous pterygium surgery, a lamellar keratoplasty may be indicated to restore the normal ocular surface integrity. Additionally, various authors have recommended a lamellar keratoplasty as a barrier to pterygium regrowth.[53] While the reported series are small, recurrence rates after lamellar keratoplasties have been reported between 0%[54] and 60%.[38] The successful use of lyophilized donor tissue has been described in the treatment of recurrent pterygia with only one recurrence in 13 eyes.[55] In severe cases where the visual axis is affected by thinning and scarring, a penetrating keratoplasty may be indicated to visually rehabilitate the eye.[34]

Mucous membrane grafts and skin grafts

In cases in which sufficient conjunctiva is not available for a pedicle graft, Trivedi et al[56] recommend the use of a mucous membrane graft from the lower lip tainty. Indeed, reports have been published to the contrary. Yamanouchi et al[75] reported on 15 patients with severe scleral complications following topical mitomycin instillation after pterygium excision. Hayasaka et al noted two cases of late-onset scleral ulceration after 0.4 mg/ml mitomycin drops three times a day for 1 week after primary pterygium excision.[69] Additionally, a recent article by Rubinfeld et al[76] described the findings in 10 patients who experienced serious, vision-threatening complications associated with the use of mitomycin after pterygium surgery. These complications included severe secondary glaucoma (four patients), corneal edema (three patients), corneal perforation (one patient), correctopia (two patients), iritis (eight patients), sudden onset mature cataract (two patients), scleral calcification (one patient), and incapacitating photophobia and pain (eight patients). Six patients required twenty operative procedures as a consequence of their complications. Five eyes had a final visual acuity of 20/200 or worse. Since three of the six patients with the most severe complications had concomitant chronic external diseases, Rubinfeld[77] stated that mitomycin C after pterygium excision is contraindicated in patients with keratitis sicca, Sjögren's syndrome, neurotrophic keratitis, or severe meibomian gland dysfunction blepharitis. A review of the Japanese literature by Rubinfeld et al[76] revealed reports of scleral ulceration, necrotizing scleritis, perforation, iridocyclitis, cataract, infection, glaucoma, scleral calcification, and loss of an eye after pterygium excision with adjunctive mitomycin therapy. While the exact incidence of these complications is unknown, the contention that mitomycin C therapy is safe remains to be determined with future long-term trials.

Unfortunately, the optimum dosage and treatment length of topical mitomycin to maximize both effectiveness and safety are not precisely known. Clues to the optimum dosage of mitomycin C may be inferred from a study on the inhibitory effects of mitomycin C on human Tenon's capsule fibroblasts in cell culture: cell colony formation was inhibited at mitomycin concentrations of 0.1 mg/ml, cell death ensued at mitomycin C concentrations of 0.3 mg/ml, and the LD_{50} for these fibroblasts was 0.2 mg/ml.[63] Other investigators are currently evaluating the effects of various mitomycin C concentrations and application times on vascular endothelium and limbal stem cells in rabbits to ascertain a dose-response curve.[77] Regarding stability of the topical solution, reconstituted mitomycin has a pH of 6 to 8 and is stable for 2 weeks when refrigerated at 2° to 8° C.[68]

Radiation therapy

Until the 1950s, radon bulbs, radium plaques, Grenz rays, and x-rays were employed in the treatment of pterygia with variable success.[34,78] In 1952 strontium 90 was introduced for the treatment of neoplastic disease and has been used extensively for the treatment of pterygia since that time. Strontium 90 is produced in the fission of uranium 235 and has a half-life of 28 years. Strontium 90 decays to yttrium 90, with a half-life of 64 hours, which, in turn, decays to zirconium 90, which is stable.[79] Beta rays from strontium 90 have an average energy of 0.21 MeV per disintegration while beta rays from yttrium 90 have an average energy of 0.89 MeV per disintegration.[79] Beta rays expend their energy maximally within the superficial 2 mm of tissue as the dose drops to 41% at 1 mm, 19% at 2 mm, 9% at 3 mm, and 1% at 5 mm.[34] This low penetration profile for strontium 90 is important, since cataracts may develop should the dose to the crystalline lens approach 1500 to 2500 rep (1 rep = 1.08 rad).[34]

Recurrence rates after pterygium excision with beta irradiation have varied widely, with a low of 0%[80] to a high of 80%[81] reported in the literature. Of the larger series reported, recurrence rates vary between 1.7% (825 cases),[82] 6% (975 cases),[83] and 12% (764 cases).[84] Direct comparison of the various studies is difficult because of the variations in the populations studied, follow-up intervals, dosage regimens, and definition of a recurrence. The mechanism of action of beta irradiation in reducing recurrences is thought to be through the inhibition of mitosis in rapidly dividing cells such as vascular endothelial cells.[35]

Various investigators report different opinions on the total dosage required, the need for fractionation, or the optimal time for delivery of beta irradiation after pterygium excision. A recent literature review by Paryani et al[82] disclosed that the total dose of beta irradiation has varied from 1800 to 6000 rad given in one to six fractions in different reports. Apparently there is some degree of flexibility in the total dose and the fractionation of beta irradiation delivered after pterygium excision, with different investigators reporting efficacy with widely varying protocols. Most investigators, however, hold that the optimal dose is between 1000 and 3000 rad given at the time of surgery or within a few days of surgery.[35] Aswad and Baum[85] reported that a single 2000 rad dose given in the immediate postoperative period had a lower recurrence rate than a similar dose given 4 days postoperatively in patients with secondary recurrent pterygia. No statistically significant difference in the timing of the beta irradiation was found in patients with primary pterygia. Furthermore, applying the beta irradiation at the time of surgery may also allow better control and localization of the treatment and may save the patient additional time and expense.[34,85]

While beta irradiation lowers the recurrence rate of pterygia, significant long-term complications have

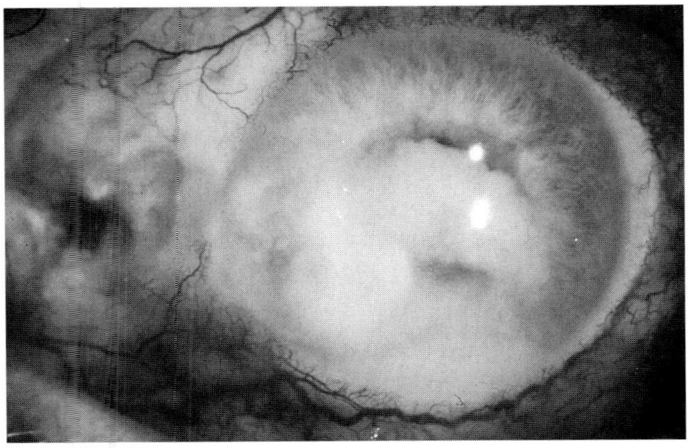

FIGURE 153-4 Necrotizing scleritis and secondary *Pseudomonas* sclerokeratitis occurring 17 years after beta irradiation for pterygium.

been reported, including cataract formation and scleral necrosis (Figure 153-4). MacKenzie et al[84] reported a 13% rate of scleromalacia with a 4.5% rate of severe scleral thinning in a large population-based study with 10 years' follow-up. Additionally, endophthalmitis as a consequence of the scleral necrosis was seen in two patients. Tarr and Constable[86] reported on 63 eyes with complications after pterygium excision with beta irradiation evaluated from 3 to 20 years postoperatively. Scleral ulceration was reported in 51 eyes, and nonvisually disabling sectoral lens opacities were identified in 19 eyes. Reduced vision secondary to a radiation-induced cataract occurred in three eyes. *Pseudomonas* endophthalmitis occurred in four patients with scleral necrosis. Other less frequently encountered complications included corneal ulcers, symblepharon, iris atrophy, ptosis, and thinned conjunctival tissue. Dusenbery et al[87] reported that 13 of 36 eyes treated with beta irradiation developed complications that included epithelial defects or corneal thinning, symblepharon, cataract, and corneal ulceration with an associated *Pseudomonas* keratitis. Four of the five eyes that were previously irradiated had an 80% complication rate. Moriarty et al[88] reported 11 cases of secondary fungal or bacterial infections as a consequence of beta irradiation–induced scleral necrosis. The average latency between the beta irradiation and the onset of the complications was 14.5 years. Seven patients required a penetrating keratoplasty to remove the associated infection or treat a full-thickness or incipient perforation.

Because conjunctival autografting offers a low rate of pterygium recurrence and is free from long-term sight-threatening complications, it appears that autografting offers patients a safer alternative when compared to beta irradiation.[88] Because scleral necrosis and possible late infectious complications occur years after the original surgery, it is not surprising that numerous short- and intermediate-term studies deemed beta irradiation safe. While it is debatable whether the reported complications from beta irradiation or mitomycin therapy are at an acceptably low rate, the serious nature of these untoward late effects make conjunctival autografting a viable alternative in the treatment of both primary and secondary pterygia.

REFERENCES

1. Barraquer-Somers E, Chan CC, Green WR: Corneal epithelial iron deposition, *Ophthalmology* 90:729, 1983.
2. Hansen A, Norn M: Astigmatism and surface phenomena in pterygium, *Acta Ophthalmol* 58:174, 1980.
3. Youngson RM: Ptergyium in Israel, *Am J Ophthalmol* 74:954, 1972.
4. Detels R, Dhir SP: Pterygium: a geographical study, *Arch Ophthalmol* 78:485, 1967.
5. Oldenburg JB et al: Conjunctival ptergia: mechanism of corneal topographic changes, *Cornea* 9:200, 1990.
6. Gridley MJ, Perlman EM: A form of variable astigmatism induced by pseudopterygium, *Ophthalmic Surg* 17:794, 1986.
7. Lin S et al: The effect of pterygia on contrast sensitivity and glare disability. *Am J Ophthalmol* 107:407, 1989.
8. Sivasubramaniam P: Pterygium in Ceylon, *Br J Ophthalmol* 55:55, 1971.
9. Norn MS: Prevalence of pinguecula in Greenland and in Copenhagen, and its relation to pterygium and spheroid degeneration, *Acta Ophthalmol* 57:96, 1979.
10. Rasanayagam RT: The incidence and racial distribution of pterygium in West Malaysia, *Trans Ophthalmol Soc NZ* 25:56, 1973.
11. Rojas JR, Malaga H: Pterygium in Lima, Peru, *Ann Ophthalmol* 18:147, 1986.
12. Hilgers JHC: Pterygium: its incidence, heredity, and etiology, *Am J Ophthalmol* 50:635, 1960.
13. Cameron ME: *Pterygium throughout the world,* Springfield, IL, 1965, Charles C Thomas.
14. Mackenzie FD et al: Risk analysis in the development of pterygia, *Ophthalmology* 99:1056, 1992.
15. Coroneo MT: Pterygium as an early indicator of ultraviolet insolation: a hypothesis, *Br J Ophthalmol* 77:734, 1993.
16. Hill JC, Maske R: Pathogenesis of pterygium, *Eye* 3:218, 1989.
17. Taylor, HR: Aetiology of climatic droplet keratopathy and pterygium, *Br J Ophthalmol* 64:154, 1980.
18. Karai I, Horiguchi S: Pterygium in welders, *Br J Ophthalmol* 68:347, 1984.
19. Moran DJ, Hollows FC: Pterygium and ultraviolet radiation: a positive correlation, *Br J Ophthalmol* 68:343, 1984.
20. Sevel D, Sealy R: Pterygia and carcinoma of the conjunctiva, *Trans Ophthalmol Soc UK* 88:567, 1968.
21. Dushku N, Tyler N, Reid TW: Immunohistochemical evidence that pterygia arise from altered limbal epithelial basal stem cells, *Invest Ophthalmol Vis Sci* 34:1013, 1993.
22. Tseng SCG et al: Classification of conjunctival surgeries for corneal diseases based on stem cell concept, *Ophthalmol Clin North Am* 3:595, 1990.
23. Goldberg L, David R: Pterygium and its relationship to the dry eye in the Bantu, *Br J Ophthalmol* 60:720, 1976.
24. Wong WW: A hypothesis on the pathogenesis of pterygiums, *Ann Ophthalmol* 10:303, 1978.
25. Pinkerton OD, Hokama Y, Shigemura LA: Immunologic basis for the pathogenesis of pterygium, *Am J Ophthalmol* 98:225, 1984.
26. Hect F, Shoptaugh MG: Winglets of the eye: dominant transmis-

sion of early adult pterygium of the conjunctiva, *J Med Genet* 27:392, 1990.
27. Austin, P, Jakobiec FA, Iwamoto T: Elastodysplasia and elastodystrophy as the pathologic bases of ocular pterygia and pinguecula, *Ophthalmology* 90:96, 1983.
28. Hogan, MJ, Alvarado J: Pterygium and pinguecula: electron microscopic study, *Arch Ophthalmol* 78:174, 1967.
29. Ansari MW, Rahi AHS, Shukla BR: Pseudoelastic nature of pterygium, *Br J Ophthalmol* 54:473, 1970.
30. Cameron ME: Histology of pterygium: an electron microscopic study, *Br J Ophthalmol* 67:604, 1983.
31. Raizada IN, Goswami AP, Bhatnagar NK: Histopathology of pterygium, *Eye Ear Nose Throat Monthly* 47:340, 1968.
32. Rich AM et al: A simplified way to remove pterygia, *Ann Ophthalmol* 6:739, 1974.
33. Rosenthal JW: Chronology of pterygium therapy, *Am J Ophthalmol* 36:1601, 1953.
34. Jaros PA, DeLuise VP: Pingueculae and pterygia, *Surv Ophthalmol* 33:41, 1988.
35. Adamis AP, Starck T, Kenyon KR: The management of pterygium, *Ophthalmol Clin North Am* 3:611, 1990.
36. Kenyon KR, Wagoner MD, Hettinger ME: Conjunctival autograft transplantation for advanced and recurrent pterygium, *Ophthalmology* 92:1461, 1985.
37. Small RG: A technique for removal of pterygium, *Ann Ophthalmol* 9:349, 1977.
38. Youngson RM: Recurrence of pterygium after excision, *Br J Ophthalmol* 56:120, 1972.
39. Sen DK: Surgery of pterygium. Modified McGavic's technique, *Br J Ophthalmol* 54:606, 1970.
40. Escapini H: Pterygium excision, *Am J Ophthalmol* 6:879, 1958.
41. Krag S, Ehlers N: Excimer laser treatment of pterygium, *Acta Ophthalmol* 70:530, 1992.
42. Zauberman H: Pterygium and its recurrence, *Am J Ophthalmol* 63:1780, 1967.
43. Anduze AL: Merest sclera technique for primary pterygium surgery, *Ophthalmic Surg* 20:892, 1989.
44. Aratoon V: Surgery of pterygium by conjunctival pedicle flap, *Am J Ophthalmol* 63:1778, 1967.
45. Wilson SE, Bourne WM: Conjunctival Z-plasty in the treatment of pterygium, *Am J Ophthalmol* 106:355, 1988.
46. Stocker FW: Operation for removal of pterygium, *Arch Ophthalmol* 27:925, 1942.
47. McCoombes JA, Hirst LW, Isbell GP: Sliding conjunctival flap for the treatment of primary pterygium, *Ophthalmology* 101:169, 1994.
48. Lewallen S: A randomized trial of conjunctival autografting for pterygium in the tropics, *Ophthalmology* 96:1612, 1989.
49. Allan BDS et al: Pterygium excision with conjunctival autografting: an effective and safe technique, *Br J Ophthalmol* 77:698, 1993.
50. Starck T, Kenyon KR, Serrano F: Conjunctival autograft for primary and recurrent pterygia: surgical technique and problem management, *Cornea* 10:196, 1991.
51. Vrabec MP, Weisenthal RW, Elsing SH: Subconjunctival fibrosis after conjunctival autograft, *Cornea* 12:181, 1993.
52. Singh G: Pterygium in the tropics, *Ophthalmology* 97:542, 1990.
53. Laughrea PA, Arentsen JJ: Lamellar keratoplasty in the management of recurrent pterygium, *Ophthalmic Surg* 17:106, 1986.
54. Poirier RH, Fish JR: Lamellar keratoplasty for recurrent pterygium, *Ophthalmic Surg* 7:38, 1976.
55. Busin M et al: Precarved lyophilized tissue for lamellar keratoplasty in recurrent pterygium, *Am J Ophthalmol* 102:222, 1986.
56. Trivedi LK, Massey DB, Rohatgi R: Management of pterygium and its recurrence by grafting with mucous membrane from the mouth, *Am J Ophthalmol* 68:353, 1969.
57. Wong WW: Behavior of skin grafts in treatment of recurrent pterygium, *Ann Ophthalmol* 9:352, 1977.
58. Olander K, Haik HG, Haik GM: Management of pterygia: should thiotepa be used? *Ann Ophthalmol* 10:853, 1978
59. Ehrlich D: The management of pterygium, *Ophthalmic Surg* 8:23, 1977.
60. Gerde LS: Management of pterygium along the mexican border, *South Med J* 79:782, 1986.
61. Kleis W, Pico G: Thio-tepa therapy to prevent postoperative pterygium occurrence and neovascularization, *Am J Ophthalmol* 76:371, 1973.
62. Asregadoo ER: Surgery, Thio-tepa, and corticosteroids in the treatment of pterygium, *Am J Ophthalmol* 74:960, 1972.
63. Chen CW et al: Trabeculectomy with simultaneous topical application of mitomycin-C in refractory glaucoma, *J Ocular Pharmacol* 6:175, 1990.
64. Dorr RT: New findings in the pharmacokinetic, metabolic, and drug-resistance aspects of mitomycin C, *Semin Oncol* 15:32, 1988.
65. Kunitomo N, Mori S: Studies on the pterygium. Part 4. A treatment of the pterygium by mitomycin-C instillation, *Acta Soc Ophthalmol Jpn* 67:601, 1963.
66. Singh G, Wilson MR, Foster CS: Mitomycin eye drops as treatment for pterygium, *Ophthalmology* 95:813, 1988.
67. Singh G, Wilson MR, Foster CS: Long-term follow-up study of mitomycin eye drops as adjunctive treatment for pterygia and its comparison with conjunctival autograft transplantation, *Cornea* 94:331, 1990.
68. Mahar PS, Nwokora GE: Role of mitomycin C in pterygium surgery, *Br J Ophthalmol* 77:433, 1993.
69. Hayasaka S et al: Postoperative instillation of low-dose mitomycin C in the treatment of primary pterygium, *Am J Ophthalmol* 106:715, 1988.
70. Hayasaka S et al: Postoperative instillation of mitomycin C in the treatment of recurrent pterygium, *Ophthalmic Surg* 20:580, 1989.
71. Rosenthal G et al: The use of mitomycin in pterygium surgery, *Ann Ophthalmol* 25:427, 1993.
72. Chayakul V: Mitomycin in treating pterygium, *Ophthalmology* 96:399, 1989.
73. Sugar A: Who should receive mitomycin-C after pterygium surgery? *Ophthalmology* 99:1645, 1992.
74. Kloess PM, Yee RW, Hopp LM: Mitomycin C after pterygium excision, *Ophthalmology* 100:292, 1993.
75. Yamanouchi U et al: Scleromalacia presumably due to mitomycin C instillation after pterygium excision, *Jpn J Clin Ophthalmol* 33:139, 1979.
76. Rubinfeld RS et al: Serious complications of topical mitomycin-C after pterygium surgery, *Ophthalmology* 99:1647, 1992.
77. Rubinfeld RS: Mitomycin-C after pterygium excision, *Ophthalmology* 100:977, 1993.
78. Tong ECK, Zaret MM, Rubenfeld S: Cellular changes in the conjunctiva after strontium 90 treatment for pterygium, *Am J Roentgenol Radium Ther Nucl Med* 106:848, 1969.
79. Bahrassa F, Datta R: Postoperative beta radiation treatment of pterygium, *Int J Radiation Oncol Biol Phys* 9:679, 1983.
80. Herbstein AU, Donovan JK: Pterygium removal. A technique to prevent recurrence, *Br J Ophthalmol* 52:162, 1968.
81. Sinha A: Combined surgical and beta radiation treatment of pterygium, *Indian Pract* 20:255, 1967.
82. Paryani SB et al: Management of pterygium with surgery and radiation therapy, *Int J Radiation Oncol Biol Phys* 28:101, 1994.
83. Pinkerton OD: Surgical and strontium treatment of pterygium: recurrence and lens changes. Age statistics, *Ophthalmic Surg* 10:44, 1979.

84. MacKenzie FD et al: Recurrence rate and complications after beta irradiation for pterygia, *Ophthalmology* 98:1776, 1991.
85. Aswad MI, Baum J: Optimal time for postoperative irradiation of pterygia, *Ophthalmology* 94:1450, 1987.
86. Tarr KH, Constable IJ: Late complications of pterygium treatment, *Br J Ophthalmol* 64:496, 1980.
87. Dusenbery KE et al: Beta irradiation of recurrent pterygia: results and complications, *Int J Radiation Oncol Biol Phys* 24:315, 1992.
88. Moriarty AP et al: Severe corneoscleral infection. A complication of beta irradiation scleral necrosis following pterygium excision, *Arch Ophthalmol* 111:947, 1993.

CHAPTER 154

KENNETH R KENYON MICHAEL D WAGONER JOHN W SHORE

Ocular Surface Transplantation

Problems of the ocular surface are diverse with respect to etiology, symptoms, and prognosis. They range from relatively minor irritations of recurrent corneal epithelial erosions with preservation of excellent vision to the devastating and potentially blinding consequences of chemical injury with persistent epithelial defects and stromal ulceration. While various medical therapies may be applied appropriately to the management of this spectrum of disorders, increasing clinical experience and laboratory investigation support the surgical management of ocular surface problems that have proven recalcitrant to conventional therapy. In particular, this chapter will focus on the roles of conjunctival, limbal, and mucous membrane transplantation as applied to specific ocular surface diseases.

Principles of Ocular Surface Replacement

The ocular surface describes the entire epithelial surface of the external eye, encompassing the corneal epithelium as well as the bulbar and palpebral conjunctival epithelium. Initially considered only as an *anatomic* classification, which recognized the physical continuity of the stratified nonkeratinizing epithelium of the conjunctiva, limbus, and cornea, the clinical and research insights of Friedenwald,[1-2] Thoft et al,[3-17] and many others[16-31] have offered compelling evidence of important *functional* relationships within this anatomic continuity. This crucial concept of the *ocular surface as a functional unit* has stimulated a complete reorganization of our approach to and management of surface disease (Table 154-1).

Although the conjunctiva and especially the limbus perform several functions, their contributions to proper corneal epithelial maintenance and integrity are critical. For example, a smooth palpebral conjunctiva permits the eyelid to move atraumatically over the cornea, thereby affording protection, distribution of the tear film, and debridement of foreign matter. Diseases that produce keratinization of the palpebral conjunctiva (e.g., Stevens-Johnson syndrome) can induce significant corneal epithelial damage mechanically. Flexible conjunctival folds are essential for proper movements of the globe and maintenance of normal lid-globe relationships. Thus conditions that produce conjunctival scarring (e.g., ocular cicatricial pemphigoid) can obliterate the normal forniceal anatomy, creating cicatricial entropion, trichiasis, and secondary corneal erosion and scarring. Such keratinizing disorders of the conjunctiva or obliteration of the fornix by cicactricial diseases can be managed by replacement of the abnormal ocular surface tissue using normal conjunctival autografts if available[32-38] or, alternatively, buccal mucosal grafts.[39-43]

Mucus secreted by conjunctival goblet cells comprises the inner portion of the precorneal tear film and is essential for proper ocular surface wetting. When this function is deficient (e.g., Stevens-Johnson syndrome or after severe chemical injury), poor wetting of the corneal surface with subsequent desiccation and epithelial damage may occur, even in the setting of sufficient aqueous tear production. Conjunctival blood vessels near the limbus provide nourishment for the limbal epithelial "stem cells" (see later discussion). In pathologic circumstances these vessels transport inflammatory cells for combating infection (e.g., infectious keratitis) or anticollagenolytic enzymes for preventing stromal degradation (e.g., peripheral ulcerative keratitis). In situations in which the conjunctiva is relatively normal in the involved eye (e.g., neurotrophic keratitis or after microbial keratitis), a conjunctival flap[44,45] may supply the necessary corneal vascularity to prevent stromal ulceration and support repair. In situations of sterile stromal ulceration related to a severe chemical burn involving cornea, limbus, and conjunctiva with vascular ischemia, advancement of conjunctiva or Tenon's tissue[46] or autologous limbal transplantation[47] may reestablish the necessary vascular supply to reverse such ischemia-related complications.

Finally, healthy conjunctival epithelium has the ability to replace directly damaged corneal epithelium and possibly to maintain normal corneal epithelium.* Anecdotal clinical observations were responsible for

*References 1, 2, 4, 9, 16, 18, 20-22.

Table 154-1. Specific indications for ocular surface replacement

Conjunctival autograft	Limbal autograft or allograft*	Mucous membrane transplantation
Recurrent pterygium	Chemical injury* (acute and chronic)	Fornix reconstruction (bilateral)
Cicatricial strabismus	Thermal burn* (acute and chronic)	Chemical injury† (bilateral)
Fornix reconstruction (unilateral)	Contact lens keratopathy*	
Post-excision of conjunctival tumor	Persistent epithelial defect (various etiologies)	
	Post-multiple surgery limbal depletion	
	Chronic medication toxicity*	
	Stevens-Johnson syndrome*	
	Ocular cicatricial pemphigoid*	
	Aniridia*	
	Atopy*	

*Limbal autograft preferable in unilateral or asymmetrical cases.
Limbal allograft reserved for bilateral cases.
†Indicated for fornix reconstruction after cicatricization.

initial notions that conjunctival epithelium could resurface the cornea. Following complete traumatic loss of corneal epithelium with only conjunctival epithelium remaining, it is common clinical experience to observe that the resurfacing corneal epithelium is derived from an advancing wave of adjacent conjunctiva. Because the normal phenotype of conjunctival epithelium is that of columnar epithelium with numerous goblet cells, the transformation to normal stratified squamous corneal epithelium without goblet cells implies that the conjunctival epithelium retains the capability of phenotypic change to that of corneal epithelium. Such *epithelial differentiation* involves not only morphologic change but the acquisition of the biochemical and physiologic properties of corneal epithelium as well.[1,5,9]

In the mechanically abraded cornea (e.g., total epithelial debridement during vitrectomy surgery), reepithelialization and restoration of relatively normal corneal epithelial appearance and function almost invariably occur. In chemically injured eyes, however, the new corneal epithelium often maintains conjunctival characteristics, with goblet cells and neovascularization, suggesting that the regulatory processes controlling proper differentiation are abnormal. Based on these observations, Thoft[10] proposed the use of autologous conjunctival transplantation for resurfacing the unilateral or asymmetrically chemically injured eye. The success of this procedure is contingent on the ability of the transplanted conjunctival epithelium to migrate across the stromal tissue of the recipient eye, to adhere firmly, and to assume and maintain the biochemical and morphologic features of normal corneal epithelium. With the initial success of this technique for chemical injury, the indications for autologous conjunctival transplantation were expanded to include other ocular surface disorders, including recurrent pterygium, fornix reconstruction, and cicatricial strabismus (chronic postoperative inflammation, persistent epithelial defects, and contact lens–related keratopathy).*

Although conjunctival transplantation can certainly provide many of the functions essential to the reestablishment of a more normal and stable ocular surface with resultant improved corneal function (e.g., intact corneal epithelium, normal conjunctival surface and motility, reestablishment of limbal vasculature), it does not address the issue of the complete restoration of a phenotypically normal ocular surface after those injuries in which there is a complete loss of both corneal and limbal epithelial cells. Although the corneal reepithelialization derived from conjunctival epithelium posterior to the limbus can occur either spontaneously or after conjunctival transplantation, it is well known that such wound healing is often less efficient, may be associated with recurrent corneal erosions, and often fails to assume completely the functional characteristics of the normal corneal epithelium.† In particular, if corneal resurfacing is required from more than 2 mm posterior to the limbus, there is often delayed corneal reepithelialization, stromal neovascularization, persistence of conjunctival goblet cells within the corneal epithelium, and other evidences of incomplete epithelial differentiation.[23]

Observations of the normal replacement process of corneal epithelium provide valuable insights into the rationale for various ocular surface replacement techniques. Since the corneal epithelium is a highly differentiated cell type with rapid self-renewal, its *stem cells* should be available and responsive to the need for epithelial replacement and migration. Davanger and Evenson[20] were possibly the first to postulate that the limbal papillary structure serves as the generative

*References 8, 10, 13, 14, 32, 33, 36, 37
†References 4, 5, 11, 22, 23, 28, 29

organ for corneal epithelial cells. Using tritiated thymidine to label the mitotic basal cells, the mitotic index of the corneal epithelium tends to be higher toward the periphery,[2,21] suggesting that the peripheral corneal basal cells are more active in DNA synthesis. After experimental chemical injury, the limbal epithelial cells have increased cytochrome oxidase activity, reflecting increased metabolic activity.[48] Thus numerous studies[2,5,21,25] have supported the hypothesis that the source of cellular migration and proliferation comes from the peripheral cornea, with centripetal replacement of epithelial cellular attrition from either normal turnover[18] or traumatic loss.[49] Based on these observations, Thoft and Friend[16] proposed the XYZ hypothesis to explain how central corneal epithelial mass is maintained by continued centripetal movement of peripheral corneal epithelium toward the visual axis, as well as by anterior movement from the basal epithelial cells. Subsequent work has supported the limbal location of the stem cells of the cornea.[19,26,27] Kenyon and Tseng[47] postulated that these stem cells are the most qualified cells to differentiate into normal corneal epithelium after those injuries (e.g., chemical) where there is widespread loss of corneal, limbal, and conjunctival epithelium, and they developed the technique of limbal autograft transplantation for the management of these disorders.

In bilateral disease the options for ocular surface transplantation are more limited. Once again, the appropriate selection of procedures depends on the relative health of the stem cell population in the prospective donor eye. If the stem cells are damaged in both eyes, such as following bilateral chemical injury, then stem cells may be obtained from appropriate nonautologous donor material. Although keratoepithelioplasty[15,50] has been advocated as a means of transferring donor corneal epithelium from eye bank eyes to the recipient eye, the combination of technical difficulties, poor epithelial viability, and rejection problems have limited the usefulness of this modality. Unfortunately, the use of cultured limbal epithelium,[51] while technically feasible, is largely investigational and its practicality remains to be proven. Hence for cases involving bilateral stem cell loss, the most promising technique for transferring donor stem cells is limbal allograft transplantation. This approach is technically similar to limbal autograft transplantation, but it is limited in application by the requirement of either a tissue-matched donor, close relative, and/or use in combination with concomitant systemic immunosuppression.[52]

If the stem cells are normal and the goal of surgery is the restoration of a more functional conjunctival mucosal surface, as in bilateral conjunctival cicatricial disorders, a buccal mucosal graft may be employed. In such cases the procedure is used to restore more normal forniceal architecture and to diminish ocular surface inflammation and corneal damage resulting from abnormal globe cornea relationships (e.g., entropion, trichiasis), chronic exposure (lagophthalmos), and direct corneal trauma (palpebral conjunctival keratinization). In advanced cases, complications caused by recurrent corneal epithelial breakdown, secondary infectious keratitis, vascularization, and scarring may lead to the final common pathway of corneal blindness. Mucosal membrane grafting is not, however, effective in repopulating the cornea with normal stem cells and in directly normalizing a better corneal epithelial surface. Its benefits are to improve ocular surface wetting by narrowing the palpebral fissure and thereby reducing exposure and evaporation, as well as by improving eyelid movement and distribution of the tear film over the cornea.

Conjunctival Transplantation

We currently use the technique of conjunctival autograft transplantation for those situations in which abnormalities of conjunctival inflammation, scarring, or loss are *not* complicated by extensive damage or destruction of the limbal epithelial stem cells (see Table 154-1). As such, this technique is essentially an ocular surface *patch graft* designed to replace either a focal or localized defect in the conjunctiva (such as after pterygium excision), to relieve the mechanical extraocular movement restrictive abnormalities caused by conjunctival and Tenon's tissue scarring (after pterygium removal, strabismus surgery, or bulbar tumor excision), or to eliminate problems of conjunctival fornix obliteration (localized chemical injury with conjunctival scarring but limbal and corneal sparing).

The management of *advanced primary and recurrent pterygium* remains our most common indication for conjunctival transplantation.[33] Given the success of conjunctival surface replacement for other disorders, as well as a number of reports of using this technique in the setting of advanced primary or recurrent pterygia,[36,53,54] we adapted this technique as a means of restoring normal ocular surface covering in the area of bare sclera excision, eliminating the frequently encountered restriction of extraocular muscle function, and, most importantly, greatly reducing the incidence of pterygium recurrence to approximately 5%. In this situation the superior bulbar conjunctiva is usually normal and undamaged, permitting use of a conjunctival autograft from the same eye.

The technique as applied to pterygium excision is illustrated in Figure 154-1. The procedure is performed on an outpatient basis, using topical plus peribulbar or retrobulbar anesthesia (the latter especially in recur-

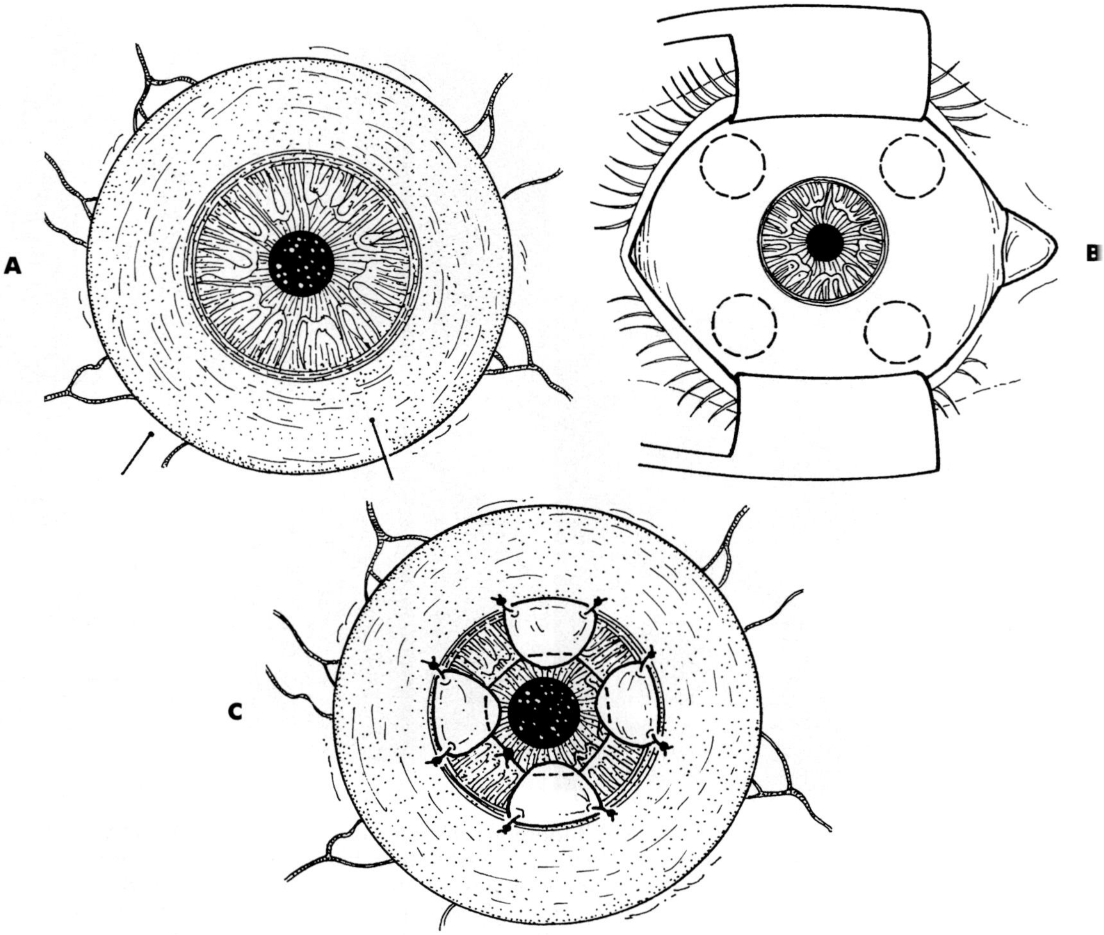

FIGURE 154-3 Thoft's original technique of conjunctival autograft transplantation for unilateral chemical injury. **A,** Extensive (5 mm) conjunctival resection and superficial keratectomy. **B,** Harvesting four pieces of conjunctiva, 4 to 5 mm in diameter, from the fellow eye. **C,** Grafts pictured in place. (Reproduced courtesy of J. Fogle, MD.)

conjunctival character. Therefore, as previously noted, we no longer perform conjunctival autografts for this indication and instead favor limbal transplantation.

Limbal Transplantation

Limbal autografts are employed to restore a more normal ocular surface epithelium in situations in which widespread destruction of the limbal stem cells has occurred (see Table 154-1). The transfer of the limbal stem cells optimizes the rehabilitation potential of corneas with the total loss or permanent damage of the corneal and limbal epithelium such as occurs in severe chemical or thermal burns, contact lens–induced keratopathy, chronic medication toxicity, postsurgical limbal depletion, radiation keratitis, and some cases of persistent epithelial defects.[47]

Chemical injury remains the most common indication for which we perform limbal autografts (Figures 154-4 to 154-6). Severe chemical injuries may result in the complete loss of corneal epithelium and stem cells, as well as conjunctival epithelium, thereby requiring resurfacing from the forniceal conjunctiva. Such corneal epithelial defects may persist for weeks or months, and if reepithelialization does occur, the conjunctivally derived epithelium may never fully differentiate into healthy corneal epithelium. These eyes remain chronically inflamed and irritated with persistent epitheliopathy, recurrent erosions, late stromal vascularization and scarring, poor visual acuity, and an extremely poor prognosis for penetrating keratoplasty.[58-60] Even if such poor quality surface healing does not occur, the persistence of epithelial defects particularly in the presence of limbal ischemia predisposes to proteolytic degradation of the stroma ("melting") with the potential for perforation and even more severe consequences. Such tenuous situations often require emer-

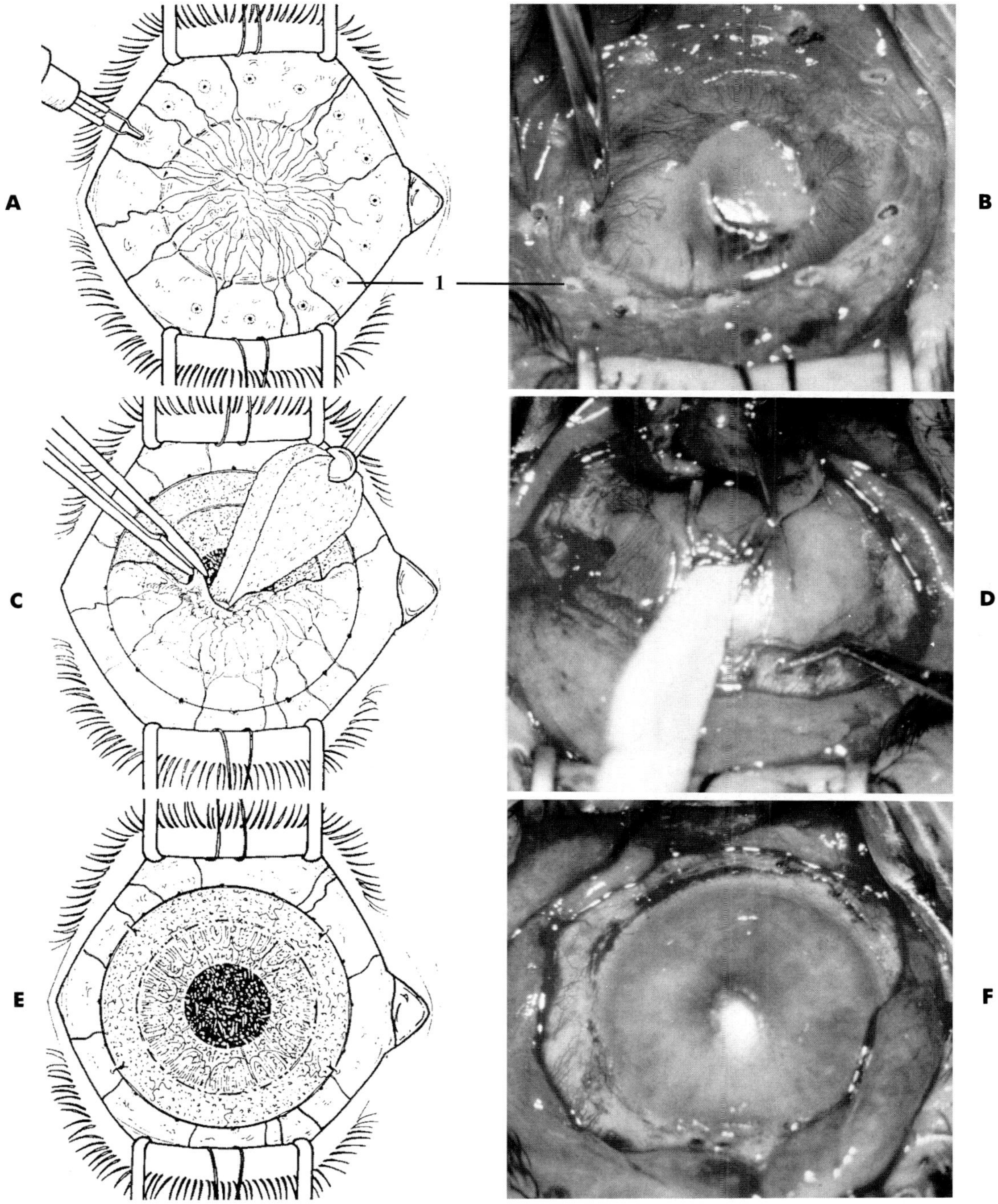

FIGURE 154-4 Technique of limbal autograft transplantation. **A** and **B**, Recipient eye preparation. Using Castroviejo calipers and disposable cautery, the area of bulbar conjunctiva to be resected is marked *(1)* approximately 2 mm posterior to the limbus. **C** and **D**, After conjunctival resection, abnormal corneal epithelium and fibrovascular pannus are stripped by blunt dissection using cellulose sponges and tissue forceps and/or superficially dissected with Martinez spatula or disposable scarifier **E** and **F**, Additional surface polishing smooths the stromal surface and improves clarity. The conjunctival margins are secured with four interrupted sutures of 8-0 Vicryl.

Continued.

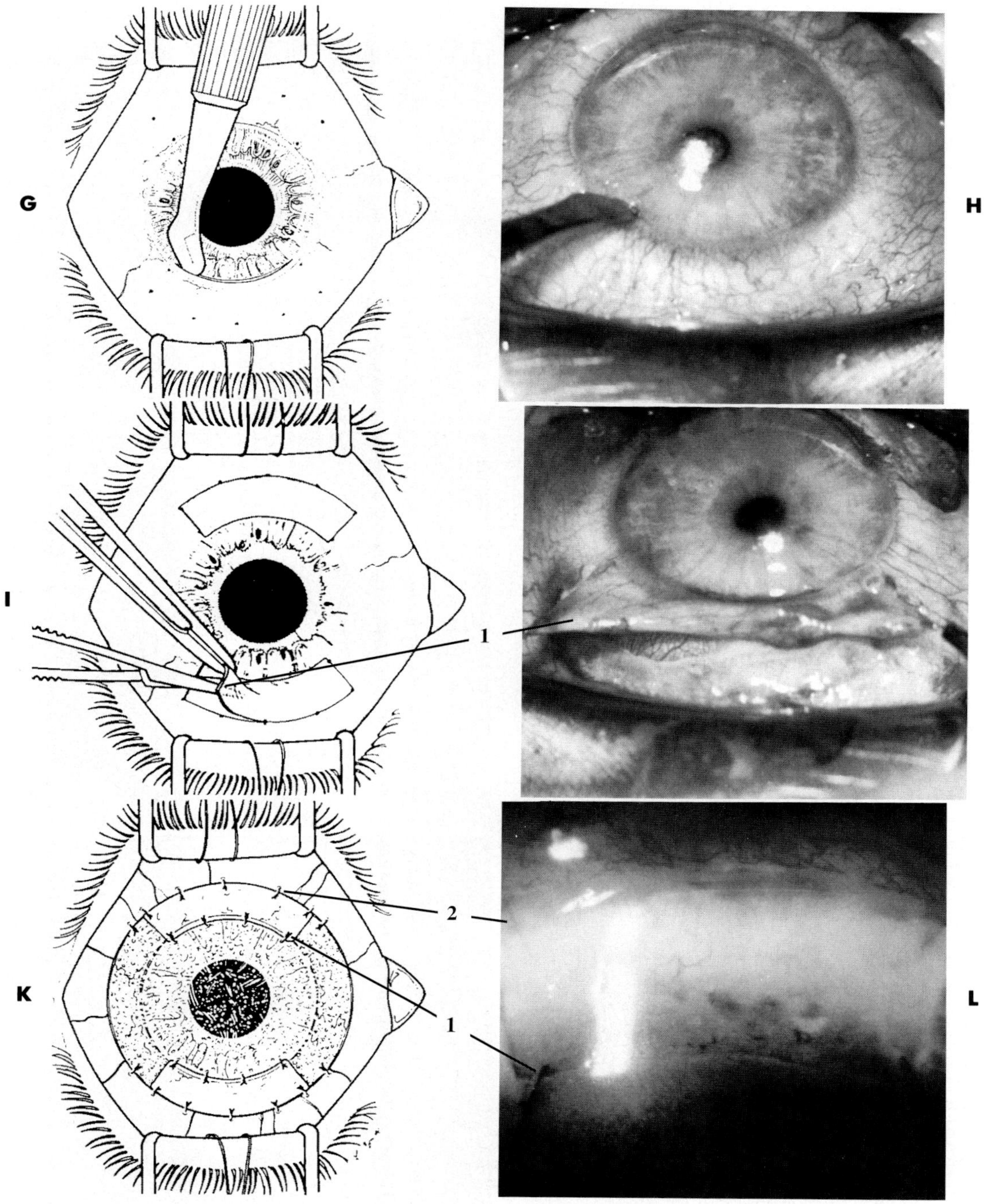

FIGURE 154-4, cont'd. Technique of limbal autograft transplantation. **G** and **H,** Donor eye preparation. Superior and inferior limbal grafts are delineated with focal applications of cautery approximately 2 mm posterior to the limbus. Each graft site extends circumferentially about three clock hours or approximately 10 mm. The initial incision is made superficially about 0.5 mm into clear cornea using a disposable scarifier. **I** and **J,** The bulbar conjunctival portion of the graft *(1)* is undermined and thinly dissected free from its limbal attachment. **K** and **L,** The limbal grafts are transferred to their corresponding sites in the recipient eye and are secured with interrupted sutures, 10-0 nylon at the corneal edge *(1)* and 8-0 polyglactin (Vicryl) at the conjunctival margin *(2)*. (**A** to **K** reproduced with permission from Kenyon KR, Tseng SCG: *Ophthalmology* 96:718-719, 1989. **L,** courtesy R Tan, MD.)

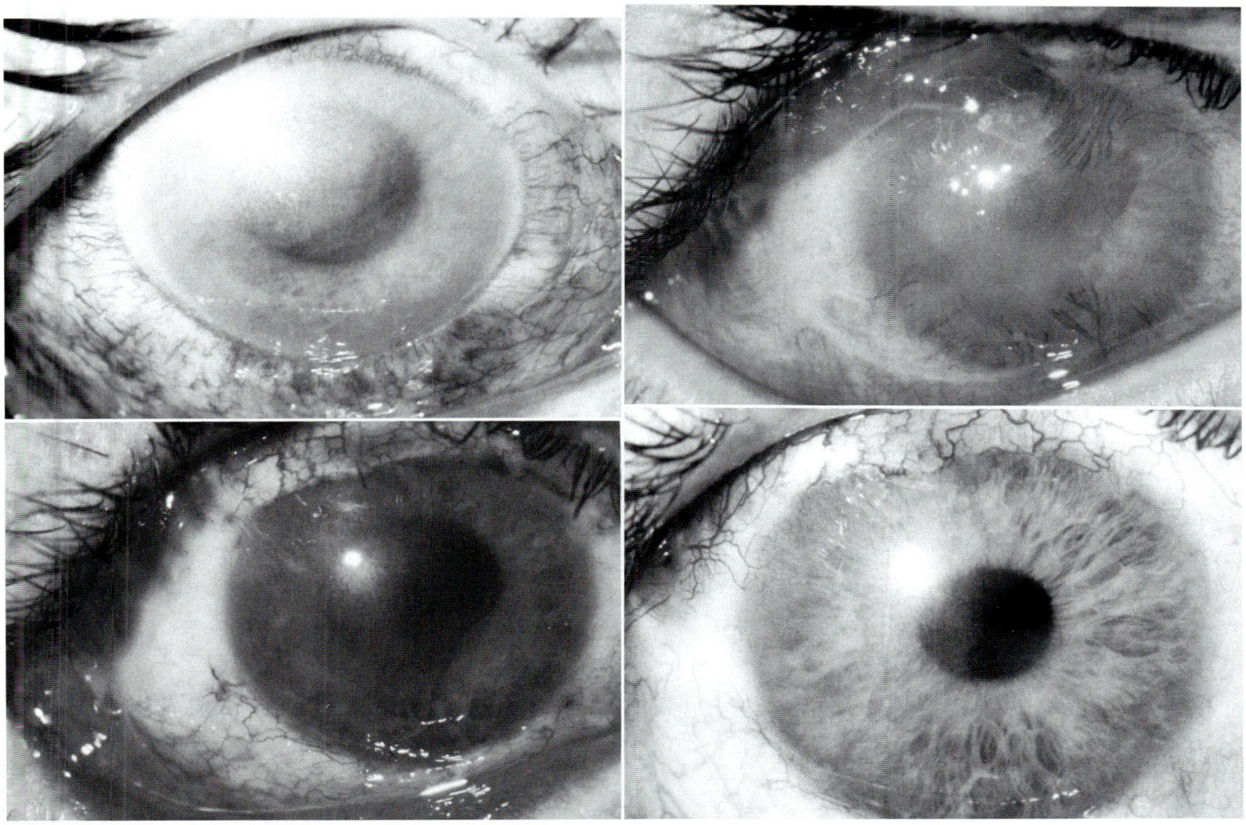

FIGURE 154-5 Early limbal autograft transplantation for persistent epithelial abnormality after severe chemical injury. **A,** One week after alkali injury, extensive conjunctival ischemia persists, as does an 80% corneal epithelial defect. **B,** One month later the healed corneal epithelium is of poor quality, irregular, and vascularized, as vision is reduced to "counting fingers." **C,** Within 3 weeks after limbal autograft transplantation, corneal reepithelialization is complete. **D,** Two years postoperatively, the ocular surface remains stable and the visual acuity is 20/25.

gency application of cyanoacrylate tissue adhesive, glued-on contact lens, or tectonic keratoplasty.[61] In either circumstance the natural healing course leads to extreme difficulty with future penetrating keratoplasty and other efforts at visual rehabilitation.

The original Thoft technique was designed as a late (more than 6 months after injury) means of rehabilitating the ocular surface following the unfortunately disasterous evolution of aberrant natural host healing mechanisms. With the advent of limbal autograft transplantation, however, came the important realization that it is possible not only to be more "physiologically correct" in late stage rehabilitation, but also to employ early intervention strategies that greatly improve the recovery process and reduce complications, eliminating much of the need for subsequent procedures. Although we advocate aggressive medical management (including topical corticosteroids or medroxyprogesterone, topical and systemic ascorbate, and prophylactic antibiotics) for several weeks in the hope that the limbus will revascularize and that the conjunctival and corneal epithelial defects will heal, we now recognize that the absence or cessation of progressive reepithelialization by 2 to 3 weeks after injury is an ominous prognostic sign and is therefore a compelling indication for early limbal autograft transplantation.

If the persistent epithelial defect is accompanied by limbal ischemia, then limbal autograft transplantation can also restore limbal vascularization (Figure 154-5), which in turn will assist in the prevention of subsequent sterile corneal ulceration. In such cases, although corneal neovascularization often occurs, as inflammation subsides and the corneal epithelium stabilizes, the stromal vessels regress remarkably or involute altogether (Figure 154-5). This combination of factors improves the prognosis for subsequent lamellar or penetrating keratoplasty (Figure 154-5), which may be performed for definitive visual rehabilitation no earlier than 6 months after limbal autografting.

Late application of limbal autograft transplantation

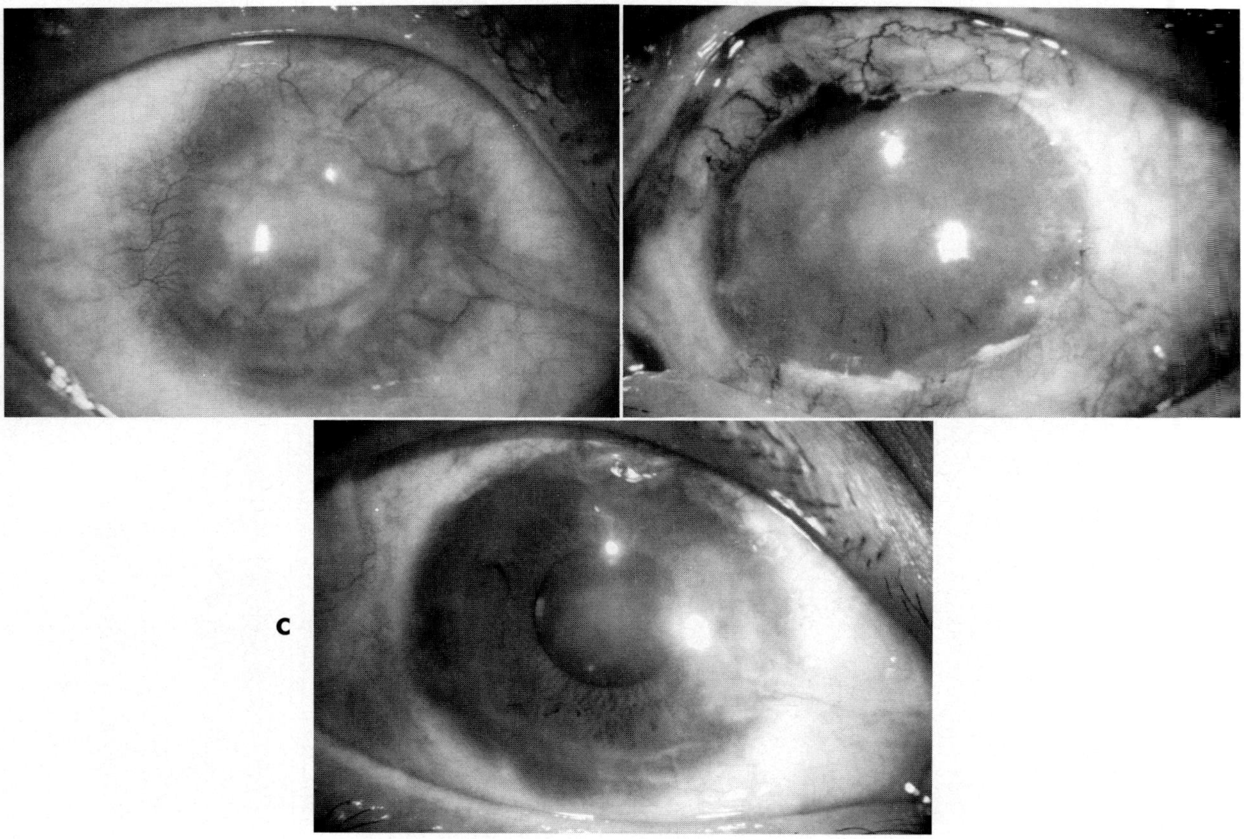

FIGURE 154-6 Late limbal autograft for severe corneal pannus after unilateral chemical injury. **A,** Scarred, vascularized cornea with visual acuity of CF 2 feet. **B,** One week after limbal autograft and superficial keratectomy, the cornea is clear and reepithelialization is complete. The limbal autografts are well vascularized. **C,** Six months later the ocular surface remains stable and the visual acuity is 20/40.

(months to years after injury) can be used to restore a more normal ocular surface in those situations in which reepithelialization had spontaneously occurred, but in which the persistent conjunctival nature of the new corneal surface produces either visual and/or cosmetic disturbance (Figure 154-6). If the extent of corneal scarring proves to be only superficial, both cosmesis and good function can often be restored with this procedure alone,[6] and keratoplasty is obviated. However, if stromal vascularization and scarring are dense, penetrating or lamellar keratoplasty may be subsequently performed with much improved prognosis.

The surgical technique, as illustrated in Figure 154-4, usually involves the transfer of two free grafts of limbal tissue from the uninjured or less injured eye to the severely injured eye. Surgery is usually performed in the major operating room, with the operating microscope, and usually under general anesthesia, although in some instances with only peribulbar or retrobulbar for the recipient eye and/or topical anesthesia for the donor eye. Attention is first directed to the injured eye, which is cleared of superficial vascularized scar tissue with a complete conjunctival peritomy approximately 2 mm posterior to the limbus. This entire ring of tissue is circumcised by bare sclera dissection to the limbus. The margins of the resected conjunctiva are then secured to the sclera with one 8-0 polyglactin (Vicryl) suture in each quadrant. The abnormal corneal polyglactin epithelium and fibrovascular pannus can be dissected superficially with a disposable scarifier (Grieshaber 681.01 or Beaver 57) and/or can be simply peeled by blunt dissection using cellulose (Weckcel) sponges and tissue forceps. Occasionally, additional scraping or polishing will be required to smooth the stromal surface, but a sharp lamellar stromal dissection is almost never appropriate, since it carries the risks of corneal perforation and postoperative optical distortion from surface irregularity. Attention is next directed to the donor eye, where two approximately 90° sectors of limbus are delineated with cautery, extending about 0.5 mm into clear corneal centrally and approximately 2 mm into bulbar conjunctiva. In cases involving extensive persistent conjunctival epithelial defects, additional segments of bulbar conjunctiva as large as 10 mm by 15 mm may be included with the limbal graft. Whatever the specific graft size, focal cautery applications are useful to mark the graft margins, thereby assuring appropriate sizing and correct reorientation in the recipient site. The initial incision is performed in clear cornea just in advance of the limbal vascular arcades, using the disposable scarifier. The second incision is made along the conjunctival margin, and the intervening strip of tissue is dissected free using spring-action scissors. The donor sites are closed with two sutures of 8-0 polyglactin (Vicryl) so that the donor eye remains comfortable and does not require patching. Autografts are then transferred to the recipient eye and secured in their anatomically appropriate positions using three sutures of 10-0 nylon at the corneal margin and four sutures of 8-0 polyglactin (Vicryl) at the conjunctival margin. Either a bandage soft contact lens or a marginal tarsorrhaphy is used to protect the grafts and the resurfacing epithelium. Topical corticosteroids and antibiotics in moderate doses are applied and continued until reepithelialization is complete and inflammation has subsided.

Among the initial reported results of limbal autograft transplantation in 26 cases,[47] the majority comprised both acute and chronic chemical or thermal burns (22 cases), three cases of contact lens–induced keratopathy (presumably a form of chronic chemical keratitis), and one case of ocular surface failure after multiple anterior segment surgical procedures. The clinical results in 21 of these patients with greater than 6 months follow-up consistently demonstrated improved visual acuity (17 cases), rapid surface healing (19 cases), stable epithelial adhesion without recurrent erosion or persistent epithelial defect (20 cases), and arrest or regression of corneal neovascularization (15 cases). Particularly encouraging was the success of all subsequently performed lamellar (2 cases) and penetrating keratoplasties (6 cases). Given the notoriously poor prognosis in these clinical situations, improved outcomes are seemingly attributable to the stability of the ocular surface epithelium, the suppression of neovascular activity, and the subsidence of chronic inflammation. Since these original observations, more than 50 cases have been performed with equally encouraging results. In particular, although we remain enthusiastic about the application of limbal transplantation for the management of chronic disease after chemical burns, it is perhaps even more compelling to employ this approach in the acute situation, to interrupt a persistent epithelial defect, to arrest sterile ulceration of the corneal or scleral stroma, and to avoid development of severe vascular pannus.

Although cases of contact lens–induced superficial pannus are relatively rarely caused by the recent generations of lens care solutions and their preservatives, the ability to use autografts of limbal tissue from the less affected portions of the same or the fellow eye has improved vision, avoided and, in at least one case, preserved corneal transplantation, and facilitated resumption of contact lens wear. We have also managed five cases in which the ocular surface was depleted by multiple anterior segment surgical procedures (cataract, glaucoma, keratoplasty) with resulting chronic inflammation, epithelial instability and stromal vascularization, either as a direct effect of surgery or possibly from chronic topical medication use. In these cases as well, limbal autograft transplantation has afforded restoration of a stable ocular surface with prompt resolution of persistent epithelial defects and improved success of subsequent keratoplasty.

The most challenging cases are patients with bilateral ocular surface injury or disease, which, pending adequacy of tear and lid function, should also potentially benefit from ocular surface transplantation, despite the major limitation of suitable limbal donor tissue. For such situations, Thoft[15] devised *keratoepithelioplasty,* in which lenticules of peripheral corneal epithelium with superficial stroma are harvested from fresh donor eyes and are sutured to the corneoscleral limbus of the recipient (Figure 154-7). Although some, notably Kinoshita,[50] have reported success with this approach, others[62] have encountered graft failure after keratoepithelioplasty. More recently, Thoft et al,[17] perhaps recognizing the importance of limbal stem cells, modified the surgical technique to include limbal tissue. Keratoepithelioplasty has been recently reviewed by Holland,[63] who confirmed that the long-term success of this procedure is limited in some cases, since the donor corneal epithelium may be eventually replaced by host conjunctiva. Therefore, for selected bilateral cases, we have used limbal *allograft* transplantation from related donors[52] (Figure 154-8). HLA typing is performed on family members to determine the most favorable match, and the procedure is performed, as previously detailed using tissue from the related donor. In instances of poor antigen matching, topical and systemic immunosuppression with cyclosporine-A is used. Others[64,65,66] have adopted similar technique but obtain limbus from the peripheral rims of keratoplasty donor tissue. Despite the additional management requirements imposed by immunosuppression and constant surveillance of ocular surface integrity, our early experience in selected cases has been notable for dramatic success in these desperate situations.

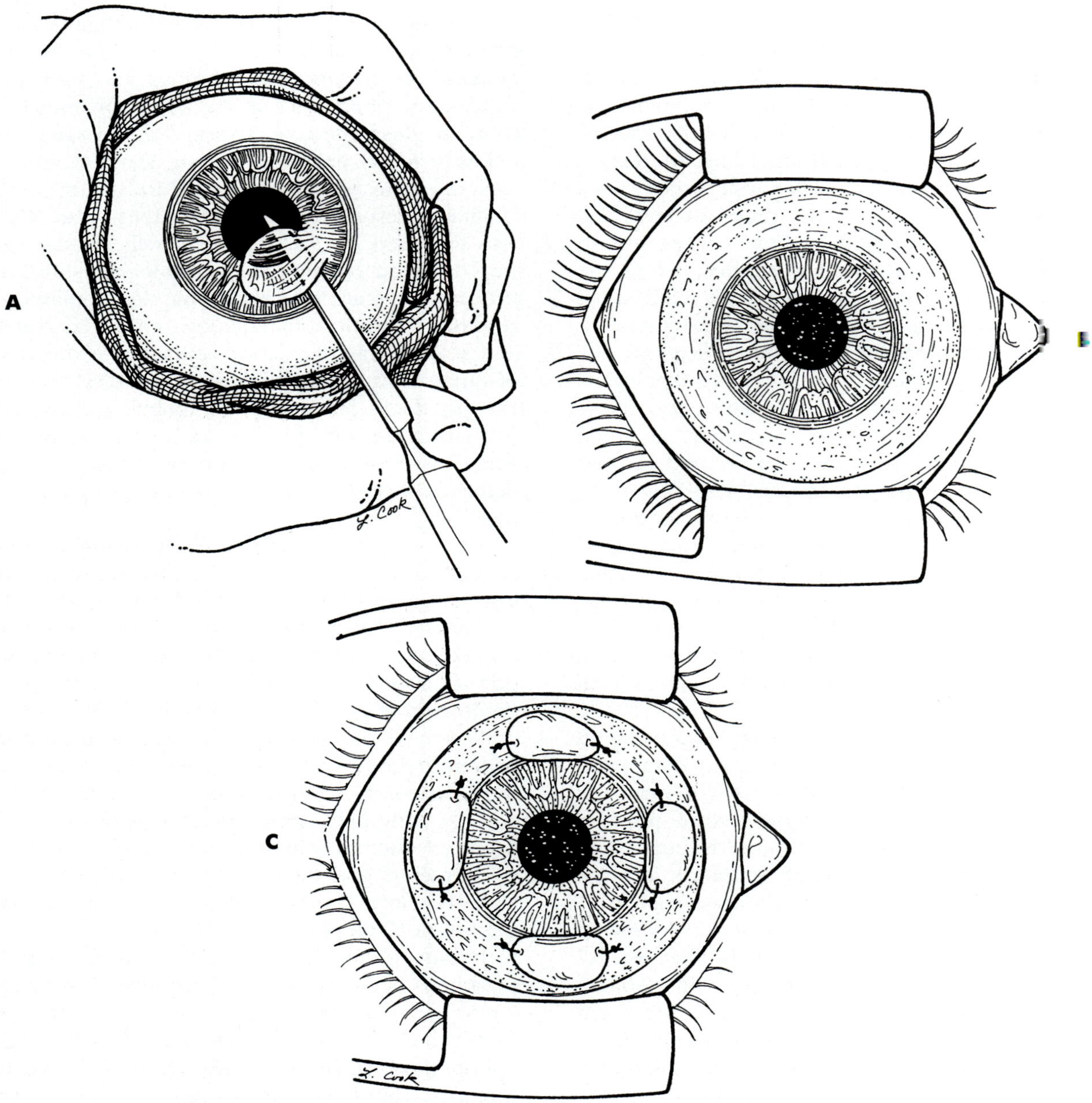

FIGURE 154-7 **Keratoepithelioplasty. A, A whole fresh donor eye with intact epithelium is used to provide usually four thin stromal lenticules with intact epithelium. B, Removal of corneal and conjunctival pannus by superficial keratectomy. C, The lenticules are secured at the limbus of the recipient. [NOTE: Although Thoft's original technique is depicted, current modification favors lenticules obtained from the limbal region.]**

Mucous Membrane Transplantation

We currently use buccal mucosal membrane grafting for reconstruction of bilateral fornix obliteration[42] or eyelid margin keratinization,[41] usually in relationship to cicatricial conjunctival disorders such as Stevens-Johnson syndrome or ocular cicatricial pemphigoid (Table 154-1). As previously discussed, this technique has been largely abandoned as a treatment for unilateral chemical injury and is used only in desperate cases of bilateral injury where advancement of Tenon's capsule is not possible and where homograft tissue is not available.

Mucosal membrane grafting has long been a popular technique of correcting eyelid position abnormalities caused by cicatrizing conjunctival disorders.[40,43,67-71]

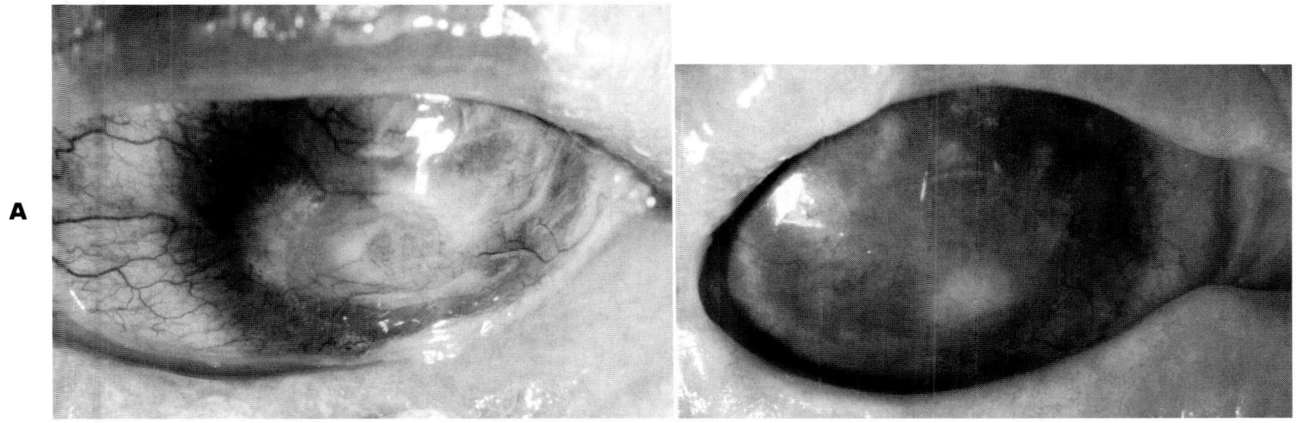

FIGURE 154-8 Limbal allograft transplantation after severe erythema multiforme. **A,** Severe corneal scarring and vascularization limits vision to "counting fingers." **B,** Improved quality of ocular surface 3 months after limbal allograft transplantation from HLA-identical sister. One year after limbal allograft, a penetrating keratoplasty was performed, and 6 months postoperatively, vision is improved to 20/50.

Although good results have been reported for indications not related to active cicatricial disorders of the conjunctiva (e.g., late stage, nonprogressive Stevens-Johnson syndrome), there has been some reluctance to apply this technique to advanced (stage III or IV) ocular cicatricial pemphigoid for fear of exacerbating this already relentlessly progressive inflammatory disorder.[72-74] With the critically important advances in immunosuppressive treatment of this immune-mediated ocular surface disorder[75,76] it is now recognized that control of mechanical eyelid complications is also essential to the successful overall management of these patients. Indeed, with appropriate systemic control of ocular surface inflammation, we have encountered substantial success in mucous membrane grafting for the eyelid abnormalities associated with late stage ocular cicatricial pemphigoid.

The technique of mucosal grafting is demonstrated in Figure 154-9.[42] In a series of 17 patients (23 eyes, 42 eyelids) with stage III or IV ocular cicatricial pemphigoid, we graded the results as improvement in 12 patients (16 eyes), satisfactory in two patients (2 eyes), and poor in five patients (5 eyes). Visual acuity improved in 14 eyes, remained within two lines of preoperative acuity in five eyes, and deteriorated in four eyes. The improvement in 14 eyes was felt to result from improved ocular tear film quality or increased corneal clarity. Not surprisingly, poor results occurred in patients who had active disease (2 patients) at the time of surgery, a flare-up of immune-mediated inflammation in the postoperative period (1 patient), or mechanical problems related to graft complications such as recurrent trichiasis, incomplete blinking, or surface keratinization, leading to continued corneal insult (2 patients). Not all patients with active inflammation, however, had poor results. Three patients with ocular surface inflammation despite maximum medical management did improve. Conversely, lack of inflammation did not always prevent complications, including breakthrough trichiasis, surface keratinization of the graft, blepharoptosis, phimosis, depressed eyelid blink, incomplete eyelid closure, submucosal abscess formation, and persistent nonhealing epithelial defects of the cornea.

Naumann et al[57] have recently described grafting of nasal mucosa taken from the middle concha to the globe and eyelids. This procedure offers the potential advantage of transfer of goblet cells (although this has not been established) but is not useful for reestablishing limbal stem cell populations. Either the technique of Shore or Naumann can be used effectively to reduce or eliminate problems associated with the mechanical disturbance of the normal function of the forniceal conjunctiva, but, as previously emphasized, cannot replace the abnormalities related to stem cell depletion or damage.

In summary, it is now feasible to tailor ocular surface transplantation to meet the specific ocular surface needs of the individual situation. As specified in Table 154-1, the conjunctival autograft is recommended as a free graft of healthy ocular surface tissue for those circumstances where there is a localized need to replace abnormal or absent conjunctival tissue (e.g., after pterygium excision) or to restore more normal conjunctival anatomy and function (e.g., cicatricial strabismus, fornix reconstruction). In bilateral cases (e.g., cicatricial pemphigoid), where normal conjunctival tissue is not available for such purposes, buccal mucosal membrane grafting may be substituted.

In situations of widespread ocular surface destruc-

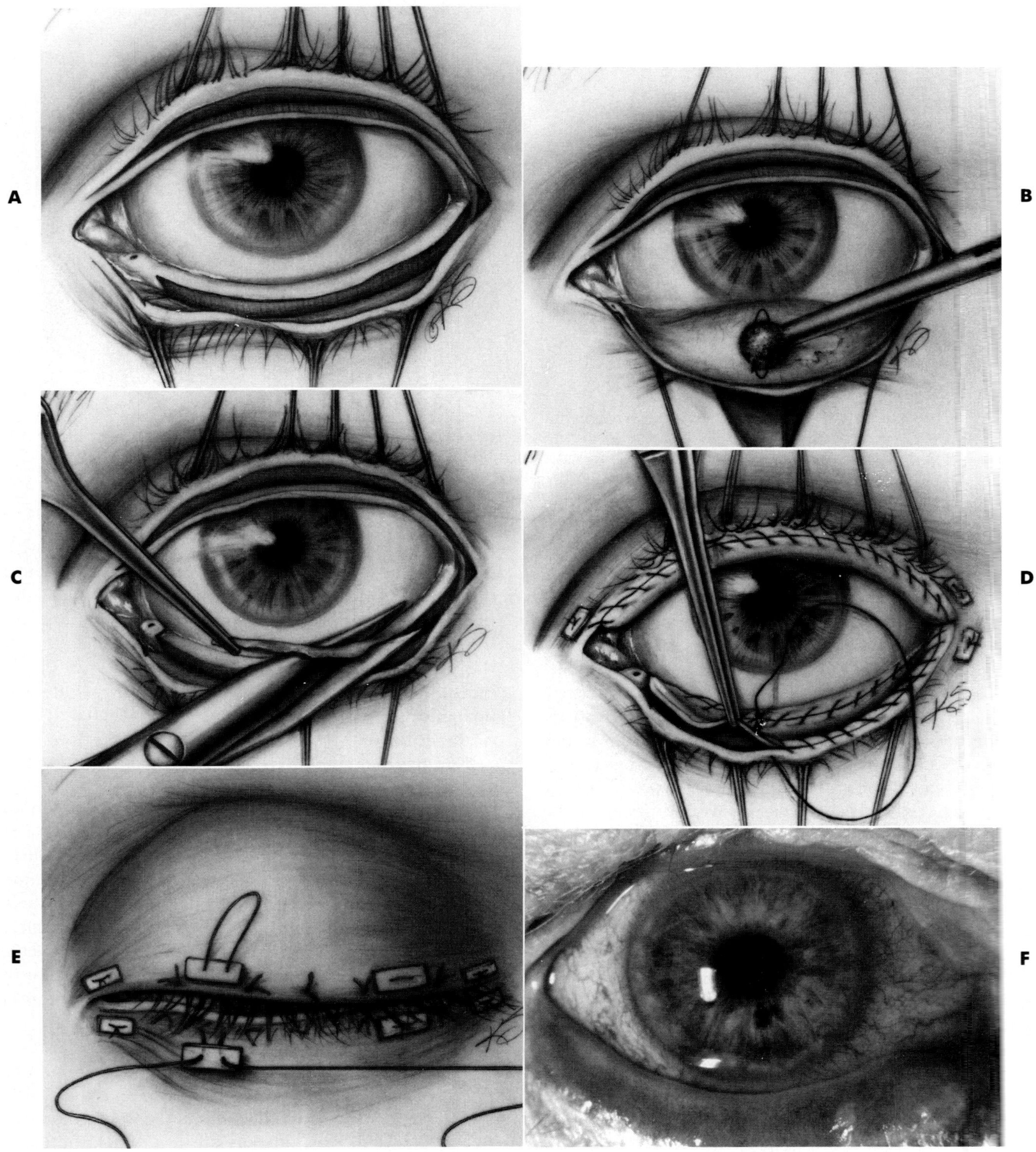

FIGURE 154-9 Technique of buccal mucosal graft for cicatricial obliteration of the inferior fornix. **A,** After the eyelid has been split at the gray line, the anterior lamella is recessed and secured to the posterior lamella with interrupted, 4-0 silk sutures. **B,** A diamond-tipped burr is used to smooth the margin and the posterior tarsal surface. **C,** Using spring-action scissors, the entire conjunctiva is removed from the tarsal conjunctival surface. A full-thickness lip mucosal graft is hydraulically dissected (technique not shown) and excised with freehand dissection at least 1 cm posterior to the vermilion border. Care is taken not to "buttonhole" the graft as the posterior surface of the graft is trimmed with sharp scissors. **D,** The graft is draped over the margin of the eyelid and sutured in position with a running, double-armed 8-0 nylon suture tied externally over silicone foam pledgets. **E,** Suture tarsorrhaphies placed through the center of the grafts hold the grafts in position and prevent graft movement caused by blinking during the first postoperative week. **F,** The healed eyelid margin has been completely resurfaced. (Reproduced by permission from Shore JW et al: *Ophthalmology* 99:383-395, 1992.)

tion, especially involving the critically important limbal stem cell population (e.g., severe chemical injury), either limbal autograft transplantation (in unilateral cases) or limbal allograft transplantation (in bilateral cases) is the procedure of choice.

REFERENCES

1. Friedenwald JS: Growth pressure and metaplastia of conjunctival and corneal epithelium, *Doc Ophthalmol* 5-6:184-192, 1951.
2. Friedenwald JS, Buschke W: Some factors concerned in the mitotic and wound-healing activities of the corneal epithelium, *Trans Am Ophthalmol Soc* 42:371-83, 1944.
3. Ebato B, Friend J, Thoft RA: Comparison of central and peripheral human corneal epithelium in tissue culture, *Invest Ophthalmol Vis Sci* 28:1450-1456, 1987.
4. Friend J, Thoft RA: Functional competence of regenerating ocular surface epithelium, *Invest Ophthalmol Vis Sci* 17:134-139, 1978.
5. Kinoshita S et al: Limbal epithelium in ocular surface wound healing, *Invest Ophthalmol Vis Sci* 23:73-80, 1982.
6. Kinoshita S, Friend J, Thoft RA: Biphasic cell proliferation in transdifferentiation of conjunctival to corneal epithelium in rabbits, *Invest Ophthalmol Vis Sci* 24:1008-1014, 1983.
7. Kinoshita S et al: Keratin-like proteins in corneal and conjunctival epithelium are different, *Invest Ophthalmol Vis Sci* 24:577-581, 1983.
8. Reat MI, Thoft RA: Ocular surface epithelial transplantation, *Int Ophthalmol Clin* 28:169-174, 1988.
9. Shapiro MS, Friend J, Thoft RA: Corneal re-epithelialization from the conjunctiva, *Invest Ophthalmol Vis Sci* 21:135-142, 1981.
10. Thoft RA: Conjunctival transplantation, *Arch Ophthalmol* 95: 1425-1427, 1977.
11. Thoft RA, Friend J: Biochemical transformation of regenerating ocular surface epithelium, *Invest Ophthalmol Vis Sci* 16:14-20, 1977.
12. Thoft RA, Friend J, Murphy HS: Ocular surface epithelium and corneal neovascularization in rabbits. I. The role of wounding, *Invest Ophthalmol Vis Sci* 18:85-92, 1979.
13. Thoft RA: Conjunctival transplantation as an alternative to keratoplasty, *Ophthalmology* 86:1084-1091, 1979.
14. Thoft RA: Indications for conjunctival transplantation, *Ophthalmology* 89:335-339, 1982.
15. Thoft RA: Keratoepithelioplasty, *Am J Ophthalmol* 97:1-6, 1984.
16. Thoft RA, Friend J: The XYZ hypothesis of corneal epithelial maintenance, *Invest Ophthalmol Vis Sci* 24:1442-1443, 1983.
17. Turgeon PW et al: Indications for keratoepithelioplasty, *Arch Ophthalmol* 108:233-236, 1980.
18. Buck RC: Measurement of centripetal migration of normal corneal epithelial cells in the mouse, *Invest Ophthalmol Vis Sci* 26:1296-1299, 1985.
19. Cotsarellis G et al: Differential response of limbal and corneal epithelia to phorbol myristate (TPA), *Invest Ophthalmol Vis Sci* 28(Suppl):1, 1987.
20. Davanger M, Evensen A: Role of the pericorneal papillary structure in renewal of corneal epithelium, *Nature* 229:560-561, 1971.
21. Hanna C, O'Brien JE: Cell production and migration in the epithelial layer of the cornea, *Arch Ophthalmol* 64:536-539, 1960.
22. Harris TM et al: Biochemical transformation of bulbar conjunctiva into corneal epithelium: an electrophoretic analysis, *Exp Eye Res* 41:597-606, 1985.
23. Huang AJW, Tseng SCG: Corneal epithelial wound healing in the absence of limbal epithelium, *Invest Ophthalmol Vis Sci* 29(Suppl):190, 1988.
24. Tseng SCG: Concept and application of limbal stem cells, *Eye* 3:141-157, 1989.
25. Kuwabara T, Perkins DG, Cogan DG: Sliding of the epithelium in experimental corneal wounds, *Invest Ophthalmol* 15:4-14, 1976.
26. Lavker RW et al: Limbal basal epithelial cells display characteristics consistent with stem cells from various stratifying epithelia, *Invest Ophthalmol Vis Sci* 29(Suppl):191, 1988.
27. Schermer A, Galvin S, Sun TT: Differentiation-related expression of a major 64K corneal keratin in vivo and in culture suggests limbal location of epithelial stem cells, *J Cell Biol* 103:49-62, 1986.
28. Srinivasan BD et al: The reepithelialization of rabbit corneal following partial and complete epithelial denudation, *Exp Eye Res* 25:343-351, 1977.
29. Tseng SCG et al: Goblet cell density and vascularization during conjunctival transdifferentiation, *Invest Ophthalmol Vis Sci* 25: 1168-1176, 1984.
30. Tsai RJ, Sun TT, Teng SCG: Comparison of limbal and conjunctival autograft transplantation in corneal surface reconstruction in rabbits, *Ophthalmology* 97:446-455, 1990.
31. Zieske JD, Bukusoglu G, Yankauckas MA: Characterization of a potential marker of corneal epithelial stem cells, *Invest Ophthalmol Vis Sci* 33:143-152, 1992.
32. Herman WK, Doughman DJ, Lindstrom RL: Conjunctival autograft transplantation for unilateral ocular surface diseases, *Ophthalmology* 90:1121-1126, 1983.
33. Kenyon KR, Wagoner MD, Hettinger ME: Conjunctival autograft transplantation for advanced and recurrent pterygium, *Ophthalmology* 92:1461-1470, 1985.
34. Serrano F: Plastia conjunctival libre en la cirugia del pterigion, *Arch Soc Am Oftalmol Optom* 2:12-17, 1977.
35. Starck T, Kenyon KR, Serrano F: Conjunctival autograft for primary and recurrent pterygia: surgical technique and problem management, *Cornea* 10:196-202, 1991.
36. Vastine DW, Stewart WB, Schwab IR: Reconstruction of the periocular mucous membrane by autologous conjunctival transplantation, *Ophthalmology* 89:1071-1081, 1982.
37. Wagoner MD, Kenyon KR: Conjunctival transplantation for pterygium and other ocular surface disorders. In Bruner W, Stark W, Maumenee A, editors: *A manual of corneal surgery,* New York, 1987, Churchill Livingstone.
38. Weise RA et al: Conjunctival transplantation, *Arch Ophthalmol* 103:1736-1740, 1985.
39. Ballen PH: Mucous membrane grafts in chemical (lye) burns, *Am J Ophthalmol* 55:302-312, 1963.
40. Leone CR Jr: Mucous membrane grafting for cicatricial entropion, *Ophthalmic Surg* 5(2):24-28, 1974.
41. McCord CD Jr, Chen WP: Tarsal polishing and mucous membrane grafting for cicatricial entropion, trichiasis and epidermalization, *Ophthalmic Surg* 14:1021-1025, 1983.
42. Shore JW et al: Results of buccal mucosal grafting for patients with medically controlled ocular cicatricial pemphigoid, *Ophthalmology* 99:383-395, 1990.
43. White JH: Correction of distichiasis by tarsal rejection and mucous membrane grafting, *Am J Ophthalmol* 80:507-508, 1975.
44. Gunderson T: Conjunctival flaps in the treatment of corneal disease with reference to a new technique of application, *Arch Ophthalmol* 60:880-888, 1958.
45. Thoft RA: Conjunctival surgery for corneal disease. In Smolin G, Thoft R, editors: *The cornea: scientific foundation and clinical practice,* ed 2, Boston, 1987, Little, Brown.
46. Reim M: A new treatment concept in severe caustic injuries and burns of the eye, *Fortschr Ophthalmol* 86:722-726, 1989.
47. Kenyon KR, Tseng SCG: Limbal autograft transplantation for

ocular surface disorders, *Ophthalmology* 96:709-722, 1989.
48. Hayashi K, Kenyon KR: Increased cytochrome oxidase activity in alkali burned corneas, *Curr Eyes Res* 7:131-138, 1988.
49. Kaye DB: Epithelial response in penetrating keratoplasty, *Am J Ophthalmol* 89:381-387, 1980.
50. Kinoshita S et al: Long-term results of keratoepithelioplasty in Mooren's ulcer, *Ophthalmology* 98:438-445, 1991.
51. Lindberg K et al: In vitro propagation of human ocular surface epithelial cells for transplantation, *Invest Ophthalmol Vis Sci* 34:2672-2679, 1993.
52. Kenyon KR, Rapoza PA: Limbal allograft transplantation for ocular surface reconstruction, *Ophthalmology.* In press.
53. Barraquer JL: Etiology, pathogenesis, and treatment of pterygium. In Symposium on medical and surgical diseases of the cornea, *Trans N Orleans Acad Ophthalmol* 167-178, 1980.
54. Lewallen S: A randomized trial of conjunctival autografting for pterygium in the tropics, *Ophthalmology* 96:1612-1614, 1989.
55. Singh G, Wilson MR, Foster CS: Mitomycin eye drops as treatment of pterygium, *Ophthalmology* 95:813-821, 1988.
56. Reubenfeld RS et al: Serious complications of topical mitomycin-C after pterygium surgery, *Ophthalmology* 99:1647-1654, 1992.
57. Naumann GOH et al: Autologous nasal mucosa transplantation in severe bilateral conjunctival mucus deficiency syndrome, *Ophthalmology* 97:1011-1017, 1990.
58. Abel R Jr et al: The results of penetrating keratoplasty after chemical burns, *Trans Am Acad Ophthalmol Otolaryngol* 79:584-595, 1975.
59. Brown SI, Tragakis MP, Pearce DB: Corneal transplantation for severe alkali burns, *Trans Am Acad Ophthalmol Otolaryngol* 76:1266-1274, 1972.
60. Brown SI, Bloomfield SE, Pearce DB: A follow-up report on transplantation of the alkali-burned cornea, *Am J Ophthalmol* 77:538-542, 1974.
61. Wagoner MD, Kenyon KR: Chemical injuries. In Shingleton BJ, Hersh PS, Kenyon KR, editors: *Ocular trauma,* St Louis, 1991, Mosby.
62. Thoft RA, Sugar J: Graft failure in keratoepithelioplasty, *Cornea* 12:362-365, 1993.
63. Holland E: Severe ocular surface trauma. In Roy FH, editor: *Master techniques in ophthalmic surgery,* Baltimore, 1995, Williams & Wilkins.
64. Tsai RJF, Tseng SCG: Human allograft limbal transplantation for corneal surface reconstruction, *Cornea* 13:389-400, 1994.
65. Tsubota K, Toda I, Saito H, Shinozaki N, Shimizaki J: Reconstruction of the corneal epithelium by limbal allograft transplantation for severe ocular surface disorders, *Ophthalmology* 1[illegible]:1486-1496, 1995.
66. Tan D, Ficker L, Buckley R: Limbal transplantation, *Ophthalmology* 103:29-36, 1996.
67. Weis FA: Surgical treatment of entropion, *J Int Coll Surg* 21:758-760, 1954.
68. Sullivan GL: Repair of cicatricial entropion, *Arch Ophthalmol* 77:232-233, 1967.
69. Tenzel RR: Repair of entropion of the upper lid, *Arch Ophthalmol* 77:675, 1967.
70. Dortzbach RK, Callahan A: Repair of cicatricial entropion of the upper eyelids, *Arch Ophthalmol* 85:82-89, 1971.
71. Baylis HI, Hamako C: Tarsal grafting for correction of cicatricial entropion, *Ophthalmic Surg* 10:42-48, 1979.
72. Foster CS: Cicatricial pemphigoid, *Trans Am Ophthalmol Soc* 84:527-663, 1986.
73. Mondino BJ et al: The acute manifestations of ocular cicatricial pemphigoid: diagnosis and treatment, *Ophthalmology* [illegible]6:543-552, 1979.
74. Mondino BJ, Brown SI: Ocular cicatricial pemphigoid, *Ophthalmology* 88:95-100, 1981.
75. Foster CS, Wilson LA, Ekins MB: Immunosuppressive therapy in ocular cicatricial pemphigoid, *Ophthalmology* 89:34[illegible]-35[illegible], 1982.
76. Mondino BJ, Brown SI: Immunosuppressive therapy in ocular cicatricial pemphigoid, *Ophthalmol* 96:453-459, 19[illegible]3.

CHAPTER 155

BRUCE D. NICHOLS

Conjunctival Flaps

Conjunctival flaps have been used by ophthalmologists for over 100 years in the management of challenging disorders of the ocular surface. German publications dating back to the 1870s and 1890s describe the first techniques using this surgical approach.[1,2] In 1958 Gundersen described a technique using conjunctiva without Tenon's capsule as a flap for a number of applications.[3] This procedure gained popularity and has remained a fundamental surgical technique with specific indications. With the development of refinements in penetrating keratoplasty as well as the advent of bandage soft contact lenses and collagen shields, the conjunctival flap procedure has become less frequent in the management of ocular surface disease. Similarly, new antibiotics and antiviral agents as well as therapy directed toward immunologic suppression of disease activity, have undoubtedly had an impact on the need for a surgical approach to manage infection and ulceration of the anterior segment. Nonetheless, there are still patients in whom a conjunctival flap remains the management procedure of choice. Patients with little visual potential and a chronically irritated anterior segment often respond well, and the resultant need for continued medication and bandage lenses is eliminated. Furthermore, this procedure can be reversed and an optical surgery performed at a later date should the situation and conditions at the time apply.

Indications

In 1958 Gunderson reported on the benefit of the conjunctival flap procedure for a wide range of conditions, many of which are treated by other means routinely today.[3]

Included in his indications were patients with recurrent corneal erosions, filamentary keratitis, and bullous keratopathy. Clearly then, and today, herpes simplex corneal ulceration remains an indication for a conjunctival flap. Herpetic ulceration is a serious complication in both the active and inactive phase of viral replication in patients with this sight-threatening disease. Penetrating keratoplasty has not enjoyed a universally favorable role in the management of this disease with a low probability of graft survival, especially after multiple grafts.[4] Newer grafting and management techniques, however, are improving the success of keratoplasty as reported by Ficker et al who described a 70% long-term survival rate of first grafts for herpes simplex virus keratitis.[5]

Conjunctival flaps have, nonetheless, been useful in managing corneal disease in patients with keratolysis secondary to herpes simplex and also in cases of herpetic keratouveitis.[6] It is important to realize that active disease may persist postoperatively despite antiviral therapy in these patients. Similarly, a case of recurrent herpes simplex infection in a conjunctival flap was recently described.[7] Patients often remark on the degree of relief of their symptoms after a conjunctival flap for herpes simplex. Subsequently, a penetrating graft can be performed in the absence of inflammation with or without removal of the flap.

Neuroparalytic keratitis is another important indication for a conjunctival flap.[8] Hypesthesia, epithelial breakdown, and ulceration typify this condition, which often follows operations on the gasserian ganglion or middle fossa.

The management of keratomycoses is by medical means if at all possible. Topical and systemic antifungal treatment is often protracted, and the response is sometimes limited. Surgical management may be required, and various techniques have been described, including the combination of lamellar keratoplasty and conjunctival flaps.[9] Recalcitrant ulceration unresponsive to medical management may also respond to flap surgery.

Other indications for a conjunctival flap include severe unresponsive keratitis sicca, chronic ulceration from exposure (Figure 155-1), peripheral marginal ulcerations, neurotrophic ulcers (Figure 155-2), and bullous keratopathy in patients with little or no useful visual potential. An interesting single case of sterile keratitis after radial keratotomy responding to treatment with a conjunctival flap has been reported.[10]

Conjunctival flaps should not be used as primary management for ocular perforations or in cases of bacterial necrotizing keratitis. The procedure has been used, however, to stabilize patients with refractory *Pseudomonas* corneal abscesses.[11]

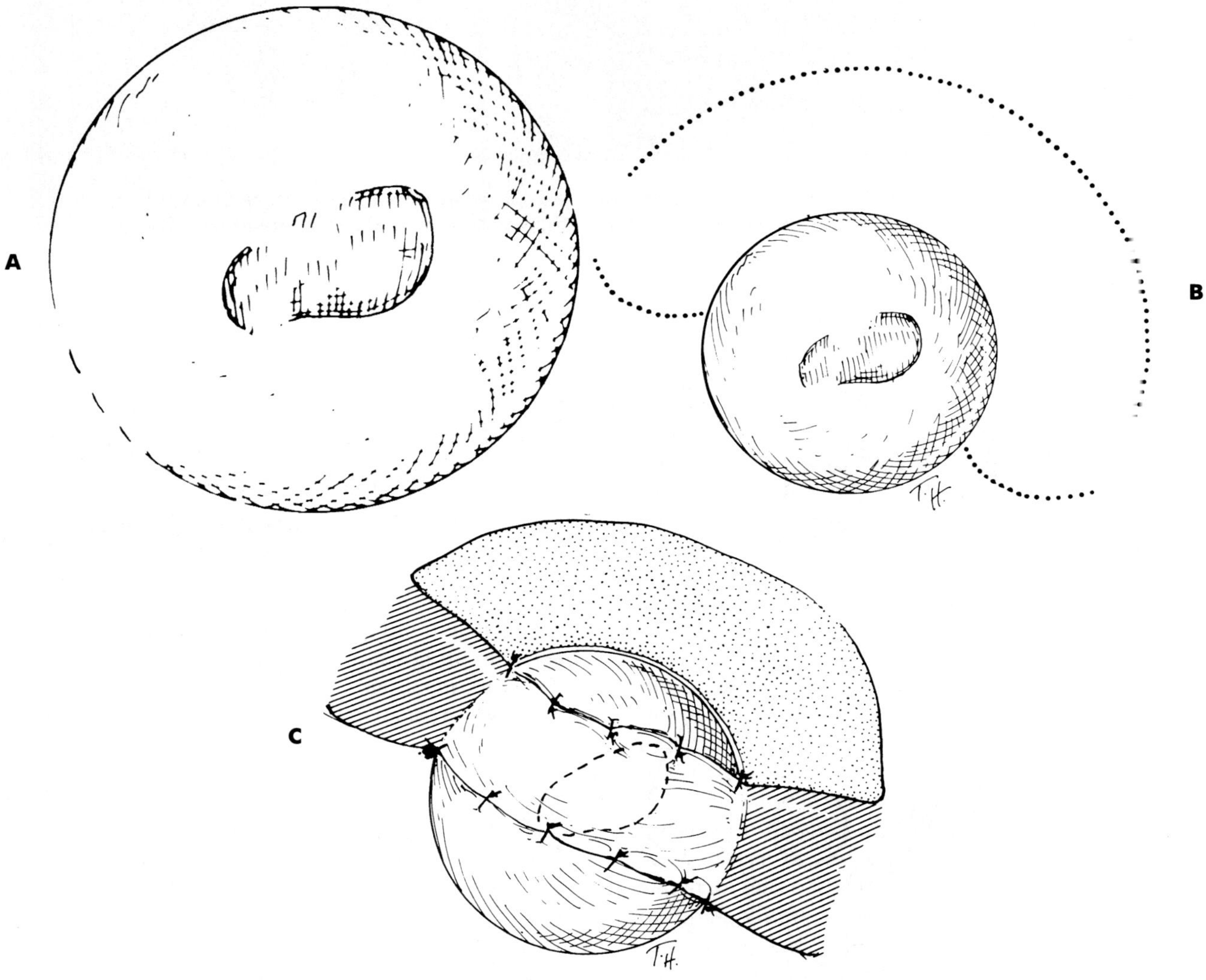

FIGURE 155-4 Bipedicle conjunctival flap (bucket handle). **A,** Examine the lesion to determine width of pedicle. **B,** Flap should be 1.3 to 1.5 times the width of the lesion. **C,** Flap secured in place. (From Reinhart WJ: *Conjunctival flap surgery.* In Bruner WE, Stark WJ, Maumenee AE, editors: *Manual of corneal surgery,* New York, 1987, Churchill Livingstone.)

A

B

C

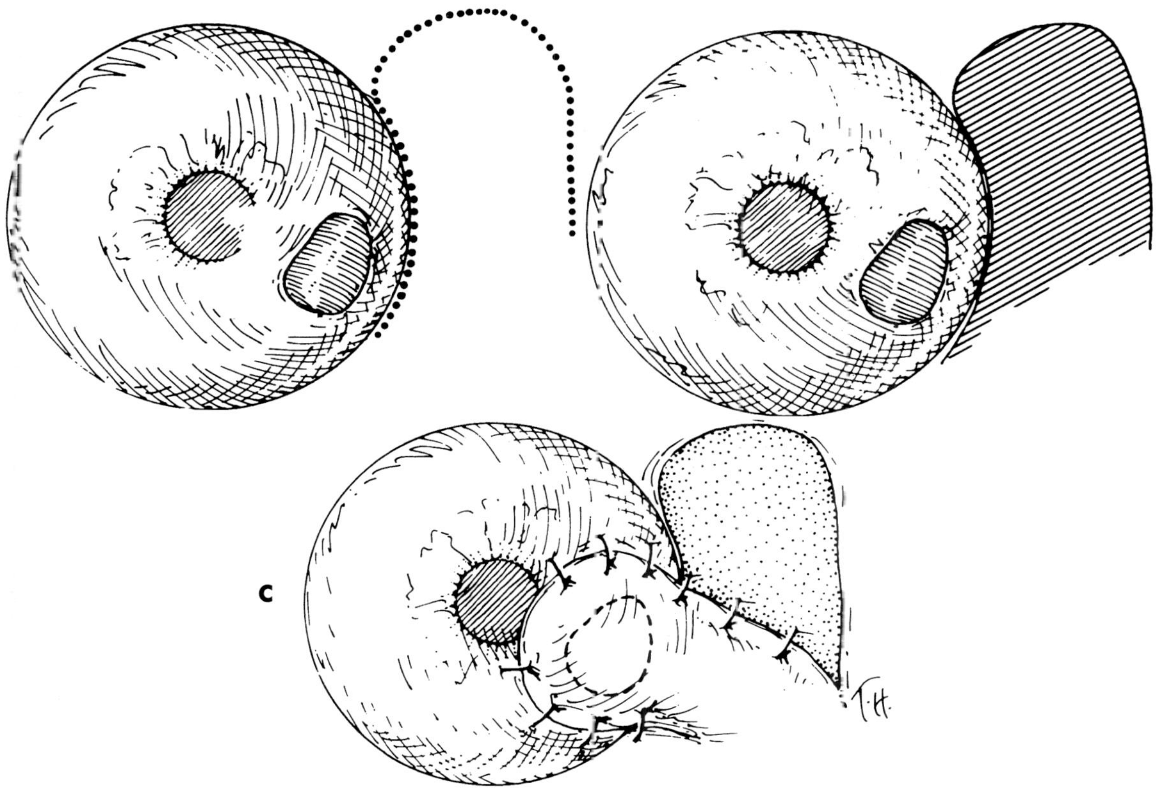

FIGURE 155-5 Single pedicle (racquet) conjunctival flap. **A,** Measure lesion and length of flap. **B,** Undermine conjunctiva. **C,** Suture flap after epithelium removed. (From Reinhart WJ: *Conjunctival flap surgery.* In Bruner WE, Stark WJ, Maumenee AE, editors: *Manual of corneal surgery.* New York, 1987, Churchill Livingstone.)

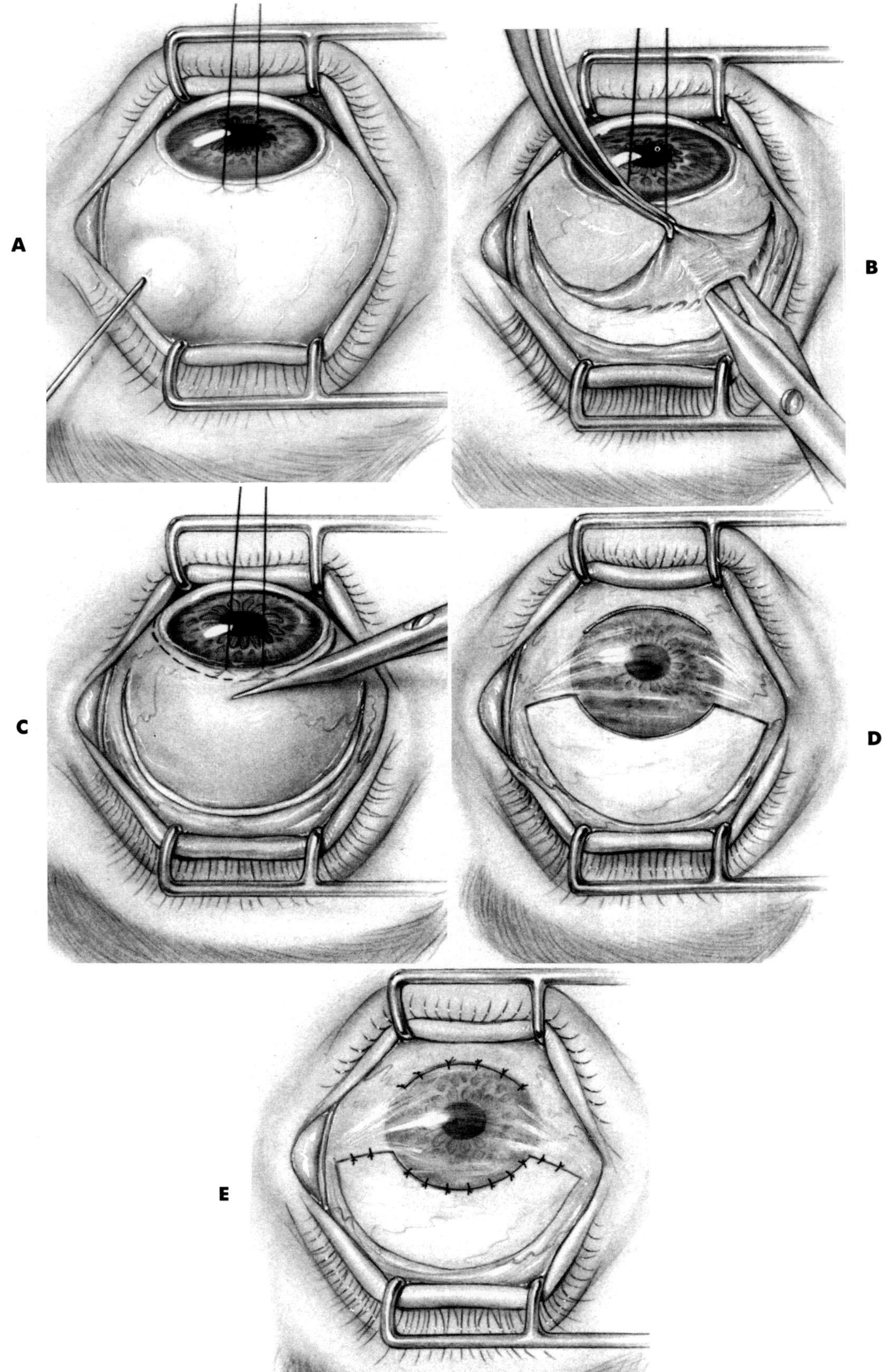

FIGURE 155-6 **A,** Ballooning of the conjunctiva with 2% lidocaine with 1:100,000 epinephrine. **B,** Blunt dissection of the superior conjunctiva. **C,** Undermined conjunctiva and 360-degree peritomy. **D,** Conjunctival flap placed over the debrided corneal surface. **E,** Multiple 7-0 silk sutures in place. (From Nelson JD: *Surgery of the ocular surface.* In Lindquist TD, Lindstrom RL, editors: *Ophthalmic surgery—looseleaf and update service,* Chicago, 1990, Year Book.)

enlarge postoperatively, creating an unacceptable result. These defects are best avoided by painstaking care not to create them. If, however, they occur, 10-0 nylon sutures can be used to close them. An additional flap may be fashioned from inferior conjunctiva if needed, especially in the presence of a large defect.[15] Ptosis may develop postoperatively in cases with excessive superior fornix dissection. The ptosis is usually of a minor degree, although occasionally plastic repair is required. Retention conjunctival cysts may form because of infolding of incised edges during the procedure.[16] These cysts may require excision but are rarely of significant concern.

Summary and the Future

Conjunctival flaps are useful when indicated for the management of pain, indolent ulceration, and in some cases of infective keratitis. Successful keratoplasty in eyes that have previously undergone conjunctival flap surgery is possible and may allow for the restoration of vision in an otherwise unsalvageable situation. For future consideration an innovative approach to conjunctival flap surgery has recently been described using the argon laser to obliterate the marginal flap vessels 1 month postoperatively.[17] This effectively creates an "ischemic central window," which, in addition to the therapeutic effect of the flap, potentially improves the vision in patients awaiting definitive optical surgery. This and other possible refinements to the technique may serve to further enhance the usefulness and role of the conjunctival flap procedure in the management of ocular surface disease.

REFERENCES

1. Schöler KW: *Jahresberichte uber die Wirksamkeit der Augen-Klinik, in den Jahren 1874-1880,* Berlin, 1975-1881, H. Peters.
2. Kuhnt H: Uber die Verwertbarkeit der Bindehaut in der prakischen und operativen Heilkunde, Monogram. Weisbaden, 1898, Bergmann.
3. Gundersen T: Conjunctival flaps in the treatment of corneal disease with reference to a new technique of application, *Arch Ophthalmol* 60:880-887, 1958.
4. Epstein RJ et al: Penetrating keratoplasty for herpes simplex keratitis and keratoconus. Allograft rejection and survival, *Ophthalmology* 94(8):935-944, 1987.
5. Ficker LA et al: The changing management and improved prognosis for corneal grafting in herpes simplex keratitis, *Ophthalmology* 96(11):1587-1596, 1989.
6. Brown DD et al: The use of conjunctival flaps in the treatment of herpes keratouveitis, *Cornea* 11(1):44-46, 1992.
7. Rosenfeld SI, Alfonso EC, Gollamudi S: Recurrent herpes simplex infection in a conjunctival flap, *Am J Ophthalmol* 116(2):242-244, 1993.
8. Lugo M, Arentsen JJ: Treatment of neurotrophic ulcers with conjunctival flaps, *Am J Ophthalmol* 103(5):711-712, 1987.
9. Sanituto JJ, Kelley CG, Kaufman HE: Surgical management of fungal keratitis (keratomycosis), *Arch Ophthalmol* 102(10): 1506-1509, 1984.
10. Mackman G: Delayed sterile keratitis following radial keratotomy successfully treated with conjunctival flap, *Refract Corneal Surg* 8(2):122-124, 1992.
11. Buxton JN, Fox ML: Conjunctival flaps in the treatment of refractory *Pseudomonas* corneal abscess, *Ann Ophthalmol* 18(11):315-318, 1986.
12. Reinhart WJ: Conjunctival flap surgery. In Bruner WE, Stark WJ, Maumenee AE, editors: *Manual of corneal surgery,* New York, 1987, Churchill Livingstone.
13. Cies WA, Odeh-Nasrala N: The racquet conjunctival flap, *Ophthalmic Surg* 7:31-32, 1976.
14. Nelson JD: Surgery of the ocular surface. In Lindquist TD, Lindstrom RL, editors: *Ophthalmic surgery—looseleaf and update service,* Chicago, 1990, Year Book.
15. Townsend WM: Conjunctival flaps. In Kaufman HE et al, editors: *The cornea,* New York, 1988, Churchill Livingstone.
16. Thoft RA: Conjunctival and limbal surgery for corneal disease. In Smolin G, Thoft RA, editors: *The cornea scientific foundations and clinical practice,* ed 3, Boston, 1994, Little, Brown.
17. Naval CI: Argon laser modified conjunctivo-plasty for bullous keratopathy. Presented at the International Anterior Segment Congress, Toronto, Ontario, Canada, June 1994, *Ophthalmic Pract Suppl* p. 25, June 1994.

CHAPTER 156

GARY S. SCHWARTZ EDWARD J. HOLLAND

Management of Conjunctival and Corneal Neoplasia

Tumors of the conjunctiva and cornea range from the benign to the sight-threatening and even life-threatening. Management depends on the proper diagnosis and treatment of these lesions. A fundamental knowledge of the anatomy and embryology of the cornea, conjunctiva, and limbus is exceptionally important if proper diagnosis and treatment are to be performed. Both biopsy and treatment strategies alike are constantly being updated as new techniques are developed and old ones allowed to resurface.

The basic technique for obtaining diagnostic material from a conjunctival neoplasm is the excisional biopsy. Because of the redundancy, elasticity, and regenerative properties of the conjunctiva, even large excisions often can be performed without significant scarring or loss of conjunctival function. The role of the excisional biopsy is twofold: diagnosis and treatment. In addition to providing tissue for pathologic diagnosis, the excision alone is often curative. In cases in which, historically, excisional biopsy alone has led to unacceptable rates of recurrence or metastasis, adjunctive therapies such as cryotherapy, chemotherapy, or radiation therapy have been developed.

Communication with the pathologist is imperative when performing a biopsy of a conjunctival lesion. The pathologist should be consulted before the procedure to establish the ideal technique for excision, storage, and transportation of the tissue. If not prepared properly, excised conjunctival tissue will curl in the fixative, making histologic diagnosis difficult. To prevent this from occurring, the following technique should be performed (Figure 156-1): A 4 cm × 4 cm square of paper should be cut from the packaging of a sterile pair of surgical gloves and wetted with balanced salt solution. When the tissue is excised, it should be laid flat on the moistened, sterile paper epithelial side up. Orientation should be maintained using the snipped upper right corner of the paper as a landmark. If a map is to be drawn on the paper, it should be done with a graphite pencil, since ink will run in the fixative. The paper is then floated on top of fixative in a specimen cup. It will eventually sink on its own as it absorbs the fixative, and the specimen container, complete with fixative, paper, and specimen, should be sent for pathologic evaluation. The specimen should be labeled clearly with the patient's name, hospital number, and biopsy source and should be sent to pathology with paperwork that includes the history, description, and likely diagnosis. The fixative most commonly used is 10% neutral buffered formalin, but the pathologist should be consulted before the procedure if there is any doubt as to which fixative to use (e.g., formalin should never be used as the sole fixative if lymphoma is the suspected diagnosis). Frozen sections should only be performed if intraoperative decisions depend on the biopsy results.

The anatomy and function of the cornea and conjunctiva are quite different, but neoplasms of the conjunctiva and cornea are closely linked because the stem cells for both the cornea and conjunctiva are found at the limbus. Lesions of the conjunctiva are much more common than lesions of the cornea, and it is unusual for a corneal lesion to exist without a concomitant conjunctival abnormality. Most lesions found on the cornea, therefore, can be thought of as extensions of conjunctival lesions and be treated as such.

For the sake of management, a conjunctival neoplasm may be thought of as belonging to one of three groups, depending on its cell of origin and location within the conjunctiva. The first group is made up of the melanocytic neoplasms. Even the noninvasive forms of these lesions can occur anywhere in the conjunctiva from the epithelium to the substantia propria. They stem from conjunctival melanocytes, which in turn are derived from the embryologic neural crest and include the nevus, primary acquired melanosis, and malignant melanoma. The second group includes the epithelial neoplasms. Aside from the invasive squamous cell carcinoma, they all reside within the corneal and conjunctival epithelium, superficial to the basement membrane. These lesions typically arise from the epithelial stem cells located at the limbus and include squamous cell papilloma,

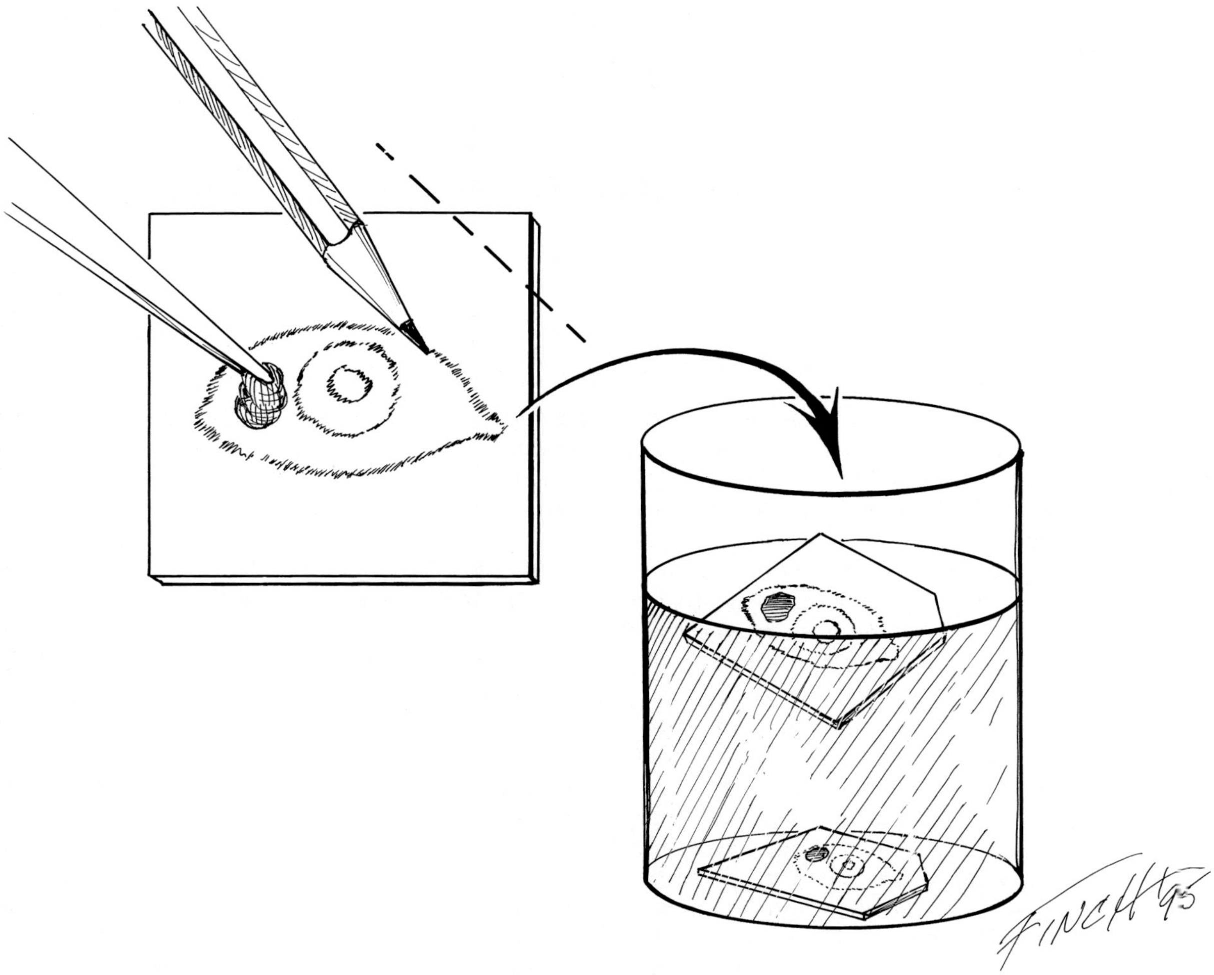

FIGURE 156-1 A 4 cm × 4 cm square is cut from the packaging of sterile surgical gloves. The upper right-hand corner is snipped to maintain orientation, and the paper is moistened with sterile balanced salt solution. The tissue specimen is laid on the paper, and a map of the surgical site is drawn with a graphite pencil. The glove paper with the specimen is then gently laid on the surface of fixative in a sterile container. The specimen is fixed immediately on the paper touching the fixative, and over the next few minutes, it will sink to the bottom of the container.

conjunctival/corneal intraepithelial neoplasia, and squamous cell carcinoma. The third group includes tumors of the substantia propria. This is the most diverse group of lesions and includes benign and malignant lymphoid proliferations and the conjunctival dermoid. The nature of each of these lesions is outlined more fully in Chapters 59 to 61; what follows is a description of their management.

Melanocytic Neoplasms

Melanocytic lesions of the conjunctiva behave more like melanocytic lesions of the skin than those of other parts of the eye. The reasons for this are embryologic. Like the melanin-containing cells of the skin, those of the conjunctiva are derived from embryologic neural crest cells that migrate to the basal layers of an epithelium. Melanocytic cells of the choroid, on the other hand, are cells of neural crest origin that migrate to reside in a connective tissue. Melanocytic cells of the retinal pigment epithelium, iris, and ciliary body are not derived from the neural crest but are derived from the neuroectoderm. Once these fundamental differences are understood, one can see why the classification, clinical course, and treatment of melanocytic lesions of the conjunctiva are so much different from those of the choroid, iris, and ciliary body and so alike those of the skin.

The most clinically important melanocytic lesions of

the conjunctiva are the nevus, primary acquired melanosis, and malignant melanoma. The treatments of these lesions are presented in detail later. The management of other melanocytic lesions such as racial melanosis and oculodermal melanocytosis (nevus of Ota) are presented along with their descriptions in Chapter 60.

NEVUS

Nevi are the most common melanocytic conjunctival neoplasms of infancy and childhood, and most occur during puberty or shortly thereafter.[1] They usually appear in the interpalpebral space near the limbus, semilunar fold, or caruncle and follow a typical developmental pattern. Nevi initially form nests of cells at the epithelial and subepithelial junction and spread superficially without breaching the basement membrane of the epithelium.[2] These "junctional" nevi clinically appear discrete, flat, and variably pigmented.[3] Folberg et al[1] have observed that pure junctional nevi are seen only in children and feel that these lesions represent a temporary stage that progresses to the next when the nevus cells descend into the superficial substantia propria. Here the lesion develops clinical thickness and can appear cystic. Eventually the junctional part of the nevus may regress, leaving only the subepithelial part. As the nevus goes through different stages of development, it changes shape, nodularity, and color.

Nevi of the conjunctiva, in and of themselves, are benign entities. It has been observed, however, that 14% to 35% of malignant melanomas of the conjunctiva are derived from nevi,[4-8] making the decision of whether or not to remove a nevus an important one. Pigmented conjunctival lesions in children are almost exclusively nevi. Only a handful of cases of malignant melanomas in patients under the age of 20 years have been reported.[8-10] The peak age of presentation of malignant melanomas is 49 to 55 years.

The occurrence of a nevus in childhood often poses a management dilemma. Because of its benign nature, the management of a nevus usually involves recording its size and position through photographs or detailed drawings, and then following its course periodically. A nevus can be removed if it has become a cosmetic problem. Although malignant melanotic lesions in children are exceedingly rare, and benign lesions must change in shape, thickness, and pigmentation over their natural history, it is acceptable for a changing nevus to be removed in a child if the parents are overly concerned about malignant change. Because benign nevi of the forniceal and tarsal conjunctiva are rare, pigmented lesions found here should be biopsied regardless of the patient's age.[1]

If the choice is made to remove a nevus, an excisional biopsy should be performed.[11] Care should be taken to avoid handling the lesion with toothed forceps or any instrument that will cause crush artifact and make it difficult for the pathologist to make a definitive reading on the tissue. After instillation of topical anesthetic and placement of a lid speculum, the lesion and neighboring tissue are ballooned up with a subconjunctival injection of 1% lidocaine with epinephrine. The lesion, along with a 1 to 2 mm nonpigmented margin of conjunctival tissue, should then be excised with a blade or small pair of scissors. Subconjunctival tissue is left in place, and the conjunctiva is left to reepithelialize without the placement of sutures. The tissue is sent to the pathology department in formalin in the aforementioned fashion. If the lesion is large, a map of its location and orientation should be drawn on the glove paper and in the patient's chart to facilitate excision of any remaining tissue if the pathologist notes that the surgical margins are not free of tumor. The patient is covered with topical antibiotics until the epithelial defect is healed.

PRIMARY ACQUIRED MELANOSIS

Primary acquired melanosis (PAM) presents as a unilateral, diffuse, patchy area of pigmentation in the conjunctiva of middle-aged Caucasians.[3,12] It usually occurs at the limbus but may occur in the forniceal or palpebral conjunctiva and can spread to the corneal epithelium. The classification system for PAM has been confusing and has changed considerably over the years. It was originally subclassified as either precancerous or cancerous melanosis.[6] The more recent system classifies PAM as either with or without atypia, depending on histopathologic study. Folberg et al have noted that the average age at diagnosis of PAM without atypia is 40 years, while the average age at diagnosis of PAM with atypia is 47 years. Investigators have concluded, therefore, that PAM with atypia likely evolves from PAM without atypia. PAM with atypia has been found to lead to malignant melanoma anywhere from 2½ to 10 years after biopsy.[13-15] Because PAM without atypia and PAM with atypia appear identical at the slit lamp, yet have such different malignant potentials, many authors feel all cases of unilateral, acquired, conjunctival melanosis in middle-aged Caucasians should be biopsied.[11,14,16,17] One study, however, has indicated that one third of Caucasian patients have unilateral, acquired, conjunctival melanosis to some degree, thus recommending against biopsy of every case.[18]

Histologically, PAM with atypia may appear identical to a junctional nevus. Both may be composed of intraepithelial atypical cells extending beyond the lateral edge of the subepithelial component or arranged in confluent nests. These histologic similarities pose a difficult problem for the pathologist because a junctional nevus is a benign lesion whereas PAM with atypia is premalignant. The proper diagnosis often depends on the clinical course and the patient's age. Junctional nevi occur in children and change to compound nevi in adolescence, while PAM with atypia occurs in middle age.

If the decision is made to biopsy a small area of PAM, an excisional biopsy may be performed as outlined for a conjunctival nevus. Care must be taken to examine the forniceal and palpebral conjunctiva carefully whenever PAM is to be biopsied. If a larger area of PAM is to be biopsied, multiple small areas should be mapped out and biopsied rather than the whole area of conjunctiva being removed. Topical anesthetic is used, and a lid speculum is placed between the lids. An outline is drawn around the lesion that maps a 2 mm tumor-free margin. The lesion is then ballooned with a subconjunctival injection of 1% lidocaine with epinephrine. Each small area to be biopsied is approached separately. The free margin is grasped with a nontoothed forceps, and the dissection is carried out in the subconjunctival space. After complete excision, wet-field cautery can be used for hemostasis. Each small specimen is placed into a separate bottle of 10% formalin and sent for pathologic evaluation. A map should be made in the patient's chart showing the anatomic location of each biopsy site. The incisions are not closed with sutures. Topical antibiotics are applied to the eye until the epithelial defects are healed.

If the biopsy results show PAM without atypia, the patient is followed periodically. If the pathology shows PAM with atypia, however, more definitive treatment in the form of excision and cryotherapy is necessary to eradicate the lesion and prevent progression to malignant melanoma.[14] Importantly, whenever PAM with atypia is diagnosed, preauricular and cervical lymph nodes should be palpated at all subsequent office visits to look for the progression to metastatic disease.

For cryotherapy of PAM with atypia, topical anesthetic drops are used and a lid speculum is placed between the lids. The area to be treated is ballooned up with a subconjunctival injection of 1% lidocaine with epinephrine (Figure 156-2). This step is an important one; adequate ballooning of the conjunctiva is important in ensuring that the conjunctiva is properly treated while damage to the subconjunctival tissue is avoided. Cryotherapy of the sclera should always be avoided. The goal of cryotherapy is to treat the lesion, surrounding conjunctiva, and the subconjunctival tissue; treatment to the sclera is not only unnecessary, but will cause damage to the sclera, iris, and ciliary body. Because the areas of atypia cannot be identified during slit lamp examination, all areas of pigmentation should be treated with cryotherapy. However, only one quadrant is normally treated per session,[16] although two quadrants may be treated with adequate reepithelization of the conjunctiva in younger patients. A flat-tipped nitrous oxide cryoprobe is used. Balanced salt solution can be used to free the probe tip from tissue should the two become frozen together. The cryoprobe is allowed to freeze to the desired temperature before it is touched to the tissue. Tissue should be frozen for 3 to 10 seconds before the cryoprobe is removed and the next area is frozen similarly.[11,16] Tissue should be frozen to an area 1 to 2 mm outside of the visible region of pigmentation. After an area has been allowed to thaw, it is refrozen in the same manner. This "double freeze-thaw" technique allows for the formation of larger ice crystals and better cell destruction than a "single freeze" technique.[16] Pigmented cells are destroyed at −20° C, while other epithelial cells are destroyed at −30° to 40° C, allowing for selective destruction of melanocytic cells using this method.[19]

All pigment found on the cornea should also be removed during the procedure to prevent future limbal nodular disease.[14] The epithelium should be scraped with a blade, then the exposed Bowman's layer should be scrubbed with absolute alcohol on a sterile cotton-tipped applicator. Gentle cryotherapy or carbon dioxide laser treatment may be performed if necessary to remove all remaining pigmented areas.

After cryotherapy, the patient should be treated with topical antibiotics until the epithelium has healed. Most eyes are inflamed after treatment, and patients do well with a 1- to 3-week course of topical steroids. Side effects of cryotherapy include symblepharon, lid swelling, loss of lashes, ptosis, pseudopterygium, and anterior segment necrosis.[14]

Recurrences of PAM with atypia are common. All recurrent lesions should be biopsied before cryotherapy. Normal macrophages in the substantia propria often engulf melanin, which may persist at the site of the biopsy. This pigment deposition, which is flat, should not be confused with recurrence of the neoplasm. True recurrence is associated with a thickened area of pigmentation.[11]

MALIGNANT MELANOMA

Malignant melanoma of the conjunctiva is rare. It makes up less than 2% of ocular melanomas and less than 1% of malignant tumors of the eye.[20] It tends to affect people in their fourth to seventh decades of life, being exceptional in children, and has been shown to have a higher incidence in females.[14,21] Malignant melanoma of the conjunctiva appears as a variably pigmented mass, most commonly in the interpalpebral area near the limbus, but it may occur in the tarsal or forniceal conjunctiva, the lid margin, or the caruncle as well. Prognosis depends on the depth and location of the lesion, multifocality, intralymphatic spread, amount

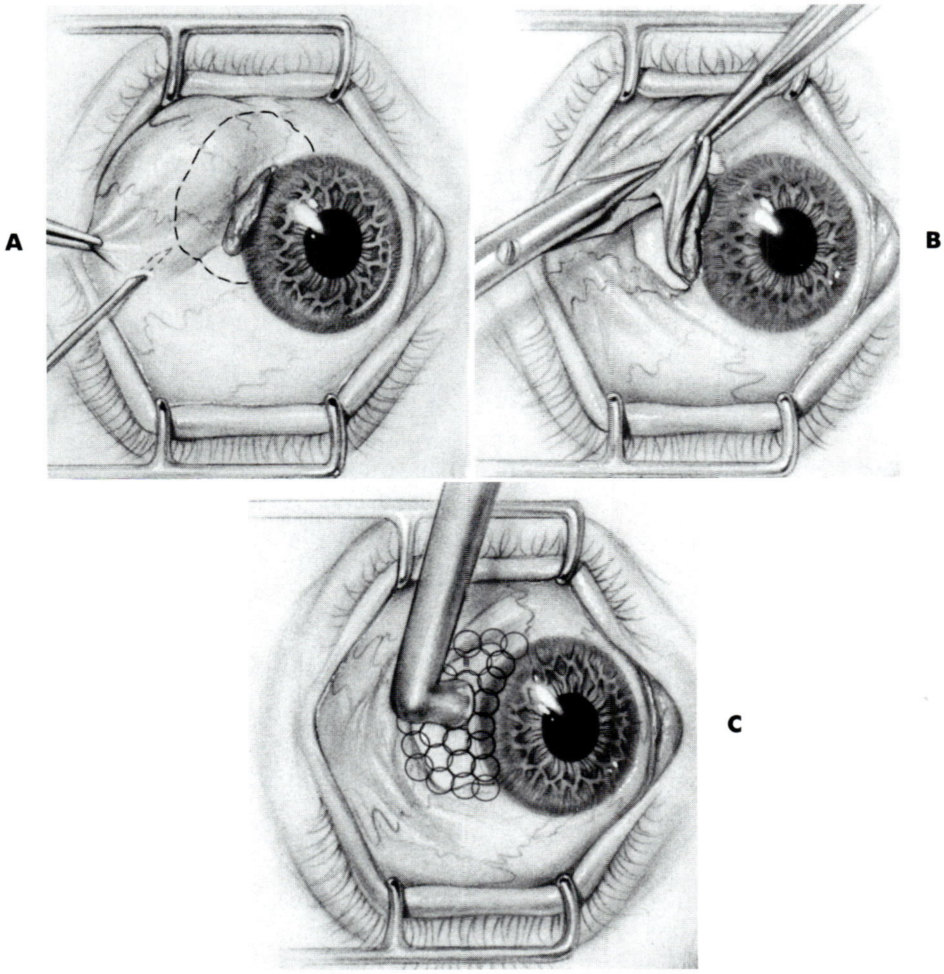

FIGURE 156-2 **A,** After the area to be excised is marked with a gentian violet pen, the lesion and surrounding conjunctiva are ballooned with a subconjunctival injection of lidocaine with epinephrine. **B,** While the lesion is grasped with untoothed forceps, it is excised with a blade or small pair of scissors. **C,** Cryotherapy of the surgical bed and conjunctival edge is then performed with a double freeze-thaw technique.

of inflammation, rate of mitosis, and presence of PAM sine pigmento,[20-22] and it is not dependent on degree of pigmentation, sex, age, or tumor origin (nevus, PAM, or de novo).[11,21] Paridaens et al, in a study of 256 patients with primary malignant melanoma of the conjunctiva, described survival rates of 82.9% at 5 years, 69.6% at 10 years, and 67.7% at 15 and 20 years.[21]

It was realized long ago that local excision of malignant melanoma is an inadequate treatment with an unacceptable rate of recurrence, metastatic spread, and patient mortality.[7] For years the treatment of choice for conjunctival malignant melanoma was orbital exenteration,[15] although removal of the eye has never been found to influence the rate of metastasis,[13] with metastases showing up even 15 years after surgery.[14] Brachytherapy,[13] external beam irradiation, and local excision with either external beam irradiation[23] or cryotherapy[14,16,22,24] have all been tried as alternate treatments to exenteration. Local excision with cryotherapy, as first described by Jakobiec et al in 1980,[22] has emerged as the treatment of choice for malignant melanoma of the conjunctiva.

When a tumor of the conjunctiva is suspected of being a melanoma, an excisional biopsy of the nodular part of the lesion should be performed along with cryotherapy of the surrounding tissue. After instillation of topical anesthetic, a lid speculum is placed between the lids and the lesion is ballooned up with a subconjunctival injection of 1% lidocaine with epinephrine. If the lesion does not lift up easily with this injection, the possibility of scleral invasion must be considered. If this is the case, partial thickness dissection must be undertaken with specific attention to tissue planes so as not to inadvertently enter the eye.

Care should be taken not to handle the lesion with toothed forceps because this may cause crush artifact and make it difficult for the pathologist to read the specimen. Also, separate instruments should be used for the pigmented and nonpigmented parts of the conjunctiva to avoid implantation of tumor cells into otherwise tumor-free tissue.[11] A 6-0 silk suture should be passed through the nodular area of the tumor and left untied. By pulling up on this suture, the tissue is tented up, allowing for easy excision of the lesion with a blade or small scissors. After excision, the suture should be trimmed but not tied, and the lesion should be placed onto a sterile piece of glove paper. A map of the excised area should be drawn on the paper and onto the patient's chart. The lesion, on the glove paper, should then be placed in formalin and sent for pathologic evaluation. Cryotherapy of the surrounding conjunctiva should then be performed to a distance of 2 mm outside the area of visible pigmentation. The tissue edge should be picked up with forceps during cryotherapy to avoid damage to the underlying structures. As with treatment of PAM with atypia, a double freeze-thaw technique should be used. A bottle of balanced salt solution can be used to free the probe tip from tissue should the two become frozen together. The liquid nitrogen cryoprobe is activated and allowed to reach the proper temperature before it is applied to the tissue. It is held in place on the tissue for at least 3 seconds. Each area is allowed to thaw, then it is refrozen to allow for maximum tumor cell destruction. The subconjunctival surgical bed is frozen similarly. If greater than half of the conjunctiva of the treated eye exhibits melanosis, the entire area should be treated in more than one session.

All pigment found on the cornea should also be removed during the procedure, as with the treatment of PAM with atypia mentioned earlier. The epithelium should be scraped with a blade; then the exposed Bowman's layer should be scrubbed with absolute alcohol on a sterile cotton-tipped applicator. Gentle cryotherapy or carbon dioxide laser may be performed if necessary to remove all pigment.

No sutures are placed in the surgical wound, and it is allowed to close by secondary intent. Because the substantia propria is not damaged by the cryotherapy, it acts as a scaffolding for reepithelialization of the conjunctiva. As long as less than half of the conjunctiva is treated at one time, it should reepithelialize quickly. After cryotherapy the patient is treated with topical antibiotics until the epithelial defect has healed. Most eyes are inflamed after treatment, and patients do well with a 1- to 3-week course of oral steroids. Some also benefit from topical cycloplegics.[16] Side effects of cryotherapy include symblepharon, lid swelling, loss of lashes, ptosis, pseudopterygium, and anterior segment necrosis.[14] Patients should be followed carefully, and preauricular and cervical lymph nodes should be palpated at each subsequent visit.

Recurrence of conjunctival melanoma must be rebiopsied and treated. In one study, local recurrence was found to be the only statistical risk factor for distal metastasis.[20] Recurrence should be treated with wider excision, cryotherapy, irradiation, or, if advanced, exenteration. Exenteration is sometimes the only way to achieve local control of large tumors, yet may not affect metastasis or patient mortality.[14] Multinodular disease meets with the worst success, and best results are often obtained if patients are referred to ophthalmic oncology centers early, before recurrent disease has occurred. Even when regional metastasis has occurred, many patients can be saved with parotidectomy and cervical node dissection.

Squamous Neoplasms

Since first described by Bowman in 1849,[25] the classification system for squamous neoplasms of the conjunctiva and cornea has changed considerably. In 1912 Bowen described carcinoma in situ of the skin, and this entity was soon named Bowen's disease after him. McGavic[26] in 1942, while studying intraepithelial squamous lesions of the conjunctiva, noted the similarities of these lesions to the skin lesions previously described by Bowen. McGavic recommended the name *Bowen's disease of the conjunctiva* for these lesions. Pizzarello and Jakobiec in 1984 emphasized that epithelial dysplasias, carcinoma in situ, and squamous cell carcinoma represent not three separate entities as previously written, but three parts of a continuous spectrum of diseases known as intraepithelial neoplasia.[27] They noted that squamous lesions of the conjunctiva appear more like intraepithelial neoplasia of the cervix than like lesions of the skin and recommended usage of the term *conjunctival intraepithelial neoplasia* (CIN) over Bowen's disease of the conjunctiva. Although, histologically, conjunctival intraepithelial neoplasia resembles cervical intraepithelial neoplasia, it must be borne in mind that while 50% of the cervical type will lead to invasive carcinoma, only 5% of conjunctival intraepithelial neoplasia will undergo this transformation.[28]

In the most recent classification system, the labels *mild CIN* and *severe CIN* replace the previously used *dysplasia* and *carcinoma in situ*.[3] Mild CIN represents the stage at which abnormal epithelial cells only make up partial thickness of the epithelium. Severe CIN occurs when the abnormally immature cells make up the entire epithelial thickness. In both forms of CIN, all abnormal cells are superficial to an intact basement membrane. If the basement membrane is breached by dysplastic cells, the lesion is labeled a *squamous cell carcinoma.* Squamous cell carcinoma is felt to arise from severe CIN, which in turn is felt to arise from mild CIN; thus mild and severe CIN should both be thought of as premalignant lesions.[29]

It is believed that squamous neoplasms of the conjunctiva originate from the dividing limbal stem cell populations. For this reason, squamous neoplasms are almost invariably found at the limbus, although they can be found in the forniceal, bulbar, and palpebral areas also. The pathology, history, and behavior of squamous neoplasms of the conjunctiva and cornea are presented more fully in Chapter 59. What follows is a guide to the management of these lesions.

SQUAMOUS CELL PAPILLOMA

Squamous cell papillomas of the conjunctiva are benign tumors that are composed of mature epithelial cells and have been associated with the human papilloma virus, especially in the pediatric population.[3,11,30] They are translucent lesions with frondlike vascular projections radiating from a central core.[31] Lesions in the pediatric age group tend to be small and located in the inferior fornix, caruncle, and limbus. Tumors in adults can be much larger and may cover the entire cornea. Small, sessile conjunctival papillomas in children may resolve with topical corticosteroids. Papillomas that are simply excised frequently recur. Recurrences are typically much more extensive than the original tumors and can involve the fornices, lid margins, and puncta.[32] Excision combined with cautery, radiation therapy, and topical silver nitrate or dinitrochlorobenzene[33] have all been advocated in the past to prevent recurrence. Carbon dioxide laser ablation, which is an accepted treatment for laryngeal papillomata, has also been advocated by some for conjunctival papillomas.[32] The current treatment of choice is excision and local cryotherapy.[34] It should be borne in mind, however, that most papillomas resolve on their own over 2 years.

Papillomas may be excised if lid function is impaired, malignant transformation is suspected, or a better cosmetic appearance is desired.[11] Because most papillomas occur in the pediatric population, excisions are normally performed with the patient under general anesthesia. A lid speculum is placed between the lids and the subconjunctival tissue is infiltrated with lidocaine with epinephrine. The lesion is grasped with a pair of forceps and excised with a blade or small pair of scissors. It is immediately placed on a sterile piece of glove paper, put into formalin, and sent for pathologic evaluation. A map of the incision site should be drawn on the glove paper and in the patient's chart. Cryotherapy at $-25°$ C should be applied to the surrounding conjunctival tissue using the double freeze-thaw method described in the section on PAM. In the case of small lesions, the surgical wound can be left open and allowed to reepithelialize. Larger wounds should be closed with absorbable suture and, occasionally, in the case of excessively large wounds, a mucous membrane graft may be needed. The patient is treated with topical antibiotics until the epithelial defect has healed. Topical cycloplegics and corticosteroids may be used to prevent inflammation.

CONJUNCTIVAL INTRAEPITHELIAL NEOPLASIA

Conjunctival intraepithelial neoplasia (CIN) most often occurs in the fifth to sixth decades of life, with a male to female ratio of roughly 6:1. It is usually found at the limbus in the interpalpebral space and has been linked to exposure to petroleum products, cigarette smoke, sunlight, and the human papilloma virus.[35,36] When the cornea is involved, the neoplasm is referred to as *corneal intraepithelial neoplasia,* which, like both cervical intraepithelial neoplasia and conjunctival intraepithelial neoplasia, is abbreviated *CIN.* Corneal lesions usually present as a slightly elevated, gelatinous, gray plaque. The leading edge characteristically has fimbriated, "finger-shaped" extensions that appear to reach toward the visual axis. These lesions are often associated with small isolated islands of abnormal gray or white tissue.[27,29,37-40] They are almost always associated with chronic conjunctivitis or conjunctival lesions such as papillomas, leukoplakia, pterygia, or pingueculae.[28] Cases of corneal intraepithelial neoplasia without associated conjunctival involvement, although rare, have been described.[28,29]

Recurrence rates of 30% to 40% were found after simple excision of these lesions,[27,29,38,41] and it was realized early on that some type of adjunctive treatment was needed to prevent recurrence. In 1983 Fraunfelder and Wingfield showed that cryotherapy used in combination with surgical excision results in a significantly lower recurrence rate than excision or cryotherapy alone,[42] and this technique has emerged as the current treatment of choice for CIN.

The extent of tumor may be more than that seen at examination under either the slit lamp or the surgical microscope. Rose bengal can be used to stain abnormal, devitalized, or dead epithelium and thus give a better idea of the tumor margins.[43] For the most accurate results, rose bengal should be applied before the topical anesthetic because the anesthetic is toxic to the epithelium and will increase the area of rose bengal staining if applied first. After the instillation of topical anesthetic, a lid speculum is placed between the lids and the lesion is elevated with 1% lidocaine with epinephrine, thus separating the conjunctiva from the underlying tissue. A separate set of instruments is used for the normal tissue and tumor to avoid seeding tumor cells into previously tumor-free conjunctiva. Instillation of topical anesthetic should be repeated many times to weaken epithelial attachments and allow for easier corneal epithelial debridement.

A gentian violet felt-tipped pen is used to mark an incision line in normal conjunctiva 1.5 mm distal to what is felt to be the farthest extent of the lesion. Although some advocate using cautery to mark this line, cautery probably causes unnecessary tissue damage to the conjunctiva. The line is cut with Westcott scissors down to bare sclera, and the conjunctiva below the tumor is dissected from underlying sclera, while the conjunctival edge is lifted with forceps.

If tumor extends to the cornea, it is usually removed by scraping toward the limbus with a blade (Figure 156-3). A 1 to 1.5 mm cuff of apparently normal corneal epithelium should be removed with the lesion to ensure clean margins. Bowman's layer should never be breached during this part of the procedure. Because of the nature of the lesion, it is thought that Bowman's layer acts as a natural barrier to downward extension of the tumor.[44] Thus an intact Bowman's layer must be preserved to avoid intraocular spread of the disease.

After the lesion and rim of normal conjunctiva are removed, they should be placed on a sterile piece of glove paper. A map of the area should be drawn on the glove paper and into the patient's chart. The specimen should be placed into formalin and sent to pathology for evaluation while still on the glove paper. All adjacent tissue and the scleral bed are then treated with double freeze-thaw cryotherapy. First the cut edges of conjunctiva are treated. To avoid damage to underlying tissue, each area of conjunctiva to be treated is lifted from the underlying tissue while undergoing freezing. The cryoprobe is always activated while held away from tissue and allowed to reach the desired freezing temperature before being held to the tissue. Balanced salt solution can be used to free the cryoprobe from the tissue should they become stuck together. The tissue is rapidly frozen to a temperature of $-25°$ C. It is allowed to thaw and then refrozen in a similar manner. This technique allows for maximum epithelial cell damage with minimum damage to the substantia propria, which can then act as a scaffolding for conjunctival reepithelialization. Care must be taken to treat the involved limbus completely because improper treatment here may lead to recurrence.[11] Peripheral cornea should only be frozen to 1 to 1.5 mm central to the limbus to avoid scarring and astigmatism.

The surgical wound can be left open and allowed to reepithelialize. The patient is treated with topical antibiotics until the epithelial defect has healed. Topical cycloplegics and corticosteroids may be used to decrease postoperative inflammation. Success with autologous limbal transplants has been described for cases where the epithelial defect was felt to be too large for primary reepithelialization.[45]

Excision combined with cryotherapy as described previously carries with it an 8% recurrence rate.[42] Tumor may recur at the operated site or at a separate site. Repeated excision and cryotherapy of recurrences may result in loss of the limbal stem cell population and subsequent corneal epitheliopathy. Extensive loss of corneal stem cells may also lead to conjunctivalization of the cornea and permanent ocular surface disease. The epitheliopathy may be misdiagnosed as tumor recurrence and occasionally requires biopsy to make the proper diagnosis.

Alternate treatments to excision with cryotherapy have recently been described in the ophthalmic literature. In 1994 Frucht-Pery and Rozenman described tumor regression without recurrence at 4, 12, and 16 months in three patients treated with topical mitomycin C.[46] Mitomycin C 0.02% was applied four times a day for 14 to 22 days. The medicine was tolerated in all patients for the first 2 weeks of treatment, but photophobia and blepharospasm developed after 2 weeks of use. We have successfully used a 2-week course of topical mitomycin C after this protocol to treat a patient with multiple recurrences of CIN.

In 1991 Jones et al described successful treatment of recurrent CIN with excision and beta irradiation.[47] Maskin in 1994 described the successful use of topical interferon α_{2b}, 1 million U/ml twice a day in a 55-year-old woman with recurrent "epithelial dysplasia." Regression was seen at 1 week; the medicine was tapered over 2 months, and the patient was tumor free at 11 months.[48]

SQUAMOUS CELL CARCINOMA

Squamous cell carcinomas are thought to derive from CIN, and like CIN, they are found most commonly in the interpalpebral space at the limbus.[49] Like CIN, isolated cases of squamous cell carcinoma that do not involve the limbus have been described.[37] A review of the Mayo Clinic's experience with epithelial conjunctival and corneal tumors from 1920 to 1983 found 22 cases of squamous cell carcinomas and 98 cases of CIN.

Clinically, it is difficult to differentiate CIN from squamous cell carcinoma of the conjunctiva because location, growth pattern, and overall appearance are similar. In some studies, it has been suggested that squamous cell carcinomas are larger than CIN and are usually associated with large, dilated feeder vessels.[28,37,50] However, the definitive diagnosis of squamous cell carcinoma of the conjunctiva is made histologically.

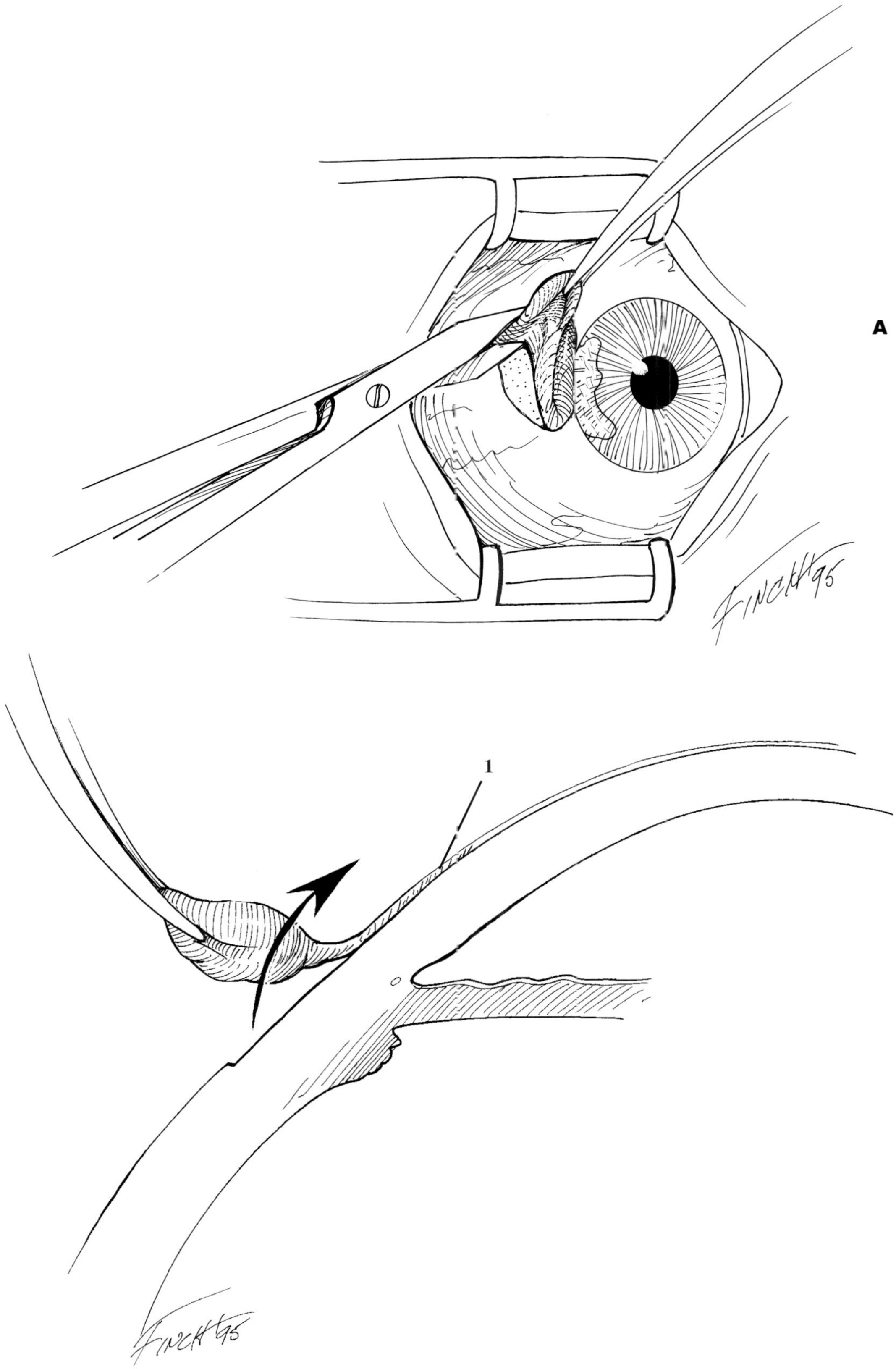

FIGURE 156-3 **A,** The conjunctival aspect of CIN is first excised with scissors. **B,** An attempt is made to lift off the corneal pathology *(1)* while grasping the conjunctival portion so that the whole tumor comes off in one piece. *Continued.*

C

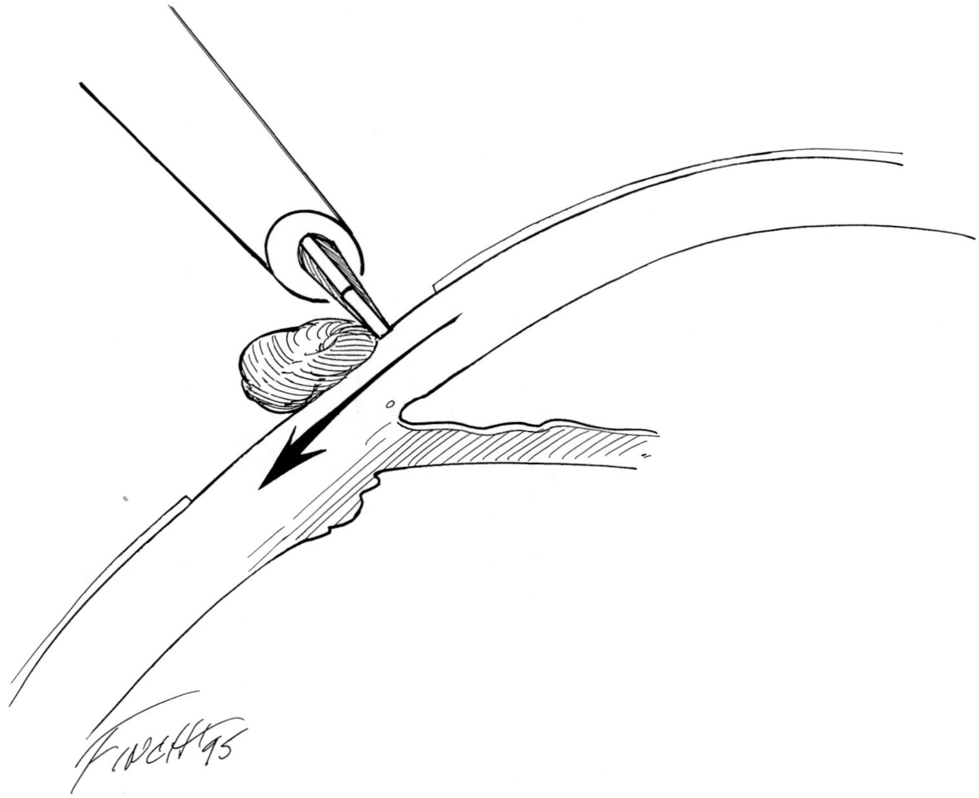

FIGURE 156-3, cont'd. **C,** Usually the corneal aspect of the lesion is removed by scraping with a knife. It is imperative not to penetrate Bowman's membrane while performing this maneuver, as Bowman's membrane acts as an important natural barrier to intraocular spread of the tumor.

Squamous cell carcinomas are not typically aggressive tumors, but they do have the potential for intraocular as well as lymphatic spread.[51,52] Lymph node metastasis occurs with a rate of less than 10% in patients with invasive squamous cell carcinoma.[53] Intraocular spread may occur as a recurrence after the attempted excision of a primary lesion.[50,54] Squamous cell carcinoma of the conjunctiva initially presenting with intraocular spread has also been described.[55,56]

Mucoepidermoid carcinoma is a rare and particularly invasive form of squamous cell carcinoma. It develops in older individuals and contains mucus-secreting cells, giving it a yellow color. It commonly metastasizes to local lymph nodes. Because of its invasive nature, it should have wider and more careful excision and more diligent follow-up than the less aggressive forms of squamous cell carcinoma of the conjunctiva.[3]

Squamous cell carcinomas of the conjunctiva that do not have obvious intraocular or lymphatic involvement should be treated with excisional biopsy and cryotherapy as described for CIN.[42,57] The rate of recurrence is associated with tumor in the surgical margins and not with cell type, clinical appearance, or degree of dysplasia,[29] so careful surgery is the most important factor in ensuring a good prognosis.

When the palpebral conjunctiva is involved, wide excisions must be performed.[3] Care must be taken if the tumor involves the fornix, as it tends to extend along the globe into the posterior orbit. In these cases, imaging studies must be performed to evaluate the posterior extent of the tumor. If the lesion is not locally resectable or lymphatic spread has occurred, orbital exenteration should be considered.[11]

Enucleation has been the standard therapy when intraocular spread of squamous cell carcinoma is discovered. In 1980 Li et al described en bloc excisions in two patients with intraocular tumors who had had previous conjunctival excisions for squamous cell carcinoma. Both patients eventually needed enucleations for persistent intraocular tumor.[50]

Lymphoid Proliferations

Lymphoid tumors of the conjunctiva most often affect patients in their sixth and seventh decades of life.[58] They tend to be slow growing and asymptomatic, being diagnosed on routine examinations.[59,60] Typically, they present as unilateral, smooth, salmon-colored patches within the substantia propria of the conjunctiva. Knowles et al described 108 patients with ocular adnexal lymphoid proliferations in whom orbital involvement was seen in 69 patients, conjunctival involvement in 30, and anterior lamellar eyelid involvement in 9. Of those with conjunctival involvement, forniceal and epibulbar lesions were most common.[60] Prognostic significance was found with extent of disease at presentation and not with age, sex, or duration of symptoms.

The majority of patients with ocular adnexal lymphoid proliferation do not show systemic disease at presentation, and neither bilaterality, lymph node involvement, nor recurrence after treatment is an indication of malignancy.[59,61,62] Studies have shown that 10% to 25% of non-Hodgkins lymphomas arise in extranodal sites[63] with frequent involvement of ocular adnexal tissues. Roughly one third of ocular adnexal manifestations of systemic lymphoma involve the conjunctiva.[60,64]

Lymphoid tumors of the conjunctiva may represent either benign lymphoid hyperplasia or lymphoma. Some studies suggest that benign tumors present more often as multifocal lesions with a "pebbly," follicular surface,[59] but clinically, it is difficult to distinguish between benign and malignant proliferations, so all such lesions should be biopsied. Cytomorphologic features of these lesions must be studied for the proper diagnosis to be made.[62] Benign tumors tend to be polymorphic proliferations, whereas malignant lymphomas are typically monoclonal collections of B-cells.

When a tumor of the conjunctiva is suspected of being a lymphoid proliferation, a biopsy of the lesion should be performed. Because of the relationship of the conjunctiva to underlying tissues, biopsies of bulbar lymphoid proliferations are easier to perform than palpebral ones. If the lesion involves the palpebral conjunctiva, an incisional biopsy should be performed, and if isolated to the bulbar conjunctiva, an excisional one. After instillation of topical anesthetic, a lid speculum is placed between the lids and a gentian violet marking pen is used to mark a conjunctival incision 1 mm distal to the apparent edge of the lesion. The surrounding conjunctiva is then infiltrated with 1% lidocaine with epinephrine. Westcott scissors are used to cut along the incision down to bare sclera. Because the lesion is located in the substantia propria of the conjunctiva, blunt dissection with Westcott scissors can be performed under it to separate the tumor from the underlying sclera. If the tumor abuts the limbus, dissection here should be performed last. The lesion and surrounding conjunctiva should then be placed onto a sterile piece of moistened glove paper and put into a moist chamber made from a specimen cup that has sterile gauze soaked in buffered balanced salt solution on the bottom. The surgeon should communicate directly with the pathologist to decide which special studies may be necessary to make the proper diagnosis. These special studies include immunohistochemistry, DNA rearrangement studies, electron microscopy, "touch" impression, mercury-based fixatives, and others. Most of these studies can be performed on tissue that has been transported in a moist chamber, as described earlier. The incision is not sutured closed but is left to heal by secondary intention. The lid speculum is removed, and the patient is treated with topical antibiotics until the epithelial defect has healed.

If the pathology results show that the lesion is a benign lymphoid proliferation, many advocate observation after excision alone or excision and cryotherapy.[11,65] The patient should have a systemic evaluation every 6 months for at least 5 years. Knowles et al recommend adjunctive radiation therapy of 1500 to 2000 cGy for a benign lymphoid proliferation.[60]

If the pathology shows lymphoma, it may represent either the extranodal origination of lymphoma, or the extranodal spread of systemic lymphoma,[66-68] and the patient should be referred to an internist or oncologist. Workup of this patient includes a complete physical examination with attention to the lymph nodes, spleen, and liver; a chest x-ray; complete blood count; serum electrophoresis; bone marrow biopsy; abdominal computed tomography (CT); and liver function tests. A patient with systemic disease should be treated with systemic chemotherapy.[60]

If the biopsy reveals lymphoma, but no systemic involvement is found, radiation therapy should be undertaken. The typical dosage for localized conjunctival lymphoma is 3000 to 6000 rad.[11,69] However, Eichler and Fraunfelder in 1994 showed a 98% eradication rate for lymphoid lesions, including five lymphoid hyperplasias and 37 lymphomas, when treating with excision and cryotherapy rather than excision and radiation therapy. Their range of follow-up was 26 to 139 months, with a mean follow-up time of 75 months, and only one of their patients subsequently required chemotherapy for systemic lymphoma.[70]

Limbal Dermoid

Limbal dermoids are choristomas.[71,72] They are congenital tumors of the cornea and sclera made up of persistent primitive tissue.[73] They tend to be white tumors, located at the limbus, and are made up of collagenous connective tissue covered with stratified squamous epithelium and fine hairs.[15] Dermal append-

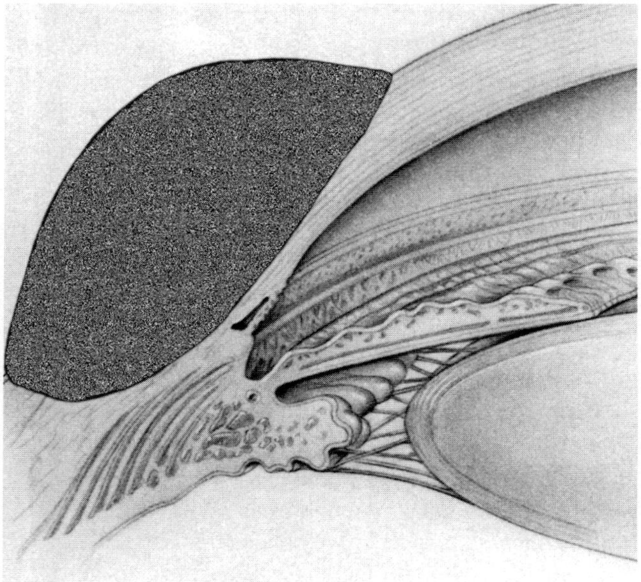

FIGURE 156-4 Limbal dermoids often extend to deep layers of the limbus. Care must be taken when removing one that the anterior chamber is not inadvertently entered. The defect left behind after removal of a limbal dermoid often must be repaired with a corneal or scleral patchgraft.

ages such as sebaceous glands, in addition to fat, nerve bundles, and lacrimal tissue, can also be seen within limbal dermoids.[72] They have been associated with staphyloma,[73] microcornea, ptosis, microphthalmia, corneal anesthesia, strabismus, and colobomata of all structures from the lids to the optic nerve.[74,75]

Limbal dermoids have been associated with Goldenhar's syndrome.[75] In one study, limbal dermoids were found to be unilateral in 53% and bilateral in 23% of patients with Goldenhar's syndrome.[74] They were found most often at the inferotemporal limbus and associated with the facial abnormalities typical of the syndrome.

Limbal dermoids grow slowly and are usually well tolerated. They may, however, cause irregular astigmatism, chronic irritation from surface hairs, abnormal pupillary extension,[72] or an unacceptable cosmetic appearance. When any of these are the case, excision may be considered. The surgeon must bear in mind, however, that limbal dermoids are often associated with scleral or corneal thinning[15,73] and occasionally with intraocular extension.[72,76] Therefore a complete examination including gonioscopy, must be performed. Great care must be undertaken when removing a limbal dermoid to avoid inadvertent entry into the globe.

Because limbal dermoid excision is usually performed on children, the procedure is typically done under general anesthesia. A lid speculum is placed between the eyelids. The outer limits of the tumor are marked with a gentian violet felt-tipped pen. The conjunctival edge of the tumor is grasped with forceps, and a knife is used to find a plane of normal sclera under the tumor. Lamellar sclerectomy is then performed toward the limbus. When the limbus is reached, the excision is completed with a lamellar keratectomy. If the remaining tissue is felt to be thin, a patch graft can be performed using donor cornea or preserved sclera (Figure 156-4). The specimen is then placed on a sterile piece of glove paper, put into formalin, and sent to the pathology laboratory for evaluation. The patient is treated with topical antibiotics until the epithelial defect has healed.

REFERENCES

1. Folberg R et al: Benign conjunctival melanocytic lesions. Clinicopathologic features, *Ophthalmology* 96:436-461, 1989.
2. Jakobiec FA: The ultrastructure of conjunctival melanocytic tumors, *Trans Am Ophthalmol Soc* 87:599-752, 1984.
3. Shields JA, Shields CL: Tumors of the conjunctiva and cornea. In Smolin G, Thoft RA, editors: *The cornea,* ed 2, Boston, 1994, Little, Brown.
4. Jay B: Naevi and melanomata of the conjunctiva, *Br J Ophthalmol* 49:169-204, 1965.
5. Zimmerman LE: The histogenesis of conjunctival melanomas the First Algernon B. Reese Lecture. In Jakobiec FA, editor *Ocular and adnexal tumors,* Birmingham, 1978, Aesculapius Publishing Co.
6. Reese AB: Precancerous and cancerous melanosis, *Am J Ophthalmol* 61:1272-1277, 1966.
7. Liesegang TJ, Campbell RJ: Mayo clinic experience with conjunctival melanomas, *Arch Ophthalmol* 98:1385-1389, 1980.
8. Croxatto JO et al: Malignant melanoma of the conjunctiva. Report of a case, *Ophthalmology* 94:1281-1285, 1987.
9. McDonnell JM et al: Conjunctival melanocytic lesions in children, *Ophthalmology* 96:986-993, 1989.
10. Bernardino VB Jr, Naidoff MA, Clark WH Jr: Malignant melanomas of the conjunctiva, *Am J Ophthalmol* 82:383-394, 1976.
11. Grutzmacher R, Fraunfelder FT, Lindquist TD: Corneal and bulbar conjunctival tumors. In Lindquist TD, Lindstrom RL, editors: *Ophthalmic surgery,* Boston, 1994, Mosby.
12. Folberg R, McLean I, Zimmerman L: Primary acquired melanosis of the conjunctiva, *Hum Pathol* 16:129, 1985.
13. Lederman M, Wybar K, Busby E: Malignant epibulbar melanoma: natural history and treatment by radiotherapy, *Br J Ophthalmol* 68:605-617, 1984.
14. Jakobiec FA et al: Cryotherapy for conjunctival primary acquired melanosis and malignant melanoma. Experience with 62 cases, *Ophthalmology* 95:1058-1070, 1988.
15. Reese AB: *Tumors of the eye,* ed 3, New York, 1976, Harper & Row.
16. Jakobiec FA et al: The role of cryotherapy in the management of conjunctival melanoma, *Ophthalmology* 89:502-515, 1982.
17. Jakobiec FA: Conjunctival melanoma. Unfinished business, *Arch Ophthalmol* 98:1378-1384, 1980.
18. Gloor P, Alexandrakis G: Clinical characterization of primary acquired melanosis, *Invest Ophthalmol Vis Sci* 36:1721-1729, 1995.
19. Jakobiec FA, Iwamoto T: Cryotherapy for intraepithelial conjunctival melanocytic proliferations. Ultrastructural effects, *Arch Ophthalmol* 101:904-912, 1983.
20. De Potter P, Shields CL, Shields JA: Malignant melanoma of the

conjunctiva. In Shields JA, editor: *International ophthalmology clinics. Update on malignant ocular tumors,* Boston, 1993, Little, Brown.

21. Paridaens ADA et al: Prognostic factors in primary malignant melanoma of the conjunctiva: a clinicopathological study of 256 cases, *Br J Ophthalmol* 78:252-259, 1994.
22. Jakobiec FA et al: Combined surgery and cryotherapy for diffuse malignant melanoma of the conjunctiva, *Arch Ophthalmol* 98:1390-1396, 1980.
23. Lommatzsch PK et al: Therapeutic outcome of patients suffering from malignant melanomas of the conjunctiva, *Br J Ophthalmol* 74:615-619, 1990.
24. Jakobiec FA, Iwamoto T: Cryotherapy for intraepithelial conjunctival melanocytic proliferations. Ultrastructural effects, *Arch Ophthalmol* 101:904-912, 1983.
25. Bowman, W: *Lectures on the parts concerned in the operations of the eye and on the structures of the retina,* London, 1849, Longman, Brown, Green & Longman.
26. McGavic J: Intraepithelial epithelioma of cornea and conjunctiva (Bowen's disease), *Am J Ophthalmol* 25:167, 1942.
27. Pizzarello LD, Jakobiec FA: Bowen's disease of the conjunctiva: a misnomer. In Jakobiec FA, editor: *Ocular and adnexal tumors,* Birmingham, 1978, Aesculapius.
28. Waring GO, Roth AM, Ekins MB: Clinical and pathologic description of 17 cases of corneal intraepithelial neoplasia, *Am J Ophthalmol* 97:547-559, 1984.
29. Erie JC, Campbell RJ, Liesegang TJ: Conjunctival and corneal intraepithelial and invasive neoplasia, *Ophthalmology* 93:176-183, 1986.
30. Lass JH et al: Detection of human papillomavirus DNA sequences in conjunctival papilloma, *Am J Ophthalmol* 96:670-674, 1983.
31. Jakobiec FA: Corneal tumors. In Kaufman HE et al, editors: *The cornea,* New York, 1988, Churchill Livingstone.
32. Bosniak SL, Novick NL, Sachs ME: Treatment of recurrent squamous papillomata of the conjunctiva by carbon dioxide laser vaporization, *Ophthalmology* 93:1078-1082, 1986.
33. Ferry AP, Meltzer MA, Taub RN: Immunotherapy with dinitrochlorobenzene (DCNB) for recurrent squamous cell tumor of conjunctiva, *Trans Am Ophthalmol Soc* 74:154-171, 1976.
34. Harkey ME, Metz HS: Cryotherapy of conjunctival papillomata, *Am J Ophthalmol* 66:872-874, 1968.
35. Napora C et al: Factors associated with conjunctival intraepithelial neoplasia: a case control study, *Ophthalmic Surg* 21:27-30, 1990.
36. Grossniklaus HE et al: Conjunctival lesions in adults. A clinical and histopathologic review, *Cornea* 7:79-86, 1988.
37. Cameron JA, Hidayat AA: Squamous cell carcinoma of the cornea, *Am J Ophthalmol* 111:571-574, 1991.
38. Winter FC, Kleh TR: Precancerous epithelioma of the limbus, *Arch Ophthalmol* 64:208-215, 1960.
39. Wise G: A case of Bowen's disease of the cornea, *Am J Ophthalmol* 26:167-171, 1943.
40. Dark AJ, Streeten BW: Preinvasive carcinoma of the cornea and conjunctiva, *Br J Ophthalmol* 64:506-514, 1980.
41. Carroll JM, Kuwabara T: A classification of limbal epitheliomas, *Arch Ophthalmol* 73:545-551, 1965.
42. Fraunfelder FT, Wingfield D: Management of intraepithelial conjunctival tumors and squamous cell carcinomas, *Am J Ophthalmol* 95:359-363, 1983.
43. Wilson FM II: Rose bengal staining of epibulbar squamous neoplasms, *Ophthalmic Surg* 7:21-23, 1976.
44. Char DH et al: Squamous cell carcinoma of the conjunctiva. In Shields JA, editor: *International ophthalmology clinics; update on malignant ocular tumors,* Boston, 1993, Little, Brown.
45. Copeland RA Jr, Char DH: Limbal autograft reconstruction after conjunctival squamous cell carcinoma, *Am J Ophthalmol* 110:412-415, 1990.
46. Frucht-Pery J, Rozenman Y: Mitomycin C therapy for corneal intraepithelial neoplasia, *Am J Ophthalmol* 117:164-168, 1994.
47. Jones DB, Wilhelmus KR, Font RL: Beta irradiation of recurrent corneal intraepithelial neoplasia, *Trans Am Ophthalmol Soc* 89:285-298, 1991.
48. Maskin SL: Regression of limbal epithelial dyspalasia with topical interferon, *Arch Ophthalmol* 112:1145-1146, 1994.
49. Freedman J, Rohm G: Surgical management and histopathology of invasive tumours of the cornea, *Br J Ophthalmol* 63:632-635, 1979.
50. Li WW, Pettit TH, Zakka KA: Intraocular invasion by papillary squamous cell carcinoma of the conjunctiva, *Am J Ophthalmol* 90:697-701, 1980.
51. Stokes JJ: Intraocular extension of epibulbar squamous cell carcinoma of the limbus, *Ophthalmology* 59:143-146, 1963.
52. Nicholson DH, Herschler J: Intraocular extension of squamous cell carcinoma of the conjunctiva, *Arch Ophthalmol* 95:843-846, 1977.
53. Iliff WJ, Marback R, Green WR: Invasive squamous cell carcinoma of the conjunctiva, *Arch Ophthalmol* 93:119-122, 1975.
54. Glasson WJ et al: Invasive squamous cell carcinoma of the conjunctiva, *Arch Ophthalmol* 112:1342-1345, 1994.
55. Wexler SA, Wallow IHL: Squamous cell carcinoma of the conjunctiva presenting with intraocular extension, *Arch Ophthalmol* 103:1175-1177, 1985.
56. Lindenmuth KA et al: Invasive squamous cell carcinoma of the conjunctiva presenting as necrotizing scleritis with scleral perforation and uveal prolapse, *Surv Ophthalmol* 33:50-54, 1988.
57. Peksayar G, Soyturk MK, Demiryont M: Long-term results of cryotherapy on malignant epithelial tumors of the conjunctiva, *Am J Ophthalmol* 107:337-349, 1989.
58. Jakobiec FA, McLean I, Font RL: Clinicopathologic characteristics of orbital lymphoid hyperplasia, *Ophthalmology* 86:948-966.
59. Sigelman J, Jakobiec FA: Lymphoid lesions of the conjunctiva: relation of histopathology to clinical outcome, *Ophthalmology* 85:818-843, 1978.
60. Knowles DM, Jakobiec FA, McNally L, Burke JS: Lymphoid hyperplasia and malignant lymphoma occurring in the ocular adnexa (orbit, conjunctiva and eyelids), *Hum Pathol* 21:959-973, 1990.
61. Specht CS: Benign and malignant lymphoid tumors, leukemia and histiocytic lesions. In Albert DM, Jakobiec FA, editors, *Principles and practice of ophthalmology,* Philadelphia, 1994, WB Saunders.
62. McNally L, Jakobiec FA, Knowles DM: Clinical, morphological, immunophenotypic, and molecular genetic analysis of bilateral ocular adnexal lymphoid neoplasms in 17 patients, *Am J Ophthalmol* 103:555-568, 1987.
63. The non-Hodgkin's lymphoma pathologic classification project. National Cancer Institute sponsored study of classifications of non-Hodgkin's lymphomas: summary and description of a working formulation for clinical usage, *Cancer* 49:2112-2135, 1982.
64. Ellis JH et al: Lymphoid tumors of the ocular adnexa; clinical correlation with the working formulation classification and immunoperoxidase staining of paraffin sections, *Ophthalmology* 92:1311-1324, 1985.
65. Conlon MR et al: Tumors of the cornea and conjunctiva. In Albert DM, Jakobiec FA, editors. *Principles and practice of ophthalmology,* Philadelphia, 1994, Saunders.
66. Leff SR et al: Unilateral eyelid, conjunctival and choroidal tumours as initial presentation of diffuse large-cell lymphoma, *Br J Ophthalmol* 69:861-864, 1985.

67. Meekins B, Proia AD, Klintworth GK: Cutaneous T-cell lymphoma presenting as a rapidly enlarging ocular adnexal tumor, *Ophthalmology* 92:1288-1293, 1985.
68. Mamalis N et al: Simultaneous bilateral conjunctival and orbital lymphoma presenting as a conjunctival lesion, *Ophthalmic Surg* 19:662-663, 1988.
69. Dunbar SF et al: Conjunctival lymphoma: results and treatment with a single anterior electron field. A lens sparing approach, *I J Radiat Oncol* 19:249-257, 1989.
70. Eichler MD, Fraunfelder FT: Cryotherapy for conjunctival lymphoid tumors, *Am J Ophthalmol* 118:463-467, 1994.
71. Grove AS Jr: Dermoid. In Fraunfelder FT, Roy FH, editors: *Current ocular therapy,* ed 3, Philadelphia, 1990, WB Saunders.
72. Schulze RR: Limbal dermoid tumor with intraocular extension, *Arch Ophthalmol* 75:803-805, 1966.
73. Hutchison DS, Green WR, Iliff CE: Ectopic brain tissue in a limbal dermoid associated with a scleral staphyloma, *Am J Ophthalmol* 76:984-986, 1973.
74. Baum JL, Feingold M: Ocular aspects of Goldenhar's syndrome, *Am J Ophthalmol* 75:250-257, 1973.
75. Gorlin RJ, Cohen MM Jr, Levin LS: *Syndromes of the head and neck,* ed 3, New York, 1990, Oxford University Press.
76. Garner LL: Dermoid of the limbus involving the iris angle and lens, *Arch Ophthalmol* 46:69-72, 1951.

CHAPTER 157

MARIAN S. MACSAI

Surgical Management of Anterior Segment Trauma

Patient Evaluation

The initial evaluation of the patient with ocular trauma is critical, since it will determine subsequent diagnostic and therapeutic decisions that may require swift intervention. The initial examiner may be the only one to obtain a clear view of the posterior pole and optic nerve, which may later be obscured by cataract formation or intraocular hemorrhage. Therefore the examiner must adopt a logical, methodical, thorough approach to each trauma patient. The goals of the initial evaluation should be as follows:

1. Recognition of life-threatening injuries
2. Complete evaluation of the eye and ocular adnexa
3. Identification of other non–life-threatening injuries
4. Identification of concurrent medical conditions
5. Localization of foreign bodies
6. Development of a therapeutic plan

The initial examination is usually performed in the emergency department with the assistance of qualified emergency medical personnel. Stabilization of any potentially life-threatening injuries should obviously take precedence over any ocular injury.

HISTORY

Because the patient frequently is not able to provide a careful history, any available family members or witnesses to the injury should be interviewed. For example, the patient with concomitant head injuries may be unable to cooperate, or the victims of assault may be suffering from shock secondary to the trauma. Children may also be reluctant to discuss the circumstances of an injury because of lack of familiarity with the examining physician or fear of punishment.[1] However, the importance of understanding the circumstances surrounding the trauma cannot be overemphasized. The history obtained should allow the examiner to reconstruct the circumstances of the injury. One must ascertain the activity of the patient at the time of injury, the involved parties, exactly how the injury occurred, and how events progressed after the injury. Specific questions should determine whether the patient was wearing protective eye wear, spectacles, or contact lenses. Samples should be obtained from any possible sources of injury, including foreign bodies or weapons, to allow the examiner to mentally reconstruct the injury. Detailed documentation of all the information obtained, including the source of the information, is critical. Many of these cases result in legal action years after the initial injury. The patient record may become a legal document. In addition, the notes of the initial examiner may be the only source of recall available before legal testimony.

Foreign bodies should always be suspected when examining a patient with anterior segment trauma.[2] If there is any suspicion that there may be a foreign body involved in the trauma, a methodical approach to obtaining key information about the foreign body must be followed (see box).

Determination of the source and composition of the foreign body is critical. It not only determines the potential for ocular toxicity (iron or copper versus glass or plastic) but also influences imaging techniques used to determine the location of a possible intraocular foreign body. A metallic foreign body resulting from metal striking metal is usually sterile because of the heat generated by the striking force. On the other

Foreign body check list

1. Source material
   a. Composition
   b. Activity at time of injury
2. Origin
   a. Size and shape
   b. Energy
   c. Temperature
3. Probable trajectory
4. Risk of microbial contamination

Modified from Freeman HM: Examination of the traumatized eye. In Miller D, Stegman R, editors: *Treatment of anterior segment ocular trauma,* Montreal, 1986, Medicopea.

hand, a tree branch, vegetable matter, or farm instrument carries a high risk for microbial contamination.

In the event of blunt trauma, the examiner must remain alert for possible rupture of the globe. The amount of energy transferred to the globe and orbit, and the physical characteristics of the object, may determine the degree of ocular damage after blunt trauma.[3,4] The globe may rupture externally with a scleral rupture. Scleral rupture occurs most commonly behind the insertions of the rectus muscles. However, in a patient who has undergone incisional keratotomy (radial or astigmatic), the areas of the previous incisions are the most likely point of rupture (Figure 157-1). Internal rupture of the globe may also occur in blunt trauma with or without external rupture. Tears in the ciliary body may result in a hyphema or angle recession. Rupture of the iris sphincter may result in traumatic mydriasis. In the absence of obvious ocular damage, optic nerve contusion may result from blunt trauma to the forehead area.[5] If head and neck injuries are present, risk estimates can be made for associated ocular involvement.[6]

Past ocular and medical history must also be obtained, including any previous ophthalmic surgery or prior ophthalmic medical conditions such as glaucoma or amblyopia, or other conditions associated with diminished visual acuity. Previously decreased vision in a traumatized eye may, in part, explain how the initial trauma could have occurred and be an important prognostic indicator of visual potential.

General medical history must also be reviewed to determine hematologic conditions or anticoagulation medications, the possibility of pregnancy, or any other condition that may influence the choice or use of medications or other types of therapy. The patient's condition immediately before the injury, including the possibility of alcohol or drug ingestion, is important. A blood alcohol level and/or a toxicology screen may be necessary to document the patent's status at the time of the injury. All medications currently being taken by

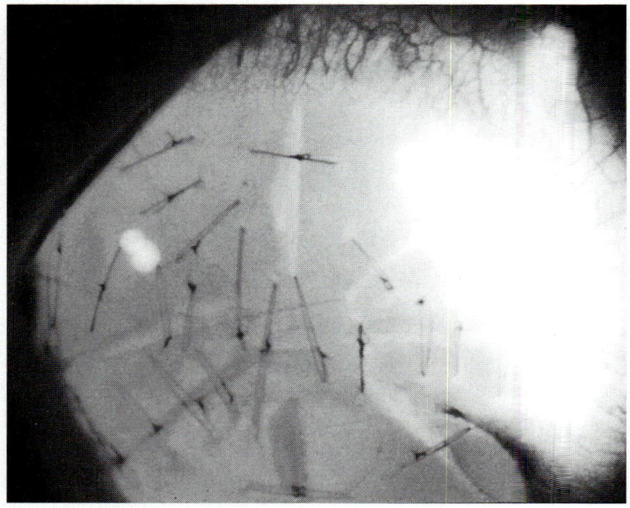

FIGURE 157-1 Indirect illumination of surgically repaired rupture of radial keratotomy incisions after blunt trauma. (Courtesy Stephen S. Lane, MD.)

the patient should be identified. In addition, any medication allergies must be recorded. The patient's tetanus immunization status should be determined and, when necessary, tetanus prophylaxis administered, and one should document any prior treatment received by the patient, including the name and location of the practitioner. The patient should always be questioned about the amount and time of recent food intake, since this information may influence the choice and timing of anesthesia in patients requiring surgery.

External Examination

In any trauma setting, the examiner must remain alert for occult or unsuspected injury. At the same time, one must take care to prevent further injury during the course of the examination. Ideally, the trauma patient should be evaluated in a fully equipped eye examination room. However, this is frequently impractical. Regardless of the physical setting, a complete examination should be obtained if at all possible. With every trauma patient the potential exists for a future medical/legal case in which the examiner may be called to testify. Careful documentation of both the history and physical examination is always necessary. External examination of the face and lids should include documentation of any external injury or laceration. Any abnormal position of the globe relative to other bony structures should be recorded, as should the presence of subcutaneous emphysema. Lid position and function should be recorded. Any particulate matter on the lids or face should alert the examiner to the possibility of a foreign body injury.

VISUAL ACUITY

In the face of any ocular trauma the goal is to obtain the best objective estimate of visual function. This may be performed with the near vision card and a pinhole or standard +2.00 diopter lens. When these are not available any printed material may be used. A newspaper or the examining physician's name tag, finger counting, hand movement, and light perception are all acceptable measurements of initial visual acuity. Desmarres retractors or a lid speculum may be needed to elevate severely swollen lids and evaluate the vision. Topical anesthetic should be used before any retractors or specula, and undue pressure should be avoided to prevent iatrogenic injury in a possible open globe. The patient may require a facial nerve block to avoid squeezing during examination of a ruptured globe, but visual acuity should always be determined before any manipulation. The importance of a baseline visual acuity and pupil examination cannot be overemphasized, since the baseline visual acuity may become an important prognostic indicator in the face of increasing media opacities.

PUPILS, EXTRAOCULAR MOTILITY, AND VISUAL FIELDS

Evaluation of pupillary function should be part of the initial examination of every trauma patient. Pupil examination may indicate intracranial pathology or direct injury to the optic nerve and in the unconscious patient may be the only indicator of visual system function. The presence or absence of a relative afferent pupillary defect must be documented, as should the pupil shape, location, and size. In anterior segment trauma, assessment of relative afferent pupillary defect may require reverse testing. Slit lamp examination may determine the location of iris sphincter tears or an iridodialysis, either of which may account for an aberrant pupil shape or reaction. If there is no evidence of a ruptured globe, extraocular motility may be assessed but may be limited because of periocular tissue swelling. If possible, all patients with ocular trauma should undergo examination of confrontation visual fields at the time of initial examination. This may be difficult in the somnolent or shock patient. As always, the judgment of the initial examiner must be used in assessing the necessity of tests beyond the baseline visual acuity and pupil examination in the triage of trauma victims.

SLIT LAMP EXAMINATION

Ideally, a slit lamp examination should be performed on every injured patient. A portable slit lamp may be necessary for children and patients in cervical collars. Examination should begin with inspection of the lids and conjunctiva. The area and extent of subconjunctival hemorrhage should be recorded, as should the presence of conjunctival chemosis. The presence of corneal lacerations or foreign bodies may raise the suspicion of possible globe perforation. The upper lid should be everted when the globe is thought to be intact in order to remove any retained foreign material that may become embedded in the upper tarsal conjunctival surface. Slit lamp examination of the cornea should note the presence or absence of corneal epithelium. The position and depth of corneal foreign bodies must be documented. If a laceration is noted, the depth and extent of the injury should be documented (Figure 157-2). Seidel testing may be necessary to determine whether a full thickness corneal laceration exists. If no leakage of aqueous is present, gentle pressure should be applied to the globe to delineate any self-sealing perforations. If leakage of aqueous is present, the remainder of the anterior segment should be examined with minimal trauma (Figure 157-3), and no topical medication should be placed in the eye for fear of entry into the anterior chamber. Corneal stromal edema may be present after blunt trauma. However, corneal swelling may also be associated with lacerating injuries of the stroma, and, for this reason, all areas of edema should be carefully inspected.

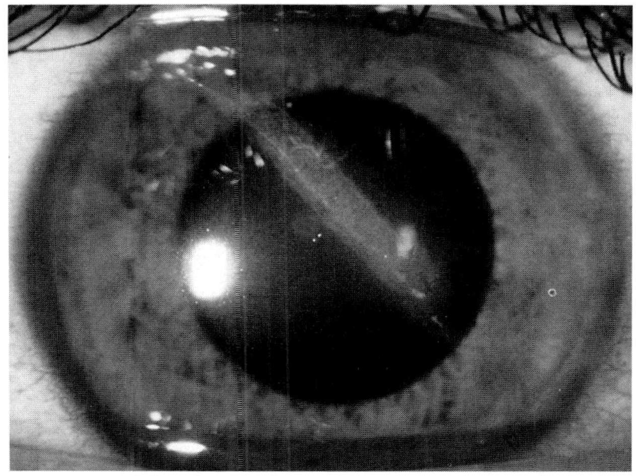

FIGURE 157-2 Slit lamp photograph of an oblique shelved partial thickness corneal laceration. (Courtesy Steven B. Koenig, MD.)

ANTERIOR CHAMBER

Initial examination of the anterior chamber should assess the anatomy of the chamber and contents of the space. The presence of blood in the anterior chamber should be documented in all cases of blunt or penetrating injury. Lens fragments, vitreous, or foreign bodies should also be documented. Foreign bodies that penetrate the anterior chamber but fail to embed in the iris or lens may fall to the 6 o'clock position in

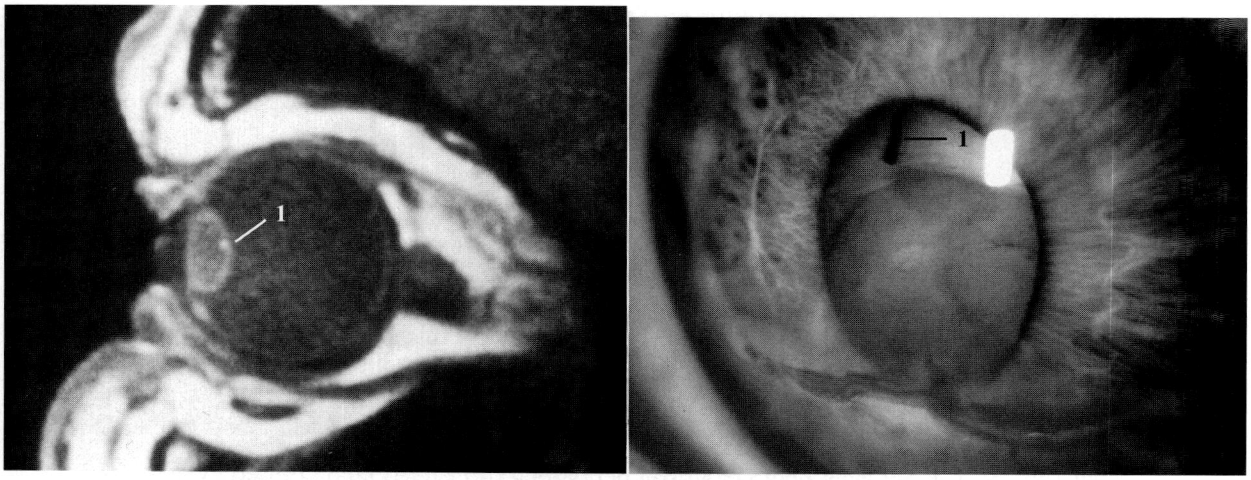

FIGURE 157-6 **A,** Magnetic resonance imaging using surface coils demonstrates an intralenticular foreign body *(1),* which is seen as a small, white hyperintense signal in the vicinity of the posterior capsule. **B,** Slit lamp examination of the same patient as in **A** with a corneal laceration. Oblique view through the lens demonstrates the same intralenticular foreign body *(1).* (Courtesy Steven B. Koenig, MD.)

out concomitant trauma. Conjunctival hemorrhage or chemosis may be the only damage from blunt trauma to the anterior segment. However, one must always suspect an occult ruptured globe in the face of low intraocular pressure, vitreous hemorrhage, conjunctival chemosis, limited ocular motility, or diagnostic imaging suggestive of a ruptured globe, and, if present, exploration of the globe is indicated. Treatment of blunt trauma to the conjunctiva resulting in subconjunctival hemorrhage includes observation and lubrication. A direct blow to the cornea may result in a corneal abrasion. Treatment of corneal abrasions includes application of a broad-spectrum antibiotic drop or ointment, the use of a cycloplegic agent, and pressure patching or the application of a bandage contact lens.[15,16] Recent studies have suggested that occlusive patching may not be necessary in the management of corneal abrasions; topical antibiotics with a collagen shield may be adequate.[17] Localized corneal contusions may result from direct focal mechanical deformation of the cornea and cause localized corneal edema. For example, a BB gun injury may cause a ring of corneal edema.[18] The acute appearance of corneal edema may be alarming. However, the injured corneal endothelium usually recovers or is replaced by adjacent endothelium. Depending on the size of the edematous area, visual recovery may take weeks to months. Numerous therapeutic modalities, including topical corticosteroids, topical pressure lowering agents, and hypertonic salt preparations, have been suggested but remain of uncertain usefulness.

Hyphemas

Hyphemas may result from blunt or penetrating injury. Most hyphemas (up to 90%) result from tears in the anterior face of the ciliary body with disruption of the major arterial circle and its branches.[19] Other sources include ruptured iris vessels, cyclodialyses, iridodialyses, or direct severing of the ocular vasculature in penetrating trauma.[20] Maximum clot formation is usually achieved at 4 to 7 days after injury. Fibrinolysis then begins leading to clot dissolution. Red blood cells and the by-products of fibrinolysis exit the anterior chamber through the trabecular outflow pathways. The major complications of traumatic hyphema are glaucoma and corneal blood staining. Patients with sickling hemoglobinopathies (AS, SC, and others) may develop glaucoma after a relatively small hyphema and are highly susceptible to optic nerve damage and occlusion of the central retinal artery with mild or moderate elevations of intraocular pressure. Corneal blood staining is associated with larger hyphemas, recurrent hemorrhage, and long-term increase in intraocular pressure.

After a careful history and complete eye examination are performed, laboratory studies should be performed as dictated by the history. African American patients should have a sickle-cell preparation and hemoglobin electrophoresis, and patients with bleeding disorders may require liver function tests or coagulation studies. Before using aminocaproic acid (Amicar), baseline blood urea nitrogen (BUN) and creatinine levels should be determined.

Numerous pharmacologic agents have been suggested in the medical management of hyphemas, including cycloplegic agents, topical steroids, and antifibrinolytic agents such as aminocaproic acid. Cycloplegics are generally used to help with patient comfort. Topical steroids do not reduce secondary hemorrhage but are used to treat the associated traumatic iritis. Aminocaproic acid is a synthetic derivative of lysosine and acts as a competitive inhibitor of the factor that converts plasminogen to plasmin. This drug slows fibrin degradation and clot breakdown through inhibition of the production of plasmin. Theoretically, secondary hemorrhage is less likely to occur if clot breakdown is prolonged. In urban populations with high rates of secondary hemorrhage, it has been shown to be effective in reducing the risk of secondary hemorrhage.[21-25] However, Volpe et al found that aminocaproic acid did not significantly lower the rate of secondary hemorrhage in a predominately Caucasian population.[26] Volpe also found that visual outcome in the Caucasian population depended more on concurrent injuries than on recurrent hemorrhage, and, therefore he does not advocate the routine use of aminocaproic acid for uncomplicated cases in similar populations.

Oral prednisone (40 mg/day) has been shown to be as effective as aminocaproic acid in lowering the rate of secondary hemorrhage in one recent study.[27] Aminocaproic acid (50 mg/kg by mouth every 4 hours, up to 30 g/day for 5 days) is associated with side effects, including nausea, vomiting, and postural hypotension. Contraindications include clotting disorders, pregnancy, cardiac, liver, and renal disease. None of these studies have successfully demonstrated a decreased risk in the acute rise in intraocular pressure from rapid clot lysis. Controversy also exists regarding a need for hospitalization of these patients. Several studies have demonstrated no significant difference with the respect to rate of secondary hemorrhage or clinical outcome when patients were treated on an ambulatory basis.[28,29]

Currently, outpatient care is recommended for most patients with uncomplicated traumatic hyphemas with minimal associated systemic or ocular trauma. Medical treatment of traumatic hyphemas must be individualized, because certain populations appear to be at greater risk for developing complications. Treatment protocols should consist of eye protection with a metal shield, avoidance of salicylates and nonsteroidal antiinflammatory agents, activity restriction, elevation of head position, and use of a topical cycloplegic and steroid agent (prednisolone acetate every 2 hours while awake). If risk factors are present, the patient should be admitted to the hospital and given aminocaproic acid.

Despite medical management, up to 5% of hyphemas may require surgical intervention.[30] Surgical intervention for hyphemas may be fraught with complications and should be avoided whenever possible. Major complications include iris or corneal damage, lens injury, and the creation of additional bleeding.[31] The indications for surgical intervention include elevated intraocular pressure, blood staining of the cornea, or total hyphemas for more than 10 days' duration. The actual timing of the operation is controversial. However, clot evacuation is most easily performed after clot retraction (4 to 7 days). To prevent optic atrophy, surgical treatment may be indicated if the intraocular pressure averages greater than 50 mg Hg for 5 days or greater than 35 mm Hg for 7 days. If the blood is in direct apposition with the endothelium, corneal blood staining may occur with an average intraocular pressure greater than 25 mg Hg for 6 days. However, patients with sickling hemoglobinopathies may require earlier intervention, and optic atrophy may occur after 24 hours if the intraocular pressure is greater than 24 mm Hg.

The goal of surgical intervention is to remove circulating red blood cells that may be obstructing the trabecular meshwork and to remove as much of the clot as possible. A paracentesis and anterior chamber washout is the simplest and most effective procedure. Two small perilimbal paracentesis tracts are made in the 2 and 10 o'clock meridians, while an irrigation cannula is placed through one paracentesis track with the intention of washing out the clot through the other paracentesis track. The second paracentesis tract may be enlarged and an automated irrigating, cutting, and aspiration instrument (mechanical vitrector) may be introduced into the anterior chamber. This instrument may be used to surgically remove the clot by both cutting and aspiration. The use of an irrigation sleeve will keep the anterior chamber formed during this procedure. This is the most atraumatic and effective method for removing the entire clot.

Other techniques involving an irrigation and aspiration unit without cutting have been recommended. However, most clots are too thick to be removed by this method. Clot expression through a large limbal wound is also possible. However, this requires a large limbal incision, and the clot frequently must be expressed by placing undue pressure on the anterior segment. Filtration surgery may be necessary to control the intraocular pressure at a later date. Therefore care should be taken to avoid manipulation of the conjunctiva during this procedure. Active intraoperative bleeding may be controlled with tamponade to elevate the intraocular pressure, or direct tamponade may be achieved using cold sodium hyaluronate injected into the anterior chamber in the area of bleeding. Pressure should be applied until the bleeding stops and there is adequate time for clot formation. However, excessive pressure on the globe may potentiate further optic atrophy. When a viscoelastic is used for this purpose, it must be very carefully removed at the end of the procedure to prevent further postoperative intraocular pressure rises.

Corneal wounds should be closed with interrupted 10-0 nylon sutures, the knots of which should be buried in the tissue and not the wound. A no-touch technique of passing the 10-0 nylon suture will avoid unnecessary trauma to the anterior segment. Postoperatively, patients should remain hospitalized at bed rest and be carefully monitored for intraocular pressure control and recurrent bleeding.

Foreign Bodies, Conjunctival or Corneal

Patients injured by foreign bodies in their cornea or conjunctiva frequently present with signs of blurred vision, photophobia, and foreign body sensation. If the foreign body contains iron, a rust ring may be evident in the cornea. If the foreign body has been present for more than 24 hours, a stromal infiltrate, which is usually noninfectious, may appear. However, one must always suspect microbial keratitis, especially in the presence of organic foreign matter. A corneal foreign body can usually be extracted at the slit lamp using topical anesthetic. A disposable 25-gauge needle under high magnification can be used to dislodge the foreign body. Before removal, the depth of the foreign body should be ascertained to determine possible perforation into the anterior chamber. If corneal perforation is suspected, a Seidel fluorescein test for aqueous leakage should be performed at the slit lamp. Gentle digital pressure on the eyelid may be required to demonstrate aqueous leakage in the presence of a self-sealing wound.

Perforating corneal foreign bodies are best approached in the operating room, where microscopic magnification, complete instrumentation, and materials such as sutures, viscoelastic agents, and tissue glue are available. A deeply embedded corneal foreign body may be removed by extending the entry site or by extracting it via the anterior chamber using intraocular foreign body forceps through a limbal incision 90° away. The incision should be placed to avoid traversing over the anterior lens capsule with instruments if at all possible. Preoperative administration of pilocarpine 1% may facilitate this and prevent possible damage to the lens by surgical instruments or the foreign body. Any foreign body removed from the cornea should be cultured if a potentially infectious infiltrate is evident, or if the foreign body is organic matter.

In the absence of perforation, a cycloplegic and broad-spectrum antibiotic ointment with pressure patching is customary. However, in a partial thickness laceration or microperforation, patching does not allow frequent application of topical medication and may place unnecessary pressure on the globe.[32-36] Therapeutic soft contact lenses may be used in the management of partial thickness corneal lacerations, or minute leakage because of a microperforation. Injuries such as these may be easily sealed with a large soft contact lens, fit slightly steep. The lens should be left in place for the first 48 hours, during which time the patient should be given frequent broad-spectrum topical antibiotic drops and cycloplegia. Pharmacologic suppression of aqueous production may encourage wound healing. As long as the anterior chamber is formed, this method is acceptable. After 48 hours the lens may be removed to assess the wound seal. If the anterior chamber is not formed, application of tissue glue or a lamellar patch graft may be indicated. Long-term shallowing of the anterior chamber may result in the formation of peripheral anterior synechiae.

Tissue Adhesive

Corneal perforations less than 2 mm in diameter may require the application of tissue glue to seal the wound. This technique is especially useful when there is a microscopic area of tissue loss. Tissue glue (cyanoacrylate) has not been approved by the United States Food and Drug Administration (FDA) for use in the eye. However, it has been used extensively by corneal surgeons over the past two decades to seal small perforations. Several glues, such as Histoacryl (Brown) and Buerylate (Ethicon), polymerize on contact with liquid. After polymerization the glue creates a rough surface; therefore it must be applied sparingly. The tissue glue will only adhere to areas of the globe that are dry and devoid of epithelium. Application techniques include a drip technique or the use of a syringe. Alternatively, a polyethylene disk may be placed on the end of an applicator stick with ophthalmic ointment. The glue is then placed on the opposite side of the polyethylene disk and applied to the area of perforation.[37] Tissue glue has antibacterial properties that make corneal infection rare in its presence. However, a surrounding infiltrate is commonly seen. After the application of tissue glue, a therapeutic contact lens must be placed to avoid rubbing of the glue against the conjunctival surface and significant patient discomfort. Frequent application of broad-spectrum topical antibiotic drops is recommended while the glue remains in place. The most frequent complication with tissue glue is patient discomfort. However, tissue loss may occur if the glue comes off while adherent to part of the underlying tissue. This is most commonly seen when tissue glue is applied liberally to a descemetocele.

Surgical Management

After physical examination of the wound and diagnostic imaging to locate any possible intraocular foreign bodies, surgical management is indicated in wounds greater than 2 mm or in any area of tissue loss. Goals include restoration of optimal visual function, restoration of normal anatomic relationships, and the prevention of glaucoma, amblyopia, or posterior segment adverse outcomes. To accomplish these goals, the ophthalmologist must have a surgical plan that includes adequate preparation of the ocular surface, conservation of tissue, and minimization of iatrogenic trauma. However, the surgeon must also be prepared to abandon any preconceived plan if events during the operation warrant a change.

PREVENTION OF TRAUMATIC ENDOPHTHALMITIS

Penetrating injuries result in culture-proven endophthalmitis in 2% to 30% of all cases. These include patients with and without retained intraocular foreign bodies.[38-42] In the absence of definitive endophthalmitis at the time of presentation, prophylactic antibiotics are recommended in cases of penetrating ocular trauma. In some cases, posttraumatic endophthalmitis may be the symptom that causes the patient to seek care. In other instances, endophthalmitis becomes a complication after surgical repair of the trauma. Rates of postoperative infection after trauma vary from 2% to 17%.[39] However, rural injuries have produced endophthalmitis in up to 30% of cases.[43] *Bacillus* species are commonly identified after injuries involving farm materials and have a universally poor outcome.[44] Prevention of posttraumatic endophthalmitis is the goal. However, the diagnosis must depend on a high index of suspicion by the clinician. After trauma, endophthalmitis may be obscured by consequences of the trauma itself, such as pain, swelling, redness, media opacity, and loss of vision. A recent study by Affeldt et al demonstrated that the injury to endophthalmitis interval is shorter in more virulent species such as bacillus (1.4 days) and longer in less virulent species such as fungi (57 days).[45] This study demonstrates the importance of immediate intervention in cases of suspected endophthalmitis. Diagnosis ultimately rests with the demonstration of infective organisms in the eye by appropriate cultures and stains. Any foreign bodies or tissue removed from the wound should be cultured on blood agar, chocolate agar, and Sabouraud's agar and placed in thioglycolate broth to identify any possible organisms. Direct inoculation of blood culture bottles with aqueous and vitreous samples has documented a 90% recovery rate.[46] Traumatic endophthalmitis is frequently caused by gram-positive cocci, with *Staphylococcus epidermidis* accounting for the majority of these cases. Most gram-negative organisms are a *Proteus* species; *Pseudomonas* is less common.[47] Fungi are an uncommon cause. However, suspicion must be high in trauma involving vegetable matter. Traumatic endophthalmitis is unique because of the high incidence of *Bacillus species,* in particular *B. cereus,* as the causative organism. *B. cereus* is the single most destructive organism encountered in the eye. Clostridia are uncommon after trauma.[48,49]

SELECTION OF ANTIBIOTICS AND ROUTE OF DELIVERY

The routine use of intravenous, periocular, and topical antibiotics is indicated in virtually all cases of penetrating ocular trauma. The duration of intravenous antibiotic course has differed in recommendations varying between 3 and 5 days to between 10 and 14 days.[50] The toxicity of intravenously administered antibiotics is well characterized; appropriate monitoring of blood levels will minimize potential adverse effects. One must consider the bacteriocidal properties of the antibiotic and the spectrum of antimicrobial coverage, the potential toxicity, the patient's age, and renal function in the selection of antibiotics. In the case of trauma, *Bacillus* species must be covered. The therapeutic benefit after intravenous injection should be considered, and a drug must be selected with good ocular penetration of the blood retinal barrier. Patients with penetrating trauma should be closely followed in an inpatient setting to facilitate prompt diagnosis and intervention in the face of endophthalmitis. A combination of topical and systemic agents have been recommended by Dhaliwal and Meredith[51] (see Box). Ceftazidime is a third-generation semisynthetic cephalosporin with excellent coverage for gram-negative organisms. Ceftazidime penetrates into the vitreous cavity after intravenous administration, and concentration in the vitreous cavity of the inflamed aphakic vitrectomized eyes is nine times the MIC for *Pseudomonas* 2 hours after infusion.[52] Studies of gram-negative endophthalmitis have demonstrated that almost all organisms involved were susceptible to ceftazidime, eliminating the advantage in spectrum of coverage previously attributed to the aminoglycosides.[53]

Prophylactic antimicrobial agents in anterior segment trauma

Intraocular (optional)

Vancomycin 1 mg/0.1 ml
Ceftazidime 2 mg/0.1 ml

Periocular

Vancomycin 25 mg
Ceftazidime 100 mg

Topical

Vancomycin 50 mg/ml
Ceftazidime 50 mg/ml
Cycloplegic

Systemic

Vancomycin 1 gm IV q12h
Ceftazidime 1-2 gm IV q8h

Modified from Dhaliwal RS, Merideth TA: Endophthalmitis. In Charlton JF, Weinstein GW, editors: *Ophthalmic surgery complications: prevention and management,* Philadelphia, 1995, Lippincott.

Ceftazidime is currently the recommended drug of choice, since it does not have the systemic toxicity seen after high intravenous doses of many aminoglycosides. Gentamicin may cost less than ceftazidime and may be more cost-effective in young patients with normal renal function. However, in the elderly or patients with impaired renal function, ceftazidime is the drug of choice. If cost is not a factor, ceftazidime offers the increased benefit of penetration into the vitreous cavity with a significantly lower risk of side effects.

Vancomycin is a complex glycopeptide that inhibits cell wall assembly in addition to RNA synthesis. Vancomycin is well established as the drug of choice for gram-positive endophthalmitis because it covers essentially all staphylococcal organisms, *Streptococcus, P. acnes,* and *Bacillus.*[54] However, vancomycin has essentially no gram-negative coverage. An additional agent for initial intravenous injection is required to cover these organisms. Vancomycin may have systemic toxicity when used in high intravenous dosages. When vancomycin is used concomitantly with other aminoglycocides, such as gentamicin, it has an additive toxic effect.

While some authors recommend the routine use of intraocular antibiotics in the face of penetrating trauma, this treatment remains controversial.[55] When there is no direct evidence of endophthalmitis at the time of primary surgical repair, one must consider the possible toxicity of antibiotic injection in the face of no obvious infection. The risk of intravitreal injections, including mechanical trauma and dosage errors, may be greater than the benefits of prophylaxis.

However, the presence of an intraocular foreign body might alter this approach; Brinton et al have shown an 11% incidence of endophthalmitis in the presence of an intraocular foreign body.[39] In addition, intraocular foreign bodies carry a much higher degree of *Bacillus* endophthalmitis. Therefore an argument may be made for prophylaxis by intravitreal injection in all cases of intraocular foreign body as long as this prophylaxis is effective against *Bacillus cereus.* An intravitreal injection of ceftazidime and vancomycin will provide coverage for *Bacillus* species with good broad-spectrum coverage against other gram-positive and gram-negative organisms. Antifungal coverage is not recommended prophylactically. However, this regimen must be altered if fungi are observed on a fresh smear of vitreous or aqueous, or if a fungal culture is positive. In the case of a positive fungal culture, 5 μg of amphotericin may be injected intravitreally and added to the intravenous drug regimen.

ANESTHESIA AND PREPARATION OF THE EYE

Regardless of history or laboratory tests, all patients should be managed with safeguards appropriate for human immunodeficiency virus (HIV) infection or hepatitis. Repair of perforating ocular injuries requires general anesthesia in almost all patients, since the presence of a laceration would be a contraindication to retrobulbar anesthesia. However, if medically contraindicated, or in selected cases, topical or local anesthesia may be appropriate. Injection into the retrobulbar or peribulbar space may increase the intraocular pressure and risk extrusion of the intraocular contents. If, indeed, general anesthesia is employed, a nondepolarizing muscle relaxant is recommended to avoid the possible co-contraction of the extraocular muscles and further increase in the intraocular pressure. Patients should be brought out of general anesthesia and extubated with great care to prevent "bucking" on the endotracheal tube and emesis in the immediate postoperative period.

The eye is prepped and draped in a sterile fashion, using extreme care to avoid iatrogenic trauma or extrusion of the intraocular contents. An adherent barrier (Johnson & Johnson 1272) may be applied to the lashes and cut open along the interpalpebral fissures to simultaneously expose the globe and cover the lashes. A lid speculum should be placed cautiously to avoid pressure to the globe. Jaffe wire lid specula with rubber bands to provide fixation and the Schott wire lid speculum both provide good exposure with little or no pressure on an open globe. If a speculum cannot be placed, 4-0 silk lid retraction sutures may be used. Placement of bridal sutures can apply untoward pressure and cause chamber flattening and tissue incarceration.

In a controlled operating room setting, using an operating microscope, the surgeon must initially inspect the wound and proceed with closure.

CORNEAL LACERATION REPAIR

Corneal wounds greater than 2 mm in size or those involving any tissue loss must be closed surgically. Careful inspection of the wound should be performed initially to delineate any perpendicular versus shelved areas of the incision. At this time the laceration should be explored to remove any foreign materials. Cultures should be performed of the wound and any foreign bodies. Prompt, secure wound closure is especially important in large lacerations (greater than 2 to 3 mm), displaced wounds, or wounds with loss of corneal, iris, or lens tissue. Surgical closure should proceed in a timely manner to decrease the risk of endophthalmitis, avoid tissue necrosis, and decrease patient discomfort. The micromechanical effects of a penetrating injury may drastically alter corneal topography so that a number of different strategies must be available to repair the cornea and minimize scarring. The overall goal is to restore the native corneal contour. In doing so one must minimize the postoperative astigmatism and corneal scarring. Every corneal laceration should be approached with these concepts in mind, and the surgeon should neither preclude the future necessity of penetrating keratoplasty nor allow this eventuality to decrease the care used in primary wound closure.

The goal of corneal suturing is to make the wound watertight with minimal scarring and to reconstruct the native nonastigmatic corneal contour. Monofilament 10-0 nylon suture material on a fine spatula–designed microsurgical needle is used for corneal suturing. A bicurved needle with a small radius of curvature will aid in passing short, deep bites. A needle with a larger radius of curvature (160°) will result in larger bites or longer passes, which are needed in the corneal periphery. Corneal sutures should be approximately 90% deep in the stroma and of equal depth on both sides of the wound. Shallow sutures may cause internal wound gape, and asymmetric sutures may result in wound override. Full-thickness sutures may allow the suture material to act as a conduit for microbial invasion and subsequent endophthalmitis formation. If at all possible, suture bites through the visual axis should be avoided. If necessary, one should attempt to minimize scarring in the visual axis. This may be accomplished by using short, small suture bites.

When passing corneal sutures, the tip of the needle is placed perpendicular to the corneal surface, and the needle is rotated through the wound along its curvature exiting perpendicular to the cut surface. All knots should be trimmed short and superficially buried in the stroma, on the side away from the visual axis. The ends of the buried knot should be directed away from the surface to facilitate subsequent removal. The suture should be tied using the smallest possible knot to facilitate burying of the surgical knot in the tissue. A granny-style slip knot allows for controlled closure of the wound and is small enough to be buried easily (Figure 157-7).[56] The surgical knot should not be buried in the wound to prevent posterior wound gape.

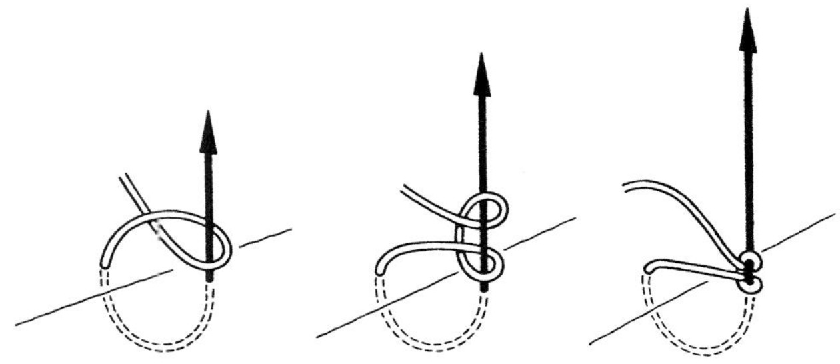

FIGURE 157-7 Slip knot for controlled suture tension. After the initial throw a slip knot may be formed. One end is pulled vertically while the other is pulled horizontally to tighten the suture to the desired tension.

Different techniques must be used when suturing a corneal laceration as opposed to a corneal incision. The surgeon must avoid override of the tissue. In perpendicular incisions, tissue override is produced if the entry and exit sites are of unequal depth, or if the suture bites on either side of the laceration are of different lengths. Therefore, deep passes of equal depth are necessary for good tissue apposition. In a perpendicular wound, the length of each suture pass should be equal as measured from the anterior surface of the cornea. In an oblique incision this technique will result in tissue override (Figure 157-8). To avoid this problem, the deepest passage of the suture should be of equal lengths from the posterior aspect of the wound, not the anterior aspect. The distance from the needle entry to the posterior edge of the oblique incision is gauged, and the needle is passed to exit the stroma, past the anterior chamber entry site. Using this technique the suture may appear to be asymmetric from the anterior or epithelial perspective. However, from the posterior perspective of the wound, the suture is symmetric.[57] If the perpendicular area of the laceration is closed first, the oblique area will appose and minimal suture tension will be required. Therefore these sutures may be tied with enough tension to appose the cut surfaces but should not be tight enough to compress the surrounding tissue.

If at all possible, the iris should always be released from incarceration in the corneal wound. The iris may be pushed posteriorly using a viscoelastic agent or iridodialysis spatula to avoid incarceration of iris stromal fibers into the corneal laceration. Iris should not remain in contact with the corneal laceration, since

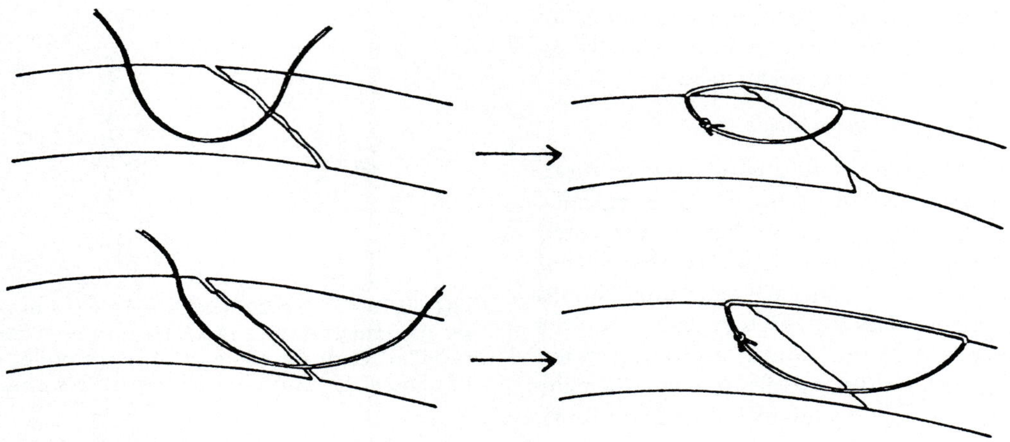

FIGURE 157-8 Suture placement for corneal lacerations. If the suture enters and emerges equal distance to the anterior wound, the stitch will be asymmetric and encompass only part of the overriding wound margin. If the entry and exit sites are equal distance to the posterior aspect of the wound, the wound will appear asymmetric from the anterior surface. The sutures should not be overly tightened because this will cause shifting of the wound margins and overriding of the tissue.

endothelial cells may slide off the cornea onto the adjacent iris, with eventual formation of corneal edema around the laceration site.

In closing any corneal wound, one must avoid tissue removal, because this will result in the need for tight sutures that have a significant torquing effect.[58] In a linear laceration the surgeon should inspect the corneal laceration for perpendicular versus shelved portions and close the perpendicular areas first (Figure 157-9). The shelved portions of the wound will then appose properly, requiring minimal suture tension. The perpendicular areas of the incision are closed first with interrupted sutures to allow for reformation of the anterior chamber. It is difficult to judge the correct tension of the initial sutures. These may be left as slip knots and then loosened or tightened after all sutures are in place. Peripheral compression sutures are then placed to close the corneal incision from the periphery toward the central cornea. This technique allows the shelved area of the incision to close spontaneously, requiring fewer sutures.[59]

Management of corneal astigmatism in the face of a corneal laceration is essential. Peripheral compression sutures may be placed to compress and flatten the corneal periphery and, conversely, to steepen the central cornea.[60] The central cornea is closed with gentle, small, short appositional sutures with minimal suture tension (Figure 157-10). If the anterior chamber is not formed, a separate limbal stab incision may be made through which a viscoelastic agent is injected to form the anterior chamber, protect the lens, and keep the iris out of the corneal laceration.

After repair, the anterior chamber may be deepened through a paracentesis track, and the wound should be checked for leaks. Fluorescein (2%) may be used to verify complete wound closure. The integrity of the wound is tested by reforming the anterior chamber with balanced salt solution. High magnification should be used while monitoring the surface of the wound for leakage. Dry cellulose sponges may be placed over the laceration to dry the surface, and areas of wound

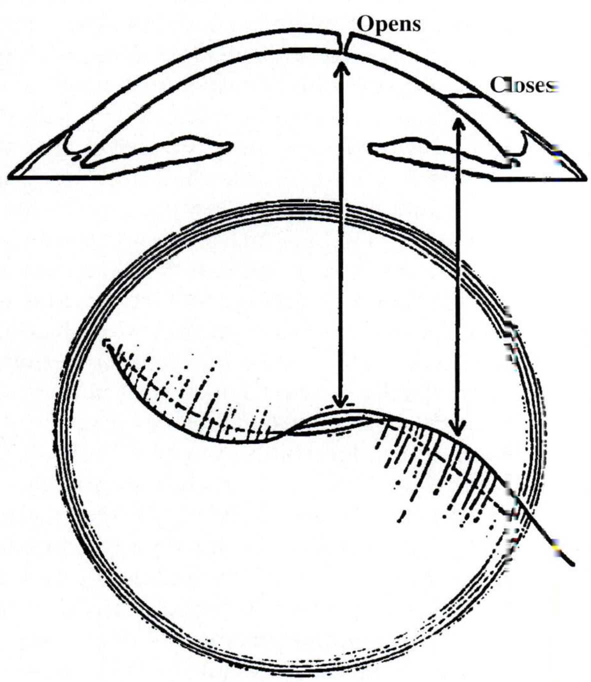

FIGURE 157-9 Perpendicular versus shelved areas of a corneal laceration. Closure of the perpendicular areas of the laceration will allow the shelved areas of the laceration to self-seal, requiring minimal suture tension.

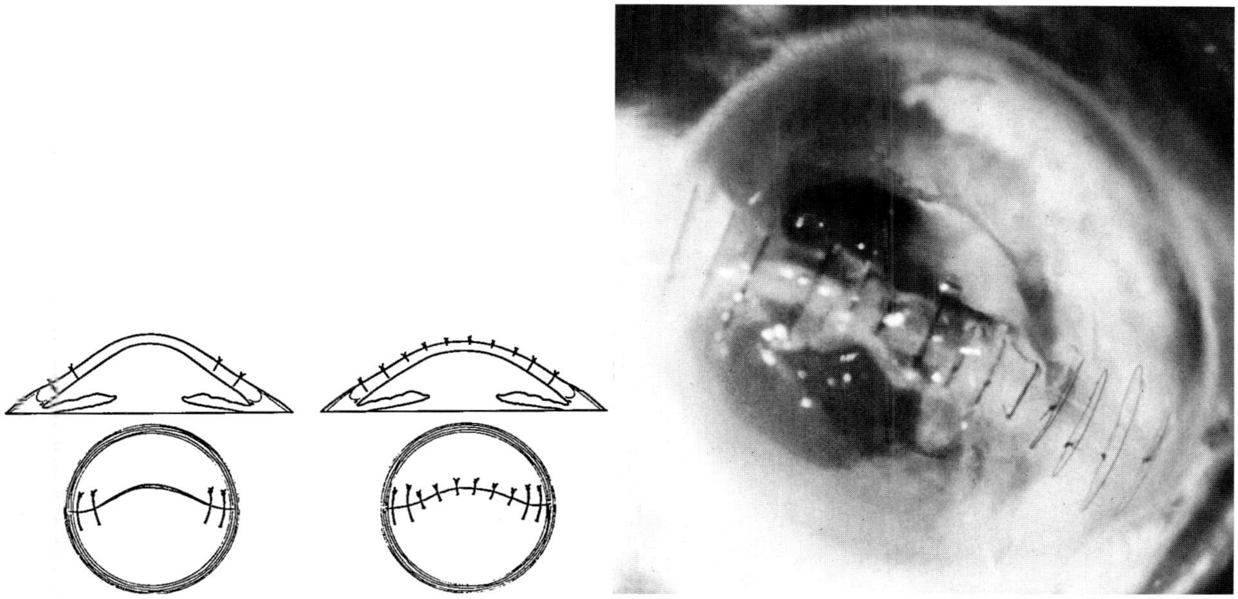

FIGURE 157-10 **A,** Peripheral compression sutures placed to flatten the peripheral cornea. NOTE: Longer bites are used in the peripheral cornea, and small, short appositional sutures with minimal tension are used in the central cornea. **B,** A corneal laceration 1 day postoperatively. Short appositional sutures have been placed centrally in the perpendicular aspect areas of the wound. The peripheral shelved areas have been closed with longer peripheral compression sutures to flatten the peripheral cornea.

leakage may be noted while pressure is applied to the globe opposite the area of the corneal wound.

Suturing the zig-zag incision

In closing a jagged incision, each linear aspect of the incision should be closed individually. It is important to avoid closing the apices first. Closing the linear aspects of the laceration first may allow the apices to self-seal, avoiding additional trauma to that tissue. The use of a slip knot may be invaluable in the repair of these lacerations. When it is necessary to close the apex of a jagged laceration, a mattress suture may be useful (Figure 157-11). A partial thickness incision is made with a guarded diamond blade set at 0.30 mm distal to the flap. The suture is passed from the base of the incision through the flap and back to the groove where it is tied

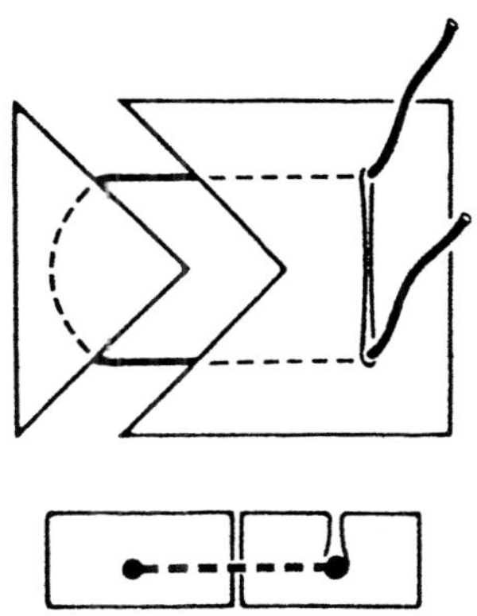

FIGURE 157-11 A purely intralamellar suture may be placed in the apex of a laceration using a mattress suture. A partial thickness incision is made with a guarded diamond blade distal to the flap. The suture is then passed from the base of this incision through the flap and back to the groove, where it is tied.

Stellate lacerations

A variation of the mattress suture technique has been suggested by Eisner to close a stellate laceration (Figure 157-12). A purse-string suture may be placed to avoid trauma to the apices of the laceration. In this technique a diamond knife is used to incise the normal corneal stroma to half stromal thickness depth. A guarded diamond knife may be set at 0.3 mm to make these incisions. A 10-0 nylon suture is then serially passed from the depth of these diamond knife incisions through the adjacent stroma and laceration, and out through the neighboring diamond knife incision. Tightening of suture will appose the central stroma and the apices of the laceration. A slip knot may be used to control the tightness of this suture, and the knot is easily buried at the predetermined depth of the diamond knife incisions. If the suture is too tight, the edges of the wound will be overly compressed, causing

A

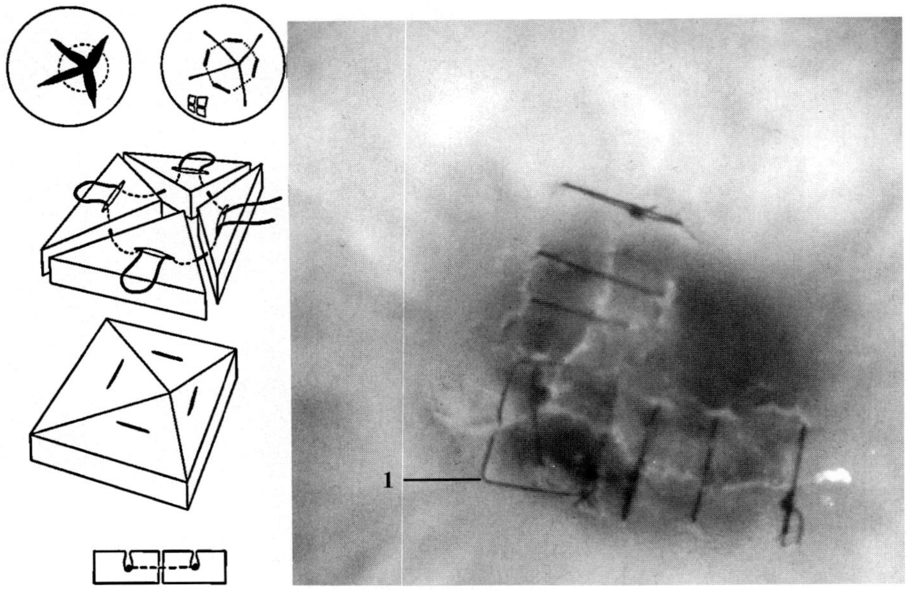

B

FIGURE 157-12 **A,** Closure of a stellate wound with an intralamellar purse-string suture. A partial thickness corneal incision is made with guarded diamond blade set at 0.3 mm. A purse-string suture is passed through these grooves and tightened to approximate the apices of the flaps. **B,** Clinical correlate of closure of a stellate wound with an intralamellar purse-string suture. A stellate laceration is closed with interrupted sutures. The apices are closed with an intralamellar purse-string suture *(1)*. (Courtesy Steven B Koenig, MD.)

forward displacement of the apices with subsequent wound leakage.

Management of tissue loss

In the face of tissue loss that cannot be sealed with tissue glue, a lamellar corneal autograft may be used (Figure 157-13).[61] This technique is useful for wounds that are less than 5 mm in diameter with nonnecrotic stroma. A circular trephine is used to trephine half corneal depth, 1 to 2 mm larger than the area of tissue loss. A corneal bed is then created by lamellar dissection of the stroma around the area of tissue loss. The same size trephine is then moved to the peripheral cornea in an area that was not involved in the injury, and a partial thickness trephination is performed. A lamellar dissection is used to free the corneal autograft, which is then placed over the area of tissue loss and secured into position with four small interrupted 10-0 nylon sutures, the knots of which are buried. If an autologous graft is not possible, donor cornea or sclera may be used. However, an autograft precludes the need for donor tissue and avoids the risk of graft rejection or disease transmission.

CORNEOSCLERAL LACERATIONS

Lacerations extending beyond the limbus and into the sclera should be carefully explored to delineate their full extent. Care must be taken at every stage to

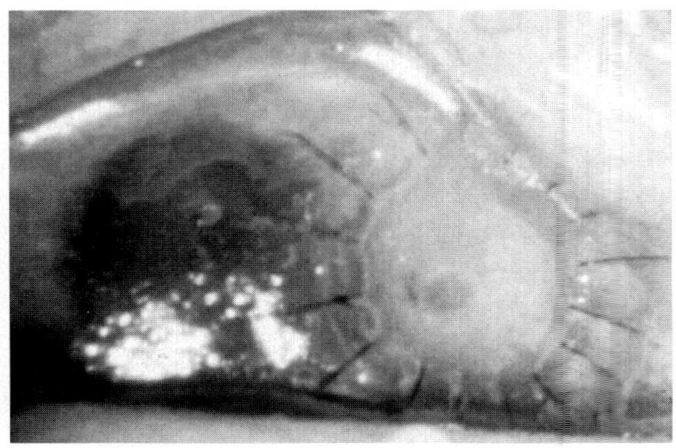

FIGURE 157-13 Use of a lamellar corneal patch graft to close an area of tissue loss. (Courtesy Steven B Koenig, MD.)

prevent iatrogenic damage or further extrusion of intraocular contents. If possible, the limbus is first reapproximated to restore anatomic relationships using 8-0 or 9-0 nylon sutures. Prolapsed iris should be reposited and the corneal wound closed. Injection of a viscoelastic agent may facilitate repositioning of the iris. A localized conjunctival peritomy is carefully made, and wound boundaries are explored, checking for foreign bodies, vitreous, or uveal prolapse. To progressively stabilize the globe and prevent uveal prolapse, scleral sutures should be placed as soon as a new area of laceration is exposed. For scleral suturing a 7-0 or 8-0 polyglactin (Vicryl-Ethicon) absorbable suture may be used. When the wound is gaping, the needle should be completely passed through one end of the wound before making the second pass to avoid distortion of the globe. A laceration that extends behind the extraocular muscles may be closed while an assistant retracts the muscle with a muscle hook. However, the muscle may be disinserted after being secured with a double arm 6-0 Vicryl suture. This may be used to retract the muscle while the full extent of the laceration is closed and to reattach the muscle at its insertion. Vitreous prolapse through the scleral wound is secured with a dry cellulose sponge and cut flush with the sclera. As always, care should be taken to avoid traction on the vitreous. One goal of surgery is to clear the wound of vitreous incarceration. If visualization is good, a vitrectomy instrument may be introduced through the wound. In the case of poor visualization, it is more important to provide a watertight closure of the globe at the time of initial surgery.

Uveal tissue may prolapse through a gaping scleral incision. If possible, uveal tissue should be reposited, since excision will cause severe bleeding. Any tissues removed from the eye should be identified histopathologically; evidence of excised retina carries an extremely poor prognosis. The preferred method of scleral closure with prolapsed uvea involves a step-by-step technique in which the wound is closed from the limbal end with interrupted sutures placed successively posteriorly as the wound is exposed. The sutures are placed closely together to close the scleral tissue over the uvea. An assistant may need to use a spatula to gently press the prolapsed tissue into the eye as the sutures are secured.

IRIS TRAUMA

Penetrating wounds of the anterior segment commonly result in iris injury, either as a consequence of iris incarceration in the wound, blunt trauma, or direct laceration. The most common patterns of iris injury after severe blunt trauma are sphincter tears and dialysis of the iris root.[62] Iridoschisis and iris atrophy may occur as more long-term sequelae. An incarcerated but nonprolapsing iris should rarely be sacrificed. As mentioned previously, during acute repair of the corneal laceration, initial suture placement should avoid incarcerated iris. The iris may be repositioned with viscoelastic material injected through a separate paracentesis track to deepen the chamber and draw the iris away from the cornea. If this technique fails, a fine cyclodialysis spatula may be used to sweep the laceration free of iris.

Prolapsed or exposed iris must be evaluated before excision. Exposed or necrotic iris may be colonized

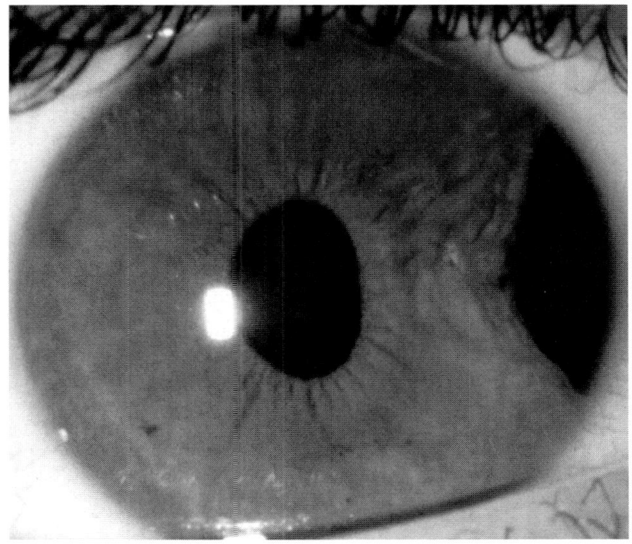

FIGURE 157-14 A traumatic iridodialysis. (Courtesy Mark J Mannis, MD.)

with microorganisms, and repositing this iris may prolong inflammation and increase the risk of endophthalmitis. Iris that has been exposed for only a few hours may be easily reposited. However, severely lacerated iris or that which has been prolapsed longer than 24 hours should be excised. If the iris is reposited, it should be irrigated with balanced salt solution to remove any adherent particulate matter.

Surgical repair of iris damage is usually deferred to a secondary procedure, if the acute corneal injury and hemorrhage reduce visualization. The principal reason for iris repair is to improve visual function, and this may not be assessed adequately until the eye heals from the initial injury and has undergone visual rehabilitation. Aggressive use of topical anti-inflammatory and cycloplegic medications postoperatively reduces the formation of anterior and posterior synechiae.[63]

IRIDODIALYSIS

A traumatic iridodialysis should be repaired only when it is large enough to cause significant, visually disabling glare or diplopia (Figure 157-14).[64,65] The peripheral iris is attached to the sclera after creation of a scleral flap, which is used to cover the external portion of the suture. A double-armed 10-0 polypropylene suture is used to repair the iridodialysis with one or more mattress sutures. The sutures are tied externally under the scleral flap. Both needles of the polypropylene suture are introduced through a paracentesis opening approximately 90° away from the iridodialysis. A long curved spatulated needle should be passed across the iris, avoiding the anterior lens capsule. A viscoelastic agent may be used to unfold the

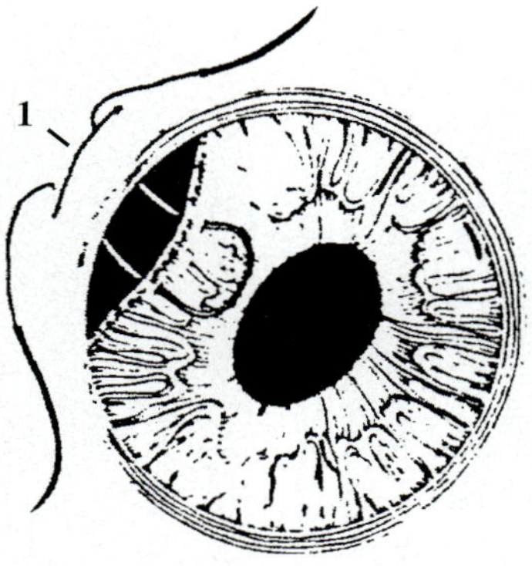

FIGURE 157-15 An iridodialysis repaired with a mattress suture of double-armed 10-0 polypropylene tied externally in a scleral groove *(1)*. Each arm of the polypropylene suture is introduced through a paracentesis tract. The dialyzed edge of the iris may be elevated with sodium hyaluronate. The dialyzed edge of the iris is engaged by each needle of the double-armed suture, and the needle is passed through the sclera into the premade scleral groove. The paracentesis wound is closed with a 10-0 nylon suture. The mattress suture is tied and rotated into the sclera. The previously recessed conjunctiva is repositioned over the buried 10-0 polypropylene suture.

retracted iris and elevate the iris off the anterior lens capsule. The torn edge of iris is engaged by each needle in turn and passed through the sclera into the bed of the scleral flap. The mattress suture is then tied in the bed of the scleral flap with a slip knot, which is then secured with a square knot. The paracentesis wound is closed with a single 10-0 nylon suture and the prolene knot of the mattress suture is rotated into the eye. The scleral flap is then closed with 10-0 nylon interrupted sutures at the corners, and the conjunctiva is closed over the scleral flap (Figure 157-7).[66,67] A scleral flap may be avoided if a groove is made in the sclera, after a conjunctival peritomy is performed (Figure 157-15). The mattress suture is tied and buried in the eye, and the polypropylene suture lies in the scleral groove. The conjunctiva is then brought over the suture and secured in position.

LENS TRAUMA

Lens injury with cataract formation frequently occurs in penetrating ocular trauma. In the absence of perforating ocular trauma, a contusion cataract or dislocated lens may result in visual problems. Initially, vision may not be decreased, although vision may decrease later (days, weeks, or months after the trauma). Fluctuating vision or decreased vision may result from a subluxed or cataractous lens. Subluxation is thought to result from equatorial expansion when blunt trauma is applied to the globe in an anterior to posterior direction, causing shortening in that meridian with concomitant equatorial stretching.[68] This equatorial expansion may cause rupture of the lens capsule in the equator, resulting in lens opacification, or zonular disruption resulting in dislocation or subluxation of the lens. Initial evaluation must include assessment of the vision and assessment of lens capsule integrity, both anterior and posterior. The presence or absence of iridodonesis and/or phacodonesis and the location of the lens will help confirm zonular integrity. If there is marked intraocular inflammation present, it is frequently difficult to separate whether infectious or lens induced. Lens-induced intraocular inflammation may result from traumatic rupture of the lens capsule with release of lens proteins into the aqueous humor. Phacolytic glaucoma may result from phagocytosis of the lens proteins by macrophages in patients with mature cataracts. Glaucoma may result from inflammation or alterations in the anterior segment angle anatomy.

If the lens capsule is intact, many dislocated or subluxated lenses do not immediately threaten vision, and surgery may be performed electively. If there is a large rupture of the lens capsule, the lens material must be removed primarily. If there is a concomitant corneal laceration, it is best to take a step-wise approach. The extent of the corneal laceration is explored, and it is repaired with reformation of the anterior chamber. The lens may then be removed through a separate limbal incision. The torn anterior capsule may be formed into a capsulorrhexis, or a can opener technique may be used. The lens should be removed using an aspiration or phacoemulsification technique, depending on the density of the lens nucleus.

The indications for surgical removal of a traumatic cataract are the same as for any cataract, with some additional indications unique to the traumatized eye. Indications include vision decreased to a level unacceptable to the patient; a need to access, treat, or follow retinal or optic nerve pathology; capsular rupture with lens swelling; lens-induced inflammation; secondary glaucoma caused by the cataract; and other trauma-related ocular conditions requiring surgical treatment. Once the decision has been made to remove the crystalline lens, one must determine whether to place a posterior chamber intraocular lens. There is considerable controversy regarding implantation of a posterior chamber lens implant at the time of primary surgical repair.[69]

In the presence of clean, full-thickness corneal laceration that permits visualization of the iris and lens with a clear laceration of the anterior lens capsule and no vitreous present, it is reasonable to place an intraocular lens if there is no evidence of posterior segment injury or foreign body. If, however, there is significant vitreous in the anterior chamber, indicating zonular rupture, or significant opacification of the

> **Management of traumatic cataract**
>
> ***Indications for staged procedure***
>
> 1. Vitreous anterior to the posterior capsular plain after anterior vitrectomy.
> 2. Corneal opacity or hyphema after repair of the laceration that obscures visualization of the lens.
> 3. Intraocular foreign body posterior to the lens iris diaphragm.
> 4. Moderate or severe posterior segment injury
> 5. Patient's age less than 18 years
>
> ***Indications for one procedure***
>
> 1. Clean full-thickness corneal laceration that permits visualization of the iris and lens.
> 2. Definite laceration or rupture of the anterior lens capsule.
> 3. Zonulocapsular integrity sufficient to support a posterior chamber lens implant.
> 4. No evidence of posterior segment injury or foreign body.

cornea, which obscures visualization of the lens, placement of a posterior chamber lens would be contraindicated. An intraocular foreign body or posterior segment injury would also contraindicate intraocular lens placement in the majority of cases (see box).

The presence of a dislocated or subluxated lens is not necessarily an indication for surgical removal. Medical therapy for a traumatically dislocated lens, including the use of dilating or constricting drugs to minimize astigmatism from the off-center lens, may be helpful. If surgical removal of a traumatic cataract or dislocated lens is necessary, vitreous loss is almost inevitable and should be considered in planning the surgical approach.[70]

Lens dislocation

If the lens is dislocated anteriorly, miotic drops are instilled to trap the lens in the anterior chamber. A soft lens may be surgically aspirated, but this technique carries the risk of losing lens material into the vitreous cavity. A limbal incision may be made through which the lens may be delivered entirely by application of minimal external pressure without introducing instrumentation into the eye. An anterior vitrectomy will invariably be necessary because vitreous is usually present with such severe dislocation. This should be performed using a fiberoptic light pipe. Traction on the vitreous should be avoided. The limbal incision is closed with interrupted 10-0 nylon sutures.

Posterior surgical approach. A posterior surgical approach (pars plana) may be preferable when the posterior capsule is ruptured or when the lens is dislocated or subluxed into the vitreous cavity. A bimanual approach is performed with the infusion line inserted nasally and the cutting and suctioning instrument inserted temporally via the pars plana. For young patients and for patients under 40 years of age, the lens may frequently be aspirated. However, for patients over 40 years of age, ultrasonic fragmentation may be necessary to remove the entire nucleus. After the removal of the nucleus, removal of the cortex and capsule is done with a suction cutter. Then a generous vitrectomy is performed.

Anterior surgical approach. An anterior or limbal approach may be used for a traumatic cataract with an intact posterior capsule and no vitreous in the anterior chamber. With hydration of the cortical material, and because most eye injuries occur in young patients with soft lenses most traumatic cataracts can be removed by an aspiration technique. This is done using a bimanual technique. The entry sites for the two instruments are made approximately 135° apart to facilitate manipulation of the globe. The vitrectomy handpiece (port 0.3 to 0.4 mm) should be placed through one port with maximum suction of 150 mm Hg while the light pipe is placed through a second port. The operating microscope illumination is turned off. The light pipe allows for easy identification of vitreous membranes. The vitrectomy handpiece may be used in a cutting mode (300 to 400 cuts/min) to incise any prolapsed vitreous into the anterior chamber or, using a slower cutting rate (50 cuts/min), the lens material can be cut after it molds into the cutting port. If possible, the vitrector may be turned to the aspiration mode to aspirate any remaining cortical remnants, if there is no surrounding vitreous. In this methodical way, vitreous may be removed from the anterior chamber as identified with the light pipe, and cortical remnants will not be left behind. The light pipe may also be used to retract the iris and inspect the equatorial region. Care should be taken to remove all remaining cortical remnants. Postoperative inflammation caused by remaining cortical remnants may be easily confused with postoperative endophthalmitis.

VITREOUS MANAGEMENT

Vitreous presentation in anterior segment trauma implies zonular rupture or rupture of the posterior capsule. In the face of a clear lens, vitreous presentation is inevitably caused by an occult zonular rupture. Regardless of the cause of presentation, vitreous should be removed from the anterior chamber at the time of primary closure, if at all possible. Vitreous incarceration in the wound may result in prolonged leakage or sliding of the endothelium over the vitreous scaffold with eventual corneal edema. Removal of vitreous may be performed manually or mechanically.

Manually, this is done using dry cellulose sponge, and the vitreous is cut flush with the surface of the eye. This technique is frequently used in corneal scleral lacerations. When the anterior chamber can be clearly visualized, in the presence of a small corneal laceration, limbal incisions may be made to introduce a vitrectomy hand piece and light pipe. The use of a light pipe as a secondary instrument for bimanual vitrectomy will allow clear identification of vitreous membranes if the operating microscope light is turned off. In this way a guillotine cutter may be used to incise the vitreous and avoid traction and at the same time excise anterior chamber membranes that may have formed. The contents of the aspiration cartridge should always be sent for culture and Gram stain.

ANTERIOR SEGMENT INTRAOCULAR FOREIGN BODIES

Most intraocular foreign bodies are magnetic and are associated with activities involving machines or striking metal against metal.[71,72] However, intraocular foreign bodies may also be glass, sand, stone, plastic, or vegetable material. Copper or iron intraocular foreign bodies require immediate and complete removal. Glass, stone, sand, and plastic foreign bodies may be inert and well tolerated. Physical examination, history, and imaging may be used to locate intraocular foreign bodies.

Metallic intraocular foreign bodies must be removed to avoid the risk of toxicity. Iron-containing intraocular foreign bodies result in siderosis.[73] Pure copper and alloys of 80% copper or less lead to chalcosis. Zinc and aluminum intraocular foreign bodies are also toxic and should be removed. When the intraocular foreign body is easily visualized in the anterior chamber, the patient should not undergo pharmacologic dilation preoperatively. General anesthesia is preferred for all patients with penetrating injuries, especially those with an intraocular foreign body. A shelved small caliber incision should be made, depending on the location and size of the intraocular foreign body.

A foreign body that is attached to the iris may be peeled loose using viscoelastic dissection and removed with a forceps. If the intraocular foreign body is metallic, it can be removed using a magnet. An 18- or 20-gauge rare earth magnet is often useful in this situation. Viscoelastic agents frequently prevent damage to the corneal endothelium and lens capsule during intracameral maneuvers with the magnet. If the intraocular foreign body is lodged in the anterior chamber angle, the incision should be made at the limbus 90° away from the foreign body to allow introduction of a forceps to retrieve the foreign body without traversing over the anterior lens capsule and causing inadvertent iatrogenic damage. If the intraocular foreign body is embedded within the lens, it is frequently preferable to remove the lens entirely with the foreign body still lodged within the lens. This technique will prevent possible loss of the foreign body into the posterior chamber. If this is necessary, a scleral fixated posterior chamber implant can be placed as a primary or secondary procedure. If the intraocular foreign body is easily visible within the lens, it may be removed using a magnet or forceps. Frequently the lens may then be aspirated through the rupture in the anterior capsule that was created by the intraocular foreign body. This anterior capsular rupture may be enlarged to form a circular capsulorhexis and allow for the surgeon to proceed with phacoemulsification and removal of the entire lens. If there is a concomitant iridodialysis from the foreign body, this may be repaired through the same incision used to remove the traumatic cataract created by the intraocular foreign body.

Postoperative Care

At the conclusion of surgery, antibiotics are injected subconjunctivally (vancomycin 25 mg, ceftazidime 100 mg). When there is a low suspicion of postoperative endophthalmitis because of penetrating injuries, subconjunctival dexamethasone (12 to 24 mg) may be given. As discussed earlier, the use of intravitreal antibiotics is controversial. For routine penetrating injuries, we currently recommend a 4-day course of intravenous antibiotics combining vancomycin 1 gm IV q12h with ceftazidime 1-2 g IV q8h. Topical fortified antibiotics (vancomycin 50 mg/ml, ceftazidime 50 mg/ml) are administered approximately every hour for the first 48 hours and then the dosage is reduced depending on the postoperative course. Antibiotic therapy is always dictated by culture results. Any sign of new infection is promptly cultured. The use of cycloplegic agents postoperatively should not be forgotten because they are key to the management of iris inflammation. Topical corticosteroids may be useful to minimize postoperative inflammation, but the advantages must be balanced against the risk of possible postoperative infection, especially in wounds contaminated with vegetable foreign matter or obtained in a rural setting. Routinely, steroids are added in moderate doses, prednisolone acetate 1% four times daily, after the potential for infection diminishes. A Fox shield is recommended over the operated eye for the entire course of hospitalization and after discharge for the first 12 weeks postoperatively. For intraocular pressure control, β blockers and carbonic anhydrase inhibitors are used as necessary. The ocular surface is treated as necessary to promote reepithelialization. Lubricants, bandage soft contact lenses, patching, or a tarsorrhaphy may be required to stabilize the ocular surface.

All patients who sustain penetrating ocular trauma should be placed in safety glasses at the time of hospital discharge (polycarbonate lenses) to prevent any possible risk of damage to the noninjured eye.

The pediatric patient presents further challenges to the surgeon in the postoperative course. Care should be taken to minimize the trauma for the child as much as possible. Every attempt should be made to have the parents stay with the child during the course of hospitalization, and the surgeon must take precautions to avoid unnecessary trauma to the child during the dressing of the wound. This may be avoided through the use of a head wrap, or a stoma dressing (stoma adhesive) may be cut and applied to the forehead and cheek. This dressing may be left in place for a number of days. The protective eye shield or patch may be taped to the protective stoma dressing, allowing for frequent removal of the shield. The tape is placed on the stoma adhesive, not the skin, reducing pain and anxiety experienced by the child. In the young child (less than 6 years of age), one must be aware of the possibility of amblyopia development from swelling of the lids or occlusion of the injured eye. These children should be cared for in conjunction with a pediatric ophthalmologist, and, when necessary, occlusion therapy should be instituted to prevent the development of amblyopia.

Suture Removal

Corneal sutures should be removed when loose to prevent possible epithelial breakdown and corneal ulcer or suture abscess formation. In addition, vascularization of the underlying stroma is an indication for suture removal. Corneal sutures may loosen as a result of wound contraction or because they were not tightened appropriately at initial placement. Loose sutures may be identified at the slit lamp and may accumulate mucus and debris. Fluorescein staining may help identify loose sutures. Otherwise, corneal sutures should be removed when fibrosis of the corneal wound is evident on slit lamp examination. In general, this takes at least 3 months. Alternate sutures should be removed initially. Topical antibiotics should be used four times a day for 5 to 7 days after suture removal. One month later, the remaining sutures may be removed. A short course of topical antibiotics should be repeated. However, in the pediatric population, wounds heal much more quickly. In an infant, sutures will need to be removed in a matter of weeks, under sedation.

Visual Rehabilitation

Visual rehabilitation may be performed using spectacles or contact lenses.[74] Initial optical correction should be attempted with spectacles. The use of computer modeling systems for the analysis of corneal topography may be useful. These may allow identification of sutures that are producing excess tissue compression and therefore corneal astigmatism. After adequate wound healing occurs, these compressive sutures can be selectively removed to correct the induced astigmatism and speed visual recovery. If visual recovery is not obtained with spectacles, and if physical examination, including potential acuity meter readings, demonstrate significantly better vision than may be obtained with spectacles, contact lenses should be tried. A rigid contact lens may be desirable after repair of anterior segment trauma because it allows for the treatment of irregular corneal astigmatism without inducing significant vascularization of the corneal lacerations. A soft contact lens has been shown to increase the risk of vascularization of the corneal scars. Penetrating keratoplasty should be viewed as a last resort in the management of corneal scars. Should penetrating keratoplasty be required, anterior segment reconstruction may be performed at that time.

Postoperative Complications

Early postoperative complications include endophthalmitis. When endophthalmitis is a possible diagnosis, aqueous and vitreous samples must be obtained for Gram stain, culture, and sensitivity. The institution of intravitreal antibiotics is the most important aspect of treating bacterial endophthalmitis.[75]

Postoperative hyphemas are more common in patients who have had manipulations of the intraocular tissues. Most hyphemas resorb slowly within the first postoperative week. Elevated intraocular pressure may result from blockage of the trabecular meshwork and may be treated with acetazolamide, β blockers, and aproclonidine. Topical and systemic steroids may also be useful to control intraocular inflammation. Anterior chamber washout is rarely indicated. However, it may be necessary to control elevated intraocular pressure and prevent corneal endothelial cell damage or corneal blood staining. Strict control of the postoperative intraocular pressure is necessary in patients with sickle cell disease or trait.

If the intraocular pressure is unrecordable during the first postoperative day, a wound leak must be suspected. A Seidel test should be performed to rule out an occult wound leak. Pressure patching, aqueous suppression, and bandage contact lenses often can be

lens overcorrection, therefore, serves not only as a potential optical correction but also as an important part of the diagnostic evaluation.

The initial choice of contact lens is dictated by the clinical situation. A large diameter (9.3 to 9.8 mm), high Dk, and increased center thickness lens is often the lens of choice. A large lens is commonly needed for stability on a highly astigmatic surface, whereas a thicker lens is required to limit unacceptable lens flexure, which is also common on irregular corneas. Because these parameters (lens diameter and thickness) limit oxygen permeability and because the traumatized cornea already has a compromised endothelium, a high oxygen-permeable lens is desirable.[1]

Conjunctiva

Before contemplating any reconstruction of the anterior segment, the surgeon should ascertain the condition of the conjunctiva, lids, lashes, and tear film. A healthy supply of corneal epithelial cells is necessary for the long-term health of the eye and for proper optical performance.[2] In anterior segment trauma caused by chemical or thermal injury, it is not uncommon to have significant destruction of both the corneal surface and the surrounding conjunctiva. In cases of depleted limbal stem cells, it is necessary to supply a new source of corneal epithelium before contemplating extensive anterior segment reconstruction.[3] Two procedures—conjunctival limbal autograft and keratoepithelioplasty—attempt to restore the corneal surface with a stable epithelial covering resembling normal corneal epithelium.[4] Donor epithelial cells are eventually replaced by the host epithelium migrating centripetally. If the host epithelium is normal, this poses no problem. When an abnormal ocular surface preexists, the normal donor epithelium is eventually replaced by the abnormal host surface predisposed to chronic epithelial breakdown and possible corneal ulceration.[3]

CONJUNCTIVAL LIMBAL AUTOGRAFT

Conjunctival limbal autograft attempts to resurface the diseased host cornea by transferring autologous limbal epithelial cells to the abnormal eye from a normal fellow eye.[5-7] The conjunctival portion of the graft acts as a carrier for the limbal stem cells. The goals of the conjunctival limbal autograft are (1) a rapidly healing and secure epithelium with minimal tendency for recurrent epithelial defects, (2) a gradual clearing of the cornea with regression of vascularization, and (3) a smoothing of the corneal surface. Use of this procedure is limited to unilateral disease because a healthy supply of autologous conjunctival limbal tissue is required. Unilateral chemical or thermal injury is the most common indication for conjunctival transplantation. Because a superficial keratectomy is necessary before conjunctival transplantation, careful preoperative evaluation with pachometry and slit lamp examination should be performed to determine whether a superficial keratectomy will remove all the significant scarring. The thinnest portion of the keratectomized cornea should rarely be less than 80% normal depth (0.4 mm). If it appears unlikely that keratectomy will yield significant optical improvement, keratectomy should be kept to a minimal depth, just exposing anterior stroma.[5] This avoids excessive graft-host edge thickness discrepancy if a penetrating keratoplasty is done at a later date.

General anesthesia is preferable, since it allows comfortable surgery on both eyes. A 360-degree, 5 mm wide limbal conjunctival resection is performed, followed by a total superficial keratectomy. A superficial keratectomy can be performed with one of many available nitrogen gas-driven drills using a large (2.5 to 5 mm) diamond burr. The nitrogen gas pressure should be kept below the normal recommended level but should be sufficient to maintain a constant smooth rotation of the burr. The drill enables the surgeon to perform a smooth, even superficial keratectomy and can also be used to smooth the sclera and limbal region. (Methods of lamellar dissection are discussed later.) Next, healthy conjunctival limbal tissue is obtained from the intermuscular quadrants of the fellow eye in areas covered by the lids.

KERATOEPITHELIOPLASTY

The clinical usefulness of the conjunctival limbal autograft procedure is limited by the requirement for healthy stem cells from the uninvolved eye. Keratoepithelioplasty uses lenticules of limbal tissue from fresh donor eyes to repopulate the corneal surface when autologous tissue is not available. In this procedure, peripheral cornea is the carrier for the stem cells. Using a disposable Graefe knife, thin saucer-like lenticules of limbal tissue are carved from a freshly enucleated donor eye (Figure 158-1, *A*). The lenticules are then positioned over the limbal region of a previously prepared recipient (as outlined for conjunctival limbal autograft). The lenticules are then sewn to the sclera with two interrupted 10-0 nylon sutures per lenticule (Figure 158-1, *B*). A bandage contact lens is placed at the conclusion of the case. Postoperative care is the same as outlined for conjunctival limbal autograft, except that low dose, long-term topical steroids are necessary to prevent rejection of the donor epithelium.[4,9]

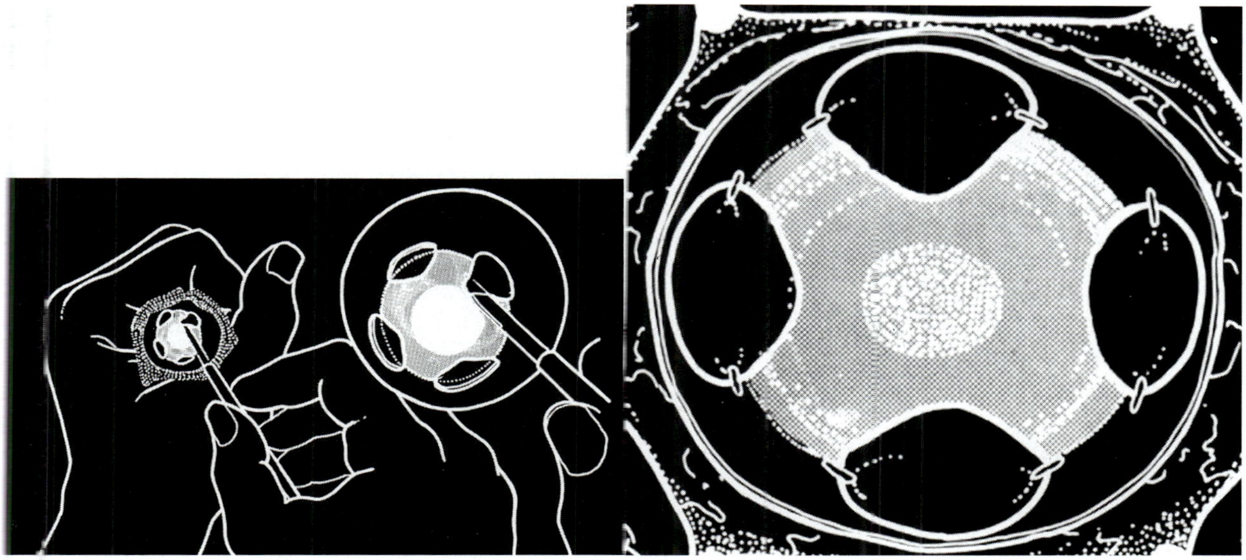

FIGURE 158-1 The keratoepithelialplasty operation is used to supply donor corneal stem cells. **A,** Lenticles are obtained from the donor globe. **B,** Lenticles are sutured into place on the recipient.

Cornea

SURGERY

Patients who do not obtain significant visual improvement with a contact lens typically require surgical intervention. If the decreased vision results from corneal scarring, a keratoplasty (penetrating, lamellar, or rotational) is indicated. If the contact lens intolerance is caused by problems with fitting (e.g., poor stability on a highly astigmatic surface), a refractive procedure (astigmatic keratotomy, wedge resection, etc.) may be indicated.

As discussed in earlier chapters, the goal of penetrating keratoplasty is to improve vision and/or allow visualization or repair of other components of the globe. While it is unusual in anterior segment trauma, it may be possible to obtain reasonable optical results with either a lamellar transplant or a rotational autograft.

ROTATIONAL AUTOGRAFT

If the opacification (scar) is focal and in the visual axis and the remaining cornea is optically clear and healthy, the scar may be rotated out of the visual axis. Preoperative photography or accurate drawings are helpful in determining whether this can be accomplished.[8] In an otherwise normal eye (central pupil), the trephination must be eccentric to move the scar out of the visual axis with rotation (Figure 158-2). The eccentric trephination must be large enough to allow for a clear visual axis after suturing. The advantage of a rotational autograft is avoiding the use of donor tissue, which eliminates the risk of immunologic rejection. Subsequently, the need for long-term immunosuppression (topical steroids) with its attendant side effects is minimal. The surgery obviously does not depend on the availability of donor tissue, and the length of time the globe is open is reduced. While useful, the procedure has several limitations. By rotating an eccentric trephined cornea, there will always be a discrepancy in the interface thickness. The portion of the cornea closer to the visual axis is naturally thinner and is subsequently placed at the thicker periphery. In addition, the normal corneal contour (asphericity) is lost for similar reasons. Finally, the major limitation to rotational autografts is that most scarred and traumatized corneas are not limited to a small central scar and therefore would not be improved with the procedure.

LAMELLAR KERATOPLASTY

Lamellar keratoplasty offers advantages when compared to full-thickness keratoplasty, but, as with rotational autografts, most patients are not appropriate candidates. Anterior segment trauma significant enough to cause visual impediment is often not limited to the anterior stroma or corneal surface. However, in patients who can obtain reasonable vision with a contact lens but who are, for other reasons, poor candidates for lens fitting (e.g., have rheumatoid arthritis or chemical burns), lamellar keratoplasty may offer a viable option. Lamellar keratoplasty is safer

A

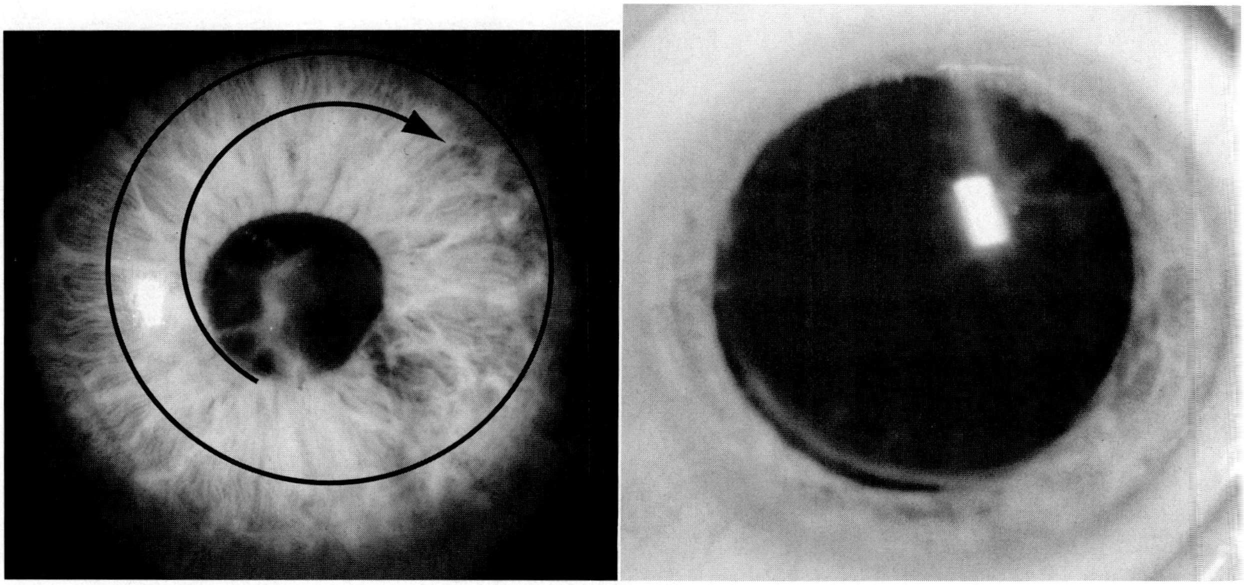

B

FIGURE 158-2 Autorotating penetrating keratoplasty is used if the pathologic area can be rotated out of the visual axis while leaving a clear and nearly distortion-free visual axis. **A,** Wound placement (*circle*) and rotation of the scar. **B,** Postoperative result.

because it is an extraocular procedure (the globe is not opened) and is less likely to present serious immunologic problems.[10] Because only the stroma (and at times the epithelium) is transplanted, the risk of rejection is lowered. The lamellar transplant does process antigenic potential, but the risks for irreversible graft rejection and subsequent endothelial dysfunction are significantly lowered. The advantage of being an extraocular procedure, however, may be lost if other additional reconstructive procedures require an open globe. In addition, lamellar keratoplasty is technically more difficult than full-thickness penetrating keratoplasty. Traditionally, lamellar surgery requires a whole globe and a freehand dissection. Although not in wide use, recent technologic advances with automated keratomes and artificial anterior chambers have eliminated this requirement.

A careful examination must be performed preoperatively to determine the depth and extent of the opacity and to search for focal areas of corneal thinning. The use of optical pachymetry is helpful in that optical pachymetry (as opposed to ultrasonic pachymetry) can measure the thickness and depth of the opacity. Surgery must be timed to the availability of fresh tissue (whole globe). Because of the possibility of inadvertent entry into the anterior chamber and the necessity of converting to a full-thickness procedure, it is advisable to prepare the recipient bed before preparing the donor tissue. The eye is prepared as for penetrating keratoplasty. Because the procedure should be extraocular, the use of a scleral support ring is not necessary. The same guidelines for centration and donor graft sizing used in full-thickness surgery apply to lamellar transplantation. An adjustable-depth trephine (e.g., adjustable obturator, Hessburg-Barron vacuum trephine, Hanna vacuum trephine) is very helpful in limiting the depth of the trephination and reducing the risk of entrance into the anterior chamber. By using a combination of preoperative optical pachymetry and an adjustable trephine, the goal of removing only the scarred stroma can often be accomplished safely. After trephination a lamellar dissection is carried out with an angled blade. The use of either a sharp or a dull blade to carry out the stromal dissection is controversial and left to the preference of the surgeon. A blunt dissection is easier to maintain in the same stromal plane and reportedly lowers the risk of inadvertent entrance into the anterior chamber. A sharp dissection, however, offers a smoother margin and the potential for an improved optical interface. After completion of the host dissection, a moist cellulose sponge or piece of the surgical instrument wipe is placed over the host bed to prevent dehydration, and attention is moved to the donor globe. The goal is to replaced the previously excised corneal tissue with a similarly sized (diameter and thickness) piece of donor tissue. Because the donor tissue is removed from the same side (epithelial) as the host tissue, the same-sized trephine is used on the donor as on the host. Before trephining, the intraocular pressure of the donor globe should be taken (or estimated). If the globe is soft, it may be reinflated with a 30-gauge needle to approximate normal pressure. An overly soft globe will deform during trephining and prevent a good host-donor match. An attempt should be made to approximate the thickness of the removed donor tissue. Unfortunately, the donor cornea is often markedly thicker than the normal cornea. A useful approach is to remove a percent of the donor cornea similar to that of the host.

The use of intraoperative ultrasound pachymetry of the donor globe allows the surgeon to estimate the depth setting of the adjustable trephine. After trephining, the donor tissue is removed as was the host. The host tissue is sutured into the recipient bed using any of the closure techniques outlined in the earlier chapters. Postoperatively, steroids and topical antibiotics are used, but steroids may be tapered more rapidly than typical for penetrating keratoplasty.[8]

PENETRATING KERATOPLASTY

While the previously mentioned techniques are useful, the majority of cases of anterior segment trauma that result in significant corneal scarring require full-thickness penetrating keratoplasty. The goal of penetrating keratoplasty is to supply a clear, optically stable surface and to allow easier access to the anterior segment. Because many cases of anterior segment reconstruction require additional concurrent surgery, the preoperative evaluation must be complete. Attention should be directed to the degree of vascularization, iris and angle abnormalities, the status of the lens, the condition of the retina and vitreous, and the intraocular pressure. Obviously the contralateral eye must be examined. Particular attention must be placed on the overall health of the other eye and knowledge of its refractive status (e.g., aphakic, pseudophakic, highly myopic) to make a logical surgical plan for the traumatized eye.

Uncontrolled intraocular pressure or borderline pressures obtained while the patient is being treated with maximal medical therapy may warrant a glaucoma procedure before further anterior segment reconstruction.[11] In cases of mild to moderate trauma, conjunctival injury, and/or corneal vascularization, a standard trabeculectomy may be attempted. When the degree of trauma precludes a trabeculectomy, an implant drainage procedure (e.g., Molteno, Barvelat, Krupin valve) should be performed. Our current technique is to perform a tube drainage procedure approximately 6 weeks before the proposed reconstruction to allow time for the implant and conjunctiva to heal and to minimize the potential for postoperative hypotony. At the time of seton placement, the tube is tied closed with a nonabsorbable intraocular suture to further reduce the chance of hypotony. This allows us to reassess the intraocular pressure 6 weeks later and determine whether a further pressure reduction is needed. If the intraocular pressure remains poorly controlled, the tube is opened at the time of penetrating keratoplasty. In addition, the absence of hypotony aids in trephination and closed chamber retinal surgery, if performed. At the time of penetrating keratoplasty the suture may be cut to allow aqueous drainage or left tied to be opened by laser lysis at a later date. Unfortunately, the long-term prognosis for maintaining functioning filtration in a trabeculectomy or the long-term graft survival with a drainage tube remains guarded.[12]

Corneal vascularization should be reduced preoperatively. Topical steroids or other immunosuppressive agents may be effective in reducing preexisting vessels. Preoperative laser photocoagulation has met with mixed results.[13,14] If extensive vascularization is present, a separate procedure may be warranted. Conjunctival recession with scleral/limbal cautery is often helpful in reducing vascularization, but it has limited effect on deep stromal vessels. Conjunctival recession and cautery can be performed before trephining (prior to securing a scleral support ring in appropriate cases). In cases of active vessels a partial-thickness trephination allows control of the bleeding vessels before entering the anterior chamber and thus minimizes bleeding into the anterior and posterior chambers. Most bleeding from the trephined bed will stop with minimal waiting. The application of topical 2.5% phenylephrine or irrigation with dilute epinephrine (1:1,000,000 dilution—comparable to intraocular usage) is often helpful.

The use of a scleral support ring, while optional in phakic cases or secure posterior chamber pseudophakic cases, is strongly recommended. Scleral support rings help position the globe, stabilize the eye during trephining, and prevent scleral collapse, particularly during deep vitrectomies. Because most cases of anterior segment reconstruction are associated with the potential for other intraocular procedures, the routine use of a ring is prudent.

The choice of donor and host trephine size is determined by the clinical setting. In most cases, however, donor openings smaller than 7.0 mm do not allow easy access into the anterior chamber and make lens removal and/or intraocular lens insertion difficult. Correspondingly, grafts greater than 8.0 mm have reportedly been associated with a greater risk of immunologic reactions and may predispose to further vascularization. The relative size of the host-donor trephines (host-donor disparity) is also determined by the clinical setting. Donor trephines have varied from the same size in cases of keratoconus (in an attempt to reduce preexisting myopia) to 0.5 mm oversized when transplanting over a retained anterior chamber intraocular lens. Same-sized grafts should probably be avoided in cases of trauma. Our routine has been to perform 0.25 mm oversized grafts (ostensibly same-sized because of the differences in the geometry of the endothelial punch compared to recipient trephining) except in cases with an anterior chamber intraocular lens. Additionally, certain trephines (i.e., Hessburg-Baron vacuum trephine) have a higher propensity to undercut the recipient and effectively produce a larger opening.

Corneal removal, placement, and suturing techniques are discussed in Chapters 130 to 133, and therefore only selected topics will be covered here. At times, corneal opacification may be severe enough to completely preclude visualization of any anterior segment details. In these instances, standard removal of the cornea with transplant scissors has a higher incidence of complications. The use of transplant scissors with a longer, lower blade allows for better visualization of the advancing scissors and may be helpful in avoiding inadvertent cutting of the iris or intraocular lens haptic. Another useful technique is to perform an initial lamellar dissection to the level of Descemet's membrane. This allows better visualization of the anterior segment, and the surgeon can plan the anterior segment reconstruction before opening the anterior chamber. Closure techniques are determined by the degree of vascularization and the preference of the surgeon.

Vitreous and Lens

Since severe ocular trauma is much more common in the young and middle-aged population, most patients will be phakic. In this population a traumatic cataract or, in severe cases, a mixture of lens material and vitreous may be present once the cornea is removed. Because the natural posterior capsule adds support to the open eye (acting like an internal supporting ring), retains the vitreous, and allows for the insertion and support of a posterior chamber intraocular lens, every attempt should be made to maintain the posterior capsule. If the posterior capsule remains intact, a standard "open sky" lens extraction can be performed. Even with a small tear in the posterior capsule, it may be possible to perform an extracapsular extraction and maintain adequate capsule for either capsular or sulcus fixation. Despite what appears to be an intact posterior capsule, it is not uncommon to have some zonular dehiscence. This may lead to anterior vitreous migration and pupillary block. Therefore, it is probably prudent to perform a peripheral iridectomy after lens extraction in all cases of anterior segment trauma.

When the posterior capsule is obviously compromised and lens and vitreous are admixed, a combination lens extraction-vitrectomy is performed. With the availability of modern vitrectomy instruments, intracapsular extraction is seldom performed. The initial attempt should be directed at delivering as much of the lens nucleus as possible. Supporting the nucleus posteriorly with a lens loop may assist in delivery and prevent the lens from dropping back into the posterior cavity. Once the nuclear material is delivered, the remaining cortex and vitreous must be removed. Direct aspiration of the residual cortex is faster than cutting and aspirating with a vitrector. However, pure aspiration can be dangerous and a potential source of vitreous traction. Aspiration, however, does allow the potential of leaving the remaining capsule, which may be adequate to support a posterior chamber intraocular lens. Each case must be evaluated individually. It is probably safe to aspirate cortex over areas of intact capsule or after vitreous removal. If doubt exists, a combination of cutting and aspiration is best. As opposed to the settings used in a posterior vitrectomy, the cutting rate is slower (approximately 240 cpm) and the aspiration higher (100 to 120 mm Hg) when working in the anterior segment. After removal of the remaining cortex, a central core vitrectomy should be performed. The vitrectomy is performed without irrigation to allow direct visualization of the vitreous cavity and to allow the iris diaphragm to drop posteriorly indicating an adequate vitrectomy. The choice of the secondary intraocular lens determines the extent of the vitrectomy. Sutured posterior chamber lenses require a more aggressive vitrectomy than an anterior chamber intraocular lens.

When the posterior capsule is not adequate for either capsular or sulcus fixation, the options for intraocular lens implantation include transsclerally sutured posterior chamber lens, iris-sutured posterior chamber lens, or anterior chamber lens. Current literature does not clearly support the superiority of one approach compared to another.[15-19] An anterior chamber lens is technically the easiest and associated with the shortest operating time. However, it is not appropriate for cases with more than minimal angle abnormalities and requires an open angle and an intact iris for support. Anterior chamber lenses have the shortest anterior chamber depths and usually require a 0.5 mm oversized graft to reduce the potential of postoperative corneal–intraocular lens touch. Sutured posterior chamber lenses offer the advantage of not requiring any anterior segment structures for support and place the intraocular lens the greatest distance from the grafted endothelium. The procedure is technically more involved, requires a deeper vitrectomy, and is potentially a source of external communication (contamination) to the posterior chamber. Iris-sutured posterior chamber lenses also place the lens behind the iris plane and do not require any transscleral sutures. However, the intraocular lens is fixated by suturing through the iris (uveal tissue).

Iris and Angle

The goals of reconstructive surgery of the iris and angle are to (1) align the visual axis of the pupil with the center of the cornea, (2) prevent further compromise of the angle, (3) minimize iris adhesion to the cornea (especially the graft-host junction), and (4) prepare the eye for possible intraocular lens implantation. Many patients with nontraumatic corectopia or updrawn pupils after cataract extraction have excellent visual acuity and minimal complaints. The reason for this is that the cornea remains clear to the periphery and the optical properties of the midperipheral cornea remain acceptable. This is not the case after anterior segment trauma and particularly after corneal transplantation. The graft-host junction causes a 360-degree circumferential scar, and suturing causes significant tissue distortion. Both combine to limit the area of the cornea with potentially acceptable optics to a small central portion. Repositioning or reconstructing the pupil to use the central cornea is therefore important.

Many cases of anterior segment trauma are associated with iridocorneal adhesions and angle compromise. The surgeon should attempt to free the adhesions and open the angle. While it is likely that the involved angle has been permanently compromised, this may prevent progressive anterior synechiae and angle closure, which are often seen after significant trauma. In addition, a taut and repositioned iris should prevent further iris adhesion to the cornea and may limit iris-induced deep corneal vascularization. Finally, a properly positioned iris, covering the edge of the intraocular lens, reduces edge-induced glare and photophobia.

After the cornea is removed (and a vitrectomy performed if necessary), the iris should be freed from any iridocorneal adhesions. A synechia or cyclodialysis spatula is useful. Care should be taken to limit the amount of traction on the angle structures, since this can cause excessive bleeding and potentially compromise the angle further. Focal areas of adhesion may require sharp dissection with the use of long angled Vannas scissors. Once the iris is freed, a blunt spatula can be used to sweep near the angle. Care should be taken to avoid direct contact with the angle structures. The iris can then be reconstructed with the goal of recentering the pupil and producing a relatively taut iris diaphragm. The iris can be sutured using either a

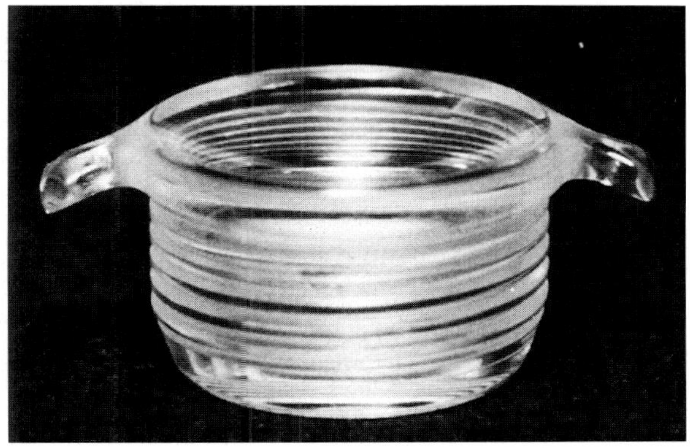

FIGURE 158-3 The Landers-Foulks keratoprosthesis.

polypropylene (Prolene*) or polyester (Mersilene*) suture. Both sutures are resistant to degradation. Polypropylene has the advantage of being offered on a tapered needle (noncutting blunt BIF-4 or taper-cutting CIF-4), which is more resistant to cutting the iris and causing the suture to pull through once tied. The iris should be closed with the goal of creating a central pupil. At times it may be necessary to make small cuts through the iris before suturing to allow the creation of a central "pupil." In patients who are pseudophakic, an attempt should be made to cover as much of the intraocular lens optic edge as possible to reduce glare and minimize the potential for iris capture.[20]

Temporary Keratoprosthesis

It is not uncommon after anterior segment trauma to have associated vitreoretinal pathologic conditions. Not only can trauma lead to direct retinal injury, but vitreous contraction and inflammation can predispose to late retinal detachment. At times the overlying corneal opacification or anterior segment derangement can be significant enough to preclude a retinal surgeon from attempting surgical repair. While a two-stage approach is possible (corneal transplantation and anterior segment reconstruction followed later by posterior pole repair), it does subject the patient to two separate procedures with the associated additional risk. A delay in repair of posterior segment trauma may further limit visual recovery. In addition, it may be months before the transplanted cornea is sufficiently clear to allow the retinal surgeon an adequate view. The subsequent retinal procedure also subjects the newly transplanted cornea to potential endothelial damage from both direct intraocular manipulation and extensive irrigation.

The use of a temporary keratoprosthesis allows the retinal surgeon to perform closed chamber poste-

*Ethicon, Somerville, NJ.

A 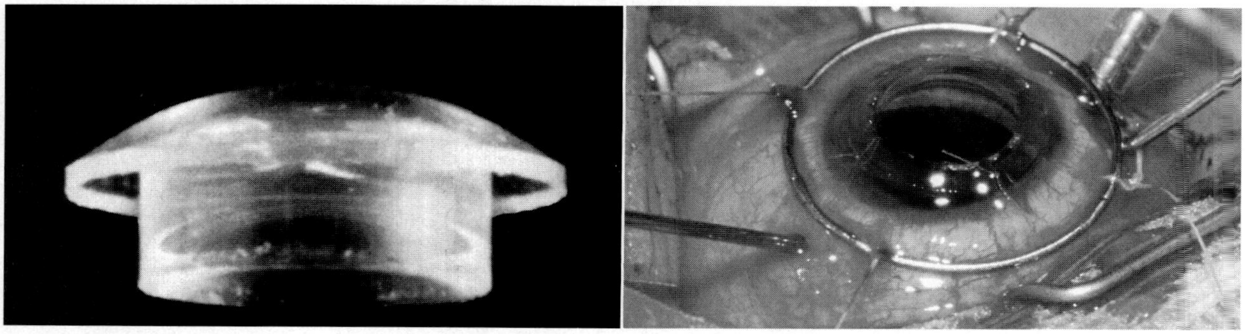 B

FIGURE 158-4 The Eckardt keratoprosthesis showing its profile (**A**) and its intraoperative application (**B**).

rior segment surgery before placement of the transplanted cornea.[21,22] Currently two types of temporary keratoprosthesis are available: (1) the Landers-Foulks keratoprosthesis* and (2) the Eckardt keratoprosthesis.†[23,24] The Landers-Foulks temporary keratoprosthesis (Figure 158-3) is readily available and is used much more commonly. The Landers-Foulks lens is a rigid polymethylmethacrylate (PMMA) lens that is available in three diameters (6.2, 7.2, and 8.2 mm). It has a screw thread on its shaft to help in placing the prosthesis into the trephined bed. The top surface of the prosthesis is a minus optical lens that allows the retinal surgeon a view of the posterior segment without the use of additional lenses.

The eye is prepared as for a penetrating keratoplasty. A scleral support ring is used in all cases because it assists in the insertion of the keratoprosthesis. Traditionally the recipient trephine is chosen 0.2 mm smaller than the associated prosthesis; however, some surgeons undersize the recipient by 0.5 mm. The largest sized prosthesis for that particular case is chosen. The larger diameter keratoprosthesis affords a superior view of the posterior segment. A partial thickness trephination is performed with the appropriately sized trephine. The prosthesis is then placed upside-down over the trephined opening, and two preplaced sutures (5-0 Dacron, T-5 or R-5 needle‡) are placed through the cornea. The anterior chamber is entered, and the cornea is removed with corneal scissors. An attempt is made to leave a positive bevel because this helps in maintaining a watertight seal. After any required anterior segment reconstruction is completed, the prosthesis is screwed into the recipient bed. It is often helpful to place a small amount of viscoelastic on the wound margin because this acts as a lubricant. The assistant fixates the scleral support ring and places gentle constant pressure on the surface of the prosthesis as the surgeon screws the lens in a clockwise direction. Often some assistance is required with a 0.12 fixation forceps to elevate the margin of the corneal wound over the beginning of the prosthesis. The lens is screwed until the wings are flush with the surface of the cornea and in position over the preplaced sutures. The sutures are then tied over the wings, securing the prosthesis in place. The scleral support ring is then removed because it interferes with the vitreoretinal surgery (some retinal surgeons prefer to place the vitrectomy ports before trephining the host). At the completion of the vitreoretinal surgery the Dacron sutures are cut and the prosthesis is removed by unscrewing in a counterclockwise direction. The donor cornea is then secured to the recipient bed in a standard fashion.[4]

While the Landers-Foulks lens gives an excellent view of the posterior pole, it does not allow an easy view of the peripheral retina and pars plana. The Eckardt keratoprosthesis (Figure 158-4, *A*) is a silicone rubber lens with a shorter intraocular cylinder[17] that allows easier access to the periphery. The lens is available in one size with a cylindrical diameter of 7.0 mm. The top or optical portion is 10 mm in diameter and is sutured directly to the corneal limbus. The lens was originally designed for single use, but it can be used a number of times. The procedure is otherwise similar to the Landers-Foulks lens. The host is trephined with a 6.5 or 6.75 mm trephine, and the lens is then placed into the opening and fixed with four interrupted sutures of 8-0 or 9-0 nylon (Figure 158-4, *B*). If a larger penetrating keratoplasty is desired, a second, larger trephine (8.0 to 8.5 mm) can be used to make a partial-thickness incision before the full-thickness trephining for the keratoprosthesis. After removal of the keratoprosthesis, the corneal tissue between the two trephine incisions can be removed with corneal scissors.[25]

*Ocular Instruments, Bellevue, WA.
†Wohlk Contactlinsen, Germany.
‡Alcon Laboratories, Fort Worth, TX.

Conclusion

Visual and anatomic reconstruction after severe anterior segment trauma represents a significant challenge to the ophthalmologist. At times a nonsurgical approach can obtain excellent visual results. Surgical intervention should be undertaken only after a careful preoperative evaluation. A multidisciplinary surgical approach may sometimes be the most appropriate choice.

REFERENCES

1. Cogger TJ: Correction with hard contact lenses. In Tasman W, Jaeger EA, editors: *Duane's clinical ophthalmology,* vol 1., Philadelphia, 1993, Lippincott.
2. Cavanagh HD, Colley A, Pihlaja DJ: Persistent corneal epithelial defect, *Int Ophthalmol Clin* 19:197, 1979.
3. Thoft RA, Friend J: Biochemical transformation of regenerating ocular surface, *Invest Ophthamol Vis Sci* 16:14, 1977.
4. Belin MW, Hannush SB: Mucous membrane abnormalities. In Abbott RL, editor: *Surgical intervention in corneal and external diseases,* Orlando, 1987, Grune & Stratton.
5. Thoft HR: Conjunctival transplantation, *Arch Ophthalmol* 95: 1425, 1977.
6. Kenyon KR, Tseng SC: Limbal autograft transplantation for ocular surface disorders, *Ophthalmology* 96:709, 1989.
7. Tsai RJ, Tseng SC: Human allograft limbal transplantation for corneal surface reconstruction, *Cornea* 13:389, 1994.
8. Karpouzas I, Pouliquen Y: Modeling and numerical optimization of corneal rotation, *J Math Appl Med Biol* 8:73, 1991.
9. Thoft RA: Keratoepithelioplasty, *Am J Ophthalmol* 97:1, 1984.
10. Arffa RC, Barron BA, McDonald MB: Optics of lamellar refractive keratoplasty. In Tasman W, Jaeger EA, editors: *Duane's clinical ophthalmology,* vol 1, Philadelphia, 1993, Lipponcott.
11. Chaplin R, Polack FM: The effect of elevated intraocular pressure on the endothelium of corneal grafts, *Cornea* 1:241, 1982.
12. Mozayeni R, Ditkoff J, Belin MW: Long-term retrospective analysis of corneal transplants with Molteno implants (abstract), Eye Association of America, Annual Scientific Program, San Francisco, 1994.
13. Baer JC, Foster CS: Corneal laser photocoagulation for treatment of neovascularization, *Ophthalmology* 99:173, 1992.
14. Nirankari VS, Baer JC: Corneal argon laser photocoagulation for neovascularization in penetrating keratoplasty, *Ophthalmology* 93:1304, 1986.
15. Schein OD et al: A randomized trial of intraocular lens fixation techniques with penetrating keratoplasty, *Ophthalmology* 100: 1437, 1993.
16. Hassan TS et al: Implantation of Kelman-style, open-loop anterior chamber lenses during keratoplasty for aphakic and pseudophakic bullous keratopathy. A comparison with iris-sutured posterior chamber lenses, *Ophthalmology* 98:875, 1991.
17. Hersh PS, Kenyon KR: Anterior segment reconstruction following ocular trauma, *Int Ophthalmol Clin* 28:57, 1988.
18. Lass JH et al: Clinical and morphometric results of penetrating keratoplasty with one-piece anterior-chamber or suture-fixated posterior-chamber lenses in the absence of lens capsule, *Arch Ophthalmol* 108:1427, 1990.
19. Davis RM, Best D, Gilbert GE: Comparison of intraocular lens fixation techniques performed during penetrating keratoplasty, *Am J Ophthalmol* 111:743, 1991.
20. Auffarth GU et al: Are there acceptable anterior chamber intraocular lenses for clinical use in the 1990s? *Ophthalmology* 101:1913, 1994.
21. Koenig SB et al: Penetrating keratoplasty after placement of a temporary keratoprosthesis during pars plana vitrectomy, *Am J Ophthalmol* 102:45, 1986.
22. Gross JG, Feldman S, Freeman WR: Combined penetrating keratoplasty and vitreoretinal surgery with the Eckart temporary keratoprosthesis, *Ophthalmic Surg* 21(1):67, 1990.
23. Landers MB et al: Temporary keratoprosthesis for use during pars plana vitrectomy, *Am J Ophthalmol* 91:615, 1981.
24. Eckardt C: A new temporary keratoprosthesis for pars plana vitrectomy, *Retina* 7:34, 1987.
25. Gallemore RP, Bokosky JE: Penetrating keratoplasty with vitreoretinal surgery using the Eckardt temporary keratoprosthesis: modified technique allowing use of larger corneal grafts, *Cornea* 14:33, 1995.

CHAPTER 159

LAWRENCE A. GANS

Cyclectomy and Iridocyclectomy

Cyclectomy and iridocyclectomy are surgical procedures intended to remove a portion of ciliary body and iris containing a tumor. A wide range of tumors can be found in the iris and ciliary body, from benign cysts to the most malignant epithelioid melanoma.[1] The potential for uveal tumors to represent the primary site of a life-threatening malignancy has historically indicated enucleation. Posterior choroidal melanomas frequently produce visual symptoms and result in poor vision from retinal detachment, hemorrhage, or tumor invasion of the choroid underlying the macula. When the vision is poor, it seems most rational to remove the eye and thus completely remove the tumor. Iris and ciliary body are accessible by virtue of their anterior location and can be partially excised without serious loss of visual function.[2-5] Thus these procedures are designed to do the following:

- Remove a tumor, which, by its growth or other effects, is threatening vision or the health of the eye
- Provide tissue for histopathologic diagnosis to determine the nature of the tumor and its malignant potential
- Preserve vision while removing a potential malignancy from the eye

Several recent surgical advancements have made cyclectomy and iridocyclectomy more successful overall and more capable of removing larger lesions than were ever thought possible. Viscoelastics maintain the anterior chamber depth while protecting the endothelium and forcing the iris containing tumor out of the limbal wound. Long-acting vitreous gases minimize postoperative bleeding, retinal detachment, and hypotony. Surgical fundus lenses for observing the anterior retinal periphery enhance the ability to determine surgical margins more accurately. Yet with all these advantages the most important factor determining the long-term success of the procedure is still the malignant potential of the tumor itself.

Indications

LOCATION AND SIZE

Because the ciliary body is not easily visualized during routine eye examination, tumors in this location can grow quite large before they are detected. Patients will not experience visual symptoms until the tumor causes lens distortion or cataract, and the appearance of the eye does not change unless the tumor extends into the iris with alterations in color and contour. Tumors may occur anywhere in the ciliary body but tend to be more frequently located inferiorly. Melanomas may grow circumferentially in a ring configuration, producing glaucoma as a presenting sign. There is no predilection for either eye, and bilateral tumors are extremely rare.

Ciliary body tumors are best seen through the widely dilated pupil using a three-mirror contact lens. The angle must be inspected for tumor invasion, and the appearance of vessels on the surface of the tumor should be noted. The size can be measured by calipers using the blockage of transillumination by tumor pigmentation.

GROWTH

The strongest indication for tumor cyclectomy is documented growth. This can be accomplished by direct observation of iris or angle portions of the tumor or measurement of blocked transillumination. Ultrasonography is difficult because the anterior location of the tumor may require a stand-off technique with a water bath to resolve the tumor from the anterior probe complex. With this technique, however, tumor growth can be very precisely documented. High resolution computed tomography (CT) and magnetic resonance (MR) scans may also provide accurate measurements of tumor size, but it is difficult to compare scans done at different times to document growth because cuts at the same level cannot consistently be obtained. As the tumor grows, it is more likely to interfere with vision, to produce cataract and/or glaucoma, to become more difficult to safely and totally excise, and to be malignant. When a tumor is large at the time of discovery, it may not be practical to wait for documented growth before considering cyclectomy. The success rate and ease of surgery are related to the size of the tumor. When a lesion already extends over 4 clock hours, waiting for additional growth constitutes a needless risk.

OCULAR STATUS AND VISUAL POTENTIAL

Enucleation is the only procedure that guarantees the eradication of the primary ciliary body tumor. Unfortunately, it also removes a precious sensory organ, and this result must be weighed to determine what is right for any individual. If vision in the involved eye is severely limited or absent and cannot reasonably be restored, enucleation is the safer option. Fine needle biopsy can yield satisfactory material for histopathologic diagnosis and avoid needless enucleation for benign tumors.

Surgical Anatomy

An understanding of the topographic anatomy and circulation of the ciliary body provides the basis for many decisions regarding the management of ciliary body tumors. The ciliary body varies in width from 4.5 to 5.0 mm nasally and from 5.5 to 6.0 mm temporally. The ora serrata is about 6.5 to 7.0 mm nasally from the limbus and 7.5 to 8.0 mm temporally. The pars plana is about 3 to 4 mm posterior to the limbus. Therefore the inferior, medial, and lateral rectus tendons normally insert about 1 mm anterior to the ora serrata, while the superior rectus tendon is about at the level of the ora. This defines the area where surgery will avoid transecting the retina.

The arterial supply to the ciliary body comes from the long posterior and anterior ciliary arteries, which join to form an episcleral network, an intramuscular network, and the arterial circle of the iris. The venous drainage goes posteriorly to the vortex system at the equator. The vascular supply to ciliary body tumors is reduced at the time of surgery by clamping the anterior ciliary arteries along with disinsertion of the rectus muscle tendon.

Uveal pigment is often seen on the inner surface of the sclera, the lamina fusca. Scleral emissary channels allow vessels through the wall and may also serve as a port for scleral and extrascleral tumor extension. In some cases, it may be difficult to differentiate the normal uveal pigment carried through emissary channels by the perforating vessels from early extension of a pigmented tumor. Suspicious areas may be treated directly during the procedure.

Procedure

PREPARATION

Medical workup (metastatic workup)

The medical evaluation of patients with intraocular tumors is intended to identify metastatic disease. Carcinomas of extraocular origin (e.g., breast, lung) may present initially as an iris or ciliary body tumor. Conversely, primary ocular malignancies may already have established metastatic foci when they are identified in the eye. This is particularly true with tumors isolated to the ciliary body, since the size of the tumor must be quite large before symptoms prompt a detailed examination to detect the tumor. Iris lesions frequently cause the patient to notice changes in the eye's appearance and are readily identified on routine examination. Since the management approach to metastic tumors rarely involves cyclectomy, a metastatic workup must be sensitive and specific. A general physical examination with blood chemistry, liver function tests, and chest x-ray film provides the initial screening. Chest and abdominal CT scans are more sensitive in detecting tumors of the lungs or liver. Positive findings indicate the direction for additional testing.

Delimiting cryopexy

The posterior margin of a cyclectomy will typically come close to the anterior edge of the retina and may occasionally transect, dialyze, or produce small tears in the adjacent retina at the time of surgery. If the tumor is large enough to extend as far as the retina or is just located posteriorly in the ciliary body, a delimiting cryopexy may reduce the risk of postoperative retinal complications. From 3 to 6 weeks before cyclectomy a single or double row of cryopexy is applied posterior to the tumor. This will provide an adhesive chorioretinal scar to minimize the risk of postcyclectomy retinal detachment and also produces a landmark to facilitate tumor localization.

ANESTHESIA

While it may be possible to perform cyclectomy under local anesthesia with long-acting agents (e.g., bupivicaine), the length of the procedure and the delicate nature of the dissection involved make general anesthesia preferable for patient comfort and safety. A typical procedure will take in excess of 2 hours. The anesthesiologist should be aware of two significant elements in the procedure. First, the rectus muscles will be manipulated to provide exposure, and an oculocardiac reflex may be stimulated. Second, intraocular gas is often used to minimize postoperative bleeding and potential retinal complications, so nitrous oxide should be turned off toward the middle of the procedure to avoid problems with diffusion into the gas bubble. Once the patient has been induced under general anesthesia, a retrobulbar injection of long-acting local anesthetic will provide the patient with postoperative analgesia and will help the anesthesiologist optimize the depth of general anesthesia during the procedure.

EXPOSURE

Maximal dilation of the pupil is essential to allow direct visualization of the tumor and to enhance transillumination for localization. Topical cyclopentolate 1% and phenylephrine 2.5% solutions are administered along with topical flurbiprofen (Ocufen) to provide sustained pupillary dilation.

The key to most successful procedures is obtaining adequate exposure of the tumor location. Many ciliary body tumors are inferior and, at least in part, underlie the rectus tendon. An adequate margin for dissection must be planned beyond the size of the tumor.

A lid speculum is selected with blades that extend into the fornix and hold the eyelids off of the globe. An expansion locking screw is preferred over a spring to prevent pressure on the globe during the procedure.

The conjunctiva is opened at the limbus and reflected into the fornix to expose a broad area for the surgical field. Bipolar cautery provides adequate hemostasis at the scleral surface with special attention to sentinel vessels, which may supply the tumor. The rectus muscles are isolated, and the intramuscular septum and bulbar facia are cleaned from the area by blunt dissection.

When the tumor is localized by the technique to be described, a scleral support ring must be positioned to stabilize the globe. While many techniques can be used to position these rings for keratoplasty, some creativity may be required to secure the ring to the globe for cyclectomy. If a standard sized ring is centered over the tumor, a portion will overlie the cornea, where sutures would produce visually significant scars. One solution is to use a very large ring (e.g., 18 to 20 mm in diameter), which would allow the opposite end to be secured to the limbus, leaving 5 to 7 mm to clear the surgical field. Most rings are somewhat malleable and can be bent into an oval or irregular shape to better expose the surgical field without requiring large sizes. Shaping one side to fit the contour of the limbus at the surgical margin often gives excellent support and exposure without straddling the cornea.

The ring is secured to the globe but must also be suspended. The structure of the ring itself prevents anterior collapse of the globe when the eye is open, but posterior collapse may still occur as the globe buckles posteriorly. To minimize this the ring is suspended with sutures (e.g., 6-0 silk) secured to the lid speculum.

LOCALIZATION

The two principal methods of tumor localization are direct visualization and transillumination. Neither method determines accurately the optimal surgical margins because of the nature of the tumor pathology. Ciliary body melanomas tend to taper at their margins, and malignant cells may extend 1 mm or more beyond the clinically apparent edges. These microscopic positive margins may be treated by cryotherapy applications at the time of cyclectomy because they are thin and easily exposed to the freeze-thaw-freeze-thaw treatment. Transillumination is often inaccurate because the microscopic extensions of the tumor will not block transillumination, but also because elevated tumor masses can produce a shadowing effect. This can falsely extend the apparent tumor margins beyond the optimal resection size. Elevated tumors can also block direct visualization of the posterior tumor margin. Therefore it is best to use a combination of both techniques, when possible, for localization (Figures 159-1 and 159-2).

Direct visualization and transillumination are both greatly enhanced by wide pupil dilation. Indirect ophthalmoscopy may be used to localize the posterior tumor margin with scleral depression, but this is a difficult technique to master and may manipulate the tumor more than is necessary. Similar problems with a gonioscopy lens make this technique awkward. It is possible to use the coaxial illumination of the indirect ophthalmoscope to visualize the tumor and localize the margins without using the indirect lens. The newer vitrectomy lenses with prisms provide excellent optics to visualize the far periphery with the surgical microscope and allow the most accurate

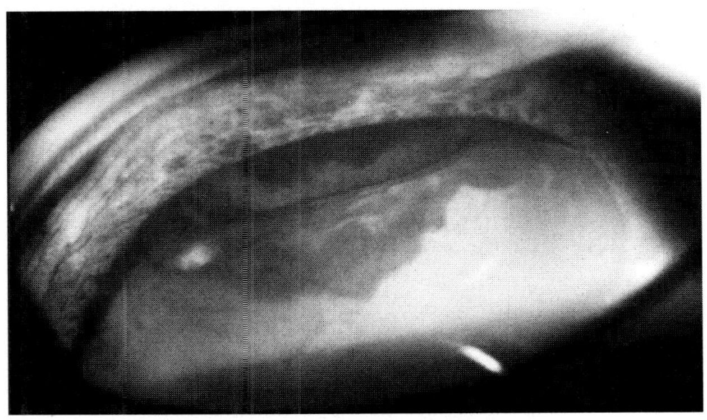

FIGURE 159-1 Iris and ciliary body epithelioid malignant melanoma. Note that the elevation of the tumor precludes direct visualization of the posterior margin for localization.

transscleral sutures, because of the tendency of the lens to migrate into the area of ciliary body resection and then further posteriorly. A flexible loop anterior chamber lens implant is an acceptable alternative if the iris root has not been disturbed. With an inferior iridocyclectomy, it is possible for an anterior chamber lens to migrate into the area of the iridectomy and then fall posteriorly.

Retinal detachment occurs in about 10% to 17% of cases, usually during the first few postoperative months. It is more common with tumors that extend posteriorly to the ora serrata but is often associated with retinal tears in the quadrant opposite the site of the cyclectomy because of traction at the vitreous base when the tumor is elevated. The histopathology of the tumor often dictates whether repair of the detachment or enucleation is indicated. With highly malignant tumors and positive surgical margins, it may be more appropriate to consider removal of the eye. At the time of reattachment surgery, vitreous fluid, subretinal fluid, and aqueous humor can all be sampled and processed cytologically to look for malignant cells.

Results

Small to moderately sized tumors of the iris and ciliary body can be successfully excised with preservation of vision.[10] The size of the tumor determines the degree of surgical difficulty involved in performing the procedure. When the tumor extends beyond 4 clock hours and/or posterior to the ora serrata, the success rate falls off sharply.[11] These eyes may remain hypotonic for a prolonged period, with resulting macular edema, mature cataract, and corneal swelling.

The tumor cell type determines the prognosis for recurrence and metastasis. No consistent clinical features distinguish between benign and malignant tumors.[12] Between 10% and 20% of eyes have a secondary enucleation because of malignant cell type with positive surgical margins, persistent hemorrhaging, or retinal detachment. Vision of 20/40 or better can be obtained in 40% to 60% of cases.[13] Some of these patients require secondary procedures (e.g., cataract extraction) to provide this final vision.

The excision of the iris portion of the tumor may leave a peripheral dialysis with occasional monocular diplopia. With larger iris excisions, patients may experience glare and photophobia (Figure 159-11).

It is common to find tumor cells at the surgical margins because of the difficulty in accurately localizing the tumor. In benign cases this may be of little consequence or may rarely result in local tumor recurrence. Most patients who manifest metastatic or recurrent tumor do so within the first 5 years after surgery, although some may take much longer. Extraocular or orbital recurrence can develop with epithelioid melanomas, and, in some cases, malignant cells can be identified on aqueous humor cytology performed at the time of secondary cataract extraction.

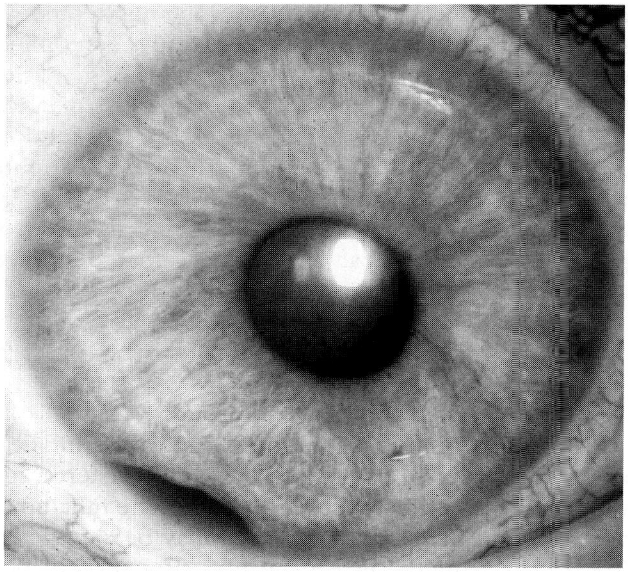

FIGURE 159-11 Postoperative appearance with a small peripheral iris dialysis/iridectomy. The tumor cell type was mixed epithelioid melanoma. The patient maintained 20/25 vision for 8 years until recurrent intraocular melanoma was diagnosed and the eye was enucleated.

REFERENCES

1. Jensen OA: Malignant melanoma of the iris. A 25-year analysis of Danish cases, *Eur J Ophthalmol* 3:181-188, 1993.
2. Malbran ES et al: Iridocyclectomy technique and results, *Ophthalmology* 86:1048-1066, 1979.
3. Peyman GA, Raichand M, Schulman J: Diagnosis and therapeutic surgery of the uvea—Part I: Surgical technique, *Ophthalmic Surg* 17:822-829, 1986.
4. Sears ML: Technique for iridocyclectomy, *Am J Ophthalmol* 66:42-44, 1968.
5. Vail DT: Iridocyclectomy. A review. Gleanings from the literature, *Am J Ophthalmol* 71(Suppl): 161-168, 1971.
6. Peyman GA et al: Role of the CO2 laser in chorioretino-iridocyclectomy, *Ophthalmic Surg* 12:426-431, 1981.
7. Barrada A, Peyman GA, Palacio MN: Limitation of iris and ciliary body resection in primates, *Retina* 4:119-122, 1984.
8. Arentsen JJ, Green WR: Melanoma of the iris: report of 72 cases treated surgically, *Ophthalmic Surg* 6:23-37, 1975.
9. Lindquist TD: Capsulorhexis, phacoemulsification, and posterior chamber lens placement following iridocyclectomy, *Ophthalmic Surg* 23:44-46, 1992.
10. Forrest AW, Keyser RB, Spencer WH: Iridocyclectomy for melanomas of the ciliary body: a follow-up study of pathology and surgical morbidity, *Ophthalmology* 85:1237-1249, 1978.
11. Gragoudas ES et al: Proton irradiation of malignant melanoma of the ciliary body, *Br J Ophthalmol* 63:135-139, 1979.
12. Burch PG, Maumenee AE: Iridocyclectomy for benign tumors of the ciliary body, *Am J Ophthalmol* 63:447-452, 1967.
13. Memmen JE, McLean IW: The long-term outcome of patients undergoing iridocyclectomy, *Ophthalmology* 97:429-432, 1990.

CHAPTER 160

M. BOWES HAMILL

Management of Scleral Perforation

Scleral perforation is fortunately rare but can present a significant management problem when it occurs. Among the difficulties encountered in the management of this condition is that it frequently arises as a result of an ongoing disease process rather than as an isolated event. This disease process generally means that the surrounding scleral tissue is involved to some degree in the same process that led to the perforation. Additionally, patients having diseases that result in scleral perforation are frequently elderly and debilitated because of their underlying medical problems. These factors work together to complicate the treatment of the scleral defect.

General Management Strategies

No single method has been universally accepted as optimal in the treatment of scleral perforation, although much has been written about this condition. The treating physician must therefore design a therapeutic approach based on the individual patient's circumstances. Because perforation of the sclera is often a manifestation of a systemic disease process, the first step in management is identification and treatment of the underlying condition, if present. Some of the conditions associated with scleral perforation are listed in the box. For perforations that result from infectious diseases, appropriate microbiologic studies and effective antimicrobial therapy should be instituted before or concurrently with surgical management. Similarly, appropriate local or systemic immunosuppression must accompany the therapy of perforations related to inflammatory conditions. If management of the underlying disease is not instituted or is not successful, the processes that led initially to the scleral defect will continue and lead either to failure of the intervention or the development of new areas of scleral disease.

Once a scleral perforation has occurred, the physician has several repair options. If there is a small scleral defect without uveal prolapse, no therapy may be necessary for the perforation per se as long as the factors that led to the process are either under control (infectious or inflammatory diseases) or no longer operative (trauma). For large perforations, surgical repair, either primary closure or patch grafting, may be required. Before surgery the patient should be examined carefully to determine the location and extent of the defect and the condition of the surrounding tissues. This evaluation permits the surgeon to determine the need for and the approximate size of the patch, if required, and permits the selection of the patch material. For example, when dealing with a perforation involving the limbus, the patch should conform to the surrounding ocular architecture to prevent dellen formation or unwanted keratorefractive sequelae. The preoperative examination should also identify potential intraoperative complications that may be encountered during the procedure, such as uveal or vitreous prolapse. The recognition of these conditions enables the surgeon to have available the equipment and assistance needed to obtain the best operative result.

Anesthesia for Scleral Perforations

The options for anesthesia must also be considered. Topical anesthesia is associated with the least systemic stress and risk of inadvertent injury to the globe. If appropriate, this method may be ideal for small, anteriorly located defects. Unfortunately these types of perforations are unusual, and most cases require more extensive conjunctival and Tenon's capsule dissection and are located too far posteriorly to allow adequate anesthesia with topical agents alone. In these cases, retrobulbar anesthesia may be more appropriate. This approach has the advantages of excellent regional anesthesia and akinesia with minimal cardiac and respiratory stress. These factors may be important in patients who are systemically ill, especially those with perforations resulting from rheumatoid arthritis. The major risks of retrobulbar injection in the setting of scleral thinning or perforation are related to the injection itself. Any volume of anesthetic agent injected

Causes of scleral perforation

Trauma

Penetrating injury
- Intraocular foreign body

Chemical injury
Radiation injury

Infectious diseases

Bacterial scleritis/sclerokeratitis
Fungal scleritis/sclerokeratitis

Inflammatory conditions

Necrotizing scleritis
Scleromalacia perforans
Mooren's ulcer

Postoperative causes

Retinal detachment surgery
- Scleral buckle erosion

Pterygium surgery
- Post-radiation application
- After mitomycin treatment

Idiopathic causes

Senile scleromalacia
Scleral coloboma—spontaneous perforation
Paralimbic/intercalcary scleromalacia of Franceschetti

into the orbital space results in increased intraorbital pressure, which is transmitted directly to the globe. This increase in intraocular pressure may cause an extension of the ruptured area or may lead to additional ruptures in areas of thinned sclera. The uvea may also be prolapsed (or further prolapsed) through a new or existing scleral defect as a result of increased intraocular pressure. In addition to the hydraulic effects of retrobulbar injection, the passage of the needle near the globe may produce complications. Patients with scleral perforation caused by necrotizing scleritis or scleromalacia may have areas of scleral thinning and staphyloma formation posteriorly, which can be injured by the retrobulbar needle. These potential problems notwithstanding, many large and complex scleral perforations have been repaired successfully using retrobulbar anesthesia.

The third anesthetic choice is general anesthesia. General anesthesia has several advantages over the other alternatives. General anesthesia results in minimal increases in intraocular pressure, produces optimal akinesia and anesthesia, and permits operative intervention at multiple sites (i.e., harvesting fascia lata or periosteum for patch materials). General anesthesia, however, is not benign in patients with a significant underlying illness. This is of special concern in patients with scleral perforation caused by rheumatoid arthritis, since these individuals may have other systemic manifestations of the disease, such as vasculitis or pulmonary involvement, which would put them at significant risk for anesthetic complications.

Surgical Repair of Scleral Perforations

PREOPERATIVE CONSIDERATIONS

For those perforations resulting from trauma, special attention must be given during the preoperative evaluation of the patient to rule out conclusively the presence of an intraocular foreign body or occult intraocular damage. In many cases where the perforation is caused by intrinsic scleral disease, however, the margins of the defect may be too tenuous to allow suture placement.

For those perforations caused by an infectious agent, one of the most important aspects of therapy is primary control of the infectious process. Surgical repair should be delayed, if possible, until appropriate antibiotic therapy has been instituted. Although scleral necrosis and melting caused by secondary inflammation may continue for a time even after control of replicating microorganisms, without antibiotic therapy any surgical intervention is destined to fail because of the progression of the disease. In infectious cases the longer the surgery can be safely delayed after institution of antibiotic therapy, the better the surgical result because of improved tissue margins and decreased tissue destruction at the perforation site. For those perforations caused by infection there may be an advantage to the use of a vascular flap (conjunctiva or tarsus and conjunctiva) versus avascular patch material (sclera) in the closure of the defect because of the beneficial effect of increasing the local blood supply. Vascularized tissue in this setting is also less likely to become infected.

In the repair of perforations caused by inflammatory disease, many of the same concerns are germane. As in infectious etiologies the initial objective is to treat the underlying condition. Additional aspects of the repair relate to the intrinsic inflammatory nature of the disease. Unlike perforations caused by infectious processes, use of a vascular graft in the repair of a perforation resulting from an autoimmune disease may be counterproductive. For the same reason, patching with sclera may not be the optimal choice, and nonscleral tissue, such as periosteum, may be preferable.[1]

Some conditions resulting in scleral perforation, such as trauma from chemical injuries and ocular cicatricial pemphigoid (OCP), are further complicated by ocular surface disease, lack of healthy conjunctiva, and epithelialization difficulties. In these situations, patch materials capable of self-epithelialization, such as split-thickness dermal grafts, may offer significant benefit over other materials.[2,3] In all cases in which patch material is to be used, the surgeon must consider the relative benefits of autologous versus donor material.

OPERATIVE CONSIDERATIONS

When faced with a scleral perforation requiring surgical closure, the physician has several alternatives, depending on the size of the defect and the underlying disease. These options include primary closure, glue or tissue adhesive, or patch grafting. Small perforations, especially those caused by trauma with good tissue margins, may be closed primarily.

Conjunctiva/Tenon's capsule

The technique of scleral patching with conjunctiva involves mobilization of a flap of conjunctiva, with or without attached Tenon's fascia, and suturing of the flap over the scleral defect. Conjunctiva has multiple advantages over other tissues for this purpose, including ready availability and technical ease of flap creation in most patients who do not have concurrent ocular surface disease. Additionally, a vascular conjunctival flap graft may be the treatment of choice in cases of small perforations resulting from infectious diseases. A conjunctival flap was used successfully by van der Hoeven to close a perilimbal scleral defect in scleromalacia perforans.[4] Rosenthal and Williams reported a similarly treated case.[5] In their patient, however, the flap retracted within 2 weeks. Over the next several months, there was progression of the disease and the eye perforated and required enucleation.[5]

When the perforation is large or significant uveal prolapse has occurred, a conjunctival patch is not appropriate, since it lacks the structural rigidity to maintain the contour of the globe and support the intraocular contents.

Tarsoconjunctival flap

Use of a tarsoconjunctival flap offers an advantage over conjunctiva alone in that this combination of tissue is significantly more rigid than conjunctiva alone and can provide structural support to thinned sclera or prolapsed uvea. The technique involves creation of a pedicle flap of tarsus and overlying conjunctiva (Figure 160-1). The bulbar conjunctiva near the scleral defect is dissected from around the area of perforation, and the perforation site is debrided of necrotic tissue. The tarsoconjunctival flap is then mobilized and sutured to cover the scleral defect. The advantages of this tissue as a patch material include the attached vascular supply and the structural strength resulting from the inclusion of tarsus in the graft. Rootman et al reported using this technique to repair scleral perforations caused by chemical injury in two patients.[6] In both patients the scleral defects healed and remained so for the duration of follow-up (4 and 6 months).

Autologous sclera

One of the materials most commonly used in patch grafts for scleral perforations is sclera. The source for this tissue can be either an unrelated donor (homologous) or the patient's own tissue (autologous). Patient-derived (autologous) sclera can be used in two forms. A "trap-door" scleral flap graft can be created in which a partial thickness sclera flap is created immediately adjacent to the defect, reflected over the defect, and sutured into place (Figure 160-2). More commonly in the repair of larger defects, an uninvolved scleral site is identified either on the affected eye or on the fellow eye and a partial-thickness scleral patch is created and lifted free. This flap is then placed over the area of scleral defect and sutured into position.

One of the benefits of using autologous sclera is that, by using the patient's own tissue, the risk of inciting a rejection reaction is eliminated. Unfortunately, in those conditions in which scleral thinning is the result of an autoimmune phenomenon the use of autologous tissue may be a liability, since autologous sclera may be more prone to involvement in the disease process than unrelated donor tissue. Additionally, there may be little uninvolved sclera available for harvesting as patch material in patients with severe disease. Autologous sclera has been used successfully, however, to treat perforations resulting from various conditions. Stilma reported his results of lamellar scleral autografts in the repair of anterior segment perforations resulting from Mooren's ulceration in 30 patients from Sierra Leone with 38 Mooren's ulcers.[7] Initially, patients with perforations were treated with conjunctival grafts, but the results were disappointing. Because of the lack of corneal donor tissue, he elected to use lamellar scleral autografts in six eyes of five patients. The grafts were harvested from the inferotemporal quadrant of the ipsilateral eye. In these reported cases, no eyes were lost and five retained useful vision. No complications were reported at the site of the donor sclera.[7] Autologous sclera was also used by Cappin to treat a patient with perilimbal scleromalacia.[8] In this case a trap-door flap was manufactured to treat the spontaneous scleral perforation successfully. A similar approach has also been reported for the treatment of senile scleromalacia.[9] In a case reported by Carroll, a free autologous lamellar sclera graft was used to treat an area of sclera thinning secondary to senile sclero-

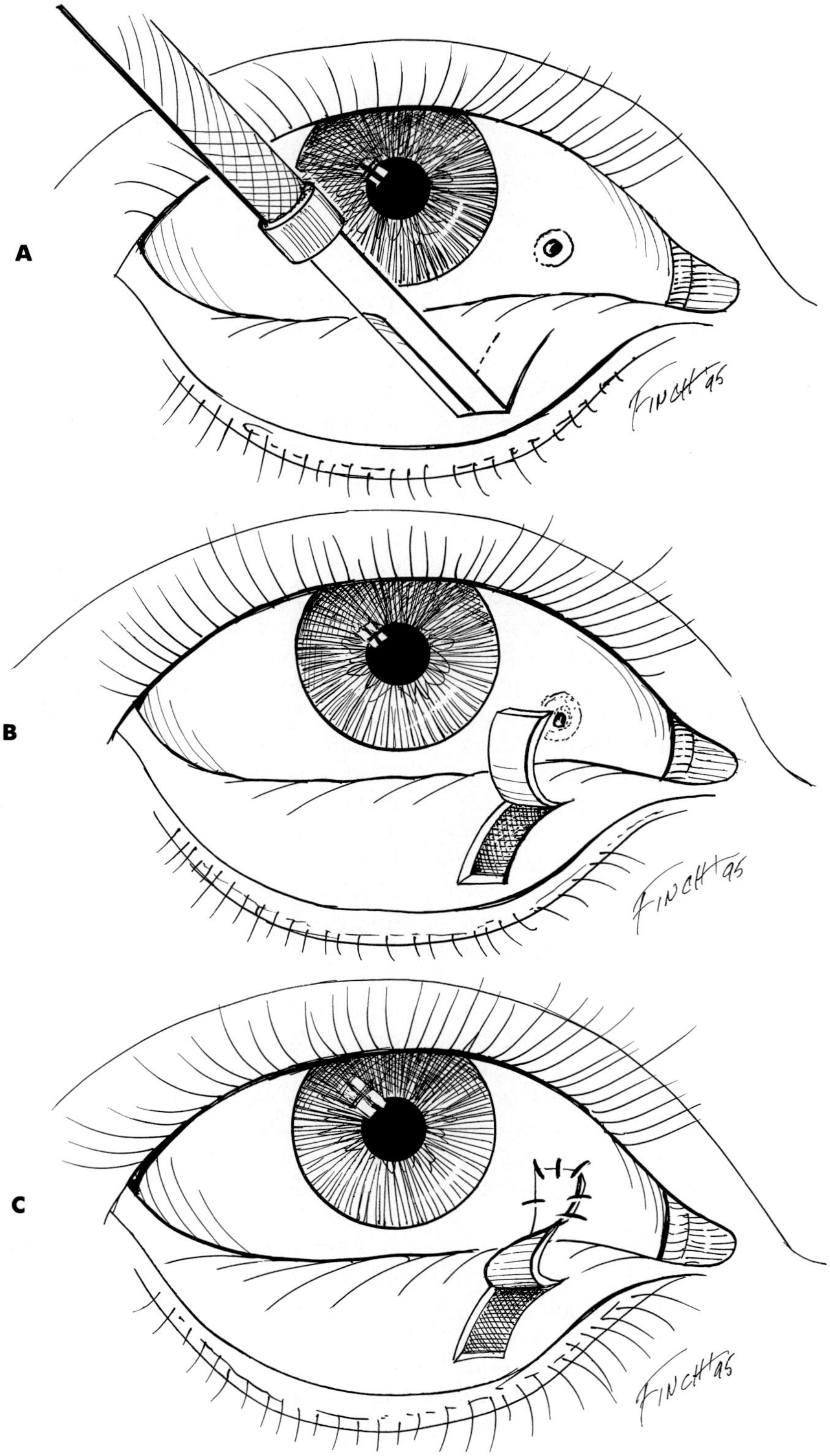

FIGURE 160-1 Tarsoconjunctival flap. **A,** The area of the perforation site is cleaned of conjunctiva and necrotic tissue to expose good tissue margins. **B,** The conjunctiva and tarsus on the palpebral surface of the lid adjacent to the scleral defect are then incised and a pedicle flap created. **C,** The flap is then rotated and sutured to cover the scleral defect. (Adapted from Rootman DS, Insler MS, Kaufman HE: *Ophthalmic Surg* 19:808-810, 1988.)

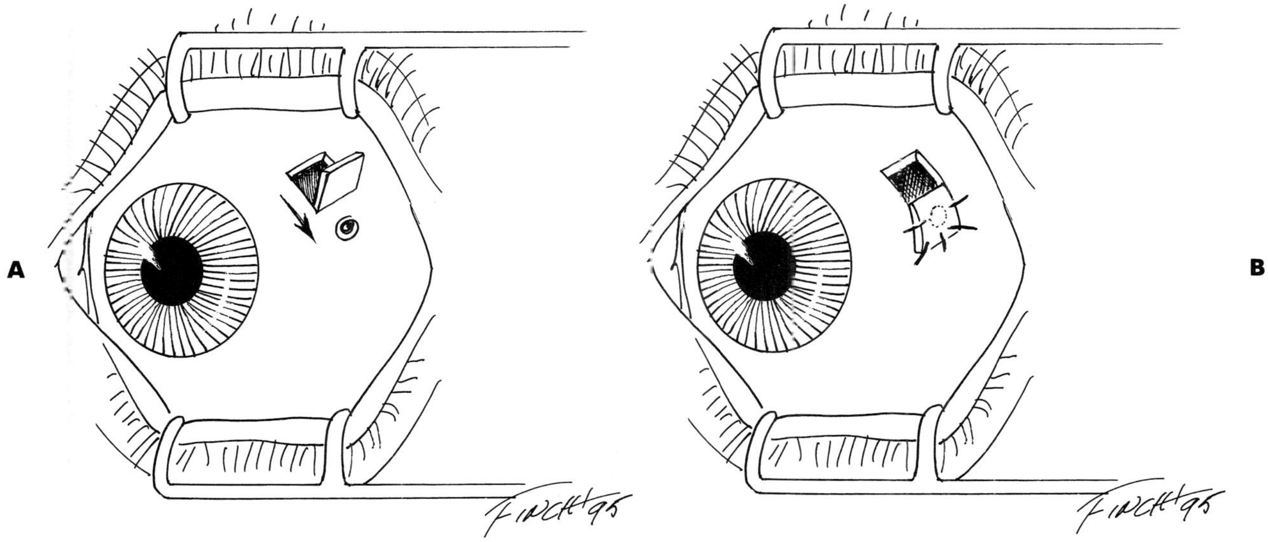

FIGURE 160-2 A "trap-door" scleral flap. **A,** This flap is created in the sclera adjacent to the defect. **B,** It is reflected over the scleral perforation and sutured. This technique requires good tissue adjacent to the defect but has the advantage of not requiring tissue removal either from a distant site or from the fellow eye.

malacia. In Carroll's patient the graft was noted to be integrating into the tissue without evidence of inflammation 15 months after the transplant. It was Carroll's opinion that autologous scleral grafting afforded several advantages over other alternatives, including no danger of an immunologic reaction, material that was easy to work with, and no danger of graft necrosis.[9]

Homologous sclera

Homologous sclera grafting is one of the most frequently reported methods in the surgical treatment of scleral perforations. Homologous sclera is derived not from the patient's own tissue but rather from donor eye material. Donor sclera can be stored either in glycerin or alcohol. When using this tissue, care must be taken to rinse the scleral patch carefully before use to avoid damaging the recipient bed with the residual preservative. In addition to rinsing, the donor sclera should be carefully cleaned of any adherent episcleral remnants and the inside wiped with gauze to remove any residual choroidal pigment left on the surface. After decantation, rinsing, and cleaning of the donor sclera the recipient bed is prepared. Any conjunctiva or necrotic sclera should be carefully dissected free and good tissue margins determined. A template is frequently helpful to determine the final size and shape of the donor scleral patch, and a piece of drape or similar material can be cut to size and used for this purpose. The template pattern is then transferred to the donor sclera, which is cut and applied over the area of the scleral defect. The patch can then be sutured into place using various suture materials, including nylon, polyglactin (Vicryl), and polyester. The choice of the suture material depends on the individual case. For example, in situations wherein sutures will be visible anteriorly and a good quality recipient bed is present, 10-0 nylon with buried knots, providing a smooth perilimbal bulbar surface, is appropriate.

Donor sclera has advantages over other materials in that it can be stored for an indefinite period of time in either glycerin or alcohol without the need for specialized technology, and therefore it is readily available throughout the world. Additionally, with the storage of entire scleral shells, there is rarely a shortage of tissue for any given patient, unlike the situation with autologous sclera. Sclera, once it has been soaked in saline solution, is supple and does not usually present technical difficulties in the fashioning and application of a patch. Clinically this tissue seems to be well tolerated. Johnson et al conducted animal studies evaluating homologous scleral patching and found that the eyes of dogs patched with freshly harvested dog sclera did well.[10] In his studies, he investigated full- and partial-thickness replacement grafts as well as full-thickness reinforcement grafts. In all cases, healing was reported to be relatively rapid, and donor sclera remained in place with little inflammatory reaction.[10] He found no sloughing of any of the homografts in the time period studied (from 4 weeks to 7 months after surgery), and microscopic examination of the eyes revealed minimal inflammatory reaction with good incorporation of the scleral graft tissue into the host bed. When full-thickness onlay grafts were applied, the overlying graft did not affect the blood supply of the underlying sclera. Interestingly, despite full- and partial-thickness lamellar bed dissections preparatory to grafting in some of these animals, there was minimal ophthalmoscopic disturbance of the underlying fundus.[10]

Homografts have also been used in human patients for various conditions, and a technique for scleral homografting has been described by Obear.[11] Obear's technique is essentially the one I currently employ with only minor modifications. The initial step is to expose the entire scleral defect by performing a conjunctival peritomy and dissection. If necessary, the conjunctival edges can be tagged with suture for ease in later reapproximation. I have found that polyglactin (Vicryl) and silk suture material in 6-0 to 7-0 sizes are excellent for this purpose, as the color differences allow the reapproximation of multiple edges without confusion. After the removal of the conjunctiva and exposure of the defect, all necrotic or suppurative tissue is debrided from the scleral margins. Care should be taken not to injure the sometimes bulging choroid in the bed of the defect. Simultaneously with debridement the edges of the defect should be evaluated to locate solid, architecturally stable sclera uninvolved in the disease process to be used as the anchoring sites for the patch graft. Once the extent of the scleral involvement is known, the graft can be cut freehand. I generally oversize the graft several millimeters beyond uninvolved sclera to allow for good edge apposition, sealing, and healing. Some authors, such as Obear, recommend significant oversizing of the graft, on the order of 5 to 10 mm.[11] Regardless of the degree, the graft should be sufficiently bigger than the defect to allow adequate suture bites into and tissue contact with normal sclera so as to provide adequate healing. The donor sclera is then placed over the scleral defect as an onlay graft, overlapping all sides of the lesion, and sewn into position. Obear recommended the use of 4-0 white silk mattress sutures to secure the graft, followed by interrupted sutures to secure the periphery.[11] While this method is successful, I prefer the use of interrupted sutures because this technique provides excellent edge apposition and needle control. Additionally, by using only interrupted sutures, the patch graft can be tightened down in a controlled manner to reposit prolapsing uvea and restore a more normal scleral contour. A wide variety of suture materials can be employed for this purpose. Rapidly reabsorbing sutures, such as chromic sutures, are not recommended because of the relatively prolonged healing times required for scleral stability. Silk and Dacron, on the other hand, are good choices because of their permanence, ease of manipulation, and lack of erosive tendencies. When securing the graft with multiple small suture bites around the perimeter of the patch,

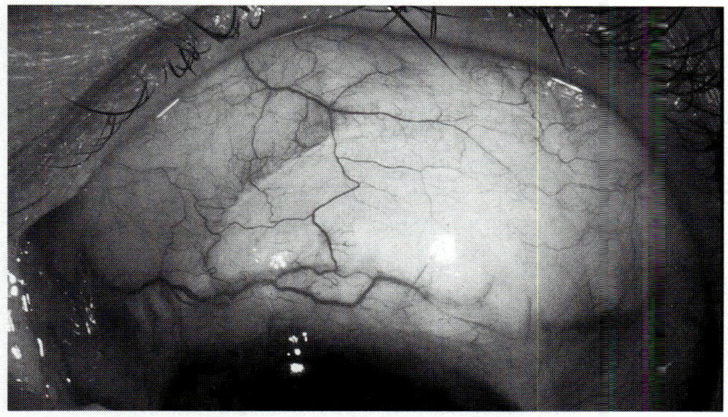

FIGURE 160-3 This patient with previous scleritis and superior scleral thinning was hit with a thrown rock, resulting in a large perilimbal scleral tear with bulging of the choroid. Because of the friability of the surrounding sclera and large size of the defect, a homologous scleral patch graft was applied. The anterior edge of the graft can be seen immediately posterior to the superior limbus. Elsewhere the graft has been well incorporated into the underlying tissue with a resultant smooth scleral contour and no evidence of recurrent scleritis.

6-0 to 10-0 suture materials are a reasonable choice, depending on the circumstances and the specific condition of the patient's recipient bed.

The only exception to these guidelines occurs when the graft abuts the limbus, as in the case of a perilimbal perforation. In this situation I recommend 10-0 nylon for the anterior sutures and for all sutures extending into the cornea. More posteriorly on the globe, larger suture materials can be used. After placement and suturing of the graft the conjunctiva is brought down into place and the edges sutured with appropriate materials.

Multiple authors have reported using scleral homografts for various conditions, and an example of a repair using a scleral homograft patch is illustrated in Figure 160-3. Sevel, in 1972, described a case of scleromalacia perforans treated successfully with homologous scleral patch grafting. The patient died 7 months later, and the eyes were obtained for examination. Histologically, the underlying tissue had been replaced with granulomatous tissue, and the graft itself was involved in the granulomatous reaction.[12] More recently, Maza et al reported results of scleral patch grafting in 12 patients with necrotizing scleritis with or without peripheral ulcerative keratitis (15 grafts in 12 eyes).[13] In the reported cases the authors used either frozen or glycerin-preserved tissue, and good long-term results (mean of 12 months follow-up) were obtained in patients without active vasculitis. In patients with untreated vasculitis the survival time of the grafts was short, with necrosis reported within 2 months of surgery. The authors recommended that immunosuppression precede or accompany scleral grafting to ensure survival of the graft.[13] Other authors have had similar problems with homologous scleral patch grafting, including Rosenthal, who reported resorption of a homologous scleral patch graft and ultimately phthisis in a patient with scleromalacia perforans.[5] In his case the graft had been preserved in paraffin. Torchia also reported scleral graft failure in a case of scleromalacia perforans, and Breslin noted a similar case of a melting scleral graft in a patient with necrotizing scleritis.[1,14] In the case reported by Torchia, pathology of the failed graft revealed infiltration with polymorphonuclear leukocytes and the presence of structures representative of necrotic bacteria, indicating the possibility that the donor tissue became infected and failed on that basis.[14] In Breslin's case the conjunctiva brought over the scleral patch graft became necrotic and avascular, and the sclera underwent subsequent spontaneous dissolution.[1]

Fascia lata

As an alternative to homologous sclera, fascia lata would seem to offer several advantages as a patching material for scleral perforation. The obvious advantages include its strength, the relative ease of harvest, and its flexibility. The source of fascia lata is the patient's lateral thigh, and the patch material is generally harvested at the same time as the patching procedure. Fascia lata is used as an onlay patch graft material in the same manner as previously described for donor sclera and has the advantages of being relatively thin and conforming well to the contour of the globe.

In 1959 Bick first reported the use of fascia lata in the American literature for the closure of scleral perforations caused by scleromalacia perforans.[15] In his case a quadrantic scleral defect was successfully repaired using autologous fascia lata. Postoperatively, Bick reported that while there was significant early overlying conjunctival edema, the graft eventually thinned and appeared to heal well to the underlying scleral tissue. A similar result was reported simultaneously by Armstrong and McGowen.[16] In Armstrong's case, multiple patch procedures were performed, during the last of which the patient unfortunately died. Histologic examination of the fascia lata graft revealed vascularization and incorporation of the grafted tissue without evidence of breakdown. After examining the photomicrographs, it was Bick's opinion that the graft was susceptible to the same process that resulted in scleromalacia, believing that the histologic specimens demonstrated a recurrence in the grafted fascia lata 4 months postoperatively.[15] Several years later Taffet reported a similar case of fascia lata grafting in scleromalacia. Examination 8 months postoperatively revealed a normal globe contour in the area of the graft without signs of recurrent disease.[17] Additional cases were reported by Blum, Torchia, and Zer.[14,18,19] Interestingly, the successful fascia lata grafting reported by Torchia followed necrosis of a previously placed homologous scleral patch graft. Zer makes the point that fascia lata autografts may be preferable to donor homografts in scleromalacia perforans in light of the underlying immunologic disturbance responsible for the ocular disease.[19]

Fascia lata is not without its problems, however; fascia lata not covered with epithelium or by conjunctiva may undergo necrosis.[3] Additionally, fascia lata requires a secondary incision on the patient's leg in order to harvest donor material, which may adversely affect the overall care of the patient.

In an interesting observation, Bick, Torchia, and Taffett each reported successful shrinkage of prolapsed uvea with the application of cautery.[14,15,17] Bick further reported that the fundus of his patient showed no abnormality 6 weeks after surgery.[15]

Periosteum

Like fascia lata, periosteum is an autologous patching material. To harvest periosteum an incision is made along the anterior tibial crest, and the preperiosteal tissues are dissected free. The periosteum is then incised and separated from its underlying attachments with a periosteal elevator. The periosteal graft is then stored under saline solution until needed for grafting. Periosteum has been used for various purposes in ophthalmology, including support of the Cardona implant.[20] Because of its usefulness in this setting, it has been employed by several authors to repair scleral defects. Periosteum is felt to be superior to other materials because it is easily harvested, has good tensile strength, and is an easily vascularized tissue.[20-22] Additionally, periosteum has been thought by some authors not to be susceptible to immunologic graft rejection.[21,22]

Multiple authors have reported patients treated with patch grafts made from autologous periosteum. Breslin in 1977 reported two cases of necrotizing scleritis with excellent results 9 months after surgery. In both cases the eyes were quiet, and areas of previous staphyloma were flat without evidence of further disease.[1] Rao reported using periosteum in a case of impending scleral perforation caused by scleromalacia.[20] In his case the periosteum was covered by a buccal mucous membrane graft derived from the patient's lower lip. Five months after surgery the graft was in position with minimal inflammatory reaction.[20] Four additional patients were reported by Koenig between 1982 and 1986.[21,22] Koenig's cases involved periosteal patch grafting for scleromalacia perforans and for corneoscleral wound dehiscence. An average follow-up of 36

PART X

REFRACTIVE SURGERY

SECTION ONE *History and Overview of Refractive Surgery*

CHAPTER 161

STEVEN C. SCHALLHORN PETER J. MCDONNELL

Refractive Surgery: Past, Present, and Future

Refractive surgery encompasses a multitude of techniques designed to correct errors of refraction and improve uncorrected visual acuity. From an unpretentious beginning over 100 years ago the field has undergone a technologic explosion with the introduction and refinement of procedures such as radial keratotomy and photorefractive keratectomy. These advances have been matched by increased public interest and by both public and professional acceptance.

Clearly, we can, and must, do better. The ophthalmic community should be skeptical of new procedures that are not supported by the following: (1) animal studies demonstrating safety and efficacy; (2) laboratory data demonstrating the principles behind the procedure and validating the clinical approach (e.g., 4 versus 8 versus 16 versus 32 incisions in radial keratotomy); and (3) frank and complete reporting of initial clinical trial results.

Historical Emergence of Refractive Procedures

The development of refractive surgical procedures has historically been characterized as involving empirical (trial and error) approaches with little, if any, preclinical testing. For example, 16- and 32-incision radial keratotomy was marketed aggressively in this country before animal and eye bank eye studies that showed that eight or even four incisions produced most of the flattening observed with large numbers of incisions. Similarly, radial thermokeratoplasty using a super-heated wire was promoted by some surgeons in the United States before animal studies of safety and efficacy and publication of clinical trial data. Only fairly recently have modern biomechanical analysis techniques, such as finite element modeling, been applied to better understand these procedures. Except when mandated by the Food and Drug Administration, laboratory studies have largely been an afterthought and have often been haphazard. Human subjects have usually served as the initial experimental animals, and office surgical suites have been the laboratories.

Evaluation of Surgical Outcomes

The development of refractive surgery has generated new issues and controversies regarding the evaluation of clinical trial results. Until recently, few procedures have been studied in a manner that clearly defines efficacy and safety. In evaluating efficacy, what are the most important measures—unaided distance acuity, magnitude of residual refractive error, level of patient satisfaction, or ability of patient to avoid the need for corrective lenses? Few studies include any measurements of the patient's postoperative functional status, such as the ability to drive an automobile without optical correction. It is clear from the few studies that have addressed this issue that many individuals with 20/40 or better uncorrected visual acuity report the need for spectacles or contact lenses for distance correction. What quantitative criteria do we use to judge the success of a refractive surgical procedure—percentage of eyes within 1 diopter of emmetropia or within 0.5 diopter? Percentage of eyes with 20/40 or better unaided acuity, or with 20/20 unaided acuity? Or do we rely on psychometric measures of visual function?

What are the important measures of safety? How much loss of best visual acuity with spectacles do we accept with refractive surgical procedures? Some of the literature suggests that a one line loss of visual acuity is within the "noise" of measurement and is best ignored.[1] In some trials, best-corrected visual acuity reductions from 20/10 to 20/20, which represents a doubling of the visual angle, were observed.[2] Does the ability of these patients to still see 20/20 on the high contrast acuity charts mean that this visual loss is not important? How do we factor in the anticipated improvement in visual acuity associated with the elimination of image minification from myopic spectacles?[3] Theoretically, virtually all patients who undergo surgical correction of myopia should experience an improvement in best-corrected visual acuity, but most do not.

What about contrast sensitivity and glare under photopic and scotopic conditions? Since we have not reached a consensus on how best to measure these variables in a clinically relevant fashion, how can we interpret and rely on data to make sure that new procedures are not causing some visual disability? Dire predictions of impaired night driving that could result in fatalities after keratorefractive surgery[4] force us to try to reassure ourselves that our new surgical procedures do not expose our patients to such risks.

What length of follow-up is sufficient? We know that radial keratotomy can cause a slowly progressive drift toward hyperopia that may be demonstrable only with large numbers of patients followed for many years. Might there also be a slight refractive change over time after excimer laser photorefractive keratectomy that may take years to become evident? We may also assume that any complications from ultraviolet irradiation of the anterior segment would not be evident immediately after surgery. What length of follow-up is adequate to address the issue of delayed complications, such as ultraviolet light–induced mutagenesis?

What complication rate is acceptable? Given projections that keratorefractive surgery will be performed by increasing numbers of comprehensive ophthalmologists and that at some future time millions of Americans each year may have the surgery, even a small risk of vision loss would translate into many patients with decreased vision as a result of surgery.

When reviewing reports of new procedures, physicians and the public alike are well-advised to ask whether the questions just asked about safety and efficacy have been adequately addressed. From such reports, surgeons bear the responsibility for distilling the important measures of safety and efficacy into a complete and comprehensible informed consent discussion that will allow surgical candidates to determine whether the potential benefits outweigh the risks of surgery.

Refractive Surgery Principles

The anterior surface of the cornea, more specifically the air to tear film interface, is responsible for 60% to 70% of the optical power of the eye; the other contribution comes from the crystalline lens. Because the shape of the cornea so profoundly affects the refractive state of the eye, most forms of refractive surgery attempt to alter its convex curvature. Myopia can be treated by increasing the central radius of curvature, making the cornea flatter with less optical power. Hyperopia treatment would be just the opposite, inducing a decrease in the radius of curvature to increase the optical power. Notable exceptions are various implants that have a higher index of refraction than does the corneal stroma (intrastromal implant) or water (intraocular lens implant). These implants rely on their own curvature to determine refractive correction.

Surgical techniques to correct refractive errors can be divided into several major categories for instructional purposes: incisional, thermal, lamellar, and intraocular. Representative techniques for these categories are illustrated in Figure 161-1. *Incisional surgery* includes radial, astigmatic, and hexagonal keratotomy. These procedures use incisions to weaken the cornea structurally, allowing intraocular pressure and biomechanical forces to induce changes in its curvature. The incisions are typically made with thin, sharp diamond blades. Major relative advantages (compared to other refractive procedures) include inexpensive instrumentation, quick visual recovery and a central clear zone that is not violated. Major relative disadvantages include limitations on the maximum refractive correction and side effects of corneal weakening, which can cause diurnal fluctuation in vision and progressive hyperopia. *Thermal-based refractive surgery* uses heat to shrink corneal collagen and includes the hot wire probe of Fyodorov and the holmium: YAG laser. A bandlike constriction occurs in the peripheral cornea by the shrinking collagen that causes central steepening. The major advantage is the ability to correct hyperopia without operating over the central optical zone. Regression, however, remains a significant disadvantage. *Lamellar procedures* include a host of varied techniques designed to alter directly the shape of the cornea with tissue addition or removal. These include keratomileusis, keratophakia, epikeratoplasty, photorefractive keratectomy, and intrastromal photoablation. These procedures were developed to

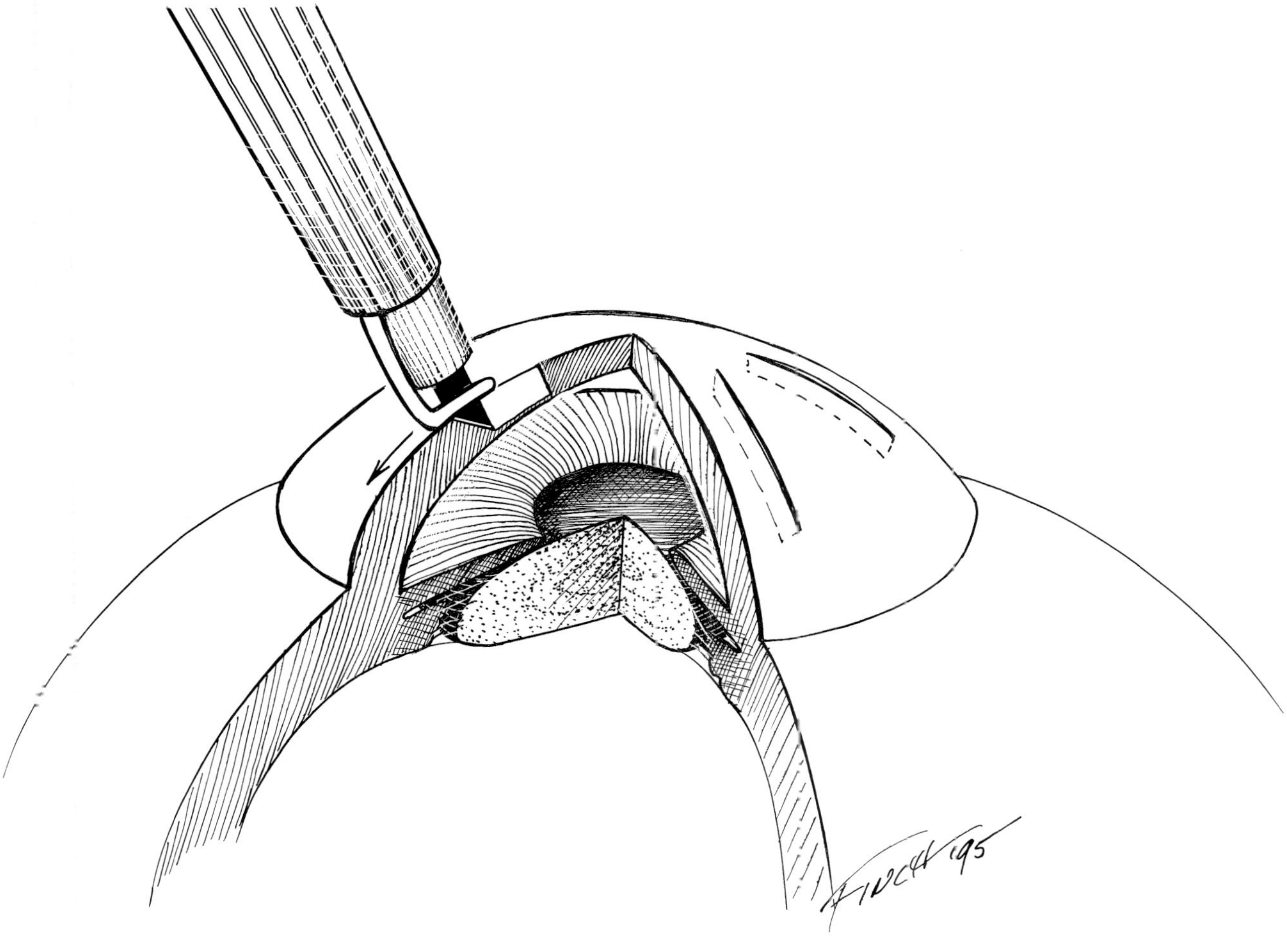

A

FIGURE 161-1 **A,** Radial keratotomy. Peripheral incisions weaken the cornea, inducing central flattening. *Continued.*

correct a wide range of refractive errors, including both myopia and hyperopia. Recently evolving techniques such as photorefractive keratectomy have at least the refractive accuracy of radial keratotomy without the disadvantage of corneal weakening. As a group, lamellar procedures are performed over the central clear zone, so the possibility of vision-threatening scarring is always present. A host of other disadvantages are procedure dependent, including surgical complexity (keratomileusis), poor predictability (myopic epikeratoplasty, keratophakia), and expensive and still investigational devices (all types of refractive lasers). Finally, *intraocular surgery* can be used to change the refractive state of the eye by either implanting high index-of-refraction artificial lenses, removing the crystalline lens, or both. Rapid rehabilitation of high refractive errors is a major advantage. However, severe intraocular complications can occur, including corneal decompensation and retinal detachment.

Each of these surgical categories has undergone major evolution since their inception. Improvements have been sought in predictability, stability, and safety. New devices, better instrumentation, and refined surgical techniques have been common denominators in the field of refractive surgery. These evolutionary changes and the future directions in each surgical category will be discussed.

Incisional Surgery

RADIAL KERATOTOMY

Radial keratotomy is a form of refractive surgery in which radial incisions (85% to 95% corneal depth) are made in the peripheral cornea with a thin, guarded blade. By weakening the cornea, peripheral steepening and central flattening correct myopia. Nomograms are used to increase the predictability of the procedure by varying the number of incisions and the diameter of the central clear zone. Radial keratotomy is commonly performed with astigmatic keratotomy to correct significant astigmatism.

B

C

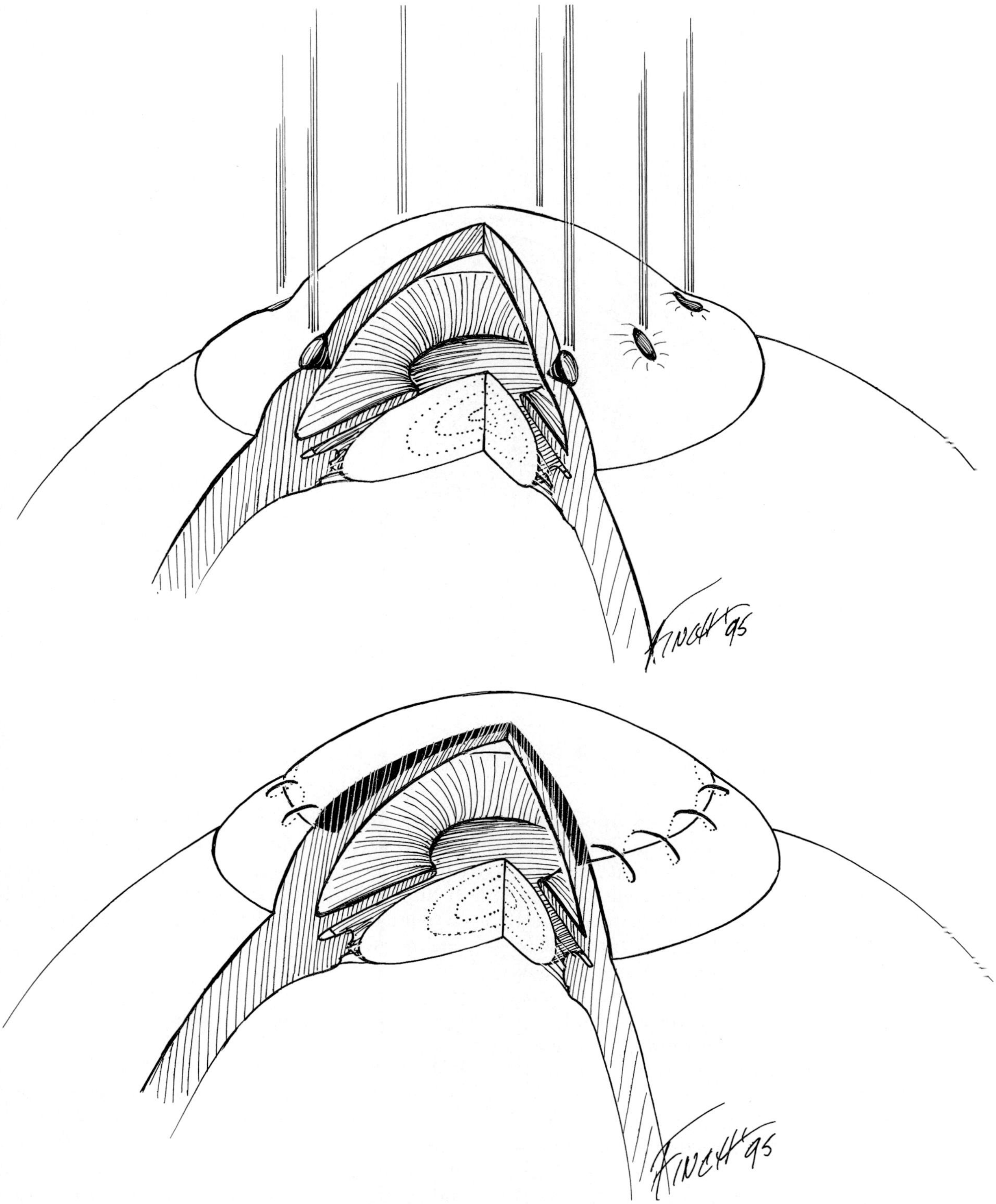

FIGURE 161-1, cont'd. **B,** Holmium: YAG laser thermokeratoplasty. Peripheral collagen shrinkage inducing central steepening. **C,** Myopic keratomileusis. Lathed lamellar lenticule sutured back onto host. *Continued.*

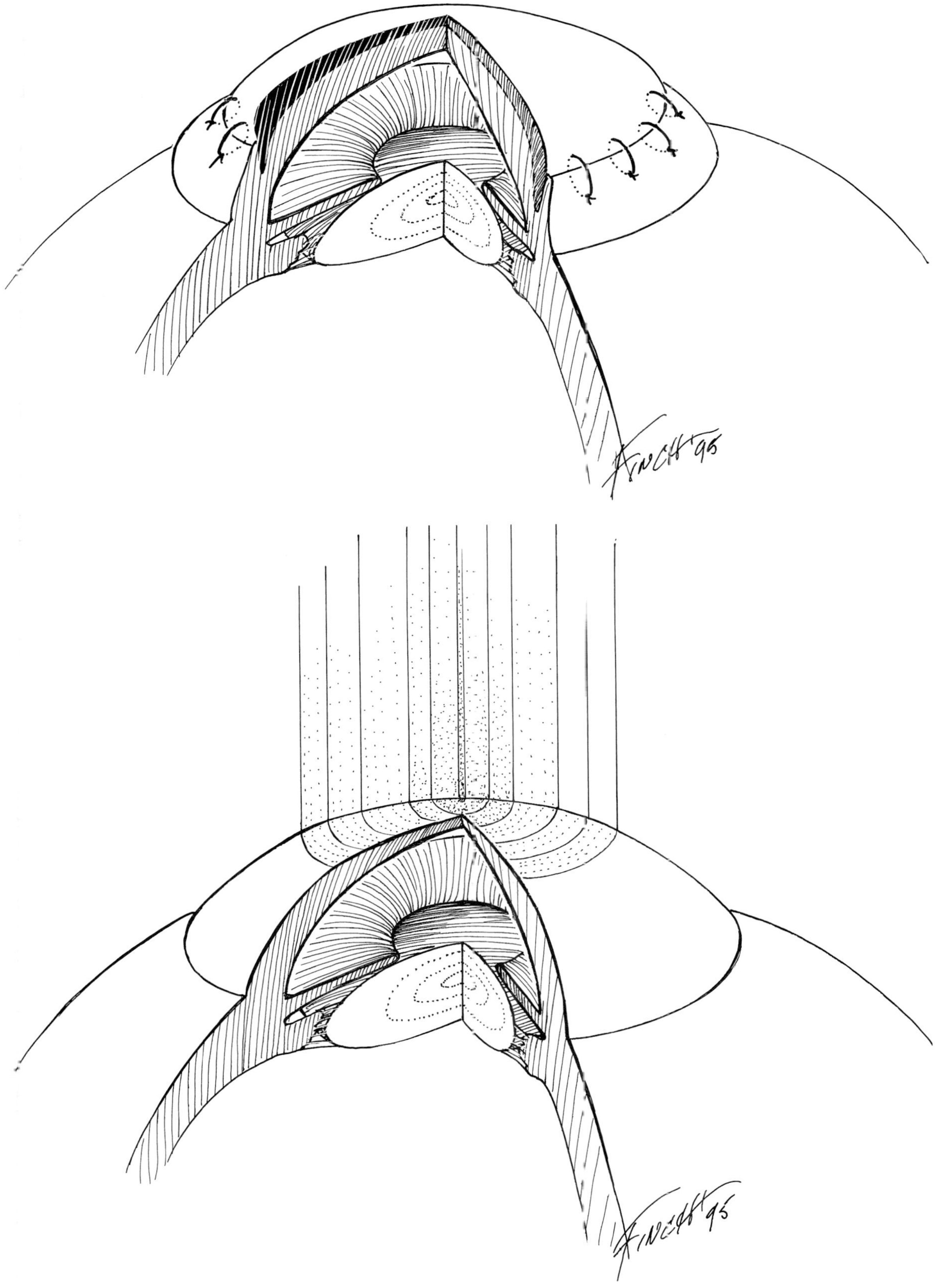

D

E

FIGURE 161-1, cont'd. **D,** Myopic epikeratoplasty. Prelathed myopic lenticule sutured onto Bowman's layer. **E,** Photorefractive keratectomy. Surface photoablation reshaping cornea using the excimer laser.

Continued.

F

G

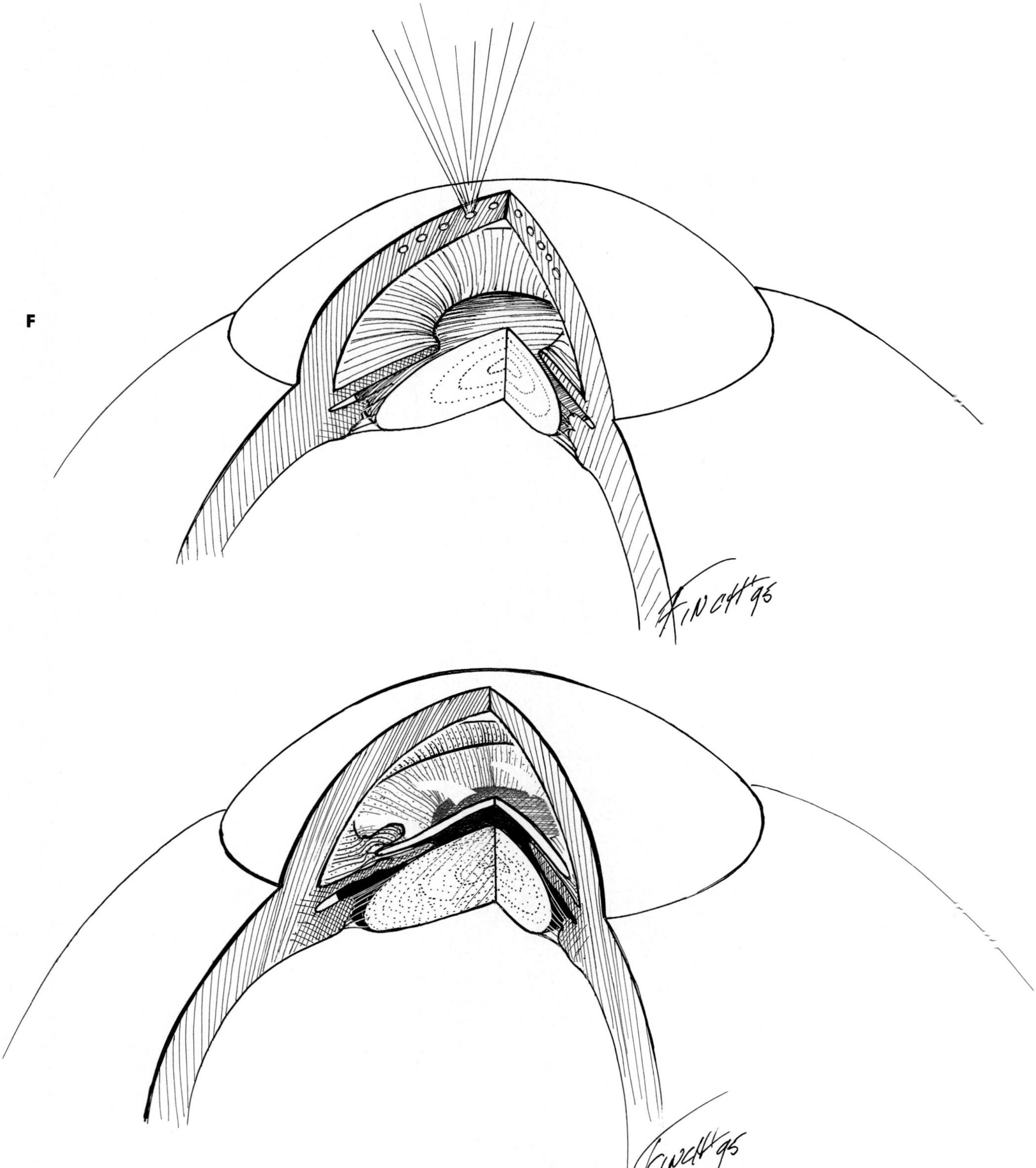

FIGURE 161-1, cont'd. **F, Intrastromal photoablation. Intrastromal cavities created by focused picosecond laser collapse, flattening central cornea. G, Minus power anterior chamber lens (iris-claw). Myopic intraocular lens is supported by iris.**

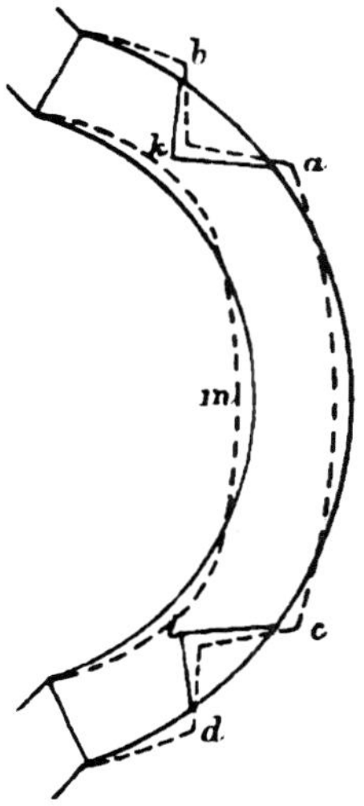

FIGURE 161-2 Drawing from Lans circa 1898 demonstrating basic principles of incisional keratotomy. Peripheral steepening and central flattening occur after partial thickness corneal incisions. (From Lans LJ: *Archiv fur Ophthalmologie* 45:122, 1898.)

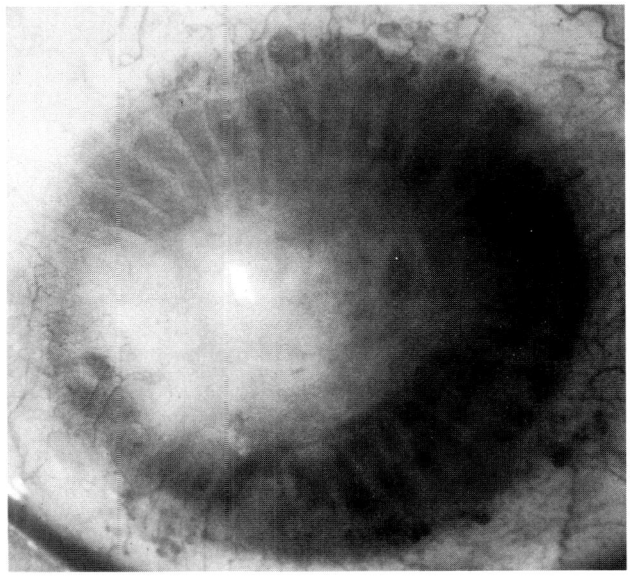

FIGURE 161-3 Posterior keratotomy using the Sato technique. Many corneas decompensate years after surgical trauma to the endothelium.

The first organized examination of incisional keratotomy is attributed to a Dutch ophthalmologist, Lendert Jan Lans.[5] Relying on early observations by Schiotz, Bates and Faber, and Lucciola, Lans examined astigmatic changes induced in rabbits after partial-thickness corneal incisions and thermal cautery.[6] In his first published report, entitled "Experimental Studies of the Treatment of Astigmatism with Non-perforating Corneal Incisions,"[7] many of the basic principles of radial and astigmatic keratotomy were established (Figure 161-2). Landmark principles he developed included (1) the fact that arcuate partial-thickness limbal incisions produce central corneal flattening in the same meridian and steepening in the perpendicular meridian and (2) the fact that the depth of the incision affects the magnitude of the refractive results.

The Japanese ophthalmologist Tutomu Sato made significant contributions to incisional refractive surgery in the 1930s and 1940s even though his long-term results in humans were disastrous. He observed central corneal flattening and improvement in vision after healing of spontaneous ruptures of Descemet's membrane (hydrops) in patients with advanced keratoconus. Sensing a potential treatment for keratoconus, he developed a technique to induce artificial ruptures of Descemet's membrane (Figure 161-3). Using a specially developed knife, he performed posterior keratotomy on keratoconus patients by making a series of incisions through the endothelium, Descemet's membrane, and posterior stroma.[8] Adding significance to this work was the fact that there was no alternative treatment available for these patients; contact lenses would not be available for another 10 to 20 years. Encouraged, Sato began to experiment with various forms of keratotomy in rabbits, which he then transferred directly to humans to correct myopia and astigmatism. On a biomechanical level, he felt that radial incisions relieved the "circular forces" of the cornea, flattening the central zone. Based on the rabbit studies, he felt that posterior radial incisions were more effective than anterior incisions for flattening the central cornea. It is now known that the rabbit is a poor model for the human cornea because of its high elasticity and lack of a Bowman's layer. The rabbit endothelium also has a much greater ability to regenerate than the human. Besides radial incisions for myopia, Sato also developed transverse posterior keratotomy to correct astigmatism.[9]

Sato performed anterior and posterior keratotomy on 281 eyes for myopia and astigmatism during an 8-year period (1943 to 1950). In 1953 he reported on 32 eyes with preoperative myopia ranging from -2.50 to -15.00 diopters (mean -10.00 diopters).[10] With early follow-up, myopia was reduced by an average of 3.00 diopters. Sato's ideas and surgical techniques never became widely accepted because contact lenses gained acceptance as a method to correct myopia. Sato died in 1960 before the important physiologic role of the corneal endothelium became apparent. Many years after posterior keratotomy a majority of his patients developed bullous keratopathy and a significant number required corneal transplantation. Kanai et al reported on 50 of Sato's patients (80 eyes) and observed that 75% of them developed corneal edema an average of 20 years after the operation.[11] In retrospect, we understand that the age-related loss of corneal endothelium, superimposed on the immediate surgically induced cell loss, resulted in the delayed corneal decompensation.

Taking lessons from the Japanese, Russian researchers investigated keratotomy techniques in the 1960s and 1970s. They first duplicated the intraocular posterior keratotomy of Sato but subsequently abandoned it in favor of an anterior approach because of the surgical problems associated with shallow anterior chambers and concerns about damage to the endothelium. Emerging as a major proponent of anterior keratotomy to correct myopia was Svyatoslav N. Fyodorov in Moscow, who is credited with laying the foundation of modern radial and astigmatic keratotomy. Fyodorov sought to improve the predictability of the procedure by deriving biomechanical formulas to account for individual corneal properties.[12] This was based on his theory of a circular corneal ligament that could be relaxed by radial incisions, similar to the model of Sato. Variables he included were the degree of myopic correction, corneal thickness, rigidity, radius of curvature, clear zone diameter, and a surgical incision depth factor. With this system, he was able to titrate the effect of the surgery and improve predictability. Through clinical and animal experimentation, he highlighted the importance of the paracentral incisions over more peripheral incisions that extended onto the sclera. He established that the diameter of the central clear zone is inversely related to the amount of refractive correction: smaller central clear zones yield greater myopic corrections. He also developed the forerunners of modern radial keratotomy instrumentation, including the micrometer blade handle with foot plate, gauge blocks for calibrating blade depth, and corneal marking devices. He developed various incisional patterns to correct myopia and astigmatism. His published reports in Western literature are limited, and his excellent results[13] have not been duplicated; others using his formulas report mixed results.[14,15] As an active proponent of radial keratotomy and a capable entrepreneur, he introduced the procedure in the United States in the late 1970s, but to the dismay of many, Fyodorov maintained tight control over his surgical techniques with proprietary rights to the nomograms and instrumentation. Few published reports exist that analyze the thousands of procedures performed in Russia.

Radial keratotomy in the United States

Refractive keratotomy had a tumultuous beginning in the United States. Bores is credited with performing the first procedure at the Kresge Institute in 1978.[16] This followed his visit to observe and perform the surgery at Moscow under the guidance of Fyodorov. Soon, many ophthalmologists were eager to learn and apply the experience of the Russians. Public interest in the procedure blossomed as the national press extolled the virtues of this surgical cure for nearsightedness. Almost as quickly, there ensued a division within the ophthalmic community over whether the procedure should be considered experimental. Clouding matters further, there were no regulatory guidelines from government agencies, such as the Food and Drug Administration, because the surgery did not involve a new drug or device. There were those who felt that by the early 1980s the procedure had established a level of safety and efficacy sufficient to be widely marketed. Others, however, were concerned about the paucity of published data with attendant critical peer review analysis. In addition, there were unanswered questions about the long-term effects of radial keratotomy, particularly in light of the devastating late consequences of posterior keratotomy. In 1979 the National Advisory Eye Council called for carefully controlled research into refractive surgery, stating, "Refractive keratoplasty as a clinical procedure is experimental."[17] Although this was initially directed at the lamellar procedures of Barraquer, the statement was later updated to include radial keratotomy. The American Academy of Ophthalmology and the International Society of Refractive Keratoplasty both adopted this position.[18] In this context, two nationwide studies were established: the Analysis of Radial Keratotomy and the Prospective Evaluation of Radial Keratotomy.

The Analysis of Radial Keratotomy (ARK) was established in 1981 with funding from the National Eye Institute as a multicenter clinical trial of radial keratotomy. Although the study was terminated in 1983, the investigators continued to publish important results of the surgery for many years afterward.

The National Eye Institute funded the Prospective Evaluation of Radial Keratotomy (PERK) study in 1980. This was a collaborative prospective study involving university-based and private practice ophthalmologists at nine clinical centers. The PERK study has produced a wealth of information about radial keratotomy and has influenced many aspects of its development. It has generally been viewed as the most critical analysis of radial keratotomy and is the benchmark by which other refractive procedures are measured.

After its introduction into the United States, radial keratotomy was modified and advanced as many researchers and clinicians sought to improve the safety and predictability. These advances included the use of better equipment (diamond blades, ultrasonic pachymetry, etc.), more accurate nomograms (incorporating variables such as patient age, intraocular pressure, etc.), and technique modification (number of incisions,

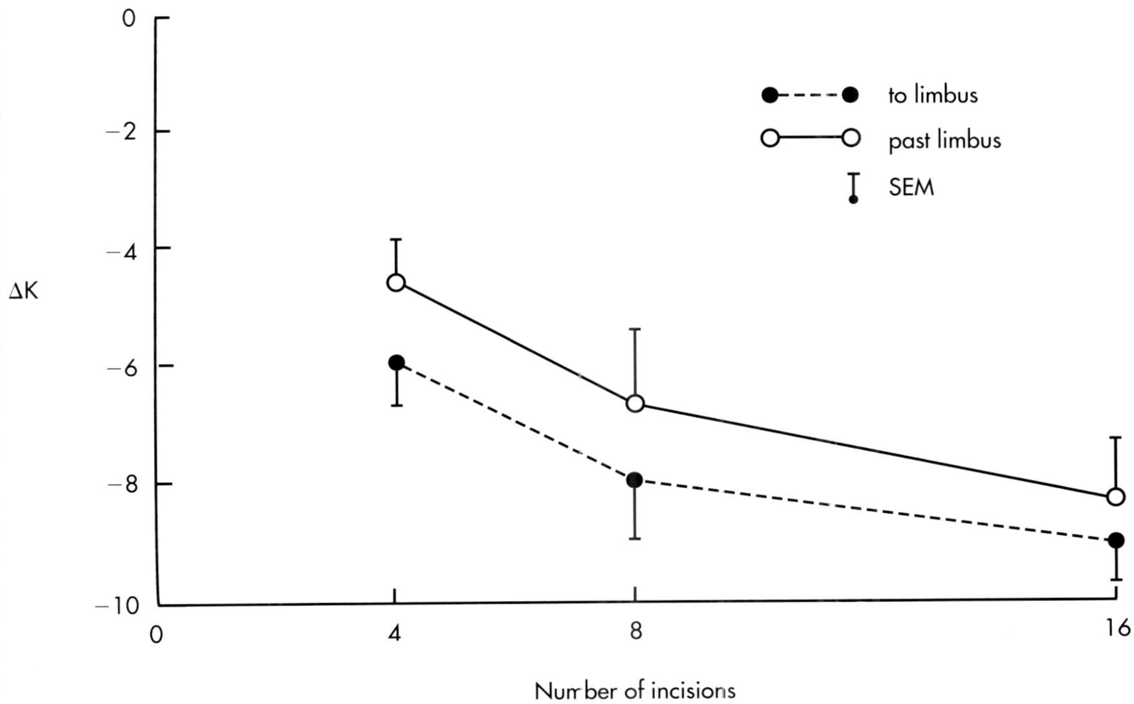

FIGURE 161-4 One of the most important trends in radial keratotomy over the last decade is that it has become less invasive. Shown are the changes in corneal curvature after four, eight, and 16 incisions in a human eye bank eye study. Between 80% and 90% of the total flattening observed with 16 incisions was achieved with only eight incisions. There was no statistical difference between the effect of incisions to the limbus versus incisions past the limbus. (From Salz J et al: *Ophthalmology* 88:744, 1981.)

mini-radial keratotomy, etc.). Computer-assisted modeling using finite element analysis has been used to study corneal changes induced by radial keratotomy in an effort to improve surgical predictability.[19-22]

The number of incisions has been gradually reduced as more knowledge about radial keratotomy has emerged. Sato used 60 anterior and posterior incisions with a 6 mm optic zone. After finding no added effect using 32 incisions, Fyodorov limited his surgery to 16. It was proposed by Schachar et al[23] in 1980 that eight incisions could produce most of the corneal flattening of radial keratotomy. This was confirmed in human cadaver eyes[24,25] and primate[26] studies. Salz et al[24] found that 80% to 90% of corneal flattening could be produced with the first eight incisions (Figure 161-4). Rowsey et al[27] analyzed the effect of eight and 16 incisions in a human clinical trial and, after matching for optic zone sizes, found no refractive difference between the two. These studies helped reduce the generally accepted practice of 16 radial incisions in the 1970s and early 1980s to eight or four. Salz and Rowsey also found that there was no refractive benefit to extending the incisions through the limbus as opposed to terminating them at the limbus.

The PERK study enrolled 427 patients (793 eyes) with preoperative myopia between −2.00 and −8.75 diopters (mean −3.875 diopters) in 1982 and 1983. The sole surgical variable was the diameter of the central clear zone (whether 3.0, 3.5, or 4.0 mm) based on the level of preoperative myopia. Ultrasonic pachymetry was used to set the depth of a diamond blade. Eight radial incisions were used for all patients; repeat surgery, if necessary, added an additional eight incisions. Ten years after the procedure,[2] 53% of patients achieved 20/20 or better uncorrected visual acuity and 85% were 20/40 or better. The mean refractive error at 10 years was +0.21 ± 1.58 diopters with 38% of eyes corrected to within 0.50 diopters of emmetropia and 60% to within 1 diopter. Of the patients who had bilateral surgery, 30% reported the use of spectacles or contact lenses for distant refractive correction at 10 years. Complications related to the procedure included a loss of best corrected visual acuity (3%), delayed bacterial keratitis, corneal scarring, irregular astigmatism, and epithelial erosions.

A major finding in the 10-year PERK study was the continuing long-term instability of the procedure, as had been previously reported.[28-30] A hyperopic shift of 1 diopter or greater was found in 43% of eyes between 6 months and 12 years. More worrisome was the lack of evidence that the amount of hyperopic shift was slowing between 5 and 10 years. It remains unknown if or when the refractive errors of this population will stabilize. There was an association between the length of the incision, as determined by the corneal diameter and the central clear zone diameter, and the amount of hyperopic shift. This association supports the theory that the more the cornea is weakened, the greater is the long-term refractive instability. It is likely that all forms of refractive surgery that act by weakening the cornea will be susceptible to some degree of instability. Two techniques have been developed in response to the hyperopic tendency after radial keratotomy: intentional undercorrection and the use of shorter incisions. "Mini-radial keratotomy" has been proposed in which the radial incisions are terminated at a peripheral diameter of 7 to 8 mm. The shorter incisions may reduce the long-term instability of the cornea, yet still provide refractive correction. In a rabbit model, short radial incisions were shown to be as effective as conventional incisions in inducing corneal flattening.[31]

As pointed out by the PERK investigators, there are numerous advantages to intentional undercorrection after radial keratotomy, such as offsetting the effects of a hyperopic shift, delaying the onset of presbyopic symptoms, and allowing repeated procedures to enhance refractive results. Titration of surgery with "enhancements" has become an important technique to improve the predictability of radial keratotomy. Werblin and Stafford[32] used additional procedures in 33% of their 205 surgical cases to achieve a 1-year postoperative refraction of $+0.27 \pm 0.58$ diopters, with 99% of patients having 20/40 or better uncorrected vision. Without the benefit of additional surgery, their accuracy was similar to the 1-year PERK results.

Despite all of the improvements since the inception of radial keratotomy, there are limits to the predictability of a procedure that relies on manual incisions. Uniform incision depth is difficult to achieve with a handheld blade. It was initially felt that the excimer laser could be used to make precise radial excisions and avoid manual incision imperfections.[33,34] However, the laser creates a wide excision of tissue (150 μm) that is unacceptable for use as a radial keratectomy procedure.[35] Even with perfect manual incisions, other problems exist that will limit the refractive outcome of radial keratotomy. Variability in the biomechanical properties of the cornea prevent prediction of the amount of corneal flattening for any given individual. Further understanding of the dynamic properties of the cornea and improved computer modeling are needed. This may make it possible to individually tailor the surgery based on preoperative measurements of material properties. There is also variability in the healing response, of which we have limited understanding.

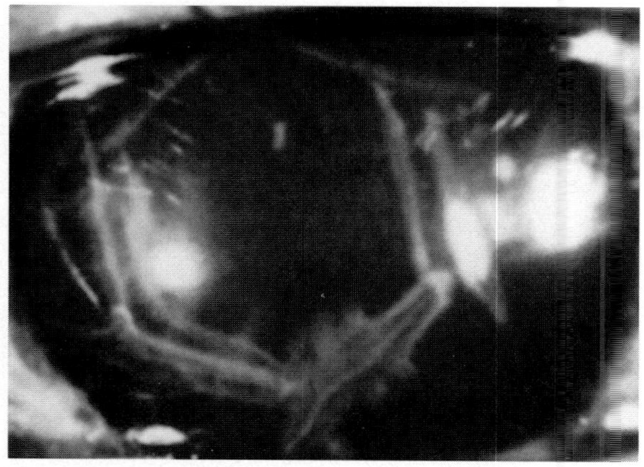

FIGURE 161-5 Slit lamp photograph of a patient who underwent bilateral hexagonal keratotomy. Note the wide scarring and wound gape. Computer-assisted videokeratography showed irregular astigmatism in both eyes with a range of refractive power overlying the entrance pupil of approximately 7.5 diopters in the right eye and 22 diopters in the left. The patient required bilateral penetrating keratoplasty for visual rehabilitation. (From Basuk WL et al: *Am J Ophthalmol* 117:42, 1994. Published with permission from the American Journal of Ophthalmology. Copyright by the Ophthalmic Publishing Co.)

There is no way to predict, at the present time, which individuals will experience a hyperopic shift after radial keratotomy.

HEXAGONAL KERATOTOMY

Hexagonal keratotomy is a refractive procedure intended to correct physiologic hyperopia, presbyopia, and postoperative hyperopia after radial keratotomy. The procedure involves making a series of paracentral incisions in a hexagonal pattern with subsequent steepening of the central cornea. This presumably occurs because the central cornea becomes mechanically "decoupled" from the rest of the cornea and bulges forward under the effect of intraocular pressure. In rabbits with hyperopia induced by radial keratotomy, Yamashita et al[36] reduced the hyperopia with hexagonal keratotomy. Early work on human cadaver and sighted eyes was encouraging and also demonstrated corneal steepening.[37,38] Initially, the hexagonal pattern was made with intersecting incisions. However, poor wound healing, corneal edema, and scarring led to the development of nonintersecting incisional patterns.[39] This was further refined to include a short transverse incision peripheral to each hexagonal apex.[40] Jensen[39] presented the results of hexagonal keratectomy in 483 eyes, of which 295 had nonintersecting incision. The average refractive change was 2.25 diopters with minimal reported complications. However, there were persistent concerns regarding the overall safety of the procedure.[41,42] Basuk et al[43]

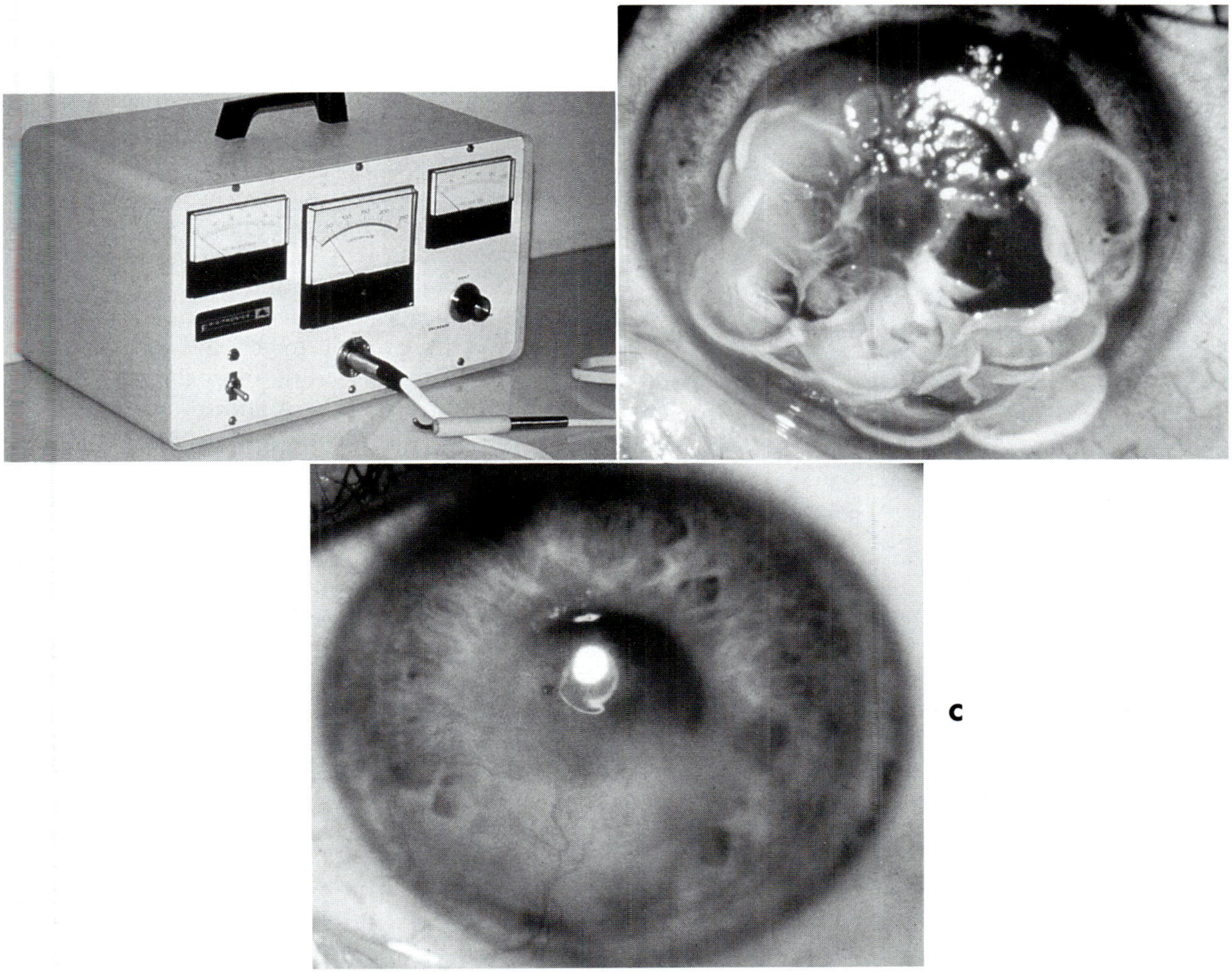

FIGURE 161-6 **A,** Thermokeratophore power unit for large area thermokeratoplasty in treating keratoconus. **B,** The probe was placed directly over the cone to induce flattening. Immediate postoperative result showing extensive sloughing of epithelium. **C,** Later scarring.

reported a series of significant complications in 15 eyes of 10 patients treated with intersecting and nonintersecting hexagonal keratotomy (Figure 161-5). These included glare, photophobia, polyopia, fluctuating vision, overcorrection, irregular astigmatism, corneal edema, corneal perforation, bacterial keratitis, cataract, and endophthalmitis. They concluded that hexagonal keratotomy should be abandoned until further studies establish its safety and efficacy.

Thermal Keratoplasty

Over the last three decades, there have been numerous attempts to correct hyperopia using heat in a procedure called thermokeratoplasty. The application of heat to the corneal stroma has long been known to effect a change in corneal curvature. In the 1890s Lans[7] demonstrated a change in corneal shape after the application of superficial thermal burns in rabbits. Gasset, Shaw, and others studied the response of mammalian corneal stroma to heat and established that the optimum temperature was approximately 65° C.[44,45] At this temperature the collagen shrinkage varied from 30% to 50%. A device called the thermokeratophore was developed to apply and regulate the application of heat (Figure 161-6). This consisted of a flat or curved probe of various sizes (3 to 7 mm) for direct thermal transfer. In the 1970s, Gasset and Kaufman[46] used this device to treat advanced keratoconus. The probe was placed over the cone, and diathermy was applied until the desired flattening occurred. The initial results were very encouraging: 46 of 50 eyes achieved 20/30 or better vision. Arentsen

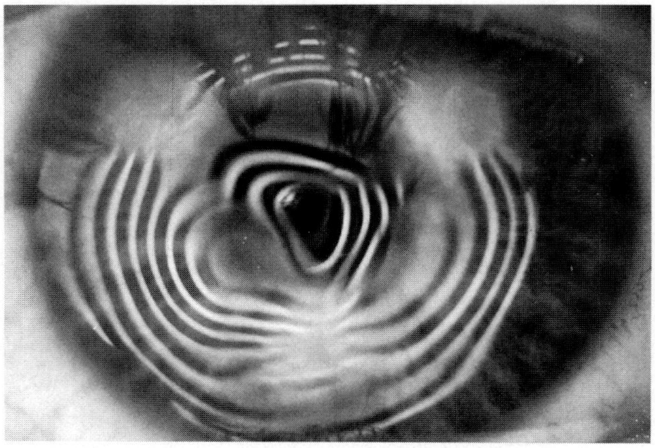

FIGURE 161-7 Keratoscopic view of patient treated with Los Alamos thermokeratoplasty. Note treatment areas and effect on keratoscopic mires.

and Laibson[47] had less favorable acuity results in a similar study of 29 eyes. Keates and Dingle[48] noted initial flattening followed by regression to pretreatment steepness in most of their keratoconus patients. Severe complications were later reported and included recurrent epithelial erosions, delayed epithelialization, stromal scarring and necrosis, iritis, hypopyon, and vascularization.[49-51] With these difficulties and the high rate of regression, externally applied, large area corneal diathermy was abandoned as a refractive procedure.

In 1979, Rowsey and Doss[52] attempted to address the problems associated with externally applied heat by using an electromagnetic delivery system (Figure 161-7). The Los Alamos keratoplasty probe was designed to heat the midstroma (200 to 400 μm) with radiofrequency to reduce damage to the epithelium and endothelium. Immediately after the procedure in keratoconus patients, significant flattening was observed. However, regression of effect and re-steepening of the cornea occurred and the Los Alamos probe was withdrawn from clinical trials.[53]

Fyodorov, in the 1980s, developed radial thermokeratoplasty. In this procedure a heated loop of wire (600° C) was driven deep into the corneal stroma (Figure 161-8).[54] The diathermy was applied in a radial fashion in the peripheral cornea, causing a beltlike circumferential tightening with central steepening. The multiple, deep paracentral burns were an attempt to eliminate the regression that had doomed previous techniques. The number and placement of the burns were determined by the desired hyperopic correction using formulas developed by Fyodorov. Unlike previous applications of diathermy, which were generally limited to treating keratoconus, radial thermokeratoplasty was intended to correct hyperopia, hyperopic astigmatism, and presbyopia (Figure 161-9). Favorable results were reported in a retrospective review of 117 procedures performed by Fyodorov.[55] Mean hyperopia was reduced from +5.27 D to +1.84 D. Schachar[56] reported similar results in 51 eyes of 41 patients. However, careful follow-up demonstrated substantial, and sometimes total, regression of effect[57] as well as damage to the corneal endothelium.[58] Complications included iritis, fibrovascular ingrowth in the peripheral burns, and microperforations.

The application of laser technology to the thermal alteration of corneal stroma was a leap ahead of previous efforts. It was developed to avoid the shortcomings of previous techniques and provide permanent refractive correction of hyperopia. The past use of metallic instruments to heat the stroma required markedly superheated devices (e.g., the 600° C hot wire of radial thermokeratoplasty) applied for long periods of time (a second or longer) because the delivery of the heat into the stroma was limited by thermal diffusion. As a result, severe coagulative necrosis was produced at the site of contact of the metal instrument with the cornea. Rather than simply shrinking the stroma, these techniques resulted in liquefaction of the collagen, followed by a marked inflammatory response. Lytic enzymes from these inflammatory cells, as well as the coagulative necrosis caused by the tremendously high temperatures used, resulted in problems such as persistent epithelial defects related to destruction of the epithelial Bowman's layer complex and probably contributed to the marked postoperative regression of corneal topographic change. With infrared lasers, such as the holmium: YAG, however, delivery of energy into the stroma is direct, rather than through thermal diffusion, the duration of treatment is measured in milliseconds, and no region of the cornea need be exposed to tremendously hot temperatures.

Seiler et al[59] used a pulsed holmium: YAG laser that emitted infrared radiation at a wavelength of 2.06 μm. The laser was focused 400 μm in front of the hand piece and concentrated the radiation in the midstroma to avoid excessive damage to the epithelium and basement membrane. Cone-shaped areas of stromal heating resulted. These were placed concentrically within the mid cornea and peripheral cornea, causing collagen shrinkage and central steepening, as in radial thermokeratoplasty. Horn et al[60] used a tunable cobalt:magnesium fluoride laser in a similar fashion. Animal eyes, human cadaver eyes, and blind eye studies demonstrated central corneal steepening after laser thermokeratoplasty.[59-61] Seiler[62] reported encouraging early results in sighted eyes with preoperative hyperopia between 2 and 4 diopters. With limited follow-up, 80% (16/20) of his patients were within 1

A

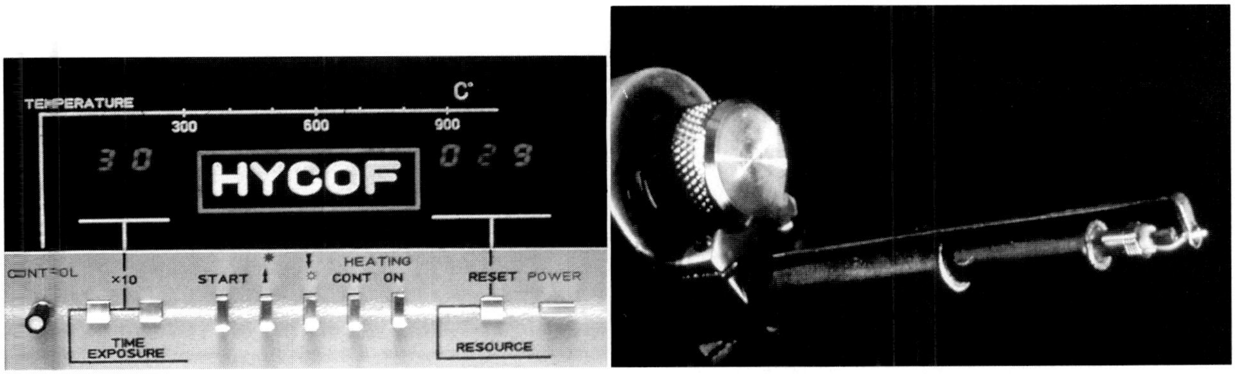

B

FIGURE 161-8 **A,** Power unit for the hot wire thermokeratoplasty technique of Fyodorov. **B,** The super-heated wire is driven into the stroma with a computer-controlled hand piece. (From Bores L: *Refractive Eye Surgery,* 1993. Reprinted by permission of Blackwell Scientific Publications, Inc.)

A

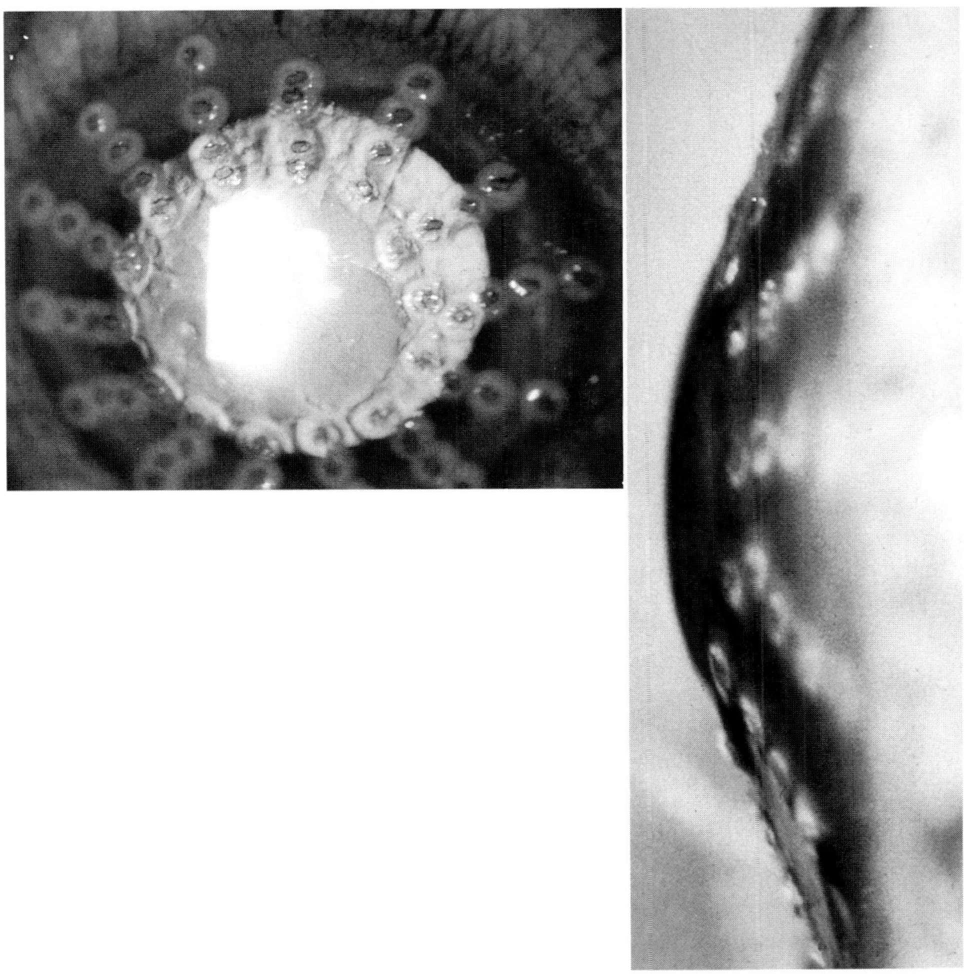

B

FIGURE 161-9 **A,** Immediate postoperative result of hot wire thermokeratoplasty showing radial pattern on frontal view. **B,** Induced central steepening on side view.

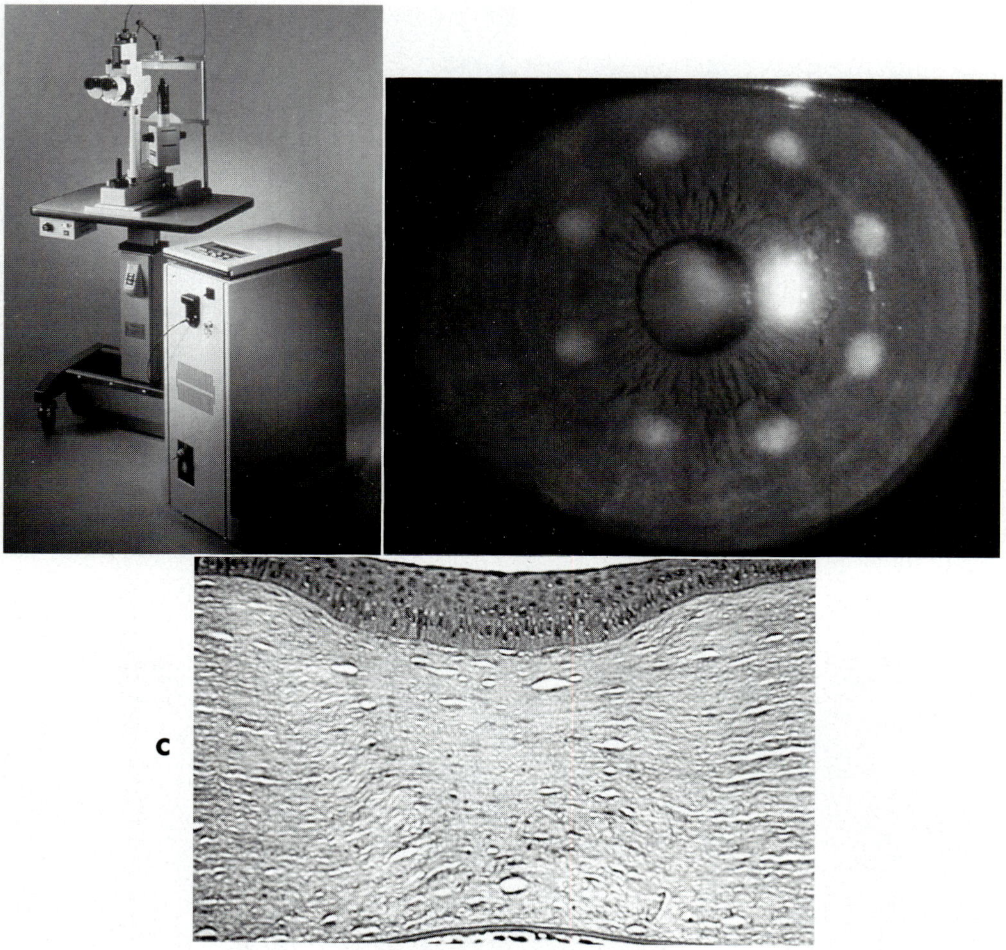

FIGURE 161-10 **A,** Slit lamp delivery system for holmium: YAG thermokeratoplasty. **B,** Immediate postoperative view showing eight peripheral applications. **C,** Histology demonstrates cone-shaped area of collagen shrinkage.

diopter of attempted correction. As with other refractive procedures that rely on collagen shrinkage, longer term analysis is needed to assess stability. Further advances for the holmium:YAG laser have included a slit lamp–based noncontact delivery system (Figure 161-10). The holmium:YAG laser for the treatment of hyperopia is currently being investigated with Food and Drug Administration approved clinical trials in the United States.

Lamellar Surgery

Lamellar procedures have evolved from techniques developed by José Barraquer in Colombia. These initially included keratophakia (corneal lens) and cryolathe keratomileusis (corneal carving), and newer techniques such as epikeratophakia, automated lamellar keratoplasty, and excimer laser photorefractive keratectomy. All of these procedures, with the exception of high-index-of-refraction intrastromal lenses, correct refractive errors by changing the curvature of the anterior surface of the cornea. They do so either by adding tissue to or removing tissue from the corneal stroma.

Techniques that require a lamellar keratectomy will be discussed first and include keratomileusis and keratophakia. Barraquer presented clinical results of cryolathe keratomileusis in 1964[63] and keratophakia in 1966.[64] Ainslie[65] used the techniques in England in the 1970s, and they were introduced in the United States by Troutman and Swinger[66] in 1977. These procedures require special lathing and keratome instrumentation and are technically complex. Lamellar keratectomies are performed with a special microkeratome that defines the diameter and depth of cut. A suction ring holds the keratome in place, and this ring can cause transient elevation of intraocular pressure to 60 mm Hg

A

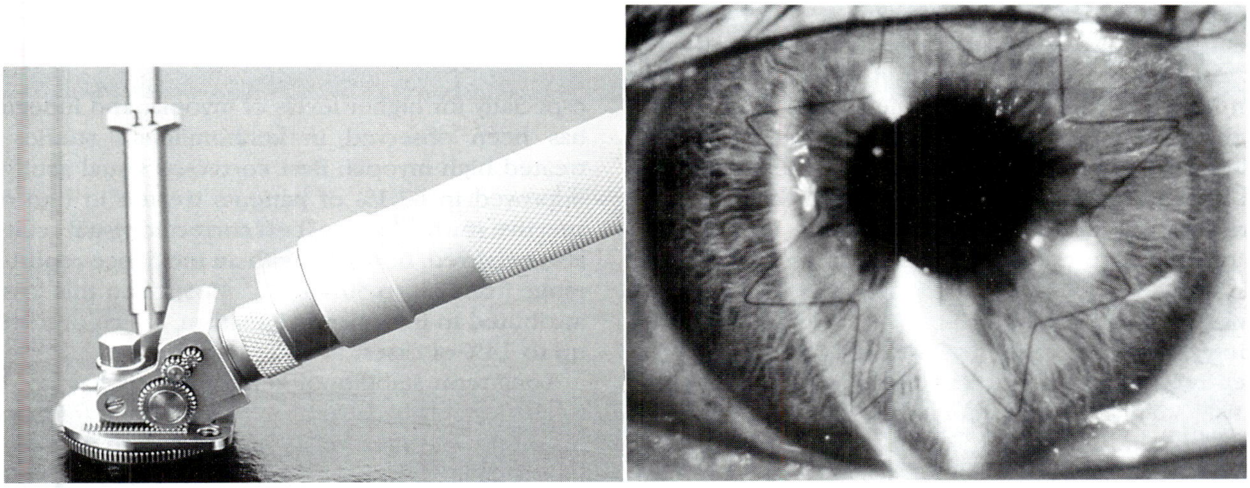

B

FIGURE 161-11 **A,** Keratomileusis lamellar dissection is performed with the technically demanding and mechanically complex microkeratome. **B,** Cryolathe myopic keratomileusis 48 hours postoperatively. (From Bores L: *Refractive eye surgery,* 1993. Reprinted by permission of Blackwell Scientific Publications, Inc.)

or higher, which in some instances is sufficient to interrupt perfusion of the retina. While the depth of the incision can reportedly be regulated to within 5% of the planned depth, inadvertent entry into the anterior chamber occurs in 1% to 2% of cases performed by experienced surgeons. Equipment failure can lead to irregular dissections or anterior chamber entry. Automated keratomes have been developed to replace the manual microkeratome and should improve the quality of the incision and reduce surgeon error.

KERATOMILEUSIS

Several variants of keratomileusis can correct either myopia or hyperopia. In the original procedure, a central lamellar keratectomy is performed and the resected disk is shaped by the Barraquer cryolathe (autoplastic keratomileusis). The shaped disk is then sutured in place. For myopic correction, more material is removed centrally, effectively flattening the central cornea (Figure 161-11). For hyperopia, more tissue is removed from the periphery of the disk, causing a compensatory steepening of the central cornea. To avoid cryo-damage to the lenticule, the Barraquer-Krumeich-Swinger (BKS) system was developed to shape the disk without freezing.[67] A donor cornea can also be used to form the lenticule (homoplastic keratomileusis). Homoplastic keratomileusis differs from epikeratoplasty in that no host lamellar dissection is performed in epikeratoplasty. The preformed lenticule is sutured directly onto Bowman's layer in epikeratoplasty instead of being placed in a lamellar pocket as in keratomileusis. In situ myopic keratomileusis is a more recent development in which a second pass of the microkeratome is used to resect a plano disk in the host bed.[68] This creates central flattening when the original lenticule is sutured back onto the host. While this obviates the need for lathing tissue, it is technically difficult to perform and may be less reversible than other forms of myopic keratomileusis because centering of the second pass is critical. In situ keratomileusis using an automated keratome has been termed automated lamellar keratoplasty (ALK). A variant of this technique involves leaving the lenticule attached to the host after the first keratome pass so it can be hinged back for the second resection pass. This ensures proper orientation of the lenticule, reduces suturing, avoids postoperative "lost" lenticules, and may speed postoperative visual recovery. Another variant of in situ keratomileusis uses the excimer laser to ablate a predetermined amount of tissue from either the host bed or the nonepithelial side of the resected anterior cap. This procedure has been termed the "flap and zap" technique or laser-assisted in situ keratomileusis (LASIK). Combining keratomileusis with photorefractive keratectomy avoids ablating Bowman's layer while using the precise tissue removal characteristics of the excimer laser. Clinical trials are under way to study this technique.

Myopic keratomileusis (MKM), the most common application of keratomileusis, is performed by a small number of experienced surgeons to treat high myopia. It has progressed from the cryolathe techniques of Barraquer, to nonfreeze lathing with the BKS system, to in situ MKM without the necessity to lathe a lenticule mechanically using either a second keratome pass or the excimer laser to achieve refractive correction. MKM has been shown to correct as much as 24 diopters of myopia with a homoplastic lenticule, and up to 16

pocket over the pupillary aperture as an alloplastic form of keratophakia. An exception is the intrastromal corneal ring, in which a plastic band is placed circumferentially around the peripheral cornea to effect a

well tolerated in cats. Meister et al[oo] had success implanting hydroxyethyl methacrylate (HEMA) lenticules in rabbits, and years later, McCarvey and Andrews used a copolymer of HEMA (Perfilcon-A) in rabbit corneas diopters using the patient's tissue (autoplastic).[69] Hyperopic keratomileusis (HKM) can correct up to 10.75 diopters of hyperopia, but this is the most

By placing myopic refractive correction at the corneal plane instead of spectacle plane, minification is reduced. Theoretically, this should improve acuity

with good tolerance. Unfortunately, nonhuman primate eyes implanted with Perfilcon-A had a high rate of failure, with epithelial ingrowth, aseptic necrosis, and progressive scarring in the majority of early cases,[89] although contamination of the lenses during preparation was postulated to be responsible for many of the failures. Werblin et al[90] studied intrastromal Perfilcon-A in five myopic patients who had a mean preoperative refraction of -14.00 diopters. Although the corneas remained clear, the refractive results were disappointing. The patients were undercorrected by an average of 5.0 diopters, and refraction had not stabilized after 18 months of follow-up. Another copolymer of HEMA, Lidofilcon-A, was reported to be well tolerated in nonhuman primate corneas.[91] High-risk aphakic patients who were implanted with this material had a mean 3-month postoperative refraction of -0.5 ± 1.8 diopters.[92] However, visual recovery was prolonged and took 12 months to return to baseline (preoperative) best corrected acuity.

Polysulfone is a nonpermeable material with excellent optical qualities and a high index of refraction (1.633). Because it can serve as an intrastromal lens, no change in anterior corneal curvature is required, as in hydrogel implants. A technically easier stromal pocket dissection can be used for insertion rather than a complete lamellar keratectomy. Attracted by these apparent advantages, Choyce[93] experimented with intrastromal polysulfone in the early 1980s. While initially the material seemed to be well tolerated in early human studies, corneal opacities, nonhealing epithelial erosions, and diurnal fluctuations in vision were later observed.[94] This led to the incorporation of microperforations into the inlay for the transfer of fluid and nutrients to the anterior cornea (Figure 161-13). Although fenestrated polysulfone (35 μm fenestrations) showed increased safety in cat corneas, it proved to be optically unsatisfactory.[95] Smaller fenestrations (10 μm) may preserve the optical properties of implanted polysulfone and still provide nourishment to the anterior cornea. Smaller diameter, high-index-of-refraction implants are also being investigated as a technique for correcting presbyopia.

EPIKERATOPLASTY

To eliminate the complexity of the lamellar dissection and intraoperative lathing of keratomileusis, Kaufman and Werblin developed epikeratoplasty (Figure 161-14).[96] This was intended as a "living contact lens" for aphakic patients unable to wear contact lenses. By eliminating the central lamellar dissection, it was hoped that the procedure would be safer, easier to perform, and reversible. In this technique, donor corneal tissue is prelathed into the proper shape and sutured onto a recipient, deepithelialized cornea in which Bowman's layer and stroma have been left intact. The change in curvature of the anterior surface produced by the lenticule provides the refractive correction. This could theoretically change the refractive status of the cornea by up to 37 diopters.[97] To prepare the host cornea the epithelium is removed, followed by an annular keratectomy with resection of a 0.5 to 1.0 mm wedge of Bowman's membrane and anterior stroma from the inner aspect of a partial thickness 7 to 8 mm trephine. A partial lamellar dissection peripheral to the trephine allows the wing of the lenticule to be tucked under the host tissue. This preparation helps to scar the lenticule to the host cornea[98] and permits repopulation of the donor with host keratocytes.[99,100] Interrupted and running 10-0 nylon sutures are used to secure the tissue and are removed 6 to 12 weeks later. Studies were conducted initially on nonhuman primates[97] and were later expanded to include human adult and pediatric aphakia,[101,102] keratoconus,[103] and myopia.[104] Plus convex lenses were used for aphakia, minus concave lenses for myopia, and plano lenses for keratoconus. Four large nationwide studies (adult and pediatric aphakia,[105,106] keratoconus,[107] and myopia[108]) were conducted after commercially prepared tissue became available in 1984. Together they comprised 1389 procedures.

In response to complications and unpredictable results, numerous changes were made during the course of these studies. Every aspect of the procedure was modified, including epithelial removal, trephination, annular keratectomy, peripheral lamellar dissection, lens design, and suture techniques.

A corneal press was developed to uniformly hydrate the donor cornea before lathing to improve refractive results.[109] Later, nonfreeze techniques were used to shape the lenticule.[110] The size of the donor lenticule relative to the recipient bed underwent refinement. It was quickly discovered that lenticules the same size as the recipient bed resulted in undercorrection of aphakia with less than intended corneal steepening. Donor lenticules were made 0.5, 1.0, and then 1.5 mm larger than the recipient. For myopia the opposite relationship was found. A donor lenticule with a 1.0 or 1.5 mm disparity resulted in under correction with less corneal flattening than desired.[104] A change was made back to a 0.5 mm difference, but this made fitting the donor onto myopic corneas more difficult. Stretching the lenticule during placement often caused folds in the underlying host, which often led to complaints of glare. A change was made back to the 1.5 mm disparity (8.5 mm tissue and 7.0 mm host bed) with the outer edge of the donor tissue tucked into a peripheral lamellar dissection.[108] Storage of the lathed lenticule changed from lyophilization to a "moist-pak" in an effort to promote more rapid epithelialization and clearing of the cornea.

Prompt reepithelialization over the graft was a major

A

B

C

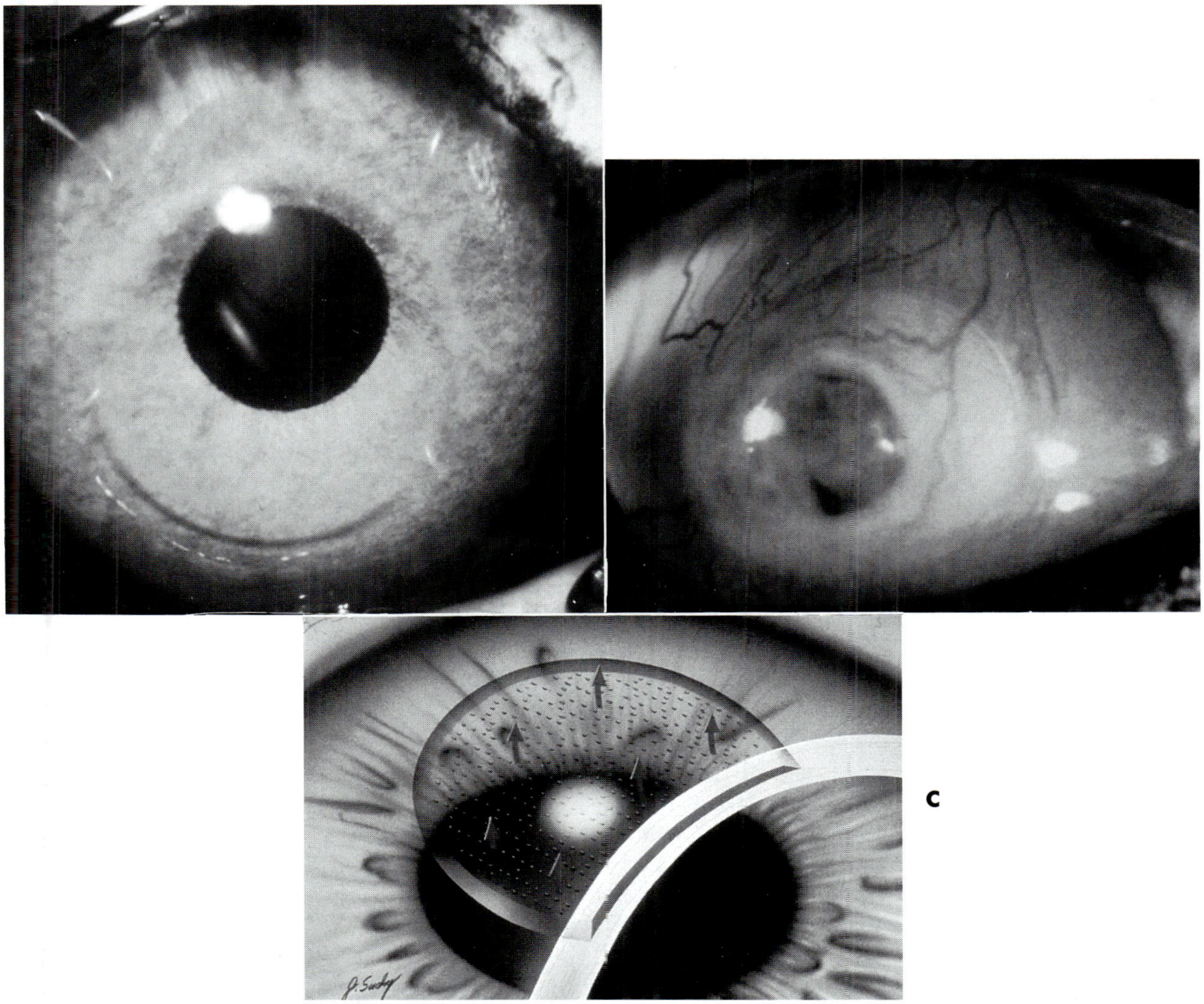

FIGURE 161-13 **A,** Successful polysulfone intracorneal lens (ICL) in a primate. **B,** Anterior stromal necrosis of ICL in the primate model led to the development of fenestrations to nourish the overlying cornea. Relatively large fenestrations (35 μm) were found to be optically unsuitable. **C,** Smaller diameter fenestrations in polysulfone lenses are being investigated as shown in this artist's rendition. (Courtesy Richard Lindstrom, MD.)

problem that was never fully solved. Bandage contact lenses, patching, temporary tarsorrhaphies,[101] and changes in lathing and preservation techniques of the lenticule were tried.[111] Topical absolute alcohol used for epithelial removal was replaced with a 4% cocaine solution. The incidence of nonhealing defects in the large nationwide series was 2.5% to 3.5%.[105,106,108] The mean time to reepithelialization was 7.1 days in adult aphakia cases, but it could take weeks to months before the epithelium had a normal histologic appearance[112] and barrier function.[113,114] The consequences of failure to reepithelialize were severe and included necrosis, infection, and melting of the graft.[99] The overall graft removal rate in the four large nationwide studies was 7.7% (105/1362), with the most common reason being a persistent epithelial defect. Other complications and causes for lenticule removal included hazy graft, infection, stromal infiltrates, melt, dehiscence, refractive error, irregular astigmatism, epithelial ingrowth and interface cysts, and severe glare symptoms.[108,115,116] After lenticule removal, 14% of patients who had undergone epikeratoplasty for myopia had a reduction of best corrected visual acuity. Central scarring of the host after donor removal was also reported, which cast doubt on the reversibility of the procedure.[117,118]

Even with all of the changes in technique, the refractive results of myopic epikeratoplasty were disappointing. With an average follow-up time of 212 days in the nationwide study, the mean spherical equivalent refractive error decreased from −12.52 to −1.38 diopters postoperatively. However, the postoperative

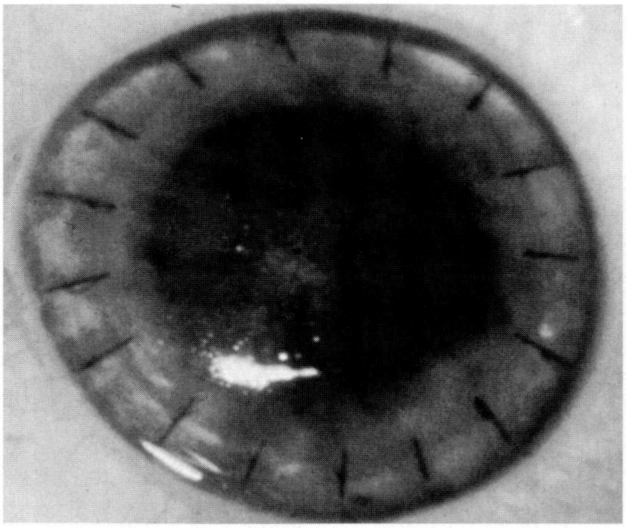

FIGURE 161-14 Epikeratoplasty lenticule sutured in place immediately postoperatively. After disappointing refractive results of myopic epikeratoplasty, commercial production of lenticules were terminated.

standard deviation was 3.64 diopters, indicating considerable variability in refractive outcome. Overall, 33% of patients attained 20/40 or better uncorrected vision, but only 35% were corrected to within 10% of emmetropia. A total of 15% of the patients lost two or more lines of best corrected visual acuity, and the mean astigmatism increased from 1.4 ± 0.8 to 2.6 ± 2.1 dipoters. Early and late regression of refractive effect was also noted.[77,108,119,120] In the nationwide myopia study, 17.6% of patients had regression of at least 2 diopters by the fifth postoperative month. This depended on the amount of preoperative myopia; in the lower range of myopia (−3.75 to −11.75), 12% regressed, compared to 32% in the high range (−18.00 to −32.50).

The results for aphakic epikeratoplasty were also less than desired. In the nationwide aphakia study the mean spherical equivalent refractive error decreased from +11.5 ± 1.92 to +0.9 ± 2.83 diopters postoperatively. Again the high postoperative standard deviation (2.83 diopters) indicated considerable variability in refractive outcome, especially when compared to the standard deviation for intraocular lens implantation, which is only 1.0 diopter.[121] Visual recovery time was also substantially more prolonged after epikeratoplasty than after intraocular lens implantation.[122] Still the procedure did offer an alternative method to correct anisometropia in the unilaterally aphakic, contact lens–intolerant patient in whom intraocular surgery was contraindicated.[116]

For keratoconus, epikeratoplasty was envisioned to provide tectonic support where severe corneal distortion and steepness made it impossible to fit contact lenses. Epikeratoplasty could then restore vision by allowing the resumption of contact lens use, while avoiding the risks of penetrating keratoplasty. The nationwide study of epikeratoplasty for keratoconus resulted in improvement in uncorrected vision in 98% (80/82) of patients. There was a higher proportion of patients who achieved 20/40 or better best spectacle-corrected visual acuity (78% after epikeratoplasty compared to 69% before surgery).[107] Astigmatism was slightly reduced from an average of 5.97 diopters before the procedure to 4.65 diopters afterward. When compared to penetrating keratoplasty, both procedures were shown to have similar results in obtaining 20/40 or better best corrected acuity.[123-125] However, penetrating keratoplasty resulted in a significantly higher proportion of eyes with 20/20 best corrected acuity (73% after penetrating keratoplasty versus 24% after epikeratoplasty).[125]

The Ophthalmic Devices Panel of the Food and Drug Administration in 1988 made the following recommendations for indications for epikeratoplasty:

1. A visually disabled monocular aphake for whom secondary intraocular lens insertion is contraindicated or who is documented to be glasses and contact lens intolerant or unsuitable for contact lens wear because of preexisting ocular disease.
2. An aphakic child over the age of 1 year who has been demonstrated to be contact lens intolerant or unsuitable for contact lens wear because of preexisting ocular disease, and who is unable to use spectacles for visual correction and in whom amblyopic therapy can be provided by a pediatric ophthalmologist or a practitioner experienced in the management of amblyopia.
3. A visually disabled patient with keratoconus who has clear corneas, who is contact lens intolerant or unsuitable for contact lens wear because of preexisting ocular disease, who is unable to achieve visual correction with spectacles, and in whom keratoplasty is contraindicated or associated with a high risk for failure.
4. A patch graft used for tectonic purposes.

In light of the disappointing results of the myopic trials, no application for myopic epikeratoplasty was submitted to the Food and Drug Administration for review. The manufacturer of the commercially prepared lenticules ceased production, and only those few centers with corneal lathe equipment have been able to continue performing this procedure.

LASER (PHOTOREFRACTIVE) KERATECTOMY

The use of lasers to sculpt the cornea has been a major advancement in the field of refractive surgery. Laser keratectomy involves remodeling the corneal stroma by tissue removal as a form of lamellar surgery.

A

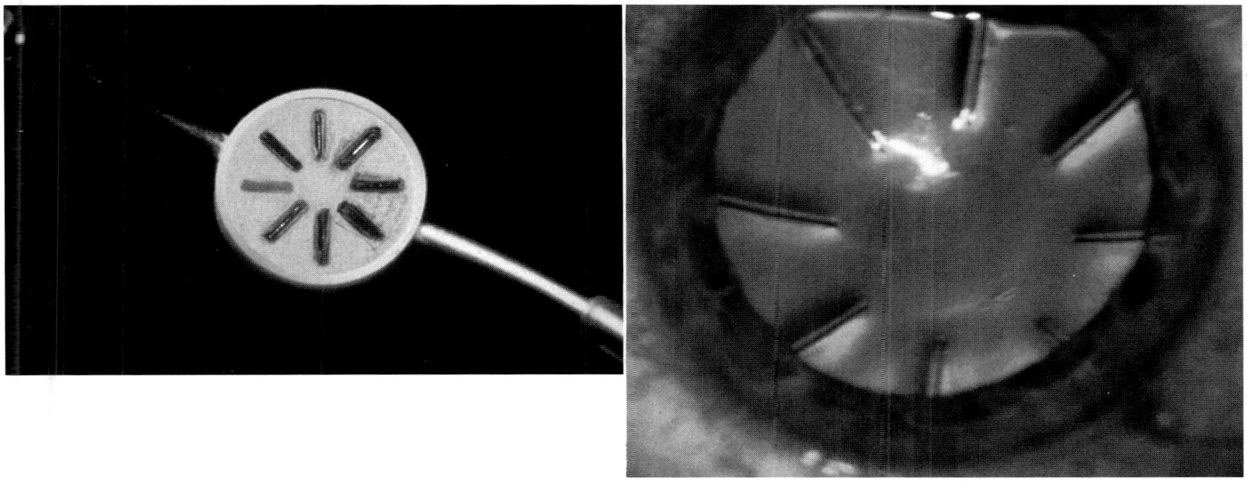

B

FIGURE 161-15 **A,** Some of the initial experiments with the excimer laser used an aperture to create radial excisions to induce central flattening. **B,** Clinically and biomechanically, these excisions could not compete with incisions made with thin diamond blades for radial keratotomy.

The overriding advantage of the laser is its ability to remove tissue with a microscopic precision that is unattainable with conventional surgery. Furthermore, the laser can alter the shape of the cornea without weakening it, unlike incisional techniques. Incisional surgery is rapidly approaching a technologic limit. The minimum amount of corneal weakening required to produce a refractive result may still lead to undesirable side effects (diurnal fluctuation in vision, progressive hyperopia, etc.).[126] However, there has not been a long-term (> 10 years) analysis of the risks and benefits of the laser procedures as there has been for radial keratotomy. Published studies have shown roughly equivalent outcomes in acuity and refraction with modern radial keratotomy and photorefractive keratectomy when treating low to moderate myopia. There is a general consensus, however, that lasers represent a future trend in refractive surgery. Laser keratectomy has evolved rapidly in the last decade and represents the major thrust of current refractive research.

With reports of epithelial sensitivity to ultraviolet lasers and precise etching properties using various substrates,[127] Trokel et al,[128] in 1983, studied the effect of the excimer laser on bovine corneas. They demonstrated that far ultraviolet laser emissions (between 150 and 200 nm) could precisely remove corneal stroma without apparent thermal trauma to the adjacent tissue This landmark report started a multitude of investigations into the use of the laser for refractive surgery. Initially these studies were directed at making radial or arcuate incisions as an alternative to incisional keratotomy (Figure 161-15). However, wide area ablation for direct resculpturing of the cornea was pursued as the precise ablative properties of the excimer became apparent. Studies were performed to establish the optimum laser wavelength from among the different gas mixtures. The 193 nm ultraviolet light from the argon fluoride laser, with the least corneal transmission, caused less adjacent tissue damage and created a smoother ablation than did longer wavelength lasers.[129,130] Argon fluoride lasers (also called excimer laser, which is short for excited dimer) were subsequently developed for keratorefractive procedures (Figure 161-16). At a wavelength of 193 nm, high energy photons break organic molecular bonds of the superficial corneal tissue in a process called ablative photodecomposition. Particles are expelled at high velocity, which helps to dissipate much of the energy.[131] Other important properties of the laser were also explored, including the optimum irradiance levels and repetition rates,[132] and optical principles for the treatment of myopia and hyperopia were developed.[133] After studies of wide area ablation in primates demonstrated satisfactory safety and optical properties, Food and Drug Administration–approved human studies were begun.

There are several ways to deliver laser energy to the cornea. The first method to be developed was wide area surface ablation with the excimer laser using an expanding or contracting iris aperture to treat spherical myopia in a procedure called photorefractive keratectomy (PRK). This corrects myopia by removing more tissue centrally, thereby flattening the cornea. The amount of correction is titrated by the number of pulses and the diameter of the ablation zone. Multizone techniques were developed to reduce regression by creating a smoother peripheral transition area for the treatment of high myopia. In all cases employing an aperture, the edge is imprinted onto the cornea with

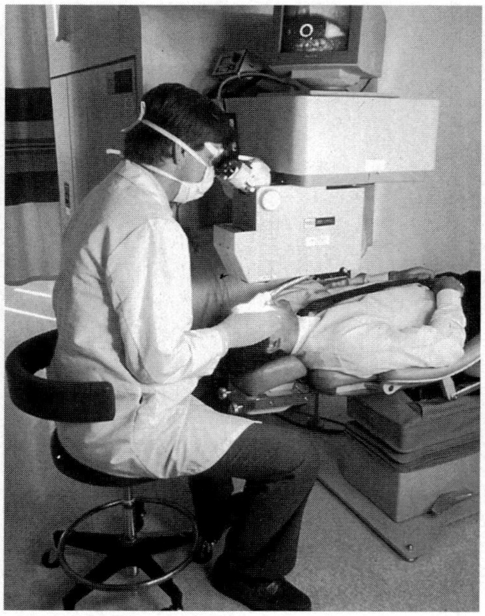

FIGURE 161-16 Excimer laser for performing photorefractive keratectomy using argon fluoride gas mixture.

each pulse, leaving a series of microscopic ridges that are normally smoothed over by the epithelium. One laser manufacturer incorporates a "wobble" into its delivery to eliminate repetitive pulse ridges. Hyperopia can be treated with wide area ablation using a ring aperture that expands centrally and removes more tissue in the periphery, thereby creating central steepening. An expanding set of parallel blades aligned to the proper axis can be used to correct astigmatism in a procedure called photoastigmatic refractive keratectomy (PARK). The erodible mask technique is one in which the shape of an ablatable mask is transposed onto the cornea to correct myopia, astigmatism, and hyperopia. A more recently developed method is by scanning a small circular ultraviolet beam or slit under computer control for precise ablation. For instance, placing a blended pattern of pulses centrally corrects myopia. Finally, picosecond infrared lasers are being developed that can perform intrastromal ablation. These differ from the previous surface ablating ultraviolet lasers in that they create tiny pockets in the stroma beneath an intact epithelium and Bowman's layer. The concept is that as the pockets collapse, it alters the shape of the anterior cornea to correct refractive errors. All of these lasers and delivery systems are under active investigation.

Initial clinical trials with the excimer laser have been made with wide area ablation. A methodical stepwise progression was made from blind eye studies to small scale-sighted eye trials to larger population studies. Concerns regarding epithelial stability over the treated area, which had plagued epikeratoplasty, were dispelled when clinical results demonstrated reepithelialization with no apparent propensity for recurrent erosions. Improvements and refinements have been incorporated into the procedure during these studies.

Initial ablation zone diameters were relatively small (4.0 to 5.0 mm) because of concerns that deeper ablations would create more corneal scarring. PRK removes Bowman's layer, and it is still not clear if this will result in any long-term complications. A reticular anterior stromal haze observed after the procedure slowly cleared in the majority of cases. With smaller ablation zones, reports of glare and halos around lights at night occurred frequently. In a European study using a 4.0 mm optical zone, 10% of the patients declined treatment in the other eye because of compromised night vision.[134] This occurred because light refracted from the unablated cornea was scattered onto the retina in a disturbing halo pattern after scotopic pupillary mydriasis. When it became apparent that scarring was not a significant problem, ablation zone diameters were gradually increased to 6.0 mm for the treatment of low to moderate myopia.

A substantial effluent plume is present during ablation.[131] Because of concerns that this might interfere with subsequent laser pulses, a removal system was developed by one manufacturer that involved the blowing of nitrogen gas across the cornea during the procedure. However, it was discovered that this created a rougher ablation surface on histopathologic examination[135] and less predictable refractive results.[136,137] Presumably this was caused by a variable amount of stromal dehydration induced by the dry gas, which affected the ablation rate. Although nitrogen blow-by was discontinued, it is still unclear what effect the effluent plume has on subsequent laser pulses. If effluent removal is necessary, humidified gas should be used to control hydration.[138]

Various topographic patterns have been observed after PRK, but the most unusual are areas of central steepening called central islands.[139] There is no clear definition of a central island, which can vary from a 1 to 3 diopter change in central corneal power with a diameter of 1 to 3 mm. Central islands can be visually significant and cause a decrease in vision, monocular diplopia, and glare at night. Fortunately, they are usually transient and resolve by 6 months after surgery in most cases. It is not clear what causes central islands, but they were first noticed after use of the nitrogen blow-by system was discontinued.[137] Perhaps interference from the effluent plume partially masks the laser beam centrally, causing steepening in this area. However, this has not been observed by other excimer lasers that do not use plume removal. It is not likely that a central "cold spot" in the laser is responsible because ablated plastic disks clearly demonstrate homogeneity of the beam. It has been proposed that shock waves from successive pulses force stromal fluid to the center of the ablation.[140] The overly hydrated central cornea would then ablate at a different rate, which could cause central steepening. Persistent central islands have been treated with repeated ablation over the steepened cornea, and new "anti–central island" software modifications have been developed to pretreat the central cornea with additional pulses in an attempt to smooth the overall contour.

Most patients in early clinical trials experienced moderate to severe pain in the immediate postoperative period until reepithelialization occurred. This typically required oral narcotics for management. Topical nonsteroidal medications were shown to reduce pain and photophobia after the procedure[141,142] and these are routinely used today for this purpose. Bandage soft contact lenses have also been used to control pain, but there have been reports of corneal infiltrates with contact lens use in the immediate postoperative period.[136,143] These were presumably caused by a microbial keratitis that responded to topical antibiotics.

Pharmacologic methods to modulate healing response are being actively pursued to improve the predictability and long-term stability of the procedure. While a highly reproducible and accurate result can be obtained by ablating a plastic disk, interindividual variation in healing results in a variable amount of regression after the procedure. This is especially prominent after treatment of higher levels of myopia. Besides the difficulty with variable regression, the healing response creates an anterior stromal haze that can interfere with vision by scattering light and reducing contrast sensitivity. This haze is made up of irregular collagen arrays that in most cases slowly organize and become optically clear as healing occurs. Topical corticosteroids have been used widely in an effort to suppress the healing response, but their benefit remains controversial; some studies have shown a beneficial effect on refractive correction, whereas others have not. Wound healing inhibitors can have serious side effects that limit their usefulness. Long-term use of corticosteroids can elevate intraocular pressure, which has been observed in approximately 10% of PRK patients, as well as lead to cataract formation. Other pharmacologic agents, such as mitomycin, plasmin inhibitors (aprotinin), and various interleukins, have undergone laboratory testing for use in PRK, but the search continues for the ideal topical wound healing modulator that has high specificity for collagen synthesis without toxic side effects such as inhibition of reepithelialization.

The excimer laser is being studied with various techniques to correct high myopia. Initial results using small diameter (3.5 to 4.0 mm) single zone ablation showed less predictability if the refractive correction were greater than 5 or 6 diopters.[144,145] A variable amount of regression was responsible for the poor results. A large ablation zone is ideal to minimize glare and halo symptoms and perhaps to reduce regression as well. However, the depth of the ablation becomes a significant factor because more tissue must be removed for higher refractive correction. In addition, as the optical zone size is increased, the depth of the ablation must be increased by the square of the diameter, and deep ablations may promote a more exuberant healing response and lead to scarring. There is a limit to how much stroma can be removed before raising concerns about corneal ectasia. An upper limit of 200 μm has been suggested, which corresponds approximately to an 18-diopter correction using a 6.0 mm optical zone. In an attempt to circumvent this problem, several strategies have been devised. Sher et al[146] used larger optical zones than did previous studies (5.5 to 6.2 mm) with a single pass ablation to treat high myopia (48 patients, mean 11.18 ± 1.89 diopters). At 1 month, the mean spherical equivalent was +0.85 ± 1.93 diopters, but this regressed to −0.33 ± 2.18 diopters by 6 months. At 6 months, 64% of the patients were corrected to within 2 diopters of emmetropia. Eleven patients required retreatment for regression between 6 and 16 months after surgery. More corneal haze was observed than with ablations for lower myopia. Heitzmann et al[147] used a multizone technique to treat 18 patients with high myopia (mean − 11.83 ± 2.92 diopters). The total myopic correction was divided into three zones: 50% of the correction was ablated with 4.0 mm, 30% with 5.0 mm, and 20% with 6.0 mm. The advantage of this approach is that it reduces the total depth of ablation and provides a more tapered transition zone. At 1 month the mean spherical equivalent was −0.40 ± 1.99 diopters, but it regressed to −1.99 ± 2.12 diopters by 6 months. At 6 months, 65% of the patients were corrected to within 2 diopters of emmetropia, but a sizable number of patients (47%) were judged to have corneal haze worse than mild. These refractive results were surprisingly similar to those of Sher and indicate the difficulty in achieving accurate and stable refractive results when treating high myopia with surface ablation. Another alternative use of the excimer laser to treat high myopia is in conjunction with keratomileusis, as discussed in that section. In this procedure a lamellar cap is created with a microkeratome, and the laser is used to sculpt either the host bed or the nonepithelial side of the lenticule for refractive correction. Combining the laser with the microkeratome results in a procedure that has both advantages (spares Bowman's layer, which may reduce

A 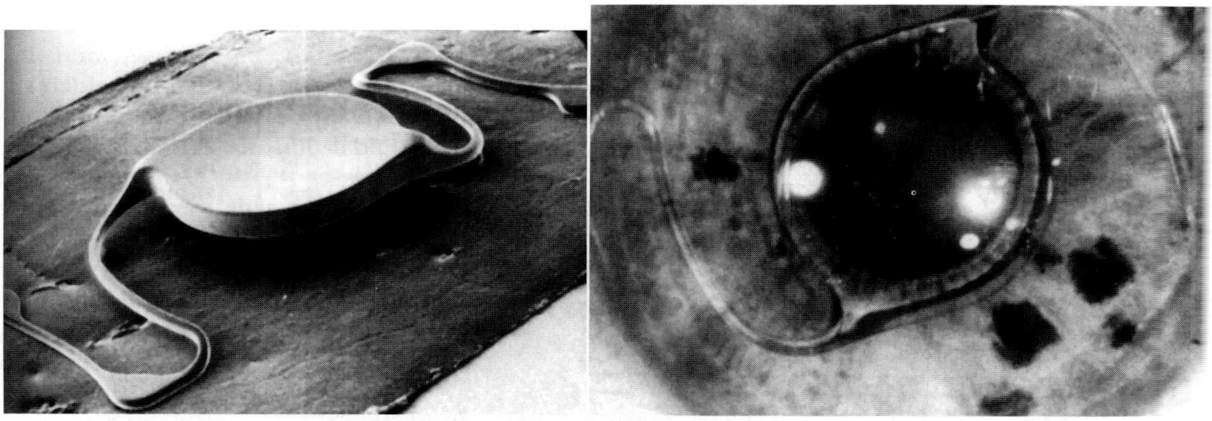 B

FIGURE 161-20 **A** and **B,** Minus powered anterior chamber intraocular lens designed by Baikoff. The high vault (25°) of the lens **(A)** was subsequently felt to be responsible for endothelial trauma. **B** demonstrates the intraocular appearance. (From Baikoff G, Joly P: *Refract Corneal Surg* 6:253, 1990.)

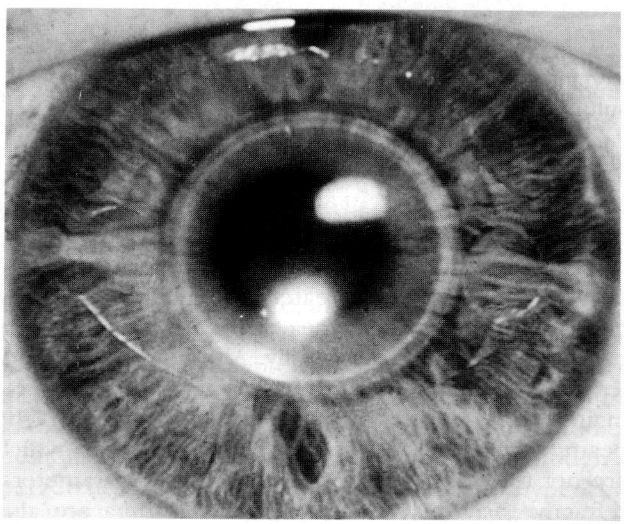

FIGURE 161-21 Worst iris-claw minus powered anterior chamber intraocular lens. (From Fechner PU, Strobel J, Wichmann W: *Refract Corneal Surg* 7:287, 1991.)

ract, and retinal detachment.[156] Given the significant risks associated with lens extraction, this procedure is generally reserved for high refractive errors.

Phakic intraocular lens insertion was initially performed by Barraquer[157] in the 1950s. He implanted hundreds of lenses, but many had to be subsequently removed because of severe corneal and intraocular complications. These early lenses were thick, poorly finished, and had sharp edges.[158] The use of phakic intraocular lenses was abandoned until recently.

In the mid-1980s, Baikhoff and Joly[159] experimented with an angle-supported anterior chamber intraocular lens (Figure 161-20). The lens was highly vaulted to ensure clearance from the iris and natural lens and had negative power to treat myopia. This procedure was compared to epikeratoplasty in a retrospective study of 62 highly myopic eyes. The anterior chamber intraocular lens was found to result in more rapid, predictable, and stable refractive correction. Similar results were found also in another retrospective study that compared phakic intraocular lenses, epikeratoplasty, and MKM.[74] However, further studies documented damage to the endothelium in a large percentage of patients. Over one third of treated eyes had a decreased central endothelial cell count of more than 20%, and over 80% of eyes had evidence of paracentral endothelial damage.[160,161] The high vault of the lens, and not the angle support, was felt to be responsible because cornea-lens touch was noted with slight pressure.[156] A less vaulted lens has been proposed.

To avoid an angle-supported lens, Worst et al[162] developed the iris-claw anterior chamber lens (Figure 161-21). This lens has pincers that incarcerate the midperipheral iris for fixation. Fechner et al[163] retrospectively analyzed 125 eyes implanted with this lens. While the refractive results were satisfactory, damage to the endothelium was observed in 10 eyes, four of which developed corneal edema. Excluding surgical trauma, endothelial damage was associated with physiologic shallow anterior chambers.

Fydorov has developed and implanted several types of intraocular posterior chamber lenses for refractive correction in phakic patients (Figure 161-22). These lenses are placed in the posterior chamber between the iris and the anterior lens capsule. No clinical results have yet been published.

It remains to be determined if intraocular procedures can offer a safe and effective alternative to other forms of refractive surgery.

A

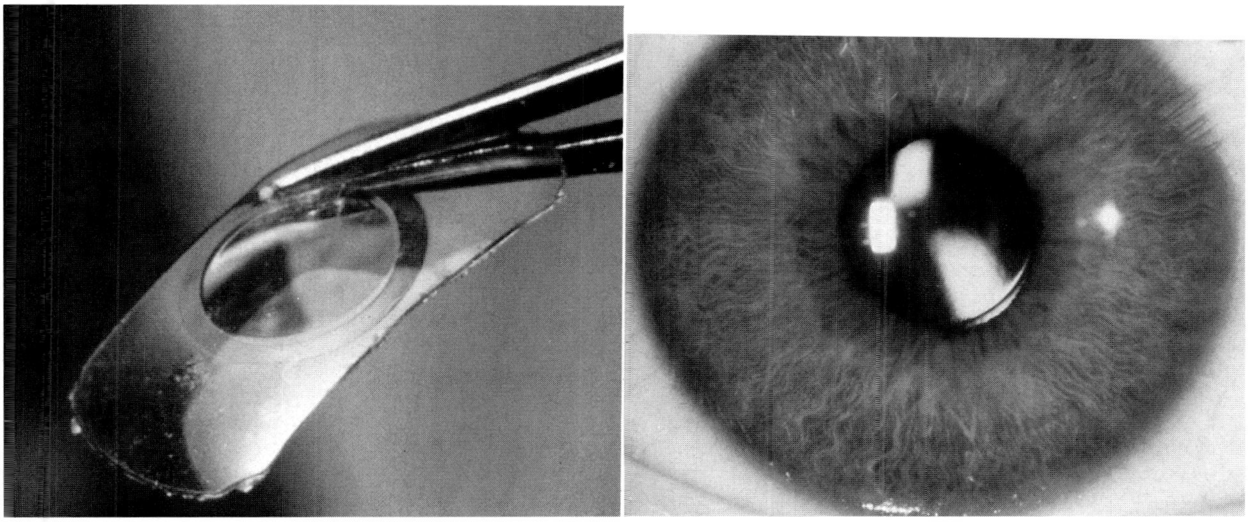

B

FIGURE 161-22 **A,** The Fyodorov silicon, phakic intraocular lens used to treat myopia. **B,** The lens is placed in the posterior chamber in front of the natural lens as shown in a postoperative result. Central vaulting is designed to prevent anterior capsule touch. (From Bores L: *Refractive eye surgery,* 1993. Reprinted by permission of Blackwell Scientific Publications, Inc.)

Conclusions

The history of refractive surgery has witnessed the reevaluation of a few basic surgical strategies (e.g., incisions, lamellar procedures, thermokeratoplasty) that have changed as new technology, such as holmium and excimer lasers, has enabled surgeons to alter the refractive state of the eye more precisely. The numerous strategies developed for the correction of refractive errors is evidence that no one procedure has conclusively demonstrated an excellent level of safety and efficacy.

Of all the lessons from past experience with refractive procedures, none may be more important than the value of unbiased, well-designed prospective studies. As new technology is developed, there is often a high level of enthusiasm that clouds objective scientific examination. Spectacular results of small, limited studies fan the lay press that seeks revolutionary technology. Caught up in the hype, there is a temptation for clinicians to "get on the bandwagon." Scientific evaluation is left behind, only to resurface after carefully controlled studies are finally performed and published. The procedure's realistic capabilities are then put into the proper risk-to-benefit context for informed patient consent or the procedure is abandoned altogether. Unfortunately this pattern has been repeated many times. Learning from the excesses and errors of the past, it is hoped that we are entering a more enlightened era of refractive surgery. The science of refractive surgery has advanced over the last 15 years, which has undoubtedly resulted in safer and more predictable procedures, but much more work is required.

REFERENCES

1. Nizam A et al: Stability of refraction and visual acuity during 5 years in eyes with simple myopia, *Refract Corneal Surg* 8:439-447, 1992.
2. Waring GO III et al and PERK Study Group: Results of the Prospective Evaluation of Radial Keratotomy (PERK) Study 10 years after surgery, *Arch Ophthalmol* 112:1298-1308, 1994.
3. Applegate RA, Howland HC: Magnification and visual acuity in refractive surgery, *Arch Ophthalmol* 111:1335-1342, 1993.
4. Maguire LJ: Keratorefractive surgery, success and the public health, *Am J Ophthalmol* 117:394-398, 1994.
5. Waring GO III: The Lans distinguished refractive surgery lecture, *J Refract Surg* 3:115-116, 1987.
6. Waring GO III: *Refractive keratotomy for myopia and astigmatism,* St Louis, 1992, Mosby.
7. Lans LJ: Experimentelle Untersuchungen über Entstehung von Astigmatismus durch nicht-perforirende Corneawunden, *Archiv fur Ophthalmologie* 45:117-152, 1898.
8. Sato T: Posterior incision of the cornea: surgical treatment for conical cornea and astigmatism, *Am J Ophthalmol* 33:943-948, 1950.
9. Sato T: Posterior half-incision of cornea for astigmatism: operative procedures and results of the improved tangent method, *Am J Ophthalmol* 36:462-466, 1953.
10. Sato T, Akiyama R, Shibata H: A new surgical approach to myopia, *Am J Ophthalmol* 36:823-829, 1953.
11. Yamaguchi T et al: Bullous keratopathy after anterior-posterior radial keratotomy for myopia and myopic astigmatism, *Am J Ophthalmol* 93:600-606, 1982.
12. Fyodorov SN, Durnev VV: Operation of dosaged dissection of corneal circular ligament in cases of myopia of mild degree, *Ann Ophthalmol* 11:1885-1890, 1979.

13. Fyodorov SN, Agranovsky AA: Long-term results of anterior radial keratotomy, *J Ocular Ther Surg* 1:217-223, 1982.
14. Hecht SD, Jamara RJ: Prospective evaluation of radial keratotomy using the Fyodorov formula: preliminary report, *Ann Ophthalmol* 14:319-330, 1982.
15. Reddy PS, Reddy PR: Anterior keratotomy, *Ophthalmic Surg* 11:765-767, 1980.
16. Cowden JW, Bores LD: A clinical investigation of the surgical correction of myopia by the method of Fyodorov, *Ophthalmology* 88:737-741, 1981.
17. Announcement: National Advisory Eye Council Meetings. Refractive keratoplasty, *Invest Ophthalmol Vis Sci* 18:882, 1979.
18. Waring GO III: Radial keratotomy in the United States: the turbulent decade, *J Refract Surg* 4:204-208, 1988.
19. Bryant MR et al: Computer-aided surgical design in refractive keratotomy, *CLAO J* 13:238-242, 1987.
20. Hanna KD, Jouve FE, Waring GO III: Preliminary computer simulation of the effects of radial keratotomy, *Arch Ophthalmol* 107:911-918, 1989.
21. Sawusch MR, McDonnell PJ: Computer modeling of wound gape following radial keratotomy, *Refract Corneal Surg* 8:143-145, 1992.
22. Sawusch MR, Wan WL, McDonnell PJ: Tissue addition theory of radial keratotomy: a geometric model, *J Cataract Refract Surg* 17:448-453, 1991.
23. Schachar RA, Black TD, Huang T: A physicist view of radial keratotomy with surgical implications. In Schachar RA, Levy NS, Schachar L, editors: *Keratorefraction. Proceedings of the Keratorefractive Society Meeting,* Denison, TX, 1980, LAL Publishing.
24. Salz J et al: Radial keratotomy in fresh human cadaver eyes, *Ophthalmology* 88:742-746, 1981.
25. Jester JV et al: A statistical analysis of radial keratotomy in human cadaver eyes, *Am J Ophthalmol* 92:172-177, 1981.
26. Steel D et al: Modification of corneal curvature following radial keratotomy in primates, *Ophthalmology* 88:747-754, 1981.
27. Rowsey JJ et al: Predicting the results of radial keratotomy, *Ophthalmology* 90:642-654, 1983.
28. Deitz MR et al: Long-term (5- to 12-year) follow-up of metal-blade radial keratotomy procedures, *Arch Ophthalmol* 112:614-620, 1994.
29. Arrowsmith PN, Marks RG: Visual, refractive, and keratometric results of radial keratotomy: five-year follow-up, *Arch Ophthalmol* 107:506-511, 1989.
30. Sawelson H, Marks R: Five year results of radial keratotomy, *Refract Corneal Surg* 5:8-20, 1989.
31. O'Donnell F: Short incision radial keratotomy: a comparative study in rabbits, *J Refract Surg* 3:102-103, 1987.
32. Werblin TP, Stafford GM: The Casebeer system for predictable keratorefractive surgery. One-year evaluation of 205 consecutive eyes, *Ophthalmology* 100:1095-1102, 1993.
33. Cotliar AM et al: Excimer laser radial keratotomy, *Ophthalmology* 92:206-208, 1985.
34. Kerr-Muir MG et al: Ultrastructural comparison of conventional surgical and argon fluoride excimer laser keratectomy, *Am J Ophthalmol* 103:448-453, 1987.
35. Tenner A et al: Excimer laser radial keratotomy in the living human eye: a preliminary report, *J Refract Surg* 4:5-8, 1988.
36. Yamashita T et al: Hexagonal keratotomy reduces hyperopia after radial keratotomy in rabbits, *J Refract Surg* 2:261-264, 1986.
37. Gilbert ML et al: Hexagonal keratotomy in human cadaver eyes, *J Refract Surg* 4:12-14, 1988.
38. Neumann AC, McCarty GR: Hexagonal keratotomy for correction of low hyperopia: preliminary results of a prospective study, *J Cataract Refract Surg* 14:265-269, 1988.
39. Jensen RP: Hexagonal keratotomy: clinical experience with 483 eyes, *Int Ophthalmol Clin* 31:69-73, 1991.
40. Gilbert ML, Friedlander M, Granet N: Corneal steepening in human eye bank eyes by combined hexagonal and transverse keratotomy, *Refract Corneal Surg* 6:126, 1990.
41. McDonnell PJ, Lean JS, Schanzlin DJ: Globe rupture from blunt trauma after hexagonal keratotomy, *Am J Ophthalmol* 104:241-242, 1987.
42. Nordan LT, Maxwell WA: Refractive surgery and informed consent. Radial keratotomy with small optical zone hexagonal keratotomy, *J Cataract Refract Surg* 18:420-421, 1992.
43. Basuk WL et al: Complications of hexagonal keratotomy, *Am J Ophthalmol* 117:37-49, 1994.
44. Gasset AR et al: Thermokeratoplasty, *Trans Am Acad Ophthalmol Otolaryngol* 77:441-454, 1973.
45. Shaw EL, Gasset AR: Thermokeratoplasty (TKP) temperature profile, *Invest Ophthalmol* 13:181-186, 1974.
46. Gasset AR, Kaufman HE: Thermokeratoplasty in the treatment of keratoconus, *Am J Ophthalmol* 79:226-232, 1975.
47. Arentsen JJ, Laibson PR: Thermokeratoplasty for keratoconus, *Am J Ophthalmol* 82:447-449, 1976.
48. Keates RH, Dingle J: Thermokeratoplasty for keratoconus, *Ophthalmic Surg* 6:89-92, 1975.
49. Aquavella JV, Smith RS, Shaw EL: Alterations in corneal morphology following thermokeratoplasty, *Arch Ophthalmol* 94:2082-2085, 1976.
50. Fogle JA, Kenyon KR, Stark WJ: Damage to epithelial basement membrane by thermokeratoplasty, *Am J Ophthalmol* 83:392-401, 1977.
51. Arentsen JJ, Rodrigues MM, Laibson PR: Histopathologic changes after thermokeratoplasty for keratoconus, *Invest Ophthalmol Vis Sci* 16:32-38, 1977.
52. Rowsey JJ, Doss JD: Preliminary report of Los Alamos keratoplasty techniques, *Ophthalmology* 88:755-760, 1981.
53. Rowsey JJ: Electrosurgical keratoplasty: update and retraction, *Invest Ophthalmol Vis Sci* 28(Suppl):224, 1987.
54. Caster AI: The Fyodorov technique of hyperopia correction by thermal coagulation: a preliminary report, *J Refract Surg* 4:105-108, 1988.
55. Neumann AC, Fyodorov S, Sanders DR: Radial thermokeratoplasty for the correction of hyperopia, *Refract Corneal Surg* 6:404-412, 1990.
56. Schachar RA: Radial thermokeratoplasty, *Int Ophthalmol Clin* 31:47-57, 1991.
57. Feldman ST et al: Regression of effect following radial thermokeratoplasty in humans, *Refract Corneal Surg* 5:288-291, 1989.
58. Feldman ST et al: Experimental radial thermokeratoplasty in rabbits, *Arch Ophthalmol* 108:997-1000, 1990.
59. Seiler T, Matallana M, Bende T: Laser thermokeratoplasty by means of a pulsed holmium: YAG laser for hyperopic correction, *Refract Corneal Surg* 6:335-339, 1990.
60. Horn G et al: New refractive method for laser thermal keratoplasty with the Co:MgF2 laser, *J Cataract Refract Surg* 16:611-616, 1990.
61. Moreira H et al: Holmium laser thermokeratoplasty, *Ophthalmology* 100:752-761, 1993.
62. Seiler T: Holmium: YAG laser thermokeratoplasty for hyperopia, *Ophthalmol Clin North Am* 5:773-780, 1992.
63. Barraquer JI: Keratomileusis for the correction of myopia, *Ann Inst Barraquer* 5:209-229, 1964.
64. Barraquer JI: Modification of refraction by means of intracorneal inclusions, *Int Ophthalmol Clin* 6:53-78, 1966.
65. Ainslie D: The surgical correction of refractive errors by keratomileusis and keratophakia, *Ann Ophthalmol* 8:349-367, 1976.
66. Troutman RC, Swinger C: Refractive keratoplasty: keratophakia

and keratomileusis, *Trans Am Ophthalmol Soc* 76:329-339, 1978.
67. Krumeich JH, Swinger CA: Nonfreeze epikeratophakia for the correction of myopia, *Am J Ophthalmol* 103:397-403, 1987.
68. Bas AM, Nano HD Jr: In situ myopic keratomileusis results in 30 eyes at 15 months, *Refract Corneal Surg* 7:223-231, 1991.
69. Swinger CA, Barraquer JI: Keratophakia and keratomileusis—clinical results, *Ophthalmology* 88:709-715, 1981.
70. Barraquer JI: Results of hypermetropic keratomileusis, 1980-1981, *Int Ophthalmol Clin* 23:25-44, 1983.
71. Barraquer JI: Keratomileusis for myopia and aphakia, *Ophthalmology* 88:701-708, 1981.
72. Swinger CA, Barker BA: Prospective evaluation of myopic keratomileusis, *Ophthalmology* 91:785-792, 1984.
73. Maxwell WA: Myopic keratomileusis: initial results and myopic keratomileusis combined with other procedures, *J Cataract Refract Surg* 13:518-524, 1987.
74. Colin J et al: The surgical treatment of high myopia: comparison of epikeratoplasty, keratomileusis and minus power anterior chamber lenses, *Refract Corneal Surg* 6:245-251, 1990.
75. Arenas-Archila E et al: Myopic keratomileusis in situ: a preliminary report, *J Cataract Refract Surg* 17:424-435, 1991.
76. Buratto L, Ferrari M, Rama P: Excimer laser intrastromal keratomileusis, *Am J Ophthalmol* 113:291-295, 1992.
77. Neumann AC, McCarty G, Sanders DR: Delayed regression of effect in myopic epikeratophakia vs myopic keratomileusis for high myopia, *Refract Corneal Surg* 5:161-166, 1989.
78. Nordan LT: Keratomileusis, *Int Ophthalmol Clin* 31:7-12, 1991.
79. Maxwell WA, Nordan LT: Myopic keratomileusis: early experience, *J Refract Surg* 1:99-103, 1985.
80. American Academy of Ophthalmology: Ophthalmic procedures assessment. Keratophakia and keratomileusis: safety and effectiveness, *Ophthalmology* 99:1332-1341, 1992.
81. Troutman RC, Swinger C, Goldstein M: Keratophakia update, *Ophthalmology* 88:36-38, 1981.
82. Troutman RC: Indications, techniques, and complications of keratophakia, *Int Ophthalmol Clin* 23:11-23, 1983.
83. Swinger CA: Comparison of results obtained with keratophakia, hypermetropic keratomileusis, intraocular lens implantation, and extended-wear contact lenses, *Int Ophthalmol Clin* 23:59-74, 1983.
84. Nosé W et al: Intrastromal corneal ring—one-year results of first implants in humans: a preliminary nonfunctional eye study, *Refract Corneal Surg* 9:452-458, 1993.
85. Barraquer JI: Modification of refraction by means of intracorneal inclusions, *Int Ophthalmol Clin* 6:53-78, 1966.
86. Knowles WF: Effect of intralamellar plastic membranes on corneal physiology, *Am J Ophthalmol* 51:1146-1156, 1961.
87. Dohlman CH, Refojo MF, Rose J: Synthetic polymers in corneal surgery. I. Glyceryl methacrylate, *Arch Ophthalmol* 77:252-257, 1967.
88. Mester U, Heimig D, Dardenne MU: Measurement and calculation of refraction in experimental keratophakia with hydrophilic lenses, *Ophthalmic Res* 8:111-116, 1976.
89. Werblin TP et al: Eight years experience with Permalens® intracorneal lenses in nonhuman primates, *Refract Corneal Surg* 8:12-22, 1992.
90. Werblin TP, Patel AS, Barraquer JI: Initial human experience with Permalens® myopic hydrogel intracorneal lens implants, *Refract Corneal Surg* 8:23-26, 1992.
91. McCarey BE et al: Refractive results of hyperopic hydrogel intracorneal lenses in primate eyes, *Arch Ophthalmol* 107:724-730, 1989.
92. McCarey BE: Current status of refractive surgery with synthetic intracorneal lenses: Barraquer lecture, *Refract Corneal Surg* 6:40-46, 1990.
93. Choyce DP: The correction of refractive errors with polysulfone corneal inlays. A new frontier to be explored? *Trans Ophthalmol Soc UK* 104:332-342, 1985.
94. Choyce DP: The correction of high myopia, *Refract Corneal Surg* 8:242-245, 1992.
95. Lane SS, Lindstrom RL: Polysulfone intracorneal lenses, *Int Ophthalmol Clin* 31:37-46, 1991.
96. Kaufman HE: The correction of aphakia, *Am J Ophthalmol* 89:1-10, 1980.
97. Werblin TP, Klyce SD: Epikeratophakia: the surgical correction of aphakia. I. Lathing of corneal tissue, *Curr Eye Res* 1:123-129, 1981.
98. Werblin TP, Kaufman HE: Epikeratophakia: the surgical correction of aphakia. II. Preliminary results in a non-human primate model, *Curr Eye Res* 1:131-137, 1981.
99. Binder PS, Zavala EY: Why do some epikeratoplasties fail? *Arch Ophthalmol* 105:63-69, 1987.
100. Googe JM et al: The histology of epikeratophakia grafts, *Invest Ophthalmol Vis Sci* 20(Suppl):8, 1981.
101. Werblin TP et al: Epikeratophakia: the surgical correction of aphakia. III. Preliminary results of a prospective clinical trial, *Arch Ophthalmol* 99:1957-1960, 1981.
102. Morgan KS et al: The use of epikeratophakia grafts in pediatric monocular aphakia, *J Pediatr Ophthalmol Strabismus* 18:23-29, 1981.
103. Kaufman HE, Werblin TP: Epikeratophakia for the treatment of keratoconus, *Am J Ophthalmol* 93:342-347, 1982.
104. McDonald MB et al: Epikeratophakia for myopia correction, *Ophthalmology* 92:1417-1422, 1985.
105. McDonald MB et al: The nationwide study of epikeratophakia for aphakia in adults, *Am J Ophthalmol* 103:358-365, 1987.
106. Morgan KS et al: The nationwide study of epikeratophakia for aphakia in children, *Am J Ophthalmol* 103:366-374, 1987.
107. McDonald MB et al: Epikeratophakia for keratoconus. The nationwide study, *Arch Ophthalmol* 104:1294-1300, 1986.
108. McDonald MB et al: The nationwide study of epikeratophakia for myopia, *Am J Ophthalmol* 103:375-383, 1987.
109. Safir A et al: The cornea press: restoring donor corneas to normal dimensions and hydration before cryolathing, *Ophthalmic Surg* 14:327-331, 1983.
110. Zavala EY, Krumeich J, Binder PS: Clinical pathology of non-freeze lamellar refractive keratoplasty, *Cornea* 7:327-330, 1988.
111. McDonald MB: The future direction of refractive surgery, *J Refract Surg* 4:158-168, 1988.
112. Werblin TP: Lamellar refractive surgery: where have we been and where are we going? *Refract Corneal Surg* 5:167-176, 1989.
113. Busin M, Schmidt J, Koch J: Physiologic analysis of corneal healing after epikeratophakia, *Ophthalmology* 99:415-417, 1992.
114. Busin M, Spitznas M, Hockwin O: Evaluation of functional and morphologic parameters of the cornea after epikeratophakia using prelathed, lyophilized tissue, *Ophthalmology* 97:330-333, 1990.
115. Busin M, Cusumano A, Spitznas M: Epithelial interface cysts after epikeratophakia, *Ophthalmology* 100:1225-1229, 1993.
116. Durrie DS, Habrich DL, Dietze TR: Secondary intraocular lens implantation vs epikeratophakia for the treatment of aphakia, *Am J Ophthalmol* 103:384-391, 1987.
117. Musco PS, Aquavella JV: Reversibility of epikeratoplasty, *J Refract Surg* 4:15-17, 1988.
118. Price FW Jr, Binder PS: Scarring of a recipient cornea following epikeratoplasty, *Arch Ophthalmol* 105:1556-1560, 1987.
119. Schlichtemeier WR, Arbegast KD: Long-term loss of effect of myopic epikeratophakia, *J Refract Surg* 3:46-49, 1987.

120. Woodhams JT: Regression of myopic epikeratophakia effects, *J Cataract Refract Surg* 13:343-344, 1987.
121. Holladay JT et al: Improving the predictability of intraocular lens power calculations, *Arch Ophthalmol* 104:539-541, 1986.
122. McDonnell PJ et al: Surgical correction of aphakia: intraocular lens implantation and epikeratophakia, *J Refract Surg* 3:209-214, 1987.
123. McDonald MB et al: A preliminary comparative study of epikeratophakia or penetrating keratoplasty for keratoconus, *Am J Ophthalmol* 103:467, 1987.
124. Steinert RF, Wagoner MD: Long-term comparison of epikeratoplasty and penetrating keratoplasty for keratoconus, *Arch Ophthalmol* 106:493-496, 1988.
125. Goosey JD et al: A comparison of penetrating keratoplasty to epikeratoplasty in the surgical management of keratoconus, *Am J Ophthalmol* 111:145-151, 1991.
126. Campos M, Lee M, McDonnell PJ: Ocular integrity after refractive surgery: effects of photorefractive keratectomy, phototherapeutic keratectomy, and radial keratotomy, *Ophthalmic Surg* 23:598-602, 1992.
127. Taboada J, Mikesell GW, Reed RD: Response of the corneal epithelium to KrF excimer laser pulses, *Health Physics* 40:677-683, 1981.
128. Trokel SL, Srinivasan R, Braren B: Excimer laser surgery of the cornea, *Am J Ophthalmol* 96:710-715, 1983.
129. Krueger RR, Trokel SL, Schubert HD: Interaction of ultraviolet laser light with the cornea, *Invest Ophthalmol Vis Sci* 26:1455-1464, 1985.
130. Marshall J et al: Photoablative reprofiling of the cornea using an excimer laser: photorefractive keratectomy, *Lasers Ophthalmol* 1:21-48, 1986.
131. Puliafito CA et al: High-speed photography of excimer laser ablation of the cornea, *Arch Ophthalmol* 105:1255-1259, 1987.
132. Krueger RR, Trokel SL: Quantitation of corneal ablation by ultraviolet laser light, *Arch Ophthalmol* 103:1741-1742, 1985.
133. Munnerlyn CR, Koons SJ, Marshall J: Photorefractive keratectomy: a technique for laser refractive surgery, *J Cataract Refract Surg* 14:46-52, 1988.
134. Gartry DS, Kerr Muir MG, Marshall J: Excimer laser photorefractive keratectomy; 18-month follow-up, *Ophthalmology* 99:1209-1219, 1992.
135. Campos M, Cuevas K, Garbus J: Corneal wound healing after excimer ablation: effects of nitrogen gas blower, *Ophthalmology* 99:893-897, 1992.
136. Maguen E et al: Results of excimer laser photorefractive keratectomy for the correction of myopia, *Ophthalmology* 101:1548-1557, 1994.
137. Piebenga LW et al: Excimer photorefractive keratectomy for myopia, *Ophthalmology* 100:1335-1345, 1993.
138. Krueger RR et al: Corneal surface morphology following excimer laser ablation with humidified gases, *Arch Ophthalmol* 111:1131-1137, 1993.
139. Lin DTC, Sutton HF, Berman M: Corneal topography following excimer photorefractive keratectomy for myopia, *J Cataract Refract Surg* 19(Suppl):149-154, 1993.
140. Krueger RR et al: Photography of shock waves during excimer laser ablation of the cornea. Effect of helium gas on propagation velocity, *Cornea* 12:330-334, 1993.
141. Eiferman RA Hoffman RS, Sher NA: Topical diclofenac reduces pain following photorefractive keratectomy, *Arch Ophthalmol* 111:1022, 1993.
142. Sher NA et al: Topical diclofenac in the treatment of ocular pain after excimer photorefractive keratectomy, *Refract Corneal Surg* 9:425, 1993.
143. Talley AR et al: Results one year after using the 193-nm excimer laser for photorefractive keratectomy in mild to moderate myopia, *Am J Ophthalmol* 118:304-311, 1994.
144. Seiler T, Wollensak J: Myopic photorefractive keratectomy with the excimer laser: one-year follow-up, *Ophthalmology* 98:1156-1163, 1991.
145. Garty DS, Kerr Muir MG, Marshall J: Photorefractive keratectomy with an argon fluoride excimer laser: a clinical study, *Refract Corneal Surg* 7:420-435, 1991.
146. Sher NA et al: 193-nm excimer photorefractive keratectomy in high myopia, *Ophthalmology* 101:1575-1582, 1994.
147. Heitzmann J et al: The correction of high myopia using the excimer laser, *Arch Ophthalmol* 111:1627-1634, 1993.
148. Thompson KP, Hanna K, Waring GO III: Emerging technologies for refractive surgery: laser adjustable synthetic epikeratoplasty, *Refract Corneal Surg* 5:46-48, 1989.
149. Thompson KP et al: Current status of synthetic epikeratoplasty, *Refract Corneal Surg* 7:240-248, 1991.
150. Maloney RK et al: A prototype erodible mask delivery system for the excimer laser, *Ophthalmology* 100:542-549, 1993.
151. Hersh PS, Patel R: Correction of myopia and astigmatism using an ablatable mask, *J Refract Corneal Surg* 10(Suppl):250-254, 1994.
152. Friedman MC et al: OmniMed II: a new system for use with the emphasis erodible mask, *J Refract Corneal Surg* 10(Suppl): 267-273, 1994.
153. Kaiser R et al: Mass spectrometry analysis of cavitation bubbles generated by intrastromal ablation with the Nd:YLF picosecond laser, *Invest Ophthalmol Vis Sci* 35(Suppl):2026, 1994.
154. Niemz MH et al: Intrastromal ablations for refractive corneal surgery using picosecond infrared laser pulses, *Lasers Light Ophthalmol* 5:149-155, 1993.
155. Coulter AH: Corneal reshaping and the intelligent surgical laser: a cautious but creative approach, *J Clin Laser Med Surg* 11:97-98, 1993.
156. Baikoff G: Phakic anterior chamber intraocular lense, *Int Ophthalmol Clin* 31:75-86, 1991.
157. Barraquer J: Anterior chamber plastic lenses. Results of and conclusions from five years experience, *Trans Ophthalmol Soc UK* 79:393-424, 1959.
158. Drews RC: The Barraquer experience with intraocular lenses: 20 years later, *Ophthalmology* 89:386-393, 1982.
159. Baikoff G, Joly P: Comparison of minus power anterior chamber intraocular lenses and myopic epikeratoplasty in phakic eyes, *Refract Corneal Surg* 6:252-260, 1990.
160. Mimouni F et al: Damage to the corneal endothelium from anterior chamber intraocular lenses in phakic myopic eyes, *Refract Corneal Surg* 7:277-281, 1991.
161. Saragoussi JJ et al: Damage to the corneal endothelium by minus power anterior chamber intraocular lenses, *Refract Corneal Surg* 7:282-285, 1991.
162. Worst JGF, van der Veen G, Los LI: Refractive surgery for high myopia. The Worst-Fechner biconcave iris claw lens *Doc Ophthalmol* 75:335-341, 1990.
163. Fechner PU, Strobel J, Wichmann W: Correction of myopia by implantation of a concave Worst-iris claw lens into phakic eyes, *Refract Corneal Surg* 7:286-298, 1991.

SECTION TWO *Preoperative Considerations*

CHAPTER 162

LARRY W. PIEBENGA   CAMILLE S. MATTA   PIERRE G. MARDELLI

Patient Selection and Evaluation

Throughout ophthalmic history, the use of surgery has been devoted almost exclusively to the restoration of visual function. In recent years the emphasis has been placed more and more on the surgical correction of ametropia with an explosive cascade of methods and devices devoted to this purpose. This represents a change in direction for ophthalmology, with the emphasis shifting from treatment of diseases that threaten sight to treatment of conditions that inherently do not.

Refractive surgery, because of its elective nature, should be approached with extreme caution and must be held to the highest standard of efficacy and safety. Accordingly, the selection, evaluation, and counseling of patients should be conducted assiduously. A cavalier approach to refractive surgery is absolutely unacceptable. This chapter will discuss the selection of procedures and patients for refractive surgery, the evaluation of patient suitability for surgery, psychologic evaluation, and informed consent.

Selection of Procedures and Patients

Refractive surgery should be bought rather than sold. Patients have high expectations from modern medicine. These are sometimes unrealistic and are encouraged by daily media coverage of real or supposed breakthroughs. The physician should be careful not to take advantage of such a mindset; every effort must be made to fully educate and appropriately counsel patients regarding results and possible complications of refractive surgery to ensure an intelligent decision is made. Patient and physician must work together to choose the most appropriate procedure for refractive correction: incisional keratoplasty, photorefractive keratectomy, in situ keratomileusis, or possibly, intrastromal implant.

A patient's interest in refractive surgery often originates in reports of the media, from experiences of friends or relatives, or from the suggestion of an eye professional. Initial screening of a patient for surgery is conducted at the first phone contact when a patient may be eliminated because of age or other specific criteria of a refractive surgery protocol (see box, top left, next page). If a patient passes the first screening, he or she is sent explanatory material and invited to attend an informational group seminar with a request to bring a pair of glasses or a copy of a recent prescription.

The first item on the agenda of the seminar is commonly a general introductory videotape outlining the basis of refractive surgery. Such videotapes are commercially available, although some surgeons prefer a custom presentation filmed in their office or surgery site to create rapport and to allow specific points to be emphasized.

After the videotape, a presentation is made by the physician, beginning with a simple explanation of visual acuity and its measurement as well as the optics of myopia, hyperopia, astigmatism, and presbyopia. The results of the proposed surgery are given in terms of visual acuity and refractive results. Graphs, tables, and scattergrams are used to particularly stress overcorrections and undercorrections. Other complications[1,2] are discussed in detail (see box, bottom left, next page). Questions are encouraged at any time.

A popular technique is the use of a series of slides to enumerate the most frequently asked questions. The presenting physician can then easily discuss and elaborate on these (see box, top right, next page). Such an approach is reassuring to the patient and gives a great amount of information in a timesaving format. If other questions from seminar audiences begin to occur frequently, they can be added to the series. After the slides, further questions are encouraged: there should be no time limit for this session. It is important to reemphasize the loss of near vision that occurs after full correction of myopia in presbyopic patients.

Before leaving the seminar, each patient's refractive

Inclusion criteria

- Age 18 years or older (in many refractive protocols, no patient is under 21 years)
- Ability to understand and sign the informed consent
- Best corrected visual acuity adequate to enhance visual function
- Stable refraction and keratometric readings taken at least 2 weeks after discontinuing soft contact lenses or 4 weeks after discontinuing hard lenses
- Available for follow-up
- Psychologically suitable

Exclusion criteria

- Unstable refraction, such as progressive myopia or keratoconus
- Residual, recurrent, or active ocular disease or corneal, conjunctival, or lid abnormalities
- Unstable central keratometric readings with irregular mires
- Systemic diseases, such as connective tissue disorders, or use of any systemic medications likely to affect wound healing, such as corticosteroids or antimetabolites
- Immunocompromised conditions
- Psychologically inclined to unrealistic expectations

Complications of refractive surgery

- Infection, including endophthalmitis
- Perforation and/or rupture
- Cataract formation
- Corneal scarring and/or astigmatism
- Fluctuating vision
- Recurrent erosions
- Ghost images
- Halos
- Glare or haze
- Starbursts
- Progressive or regressive refractive changes
- Medication side effects

error is written on a screening sheet along with demographic data. Finally, the patient may schedule an appointment for an ophthalmic examination to evaluate possible refractive surgery.

Evaluation

Once the patient has attended the seminar and has an understanding of the contemplated refractive surgery, he or she is scheduled for a complete ophthalmic examination. This includes history, external examination, visual acuity, refraction, keratometry, computed topography, contrast sensitivity, brightness acuity testing (BAT), slit lamp examination, fundus examination, tonometry, pachymetry, endothelial cell evaluation, Schirmer's test, and ocular dominance determination. These are listed in their recommended sequence in the box on the facing page.

Patients' common questions

- How bad is the pain and how long does it last?
- Are there restrictions on activity?
- When can I return to work?
- Do I wear a patch? How long?
- When will my vision improve?
- Will I use drops or medicine?
- When will I need to be seen postoperatively?
- When can I have treatment for my other eye and what do I do in the meantime?
- If my result is not satisfactory, can I resume wearing my contact lenses?
- If my correction is not right, can I be retreated?
- How do I use my operated eye and other eye together?
- How much does surgery cost? Will insurance cover it?

HISTORY

A thorough history of systemic and ocular conditions, including any allergies and use of medications, is documented.

EXTERNAL EXAMINATION

It is important to note abnormalities, particularly those conditions which may influence the outcome of surgery. These include atopic or other skin abnormalities (e.g., rosacea), blepharitis, conjunctivitis, lash or eyelid malpositions, exposure changes (e.g. sicca), strabismus, or pupillary anomalies (which may affect the treatment zone).

VISUAL ACUITY

Uncorrected visual acuity is recorded using the Snellen notation. Frequently, for investigational purposes, the Bailey-Lovie system is used to give more quantitative measurements.[3] It should be stressed that 20/20 is not the ultimate visual acuity, and patients should be encouraged to read at the 20/15 or 20/10 level.

REFRACTION

An initial manifest refraction must precede those tests that require a best corrected vision. Contrast sensitivity and BAT can then be done using the appropriate correction. While a later cycloplegic refrac-

Examination: recommended sequence

History
External examination
Visual acuity
Manifest refraction
Ocular dominance determination
Contrast sensitivity
BAT
Keratometry
Computed topography
Slit lamp examination
Cycloplegic refraction
Fundus examination
Tonometry
Pachymetry
Shirmer's test
Endothelial cell imaging

tion is essential to identify patients with latent ciliary hypertonus, keratometry and corneal topography need to precede diagnostic drops, which may distort these readings.[4] Conversely, some examinations that may disturb the epithelial surface should follow both manifest and cycloplegic refraction, such as contact endothelial imaging, tonometry, and pachymetry.

Since the refraction will dictate the magnitude of the refractive surgery, it is important to emphasize that the ophthalmologist should refrain from increasing minus lenses if no additional letters are read and should stress that the goal of refraction is to achieve the very least minus correction for best vision.

The vertex distance must be measured carefully, since surgical alterations of the corneal refraction are necessarily performed at the corneal plane. Widely available charts (usually from 8 to 15 mm vertex distance) convert power from glasses to the corneal plane measurement. For converting the vertex distances beyond the usual range, the following formula is used: $D_2 = D_1/(1 - sD_1)$, where D_2 is the power at the corneal plane, D_1 is the power at measured vertex distance, and s is the vertex distance in meters. Care should be taken to include the sign of the lens power (a minus lens will decrease in power as it moves closer to the cornea). For example, a patient with a vertex distance of 22 mm and spectacle correction of −7.00 diopters will have a corneal plane power of −6.00 diopters. With a more common 12 mm vertex distance, it would be −6.50 diopters.

KERATOMETERY

Traditional keratometric central 3.0 mm zone readings are recorded and compared to previous measurements, if available, to ensure stability. If discrepancies of greater than 0.5 diopter per year are present, serial readings should be obtained until stability is confirmed.[5]

Since only the central cornea is evaluated by keratometry, further investigation is needed before refractive surgery. This investigation could be a detailed corneal mapping by photographic recordings of the corneoscope (Placido rings) or the now infrequently used topogometer.[6] While these techniques alert the surgeon to peripheral corneal abnormalities, they have now been virtually replaced by computed topography.

COMPUTED TOPOGRAPHY

While a very detailed and careful corneal examination could be adequate for some types of refractive surgery, it is generally agreed that computed topography is necessary for more sophisticated surgery, especially surgery related to astigmatism.[7,8] Most physicians like the ease of this technology as well as the wealth of information that can be stored and retrieved for investigational and clinical purposes. A considerable literature has evolved describing the capabilities of this modality, with particular emphasis on undetected keratoconus.[9,10] In our series of over 325 myopic PRK patients, all of whom had computed topography, two were noted to have early keratoconus not suspected by other means. However, considerably higher percentages of occult keratoconus have been reported.[11,12]

There are now a multitude of Placido disk-based machines available. Other systems in development using several technologies allow the recording of actual corneal stromal thickness and curvature and promise significant improvement in approaching irregular corneal surface problems.[13-16]

CONTRAST SENSITIVITY

Contrast sensitivity is a technique that has been used in addition to Snellen visual acuity to characterize a patient's visual function. Experience in PRK at 1 year follow-up reveals that there is no change in contrast sensitivity parameters from baseline at 3, 6, and 12 cycles per degree. A slight but statistically significant change at 18 cycles per degree was reported.[17] Data were obtained using the CSV-1000E.*

BAT

As in contrast sensitivity, no preoperative abnormalities would be anticipated. Postoperatively, fewer than 1% of patients have shown a loss of one line of Snellen visual acuity with the BAT.[17,18] No correlation between this change and the magnitude of haze or subjective symptoms of glare and halos was reported.

*Vector Vision, Dayton, OH.

SLIT LAMP EXAMINATION

It is important to note any abnormalities in the conjunctiva, the lids, and the central and peripheral cornea. Particular attention should be given to the health of the tear film and lid border. Although mild sicca, by causing intolerance to contact lens wear, may be an indication for refractive surgery, more significant dryness may pose a threat to successful epithelial healing. As in any elective ophthalmic surgery, profound sicca, inflammatory processes, or infectious conditions should be addressed preoperatively.

As the cornea is evaluated, close attention should be paid to any anterior membrane dystrophy, stromal scarring, or vascularization that may influence the type of surgery or whether it should be done at all. Any variation in stromal thickness, as in pellucid or Terrien's degeneration, keratoconus, or stromal dystrophies, should alert the surgeon to reconsider performing a refractive procedure.

Descemet's membrane haze or guttae suggest an abnormality in endothelial function and should warn the examiner of possible decompensation. While a skilled clinician can obtain considerable information from specular microscopic endothelial examination, further assessment may be desired by pachymetry and statistical evaluation of endothelial images.

FUNDUS EXAMINATION

A complete dilated fundus examination should be well documented. Changes that might be related to future visual aberrations must be particularly detailed, including disk anatomy with regard to operative and postoperative intraocular pressure elevation, macular degenerative or vascular changes, and peripheral retinal thinning or holes.

TONOMETRY

Preoperative intraocular hypertension must be identified and evaluated. The success of refractive surgery can be influenced by the level of intraocular pressure.[19,20] Whitacre et al and Simon et al[21,22] showed evidence that tonometric readings, particularly with the applanation method, can be significantly underestimated postoperatively as a result of the corneal curvature and/or thickness altered by refractive surgery. Although this rarely seems to be of any clinical significance, in extreme cases it should be kept in mind.

PACHYMETRY

Accurate pachymetry readings are essential in some refractive surgeries—RK, AK, ALK—and in extreme-depth PRK. Pachymetry is correlated with dioptric effect in ablative procedures when the means in a large series are analyzed; however, present systems are of limited value in individual patients.[17] Ultrasonic pachymetry has largely supplanted optical systems because of its ease of use although both are of equal accuracy in clinical measurements.[23,24]

ENDOTHELIAL CELL EVALUATION

While initial studies have revealed little or no loss of endothelial cells 1 year after RK[25-27] or up to 55 months after PRK,[28] it might be useful for a physician performing refractive surgery to obtain endothelial images at baseline when this technology is available. It is highly recommended that endothelial readings be obtained in the evaluation of newer procedures, including ALK, LASIK, corneal intrastromal rings, and holmium laser intrastromal ablation. From an investigational point of view, baseline readings will be helpful for later evaluation of the effect of the treatment modality as well as contact lens wear, possible retreatments, or subsequent intraocular surgery.

SCHIRMER'S TEST

Schirmer's test is a readily available and inexpensive clinical test of lacrimal secretion that helps in documenting dry eye syndrome,[29] despite its recognized low sensitivity.[30] In our refractive surgery application, we use topical anesthesia and a 5-minute interval. The test is considered significant with 3 mm of wetting or less, and should alert the surgeon to possible epithelial surface problems postoperatively.[31]

OCULAR DOMINANCE DETERMINATION

Determination of ocular dominance is done preoperatively to choose the first eye to be treated. If both eyes are to be fully corrected, it is prudent to begin with the nondominant eye to allow any needed adjustments to the treatment parameters of the second eye. In low myopes with consideration of the age of the patient and the visual needs, it may be desirable to plan only to treat one eye. In this instance the treatment goal should be the full distance correction of the dominant eye.

Although there are many determinations for ocular dominance, one popular technique is the sighting test, whereby the patient is asked to fix on a large letter of the Snellen chart while viewing through a half-inch aperture at arm's length. The patient identifies the aiming eye by closing one eye or by bringing the aperture closer to the face until it is evident which eye is aiming. A second test makes use of physiologic diplopia to determine the dominant eye; the patient fixes in the distance and holds a finger about 18 inches away in the midline. This finger is perceived as two images as long as fixation is maintained in the distance. The question is then asked: Which image is more real or solid? If the left image is more "real," then the right eye is dominant and vice versa. Both methods of determination are subject to uncertainty, and sometimes little or no dominance is demonstrated. It is always wise to discuss with the patient any preference for the eye to be treated. Occasionally one eye will be quite intolerant to a contact lens, and that eye probably should be treated first.

Psychologic Evaluation

Although specific psychologic abnormalities were not identified in the Prospective Evaluation of Radial Keratotomy (PERK) study,[32,33] today's physician is aware that each patient's mental health and attitude toward the outcome of refractive surgery must be evaluated preoperatively. It is imperative that the surgeon identify those patients who might be disappointed with merely "good" results ("not so sharp" 20/20 or better) or minor aberrations in vision (halos, glare, shadow images, sunburst).[34] The patient's expectations must be rational; no surgeon can predict the result for any one individual. Similarly, it must be understood that 40% of postoperative patients wear glasses after RK, for example.[33]

While only a minority of patients undergo refractive surgery for occupational reasons, these patients must clearly understand the employer's requirements because specific visual results may not be attainable. Other considerations for the ophthalmologist include the awareness of patients who might be acting on impulse or who are emotionally labile, passive-aggressive, overtly aggressive, or possibly chronic complainers. Concern should be demonstrated for those patients who ask obsessively detailed questions, ask the same questions repeatedly, or demand unreasonable assurance. It is always prudent to emphasize that refractive surgery cannot improve vision; it can, at best, offer results comparable to an individual's preoperative best vision, now without artificial correction from lenses.

Informed Consent

The informed consent must cover the preoperative preparation, operative sequence, all the potential risks, and outcomes involved in any refractive surgical procedure. Since refractive surgery is an elective procedure on an otherwise anatomically normal organ, the physician bears the significant responsibility to emphasize to the patient all risks and complications. The ophthalmologist must be cognizant of studies in the current literature, as well as his own clinical experience, to better inform the patient of the expected results and the possible need for reoperation or retreatment. Again, it should be emphasized that although the aim is emmetropia, under correction or overcorrection can occur. The patient should have realistic expectations from the procedure.

After a review of the intended surgery, the consent must cover alternatives (e.g., glasses, contact lenses, or other procedures) and should include no treatment at all, since this is an elective option. Then the consent must delineate the potential risks and complications that might result from a surgical procedure performed on an otherwise normal eye (see previous box). The necessity for close follow-up and continued long-term observation, similar to any ophthalmic surgery, should be made clear in the consent. The surgeon, patient, and a witness should sign the document, and a copy should be given to the patient.

Conclusion

Earlier the point was made that ophthalmology is embarking on a new course, one treating inherently non–vision-threatening problems rather than vision-threatening diseases. While the endpoint is similar—useful vision—the ultimate goal is assuring useful vision to each individual patient.[35] Only then will the Hippocratic oath be well served.

REFERENCES

1. Changing practice patterns in refractive surgery: results of a survey of the American Society of Cataract and Refractive Surgery, *J Cataract Refract Surg* 20:172-178, 1994.
2. Lindquist TD: Complications of corneal refractive surgery, *Intern Ophthalmol Clinics* 32:97-114, 1992.
3. Lovie-Kitchin JE: Validity and reliability of visual acuity measurements, *Ophthalmic Physiol Opt* 8:363-370, 1988.
4. Mardelli PG et al: Corneal topographic abnormalities following the use of artificial lubricants, *Invest Ophthalmol Vis Sci* 34(Suppl):3809, 1993.
5. Wilson SE et al: Topographic changes in contact lens-induced corneal warpage, *Ophthalmology* 97:734-744, 1990.
6. Stein HA, Slatt BJ: *Fitting guide for hard and soft contact lenses*, St Louis, 1977, Mosby.
7. Lundergan MK, Rowsey JJ: Relaxing incisions. Corneal topography, *Ophthalmology* 92:1226-1236, 1985.
8. Cantera E, Cantera I, Olivieri L: Corneal topographic analysis of photorefractive keratectomy in 175 myopic eyes, *Refract Corneal Surg* 9(Suppl):S19-22, 1993.
9. Rabinowitz YS, McDonnell PJ: Computer-assisted corneal topography in keratoconus, *Refract Corneal Surg* 5:400-408, 1989.
10. Wilson SE, Lin DT, Klyce SD: Corneal topography of keratoconus, *Cornea* 10:2-8, 1991.
11. Wilson SE, Klyce SD: Screening for corneal topographic abnormalities before refractive surgery, *Ophthalmology* 101:147-152, 1994.
12. Nesburn AB et al: Computer assisted corneal topography (CACT) to detect mild keratoconus (kc) in candidates for photorefractive keratectomy, *Invest Ophthalmol Vis Sci* 33(Suppl):995, 1992.
13. Reinstein DZ et al: Corneal pachymetric topography, *Ophthalmology* 101:432-438, 1994.
14. Belin MW et al: The PAR technology corneal topography system, *Ref Corneal Surg* 8:88-96, 1992.

15. Saunders DR, Koch DD: *An atlas of corneal topography,* Thorofare, NJ, 1993, Slack.
16. Izatt JA et al: Micrometer-scale resolution imaging of the anterior eye in vivo with optical coherence tomography, *Arch Ophthalmol* 112:1584-1589, 1994.
17. Piebenga LW et al: Excimer photorefractive keratectomy for myopia, *Ophthalmology* 100:1335-1345, 1993.
18. Piebenga LW et al: Two zone photorefractive keratectomy for moderate myopia, *Ophthalmology* 102:1054-1059, 1995.
19. Sanders DR et al: Factors affecting predictability of radial keratotomy, *Ophthalmology* 92:1237-1243, 1985.
20. Feldman ST et al: The effect of increased intraocular pressure on visual acuity and corneal curvature after radial keratotomy, *Am J Ophthalmol* 108:126-129, 1989.
21. Whitacre MM et al: The effect of corneal thickness on applanation tonometry, *Am J Ophthalmol* 115:592-596, 1993.
22. Simon G et al: Effect of corneal hydration on Goldmann applanation tonometry and corneal topography, *Refract Corneal Surg* 9:110-117, 1993.
23. Nissen J et al: A clinical comparison of optical and ultrasonic pachometry, *Acta Ophthalmol* 69:659-663, 1991.
24. Giasson C, Forthomme D: Comparison of central corneal thickness measurements between optical and ultrasound pachometers, *Optom Vis Sci* 69:236-241, 1992.
25. MacRae SM, Matsuda M, Rich LF: The effect of radial keratotomy on the corneal endothelium, *Am J Ophthalmol* 100:538-542, 1985.
26. Shapiro MB, Harrison DA: Radial keratotomy for intolerable myopia after penetrating keratoplasty, *Am J Ophthalmol* 115:327-331, 1993.
27. Chiba K et al: Morphometric analysis of corneal endothelium following radial keratotomy, *J Cataract Refract Surg* 13:263-267, 1987.
28. Mardelli PG et al: Corneal endothelial status 12 to 55 months following excimer laser photorefractive keratectomy, *Ophthalmology* 102:544-549, 1995.
29. Petroutsos G et al: Diagnostic tests for dry eye disease in normals and dry eye patients with and without Sjögren's syndrome, *Ophthalmic Res* 24:325-331, 1992.
30. Lucca JA et al: A comparison of diagnostic test for keratoconjunctivitis sicca: Lactoplate, Schirmer and tear osmolarity, *CLAO J* 16:109-112, 1990.
31. Farris RL et al: Basal and reflex human tear analysis. I. Physical measurements: osmolarity, basal volumes and reflex flow rate, *Ophthalmology* 88:852-857, 1981.
32. Powers MK et al: Psychosocial findings in radial keratotomy patients two year after surgery, *Ophthalmology* 91:1193 1984.
33. Bourque LB et al: Psychosocial characteristics of candidates for the prospective evaluation of radial keratotomy (PERK) study, *Arch Ophthalmol* 102:1187-1192, 1984.
34. Bourque LB et al: Reported satisfaction, fluctuation of vision, and glare among patients one year after surgery in the prospective evaluation of radial keratotomy (PERK) study, *Arch Ophthalmol* 104:356-363, 1986.
35. Warring GO: The Hamburger Institute, *J Refract Corneal Surg* 10:495-497, 1994.

CHAPTER 163

KERRY K. ASSIL

Refractive Keratotomy—Assistive Technology and Instrumentation

When evaluating assistive technology and instrumentation for a refractive keratotomy practice, the physician should pay particular attention to the products reproducibility, durability, and affordability. Proper instrument selection may facilitate surgical outcome, efficacy, and reproducibility while promoting cost-effective practice management. Furthermore, unnecessary expenditures may adversely influence delivery of care.

There is a great variety of useful instrumentation and assistive technology for keratorefractive surgery. Any attempt at a comprehensive survey of all available systems would be futile, owing to the vast array of available instrumentation and the rapid evolution of technology. We will therefore focus instead on those features essential to any system component, hoping that our descriptions will be broad enough to encompass the majority of available systems.

Operating Room Equipment

In selecting the operating room equipment,* attention should be paid to the room's overall size limitations. Other considerations include electrical outlet availability and a surgical scrub sink.

A fully reclining, height-adjustable chair in place of a surgical bed may aid with space economy, possibly enabling use of the space for slit lamp biomicroscopy as well as refractive keratotomy. In the event that a reclining chair is selected, prominent side arms are needed (in place of side rails) for considerations of patient safety. The chair or bed should also accommodate a wrist rest to facilitate surgeon wrist support.

The surgeon's chair should be height adjustable, with a foot bar or pedal control. The chair should also[1] have a backrest and elbow rests, particularly if the surgeon wishes to forego the wrist rest.

A large array of operating microscopes is now available and specifically designed for in-office delivery of keratorefractive procedures. In selecting a microscope, particular attention should be paid to the quality of the optics, including the depth of field. A relatively large depth of field is useful in maintaining focus, as the globe is indented during the procedure. Variable magnification and light source intensity are other valuable features. Secondary procedures (enhancements) often require higher magnification and variable lighting because these procedures are often performed with the pupil dilated for better visualization of prior incisions, against the red reflex. Adjustable ocular spacing and tilt angle are also useful. Practical foot pedal features include focus and x/y control, although these may be compensated for by a lightweight microscope coupled with autoclavable handles. The microscope field illumination light source should consist of either a nearly coaxial focal beam or a concentric illumination ring. Either of these designs avoids formation of bothersome shadows in association with corneal surface markings, which can occur with significant paraxial light sources.

To assist with patient cooperation during the procedure, fixation light systems have evolved, enabling either coaxial visual axis determination and/or automated eccentric gaze globe fixation during the procedure (Figure 163-1).

Microscope designs have been described that detail the optimal features for in-office delivery of refractive procedures.[1] These proposed microscope designs include a paraxial light source in the form of a ring illumination system of relatively large diameter (concentric to the microscope head), which enables diffuse surface illumination at high intensity. Thus, the subject would not experience light-induced discomfort, since the paraxial light reflex is concentric with and peripheral to the entrance pupil. The concentric nature of the light source eliminates shadows from either corneal markings or the surgeons' hands, in the presence of paraxial illumination. By placing an infrared filter within the fiberoptic light pathway, the ocular surface is not desiccated by heat energy, enabling the diamond knife foot plates to glide

*The author has no proprietary interest in any of the technologies or equipment presented within this manuscript.

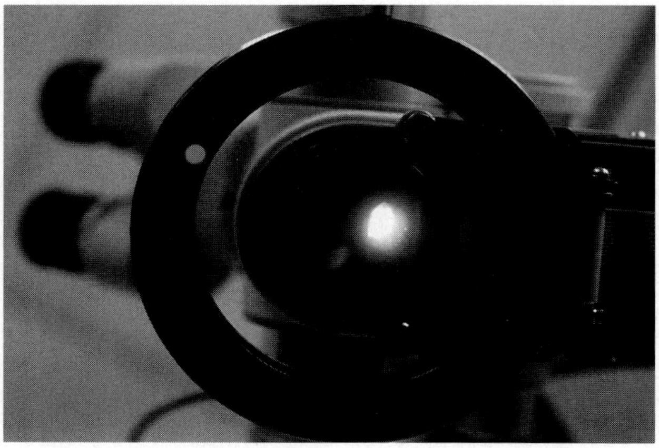

FIGURE 163-1 Accessory eccentric gaze light fixation ring mounted onto operating microscope.

smoothly along the moist epithelial surface in the presence of bright surface illumination. Within this system, a separate (flashing) coaxial fixation light source (red or green) would project from within one of the two objectives. Sighting through the complementary eyepiece, the surgeon's view will be coaxial with the patient's corneal optical center, which serves as the closest measurable landmark to the true visual axis.[2] Coaxial light fixation devices, which are either mounted onto surgical microscopes or aligned within the microscope optical system, make the precise localization of the corneal optical center readily possible. An alternative (and possibly superior) lighting system uses paraxial series of flashing red target light-emitting diodes (LED's), mounted onto the microscope head in the form of a concentric ring. Such a system enables automated eccentric gaze ocular fixation. The patient is instructed to view the selectively activated flashing LED light source, which guides the eye into an eccentric field of gaze, opposite the desired incision axis.[3] This eye position maximizes surgical site exposure and facilitates perpendicular orientation of the blade tip to the corneal surface. Such an eccentric gaze fixation system also minimizes patient discomfort from the bright operating light source, affording greater field illumination with improved visibility.

A Mayo stand should be of sufficient size for the proper display of instruments. After the procedure, instruments should be rinsed and placed into an ultrasonic cleanser. Ultrasonic cleansers with plastic fingerlike projections along the chamber base are now available, accommodating diamond knives as well as corneal markers. The chamber may be filled with either hydrogen peroxide or distilled deionized water. Cidex should not be used within a refractive surgical practice because it is extremely toxic to the eye, with its corrosive action capable of dislodging the diamond blade from its base.

After ultrasonic cleaning, the instruments are autoclaved. An autoclave, available within the operating room and capable of rapid instrument sterilization (packaged either singly or within an instrument tray), reduces interoperative time and facilitates quality assurance. In autoclaving the instruments, it is generally important that distilled and deionized water be used to avoid a build-up of crystalline precipitates on the diamond knife blade and foot plates. Modern autoclaves enable instrument sterilization in less than 10 minutes. Unless otherwise instructed by the manufacturer, simultaneous packaging of steel and titanium instruments in the autoclave should be avoided. Most titanium instruments produce acidic vapors that are caustic to steel products.

While studies determining the necessary environment for sufficiently minimizing the risk of airborne contamination during refractive keratotomy are lacking, several simple precautionary measures appear prudent. If the minor procedures are performed outside of a standard operating room setting, some consideration may be given to air purification. Other precautions include the wearing of masks by persons entering the room, the elimination of carpeting or substandard ceiling tiles, and the placement of hoods over air vents to redirect air flow away from the patient. The use of an air purification system that continuously filters particulate matter from the environment may also prove useful.

Surgical Supplies and Medications

1. Surgical mask (anti-fog) — gown and head cover are often not used.
2. Mayo stand cover — sterile field for display of surgical instruments.
3. Anxiolytics — provided before the procedure.
4. Analgesics — may include topical nonsteroidal anti-inflammatory medication.
5. Blanket or cover sheet — for patient comfort.
6. Folded towel — placed beneath patient's shoulders, facilitating the chin-up position.
7. Eye patch — occludes patient's nonsurgical eye.
8. Povidone-iodine (Betadine) skin preparation — taking care to avoid the ocular surface.
9. Sterile open eye surgical drape.
10. Topical antibiotics — broad spectrum.
11. Topical anesthetics — avoid direct instillation onto the corneal epithelium (minimizes toxicity).

12. Hand disinfecting solution.
13. Sterile surgical gloves (powderless).
14. Cellulose sponges.
15. 10-0 nylon suture—for intraoperative crossed incisions or perforation.
16. Topical analgesics, steroids, and broad-spectrum antibiotics—initiated just before the procedure; may be continued for several days thereafter.

Primary Procedure Instrumentation

Proper machining of quality materials produces durable instruments that facilitate procedure efficacy and reproducibility. In attempting to contain costs while ensuring instrument quality, for example, the surgeon may wish to avoid cosmetic packaging features that transfer the costs of instrument production to nonfunctional parameters. Gold plating, for instance, having a different coefficient of expansion than the underlying steel or titanium, tends to flake off with repeat autoclaving. In general, titanium instruments may be more desirable than steel; in addition to being of lighter weight, they may be more durable. With titanium the cross hairs and radial wing extensions may be readily machined from the same sheet of metal as the body of the instrument, thereby obviating the need for soldering and circumventing the potential for damaged alignment with repeat autoclaving.

Radial keratotomy instruments are discussed here in their most typical order of use.

Eyelid speculum. A wire eyelid speculum providing adequate globe exposure is sufficient in most cases.

Visual axis marker. A fine-tipped Sinskey hook or jeweler's forceps, for indenting the corneal epithelium, serves as a surgical centration landmark.

Optical (central clear) zone markers. These are generally provided in two varieties: those with a dull contact margin, requiring ink for corneal marking, and those with sharper contact margin, obviating the need for the use of surgical dyes. The more refined markers taper to a 4 μm wide contact margin, providing a precise and prominent surgical landmark. The central clear zone marker should be equipped with cross hairs so as to ensure precise centration, concentric to the visual axis marking (Figure 163-2). Central clear zone marker diameters ranging from 3 to 5 mm in 0.25 mm increments are generally sufficient.

Outer zone markers. The ideal outer zone diameter size remains to be determined. While recent data suggest that an outer zone diameter of 10 mm may provide a greater range of corneal flattening than does

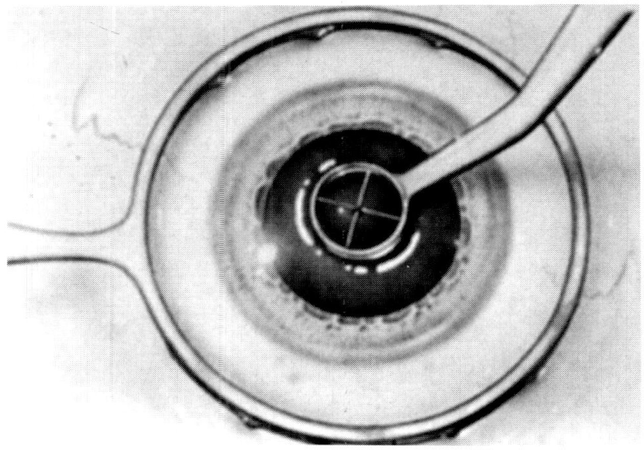

FIGURE 163-2 Artist's rendition of central clear zone marker with cross hairs. Globe is fixated using a Thornton fixation ring.

an outer zone of 8 mm,[4] longer incision lengths may be associated with a greater propensity for hyperopic drift.[5] The optimal outer zone diameter may lie somewhere between 8 and 10 mm. Furthermore, no clinical data presently available distinguish between the relative value of outer zone marking centered with respect to the corneoscleral limbus versus the central clear zone. Such studies are currently under way and will hopefully help to delineate the optimal outer zone diameter and centration site.

Radial wing markers. Radial keratotomy procedures providing greater than eight radial incisions in a single setting are now generally discouraged. Radial wing markers may be obtained for delineating three, four, six, and eight radial incision sites. The markers should be judged for durability, low profile (do not obscure corneal visualization), and sharp contact margins for prominent epithelial indentation. As with the other markers, the use of titanium enables machining of the marker head from a single sheet of metal, therefore obviating concerns of durability associated with soldering.

Forceps. Globe fixation forceps stabilize the globe and facilitate proper diamond orientation (perpendicular to the corneal surface) over the length of the incision, thereby improving procedure outcome predictability and safety. Globe fixation may also enable more predictable incision depth placement, thereby reducing the need for secondary (enhancement) procedures.[6] Typical fixation techniques include the use of 0.3 forceps, grasping the conjunctival insertion at the limbus, directly across from the radial incision site (Figure 163-3), or Kelman style (two-point fixation) forceps and Thornton 360° ring forceps (Figure 163-2), each of which also retards globe torsional motion. Continual globe pressure elevation applied by the

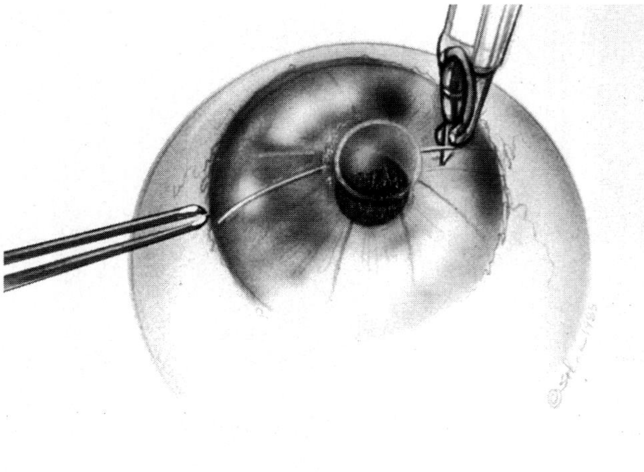

FIGURE 163-3 Artist's rendition of globe fixation, with forceps grasping conjunctival insertion across from incision site.

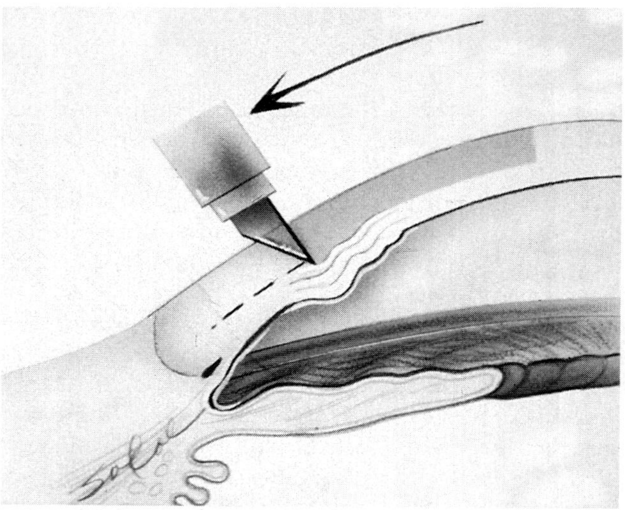

FIGURE 163-4 American incision. Artist's rendition of centrifugal incision.

Thornton ring may result in progressive corneal deturgescence during the procedure, with consequent increase in perforation incidence. Recently, ring fixation forceps with foot plate guides for more linear incision placement have been reintroduced.[7] Care must be taken to avoid chipping the diamond blade tip when using these devices.

Radial keratotomy knives. The first generation knives used for the performance of anterior surface radial keratotomy consisted of steel blades that were broken and fashioned onto scalpel handles or forceps. The introduction of diamond technology for refractive keratotomy coincided with the initiation of the Prospective Evaluation of Radial Keratotomy (PERK) study in the United States.[8,9] Traditionally the most common diamond designs were those with a cutting edge along

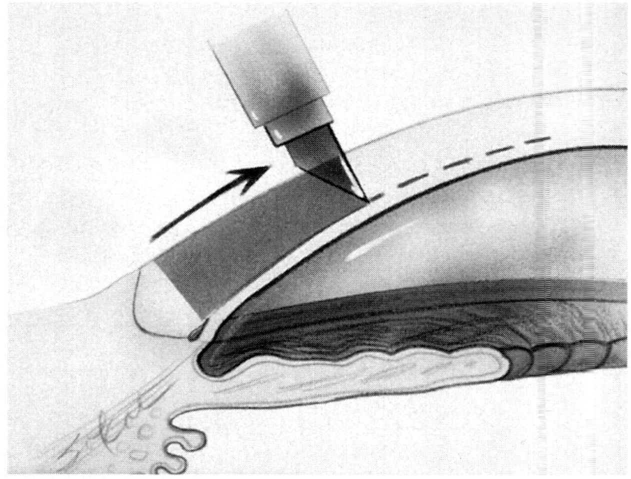

FIGURE 163-5 Russian incision. Artist's rendition of centripetal incision.

the angled margin, for performing centrifugal directed incisions (Figure 163-4) or those with a cutting edge along the vertical margin (Figure 163-5), enabling centripetally directed incisions.[10] Throughout the 1980s, numerous modifications were made to these diamond designs, including the angle subtended by the diamond's tip, the blade thickness, and even the appearance of a faceted margin along the distal portion (tri-faceted).

In 1991 the combined technique diamonds were designed, becoming generally available in 1992 (Figure 163-6).[11] These diamonds enable the surgeon to begin the incision at the central clear zone (Figure 163-7, *A*), extend out toward the limbus, and then reverse direction back toward the central zone (Figure 163-7, *B*) without the risk of central clear zone invasion. The angled margin on the front surface, which is the centrifugal cutting component is sharpened along its entire length. The vertical margin is ground sharp to a cutting edge for a distance of only 250 μm from the blade's distal tip (Figure 163-6).

The blunt superficial portion of the vertical margin prevents undesirable invasion of the central clear zone when the blade tip is initially inserted into the cornea at the clear zone margin. During the next phase, as a centrifugal incision is made toward the limbus (downhill), the diamond produces a linear radial incision groove of variable depth ranging between 55% and 80% of the corneal thickness.[11] On arriving at 1 mm of the limbus, the cutting motion is reversed centripetally toward the central clear zone, within the same groove created by the preceding centrifugal incision. Because the vertical margin of the diamond is sharp only along its distal portion (250 μm), it is difficult for the blade to escape from within the previously incised groove.

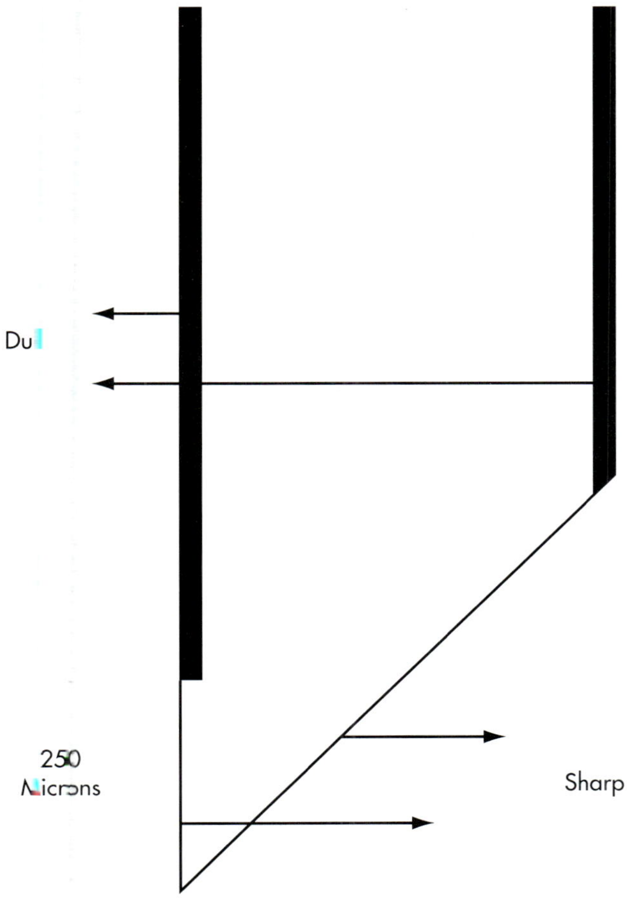

FIGURE 163-6 Schematic diagram of a combined-technique diamond blade.

This centripetally directed motion increases the incision depth uniformly to approximately 80% to 90% of corneal thickness. Once the diamond blade returns to the central clear zone margin, it is unable to advance further. Thus the ideal feature of the centrifugal radial incision method, a linear groove with minimal risk of invading the central clear zone, is combined with the ideal feature of the centripetal radial incision method, uniformly deep incision (for reproducible corneal flattening). By obviating the need to extend the diamond setting well beyond 100% of corneal thickness, as is routine among centrifugal incision protocols, the risk of globe perforation may also be reduced.[6]

In a comparative study using cadaveric eyes, the combined (Genesis) technique for radial incisions demonstrated significantly greater corneal flattening than did the centrifugal (American) method, with reduced outcome variability as compared to the centripetal (Russian) method incision.[11] Early clinical data appear consistent with these cadaveric studies.[6,12]

Other diamond-tipped designs currently being used include the undercut diamonds designed for maximizing central corneal flattening while affording relatively larger central clear zone diameters, thereby diminishing associated glare and induced astigmatism.[13]

To maximize diamond-tipped instruments' shelf life, the diamond tip should be readily retractable into a safe housing position when not in use. Cleaning of the diamond knives should be performed in balanced salt solution or hydrogen peroxide within the ultrasonic cleanser and in distilled deionized water during the autoclave cycle. The diamond-tipped knife should not come into contact with Cidex because formaldehyde is highly corrosive and may weaken the diamond's attachment at its base. As is the case with the other handheld instruments, it may be prudent to invest in quality instruments rather than choosing gold plating and other marketing expenditures aimed at cosmetic appeal.

Diamond knife foot plates. The foot plate design must be forgiving of undesirable deviations caused by the surgeon's hand by helping to maintain the diamond blade at a uniform stromal depth, over a broad range of diamond knife–corneal surface angular excursions. With knife foot plates that make minimal radial contact against the corneal surface, the blade tends to maintain uniform depth within the stroma even if the surgeon's hand rocks (Figure 163-8, *A* and *B*). The knife foot plates should also be relatively broad so as to maximize lateral support. In this way, should the surgeon's hand rock from side to side, the foot plate's lateral corneal compression maintains perpendicular blade stromal penetration (Figure 163-8, *C*).

The knife foot plates should also be designed to generate minimal resistance against the corneal epithelium over the course of the incision. The foot plate's central tip should be curved and smoothly polished, providing minimal resistance against a dry epithelium. Finally, diamond knife foot plates should be designed to readily enable simultaneous viewing of the diamond blade and the cornea, a feature referred to as having a low profile. We refer to diamond knife foot plates with this combination of features as having a universal design. The recent trend toward globe fixation rings that contain foot plate guidance tracks may facilitate improved incision quality.

Foot plate spacing also serves as a significant variable affecting incision depth. Widely spaced foot plates may cause anterior bowing of the cornea between the foot plates, resulting in relatively deeper blade penetration. Conversely, more closely spaced foot plates may cause relative posterior corneal displacement, resulting in a shallower incision. It is evident that foot plate design features are just as important determinants of incision precision and efficiency as are diamond blade design features. It may therefore be somewhat misleading to suggest that two surgeons,

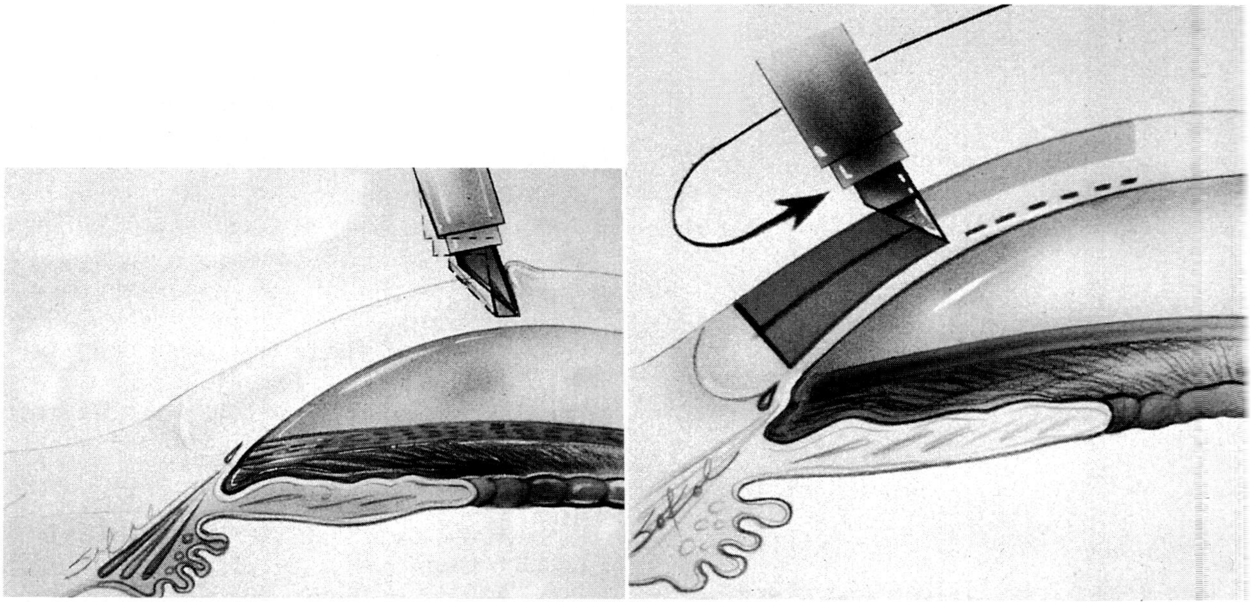

A

B

FIGURE 163-7 **A,** Genesis incision. Initiation of a combined incision with corneal penetration and undermining of central clear zone margin. **B,** Genesis incision. Artist's rendition of combined-style incision in progress. Having completed the centrifugal complement of the incision, the surgeon is now retracing centripetally within the original incision groove.

using different diamonds, should achieve identical results.

Foot plates that also serve as pachymeter probe tips are currently being developed to enable real-time diamond knife extension, precisely matching regional corneal thickness. To date the inability to design autoclavable probe tips serves as the challenge precluding clinical utility.

Needle holder. A standard curved needle holder should be readily available for primary repair of intraoperative crossed incisions or perforations or for subsequent sutured wound closure.

Irrigating cannula. Either an angled 27-gauge or a Rowsey-style irrigating cannula may be used to flush saline solution into the incision groove at the termination of the case. Many surgeons do not routinely irrigate the wounds.

Astigmatic Keratotomy Instrumentation

Several instruments unique to astigmatic keratotomy include central clear zone markers measuring 6, 7, and 8 mm in diameter. For the placement of transverse incisions, 3 mm T-cut markers are generally sufficient, since the anticipated effect of transverse incisions is titrated by varying the central clear zone size, while incision length remains constant. When employing arcuate keratotomy for the correction of astigmatic errors, the central clear zone size is generally held constant, while the arc length is varied. A set of four, six, and eight-wing radial keratotomy markers is sufficient for delineating the desired arc length in most cases. A six-wing radial keratotomy marker, for instance, will intersect the central clear zone marker at 60° intervals, whereas an eight-wing marker will do so at 45° intervals.

Diamond blade designs most commonly used for performing astigmatic keratotomy include the standard back-cutting (Russian style), double-edged, tri-faceted (Figure 163-9), or 15° diamond blade with the latter often proving most responsive. Mechanical globe fixation is essential when using these diamonds.

Secondary Procedure Instrumentation

Undercorrections may typically be addressed by either adding additional incisions or by lengthening or deepening the original ones. Instrumentation for incision addition consists of those used for the primary procedure itself, including corneal topographic analysis to guide in localizing corneal steep zones. Incision lengthening is an option, particularly during the first several weeks to months after the primary procedure, since minimal cross-linking of stromal collagen has

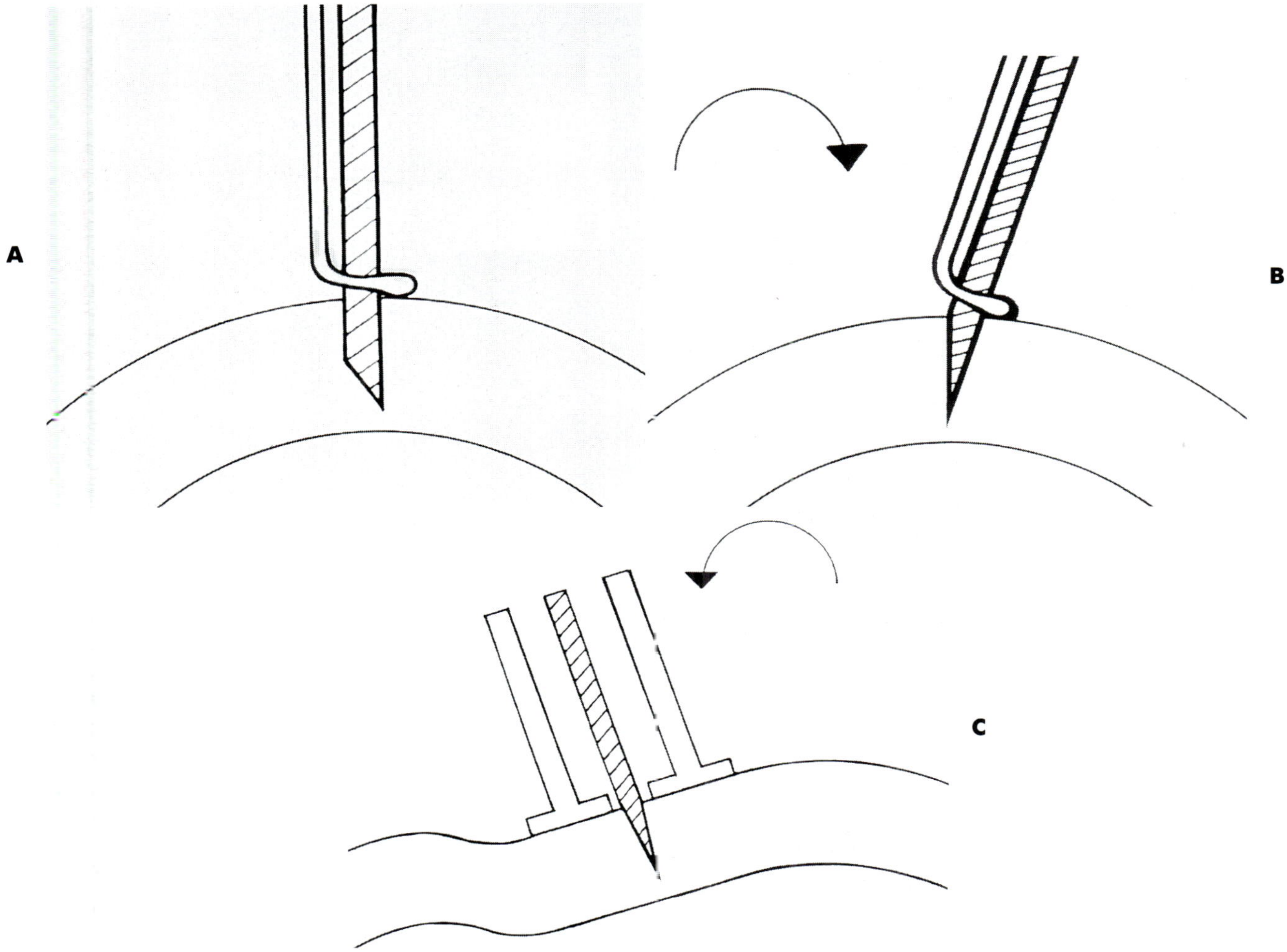

FIGURE 163-8 **A,** Foot plate design with rounded leading toe and minimal radial epithelial contact. **B,** Minimal foot plate radial contact with the epithelium enables the diamond blade to maintain a relatively uniform stromal depth, despite inadvertent rocking motion of the diamond knife. **C,** Broad lateral contact between the diamond foot plates and the corneal epithelium enables the diamond blade to maintain relative perpendicular orientation with respect to the corneal stroma despite inadvertent lateral rocking of the diamond knife.

occurred at this stage. For incision lengthening a Sinskey hook may be used to splay open the superficial (epithelial) portion of the original incisions, with a combined-style diamond used to elongate the incisions either peripherally or centrally.

Overcorrections may be addressed pharmacologically (if recognized early) or surgically, using selective sutured wound closure of incision sites topographically identified as being excessively flat. A specialized Sinskey hook with a serrated lateral wall may be used to scrape out the epithelial cysts and loose fibrous tissue from within the incision groove (Figure 163-10). Sutured closure using a needle holder and interrupted 10-0 nylon sutures at the 5, 7, and 9 mm zone diameters may then be carried out.

Additional Assistive Technology

Glare tester. A standard glare tester, including the brightness acuity tester, is a useful ancillary tool to screen for subclinical lenticular opacities and to assist in the unmasking of subtle irregular astigmatism, although corneal topography and contrast sensitivity testing may be more accurate in identifying the latter.

Auto refractor. While there is no substitute for manifest and cycloplegic refraction, automated refraction with the eye in a cycloplegic state may provide a useful starting point in refraction of a patient whose baseline error is otherwise unknown.

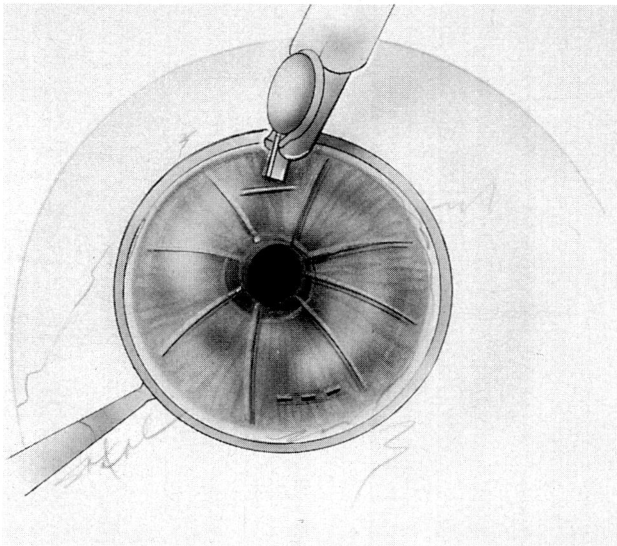

FIGURE 163-9 Artist's rendition of a tri-faceted diamond for performing astigmatic keratotomy. A fixation ring is in position, and the eye has previously undergone eight-incision radial keratotomy.

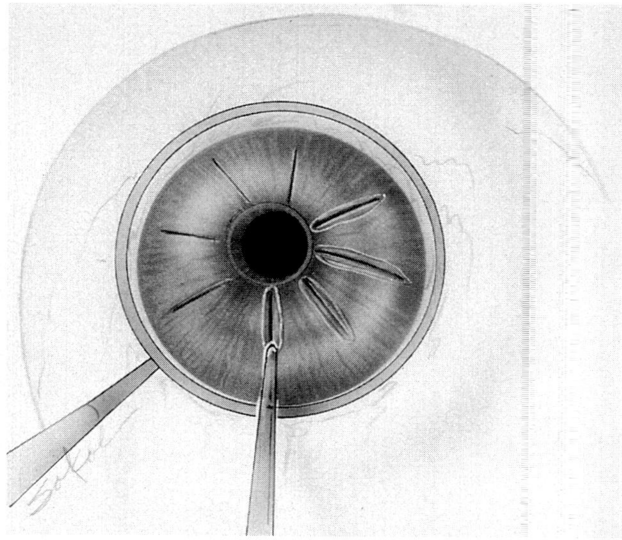

FIGURE 163-10 Artist's rendition of a modified Sinskey hook used to open a previous keratotomy incision site and to scrape free epithelial inclusion cysts and fibrous debris.

Computerized videokeratography. The improvements in keratorefractive surgical outcome would not be possible without the aid of sophisticated corneal shape analysis. With the advent of computerized videokeratography, we are now able to explain many of the previously unanswerable questions regarding corneal physiologic optics. Computerized videokeratography in the setting of a keratorefractive practice facilitates (1) patient screening, (2) surgical planning, (3) documentation of irregular astigmatism, (4) guidance of secondary procedures, and (5) surgeon feedback. Available systems clinically use Placido ring projections, with first Purkinje image capture analysis. Laser-based topographic and direct visualization imaging systems are currently under development. Such systems may provide more accurate corneal shape determination.

Ultrasonic pachymeter. The use of intraoperative, real-time, solid-state ultrasonography is critical to achieving accurate corneal pachymetry readings. It is also advisable to conduct preoperative screening pachymetry to supplement intraoperative measurements (Figure 163-11, *A* and *B*).

To reduce the risk of microperforation, intraoperative pachymetry for radial keratotomy may be conducted within a 3 mm optical zone, that is to say, 1.5 mm from the visual axis, at the inferotemporal site, and over the thinnest paracentral cornea, as previously established by the screening pachymetry. These two loci often coincide. Optimal design features for an ultrasonic pachymeter should include a solid-state probe with angled tip, contact-activated corneal measurement, semi-continuous readings, without the need for foot pedal activation, a digital display monitor, and memory for storing sequentially gathered data. To date, autoclavable pachymeter tips are not available, necessitating the soaking of the probe tip in hydrogen peroxide, coupled with an alcohol wipe, before use.

Diamond calibration microscopes. There are multiple alternative techniques available for calibrating the amount to extend a diamond tip beyond the plane of the foot plates. These include using the micrometer on the knife itself (Figure 163-12) and several alternative external validation systems. The systems of external validation include plastic blocks (Figure 163-13), coin gauges (Figure 163-14, *A* and *B*), shadowgrams, and, most recently, diamond calibrating microscopes (Figure 163-14, *C*).

A number of coaxial microscope systems are designed for precise calibration of the diamond-tipped instruments. Diamond microscopes with the least number of accessory components tend to be quite accurate in addition to being more economical. We have found that the ideal calibrating microscopes are those with (1) high quality optics that maximize depth of field while minimizing spherical aberration, (2) stages mounted on cross rollers that minimize vibrational motion, (3) motion detectors (in place of micrometers) capable of reporting any diamond tip excursion relative to the viewing system, and (4) rotatable reticle within the eyepiece for precise alignment of both foot plates relative to the vertical zero position. The calibrating microscopes also enable

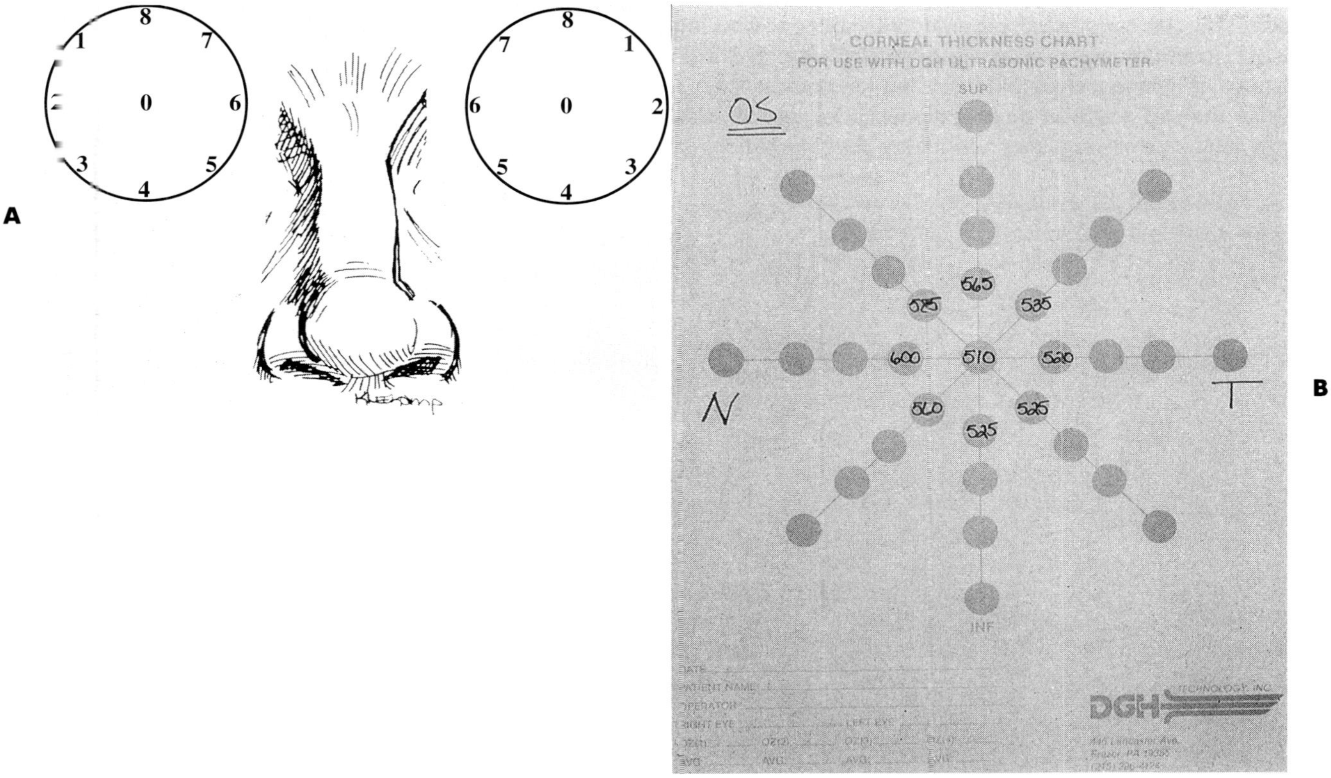

FIGURE 163-11 **A,** Schematic representation of desirable sites for pachymetric corneal measurement, including the apex (position Ø) and eight paracentral sites at an approximate 3 mm diameter. **B,** Representative pachymetric measurements at the corneal apex and eight paracentral locations.

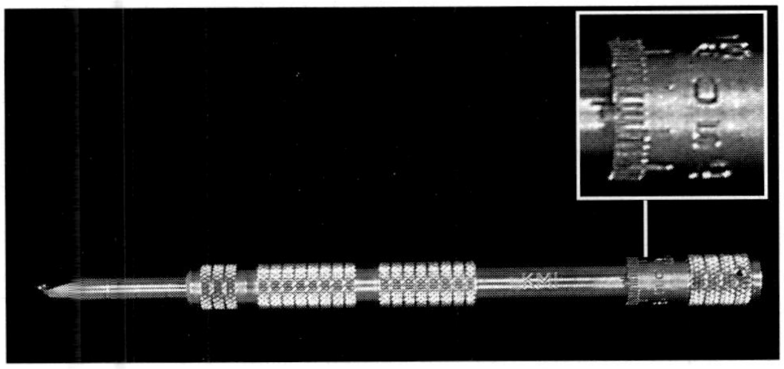

FIGURE 163-12 Standard radial keratotomy diamond knife equipped with micrometer for self-contained calibration of diamond tip extension.

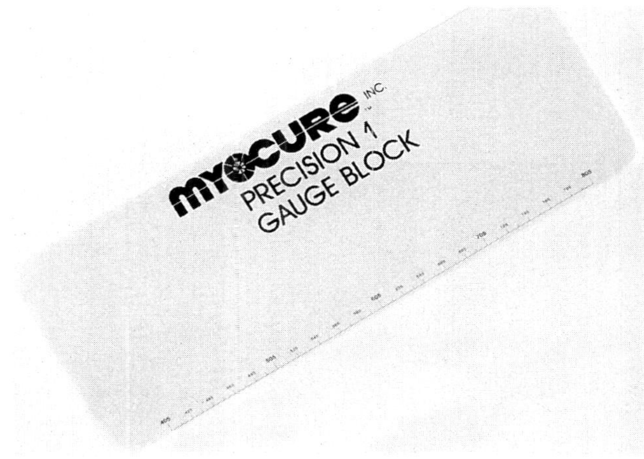

FIGURE 163-13 Plastic guage block used for measurement of diamond tip extension.

evaluation of diamond defects, including chipping or accumulation of debris (Figure 163-15).

Video monitor. The surgeon may wish to link a video monitor system to the operating microscope to enable real-time procedure viewing, aid with precise centration of the globe within the operative field, and allow for videotaping of selected procedures. While this feature is clearly not mandatory, it may lend an incremental benefit in certain clinical settings.

Data tracking software. This may be useful in providing the surgeon with outcome analysis and assisting in long-term selection between alternative viable techniques. Such systems may also assist in the tracking of costs and in surgical planning. Surgeon-specific nomograms may also be possible with the basic nomograms provided within such systems, modified by

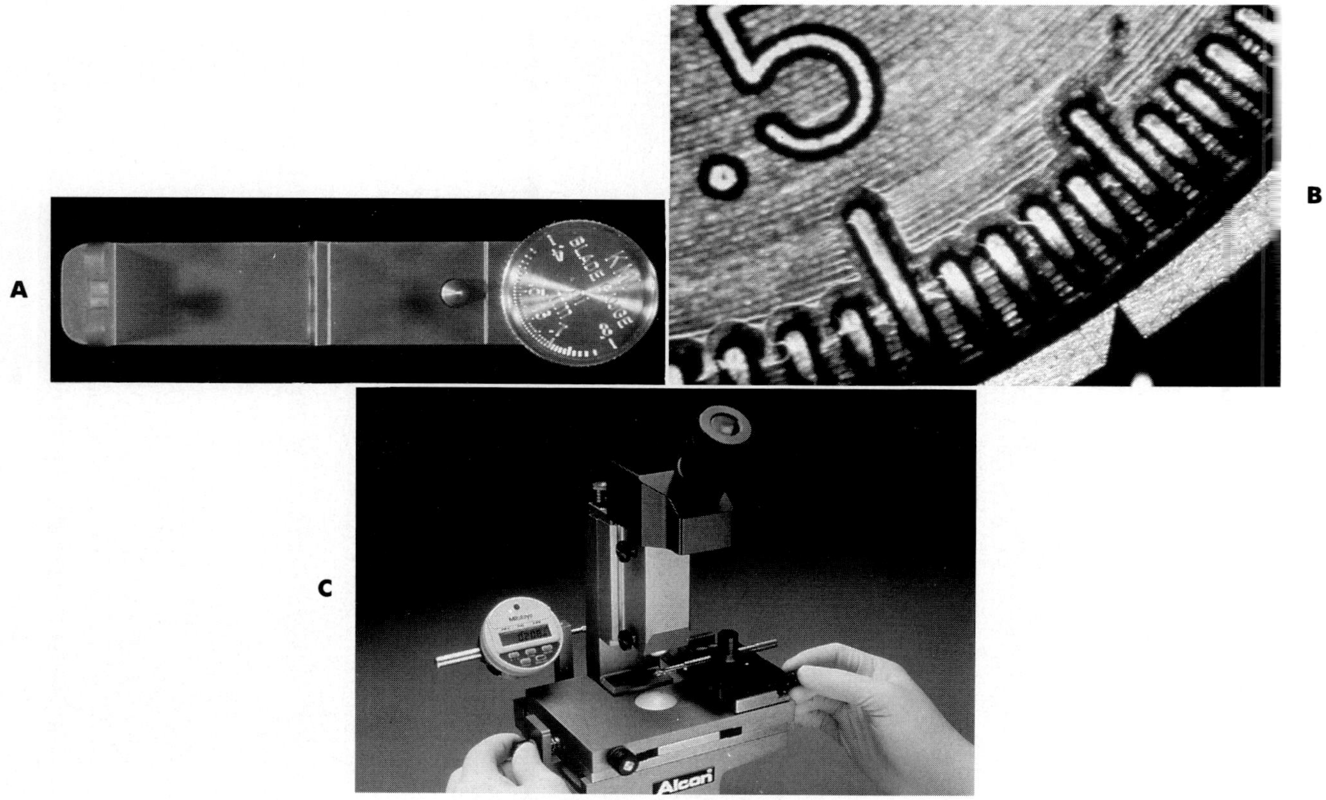

FIGURE 163-14 **A,** Standard coin gauge used for diamond tip calibration. **B,** The diamond tip has been extended approximately 530 μm. **C,** State-of-the-art diamond calibrating microscope.

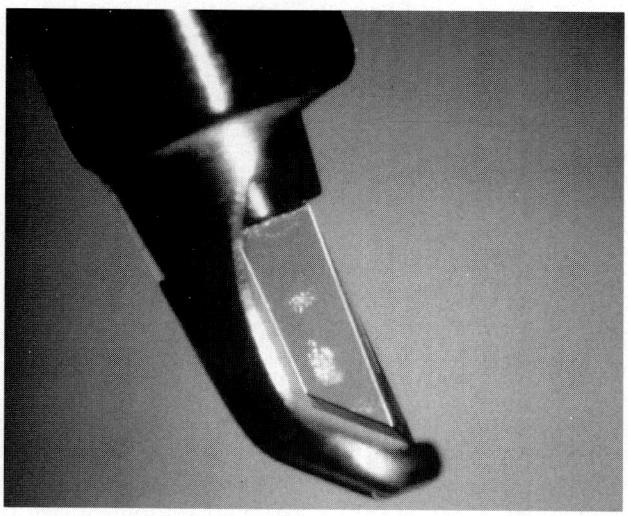

FIGURE 163-15 Debris accumulated onto diamond blade, readily observable under magnification.

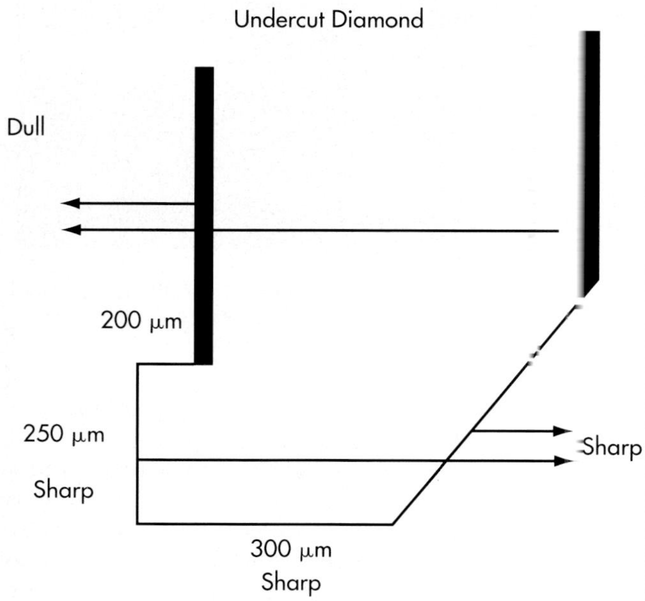

FIGURE 163-16 Schematic representation of a diamond knife blade designed for maximal undermining of the central clear zone.

A

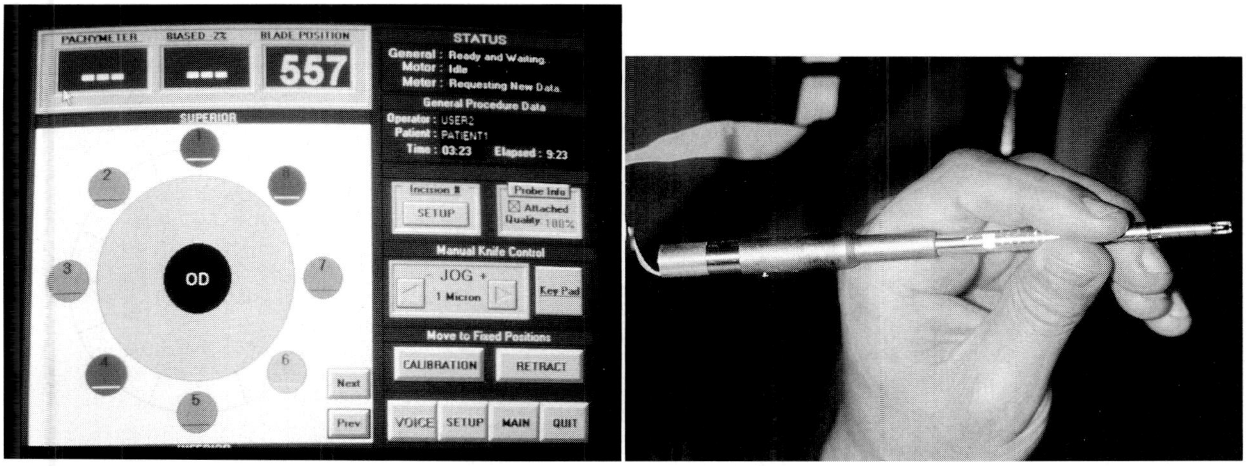

B

FIGURE 163-17 **A,** Sample computer screen displays of programmable diamond system demonstrating incision sequence programming. **B,** With inferotemporal incision site activated, diamond knife displays setting at that site.

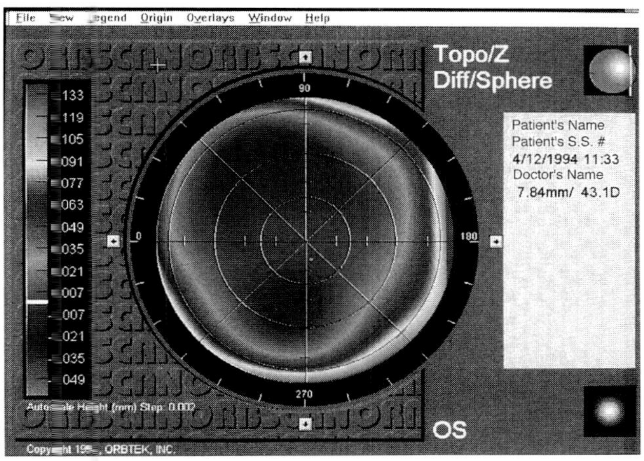

FIGURE 163-18 Topography map printout provided by the Orbscan slit beam corneal imaging system.

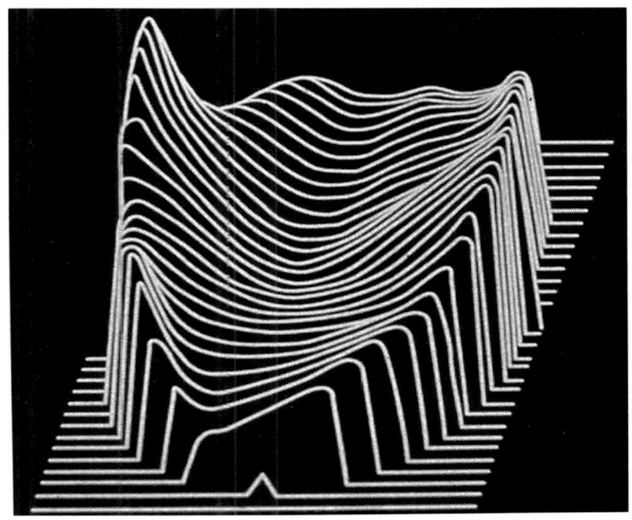

FIGURE 163-19 Holographic topography map: amplified deviations. Postoperative eye after PRK.

the program's linear regression capability, based on cumulative surgical results.

Investigative Aids

Specular or confocal scanning microscopy. Examination of the corneal endothelial layer is of critical value in studies evaluating the impact of keratorefractive procedures on corneal integrity. While to date there are no prospective studies demonstrating significant endothelial cell loss in association with anterior surface radial keratotomy, the impact of radial keratotomy coupled with other refractive procedures, or with subsequent contact lens wear, remains unclear.

Contrast acuity. This testing will likely become an increasingly important modality in keratorefraction. Because most refractive procedures alter corneal topography away from its physiologic positively aspheric shape, many are likely to adversely affect contrast sensitivity. While any adverse effect of radial keratotomy on contrast sensitivity appears to be small, this assertion may not hold true for extremely small optical zone size selections. Furthermore, contrast sensitivity data may become increasingly important in selecting between alternative keratorefractive modalities.

Aesthesiometer. This is of potential value in assessing postoperative changes in the corneal sensation of patients undergoing keratorefractive procedures.

Future Advances

Refractive keratotomy as practiced in 2 to 3 years will most likely differ significantly from our current approach. Technology presently undergoing clinical investigation includes undercut diamonds, designed for greater range of corneal flattening (Figure 163-16) and computer-assisted diamond knives, whereby real-time pachymeters adjust diamond tip extension via optically guided motor drives linked through a computer interface (Figure 163-17, *A* and *B*).[14] Corneal topographic systems may evolve to enable real-time corneal shape analysis, further aiding in the refinement of technique and diminishing the need for future enhancements (Figures 163-18 and 163-19). Automated globe fixation systems will most likely become available as well, controlling intraocular pressure and ocular movement, thereby adding to outcome predictability and procedure safety. Perhaps of greatest value, however, will be advances to our insights in the area of corneal wound healing, affording us the capability of postoperative pharmacologic corneal shape manipulation.[15]

REFERENCES

1. Assil KK, Schanzlin JD: Proposed refinements to microscope design. In *Radial and astigmatic keratotomy: a complete handbook for successful practice of incisional keratotomy using the combined technique,* Thorofare, NJ, 1994, Slack.
2. Pande M, Hillman JS: Optical zone centration in keratorefractive surgery, *Ophthalmology* 100:1230-1237, 1993.
3. Assil K, Knepshield W: *Light guided eccentric gaze fixation system,* American Society of Cataract and Refractive Surgery, annual symposium, Boston, April 1994.
4. Chayet A et al and the Refractive Keratoplasty Study Group: *8 vs. 10 mm outer zone radial keratotomy,* American Society of Cataract and Refractive Surgery symposium, Boston April 1994.
5. Waring GO III, Lynn MJ, McDonnell PJ, and the PERK Study Group: Results of the prospective evaluation of radial keratotomy (PERK) study 10 years after surgery. *Arch Ophthalmol* 112:1298-1308, 1994.
6. Verity SM et al for the Refractive Keratoplasty Study (TRKS) Group: The combined (Genesis) technique of radial keratotomy: a prospective, multi-center study. *Ophthalmology* 102:1908-1917, 1995.
7. Binder PS The Byron-Mastel guide, *J Refract Corneal Surg* (In press).
8. Bores LD, Myers W, Cowden J: Radial keratotomy: an analysis of the American experience, *Ann Ophthalmol* 13:941-948, 1981.
9. Waring GO III et al: Rationale for and design of the National Eye Institute Prospective Evaluation of Radial Keratotomy (PERK) Study, *Ophthalmology* 90:40-58, 1983.
10. Melles GRJ, Binder PS: Effect of radial keratotomy incision direction on wound depth, *Refract Corneal Surg* 6:394-403, 1990.
11. Assil K et al: A combined incision technique of radial keratotomy: a comparison to centripetal and centrifugal incision techniques in human donor eyes, *Ophthalmology* 101:746-754, 1994.
12. Chayet A, Meyer JC: The combined technique of radial keratotomy, *Semin Ophthalmol* 9:106-109, 1994.
13. Assil K et al: The undercut technique of radial keratotomy: a comparison to the combined technique. The Association for Research in Vision and Ophthalmology, annual meeting on Investigative Ophthalmology and Visual Science, Sarasota, FL, May 1994.
14. Assil KK, Knepshield W: The sentry programmable diamond for radial keratotomy, American Society of Cataract and Refractive Surgery, summer symposium, Los Angeles, Sept. 1993.
15. Assil KK, Quantock AJ: Wound healing in response to keratorefractive surgery, *Surv Ophthalmol* 38:289-302, 1993.

CHAPTER 164

THANASSIS PAPAIOANNOU JAMES J. SALZ EZRA MAGUEN

Predictive Formulas for Refractive Surgery

For over 100 years ophthalmic surgeons have been attempting to modify the cornea to correct refractive errors.[1] Various procedures involving the addition, subtraction, incision, or thermal modification of corneal tissue have been attempted. The success of all these procedures lies in their predictability and long-term stability. Quantification of the role and the interrelationship of all preoperative and operative variables involved in corneal reshaping will ensure this success. These variables include the optical, mechanical, and biologic properties of the cornea and the rest of the eye, the type and quality of the surgical tools used and the skills of the surgeon.

Modeling of such a multivariate process is by no means easy, since it involves variables such as the surgeon's skill or the uncertainty of the biologic response of the eye. As a result, only a few of these procedures have achieved some degree of predictability. In this chapter we will summarize the methods that have been used for refractive surgery in the form of predictive formulas or nomograms. We will focus specifically on three procedures: keratomileusis, radial keratotomy (RK), and photorefractive keratectomy (PRK).

Keratomileusis was pioneered by Barraquer, who provided formulas that are still applicable to many of the modern refractive surgery procedures. Since much of the later modeling work of refractive surgery, especially of the recent technique of PRK, is based on this early work, an outline of the formulas derived for myopic keratomileusis will be presented first. Within the context of Barraquer's initial keratomileusis, a number of related techniques has been devised over the years. Among them is the automated lamellar keratoplasty proposed by Ruiz. A short account of this technique will be given in the discussion of keratomileusis in this chapter.

RK is the most widely used refractive surgery today that has reasonable predictability. Applications of this technique are based on nomograms reflecting accumulated clinical experience. In the third part of this chapter a discussion of the various factors that may affect the outcome of RK, along with the most recent algorithms used in practice, are presented. The fourth and largest section of the chapter is devoted to the presentation and discussion of predictive formulas for PRK.

Keratomileusis

In 1949 José I. Barraquer began his pioneering work on the concept of modifying the corneal curvature to change the refractive power of the eye.[2,3] Keratomileusis, one of Barraquer's suggested techniques for the correction of myopia, or hyperopia, involves the removal of a lamellar corneal disk from the patient's own cornea. The resected lamellar disk is frozen, and appropriate refractive power is lathe-cut from it. The modified corneal disk is then surgically reattached to the cornea. The removal of tissue results in a positive (hyperopic correction) or negative (myopic correction) modification of the corneal power.

The goal of myopic keratomileusis is reduction of the refractive power of the cornea through flattening of the anterior corneal curvature. This is achieved by removing an intracorneal positive meniscus, thus changing the initial anterior corneal radius of curvature (R_1) to a new, longer radius of curvature (R_2). Initially a disk of thickness d is removed from the anterior part of the cornea with a microkeratome. The anterior curvature of this corneal disk is R_1, while the posterior is R_{1-d} (Figure 164-1, *A*). The resected lamella is then placed on the base of a lathe, which has already been carved to the desired final anterior corneal radius of curvature R_2, given by the following equation[2]:

$$R_2 = \frac{n-1}{D + \dfrac{n-1}{R_1}} - \frac{n-1}{n}(C_1 - C_2) \tag{1}$$

where R_1 and R_2 are the initial and final anterior corneal curvatures, (respectively), C_1 and C_2 are the initial and final thicknesses of the cornea (respectively), D is the refractive correction for emmetropia measured at the corneal vertex, and n is the index of refraction of the corneal stroma. The second term of the left-hand side of equation 1 is a corrective term attributed to Littman.[4] As the final corneal thickness is unknown, this term was replaced by the approximate term: 0.004095*D.[2]

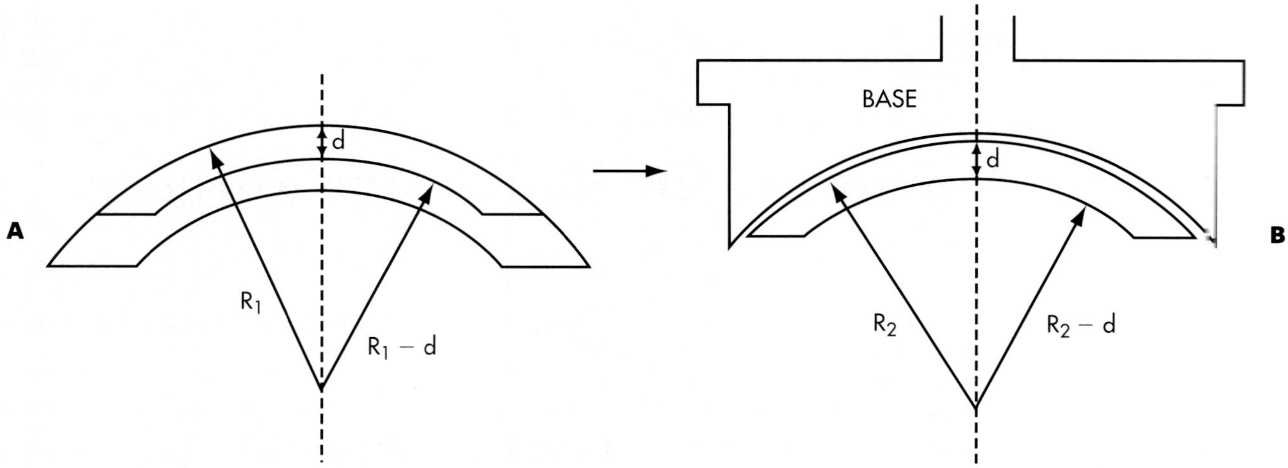

FIGURE 164-1 Keratomileusis. A corneal disk of thickness *d* is resected with a microkeratome. **A,** R_1 is the corneal anterior radius of curvature, whereas $R_1 - d$, is the radius of curvature of the interface. **B,** The corneal disk is placed on the base of a lathe, prepared to the desired final anterior radius of curvature R_2. The posterior side of the corneal disk assumes a radius of curvature $R_2 - d$.

The anterior surface of the corneal disk placed on the base, assumes the final curvature R_2, while its posterior surface assumes a radius of curvature equal to R_{2-d} (Figure 164-1, *B*). The task of the lathe is to reshape the posterior surface of the disk from R_{2-d} to the interface radius of curvature R_{1-d}, so that there is an exact match between the disk and the patient's cornea at reattachment. The effect of the lathing is the subtraction of a positive meniscus from the cornea. This reduces the corneal refractive power, resulting in correction of myopia. The central depth of tissue removal (t_O) required to achieve such a correction can be calculated from the geometry at hand, as illustrated in Figure 164-2. For a treatment zone of diameter *S*, the *h* is the line segment between the vertex of the surface with radius *R* and the chord formed at the zone (Figure 164-2, *A*). Therefore, the maximum depth t_O is the difference of AC and BC corresponding to surfaces with radii of curvature $R_1 - d$ and $R_2 - d$, respectively (Figure 164-2, *B*). Combining these sagittal calculations (Figure 164-2, *B*) with equation 1 leads to the following prediction formula for the maximum depth of cut for myopic correction:

$$t_0 = \left(R_1 - \frac{n-1}{D + \frac{n-1}{R_1}}\right) - \sqrt{(R_1 - d)^2 - \frac{S^2}{4}} + \sqrt{\left(\frac{n-1}{D + \frac{n-1}{R_1}} - d\right)^2 - \frac{S^2}{4}} \qquad (2)$$

where *d* is the thickness of the resected corneal disk and *S* is the treatment zone diameter. The rest of the variables are the same as in equation 1. The small corrective term of equation 1 has been omitted in deriving this equation.

Figure 164-3 shows a plot of the maximum depth t_O given by equation 2 versus the desired correction for two lamellar disk thicknesses of 0.25 mm (thick line) and 0.35 mm (thin line). The depth is shown to be almost directly proportional to the desired correction *D* for both thicknesses. A 6 mm optical zone was assumed because this is the usual clinically applied zone for myopia,[2] along with a nominal R_1 equal to 7.86 mm and an index of refraction equal to 1.377.[5] As shown later in this chapter, the corresponding PRK formula as it is derived by Munnerlyn et al[5] is identical to the previous formula, except for the corneal disk thickness factor *d*.

In deriving these formulas, a number of assumptions have been made:

1. All surfaces involved are spherical. This is not true in general because the cornea is aspherical in order to minimize geometric aberrations. This assumption can be considered satisfactory for the central corneal zone.
2. The surfaces of the resected disk are parallel. However, variations in microkeratome performance and cutting techniques, nonhomogeneous freezing and bending of the corneal disk during lathing, and/or torque reattachment may affect parallelism.

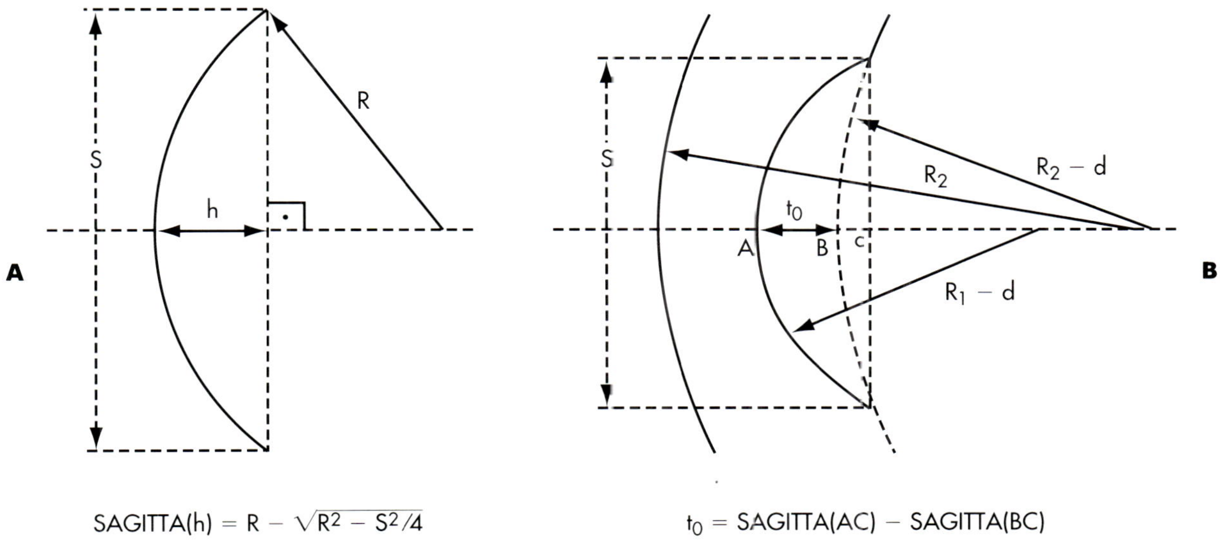

FIGURE 164-2 **A,** Barraquer's "law of thickness" expresses the sagittal depth h as a function of the radius of curvature R and the diameter of the optical zone S. **B,** In myopic keratomileusis the resected corneal disk is modified on its stromal side by removal of tissue, resulting in a myopic lenticule of anterior radius of curvature R_2 and posterior radius of curvature $R_1 - d$. The maximum thickness of the removed tissue t_0 is given by the indicated sagittal differences.

3. The posterior corneal surface remains constant.

It must be emphasized that equation 2, derived from sagittal calculations (Figure 164-2) and equation 1, reflects the ideal case of myopic keratomileusis. However, in practice, further simplifications and/or modifications must be introduced to accommodate reality. For instance, freezing changes both the diameter and the thickness of the resected corneal disk. The new thickness must either be measured during operation or a correction factor must be applied to account for central thickening and diameter reduction.[2] Similarly, since the corneal disk does not adapt well to the base curve at the desired final curvature R_2, a base with suitable curvature is required for the lamella to conform. An 8 mm base radius of curvature has been adopted through experience.[2] This calls for a sagittal transposition that incorporates the new base curvature into the equations. The final outcome of all these calculations is the equations that will set the cutting radius and displacement of the lathe cutting tool to remove the right amount of corneal tissue. A detailed account of the computational modifications, the computer programs, and other practical aspects of this technique are described by Barraquer.[2]

Much of the theoretical basis for this technique has been worked out by Barraquer,[2] while both Littman[4] and Kaplan[6,7] have contributed to theoretical refinements. The equations presented earlier are a satisfactory geometric representation of the problem at hand. However, they include neither the physician's skills nor the biologic factors (age, sex, individual variability) and other technical details (lathing) that could possibly affect the predictability of the procedure. A number of studies have shown that keratomileusis can be useful for the correction of high myopia and hyperopia.[8,9] However, most of the published studies are characterized by small series of data, short follow-up periods, and significant scatter and standard deviations of the refractive outcome.[9] So far the results indicate that the factors involved in the formulas shown earlier are only partially responsible for the predictability of the technique.

More recently, Ruiz[10] proposed an improved, nonfreeze, lamellar refractive technique termed automated lamellar keratoplasty (ALK). This technique involves the use of a mechanical microkeratome to first remove a corneal flap approximately 160 μm thick and 7.2 mm in diameter. A second corneal disk of appropriate dimensions is then removed from the exposed stroma. The unfrozen flap is finally replaced on the modified stromal surface. The removal of the second corneal disk results in corneal flattening, thus producing refractive changes. The desired refractive outcome depends, among other parameters, on the diameter and thickness of the removed disk. No predictive formulas

tory studies. Thus virtually all radial keratotomy nomograms use patient age, number of incisions, and the size of the optical clear zone to determine the appropriate surgical plan for the patient's myopic refractive error. Incision depth is assumed to be a constant for each nomogram, although the actual incision depth varies depending on the incision direction and the type of diamond blade used.

Laboratory confirmation of the importance of the major predictive factors identified in the clinical studies already cited has been reported. The study by Jester et al[20] identified incision depth as the most important factor in achieving maximum corneal flattening in a series of cadaver eyes in which optical zone size and incision number were constants. The size of the optical clear zone (4.0, 5.0, and 6.0 mm) and the number of incisions (four versus eight) were significantly correlated to the amount of corneal flattening obtained in eye bank eyes by Salz et al.[21] In this study a 3.0 mm clear zone four-incision RK achieved 7.75 diopters of corneal flattening compared to 1.23 diopters of effect from four incisions with a 6.0 mm clear zone. Eight incisions with a 3.0 mm clear zone achieved 9.06 diopters of flattening, compared to only 2.3 diopters of effect from eight incisions with a 6.0 mm clear zone. This cadaver eye study confirmed numerous clinical reports that smaller optical clear zones (and therefore longer incisions) and, to a lesser extent more incisions[20] achieved more effect than larger optical clear zones (shorter incisions) and fewer incisions.[13]

Laboratory studies by Steel[22] in primate eyes and Salz[23] in eye bank eyes showed that eight incisions were almost as effective as 16 incisions in flattening corneal curvature. This concept was confirmed in a clinical study by Rowsey,[24] in which the results of eight and 16 RK incisions were compared for several different optical clear zones. The important predictive factors in RK have been summarized by Lynn et al.[18]

Over the past 15 years these clinical and laboratory reports have provided sound scientific evidence for the evolution of contemporary RK. Most current RK systems base the surgical plan for a given amount of myopia on patient age, number of incisions (four, six, or eight), and optical clear zone (2.75 mm to 5.0 mm in 0.25 mm steps). Other modifiers based on keratometry, pachymetry, tonometry, sex, and corneal diameter have also been considered. However, there is no unanimity of opinion about the role of these modifiers, as there is about the importance of patient age, incision depth and number, and optical clear zone size. Sanders thoroughly discusses the role of the various predictive factors and many of the popular RK nomograms.[25]

Two prospective, multisurgeon studies were presented at the American Academy of Ophthalmology meeting in San Francisco in October 1994 using the Genesis blade and the Casebeer system.[[illegible]6,27] The results of these two studies are compared to the PERK study in Table 164-2. Although the important clinical results of these two systems of radial keratotomy are comparable in terms of efficacy and predictability, the Casebeer system using the DuoTrak blade required a significantly greater number of secondary and at times tertiary operations. The Genesis nomograms for four, six, and eight incisions are reproduced in Tables 164-3 to 164-5. The Casebeer system nomogram for the DuoTrak blade is shown in Table 164-6. Details of RK techniques can be reviewed in Chapter 16[illegible] on RK technique.

Table 164-2. Comparison of prospective keratotomy studies

	PERK	Casebeer	Genesis
% 20/40 (after reoperations)	88	93	[illegible]5
% 20/20 (after reoperations)	60	54	[illegible]2
% +/−1 D of emmetropia	41	89	[illegible]5
% > +1 diopter	17	2	1.3
% reoperations	12	39	[illegible]3
% reoperations > 1	0	14	1

PRK

PRK modifies the eye's refractive power by flattening (myopic correction) or steepening (hyperopic correction) the anterior curvature of the cornea. This is achieved by excimer laser ablation of a precise amount of the anterior corneal stroma. The ablated tissue is of power equal to the desired refractive correction. This is equivalent to the addition of a negative (myopic correction) or positive (hyperopic correction) lens of the same power. Corneal ablation by an ArF excimer laser has been demonstrated to be precise and largely predictable, therefore allowing for precise ablation of a lenticule of a prescribed power.[28,29]

The power (D) of the removed lenticule, considered as a thin lens, is determined by the initial (R_1) and final (R_2) anterior corneal curvatures and the index of refraction n of the corneal stroma, as follows

$$D = (n - 1)\left(\frac{1}{R_2} - \frac{1}{R_1}\right) \tag{4}$$

Munnerlyn et al[5] combined equation 4 with simple geometric calculations to the corneal model shown in Figure 164-4, *A* to deterimine how much corneal tissue

Table 164-3. Combined (Genesis) four-incision RK nomogram*

	Age (yr)	21-26	27-32	33-36	37-39	40-42	43-47	48-52	53-60
		Diopters of myopia cycloplegic spherical equivalent							
Optical zone	2.75	−3.45	−3.60	−3.90	−4.05	−4.20	−4.50	−4.80	−5.40
	3.00	−3.20	−3.25	−3.30	−3.60	−3.90	−4.30	−4.50	−5.10
	3.25	−2.70	−2.80	−3.00	−3.15	−3.45	−3.75	−3.85	−4.05
	3.50	−2.20	−2.30	−2.45	−2.90	−3.20	−3.30	−3.45	−3.75
	3.75	−1.95	−2.10	−2.30	−2.40	−2.60	−2.70	−3.00	−3.15
	4.00	−1.70	−1.75	−1.80	−1.90	−2.45	−2.55	−2.70	−2.80
	4.25	−1.45	−1.50	−1.70	−1.80	−2.25	−2.30	−2.40	−2.50
	4.50	−1.30	−1.35	−1.45	−1.50	−1.80	−1.95	−2.10	−2.15
	4.75	−1.20	−1.25	−1.30	−1.35	−1.65	−1.75	−1.95	−2.00
	5.00	−1.00	−1.10	−1.15	−1.20	−1.50	−1.65	−1.80	−1.85

*1. Assumes thinnest zones incised first/thickest last.
2. Assumes range of paracentral (3 mm optical zone) pachymetry <75 μm.
3. Assumes incision terminated 1 mm from limbus (distance from vertical edge to limbus).
4. Assumes slight undercorrection on average (≈0.50 diopter).
Blade should be set at 100% ± 20 μm of thinnest paracentral pachymetry measurement (100% on initial use and modified as needed).

Table 164-4. Combined (Genesis) eight-incision RK nomogram*

	Age (yr)	21-26	27-32	33-36	37-39	40-42	43-47	48-52	53-60
		Diopters of myopia cycloplegic spherical equivalent							
Optical zone	2.75	−5.75	−6.00	−6.50	−6.75	−7.00	−7.50	−8.00	−9.00
	3.00	−5.30	−5.40	−5.50	−6.00	−6.50	−7.20	−7.50	−8.50
	3.25	−4.50	−4.70	−5.00	−5.25	−5.75	−6.25	−6.40	−6.75
	3.50	−3.70	−3.80	−4.10	−4.80	−5.30	−5.50	−5.75	−6.25
	3.75	−3.25	−3.40	−3.80	−4.00	−4.30	−4.50	−5.00	−5.25
	4.00	−2.80	−2.90	−3.00	−3.20	−4.10	−4.25	−4.35	−4.50
	4.25	−2.40	−2.50	−2.80	−3.00	−3.75	−3.80	−3.90	−4.00
	4.50	−2.15	−2.25	−2.40	−2.50	−3.00	−3.25	−3.50	−3.60
	4.75	−2.00	−2.10	−2.15	−2.25	−2.75	−2.95	−3.25	−3.30
	5.00	−1.70	−1.80	−1.90	−2.00	−2.50	−2.75	−3.00	−3.10

*1. Assumes thinnest zones incised first/thickest last.
2. Assumes range of paracentral (3 mm optical zone) pachymetry <75 μm.
3. Assumes incision terminated 1 mm from limbus (distance from vertical edge to limbus).
4. Assumes slight undercorrection on average (≈0.50 diopter).
Blade should be set at 100% ± 20 μm of thinnest paracentral pachymetry measurement (100% on initial use and modified as needed).

must be removed to predictably modify the anterior corneal curvature and achieve the desired correction. It was found that the maximum depth of tissue removal (t_0 at the optical axis (myopic correction) is given by the following formula:

$$t_o = R_1 - \frac{(n-1)R_1}{(n-1)+R_1D} - \sqrt{R_1^2 - \frac{S^2}{4}} + \sqrt{\left(\frac{(n-1)R_1}{(n-1)+R_1D}\right)^2 - \frac{S^2}{4}} \quad (5)$$

The maximum depth of ablation is given here as a function of R_1, R_2, n, and S, the diameter of the treatment zone. This formula describes the maximum central ablation depth for myopic correction as shown in Figure 164-4, *A*. The same formula can be used for hyperopic correction. In this case the t_o is the maximum ablation depth at the periphery of the treatment zone, while no tissue removal occurs on the optical axis (Figure 164-4, *B*).

Note that the corresponding equation 2 for myopic keratomileusis reduces to equation 5 for zero corneal disk thickness ($d = 0$). This is expected because both formulas describe very similar geometries and are derived with essentially the same sagittal calculations.

Table 164-5. Combined (Genesis) six-incision RK nomogram*

		Diopters of myopia cycloplegic spherical equivalent							
	Age (yr)	**21-26**	**27-32**	**33-36**	**37-39**	**40-42**	**43-47**	**48-52**	**53-60**
Optical zone	2.75	−4.90	−5.10	−5.50	−5.75	−5.95	−6.35	−6.80	−[illegible].65
	3.00	−4.50	−4.60	−4.65	−5.10	−5.50	−6.10	−6.35	−[illegible].20
	3.25	−3.80	−4.00	−4.25	−4.45	−4.90	−5.30	−5.45	−[illegible].75
	3.50	−3.15	−3.25	−3.50	−4.10	−4.50	−4.65	−4.90	−[illegible].30
	3.75	−2.75	−2.90	−3.25	−3.40	−3.65	−3.80	−4.25	−[illegible].45
	4.00	−2.40	−2.45	−2.55	−2.70	−3.50	−3.60	−3.70	−[illegible].80
	4.25	−2.05	−2.10	−2.40	−2.55	−3.20	−3.25	−3.30	−[illegible].40
	4.50	−1.80	−1.90	−2.05	−2.10	−2.55	−2.75	−2.95	−[illegible].05
	4.75	−1.70	−1.75	−1.80	−1.90	−2.35	−2.50	−2.75	−[illegible].80
	5.00	−1.45	−1.55	−1.60	−1.70	−2.10	−2.35	−2.55	−[illegible].65

*1. Assumes thinnest zones incised first/thickest last.
2. Assumes range of paracentral (3 mm optical zone) pachymetry <75 μm.
3. Assumes incision terminated 1 mm from limbus (distance from vertical edge to limbus).
4. Assumes slight undercorrection on average (≈0.50 diopter).
Blade should be set at 100% ± 20 μm of thinnest paracentral pachymetry measurement (100% on initial use and modified as needed).

Table 164-6. Casebeer study–based comprehensive RK nomogram*

		Age (yr)									
No. of incisions	**Optical zone**	**18-20**	**21-25**	**26-30**	**31-35**	**36-37**	**38-40**	**41-45**	**46-50**	**51-60**	**61-UP**
8	3.25	−4.25	−4.50	−4.75	−5.00	−5.25	−5.75	−6.25	−6.50	−6.75	x
	3.50	−3.50	−3.75	−4.00	−4.25	−4.50	−5.00	−5.50	−5.75	−6.25	−6.[illegible]5
	3.75	−3.00	−3.25	−3.50	−3.75	−4.00	−4.25	−4.50	−5.00	−5.25	−6.[illegible]0
	4.00	−2.50	−2.75	−3.00	−3.25	−3.50	−4.00	−4.25	−4.50	−4.75	−5.[illegible]5
	4.25	−2.25	−2.50	−2.50	−2.75	−3.00	−3.50	−3.75	−4.00	−4.25	−4.[illegible]0
	4.50	−2.00	−2.25	−2.25	−2.50	−2.50	−3.00	−3.25	−3.50	−3.75	−4.[illegible]0
6	4.25	−1.75	−2.00	−2.00	−2.25	−2.25	−2.50	−2.75	−3.00	−3.25	−3.[illegible]0
	4.50	−1.50	−1.75	−1.75	−2.00	−2.25	−2.50	−2.75	−3.00	−3.00	−3.[illegible]5
4	4.00	x	x	x	x	x	x	x	−2.75	−2.75	−3.[illegible]0
	4.25	x	−1.50	−1.50	−1.50	−1.75	−2.25	−2.25	−2.50	−2.50	−2.[illegible]5
	4.50	−1.25	−1.25	−1.25	−1.25	−1.50	−1.75	−1.75	−2.00	−2.25	−2.[illegible]0
3	4.50	−0.87	−1.00	−1.12	−1.25	−1.37	−1.50	−1.62	−2.00	−2.12	−2.[illegible]5
	4.75	−0.75	−0.87	−1.00	−1.12	−1.25	−1.37	−1.50	−1.62	−1.87	−2.[illegible]0
2	4.75	−0.62	−0.75	−0.87	−1.00	−1.12	−1.25	−1.37	−1.37	−1.50	−1.[illegible]5
	5.00	−0.50	−0.50	−0.50	−0.62	−0.75	−0.87	−1.12	−1.12	−1.25	−1.[illegible]7

*Greater degrees of myopia are preferably treated with automated lamellar keratoplasty.

Binomial expansion of the third and fourth terms of equation 5 leads to the following simplified equation for t_0:

$$t_0 \cong -\frac{S^2 D}{3} \quad (6)$$

or, equivalently:

$$\frac{\text{Diopters of Myopia}}{3} \times (\text{Optical zone})^2 = \text{Ablation depth } (\mu\text{m})$$

Alternatively, this equation indicates the following:

1. The refractive outcome is roughly proportional to the depth of ablation.
2. The refractive outcome is roughly inversely proportional to the square of the treatment zone.

In Figure 164-5 the maximum central ablation depth is plotted against the desired correction for different treatment zones between 3 and 6 mm, as predicted by Munnerlyn's model. Both the exact (solid line) and the approximate (circles) formulas are shown. A nominal value of the anterior corneal curvature of 7.86 mm was used for the exact formula. As expected from the nature of the approximation, the predictions of the approximate formula are close to the ones of the exact formula for small treatment zones and low or moderate myopic corrections. This formula underestimates the ablation

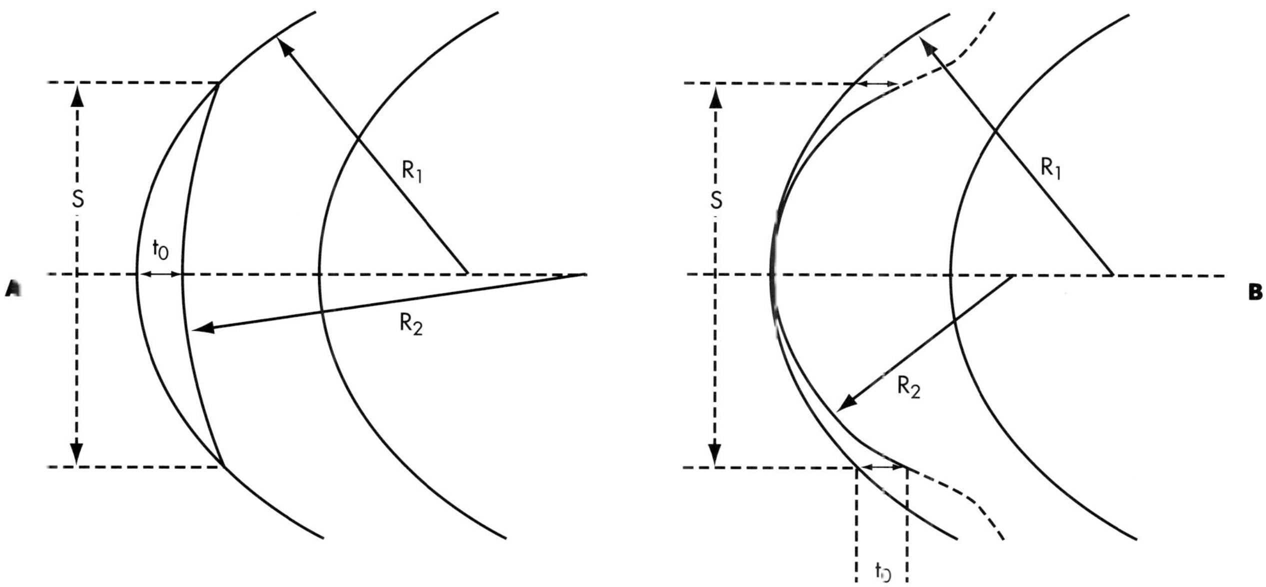

FIGURE 164-4 **A,** In myopic photorefractive keratectomy, tissue from the central part of the cornea is removed with an excimer laser, resulting in anterior corneal flattening. R_1 and R_2 are the initial and final corneal anterior radii of curvature, S is the optical zone diameter, and t_0 is the maximum depth of ablated tissue. **B,** Hyperopia is corrected by tissue ablation, resulting in anterior corneal steepening.

depth at zones of clinical importance (5 to 6 mm). The deviation of prediction becomes appreciable for corrections higher than ~ -4 diopters. However, the predictions of equation 6 follow the overall trends shown by the exact formula and thus can serve for "rule of thumb" calculations. As indicated by equation 6 the approximate central ablation depth per diopter is ~ 3, ~ 5.3, ~ 8.3, and ~ 12 μm/diopter for optical zones of 3, 4, 5, and 6 mm, respectively.

Equation 5 suggests that the required depth of ablation depends also on the initial anterior corneal curvature (R_1). However, this effect is generally small, as shown in Figure 164-6. In this figure the maximum ablation depth was calculated from the exact formula, with R_1 = 7.55 mm (solid line) and R_1 = 9.43 mm (circles). These radii represent two extreme values of the anterior corneal curvature, corresponding to ~ 50 and ~ 40 diopters of power, respectively. The true index of the corneal stroma was used for calculating these power values.[30] There is less than 5% change in the predicted maximum depth for corrections less than −6 diopters at the 6 mm treatment zone. It is therefore anticipated that the initial anterior curvature plays a small role in the predictability of the outcome. The lack of significance of the initial corneal curvature has also been discussed by Blaker,[31] and Colliac.[32]

Recently Blaker[31] derived a predictive formula for myopic correction based on geometric arguments that consider the change of sagittal depth of the central treatment zone for small ablation depths. By rearrangement of the equations derived by Blaker (equations 2 to 6 of reference 31), one can arrive at the following formula:

$$t_0 = \frac{\left(2R_1^2 - 2R_1\sqrt{R_1^2 - \frac{S^2}{4}}\right)^2}{2(n-1)\left(\frac{S^2}{2} - 2R_1^2 + 2R_1\sqrt{R_1^2 - \frac{S^2}{4}}\right)} D \qquad (7)$$

As in equation 5, this formula predicts the maximum ablation depth for a desired correction D. The depth depends on the initial anterior corneal curvature R_1, the treatment zone S, and the index of refraction of the stroma. A graphic comparison of the predictions of this formula to those of Munnerlyn's formula is shown in Figure 164-7. Here equation 5 (solid line) and equation 7 (--) are shown in a different perspective, revealing the quadratic dependence of t_0 on S. In this figure the maximum central depth has been plotted against the treatment zone for a range of corrections between −2 and −12 diopters. The true index of refraction of stroma has been used (n = 1.377), along with a

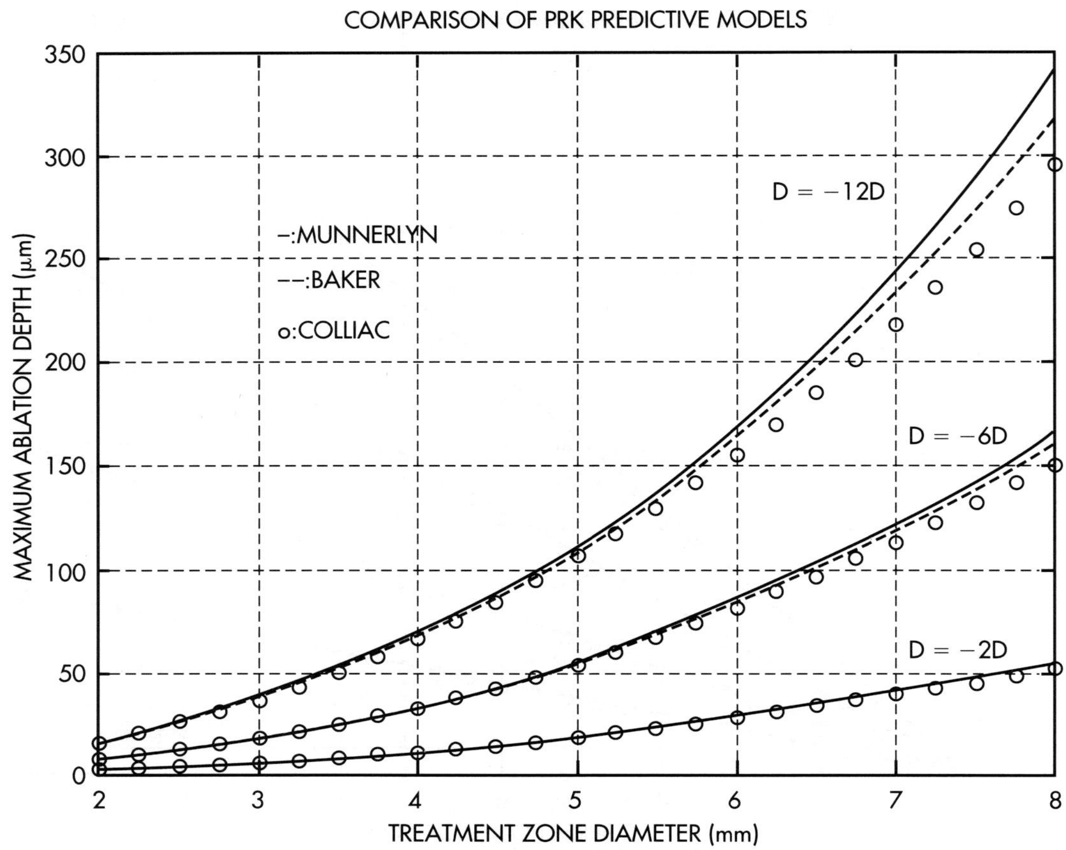

FIGURE 164-7 Comparison between the predictions of the Munnerlyn (equation 5), Blaker (equation 7), and Colliac formulas (equations 8 to 10). The maximum depth of ablation is compared to the treatment zone diameter at different values of the desired refractive correction. There is no significant difference between the three models, for low to moderate myopias, at optical zones of clinical significance.

(Figure 164-6) and also verified from clinical data by Blaker.[31] Blaker analyzed the clinical data from 599 patients with 12 months' follow-up. The patients were stratified according to their preoperative mean keratometry results. No statistically significant correlation was found between the initial keratometric readings and the outcome of PRK.

Maguen et al[39] evaluated the short-term effect of nitrogen flow from the suction ring applied to the eye during surgery. Significant improvement of the final outcome was found for the procedures that were performed without nitrogen flow compared to the procedures performed with nitrogen flow. Since the predictive formulas do not incorporate the nitrogen flow as a variable, modification of the algorithm may be necessary to correct for its effect on the outcome.

The corneal epithelium may also be a variable affecting the final outcome. A study conducted by Simon et al[40] suggests that the corneal epithelium accounts for as much as 1 diopter of the power of the eye at the central 2 mm diameter zone. There are indications of hyperplastic and/or irregular regenerated epithelium after PRK as well as other refractive surgeries. It is therefore conceivable that the optics of the regenerated epithelium—not presently accounted in the predictive formulas—could affect the final refractive correction.

One of the most appealing advantages of PRK compared to RK and to a certain degree to keratomileusis is that the desired change in corneal curvature is based on sound principles of geometric optics and the precise interaction of the excimer laser with the cornea tissue. These formulas predict that any given refractive error can be corrected by precisely removing the calculated microns of tissue from the desired optical zone of the cornea. The challenge to obtain even better results will be to further improve the algorithms and possibly to eventually modify the cornea's wound healing response.

REFERENCES

1. Villasenor RA: Introduction to and historical overview of surgical procedures for the correction of refractive errors. In Binder PS, editor: *Refractive corneal surgery: the correction of aphakia, hyperopia, and myopia, Int Ophthalmol Clin* 23(3):1-9, 1983.
2. Barraquer JI: *Queratomileusis y Queratofaquia,* Bogotá, Columbia, 1980, Instituto Barraquer de America.
3. Barraquer JI: Basics of refractive keratoplasty, *Refract Corneal Surg* 5:179-193, 1989.
4. Littman H: Optics of Barraquer's keratomileusis, *Arch Soc Oftal Optom* 6:103-110, 1967.
5. Munnerlyn CR, Koons SJ, Marshall J: Photorefractive keratectomy: a technique for laser refractive surgery, *J Cataract Refractive Surg* 14:46-52, 1988.
6. Kaplan MM et al: Refractive keratoplasty—corneal bending, *Am J Optom Arch Am Acad Optom* 45:806-820, 1968.
7. Kaplan MM: Refractive keratoplasty—vergence calculations, *Am J Optom Arch Am Acad Optom* 43:795-811, 1967.
8. Swinger CS, Barker BA: Prospective evaluation of myopic keratomileusis, *Ophthalmology* 91:785-792, 1984.
9. American Academy of Ophthalmology, Keratophakia and Keratomileusis: safety and effectiveness, *Ophthalmology* 99(8): 1332-1341, 1992.
10. Ruiz L, Rowsey J: *In situ* keratomileusis, *Invest Ophthalmol Vis Sci* 29(Suppl):392, 1988.
11. Arenas-Archila E et al: Keratomileusis *in situ:* a preliminary report, *J Cataract Refract Surg* 7:424-435, 1991.
12. Bosakis G, editor: *Refractive lamellar keratoplasty,* Thorofare, NJ, 1994, Slack, Inc.
13. Waring GO: Development of refractive keratotomy in the Soviet Union, 1960-1990. In Waring GO, editor: *Refractive keratotomy for myopia and astigmatism,* St Louis, 1992, Mosby.
14. Fyodorov S: Surgical correction of myopia and astigmatism. In Schachar RA, Levy NS, Schachar L, editors: *Keratorefraction, proceedings of the Keratorefractive Society meeting* Denison, TX, 1980, LAL Publishing.
15. Sanders DR, Deitz MR, Gallagher D: Factors affecting predictability of radial keratotomy, *Ophthalmology* 92:1237-1243, 1985.
16. Arrowsmith PN, Marks RG: Four year update on predictability of radial keratotomy, *J Refract Surg* 4:37-45, 1988.
17. Lynn MJ et al: Factors affecting outcome and predictability of radial keratotomy in the PERK study, *Arch Ophthalmol* 105:42-51, 1987.
18. Lynn MJ, Waring GO, Kutner MH: Predictability of refractive keratotomy. In Waring GO, editor: *Refractive keratotomy for myopia and astigmatism,* St Louis, 1992, Mosby.
19. Waring GO et al: Results of the prospective evaluation of radial keratotomy (PERK) study one year after surgery, *Ophthalmology* 92:177-198, 1985.
20. Jester JV et al: A statistical analysis of radial keratotomy in human cadaver eyes, *Am J Ophthalmol* 92:172-177, 1981.
21. Salz JJ et al: A study of optical zone size and incision redeepening in experimental radial keratotomy, *Arch Ophthalmol* 103:590-594, 1985.
22. Steel D et al: Modification of corneal curvature following radial keratotomy in primates, *Ophthalmology* 88:747-754, 1981.
23. Salz JJ et al: Radial keratotomy in fresh human cadaver eyes, *Ophthalmology* 88:742-746, 1981.
24. Rowsey JJ et al: Predicting the results of radial keratotomy, *Ophthalmology* 90:642-654, 1983.
25. Sanders, DR: Computerized predictability formulas for refractive keratotomy. In Waring GO, editor: *Refractive keratotomy for myopia and astigmatism,* St Louis, 1992, Mosby.
26. Verity S et al: The combined (genesis) technique of radial keratotomy: a prospective multi-centered clinical trial (abstract), *Ophthalmology* 101:1908, 1995.
27. Waring GO, Allen R, Berg JC: A prospective multicenter study of refractive keratotomy for myopia and astigmatism (abstract), *Ophthalmology* 101:1-25, 1994.
28. Kruger RR, Binder PS, McDonnell PJ: The effects of excimer laser photoablation on the cornea. In Salz JJ. McDonald MB, McDonnell PJ, editors: *Cornea laser surgery,* St Louis, 1994, Mosby.
29. Trokel SJ: History and Mechanism of action of excimer laser corneal surgery. In Salz JJ, McDonald MB, McDonnell PJ editors: *Cornea laser surgery,* St Louis, 1994, Mosby.
30. Mandell RB: Corneal correction factor for photorefractive keratectomy, *J Refract Corneal Surg* 10:125-128, 1994.
31. Blaker WJ, Hersh PS: Theoretical and clinical effects of preoperative corneal curvature on excimer laser photorefractive keratectomy for myopia, *J Refract Surg* 10:571-574, 1994.
32. Colliac JP, Shammas JH, Bart DJ: Photorefractive keratectomy for the correction of myopia and astigmatism, *Am J Ophthalmol* 117:369-380, 1994.
33. Colliac JP, Shammas JH: Optics for photorefractive keratectomy, *J Cataract Refract Surg* 19:356-363, 1993.
34. Colliac JP, Shammas JH, Bart DJ: Photorefractive keratectomy for the correction of myopia and astigmatism—Reply, *Am J Ophthalmol* 118:541, 1994.
35. Schipper I: Photorefractive keratectomy for the correction of myopia and astigmatism, *Am J Ophthalmol* 118(4):540-541, 1994.
36. Dougherty PJ, Wellish KL, Maloney RK: Excimer laser ablation and corneal hydration, *Am J Ophthalmol* 118:169-176, 1994.
37. Poirier L et al: Energy fluctuations in an excimer laser during photorefractive keratectomy, *J Refract Corneal Surg* 10 (2 Suppl) S258-261, 1994.
38. Dutt S et al: One-year results of excimer laser photorefractive keratectomy for low to moderate myopia, *Arch Ophthalmol* 112:1427-1436, 1994.
39. Maguen E et al: 193 nm excimer laser photorefractive keratectomy, short term visual rehabilitation with and without nitrogen flow, *Refract Corneal Surg* 10:321-326, 1994.
40. Simon G et al: Optics of the corneal epithelium, *Refract Corneal Surg* 9:42-50, 1993.

CHAPTER 165

STEPHEN D. KLYCE

Role of Corneal Topography in Keratorefractive Surgery

The ability to correct surgically all degrees of ametropia safely and efficaciously has been the aspiration of corneal refractive surgeons for decades. Enormous strides have been made with both incisional procedures, such as the modern rendition of radial keratotomy, and excisional procedures, such as excimer laser photorefractive keratectomy. The success of these procedures is based on the efforts of many talented clinical researchers in the traditional university research setting, in private practice, and in industry. One of the most powerful adjuncts to this success has been the revelations that computer-assisted corneal topography analysis (or videokeratography) have provided over the past decade.

Conventional outcome analysis schemes used for keratorefractive surgery have used the preoperative and final refractive status of the eye to evaluate predictability. While it is necessary to measure the change in manifest refraction, changes in axial length or accommodation over time can confound interpretation. Achieving 20/20 Snellen visual acuity does not, by itself, provide a complete assessment of visual function. The change in refraction provides no information on irregular astigmatism, the size of the treated area, or the position of the treated area relative to the center of the entrance pupil. These are all factors that may influence contrast sensitivity and produce glare or ghost images without altering the refractive status of the eye. Keratorefractive surgery achieves its effect by modifying corneal curvature. Examining the topography of the entire corneal surface permits the best evaluation of the success of the surgery. Routine keratometry is unable to measure central corneal curvature after refractive surgery, since the keratometer mires do not always fall within the treated area. Measuring curvature change with traditional keratometry is not an adequate topographic assessment for keratorefractive surgical outcome.

This chapter will explore the role of videokeratography in the development, screening, and postoperative evaluation of keratorefractive surgical patients.

This work was supported in part by US Public Health Service grants EY03311 and EY02377 from the National Eye Institute, National Institutes of Health, Bethesda, MD, and by research grants and equipment donations from Computed Anatomy, Inc., New York, NY. Dr. Klyce has been a paid consultant to Computed Anatomy, Inc., manufacturers of the TOMEY TMS-1 videokeratoscope.

The Videokeratoscope

In the past, when a refractive surgical patient had unsatisfactory spectacle-corrected vision that was improved with contact lens overrefraction, "irregular astigmatism" was often the diagnosed culprit. Considering that irregular astigmatism might be defined as any optical aberration not correctable with spherocylindrical optics, this diagnosis, with no additional detail, provided little or no guidance to the refractive surgeon. The relationship between corneal topography and visual performance is strong, with roughly 75% of the eye's vergence occurring at this interface; even subtle alterations of the surface can seriously degrade the potential visual acuity of the eye.

ORIGINS

Placido disk photokeratoscopy was the predecessor of modern corneal topography analysis. Although this procedure required manual digitization of keratoscope photographs,[1,2] an expensive and labor-intensive process, it nevertheless demonstrated that this approach was both feasible and useful. Widespread use would not have been possible, however, without the automation inherent in the videokeratoscope first developed by Computed Anatomy, Inc.,[3,4] coupled with the color-coded contour map of corneal surface powers developed at Louisiana State University (LSU) School of Medicine.[5] The earliest commercial device, the Computed Anatomy CMS, was soon succeeded by the TMS-1, as well as a number of other videokeratoscope models from various manufacturers.[6,7]

Videokeratoscopy remains the most efficient technology for measuring corneal topography, although additional technologies have been explored, such as rasterstereography,[8,9] laser holography,[10] acoustic pachymetry,[11] and scanning slit lamp devices. The accuracy and precision of videokeratoscopes are generally good,[12-16] although there are limitations in the current generation of instruments, particularly in the measurement of the peripheral cornea and the inability, in many cases, to accurately track rapid changes in curvature.[17,18] Nevertheless, the clinical usefulness and validity of videokeratography have been established in hundreds of publications.

USE

The color-coded contour map of corneal surface power has been adopted as a standard presentation scheme in videokeratography.[5] Wire-mesh three-dimensional models have been tried,[2,19] but these have not been widely accepted in the clinic. The color-coded map embodies two concepts for diagnostic use: (1) color association, in which cool colors represent lower than normal powers, greens and yellows represent powers associated with normal corneas, and warm colors represent higher than normal powers; and (2) pattern recognition, in which, for example, bow ties indicate regular astigmatism, central flat areas indicate myopic refractive surgery, and localized areas of corneal steepening can imply keratoconus.

A number of different color scales have been used since the original introduction of the *international standard* or *absolute scale.*[5] This scale spanned a range of corneal powers from 9 to over 100 diopters, with 1.5-diopter intervals in the center of the range and 5-diopter intervals at each end. Wilson et al introduced a more practical scale (the Klyce/Wilson scale),[20] which ranges from 28.0 to 65.5 diopters in equal 1.5-diopter intervals. They pointed out the need for standardization because of the dramatic increase in clinical and scientific usage and the fact that presentation of data in varying or nonstandard formats inhibits easy interpretation and precludes comparison.

It has been argued that the 1.5-diopter interval between contours is so wide that irregularities in corneal topography may be masked. Generally this is not the case, in part because the cornea is normally aspheric (i.e., steeper in the center than in the periphery), and this characteristic will expose features such as 0.75 diopter of regular astigmatism. The diagnostic adequacy of the Klyce/Wilson scale was evaluated retrospectively with a 252-examination sample that included normal corneas, contact lens–wearing corneas, early to moderate and advanced keratoconus, penetrating keratoplasties, extracapsular cataract surgery, excimer laser photorefractive keratectomy, radial keratotomy, aphakic epikeratophakia, and myopic epikeratophakia. It was found that there were no topographic characteristics that were not appreciated with the 1.5-diopter scale that could be detected with a 1.0-diopter scale.[20] Additionally, the 1.5-diopter scale proved broad enough to cover the full range of powers in the 252-cornea sample. The routine use of a fixed, standard scale showing only adequate detail and not redundant information or extraneous noise is essential for efficient and accurate clinical interpretation. A finer, higher resolution contour interval can be selected; doing so will often reveal topographic features that are not of consequence to visual acuity, but their depiction may be used, for example, to inspect the details of a refractive procedure.

The color-coded map is a qualitative diagnostic aid in the sense that it masks information unnecessary for interpretation. The size of the bowtie representing regular astigmatism in a color map cannot be used to measure the amount of corneal cylinder, although counting contours, if there are several, can give an estimate of the magnitude. Therefore, to provide the quantitative data underlying the color map, various indices have been created, from simple values that simulate standard clinical keratometry (SimK values) to more sophisticated numbers (surface regularity index [SRI]), which correlate topography with the potential visual acuity of the eye.[21-23] In this way, objective characteristics of surgical procedures can be obtained; this objectivity is necessary to use videokeratography scientifically in clinical research, as well as diagnostically in the refractive surgical arena for preoperative screening and postoperative evaluation.

ABUSE

As with many clinical tests, videokeratography has limitations and can provide misinformation if intentionally or unintentionally abused. For example, if the inner mires of the Placido disk generator are intentionally masked[24] or if the operator fails to achieve adequate focus and/or alignment,[25] artifactual information will be generated. Tear film breakup can be a source of artifact if a prolonged fixed gaze is requested by the operator; the effect is usually poor tracking with missing data and a map with the appearance of irregular astigmatism. In routine clinical workup, keratometry or videokeratography is best done as the first procedure, before instillation of topical medications, intraocular pressure measurement, refraction, or external examination, to preserve the normal corneal tear film.

As emphasized earlier, the use of a standardized scale is important for consistent evaluation of corneal topography. For example, scales that adapt themselves to the range of powers on the corneal surface can lead to confusion (Figure 165-1, *A* to *D*). In fact, adaptable scales can easily lead to the misdiagnosis

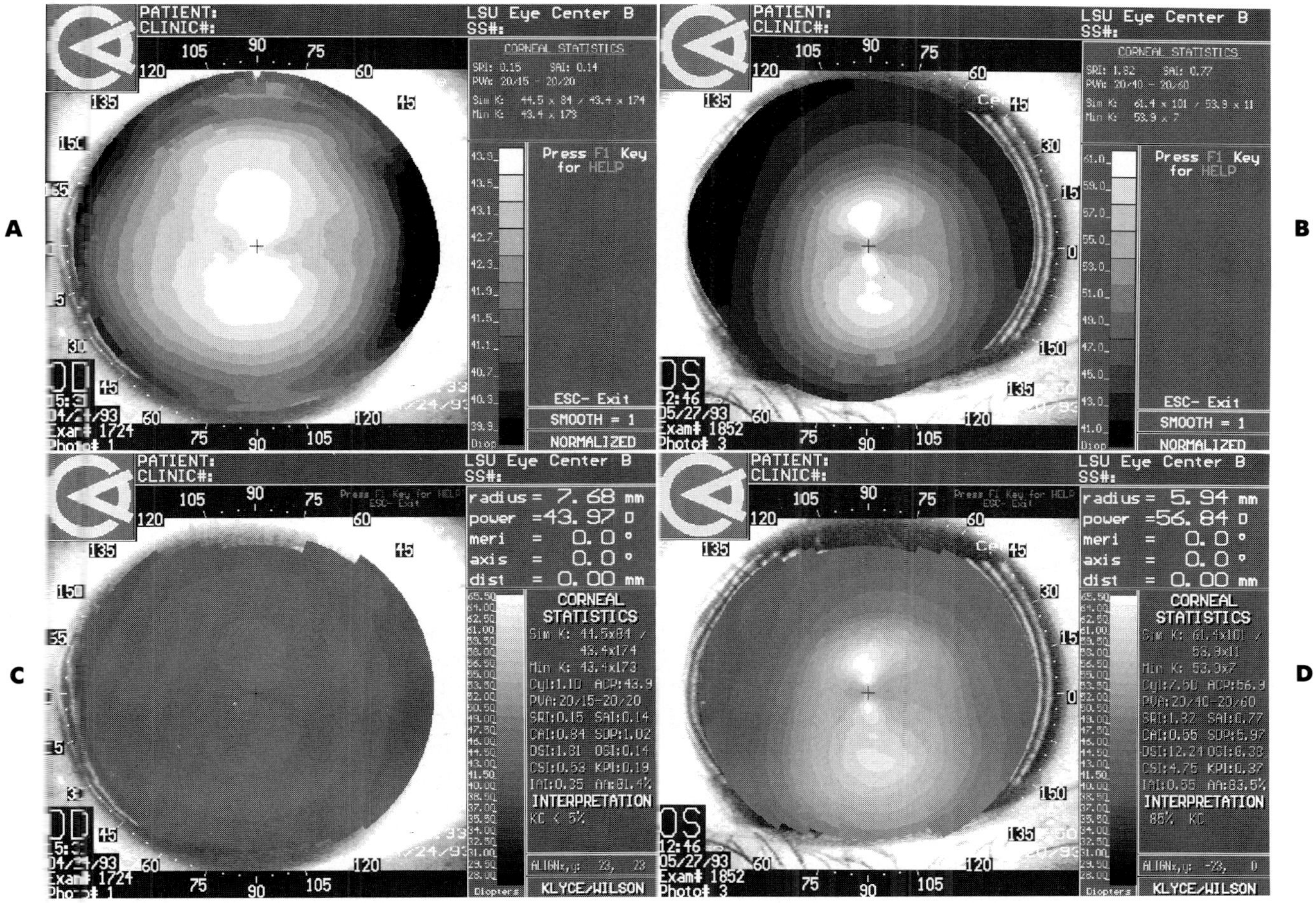

FIGURE 165-1 Use of scales with the color-coded contour map of corneal surface powers. **A and B,** Two corneas are shown with an adaptive color scale known as the normalized scale on the TMS-1. With this scale these two corneal topographies appear to be similar in many ways in that both maps show red bowtie-shaped patterns characteristic of cylinder; however, note that the contour interval in **A** is 0.4 diopter, while in **B** it is 2 diopters. There is a good deal more variation in power in **B** than **A. C** and **D,** The same two corneas shown in **A** and **B** are presented here using a standard 1.5-diopter interval scale, starting at 28.0 diopters and ending at 65.5 diopters (the Klyce/Wilson scale[20]). On this scale, it is clear that the cornea on the left (**A** and **C**) is a cornea with a mild amount of with-the-rule corneal astigmatism, whereas the cornea on the right (**B** and **D**) has moderately advanced keratoconus. **See color plate 165-1.**

of keratoconus in a cornea that simply has a modest amount of asymmetry. If a cornea has sufficient topographic radial asymmetry to indicate the possibility of keratoconus, then using a fixed, standard scale will permit the serial evaluation of individual corneal topography to determine whether the area of concern progressively steepens.

The keratometer and the videokeratoscope are often used to evaluate the change in curvature of the central cornea after refractive surgery. Aside from the well-known limitations of the keratometer (inability to measure curvature within a 3 to 4 mm diameter), both the keratometer and the videokeratoscope report corneal power by dividing the corneal front surface curvature in millimeters by the keratometric index minus the refractive index of air (1.3375 − 1.0). The keratometric index has been arranged empirically to yield total corneal power, which includes the negative refractive power of the corneal back surface. This is a convention that seemed appropriate before the development of refractive surgery, but when only the front surface curvature of the cornea is altered, the change in refractive power of the cornea, with its actual refractive index of 1.376, will in general be 11.4% (1.376/1.3375·100) greater than is calculated from the keratometric index.[26-29] Parenthetically, it is noted that one must also consider vertex distance (*VD*) if manifest refractions or power at the spectacle plane (D_s) is compared to power at the corneal plane (D_c). The conversion is as follows:

$$D_c = \frac{1}{\frac{1}{D_s} - \frac{VD}{1000}}$$

Preoperative Screening of Refractive Surgical Patients with Topographic Analysis

Every candidate for keratorefractive surgery should undergo preoperative screening with videokeratography as a routine element of the qualifying clinical tests. The detection and management of corneal shape anomalies during the screening process will improve the safety and efficacy of refractive surgery. The justification for these assertions is provided later.

BACKGROUND AND RATIONALE

The corneal topographic screening of all refractive surgical patients has been performed routinely at research institutions for over a decade, initially as a means of evaluation and improvement of the surgical techniques. Among the postoperative findings (reviewed more thoroughly later), correlations were seen between the topographic multifocality of a myopic keratomileusis procedure and the patient's refraction over a wide range of powers.[30] Also, treatment zone decentration and central islands of elevated power were demonstrated with videokeratography of excimer laser myopic photorefractive keratectomy.[31-35]

However, as experience grew with refractive surgical populations, an interesting trend began to appear. This was first noted during a training visit at a new excimer laser site overseas: 8 of the 22 corneas considered candidates for photorefractive keratectomy at that site had the topographic characteristics associated with early clinical keratoconus (with the attendant subtle clinical signs) (Klyce & McDonald, unpublished observation, 1991). Subsequently, reports in the literature[36,37] have confirmed the observation that a high percentage of candidates desiring keratorefractive surgery have clinical keratoconus. The incidence of keratoconus in the general population is quite low (1 in 2000, or 0.05%, has been reported[38]), while for keratorefractive surgical candidates the incidence is more than 100 times higher—as much as 6% to 12%. This positive correlation is not by chance; it seems reasonable to hypothesize that patients with shape anomalies like keratoconus, even those classified as "keratoconus suspect" (see Waring[39]), select themselves into alternative forms of refractive correction. With even the subtle shape changes associated with preclinical keratoconus, the vision achieved with spectacle wear may not be satisfactory. These patients may not be able to tolerate contact lenses because an adequate fit to a radially asymmetric cornea is not easily achieved.

The discussion of keratorefractive surgical screening is focused on keratoconus primarily because keratoconus is the most prevalent shape anomaly detected only with videokeratography in this patient group. Pellucid marginal degeneration and cases of Terrien's marginal degeneration are also encountered in refractive surgical screening, but these often present at a more advanced clinical stage than keratoconus. One might hypothesize that patients with keratoconus seek alternatives to refractive correction sooner than those with other ectasias because keratoconus tends to produce earlier spectacle blur owing to the usually decentered cone. Pellucid marginal degeneration and Terrien's marginal degeneration tend to produce regular astigmatism, which is more easily corrected with conventional appliances.

The etiology is still being debated, but keratoconus can be classified as a noninflammatory thinning disorder that can lead to anterior protrusion of the cornea and the development of visual impairment through irregular astigmatism and sometimes stromal scarring.[40] In retrospective studies of contact lens–wearing patients performed before the availability of refractive surgery the incidence of keratoconus was reported to be as high as 25%, and long-term contact lens wear itself was proposed as a factor that could lead to keratoconus.[41,42] While the mechanical effects of contact lens wear can produce contact lens–induced warpage, in some cases producing a keratoconus suspect–type topography,[43] finding a high incidence of clinical keratoconus among contact lens wearers demonstrates an association but does not prove causation.

Even if the patient self-selection hypothesis is incorrect, the fact remains that the incidence of clinical keratoconus among refractive surgical candidates is high. Assuming for the moment that clinical keratoconus can be correctly diagnosed, is the presence of a corneal ectasia by itself an adequate reason to exclude an eye from a refractive surgical procedure? Reports have been published of radial keratotomy being performed on eyes with "atypical inferior steepening" with "good results."[44] It has been pointed out in the past that while good initial results can be obtained with radial keratotomy on eyes with clinical keratoconus, the effect of the procedure can regress and scarring of the cone apex can occur.[45] Excimer laser astigmatic photorefractive keratectomy has been performed to "treat" keratoconus as an alternative to corneal transplantation,[46] but one cannot draw the conclusion from this study that it is safe and effective to use the excimer laser to treat myopia in a patient with keratoconus. The current generation of excimer lasers is able to correct spherocylindrical optics. However, the astigmatism that accompanies keratoconus is not usually regular, making the excimer lasers now in use generally incapable of producing good results on irregular surfaces.

NOMENCLATURE

Exclusion criteria are not easily established and require careful consideration. One might begin with a clear definition of the descriptive terms being used to designate keratoconus. Waring sought opinions for nomenclature to designate the earliest signs of keratoconus that are detectable with videokeratography before the detection of any other clinical signs. The consensus was to term such cases "keratoconus suspect," which is analogous to the rationale used for designating "glaucoma suspect."[39] "Clinical keratoconus" then can be used to indicate corneas with one or more of the classic clinical signs obtained with retinoscopy or slit lamp biomicroscopy. Videokeratography by itself may not be sufficient to make the diagnosis of clinical keratoconus because of the possible confounding influences of contact lens–induced warpage, misalignment artifact, or inadvertent external pressure on the globe, all of which can lead to a "pseudokeratoconus," that is, a topographic pattern and sometimes retinoscopic findings similar to those seen in clinical keratoconus. "Preclinical" and "subclinical" keratoconus are terms that should be reserved for hindsight observations where clinical keratoconus has been diagnosed subsequently.[39]

CONSIDERATIONS FOR EXCLUDING KERATOCONUS PATIENTS FROM REFRACTIVE SURGERY

The grounds for excluding patients with clinical keratoconus and for proceeding with caution with keratoconus suspect cases in keratorefractive surgery are straightforward. In addition to normal neural function and clear ocular media, good vision requires that the topography of the cornea be radially symmetrical and free of irregular astigmatism, particularly those areas of the cornea over the entrance pupil. Keratorefractive surgery achieves its success through the uniform flattening of the central cornea—increasing its radius of curvature for myopic corrections and decreasing its radius of curvature for hyperopic corrections. When a surgical procedure produces irregular astigmatism (lamellar and full–thickness keratoplasties are good examples), the best possible spectacle-corrected visual acuity can be suboptimal. To achieve a good visual result, radial keratotomy relies on the existence of a stable stromal thickness that is radially uniform. Performing radial keratotomy on an eye with keratoconus risks perforation in areas of stromal thinning and can induce or accelerate the onset of irregular corneal astigmatism. Performing excimer laser photorefractive keratectomy on an eye with keratoconus involves little risk of perforation, but the cornea will gain marked irregular astigmatism should the keratoconus progress. The same progression of keratoconus and onset of irregular astigmatism could have occurred without the surgery. However, the patient will generally expect the refractive result of the surgery to be stable; without this assurance there may be little justification for the procedure.

Moderate to advanced keratoconus should contraindicate keratorefractive surgery, but how should one approach cases of mild clinical keratoconus or keratoconus suspect? In an older patient with a (presumed) low chance for progression of the pathology and an eye with relatively spherical topography, refractive surgery may achieve satisfactory results. However, this conclusion needs the support of a controlled clinical trial.

An interesting hypothesis has been put forward[47] suggesting that the progressive hyperopia noted in 24% of the Prospective Evaluation of Radial Keratotomy (PERK) patients[48] might be caused by the fact that PERK patients were not screened preoperatively with videokeratography. Although the percentage of PERK patients with progressive changes is much higher than published figures for the incidence of clinical keratoconus in refractive surgical candidates, it is identical to the percentage of patients in a population of contact lens wearers who developed keratoconus.[42]

KERATOCONUS DETECTION BY VISUAL INSPECTION OF THE COLOR MAP

Keratoconus suspects are most easily detected with videokeratography; it is the most sensitive means for screening, and controversy on this issue is diminishing.[49] Previously, clinicians used distortion of keratometer or keratoscope mires and scissoring of the light reflex during retinoscopy as signs of the irregular astigmatism often present with preclinical keratoconus. Relatively rapid changes in refraction were often noted to accompany keratoconus in the progressive phase. However, with videokeratoscopy, the keratoconus suspect cornea is easily identified using the standard 1.5-diopter interval scale (Figure 165-2), even though by definition there are no other clinical signs and the only visual symptom may be spectacle blur from associated irregular astigmatism. The earliest topographic signs are recognized by a localized area of corneal steepening some two or more contour intervals above the surrounding topography. Although "atypical inferior steepening"[44] is a common finding with keratoconus suspect cases, the steepest part of the

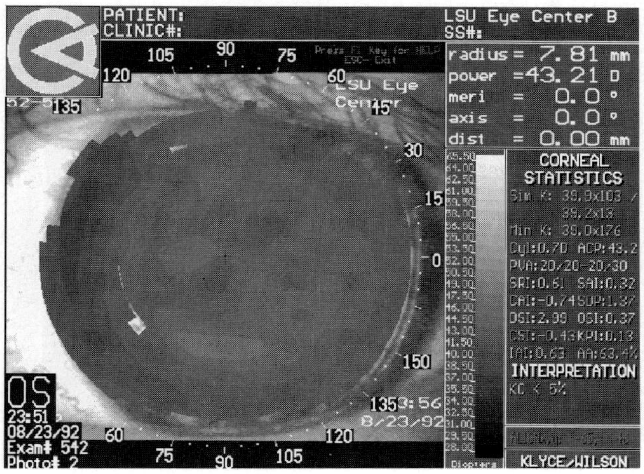

FIGURE 165-11 The topography of a hexagonal keratotomy patient referred to LSU. Note the irregular astigmatism that is consistent with the observations of Basuk et al.[82] **See color plate 165-11.**

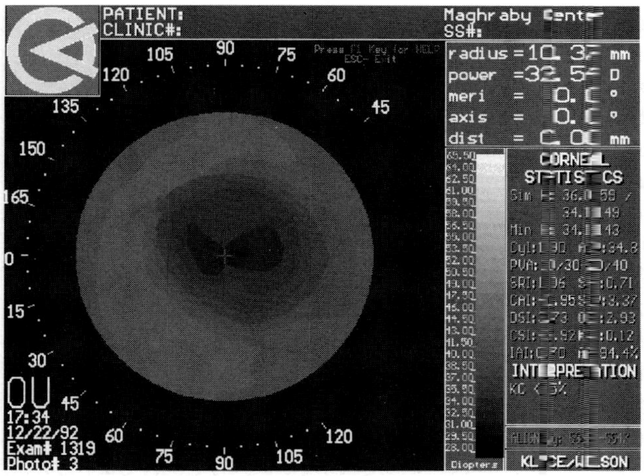

FIGURE 165-12 Example of topography after automated lamellar keratectomy (ALK) for the correction of moderate to high myopia. (Courtesy El Maghraby Eye Center, Jeddah, Saudi Arabia.) **See color plate 165-12.**

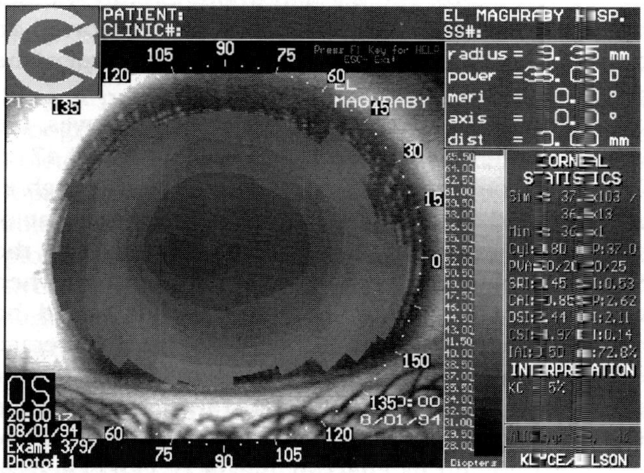

FIGURE 165-13 Example of topography after laser in situ lamellar keratectomy (LASIK) for the correction of moderate to high myopia. (Courtesy El Maghraby Eye Center, Jeddah, Saudi Arabia.) **See color plate 165-13.**

that the irregularities were revealed by sensitive videokeratography as a physical presence, which was associated with visual loss in severe cases. Precisely because these events can be captured with videokeratographs, they can be followed serially to examine changes with time, and the means to eliminate them can be prospectively developed and tested.

Some refractive surgical procedures have made their entrance and exit with little or no topographic evaluation. An example is circumferential (hexagonal) keratotomy for the management of hyperopia, which first appeared with only anecdotal information on the development of irregular astigmatism (Figure 165-11). Only after a severely critical assessment of its complications was reported[82] was this procedure condemned until such time as a controlled experimental trial could be conducted to establish safety and efficacy. The extensive list of complications[82] included glare, photophobia, polyopia, fluctuation in vision, overcorrection, irregular astigmatism, corneal edema, corneal perforation, bacterial keratitis, cataract, and endophthalmitis. There were wound healing abnormalities and anterior displacement of the central cornea adjacent to the incisions. Eight eyes lost best-corrected visual acuity of two or more Snellen lines, and three eyes required penetrating keratoplasty for visual rehabilitation. This is an example of a situation in which a carefully constructed clinical trial that included topographic evaluation might have prevented many complications and perhaps pointed the way toward improving the procedure.

Currently, automated lamellar keratoplasty (ALK), introduced by Ruiz, and excimer laser in situ keratomileusis (LASIK), introduced by Pallikaris,[83,84] are being explored to treat moderate to high myopia, as radial keratotomy and photorefractive keratectomy are most effective for myopic corrections of 6 diopters or less. Topographic examples of these procedures are shown in Figures 165-12 and 165-13. However, except for limited information on centration, there is little topographic information on these procedures for comparison, yet there are numerous anecdotal reports of ALK complications involving lost tissue and equipment problems that lead to irregular astigmatism.

Computer-assisted corneal topography has had an active and important role in the development of several refractive surgical procedures. It has been exceptionally useful to indicate limitations, so that the refractive pioneer can have a more complete indication of the

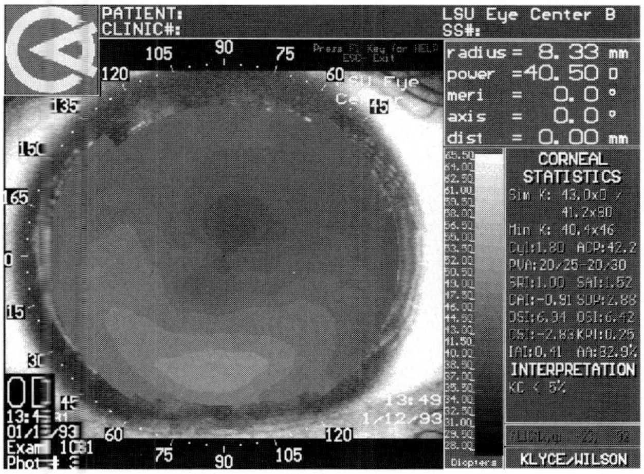

FIGURE 165-14 The topography of the right eye of a patient after radial keratotomy for the correction of myopia complicated by the presence of keratoconus. With the irregular astigmatism caused by keratoconus, there is a reduction in the best spectacle-corrected acuity in this eye and a loss of refractive stability if the keratoconus progresses. **See color plate 165-14.**

surgical effect on the cornea. The aim of refractive surgery is to correct refractive error without unduly reducing contrast sensitivity. Decentration and diameter of the treated area and irregular astigmatism can easily be visualized with videokeratography; this is the kind of information that can be used to ensure the highest quality result.

MANAGING COMPLICATIONS

Videokeratography is useful not only for improving surgical procedures, but also for the postoperative management of complications that may arise. If there is visual loss from irregular astigmatism, it is important to identify the specific type and distribution. For example, if the patient experiences a smaller-than-desired treatment zone, or one that is markedly off-center, miotics have been considered to reduce the diameter of the entrance pupil. Where the corneal surface has a large amount of irregular astigmatism over the entrance pupil, perhaps contact lens wear may be the only nonsurgical way to provide an adequate correction. Patients referred to our clinic with unsatisfactory results from radial keratotomy have been found to display a typical keratoconus topography rather than the expected central flattening (Figure 165-14).

Although cataract extraction with secondary intraocular lens implants is a refractive procedure, little attention has been directed in the past toward the irregular astigmatism that might be induced in the cornea as a result of the surgical incision. If best spectacle-corrected vision is reduced, evaluation of the corneal topography, particularly with the use of the Surface Regularity Index along with the potential visual acuity, may indicate whether the visual loss can be ascribed to corneal surface irregularities.

Similarly, videokeratography can and should be used to evaluate and manage the irregular astigmatism that can accompany other surgical procedures, including penetrating keratoplasty, lamellar keratoplasty, and excimer laser phototherapeutic keratectomy. With penetrating keratoplasty it has been suggested that rigid contact lens wear early after grafting can help to reduce the amount of irregular astigmatism in the graft, which can be assessed with videokeratography.[85]

OUTCOME ANALYSIS

As illustrated earlier, the color map is useful to distinguish normal corneas from abnormal ones and to differentiate the types of irregular astigmatism that may accompany complications in refractive surgery and to classify them as decentration, multifocality, and/or central islands. However, as with keratoconus evaluation and detection, objective criteria are needed to assess the type and magnitude of irregular astigmatism present in a cornea. For example, with the PRK "central island," measurement is essential not only to establish criteria based on elevation and extent, but also to correlate such features with possible influences on vision.

A first step in quantifying irregular astigmatism was made with the derivation of the Surface Regularity Index, noted earlier,[21,22] which is proportional to the amount of local mire-to-mire fluctuation in corneal power. This index correlates strongly with potential visual acuity in otherwise normal eyes. Another approach has been to use ray tracing analysis to produce theoretical images projected through videokeratoscope reconstructions of the central cornea. In this way, Maguire et al[81] could simulate the types of visual phenomena produced in refractive surgical patients, such as loss of contrast sensitivity and ghosts. Applegate et al[86-88] calculated the aberration structures from videokeratographic data for normal corneas and for corneas that had undergone radial keratotomy and used these calculations to show an excellent correlation between topographic irregularities and loss of best-corrected visual acuity.

One can extend the topographic index approach to determine the optical characteristics of a refractive surgical procedure by deriving expressions that capture the magnitude of certain classifications of irregular astigmatism.[89] Certainly the amount of decentration of the treatment zone from the intended position is an important measurement and can be estimated from videokeratographic data as the distance between the center of the entrance pupil to the center of the treatment zone. How this is done varies with the in-

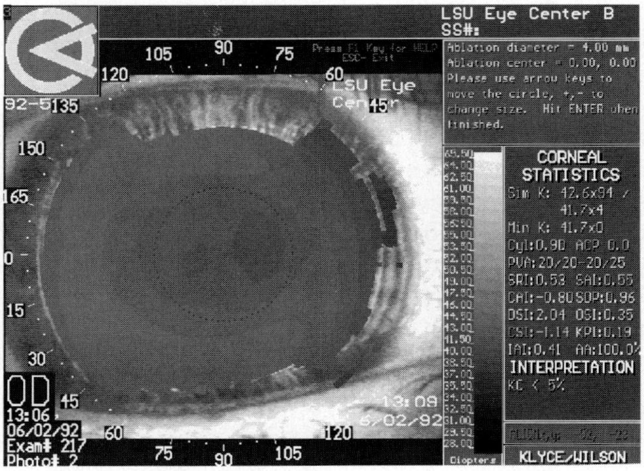

FIGURE 165-15 **Locating the treatment area of a refractive surgical case with a 4 mm diameter circular cursor (*dotted outline*) enables objective characterization, such as measurement of centration and irregular astigmatism. See color plate 165-15.**

strument used, but in a research environment, one can move a circular cursor around to indicate the center of the treated area as well as the location and size of the apparent pupil (Figure 165-15).

While the Surface Regularity Index relates to local surface irregularities, another correlate to visual acuity and contrast sensitivity in particular should be the Coefficient of Variation of corneal Powers (CVP), as this should be related to the amount of blur produced by the presence of a wide range of powers in a lens. The coefficient of variation is related to the Standard Deviation of the Power distribution (SDP) divided by the mean power ($\overline{P}$) for that group of observations, or the following:

$$CVP = \frac{SDP}{\overline{P}}$$

CVP can be calculated for the area ahead of the apparent entrance pupil as observed in a videokeratograph image to correlate individual topography with visual acuity. Alternatively, CVP can be calculated for a 4 mm diameter circle centered on the treatment zone to evaluate the optical quality of the surgery independent of decentration effects. CVP provides an estimate of the *varifocality* of the corneal topography.

Whereas multifocality has been used traditionally to describe the variability of corneal power, variations in corneal power after refractive procedures do not occur in a discrete or stepwise fashion, as with bifocal or trifocal prescription spectacle or contact lenses, but rather in a more continuous fashion, as with the Varilux* lens with poorly distinguishable or indistin-

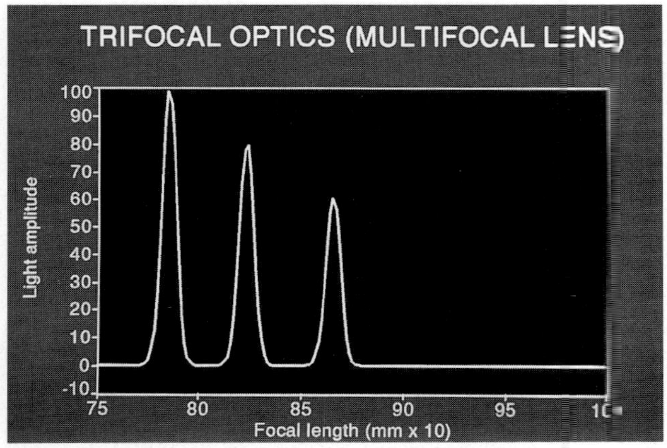

FIGURE 165-16 **Trifocal optical system. With distinct foci, adequate contrast between image planes can be maintained.**

guishable modal peaks. The use of the term *varifocal* to describe a corneal surface with a wide range of powers is usually more accurate than *multifocal*, and this can be easily illustrated. Figure 165-16 is a schematic plot of light amplitude at a point along various focal planes through an optimum trifocal optical system. The dispersion of the Gaussian distributions is similar to that seen in normal corneal power distributions. With corneal transplants, moderately advanced keratoconus, and other situations in which there is a moderate amount of irregular astigmatism and a wide range of corneal powers, discrete focal points are spread out as shown in Figure 165-17. This is an example of varifocal optics, which can be assessed statistically with the CVP.

Varifocality can take a number of forms. Varifocality becomes increasingly pronounced as keratoconus advances—a wide range of powers is created by the presence of the cone; this phenomenon can also be present in a highly decentered refractive surgical treatment, although this form tends to be bimodal and, therefore, to produce ghost images.

Corneas can also exhibit central islands after excimer laser photorefractive keratectomy for myopia as noted earlier, and it should be possible to objectively measure such features to determine their persistence and whether this specific type of irregular astigmatism correlates with loss of visual acuity. It was argued that the type of topographic feature represented by a central island should affect vision in much the same manner as a central depression in topography might, and, for this reason, algorithms were derived that would detect each equally. The result was termed the Elevation/Depression Magnitude (EDM). This algorithm calculates the product of area and power for those areas of the cornea within a 4 mm circle centered on a refractive surgical treatment zone that are more

*Varilux Corp., Oldsmar, FL.

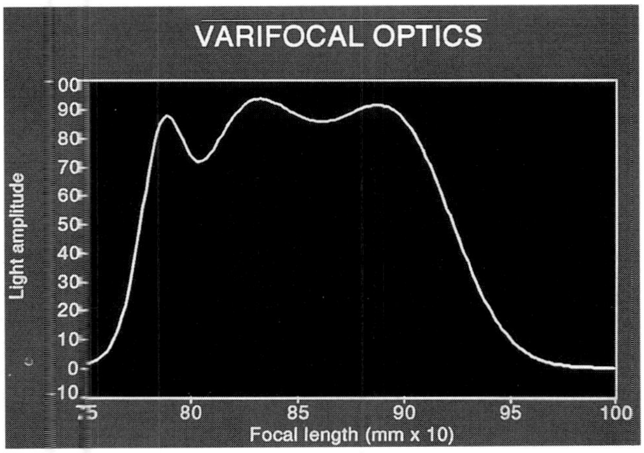

FIGURE 165-17 Varifocal optical system. With overlapping foci, inadequate contrast reduces the optical performance of the eye. Such a distribution of corneal powers has been observed in keratoconus and in corneas with irregular astigmatism.

than 1 diopter beyond the mode (most frequently occurring power). The 1-diopter window was chosen because it encompasses the range of powers seen in the central region of normal corneas, possibly representing to some extent positive spherical aberration. The areas so summed up are not necessarily contiguous, although they tend to be, since this estimate tends to assess large variations from the local power, while the Surface Regularity Index is sensitive only to local mire-to-mire changes in power.

Hence, the measure of centration, the Surface Regularity Index, the CVP, and the EDM provide four different tools with which to measure and characterize irregular astigmatism. As a preliminary evaluation of these variables, 36 eyes in the LSU Phase III excimer laser photorefractive keratectomy (PRK) for myopia study[90] with 2 years of follow-up were compared to 85 PERK corneas operated on by the same surgeon. The results are shown in Table 165-2. There was no difference in centration between PRK and PERK, even though the early PERK corneas were centered on the line of sight rather than on the center of the entrance pupil. There was also no statistically significant difference in the Surface Regularity Index between the two procedures, although both were elevated over normal values by an amount equivalent to the loss of one Snellen line. However, the CVPs within the pupil and within the treated area were both statistically significantly larger for the PERK corneas than for the PRK group ($p < 0.05$); both parameters were increased by 40% to 50% in the PERK group. These results would lead one to conclude that the excimer laser procedure yields a more spherical result. Neither group was significantly different from the normal preoperative corneas. Whereas central islands were a feature first noted with the excimer laser procedure, the quantitative estimator for these, the EDM, was nearly 50% smaller for the PRK corneas than for the PERK corneas ($p < 0.05$), and only the PERK corneas had values significantly greater than normal. These data confirm the idea that quantitative topographic measures can be used to compare refractive surgical procedures and to obtain objective information for evaluation. It is also likely that this kind of analysis will be used routinely for outcome analysis in the development of new refractive surgical procedures.

Challenges for the Future and Conclusions

Enormous strides continue to be made in the development of videokeratography. The development of artificial intelligence techniques to aid in the interpretation of corneal shape abnormalities, such as the refractive surgical screening process for keratoconus, will provide sound methods for formulating clinical decisions.[57] Neural networks will be applied to the automatic classification of corneal topography.[91,92] Unlike the approach taken with the expert system classifier for keratoconus interpretation, neural networks will be able to differentiate many classes of corneal shape, from normal to pellucid marginal degeneration. The usefulness of sound and scientifically validated discrimination systems is immense.

Classification of corneal topography brings up the issue of standards. If all topography machines provided the same data using the same color scale and derived numerical indexes, the resulting consistency would accelerate the learning phase for the user. Standardization would also enable one expert to evaluate topography independent of the machine used to capture it. There are several aspects needing attention. The most obvious beginning would be adoption of the absolute color scale introduced by Maguire et al[5] as modified by Wilson et al.[20] This color scale has been tested clinically and has been shown to provide the necessary diagnostic capability and range of coverage to be a practical presentation form. A standard scale would allow the reader or audience to judge refractive surgical outcomes easily from topography.

Several approaches are being explored to evaluate the optics of the refractive surgical eye using traditional optical methods to calculate aberration structures[86-88] as well as ray tracing methods that examine the theoretical image quality directly through a mathematical abstraction of the videokeratoscope-reconstructed corneal surface.[81] Another exciting method to evaluate

Table 165-2. Comparison of irregular astigmatism: 2-year photorefractive keratectomy (PRK) versus 10-year PERK

Group	Centration	SRI	CVP_p	CVP_t	EDH
Normal	—	0.28 ± 0.14	0.46 ± 0.17	0.39 ± 0.13	1.43 ± 1.98
PRK	0.34 ± 0.21	0.62 ± 0.20*	0.42 ± 0.14	0.33 ± 0.11	2.21 ± 2.51
PERK	0.37 ± 0.28	0.60 ± 0.23*	0.52 ± 0.26†	0.42 ± 0.21†	3.91 ± 3.85†*

Modified from Klyce SD et al: *Invest Ophthalmol Vis Sci Suppl* 36:S1, 1995.
*$p < 0.004$; value greater than normal values.
†$p < 0.05$; PERK value greater than PRK value.

refractive surgery is through the use of spatially resolved refractometry, a concept that could map the true refractive power of the eye point by point through the pupil.[93] The concept of extracting topographic characteristics from the refractive surgical treatment zone and the area overlying the pupil and correlating these with vision provides a means to compare surgical procedures as well as to follow the changes they induce over time. Collectively these approaches form the basis for an important next advance in corneal topography: understanding the full relationship between corneal topographic variations and the effect of those variations on vision.

Real-time corneal topographic analysis may find its way to the operating room to improve the accuracy of refractive surgical procedures. Initial work using projected-fringe contouring with phase-shifting algorithms has appeared.[94] While intraoperative corneal topography could be useful for various incisional procedures, it would seem to be unnecessary for computer-guided laser refractive sculpting procedures such as the area ablations used with PRK for myopia or hyperopia. However, excimer laser phototherapeutic keratectomy (PTK) would benefit greatly from real-time corneal topography analysis. An adequate smoothing agent for use in ablating surfaces with irregular astigmatism has not yet been described; therefore if real-time topographic data were available, it could be used to control a motion-stabilized laser-tracked system that could achieve the same result.

It is clear that videokeratography has a permanent home among the diagnostic capabilities of the ocular surgeon. When used appropriately, it provides a clarity of perception that makes classification of corneal topography nearly intuitive. It may be, also, that in the future, as corneal transplant surgeons gain more experience with the postoperative videokeratographic follow-up of their graft patients, better methods will be developed to reduce the visually disabling consequences of large amounts of regular and irregular astigmatism. Initial studies using contact lens molding to achieve this aim show reduction in the amount of surface irregularity.[85] Examination of the amount and axis of cylinder and the amount and nature of irregular astigmatism induced after cataract surgery, filtering procedures, and other surgeries involving ocular incisions can use videokeratography to scrutinize and improve methodology. Modern videokeratography had its origins in the refractive surgery laboratories; it has succeeded beyond expectations in its initial goal to provide topographic analysis for keratorefractive surgery. The future holds continued opportunities for videokeratography to perform an important role in clinical eye care and vision research.

REFERENCES

1. Doss JD et al: Method for the calculation of corneal profile and power distribution, *Arch Ophthalmol* 99:1261, 1981.
2. Klyce SD: Computer-assisted corneal topography: high resolution graphical presentation and analysis of keratoscopy, *Invest Ophthalmol Vis Sci* 25:1426, 1984.
3. Gormley DJ et al: Corneal modeling, *Cornea* 7:30, 1988.
4. Mammone RJ et al: 3-D corneal modeling system, *IEEE Trans Biomed Engineer* 37:66, 1990.
5. Maguire LJ, Singer DE, Klyce SD: Graphic presentation of computer-analyzed keratoscope photographs, *Arch Ophthalmol* 105:223, 1987.
6. El Hage SG: A computerized corneal topographer for use in refractive surgery, *Refract Corneal Surg* 5:418, 1989
7. Koch DD et al: The Corneal EyeSys System: accuracy analysis and reproducibility of first generation prototype, *Refract Corneal Surg* 5:424, 1989.
8. Arffa RC, Warnicki JW, Rehkopf PG: Corneal topography using rasterstereography, *Refract Corneal Surg* 5:414, 1989.
9. Belin MW et al: The PAR technology corneal topography system, *Refract Corneal Surg* 8:88, 1992.
10. Baker PC: Holographic contour analysis of the cornea. In Masters BR, editor: *Noninvasive diagnostic techniques in ophthalmology,* New York, 1990, Springer-Verlag.
11. Reinstein DZ et al: Corneal pachymetric topography, *Ophthalmology* 101:432, 1994.
12. Hannush SB et al: Accuracy and precision of keratometry, photokeratoscopy, and corneal modeling on calibrated steel balls, *Arch Ophthalmol* 107:1235, 1989.
13. Wang J, Rice DA, Klyce SD: Analysis of the effects of astigmatism and misalignment on corneal surface reconstruction from photokeratoscopic data, *Refract Corneal Surg* 7:129 1991.
14. Koch DD et al: Comparison of the accuracy and reproducibility of the keratometer and the EyeSys Corneal Analysis System Model I, *J Cataract Refract Surg* 18:342, 1992.
15. Wilson SE, Verity SM, Conger DL: Accuracy and precision of the corneal analysis system and the topographical analysis system, *Cornea* 11:28, 1992.
16. Roberts C: Characterization of the inherent error in a spherically-

biased corneal topography system in mapping a radially aspheric surface, *J Refract Corneal Surg* 10:103, 1994.
17. Wang J, Rice DA, Klyce SD: A new reconstruction algorithm for improvement of corneal topographical analysis, *Refract Corneal Surg* 5:379, 1989.
18. Roberts C: The accuracy of 'power' maps to display curvature data in corneal topography systems, *Invest Ophthalmol Vis Sci* 35:3525, 1994.
19. Young JA, Siegel IM: Corneal contour mapping: an isomorphic approach, *CLAO J* 19:182, 1993.
20. Wilson SE, Klyce SD, Husseini ZM: Standardized color-coded maps for corneal topography, *Ophthalmology* 100:1723, 1993.
21. Dingeldein SA, Klyce SD, Wilson SE: Quantitative descriptors of corneal shape derived from computer-assisted analysis of photokeratographs, *Refract Corneal Surg* 5:372, 1989.
22. Wilson SE, Klyce SD: Quantitative descriptors of corneal topography: a clinical study, *Arch Ophthalmol* 109:349, 1991.
23. Maeda N, Klyce SD, Hamano H: Alteration of corneal asphericity in RGP contact lens-induced warpage, *CLAO J* 20:27, 1994.
24. Legeais JM et al: Computer-assisted corneal topography: accuracy and reproducibility of the topographic modeling system, *Refract Corneal Surg* 9:347, 1993.
25. Hubbe RE, Foulks GN: The effect of poor fixation on computer-assisted topographic corneal analysis. Pseudokeratoconus, *Ophthalmology* 101:1745, 1994.
26. Swinger CA, Barker BA: Prospective evaluation of myopic keratomileusis, *Ophthalmology* 91:785, 1984.
27. Arffa RC, Klyce SD, Busin M: Keratometry in epikeratophakia, *J Refract Surg* 2:61, 1986.
28. Munnerlyn CR, Koons SJ, Marshall J: Photorefractive keratectomy: a technique for laser refractive surgery, *J Cataract Refract Surg* 14:46, 1988.
29. Mandell RB: Corneal power correction factor for photorefractive keratectomy, *J Refract Corneal Surg* 10:125, 1994.
30. Maguire LJ et al: Visual distortion after myopic keratomileusis: computer analysis of keratoscope photographs, *Ophthalmic Surg* 18:352, 1987.
31. Wilson SE et al: Changes in corneal topography after excimer laser photorefractive keratectomy for myopia, *Ophthalmology* 98:1338, 1991.
32. Cavanaugh TB et al: Centration of excimer laser photorefractive keratectomy relative to the pupil, *J Cataract Refract Surg Suppl* 19:144, 1993.
33. Lin DT, Sutton HF, Berman M: Corneal topography following excimer photorefractive keratectomy for myopia, *J Cataract Refract Surg Suppl* 19:149, 1993.
34. Parker PJ et al: Central topographic islands following photorefractive keratectomy, ARVO abstract, *Invest Ophthalmol Vis Sci Suppl* 34:803, 1993.
35. Lin DT: Corneal topographic analysis after excimer photorefractive keratectomy, *Ophthalmology* 101:1432, 1994.
36. Nesburn AB et al: Computer assisted corneal topography (CACT) to detect mild keratoconus (KC) in candidates for photorefractive keratectomy, ARVO abstract, *Invest Ophthalmol Vis Sci Suppl* 33:995, 1992.
37. Wilson SE, Klyce SD: Screening for corneal topographic abnormalities prior to refractive surgery, *Ophthalmology* 101:147, 1994.
38. Kennedy RH, Bourne WM, Dyer JA: A 48-year clinical and epidemiologic study of keratoconus, *Am J Ophthalmol* 101:267, 1986.
39. Waring GO III: Nomenclature for keratoconus suspects, *Refract Corneal Surg* 9:220, 1993.
40. Krachmer JH, Feder RS, Belin MW: Keratoconus and related noninflammatory corneal thinning disorders, *Surv Ophthalmol* 28:293, 1984.
41. Gasset AR, Houde WL, Garcia-Bengochea M: Hard contact lens wear as an environmental risk in keratoconus, *Am J Ophthalmol* 85:339, 1978.
42. Macsai MS, Varley GA, Krachmer JH: Development of keratoconus after contact lens wear: patient characteristics, *Arch Ophthalmol* 108:534, 1990.
43. Wilson SE et al: Topographic changes in contact lens-induced corneal warpage, *Ophthalmology* 97:734, 1990.
44. Grandon SC, Weber RA: Radial keratotomy in patients with atypical inferior steepening, *J Cataract Refract Surg* 20:381, 1994.
45. Ellis W: Radial keratotomy in a patient with keratoconus, *J Cataract Refract Surg* 18:406, 1992.
46. Mortensen J, Ohrstrom A: Excimer laser photorefractive keratectomy for treatment of keratoconus, *J Refract Corneal Surg* 10:368, 1994.
47. Saragoussi JJ, Pouliquen YJM: Does the progressive increasing effect of radial keratotomy (hyperopic shift) correlate with undetected early keratoconus? *Refract Corneal Surg* 10:45, 1994.
48. Waring GO, Lynn MJ, Kutner MH: Stability of refraction after refractive keratotomy. In Waring GO, editor: *Refractive keratotomy for myopia and astigmatism,* St Louis, 1992, Mosby.
49. Rabinowitz YS et al: Opinions. Keratoconus, videokeratography, and refractive surgery, *Refract Corneal Surg* 8:403, 1992.
50. Wilson SE, Klyce SD: The corneal topography of keratoconus, *Cornea* 10:2, 1991.
51. Maguire LJ, Lowry JC: Identifying progression of subclinical keratoconus by serial topographic analysis, *Am J Ophthalmol* 112:41, 1991.
52. Dingeldein SA, Klyce SD: The topography of normal corneas, *Arch Ophthalmol* 107:512, 1989.
53. Bogan SJ et al: Classification of normal corneal topography based on computer-assisted videokeratography, *Arch Ophthalmol* 108: 945, 1990.
54. Rabinowitz YS, McDonnell PJ: Computer-assisted corneal topography in keratoconus, *Refract Corneal Surg* 5:400, 1989.
55. Maeda N et al: Comparison of three keratoconus detection schemes with videokeratography, ARVO abstract, *Invest Ophthalmol Vis Sci Suppl* 35(4):2078, 1994.
56. Rabinowitz YS, Wilson SE, Klyce SD: *Atlas of corneal topography,* New York, 1993, Igaku-Shoin.
57. Maeda N et al: Automated keratoconus screening with corneal topography analysis, *Invest Ophthalmol Vis Sci* 35:2749, 1994.
58. Waring GO: *Refractive keratotomy for myopia and astigmatism,* St Louis, 1992, Mosby.
59. Rowsey JJ et al: Corneal topography as a predictor of refractive change in the prospective evaluation of radial keratotomy (PERK) study, *Ophthalmic Surg* 22:370, 1991.
60. Wyzinski P, O'Dell LW: Diurnal cycle of refraction after radial keratotomy, *Ophthalmology* 94:120, 1987.
61. Santos VR et al: Morning-to-evening change in refraction, corneal curvature, and visual acuity 2 to 4 years after radial keratotomy in the PERK study, *Ophthalmology* 95:1487, 1988.
62. MacRae S et al: Diurnal variation in vision after radial keratotomy, *Am J Ophthalmol* 107:262, 1989.
63. Maloney RK: Effect of corneal hydration and intraocular pressure on keratometric power after experimental radial keratotomy, *Ophthalmology* 97:927, 1990.
64. McDonnell PJ, McClusky DJ, Garbus JJ: Corneal topography and fluctuating visual acuity after radial keratotomy, *Ophthalmology* 96:665, 1989.
65. Moreira H et al: Corneal topographic changes over time after radial keratotomy, *Cornea* 11:465, 1992.
66. Waring GO et al: Results of the prospective evaluation of radial keratotomy (PERK) study 10 years after surgery, *Arch Ophthalmol* 112:1298, 1994.

67. Santos VR et al: Relationship between refractive error and visual acuity in the Prospective Evaluation of Radial Keratotomy (PERK) study, *Arch Ophthalmol* 105:86, 1987.
68. Applegate RA, Howland HC: Magnification and visual acuity in refractive surgery, *Arch Ophthalmol* 111:1335, 1993.
69. McDonnell PJ, Garbus J, Lopez PF: Topographic analysis and visual acuity after radial keratotomy, *Am J Ophthalmol* 106:692, 1988.
70. Hemenger RP, Tomlinson A, McDonnell PJ: Explanation for good visual acuity in uncorrected residual hyperopia and presbyopia after radial keratotomy, *Invest Ophthalmol Vis Sci* 31:1644, 1990.
71. Kaufman HE: The correction of aphakia, *Am J Ophthalmol* 89:1, 1980.
72. Werblin TP, Klyce SD: Epikeratophakia: the surgical correction of aphakia. I. Lathing of corneal tissue, *Curr Eye Res* 1:123, 1981.
73. Maguire LJ et al: Corneal topography in myopic patients undergoing epikeratophakia, *Am J Ophthalmol* 103:404, 1987.
74. Werblin TP, Klyce SD: Epikeratophakia: the surgical correction of myopia. I. Lathing of corneal tissue, *Curr Eye Res* 1:591, 1982.
75. McDonald MB et al: Refractive surgery with the excimer laser, *Am J Ophthalmol* 103:469, 1987.
76. McDonald MB et al: One year refractive results of central photorefractive keratectomy for myopia in the nonhuman primate cornea, *Arch Ophthalmol* 108:40, 1990.
77. McDonald MB et al: Central photorefractive keratectomy for myopia: the blind eye study, *Arch Ophthalmol* 108:799, 1990.
78. Klyce SD, McDonald MB: Computerized corneal topography of surface ablations with the Tomey TMS-1. In Salz JJ, McDonnell PJ, McDonald MB, editors: *Corneal laser surgery,* St Louis, 1995, Mosby.
79. Uozato H, Guyton DL: Centering corneal surgical procedures, *Am J Ophthalmol* 103:264, 1987.
80. Maloney RK: Corneal topography and optical zone location in photorefractive keratectomy, *Refract Corneal Surg* 6:363, 1990.
81. Maguire LJ et al: Topography and raytracing analysis of patients with excellent visual acuity 3 months after excimer laser photorefractive keratectomy for myopia, *Refract Corneal Surg* 7:122, 1991.
82. Basuk WL et al: Complications of hexagonal keratotomy, *Am J Ophthalmol* 117:37, 1994.
83. Pallikaris IG: Laser in situ keratomileusis, *Lasers Surg Med* 10:463, 1990.
84. Pallikaris IG et al: A corneal flap technique for laser in situ keratomileusis: human studies, *Arch Ophthalmol* 109:1699, 1991.
85. Wilson SE, Friedman RS, Klyce SD: Contact lens manipulation of corneal topography after penetrating keratoplasty: a preliminary study, *CLAO J* 18:177, 1992.
86. Applegate RA et al: Changes in the aberration structure of the RK cornea from videokeratographic measurements, ARVO abstract, *Invest Ophthalmol Vis Sci Suppl* 35:1740, 1994.
87. Applegate RA et al: Corneal aberrations before and after radial keratotomy (RK) calculated from videokeratometric measurements. In *Vision science and its applications,* Technical Digest Series, Vol 2, Washington, DC, 1994, Optical Society of America.
88. Howland HC, Beuttner J, Applegate RA: Computation of the shapes of normal corneas and their monochromatic aberrations from videokeratographic measurements. In *Vision science and its applications,* Technical Digest Series, Vol 2, Washington, DC, 1994, Optical Society of America.
89. Klyce SD et al: Evaluating refractive surgery with corneal topography, ARVO abstract, *Invest Ophthalmol Vis Sci Suppl* 36:S1, 1995.
90. McDonald MB et al: Central photorefractive keratectomy for myopia: partially sighted and normally sighted eyes, *Ophthalmology* 98:1327, 1991.
91. Klyce SD, Maeda N, Smolek MK: Use of neural networks for interpretation of corneal topography: I. Initial demonstration, ARVO abstract, *Invest Ophthalmol Vis Sci Suppl* 35:2079, 1994.
92. Smolek MK, Klyce SD, Maeda N: Use of neural networks for interpretation of corneal topography: II. A data simulation paradigm for optimization, ARVO abstract, *Invest Ophthalmol Vis Sci Suppl* 35:2079, 1994.
93. Webb R, Penney CM, Thompson KP: Measurement of ocular local wave front distortion with a spatially resolved refractometer, *Appl Optics* 31:3678, 1992.
94. Thall EH, Lange SR: Preliminary results of a new intraoperative corneal topography technique, *J Cataract Refract Surg Suppl* 19:193, 1993.

SECTION THREE *Radial Keratotomy*

CHAPTER 166

STEPHEN S. LANE

Radial Keratotomy Surgical Techniques

The goal of radial keratotomy (RK) surgery is to develop a series of reproducible steps that will achieve accurate and predictable results to meet the expectations of the patient.

As refractive surgeons, our desire is to achieve outcomes equal to or better than spectacle or contact lens correction. At the present stage of development, RK cannot predictably do this. Thus current RK surgeons are confronted with a group of techniques based on science and art. It is science because of the precision and reproducibility of current instrumentation[1]; studies (Prospective Evaluation of Radial Keratotomy [PERK]),[2-6] which have enlightened surgeons to the concepts of progressive hyperopia and variation of effect with regard to age and optical zone size; and improved understanding of corneal topographic changes and their complications borne by the introduction and proliferation of corneal videokeratography. It is art because of the tremendous individual variability and idiosyncrasies among surgeons based on their own personal experiences and that learned from colleagues. Waring has proposed a number of the variables that may affect the outcome of the procedure. These include the following[7]:

1. Cooperation of the patient during surgery
2. Use of topical versus peribulbar anesthesia
3. Method of determining the center of the clear zone
4. Surgical plan—the relationship between the amount of myopia, patient age, clear zone diameter, and number and depth of incisions[8]
5. Selection of the area to measure the corneal thickness that is used as the reference value for setting the knife blade
6. Pachymeter used to measure corneal thickness and the method of calibration
7. Design and configuration of the knife blade (width, blade angle, sharpness) and the foot plates
8. Percent bias that the length of the knife blade is set and the method by which it is verified
9. Hydration of the cornea during the procedure
10. Method of fixation of the eye and the level of the intraocular pressure during the incision
11. Method of spacing the incisions
12. Sequence in which the incisions are made
13. Direction in which the incisions are cut: centrifugal versus centripetal versus combined
14. Manual kinesthetic techniques of executing the incision, including the perpendicularity of the knife blade and the pressure exerted on the knife during the incision
15. Speed at which the incisions are made
16. Length of the incisions, as determined by their termination near the limbus and the clear zone[9,10]
17. Achieved depth of the incisions, including redeepening incisions[11,12]
18. Frequency and size of corneal perforations
19. Amount of manipulation and irrigation of the incisions
20. Types of postoperative medications used, for example, corticosteroids

If outcomes that are equal to or better than spectacle or contact lens correction are to be realized, the individual idiosyncrasies of art must be carefully studied and elucidated. Combined with our present knowledge, RK surgeons will then have a procedure with a substantial scientific basis.

Given these limitations, the text, photographs, and drawings that follow will demonstrate techniques that represent the current "state of the art" and science. As with all surgical training, there can be no substitute for taking a course, practicing, and training with someone who has developed the artistic and scientific surgical skills of radial keratotomy.

PATIENT NAME: ______________________ AGE: __________

OPERATIVE PLAN

	OD	OS
PRIMARY PROCEDURE:	________	
ENHANCEMENT:	________	

ATTEMPTED CORRECTION		PLAN	
SE: ______		# INCISIONS	______
		SPHERE OZ	______
CYLINDER: ______		CYLINDER OZ	______
REFRACTIVE GOAL: ______		LZ	______

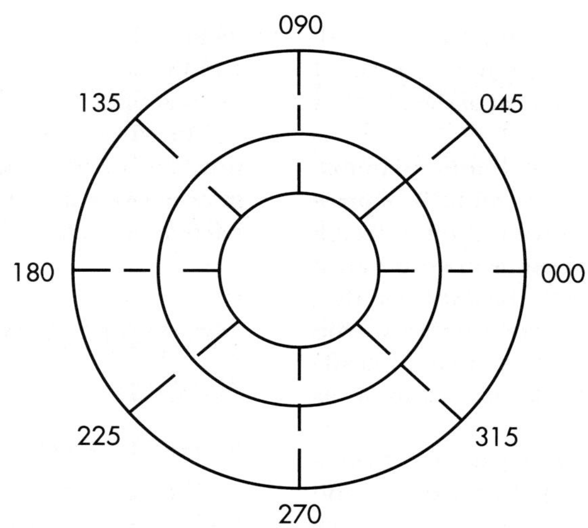

SIGNATURE: DATE:

FIGURE 166-2 Operative planning sheet. The surgical procedure is planned on this preoperatively, and it is brought to the operating and reviewed before surgery and/or referred to during surgery.

Full draping is unnecessary for keratotomy surgery. A fenestrated plastic drape is commonly used. Reassurance from the surgeon, elevation of the plastic drape over a support, and a good flow of air or oxygen under the drape or through a nasal cannula make it easy for the patient to breathe, ease patient apprehension, and lessen the claustrophobic sensation some experience. Taping the nonoperative eye closed is recommended to optimize fixation of the operative eye on the microscope light.

From this point on, it is important to avoid corneal surface desiccation, which can cause excessive diamond knife foot plate drag against the epithelium during attempted corneal incising. Frequent blinking by the patient or asking the patient to close his or her eyelids until directed to reopen them accomplishes adequate lubrication.

Before beginning surgery the surgeon, double-gloved with powder-free gloves or gloves that have been rinsed to remove the powder, instills a third and final drop of 0.5% tetracaine onto the conjunctiva.

A light wire eyelid speculum, such as a Barraquer speculum, holds the drape in place and retracts the lid without excessive pressure. The lid speculum should provide adequate exposure without placing undue tension on the eyelid, which may damage the levator palpebrae aponeurosis and produce postoperative ptosis. An open blade speculum without a cross wire allows room for the knife handle when making the 6 o'clock and 12 o'clock incisions. On the other hand, a blade speculum helps isolate the eyelashes when using a fenestrated plastic drape. The cornea is kept moist with topical balanced salt solution (BSS) to prevent drying and thinning. A wrist rest is recommended by some surgeons to help steady the wrists and hands.

MANIPULATION OF THE MICROSCOPE

As the microscope is swung into position, the light is dimmed to the minimum brightness necessary by adjusting the rheostat. A warning ("you'll notice a bright light like on a sunny day") is helpful to minimize the avoidance reflex and Bell's phenomenon that invariably occurs. The patient is then asked to fixate on the microscope light filament. The rheostat can be alternately adjusted higher and lower to confirm fixation for both the patient and the surgeon.

Operative Procedure

VISUAL AXIS DETERMINATION AND MARKING

The goal of marking the visual axis is to mark the center of the uncut clear optical zone to minimize glare and irregular astigmatism over the entrance pupil. It should be realized that using a corneal light reflex to guide procedure centration serves only as an approximation of the true visual axis location, since the light reflex corresponds to the center of the corneal optical system and not the true visual axis. Using the corneal light reflex, visual axis determination may be carried out by one of several techniques.

Light filament reflex centration

The PERK study group recommended that the patient fixate on the microscope light filament while the lower margin of the reflex is marked on the cornea. This is accomplished by the surgeon looking through

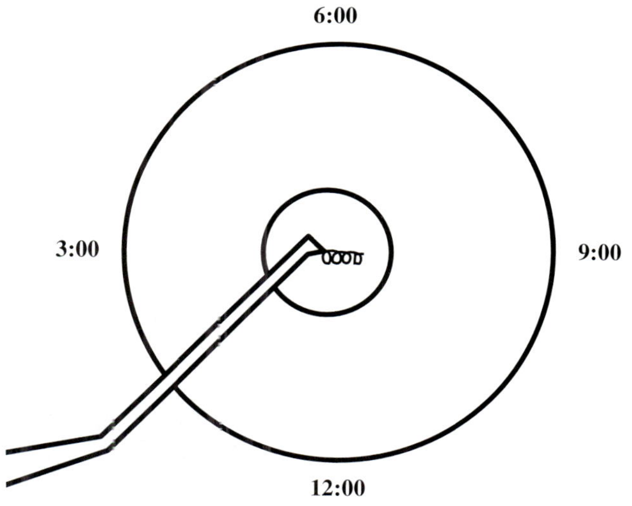

FIGURE 166-3 Visual axis marking. The recommended method of visual axis marking from the PERK Study group. With the patient fixating on the microscope filament, the surgeon fixates with the right eye, and a mark is made with an IOL hook at the left inferior edge of the filament reflex on the corneal epithelium.

one eyepiece and marking along the opposite inferior border of the light filament reflex. For example, if the surgeon views through the right ocular, the mark is placed along left lower border of the microscope filament reflex (Figure 166-3). This method compensates for the prism displacement of the light and for parallax. A fine, blunt instrument, such as a intraocular lens hook (Sinsky) or Grene marker, should be used. These will indent the corneal epithelium, leaving a mark that will last throughout the procedure and will not lacerate Bowman's layer as a sharp needle might. The administration of a drop of fluid (BSS) over the corneal apex may enhance an otherwise dull corneal light reflex.

Miotic pupil centering

An alternative approach is to place the center of the clear zone over the center of the pupil (either miotic or natural), not over the corneal light reflection, which is displaced somewhat nasally.

Coaxial light source

The optimal technique for centration of the optical clear zone is the use of a coaxial light source mounted onto or within the microscope optical system. This provides the patient with a light target that is nearly coaxial with the viewer. It is important that the surgeon mark the center of the entrance pupil and not the corneal light reflex. Alternatively, a 1 to 2 mm fixation spot can be placed over the exact center of one of the viewing tubes of the microscope where it will not

temperature. For consistency the knife is best calibrated after cooling to room temperature.

The use of a compound microscope fitted with a movable micrometer stage has found widespread acceptance as the method of choice for diamond knife calibration (Figure 166-9, *A*). The microscope offers a number of advantages. It allows magnification up to 150 times, so the surgeon can inspect the blade and foot plates and identify any damage. Chips on the blade's tip or breaks in the cutting edge are easily identified as well as excess debris on the blade (Figure 166-9, *B*). Alignment and symmetry of the foot plates can be checked as well as centration of the blade between the foot plates and wobble of the blade with advancement. The foot plates can also be inspected for defects such as scratches or debris (Figure 166-9, *C*). With such high magnification and absence of parallax, the microscope also ensures that the knife blade is set accurately at the desired length. Finally, use of the compound microscope almost eliminates the possibility of blade damage, which occurs more easily using calibrating coin gauges or gauge blocks.

There are three approaches to using the microscope gauge. The first is to use the knife micrometer handle to set the length of the knife blade to a known length as it is mounted on the microscope stage. The blade is then brought into focus, and the foot plates are aligned on the zero line at cross hairs of the reticule (Figure 166-9, *C*). With the microscope micrometer set at zero, the micrometer stage is moved until the tip of the knife blade is on the reticule line. The length of the blade is measured as the distance the micrometer stage has

A

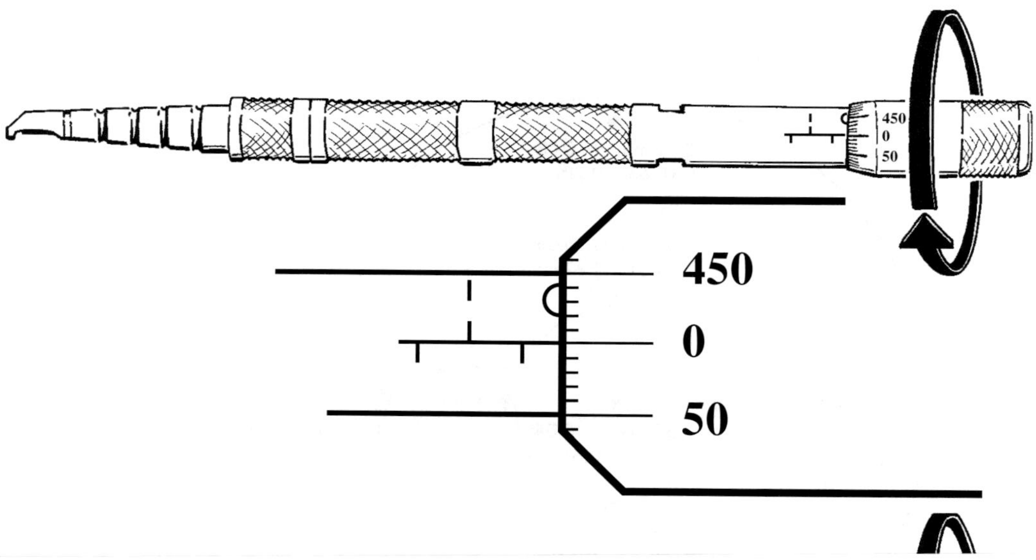

A
B
C

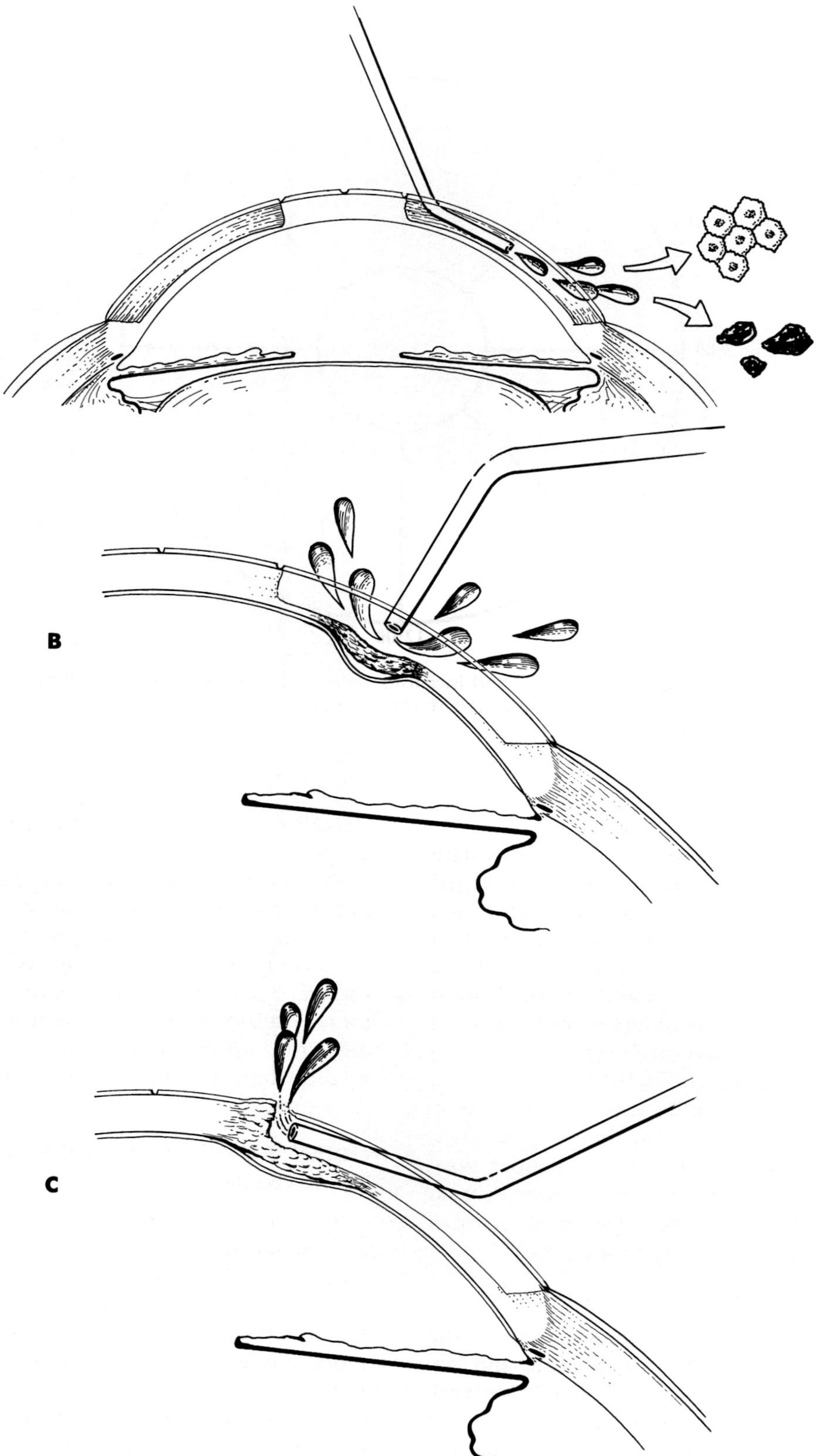

FIGURE 166-22 **A,** Irrigation of the wound with BSS is performed with a blunt 26- to 30-gauge cannula. The tip of the cannula is placed in the wound parallel to the surface at the clear zone. Foreign material, epithelial cells, and blood are removed. **B** and **C,** Care should be taken to avoid irrigating with the cannula perpendicular to the surface to prevent damage to Descemet's membrane or the endothelium. Fluid should also not be directed at the optical clear zone to avoid hydration into the clear zone stroma. (From Waring GO: *Refractive keratotomy,* St Louis, 1992, Mosby.)

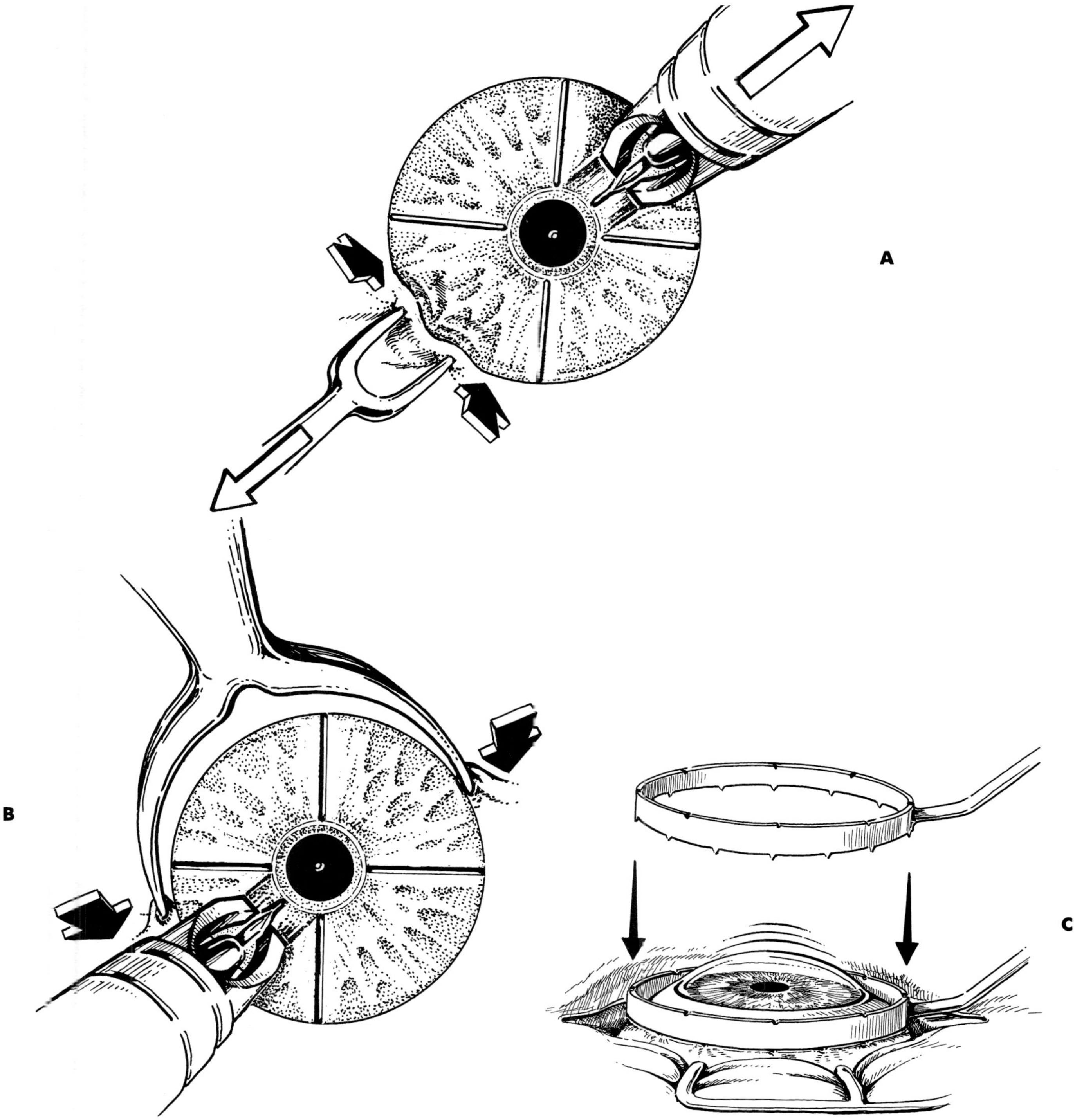

FIGURE 166-23 Fixation of the globe can be accomplished with several instruments. **A**, Stabilization and fixation of the globe during RK with a double-point fixation forceps. **B**, Stabilization and fixation of the globe during RK with a double-point spanning forceps. **C**, Stabilization and fixation of the globe during RK with a compression ring. (From Waring GO: *Refractive keratotomy,* St Louis, 1992, Mosby.)

scribed.[10] This technique involves incisions that extend from the desired optical zone to a 7 mm optical zone. This results in incision lengths of 2 to 4 mm. It has been postulated that these shorter incisions will enhance corneal stability, thus reducing diurnal fluctuation, refractive instability, and postoperative long-term hyperopic shift. Prospective clinical trials that require a minimum 5-year follow-up are now under way to fully analyze these potential benefits.

CONTROL OF MICROTREMORS IN RK

Microtremors that are greatly magnified under the microscope are an unnerving annoyance to the early RK surgeon. A number of techniques that may help the surgeon alleviate these microtremors include using both hands on the diamond knife (using a combined diamond blade); using a wrist rest or resting both hands on the patient's face; relaxing the shoulders and slowly exhaling; or holding the breath by using a mild Valsalva maneuver. If not contraindicated by a medical condition, some surgeons have used systemic nonselective β-blockers orally or topically. Over time, however, with increasing surgical experience and skill, methods to reduce microtremors will be unnecessary.

The art and science of radial keratotomy are in continual evolution.[16] Thus RK will remain a dynamic discipline in which sound, well-conceived studies will be performed based on the current state of the art.

REFERENCES

1. Werblin TP, Stafford EM: The Casebeer system for predictable keratorefrative surgery, *Ophthalmology* 100:1095-1102, 1991.
2. Waring GO et al and PERK Study Group: Results of the Prospective Evaluation of Radial Keratotomy (PERK) study 10 Years after surgery, *Arch Ophthalmol* 112:1308, 1994.
3. Arrowsmith P, Marks R: Visual refractive and keratometric results of radial keratotomy, *Arch Ophthalmol* 107:506-511, 1989.
4. Lavery FL: Comparative results of 200 consecutive radial keratotomy cases using three different nomograms, *J Refract Surg* 3:88-91, 1987.
5. Salz JJ, Salz MS: Results of four and eight incision radial keratotomy for 6 to 12 diopters of myopia, *J Refract Surg* 4:46-50, 1988.
6. Villasenor RA, Cox KC: Radial keratotomy: reoperations, *J Refract Surg* 1:35-57, 1985.
7. Waring GO: *Refractive keratotomy,* St Louis, 1992, Mosby.
8. Moreira H et al: Retrospective comparison of simultaneous and non-simultaneous bilateral radial keratotomy, *J Refract Corneal Surg* 10:545, 1994.
9. Casebeer JC: Corneal stability and avoidance of hyperopia following incisional keratotomy, *J Refract Corneal Surg* 10:153-154, 1994.
10. Lindstrom RL: *Mini RK. Current research: refractive and corneal surgery symposium,* Chicago, 1992, Pre-American Academy of Ophthalmology.
11. Poirier L et al: Effect of peripheral deepening of radial keratotomy incisions, *J Refract Corneal Surg* 10:621, 1994.
12. Binder PS et al: An ultrastructural and histochemical study of long-term wound healing after radial keratotomy, *J Ophthalmol* 103:432-440, 1987.
13. Assil KK, Schanzil DJ: *Radial and astigmatic keratotomy,* Thorofare, NJ, 1994, Slack.
14. Sher NA et al: Topical diclofenac in the treatment of ocular pain after excimer photorefractive keratectomy, *J Refract Corneal Surg* 9:425, 1993.
15. Cher V, Lindstrom RL: Oblique orientation of incisions in four incision radial keratotomy, *Ophthalmalmic Surg* 23(5):359, 1992.
16. Hoffman RF et al: *Radial keratotomy surgical techniques,* NJ, 1986, Slack.

CHAPTER 167

MICHAEL P. VRABEC SOOHYUNG KIM

Results of Radial Keratotomy

It is estimated that more than 10% of ophthalmologists in the United States are actively involved in radial keratotomy and that 250,000 Americans undergo radial keratotomy surgery each year.[1,2] Thus radial keratotomy is currently the most commonly performed refractive surgical procedure.

The goal of radial keratotomy is the safe, stable, and predictable reduction or elimination of myopia or myopic astigmatism, resulting in elimination or a reduced dependency on spectacles or contact lenses for activities of daily living. Because of improvements in spectacle and contact lens design and materials (with an accuracy of ± .50 diopters), it is important that the results of radial keratotomy be outstanding. Because radial keratotomy is an elective surgical procedure, patient satisfaction postoperatively should be high. Most patients undergoing radial keratotomy are in the prime of their lives, and their livelihood depends on good visual acuity. In addition, a patient's functional visual acuity after radial keratotomy is important to consider. For example, after radial keratotomy if a patient is bothered by glare during night driving the safety of both the patient and the general public may be at risk.[3]

This chapter examines published results of radial keratotomy, reviewing its safety, stability, and predictability. The results of radial keratotomy are reviewed when the procedure is performed in both eyes at the same time, when it is performed by beginning refractive surgeons, and when it is intentionally staged to avoid overcorrections. Newer trends such as "mini-RK" and hexagonal keratotomy are discussed, and comparative results with photorefractive keratotomy are also reported.

Results of Radial Keratotomy

As the number of radial keratotomy operations performed has grown tremendously over the last several years, so have the number of published reports on surgeon's results. We have included studies for review (Table 167-1) that meet the following criteria:

1. The report was a study in a peer-reviewed journal; no anecdotal reports were included.
2. There was close to at least 1 year of follow-up on most patients.
3. An adequate number of patients were included for statistical significance, with a relatively high follow-up rate (which in general was lower than that found in other areas of clinical research). Prospective studies were favored over retrospective studies.
4. Only those studies that used diamond blades with micrometer handles were included.
5. There was a clear description of the intraoperative parameters (e.g., clear zone diameter, number of incisions, blade setting, and incision direction).

When possible the percentage of patients with an uncorrected visual acuity of 20/40 or better is reported, because this has generally been accepted as the level of vision to qualify the operation as being a "success." It is important to note, however, that this level of vision does not necessarily equate to a total independence of spectacles and contact lenses. As an example, in the 6-year follow-up study of patients undergoing radial keratotomy in the Prospective Evaluation of Radial Keratotomy (PERK) study, only 34% of patients with an uncorrected visual acuity of 20/25 to 20/40 wore no correction.[4]

Complications other than a loss of best corrected visual acuity, glare, and vision fluctuation (the last two probably better classified as side effects of the surgery) have been omitted and are covered in Chapter 168.

Table 167-1 condenses and summarizes the results of 14 studies that meet these criteria. More exhaustive study results are detailed elsewhere.[5,6] The table is in chronologic order, with the more recent reports listed first. When not specified, the amount of myopia in these studies is categorized around the following groupings:

Low myopia	1.5 to 3.00 D
Moderated myopia	3.25 to 4.50 D
High myopia	4.75 to 6.00 D

Salient points of the studies cited in Table 167-1 are discussed below.

Text continued on p. 2094.

Table 167-1. Results of radial keratotomy

	Authors and publication			
	Werblin TP, Stafford MS: The Casebeer system for predictable keratorefractive surgery. One year evaluation of 205 consecutive cases, *Ophthalmology* 100:1095-1102, 1993	Friedberg ML et al: Results of radial and astigmatic keratotomy by beginning refractive surgeons, *Ophthalmology* 100:746-751, 1993	Bauerberg J, Sterzorsky M, Brodsky M: Radial keratotomy in myopia of 6 to 12 diopters using full-length deepening incisions, *Refract Corneal Surg* 5: 150-154, 1989	Arne JL, Bourdiol AM: Results of 350 anterior radial keratotomies in myopia: postoperative follow-up of more than 1 year, *J Implant Refract Surg* 5:94-103, 1987
Study design	Prospective	Retrospective	Prospective	Retrospective
Consecutive eyes	Yes	No	Yes	NR
Selection criteria specified	No	No	Yes	NR
Independent statistical analysis	No	No	NR	No
Study parameters				
Surgery date	9/1990-9/1991	10/1985-1991	4/1985-4/1988	1983-1984
Follow-up time: (range/average)	1 month to 1 year/1 year	0.25 to 2 year	NR	NR/1 year
Number of eyes operated	205	79	409	350
Number of patients operated	125	70	364	198
Age of patients: (range/average)	22-62 yr/38.4 ±8.6 years	23-63 yr/35 years	22-64 yr/35.77 yr	20-41
% eyes followed up	100%	66%	65% at 6 months 41% at 12 months	NR
Instrumentation				
Ultrasonic pachometry	Yes	Yes	Yes	Yes
Micrometer	Yes	Yes-handle	Yes-handle	Yes-handle
Surgery				
Preoperative variables considered in nomogram (e.g., myopia amount, sex, age, corneal thickness, keratometry, IOP, ocular rigidity, corneal diameter)	Casebeer nomogram	Salz nomogram	Refraction, corneal thickness	Refraction, age
Clear zone diameters	2.75 to 5.0 mm		NR	3 to 4 mm
Number of incisions	4, 8, 16	4 to 8	8 (100%)	4, 8
Incision direction	Centripetal	Centrifugal	Centrifugal	Centrifugal
Blade setting	100% of pachymetry reading measured 1.5 mm temporal to the corneal light reflex	110% thinnest paracentral reading	110% of central reading for initial incisions; 115% of central for deepening-full length recut in centrifugal direction	100% of central reading
Single or dual pass	Single	Single	100% recut using full-length deepening incisions	Single with peripheral redeepening

Transverse incisions for astigmatism	Yes	Yes	No	No
Enhancements included in data (% of eyes)	Yes, 33%	Yes	No	Yes
Postoperative steroids	Yes	Yes	Yes	NR
Results				
Type of refraction	Cycloplegic	Manifest	Manifest	Cycloplegic
% of eyes between ± 1.00 D	NR	85%	58%	NR
% of eyes that had mild myopia (−1.00-3.00 D) preoperatively that were between ± 1.00 D postoperatively	(−2.00) − (−3.12): 30% were +0.19 ± 0.55 D	96%	65% @ 6 months 69% @ 1 year	NR
% of eyes that had moderate myopia (3.25 − 6.00) that were between ± 1.00 D	(−3.25) − > (−4.37): 20% were +0.15 ± 0.52 D	81%	39% @ 6 months 33% @ 1 year	NR
% of eyes that were highly myopic (6.25 − 10.00) that were between ± 1.00 D	(−4.50) − > (−8.00): 32% were +0.25 ± 0.58 D	67%	–	NR
% overcorrected by >1.00 D	Shift of 0.22 D @ 1 yr	19%	3%	NR
% undercorrected by >1.00 D	NR	NR	NR	NR
% of eyes with VA ≥20/40	99% (86% were 20/25 45% were 20/20)		38%	See below
% of eyes with low myopia ≥20/40 postoperatively	(−2.00) − (−3.21) mean 20/25 (0.88)	96%	48% @ 1 year	89% ≥20/30 1.5-3
% of eyes with moderate myopia ≥20/40 postoperatively	(−3.25) − (−4.37) mean 20/25 (0.85)	97%	14% @ 1 year	68% ≥20/30 3.25-4.50
% of eyes with high myopia ≥20/40 postoperatively	(−4.50) − (−8.00) mean 20/25 (0.84)	67%	NR	14% ≥20/30 4.75-6.00
% of eyes not needing contact lens or glasses	NR	NR	NR	NR
Predictability				
% of patients around a predicted outcome of: ±1.00 D ±1.50 D ±2.00 D	+0.27 ± 0.58 D residual refractive correction. Range (−0.88) to +2.50 D	NR	NR	NR
Width of 90% prediction interval	NR	NR	NR	NR
Stability				
Time interval	1 yr	NR	NR	NR
# of eyes	163	NR	NR	NR
% of eyes with refraction change ≥1 D	4%	NR	NR	NR
% of eyes with continued surgical effect (hyperopic shift)	21%	NR	NR	NR

Continued.

Table 167-1. Results of radial keratotomy—cont'd.

	Authors and publication			
Complications				
Loss of ≥2 lines of BCVA (Snellen)	NR	None	25% lost one Snellen line	NR
Loss of VA ≤20/20	NR	NR	NR	NR
% of patients with moderate to severe glare	NR	NR		
% of patients with moderate to severe vision fluctuation	3%	NR	NR	25%
Patient satisfaction				
Level of patient satisfaction:				
high	High	NR	NR	95%
medium				
low				
	Spigelman AV, Williams PA, Lindstrom RL: Further studies of four incision radial keratotomy, *Refract Corneal Surg* 5:292-295, 1989	Waring GO, Lynn MJ, McDonnell PJ, PERK Study Group: Results of the prospective evaluation of radial keratotomy (PERK) study 10 years after surgery *Arch Ophthalmol* 112:1298-1308, 1994	Kim JH: A prospective clinical study of radial keratotomy in Koreans, *J Korean Ophthalmol Soc* 2:13-21, 1988	Dietz MR, Sanders DR, Raanan MS: A consecutive series (1982-1985) of radial keratotomies performed with the diamond blade, *Am J Ophthalmol* 103:417-422, 1987
Study design				
	Retrospective	Prospective	Prospective	Prospective
Consecutive eyes	Yes	Yes	NR	Yes
Selection criteria specified	No	Yes	NR	Yes
Independent statistical analysis	No	Yes	NR	Yes
Study parameters				
Surgery date	Before 9/1986	3/1982-10/1983	2/1982-12/1986	1/1982-5/1985
Follow-up time: (range/average)	1 to 3 year/1 year	10 years	6 months-4 years/12 months	9 to 15 months/1 year
Number of eyes operated	52	681	348	972
Number of patients operated	30	374	246	458
Age of patients: (range/average)	NR	21 to 58 year/33.5 year	16 to 44 years/26 years	18 to 62 years/34.2 years
% of eyes followed up	62%	86%	NR	68%
Instrumentation				
Ultrasonic pachometry	Preoperative	Yes	Yes	Preoperative
Micrometer	Yes-handle	Yes-handle	Yes-handle	Yes-handle

Surgery				
Preoperative variables considered in nomogram (e.g., myopia amount, sex, age, corneal thickness, keratometry, IOP, ocular rigidity, corneal diameter)	Refraction, age	Myopia, corneal thickness	Refraction	Myopia amount, sex, age, corneal thickness, keratometry, IOP
Clear zone diameters	3.0 to 5.0 mm	3, 3.5, 4 mm	3 to 4 mm	2.7 to 6.0 mm
Number of incisions	4 (100%)	8 (100%)	8 (92%) 16 (5%) >30 (3%)	8 (89%) 16 (6%) Other (5%)
Incision direction	Centrifugal	Centrifugal	Centripetal	Centrifugal
Blade setting	100 to 115% of thinnest paracentral	100% of thinnest paracentral	95% of mid periphery	108% of central thickness
Single or dual pass	Single pass	Single pass	Single pass with peripheral redeepening	Majority single with recuts for >6.00 D myopes
Transverse incisions for astigmatism	No	No	Yes	Yes
Enhancements included in data (% of eyes)	No	Yes	Yes	No
Postoperative steroids	Yes	No	Yes	Yes
Results				
Type of refraction	Cycloplegic	Cycloplegic	Cycloplegic	Cycloplegic
% of eyes between ± 1.00 D	91% (range of preoperative myopes was −1.50 to −4.75 D with one eye −8.37 D)	60%	NR	76%
% of eyes that had mild myopia (−1.00-3.00 D) preoperatively that were between ± 1.00 D postoperatively	NR	−1.50 to 3.22 67%	NR	(1.5-3.0 D) 90%
% of eyes that had moderate myopia (3.25 − 6.00) that were between ± 1.00 D	NR	−3.25 to 4.37 62%	NR	(3.10-6.0 D) 76%
% of eyes that were highly myopic (6.25 − 10.00) that were between ± 1.00 D	NR	−4.50-8.87 54%	NR	(6.12-9.0 D) 53%
% overcorrected by >1.00 D	NR	23%	2%	13%
% undercorrected by >1.00 D	3%	17%	1%	12%
% of eyes with VA ≥20/40	88%	65%	(≥20/40) 56% (≥20/20) 22%	(≥20/40) 88% (≥20/20) 47%
% of eyes with low myopia ≥20/40 postoperatively	NR	92%	79% 47%	(0-3D) 96%/ 65%
% of eyes with moderate myopia ≥20/40 postoperatively	NR	86%	73% 36%	(3.12-6D) 89%/ 44%
% of eyes with high myopia ≥20/40 postoperatively	NR	77%	34% 50%	(6.12-9D) 77%/ 30%

Continued.

Table 167-1. Results of radial keratotomy—cont'd.

	Authors and publication			
% of eyes that had moderate myopia (3.25-6.00) that were between ± 1.00 D	NR	NR	(3.10-5.80) 81%	NR
% of eyes that were highly myopic (6.25-10.00) that were between ± 1.00 D	NR	NR	(6.00-11.60) 45%	NR
% overcorrected by >1.00 D	NR	7.7%	3%	13% in 16 incision group 3% in 8 incision group
% undercorrected by >1.00 D	NR	11.3%	24%	NR
% of eyes with VA ≥20/40	20/20: 100% @ 6 months 23% @ 12 months	86.1%	69%	50% in 16 incision group 65% in 8 incision group
% of eyes with low myopia ≥20/40 postoperatively	NR	NR	100%	NR
% of eyes with moderate myopia ≥20/40 postoperatively	NR	NR	73%	NR
% of eyes with high myopia ≥20/40 postoperatively	NR	NR	47%	NR
% of eyes not needing contact lens or glasses	6% wore lenses part time after RK	NR	NR	NR
Predictability				
% of patients around a predicted outcome of:	NR	NR		NR
±1.00 D			NR	
±1.50 D			NR	
±2.00 D			NR	
Width of 90% prediction interval	NR	NR	NR	NR
Stability				
Time interval	NR	NR	24 to 110 months	NR
# of eyes	NR	NR	100	NR
% of eyes with refraction change ≥1 D	NR	NR	23%	NR
% of eyes with continued surgical effect (hyperopic shift)	NR	NR	17%	NR
Complications				
Loss of ≥2 lines of BCVA (Snellen)	None	NR	1%	NR
Loss of VA ≤20/20	None	NR	2.5%	NR
% of patients with moderate to severe glare	NR	NR	NR	NR
% of patients with moderate to severe vision fluctuation	NR	NR	NR	NR

Patient satisfaction				
Level of patient satisfaction:	NR	NR	NR	NR
high				
medium				
low				
	Lavery FL: Comparative results of 200 consecutive radial keratotomy cases using three different nomograms. *J Refract Surg* 3:88-91, 1987		Nirankari VS et al: Ongoing prospective clinical study of radial keratotomy, *Ophthalmology* 90:637-641, 1983	
Study design	Retrospective		Prospective	
Consecutive	Yes		Yes	
Selection criteria specified	No		Yes	
Independent statistical analysis	No		No	
Study parameters				
Surgery date	NR		NR	
Follow-up time: (range/average)	NR/6 months		6 to 38 months/19 months	
Number of eyes operated	200		58	
Number of patients operated	NR		NR	
Age of patients: (range/average)	NR		19 to 57 years/32 years	
% eyes followed up	100%		100% @ 6 months	
Instrumentation				
Ultrasonic pachometry	NR		Yes	
Micrometer	Yes-handle		Yes-handle	
Surgery				
Preoperative variables considered in nomogram (e.g., myopia amount, sex, age, corneal thickness, keratometry, IOP, ocular rigidity, corneal diameter)	Used other published nomograms of Sawelson, Ellis and Thorton		NR	
Clear zone diameters	NR		3 mm only	
Number of incisions	4 to 16		8, 16 (76%)	
Incision direction	Centrifugal		Centrifugal	
Blade setting	Central optical pachometer reading plus 15%		100% of central	
Single or dual pass	Single with peripheral redeepening		Single with peripheral redeepening	
Transverse incisions for astigmatism	Yes		NR	
Enhancements included in data (% of eyes)	No		Yes	
Postoperative steroids	Yes		Yes	
Results				
Type of refraction	Cycloplegic		NR	
% of eyes between ± 1.00 D	NR		43%	

Continued.

Table 167-1. Results of radial keratotomy—cont'd.

	Authors and publication		
% of eyes that had mild myopia (−1.00-3.00 D) pre-op that were between ± 1.00 D postoperatively	70% to 92%		NR
% of eyes that had moderate myopia (3.25-6.00) that were between ± 1.00 D postoperatively	77% to 100%		NR
% of eyes that were highly myopic (6.25-10.00) that were between ± 1.00 D	27% to 70%		NR
% overcorrected by >1.00 D	10% to 25%		NR
% undercorrected by >1.00 D	0 to 55%		61%
% of eyes with VA ≥20/40	≥20/40 25-44%	≥20/20 39-57%	48%
% of eyes with low myopia ≥20/40 postoperatively	NR	69% to 100% 1.5 to 3.0	<5.00 D 65%
% of eyes with moderate myopia ≥20/40 postoperatively	NR	54% to 75% 3.25 to 4.50	
% of eyes with high myopia ≥20/40 postoperatively	NR	30% to 44% 4.75 to 9.95	>5.00 D 19%
% of eyes not needing contact lens or glasses	NR		NR
Predictability			
% of patients around a predicted outcome of: ±1.00 D ±1.50 D ±2.00 D	NR		NR
Width of 90% prediction interval	NR		NR
Stability			
Time interval	1 year		NR
# of eyes	NR		NR
% of eyes with refraction change ≥1 D	NR		NR
% of eyes with continued surgical effect (hyperopic shift)	NR		NR
Complications			
Loss of ≥2 lines of BCVA (Snellen)	NR		NR

Loss of VA $\leq 20/20$	NR	NR
% of patients with moderate to severe glare	NR	NR
% of patients with moderate to severe vision fluctuation	NR	NR
Patient satisfaction		
Level of patient satisfaction:	NR	NR
high		
medium		
low		

IOP, intraocular pressure; *NR,* not reported; *BCVA,* best corrected visual acuity; *VA,* visual acuity.

Published Studies

WERBLIN ET AL.

In the early 1990s, the Casebeer system for keratorefractive surgery was developed and marketed to ophthalmologists as a way to achieve precise results with radial keratotomy. "The system" involved all aspects of radial keratotomy including preoperative screening, intraoperative equipment, and postoperative care. The reported results in the study by Werblin et al. were outstanding, with 99% of patients achieving 20/40 or better vision, and 86% achieving 20/25 or better. Individual postoperative refractive errors ranged from − 0.88 to + 2.50 diopters. Follow-up at 1 year was 100%, a rarity in most clinical reports on the results of radial keratotomy. The high success rates were attributed to better instrumentation, nomograms, and a high enhancement rate. Six patients required resuturing of incisions to decrease the effect (suture enhancement). Incisions were made toward the optical zone from the limbus, which are generally deeper than incisions beginning at the optical zone and directed toward the limbus. Twenty-one percent of eyes did show a hyperopic drift with time. These results have not been matched by other reported series. Three-year follow-up data on 128 patients showed that the amount of hyperopic shift slowed over 3 years (from + 0.34 D/year to + 0.12 D/year). Ninety-six percent of eyes had an uncorrected visual acuity of 20/40.

Results of other surgeons using the Casebeer system have been reported. These studies were not as complete as the Werblin study, but do allow for at least some comparison to see if "the system" can potentially remove the surgeon factor in predicting results. A retrospective study of surgery performed by Gordon et al.[8] reported 20/40 or better uncorrected vision in 98% of eyes, with 85% within ± 1 diopter of emmetropia. An enhancement rate of 43% was reported. A study by Robin et al.[9] on results with "the system" reported 20/40 or better uncorrected vision in 79% of patients, with 3 to 9 months of follow-up and an enhancement rate of 29%.

FRIEDBERG ET AL.

This retrospective study examined the results of radial keratotomy performed by novice refractive surgeons, namely corneal fellows. It is generally assumed that there is a significant learning curve in performing radial keratotomy, but this study demonstrated that good results (96% of patients with mild myopia and 97% of patients with moderate myopia achieved a postoperative visual acuity of 20/40 or better) were possible by inexperienced refractive surgeons.

BAUERBERG ET AL.

The overall results of this study were not as good as others. In fact, only 38% of eyes had an uncorrected visual acuity of 20/40 or better. The authors were able to correct larger amounts of myopia than is generally thought to be safely correctable (up to 12 diopters) by using a double pass technique in which the blade was reset 5% deeper during a second full-length pass. The rate of corneal perforation was not mentioned.

ARNE ET AL.

A majority of patients with low myopia (89%) and moderate myopia (68%) achieved vision of approximately 20/30 postoperatively, but only 14% of high myopes reached this level.

SPIGELMAN ET AL.

The overall percentage of patients with an uncorrected postoperative vision of ≥ 20/40 was 88%. This study involved the use of only four incisions and the range of preoperative myopia was smaller (1.5 to 4.75 diopters) than most other published studies. Despite limiting the number of radial incisions to four, however, 23% of patients noted moderate to severe glare postoperatively, and 30% of patients noted vision fluctuation. In most cases, these symptoms improved with time. No patients, however, experienced a loss of best corrected vision, suggesting that a four-incision approach is safer than nomograms calling for 8, 12, or 16 incisions.

WARING ET AL. (PERK 10-YEAR RESULTS)

The PERK study is considered the gold standard when judging the results of radial keratotomy. Unlike other studies, the PERK study was prospective, had specified selection criteria, reported the results of consecutive eyes, was independently funded, and used independent statistical analysis. Eighty-six percent of patients were seen at the 10-year follow-up, a high successful follow-up rate compared to other studies. Eighty-five percent of all eyes achieved 20/40 or better visual acuity. Sixty-three percent of patients less than 40 years of age were totally spectacle independent. However, the 90% prediction interval was a wide 4.42 diopters. Three percent of patients lost two or more lines of best corrected visual acuity, but 35% gained one to two lines of best corrected vision. PERK was the only study to report the percentage of postoperative anisometropia (another measure of predictability), with 88% of eyes having 2 diopters or less.

Perhaps the finding of most interest to ophthalmologists was the phenomenon of progressive hyperopia. Forty-three percent of eyes showed a refractive change of ≥ 1 diopter, and 81% of eyes showed some movement toward hyperopia after surgery. Of concern is the fact that the PERK nomogram was not a particularly aggressive method of radial keratotomy (eight incisions maximum, centrifugal incisions, one pass with no redeepening). Because most other studies either ignore the phenomenon of hyperopic progression or do not have sufficient follow-up to detect it, the finding is important in assessing radial keratotomy's long-term stability and predictability.

The results of the PERK study are often criticized for several reasons. The nomogram did not evaluate the age of the patient, which is now considered to be an important variable in determining how a patient will respond to surgery (the older the patient, the more response); enhancement procedures were discouraged; and multiple surgeons with varying experience operated at multiple sites. These factors might be important in the percentage of patients achieving 20/40 or better vision, but would not be expected to play a role in the phenomenon of progressive hyperopia.

KIM

The overall percentage of patients with ≥20/40 vision was a relatively low 56%. Of interest, centripetal incisions were made, and 3% of patients had more than 30 incisions. It is generally believed that one can expect 90% to 95% effect of surgery with eight incisions, and that additional incisions have little effect on the refractive outcome.

DEITZ ET AL.

Eighty-eight percent of all patients had a postoperative acuity of 20/40 or better. Progressive hyperopia of 1 or more diopters was also noted in 35% of cases.

VAUGHAN ET AL.

This study evaluated four-incision radial keratotomy in low myopia (<3 diopters). Ninety-three percent of those seen at the 12-month follow-up had 20/20 visual acuity and 100% of those followed for 3.5 years achieved 20/20 vision without correction. However, only 10 of the original 86 patients in this study were examined (12%) at this time.

SHEPARD ET AL.

The overall percentage of patients with 20/40 or better vision postoperatively was 86.1%, with no further breakdown of results. With 1,058 cases reported, this was the largest published series on the results of radial keratotomy. Various surgical techniques were used, and 72% of patients had bilateral simultaneous surgery. Follow-up time for some of the patients was shorter than 1 year. The authors commented that contrary to conventional teaching, the depth of the incisions was probably not important.

SALZ ET AL.

This study suggested that radial keratotomy could be titrated, making four incisions initially and adding incisions as necessary. With this approach, the overall percentage of patients achieving 20/40 or better visual acuity postoperatively was 69% (less than other reports), but the percentage of patients overcorrected by more than 1 diopter was small (3%). Because radial keratotomy can result in wildly unpredictable results in individual patients, this approach has its merits. Even though patients were more likely to remain somewhat undercorrected compared to those who underwent other more aggressive techniques, this approach had several advantages:

1. The potential for progressive postoperative hyperopia in the future is lessened.
2. Better toleration of postoperative myopia than postoperative hyperopia.
3. Less dependency on reading spectacles (delayed onset of symptomatic hyperopia).

HOFFER ET AL.

This series examined the results of 16- and 8-incision radial keratotomy. Interestingly, the overall percentage of patients with uncorrected visual acuity of ≥20/40 was higher in the 8-incision group (65% versus 50%). There was also a higher percentage of patients with a refractive error of ≥1.00 diopters in the 16-incision group. This is one of the earlier studies reported using diamond blades.

LAVERY

This study was undertaken by one surgeon reporting his results over time with three different nomograms. His results varied from 25% to 44% of patients visible acuity ≥20/40. However, the three different techniques were performed in sequence; therefore, his finding that the Thornton nomogram was the best of the three may have been partially due to his increased surgical experience.

NIRANKARI ET AL.

Some metal blades were used in this study. Interestingly, the authors also reported that results did not differ whether 8 or 16 incisions were made.

RESULTS AND PREDICTABILITY OF RADIAL KERATOMETRY

From a review of the data presented in Table 167-1, it is clear that the results of radial keratotomy have improved over time. One can conclude that patients in the low to moderate myopia group had an excellent chance of having 20/40 or better uncorrected visual acuity (in the 80% to 90% range). This percentage

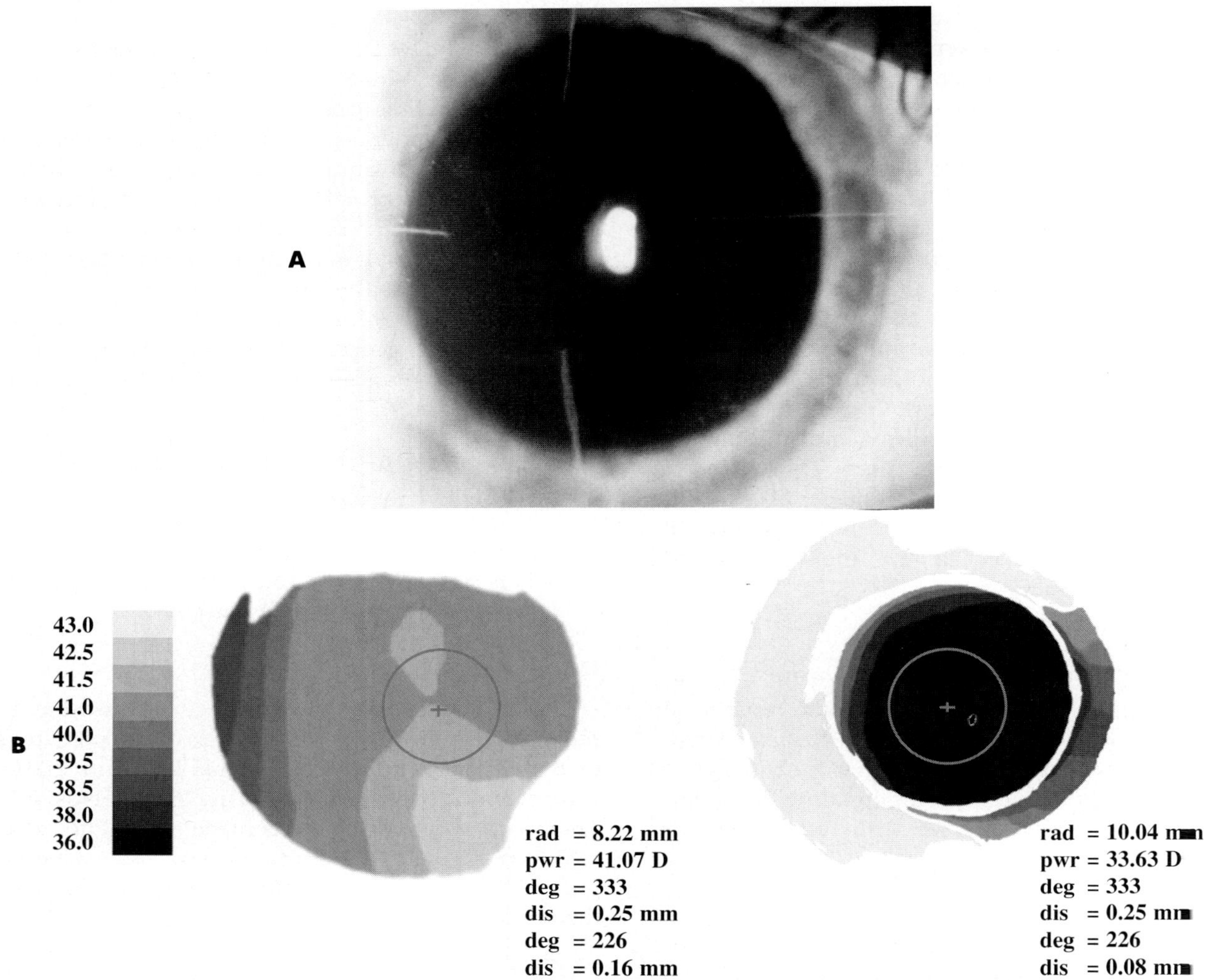

FIGURE 167-1 Eight diopters of corneal flattening achieved after a 4 incision radial keratotomy with a 3 mm optical zone. **A,** Postoperative clinical appearance. **B,** Topographic maps before surgery (*left*) and 1 week after surgery (*right*).

drops off significantly after −6.00 diopters of preoperative myopia. Perioperative medications, especially topical corticosteroids also play an important role in the final visual outcome. For patients with low amounts of myopia, four incision radial keratotomy appears to be predictable. However, the trend of progressive hyperopia is worrisome. For this reason, surgeons may wish to aim for a postoperative result slightly less than emmetropia. The risk of a loss of best corrected visual acuity is small as are severe vision-threatening complications.

The predictability of radial keratotomy is more difficult to ascertain. Few of the reports give a range of refraction around a predicted outcome. Many times, one can only assume the intended postoperative refractive goal was emmetropia when in fact a monovision correction might have been attempted. A summary of results from published reports (some of the papers have been included in Table 167-1) found that the percentage of eyes that achieved a refraction between −1.00 and +1.00 diopters at 6 to 12 months postoperatively varied from 39% to 100%.[10] Individual cases of larger overcorrections have been reported.[11] Figure 167-1 demonstrates one example from the author's experience in which 8 diopters of corneal flattening (demonstrated by computed topography) resulted after four centrifugal incisions with a 3.0 mm optical zone. For this reason, a conservative, titratable approach toward radial keratotomy seems reasonable.

Symmetry of Results

One must consider the final refractive error of both eyes, not simply that vision is "20/40 or 20/25 uncorrected." In a case in which a patient's right eye was

−1.25 diopters and the left was +2.25 diopters and both eyes saw 20/25, patient satisfaction would most likely be low because of anisometropia and aniseikonia. Most reports do not mention symmetry of results in their data. The PERK study, however, reported that 1 year after surgery on the second eye, the median difference between the two eyes was 0.62 diopters, with a range of 0 to 6.87 diopters. Ninety percent of the patients had a difference of 2 D or less, and 2% had refractive differences between the two eyes that were greater than 3.00 diopters.[12]

Other Trends in Radial Keratotomy

In recent years, newer instrumentation and techniques have evolved that affect the overall outcome of radial keratotomy.

COMPUTED TOPOGRAPHY AND RADIAL KERATOTOMY

There is no question that computed topography systems have aided refractive surgeons in the preoperative and perioperative management of patients undergoing radial keratotomy. It provides more information on more of the cornea than is possible with keratometry. Studies have suggested that some of the aberrant results in radial keratotomy and progressive hyperopia have been due to surgeons operating on subclinical keratoconus, which was previously undetected by standard keratometry.[13] Using computed topography as a screening device, we have not created one patient with hyperopia of more than 0.25 diopters in 2 years of performing radial keratotomy. Since 1994, most surgeons would hesitate to perform refractive surgery on a patient without preoperative topography. It will take several years, however, for published reports to demonstrate whether the overall results are better with this relatively new technology.

SIMULTANEOUS BILATERAL RADIAL KERATOTOMY

Some surgeons recommend performing radial keratotomy in both eyes at the same surgical setting. The rationale for this technique includes an attempt to decrease the possible variations in technique that might occur between operations (e.g., blade sharpness, the steadiness of the surgeon's hand) and not subjecting a patient to the expense or inconvenience of two operations. A retrospective study by Moreira et al.[14] compared results obtained by one surgeon who operated both eyes in one setting and cases in which the patient underwent the procedures on different occasions. The average postoperative refractive errors for eye 1 and eye 2 in both groups were not statistically significant. The overall overcorrection rate in both groups were similar. Thus, performing simultaneous radial keratotomy did not improve the overall outcome.

The potential benefits of simultaneous bilateral radial keratotomy must be weighed against the potential disadvantages. First, and most important, there is the increased potential for bilateral infectious keratitis, which has been reported.[15] In addition, simultaneous surgery eliminates the opportunity to use the result in the first eye to modify the procedure in the second eye. Finally, some patients choose not to have surgery on the second eye, and this technique prevents that decision.

MINIMALLY INVASIVE OR "MINI-RK"

In this technique, incisions are intentionally stopped well short of the limbus (at a 7 or 8 mm optical zone), and no more than eight incisions are used in an attempt to increase predictability and safety. No large studies have been published comparing this technique to other methods of radial keratotomy techniques, but Lindstrom[16] has reported results of a pilot clinical study, retrospectively reviewing 100 eyes undergoing 4- or 8-incision "mini-RK." The range of preoperative myopia was −1.00 to −6.00 diopters. At 6 months, 92% of eyes were within 1 diopter of emmetropia, and 94% had 20/40 or better uncorrected visual acuity with no enhancements. No patient was overcorrected by more than 1 diopter. Eight eyes had enhancements; and when these eyes were included in the data, 98% were within 1 D of emmetropia and 100% had 20/40 or better uncorrected vision.

HEXAGONAL KERATOTOMY

This incisional surgical approach is used to correct hyperopia, whether it existed preoperatively or as a result of previous refractive surgery. The refinement of this procedure has been largely one of trial and error. These refinements have included the size and pattern of the hexagonal keratotomy, as well as additions such as the "Hex T."[17] It is a controversial procedure because of its questionable safety and predictability and is not widely accepted by refractive surgeons.

Results of Excimer Laser Photorefractive Keratectomy

Studies with the excimer laser for the correction of myopia have been ongoing in the United States during the last 3 years, compared to more than 10 years of

Table 167-2. Excimer laser photorefractive keratectomy results

Study	Epstein et al	Maguen et al	Talley et al	Dutt et al
Follow-up period	2 years	3 years	1 year	1 year
Eyes treated	495	240	91	47
Preoperative refraction	−1.25 → −7.50 D	−1.00 −> −7.75 D	−1.00 −> −7.50 D	−1.50 −> −6.10 D
% of eyes ≥ 20/40 uncorrected	91%	@ 3 months 88% @ 1 year 89% @ 3 years 90%	@ 6 months 95% @ 1 year 98%	94%
% of eyes within ± 1D of goal	87.5%	@ 3 months 86% @ 1 year 79% @ 3 years 90%	@ 6 months 93% @ 1 year 85%	80%
% of eyes ≥ 1D hyperopia	1%	2.5%	3.3%	15%
% of eyes with 2 diopter loss of BCVA	0%	@ 3 months 10% @ 1 year 4%	1 patient lost 3 lines	0%

BCVA, best corrected visual acuity.

studies on radial keratotomy. These results are being carefully watched by refractive surgeons. Some have predicted that excimer laser photorefractive keratectomy may completely replace radial keratotomy as the primary surgical means to correct myopia.

Table 167-2 summarizes four excimer studies with at least 1 year of follow-up.[18-21] Studies in which larger amounts of myopia were treated are not included.[22] Data reported in these studies tend to be presented in a much more unified manner, as compared to data on radial keratotomy, perhaps because many of these procedures were performed as part of a clinical trial monitored by the Food and Drug Administration. Based on these data, the following conclusions can be reached:

1. The overall percentage of patients with an uncorrected visual acuity of 20/40 or better averages more than 90%. For correction of low amounts of myopia, the percentage is often well above 90%, with a tight predictability range. With moderate myopia, the percentages decrease with a wider predictability range. The same phenomenon is seen in radial keratotomy. However, the predictability range is wider in radial keratotomy in the moderate myopia group. Only 71% of cases in the Werblin Radial Keratometry study achieved 20/40 uncorrected visual acuity after one operation, whereas in most cases, excimer patients need only one treatment.
2. There is a small but clinically significant number of patients who, as in radial keratotomy, will overrespond to the surgery, and others who will underrespond to the surgery.
3. The number of eyes left with a refraction of 1 or more diopters of hyperopia is less (especially if the study by Dutt[22] is excluded) than with radial keratotomy (e.g., 1% in the Epstein study versus 23% in the PERK study).
4. There appears to be a regression of effect with the excimer that stabilizes after 12 to 24 months. No reports of progressive hyperopia have been published to date. The advantages of leaving patients slightly myopic after surgery have been discussed previously.
5. The percentage of patients with a loss of best corrected visual acuity is probably similar between the two operations. More excimer patients have reported an improvement in best corrected visual acuity compared to radial keratotomy.
6. There is less variability in results obtained by the various investigators between excimer laser reports and radial keratotomy results.

It is not clear whether excimer laser is better than radial keratotomy because of the multiplicity of variables involved in their evaluation. However, from the single perspective of visual results, early reports suggest that the excimer is a more accurate refractive tool for the correction of moderate amounts of myopia.

Summary

Radial keratotomy can safely reduce myopia. It has withstood the test of time as an effective refractive surgical technique. Further refinements may produce even better results.

REFERENCES

1. Waring GO: *Refractive keratotomy for myopia and astigmatism,* St Louis, 1992, Mosby.
2. Leaming DV: Practice styles and preferences of ASCRS members: 1993 survey, *J Cataract Refract Surg* 20:459-467, 1994.
3. Maguire LJ: Keratorefractive surgery, success, and the public health, *Am J Ophthalmol* 117:394-398, 1994.
4. Bourque LB, Lynn MJ, Waring GO, Cartwright C: Spectacle and contact lens wearing six years after radial keratotomy in the prospective evaluation of radial keratotomy study, *Ophthalmology* 101:421-431, 1994.

5. Waring GO: *Refractive keratotomy for myopia and astigmatism,* St Louis, 1992, Mosby.
6. Committee on Ophthalmic Procedures Assessment, American Academy of Ophthalmology: Radial keratotomy for myopia, *Ophthalmology* 100:1103-1115, 1993.
7. Werblin TP, Stafford GM: Should progressive hyperopia be a serious concern after routine refractive keratotomy procedures. Submitted for publication, Nov. 1994, Ophthalmology.
8. Gordon JF et al: A retrospective study of the Casebeer system for incisional keratorefractive surgery, *Invest Ophthalmol Vis Sci* 34: 1243, 1993.
9. Robin SB, Epstein RJ, Robin JB: Casebeer-system refractive keratotomy: a multi-surgeon retrospective evaluation, *Invest Ophthalmol Vis Sci* 34:1243, 1993.
10. Committee on Ophthalmic Procedures Assessment, American Academy of Ophthalmology: Radial keratotomy for myopia, *Ophthalmology* 100:1106, 1993.
11. Waisberg Y: Bilateral high hyperopia after radial keratotomy, *J Cataract Refract Surg* 19:88-89, 1993.
12. Lynn MJ et al: Symmetry of refractive and visual acuity outcome in the Prospective Evaluation of Radial Keratotomy (PERK) study, *J Refract Corneal Surg* 5:75-81, 1989.
13. Saragoussi JJ, Pouliquen YJ: Does the progressive increasing effect of radial keratotomy correlate with undetected early keratoconus, *J Refract Corneal Surg* 10:45-48, 1994.
14. Moreira H et al: Retrospective comparison of simultaneous and non-simultaneous bilateral radial keratotomy, *J Refract Corneal Surg* 10:545-549, 1994.
15. Szerenyi K et al: Keratitis as a complication of bilateral, simultaneous, radial keratotomy, *Am J Ophthalmol* 117:462-467, 1994.
16. Lindstrom RL: Minimally invasive radial keratotomy: "mini-RK", *J Cataract Refract Surg* 21:27-34, 1995.
17. Neumann AC, McCarty GR: Hexagonal keratotomy for the correction of low hyperopia: preliminary results of a prospective study, *J Cataract Refract Surg* 14:265-269, 1988.
18. Epstein D, Fagerholm P, Hamberg-Nystrom H: Twenty-four month follow up of excimer laser photorefractive keratectomy for myopia, *Ophthalmology* 101:1558-1564, 1994.
19. Maguen E et al: Results of excimer laser photorefractive keratectomy for the correction of myopia, *Ophthalmology* 101: 1548-1557, 1994.
20. Talley AR et al: Results one year after using the 193-nm excimer laser for photorefractive keratectomy in mild to moderate myopia, *Am J Ophthalmol* 118:304-311, 1994.
21. Dutt S et al: One-year results of excimer laser photorefractive keratectomy for low to moderate myopia, *Arch Ophthalmol* 112: 1427-1436, 1994.
22. Sher NA et al: 193-nm excimer photorefractive keratectomy in high myopia, *Ophthalmology* 101:1575-1582, 1994.

CHAPTER 168

SCOTT X. STEVENS DOUGLAS A. YOUNG PETER J. POLACK JULIE C. TSAI
BRADLEY D. FOURAKER J. JAMES ROWSEY

Complications of Radial Keratotomy

Complications of radial keratotomy can be reduced by careful attention to detail. In this chapter we review complications of radial keratotomy and efficacious methods for avoiding them and for correcting surgical problems.

Intraoperative Complications

ANESTHESIA

Complications associated with peribulbar or retrobulbar anesthesia were reported in the early development of radial keratotomy. These complications included superficial blood staining of the cornea from subconjunctival hemorrhage,[1] retrobulbar hemorrhage,[2] and perforation of the globe[3] or optic nerve[4] with resultant optic atrophy. A few cases of retinal detachment following radial keratotomy complicated by microperforation or macroperforation have been attributed to rapid decompression of eyes with preexisting retinal pathology.[5]

Today most refractive surgeons use topical anesthesia in one form or another. Immediate toxic reactions to topical anesthetics are rare, and cross-allergy phenomena are unlikely. History of previous allergic reactions is obviously helpful. We currently use a combination of topical 0.5% proparacaine hydrochloride followed by topical 0.75% bupivicaine hydrochloride for most refractive surgical procedures.

In cases involving general anesthesia, most surgeons advocate the use of a mild sedative or anxiolytic. However, an overly sedated patient may be uncooperative and may not maintain fixation, causing a decentered optical zone. In addition there are risks of respiratory and cardiac depression.

PROCEDURE-RELATED

Perforations of the globe by the blade have been divided into microperforations (efflux of aqueous without shallowing of the anterior chamber) or macroperforations (resulting in shallowing of the anterior chamber and requiring placement of sutures).[6] Early studies referred to any entry into the anterior chamber as a microperforation even if sutures were ultimately placed. More recent studies distinguish between microperforations and macroperforations, especially when comparing differing techniques of radial keratotomy. Higher rates of perforation in early radial keratotomy studies may be attributed to the use of metal blades, less accurate methods of determining blade cutting depth, redeepening procedures, and less accurate pachometry techniques and instrumentation.[7] American or downhill cutting technique appears to have a lower rate of perforation than the Russian or up-hill cutting technique, especially when pressure is applied to the eye.[8]

Today microperforations are the most common intraoperative complication. Nevertheless, many surgeons believe that microperforations are not only acceptable to a degree but also are desirable because they indicate an adequate depth of incisions. Earlier (before 1984) studies reported microperforation rates approaching 40% (0%,[9] 19%,[10] 30%,[7] 15%,[11] 37%,[12] 30%,[13] 10%,[14] 35%,[15] and 10%[16]) and macroperforation rates up to 10% (5%[16]). Sometimes the distinction between microperforation and macroperforation was not made. Later studies, which the use of micrometer diamond knives and ultrasonic pachometry, reported lower microperforation rates[8,17] and macroperforation rates.[17] In a study probably bridging both these periods, Marmer[18] reported a microperforation rate of 7.4% and a macroperforation rate of 0.16%.

Microperforations are associated with an increased risk of complications and should be avoided. A barely moist cornea is important to prevent corneal perforation by permitting smooth movement of the footplates during incision-making and decreasing dessication, resulting in thinning of the cornea. Microperforation should be carefully noted to prevent the development of a macroperforation. Even so, entry into the anterior chamber may not be evident clinically at the time of the procedure.[19] Entry into the anterior chamber increases the risk of endophthalmitis,[14,20] epithelial ingrowth, asymmetric astigmatism,[21] and decreased structural integrity. Persistent iritis associated with perforation has also been implicated in the development of cystoid

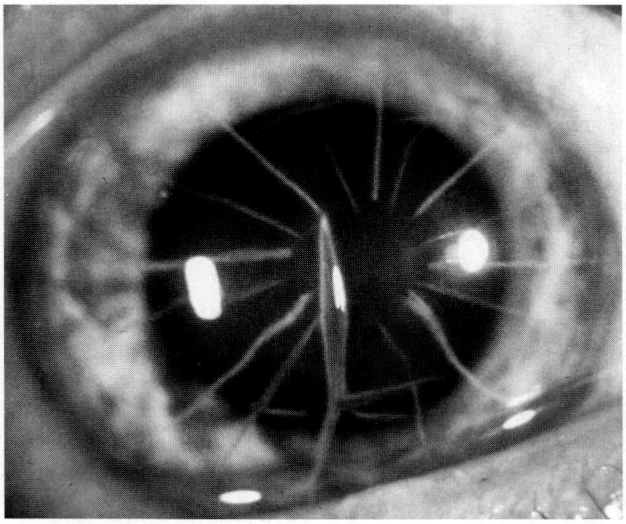

FIGURE 168-1 A radial incision passes through the visual axis, resulting in marked reduction of visual acuity.

macular edema.[22] Patients should be forewarned of the perforation potential and should be seen the day after any perforation to delineate signs of infection. The patient should be informed of any perforation and the necessary vigilance for pain or decreasing vision, both harbingers of infection.

Cataract formation has been associated with perforating radial incisions[14] or aggressive steroid treatment of persistent iritis following a presumed wound leak.[20,23] Cataracts may also occur if the chamber shallows from lack of high intraocular pressure maintenance as the cornea bends posteriorly beneath the diamond knife. Other cases of cataract formation and loss of anterior chamber with development of synechiae and secondary glaucoma have been more obvious, with gross negligence a major factor.[24]

Errant incisions include deviation into the optical zone, incorrect number of incisions, curvilinear incisions, incorrect meridian of incisions, incisions across the limbus, and intersecting incisions (Figure 168-1). Except for symptoms of glare, a single incision breaching the visual axis, more common in centripetal or Russian techniques, may cause no other sequelae. However, glare and other symptoms such as ghost images, starburst, or monocular diplopia can often be quite debilitating. The likelihood of placing an incorrect number of incisions increases with the number of incisions in the surgical plan. Curvilinear incisions, commonly seen with the Russian technique, may also be due to patient movement, excessive resistance to gliding of the knife across the corneal surface, use of a very thin blade, cutting an eye with low intraocular pressure, or attempts to recut an existing incision. They have not been shown to significantly affect the final refractive outcome. Incisions across the limbus, part of the original Fyodorov technique, have been shown to result in vascularization of the cornea through the incisions[25] and can negate any initially beneficial refractive effect and increase the risk of irregular astigmatism. In addition, vascularization can increase the likelihood of graft rejection in complicated cases that ultimately required penetrating keratoplasty. Intersecting incisions are potentially more serious and can lead to instability of the cornea and healing difficulties, including persistent wound gape with epithelial inclusion cysts[26] and stromal melting.[27] Use of centrifugal cuts, adequate anesthesia, a blade that is not too thin, adequate fixation, a moist but not wet surface, and avoidance of overly bright illumination (which may stimulate a Bell's reflex) help decrease the chance of stray incisions.

A decentered optical zone is most often attributable to poor surgical technique and may result in glare, halos or starburst, or even astigmatism. Uozato et al.[28] have demonstrated the superiority of centering the surgery about the patient's visual axis, rather than using the geographic or geometric center of the cornea.

Early Postoperative Complications

PAIN

Most patients experience pain that may last from 24 to 72 hours after surgery.[6] The use of oral analgesics or narcotics and sedatives in the first 2 days will usually alleviate the pain. Early in the Prospective Evaluation of Radial Keratotomy (PERK) study,[29,30] most patients were patched for 12 to 24 hours after surgery; however, patching increased postoperative pain. Most surgeons have stopped using a patch. Alternatively, the use of topical nonsteroidals (Voltaren or Acular) in the eye at the end of the surgery along with antibiotic-steroid (Tobradex) eye drops frequently leads to improved patient comfort. This combination allows the patient to leave the hospital patch free. Use of a bandage contact lens can also be considered for patient comfort, although it may lead to some stromal swelling, with an enhanced surgical effect in the early postoperative period. Rowsey and Balyeat[31] found that patients whose incisions were close to or across the corneoscleral limbus experienced more discomfort for a longer period of time than those patients whose incisions were limited to clear cornea.

PHOTOPHOBIA

In the PERK study, photophobia commonly occurred for a few weeks after surgery as a result of epithelial defects, mild stromal edema and inflammation, and mild iridocyclitis.[30,32] Wearing dark glasses immediately after surgery and in the first few postoperative weeks is helpful. Topical corticosteroids used four times a day for 1 month ameliorates the stromal edema and anterior chamber inflammation.

EPITHELIAL DEFECTS AND FOREIGN BODY SENSATION

Small epithelial defects along the incision can occur. These and the incisions themselves can cause foreign body sensation and pain. Epithelial defects usually heal without difficulty in 48 hours. Artificial tears help soothe the foreign body irritation, whereas ointments should be avoided. Punctate staining may also appear over the incisions and usually disappears by 1 week after surgery. Sawelson and Marks[33] reported that one third of their patients had foreign body sensation similar to those of dry eye symptoms, which resolved after lubrication. Filaments have also been reported to occur along incision lines in patients with dry eye.[34]

FLUCTUATING VISION AND CORNEAL EDEMA

Diurnal fluctuation in vision is a common side effect reported anywhere from 1.9% to 60% of cases after radial keratotomy.* Most of the fluctuation occurs within the first few weeks after surgery and subsides by 6 months after surgery, but some patients continue to complain of vision fluctuation for years.[4,42-45] The fluctuation of vision can be caused by (1) temporary changes from surface drying and eyelid movement, (2) diurnal topographic changes, (3) long-term changes associated with wound healing, and (4) underlying undiagnosed keratoconus.[32] Several factors influence diurnal variation in vision. One factor is residual stromal edema, which occurs around incisions and enhances the effect of the surgery temporarily. As the epithelial barrier of the zonula occludens is restored and the fluid is pumped out by the endothelium, the edema gradually disappears.[2,29] Stromal edema is more pronounced in the mornings after the eyelids have been closed all night. As the day progresses, the cornea tends to deturgesce. A flatter cornea is observed in the morning than in the afternoon. Thus, patients who are overcorrected may see better in the evenings than in the mornings. On the other hand, individuals who are slightly undercorrected will be more myopic in the evenings. In the clinic, one can rapidly determine if a patient is overcorrected (better evening) or undercorrected (better morning vision). In the PERK study, 33.5% of patients reported difficulty with daily fluctuations of vision after 1 year.[30,35,46] This daily fluctuation was measured objectively by visual acuity, corneal curvature, and refractive error.[35] In a selected group of patients, 44% of treated eyes had 0.50 diopters or more of change in refractive error from morning to night.

*References 11, 12, 16, 18, 35-41.

During the first year after surgery, the vision is unstable because of the change in corneal configuration as wound healing is active. The normal pattern of wound healing after radial keratotomy surgery was studied by Waring et al.[47] using slit lamp microscopy on 84 eyes from the PERK study. They observed the incisions from 2 weeks to 3 years postoperatively. At 3 months they noted fine spicules protruding at right angles from the incisions. By 1 year, these spicules had disappeared from the anterior part of the incisions and were concentrated in the posterior parts. By 2 to 3 years, these spicules had disappeared in all but the deepest portion of the incisions. They believed that persistence of these spicules suggested that wound healing may take 2 or more years to complete. As the wound heals, vision stabilizes as the cornea tends to heal toward the evening visual acuity.[35,42,46] Variation and delays in wound healing after radial keratotomy can explain the lack of predictability of refractive outcomes and continued refractive changes long term.[32,47-50]

Another factor contributing to fluctuation of vision is variation in intraocular pressure.[35,51,52] A higher pressure flattens the corneal surface, enhancing the radial keratotomy effect. This effect may be of consequence in the overcorrected patient, as a lowering of the pressure may decrease the overcorrection.

REDUCED BEST CORRECTED VISUAL ACUITY

In the PERK study, reduced best corrected manual acuity is defined as a loss of two or more Snellen lines.[30] A decrease in best corrected visual acuity may occur in 1% to 3% of all patients after radial keratotomy.[42] In the PERK study at the 5 year follow-up, only 3% of eyes lost two or three lines of Snellen acuity.[53] After 10 years, this did not change (3% or 23 of 793 eyes).[54] Causes of decrease in vision include operative, corneal, and intraocular complications. These complications are discussed in detail later.

GLARE

Mild to moderate glare has been reported in up to 30% to 50% of cases after surgery but diminishes over time[29,43,55,56] to 0 to 4% after 1 year.* Most patients see radiating lines around light sources at night that usually do not disrupt visual function. Disabling glare is defined as that amount of glare that disrupts normal activity so that the patients have changed occupation or curtailed night driving.[4,42] In the PERK study, 17% of patients noted glare before and after radial keratotomy. Fluctuating vision was noted in 12% of 354 patients 1

*References 29, 33, 34, 51, 52, 55, 57, 58.

year after monocular surgery.[30] At 5 years, 36% of patients continued to note fluctuating vision from morning to evening.[53]

Causes of glare include a mobile or dilated pupil, or too small an optical zone (less than 3.0 mm) causing the patient to see the edges of the incisions.[31] Rowsey and Balyeat[31] observed that a 3.0 mm optical zone produced a higher incidence of glare (79% of 40 patients) compared to 20% of 10 patients with a 4.0 mm optical zone.[31] Glare also may be aggravated by inadvertent stray incisions into the optical zone. Extensive incisional scarring over the incision can produce more glare, especially in the presence of debris within the incision. An increase in glare is associated with reincising a previous incision near the optical zone with attendant enhanced scar formation. Irregular astigmatism also can produce glare, which is usually reported as a starburst pattern.

Management of glare

Oblique incision orientation in a 4-incision radial keratotomy can reduce the symptoms of glare as the incisions are covered by the eyelids. This technique may be especially advantageous during night driving.[59] Removal of incisional debris at the time of surgery also decreases scarring and glare. Treatment of glare includes use of high quality sunglasses with ultraviolet and infrared light blockage, miotics such as pilocarpine, 1% to 2%, four times a day, and topical steroids to decrease scar formation. Scar removal is also an option in cases of extensive scarring.[18] If the glare is disabling, corneal transplantation may be required.[60]

MONOCULAR DIPLOPIA

When the corneal surface has abnormal topography, irregular astigmatism and symptomatic diplopia may result.[51] One patient, 5 years into the PERK study, had bothersome monocular diplopia. Slit lamp examination revealed a hypertrophic scar, and corneal topography demonstrated surface irregularity over this area, prompting the patient to undergo scar revision.[18,51] Incisions through the visual axis and radial keratotomy in patients with keratoconus can lead to central irregular astigmatism. A gas permeable contact lenses may be a reasonable alternative to reduce astigmatism and restore vision.

Refractive Complications

Refractive complications include overcorrection, undercorrection, astigmatism, anisometropia, presbyopia, and a multifocal cornea.

OVERCORRECTION

Unplanned overcorrection is an undesirable complication of radial keratotomy. Converting a myopic patient to a hyperopic state can be quite bothersome to the patient. We advocate leaving the myopia slightly undercorrected to avoid overcorrecting the vision.[61] When the vision of a myopic patient is suddenly overcorrected by as little as 0.75 diopters, there is an increased demand for accommodation, with the accompanying accommodative-convergence of the near reflex. Fusional divergence is necessary to maintain binocularity. The required divergence produces more symptoms than the need for increased accommodation. Obviously, the greater the overcorrection induced by surgery, the greater the symptoms, especially if the patient has a high accommodative convergence/accommodation ratio.[62]

Overcorrection can be defined in several ways. The literal definition would mean any hyperopic refractive error. The PERK study defined hyperopia as a refraction greater than +1.00 diopters.[33,34,51,63] Sawelson and Marks[33,34] defined hyperopia as the level of hyperopia that generated visual symptoms. The accuracy of clinical refraction varies by 0.50 to 1.00 diopters. In this chapter, we use the PERK definition of hyperopia. The incidence of overcorrection therefore varies from 0.82% to 33%.* The PERK study reported an overcorrection rate of 17% at 5 years and 36% at 10 years. Arrowsmith et al.[63] reported that 33% of patients were overcorrected by more than 1 diopter at 5 years compared to 20% at 1 year. Deitz et al.[65] reported an increase of overcorrection (>1 diopter) of 31% at 1 year and 48% at 8.5 years.

Waring[29] defined four circumstances in which overcorrections occur. The first circumstance occurs during the immediate postoperative period and is related to corneal edema, excessive corneal incision gaping and enhanced flattening of the central cornea.[66] The hyperopic effect of these conditions resolves within 3 to 6 weeks after surgery as the radial incisions heal. The second circumstance is the result of incorrect surgery, such as using too small a central clear zone. Salz[64] has recommended using fewer incisions to reduce the possibility of overcorrections. He was able to reduce the incidence of overcorrections to 4% when using 4-incision radial keratotomy, although the first few incisions have the greatest effect. Hyperopia may also occur when the patient is an overresponder. We cannot readily identify the incidence of overresponse or which patients are likely to overrespond to surgery. Overresponse to surgery is a valid reason to delay surgery in the fellow eye for 4 to 12 weeks. The fourth circumstance is progressive hyperopia. There is significant

*References 18, 33, 34, 51, 61, 63, 64.

evidence in the Dietz study and 10-year follow-up data of PERK patients that progressive hyperopia occurs with some regularity.[54,65] The Perk study at 5 years reported that 22% of eyes had a hyperopic shift of 1 diopter or more between 6 months and 5 years postoperatively. Ten-year data indicate that 43% of operated eyes shifted by 1 diopter or more between 6 months and 10 years.[54] The true long-term incidence of hyperopia is unknown.

The best way to approach the development of hyperopia after radial keratotomy is prevention. The current trend is to undercorrect the patient intentionally, which has additional benefits in the early presbyopic population. If vision is undercorrected, one can always accomplish an enhancement procedure. Enhancements or reoperations are required in approximately 33% of patients.[67] One must be cautious with enhancements, however because the greatest risk for overcorrection and perforations is during an enhancement procedure.[67,68] Treating hyperopia after radial keratotomy often involves the use of spectacles or contact lenses. One should include a reading correction for presbyopic patients. Use of topical antiglaucoma medications have been advocated to reduce intraocular pressure and eliminate overcorrection.[61,69] No published reports have supported this theory. Miotic agents produce other effects that influence the outcome of overcorrection, including accommodative spasm and pupillary miosis. Accommodative spasm helps to reduce residual hyperopia, and pupillary miosis increases depth of field. One can often obtain a myopic shift up to 1.50 diopters using miotics.[70] Pupillary miosis can also result in decreased glare and improved contrast sensitivity. Risks of using miotics need to be discussed with the patient because phospholine iodide has the potential to cause a retinal detachment and iris pigment cysts.[4] Orthokeratology has been advocated as a means of steepening the cornea in overcorrected patients,[71] although this technique is controversial.

Patients who do not tolerate medical management of hyperopic correction may be candidates for surgical intervention. The primary goal for surgical intervention is to suture the wounds closed, thereby reversing the effect of the refractive keratotomy. Often, this technique requires opening the incision, removing the epithelial cysts and epithelium, and suturing the wound. A purse-string suture can be used to reduce the hyperopia. Several investigators have described this technique and, on average, they are able to reduce approximately 2 diopters of hyperopia.[64,72-74] Using multiple interrupted sutures to close each of the radial incisions also reduces hyperopia and makes the patient myopic again. Selective suture removal over the ensuing 6 months generally leaves the patient mildly myopic. The difficulty with this procedure is its variability and the fact that the sutures loosened unpredictably, so that the patient may have irregular steepening and flattening over time.[75] We have found that the contraction of a 10-0 nylon purse-string suture at the 8.0-mm optical zone with interrupted 11-0 mersilene sutures inside and outside of the purse-string suture is efficacious for long-term corneal stability. It is advisable to place the purse-string suture above the incisions, and intrastromally between the incisions to allow for maximum posterior compression along the knee of the dehiscence area. Keratomileusis, air-lamellar keratoplasty, and epikeratoplasty have been advocated to treat overcorrection; however, there are no published data to support these methods.

The Mendez technique, or hexagonal keratotomy, has gained popularity in the treatment of overcorrection. Hexagonal keratotomy for the correction of hyperopia after radial keratotomy may result in a corneal wound gape with scarring at the incision intersections.[76,77] Any crossing of incisions can result in corneal dehiscence and melting. A rather marked myopic shift may occur over time as the cornea undergoes ectatic change (Figure 168-2). Hexagonal keratectomy alone or after a radial keratotomy has been associated with numerous complications and is not recommended for the treatment of hyperopia.[78]

UNDERCORRECTION

Although hyperopia is an undesirable consequence of radial keratotomy, myopia may be a desired effect in patients, especially in the nondominant eye. Every patients wound healing response is different, and the patient is sometimes undercorrected. The actual incidence of undercorrection is difficult to ascertain, because each study has its own definition. The incidence of undercorrection is obviously higher in patients with greater levels of myopia.

Deitz et al. indicate a 11.8% prevalence of undercorrection at 1 year ($n = 656$).[79] Twenty-eight percent of the patients in the PERK study were undercorrected more than -0.50 diopters 4 years after the surgery.[80] Twenty-six percent of the patients in the PERK study were undercorrected more than -0.50 diopters 10 years after the surgery.[54] Patients with the greatest myopia preoperatively had the highest percentage of undercorrections.

Undercorrection occurs in three circumstances. First, patients after radial keratotomy demonstrate an initial regression in the immediate postoperative period. In most patients the amount of regression is small. Second, if there is a miscalculation in the amount of surgery necessary to correct the myopia, an undercor-

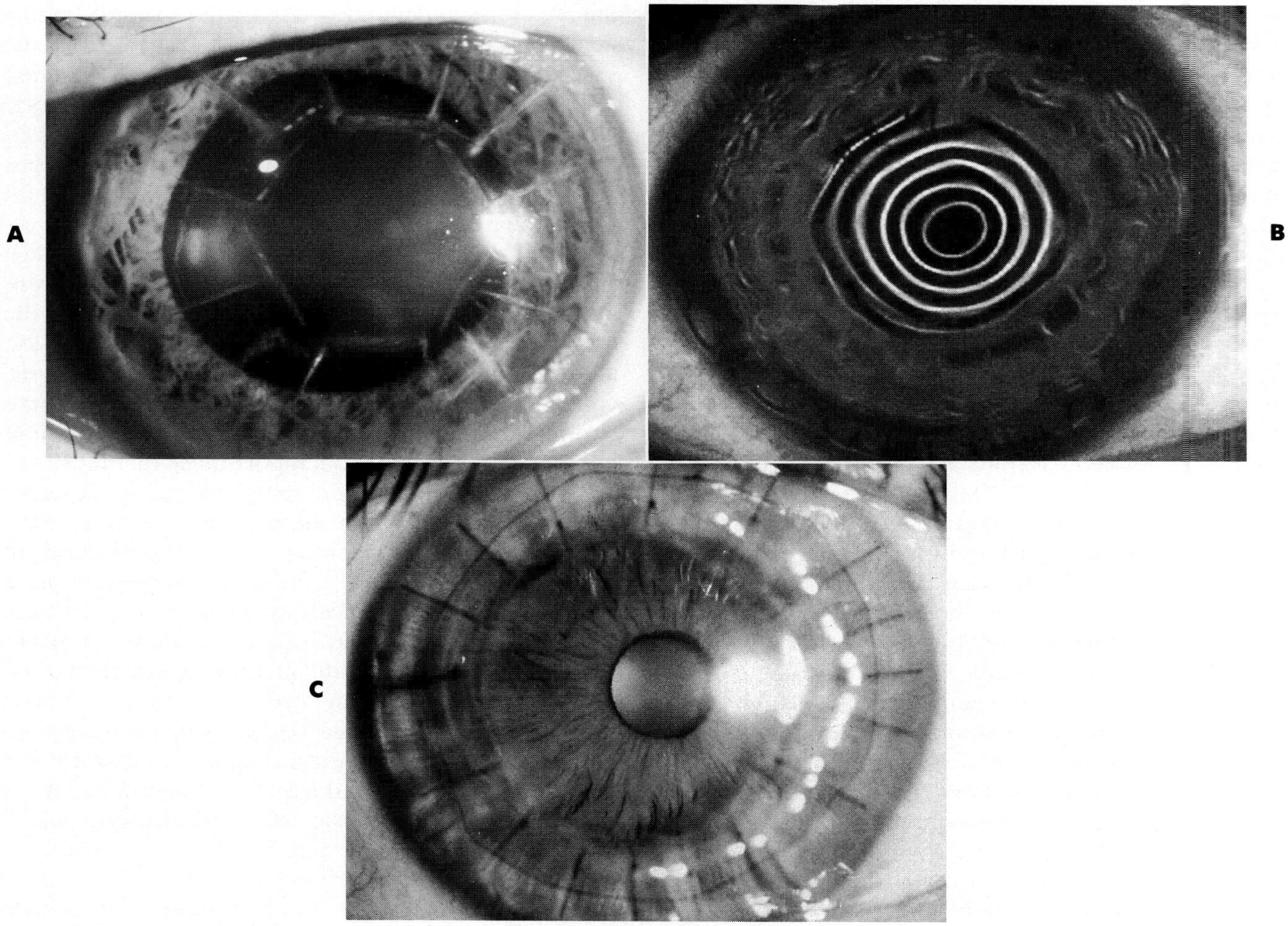

FIGURE 168-2 **A,** Slit lamp photograph of a patient who received multiple radial and tangential incisions followed by a hexagonal keratotomy. **B,** The adjacent corneoscope photograph displays the marked anterior shift of the cornea with associated irregular astigmatism. **C,** A penetrating keratoplasty was required to restore vision.

rection results. Triple checking the patient data and selected nomogram will often prevent insufficient surgery. Most refractive surgeons intentionally undercorrect to decrease the risk of hyperopia in the immediate postoperative period and progressive hyperopia in the long term. Slight undercorrection does not appear to have as great an impact on vision after radial keratotomy as it does in unoperated myopes. The third circumstance of undercorrection is the patient who remains undercorrected despite proper surgery. This loss of effect in some patients has been attributed to an aggressive wound healing response after radial keratotomy. Shallow incisions, dry eyes, lack of topical steroids, or normal wound healing may all contribute to a variable wound response. Some researchers have suggested that patients with low intraocular pressure and flatter corneas have less response to surgery.[25,61] However, flatter corneas flattened more than steeper corneas in the PERK study.[81]

Treatment of persistent undercorrection is both medical and surgical. Spectacles and contact lenses are the mainstay of therapy. Soft contact lenses can result in neovascular ingrowth into the radial incisions, causing scarring and eliminating the effect of the radial keratotomy. Postoperative topical steroids influence wound healing in the immediate postoperative period and enhance the effect of the initial surgery. Rowsey et al.[81] were able to achieve the same effect with 8-incision radial keratotomy without steroids as with 4-incision radial keratotomy with steroids in patients with the same level of myopia. Patients are placed at a greater risk for complications with topical steroids including elevated intraocular pressure and cataract formation. Fortunately, the incidence of elevated intraocular pressure has been minimal.[16]

Surgical management of undercorrection, also known as "enhancement," may become a more common method of titrating the effect of radial keratotomy. The reoperation rate of radial keratotomy for undercorrection in several initial studies (PERK, 14%;[83] Hofmann, 4.5%;[84] Franks, 23%;[85] Sawelson and Marks, 17%;[86] Villasenor, 14%;[87] Buzzard, 17%[88]) ranged from 4.5% to 23%. Werblin and Stafford,[67] in their more recent work, reported a reoperation rate of 33% within the first year of radial keratotomy. All patients should understand the relative efficacy of undercorrecting the radial keratotomy initially and adding incisions as indicated. It may also be appropriate to consider reincising shallow incisions, shortening the optical zone or performing excimer phototherapeutic keratectomy.

ASTIGMATISM

Three types of astigmatism are described: residual astigmatism, induced astigmatism, and irregular astigmatism.

Residual astigmatism is defined as preexisting astigmatism not corrected by the refractive procedure. All patients enrolled into the PERK study had less than 1.50 diopter of cylinder.[89]

Induced astigmatism is defined as an increase of astigmatism after the operative procedure. A true analysis of induced astigmatism would incorporate vector analysis. However, most reported studies did not involve vector analysis. In the PERK study at 5 years, 15% of eyes had an increase in refractive astigmatism of 1 diopter or more.[53] Repeat operations can increase the amount of induced astigmatism. It is also important to note the preoperative axis of astigmatism in each patient. Some patients will not experience an increase in astigmatism, but will have an axis shift in their astigmatism, which may result in asthenopic complaints. A 1 diopter shift from 90 degrees preoperatively to 180 degrees postoperatively is clinically significant.

Irregular astigmatism exists when a spectacle lens cannot correct the amount of astigmatism and more commonly occurs with additional surgery. Eyes that have radial incisions intersecting with transverse or circumferential incisions or with an optical zone less than 3.0 mm are especially prone to this complication. Microperforations or macroperforations may cause an uneven distribution of corneal power and result in irregular astigmatism. The combination of multiple radial and tangential incisions destabilizes the cornea and may also be associated with irregular astigmatism, marked fluctuation of vision, glare, and light sensitivity.

Mild to moderate amounts of astigmatism can be managed with a gas permeable contact lens. Large amounts of irregular astigmatism may require penetrating keratoplasty.[78] It is appropriate to gauge the wound healing response of both radial and tangential incisions. The latter are predisposed to wound gape and progressive corneal hysteresis. Suturing of tangential incisions is auspicious if the edges begin to separate suggesting wound dehiscence.

ANISOMETROPIA

Anisometropia is the difference in refractive error between a patient's two eyes. Anisometropia commonly occurs in all patients after refractive surgery is performed on one eye and before surgery on the second eye. It is imperative to discuss this "side effect" of surgery with the patient. Some refractive surgeons operate on both eyes on the same day to avoid the difficulties the patient experiences with anisometropia. However by performing bilateral simultaneous surgery, one sacrifices the information that might be obtained from the outcome on the first eye that may be used to plan surgery for the second eye. We advocate waiting at least 1 month to establish the effect of radial keratotomy on the first eye before operating on the second eye.

Another argument against bilateral simultaneous surgery is that patients may decide not to proceed with surgery on the second eye, especially if they are presbyopic. Twenty percent of the patients in the PERK study did not want surgery on their second eye. The patients were either completely satisfied with the monocular effect of the procedure or were dissatisfied with the outcome.[80] This approach also supports the concept of performing surgery on the dominant eye first. Bilateral surgery does not necessarily eliminate the incidence of anisometropia. Approximately one third of the PERK patients who had bilateral surgery demonstrated a refractive difference of greater than 1 diopter.[51] Eleven percent of the PERK patients were highly asymmetric, showing four or more lines of difference in visual acuity 1 year after surgery.

Many patients do not complain of asthenopia in the face of anisometropia because they have become accustomed to monovision and make no attempt to fuse at all. Monovision is becoming more acceptable to patients, and often the patient requests monovision. Therefore, the dominant eye is corrected to distance and the nondominant eye is intentionally undercorrected to give the patient reading capability.

Bilateral radial keratotomy that results in marked astigmatism in one eye or astigmatism of differing powers and axes in both eyes can result in anisometropia, which is especially difficult to manage. Gas permeable contact lenses, special spectacle prescriptions, and additional refractive surgery[3] are treatment options.

PRESBYOPIA

All patients will develop symptoms of presbyopia as their accommodative reserve diminishes with age. It is important to discuss the ramifications of presbyopia with the patient preoperatively. Patients who are already presbyopic and interested in radial keratotomy must understand that they will require reading glasses immediately after surgery if they are corrected to emmetropia (or mild hyperopia). Many patients would rather depend on reading glasses than on permanent distance correction. The trend today is to undercorrect the middle-aged patient's nondominant eye intentionally by −0.75 to −1.50 diopter and to correct the dominant eye to emmetropia. This monovision provides the patient with the best option of being spectacle free most of the time. This option should be presented in detail because most patients believe that they will be able to read by simply removing their glasses, as occurs preoperatively. Radial keratotomy should not be performed unless the patient understands the certainty of eventual presbyopia development.

MULTIFOCAL CORNEA

After radial keratotomy, corneas generally have a greater range of refractive power than before the refractive procedure. The normal cornea is steeper in the center and flatter toward the limbus (aspheric or prolate shape). The post-radial keratotomy cornea is flatter in the center and steeper toward the limbus (oblate shape). Irregularities in this shape can be beneficial. Occasionally the presbyopic patient who obtains excellent distance visual acuity after radial keratotomy will retain excellent near vision without the aid of a bifocal. Moreira et al.[90] reported three patients who experienced excellent unaided distance and near vision who had a wide distribution of corneal power throughout the cornea. Similarly, a multifocal cornea after radial keratotomy can produce symptoms of visual distortion or monocular diplopia.[91]

Corneal Complications of Refractive Keratotomy

HERPES SIMPLEX KERATITIS

Sunlight, trauma, fever, contact lenses, menstruation, suture removal, or any epithelial defect can induce reactivation of herpes simplex virus (HSV).[92] Marmer[18] reported two cases of herpes keratitis after radial keratotomy in a 62,814 patient survey. It is unclear whether these patients had a prior history of HSV. Additionally, a case of presumed HSV infection has been reported after refractive keratotomy in a patient with no known prior history of HSV keratitis. However, no documentary photographs or viral cultures were performed.[93] Refractive keratotomy is a form of corneal trauma that may lead to reactivation of HSV and therefore should be avoided in patients with a prior history of HSV keratitis.

CORNEAL IRON LINES

It is well recognized that iron deposits in the epithelium of the cornea occur around surface irregularities. Iron lines are often found at the base of cones in keratoconus (Fleischer ring), anterior to the head of a pterygium (Stocker's line), anterior to a filtering bleb (Ferry's line), or adjacent to other corneal irregularities.[94] Iron deposits tend to occur in areas of relative depression in the corneal contour, creating a localized change in the tear film, although the exact mechanism of deposition is unknown. These iron lines also occur after refractive keratotomy. In the PERK study, central corneal iron lines occurred in 81% of patients at 6 months, 86% of patients at 1 year, and 78% of eyes at 2 years after surgery.[95] However, the iron lines did not affect the visual outcome and are of no consequence.[30]

EPITHELIAL DISORDERS

The development of anterior basement membrane (ABM) changes after radial keratotomy was initially recognized by Rowsey and Balyeat[31] and further studied by Nelson et al.[96] Nelson et al discovered ABM changes in 33 of 71 eyes (46.5%) that underwent radial keratotomy. ABM changes were found in 20% of eyes at 3 months, 16.9% of eyes at 6 months, and 18.5% of eyes at 1 year after surgery. However, there were no episodes of recurrent erosion in any of these patients.[96] Marmer[18] found that 8 of 62,814 patients developed recurrent erosions in a national survey, but it is unclear whether these patients had any predisposing factors. In the PERK study, four patients developed recurrent erosions. One patient had evidence of map-dot-fingerprint dystrophy in the unoperated eye. This patient required a therapeutic soft contact lens that induced vascularization of the incisions.[30] Speculation has arisen that dull blades, rough knife footplates, and excessive topical anesthesia (especially cocaine) may contribute to this problem.[16,61] We have observed one patient with sufficient basement membrane changes to completely reverse the radial keratotomy effect. Removal of the epithelium and polishing of Bowman's membrane restored the initial effect of the radial keratotomy. It is important to evaluate thoroughly all patients preoperatively for ABM changes and other corneal pathology. Treatment of erosions after radial keratotomy is similar to the management of this problem in other patients.

Subepithelial fibrosis of the central cornea has been

reported after radial keratotomy. This fibrosis has occurred in the absence of keratitis, edema, epithelial disorders, or other evidence of ocular inflammation. It was recurrent after superficial keratectomy and has resulted in decreased best corrected visual acuity.[97] Polit et al.[98] have also described a patient with subepithelial reticular cicatrization after radial keratotomy who had inactive trachoma, resulting in regression of the radial keratotomy effect and need for homoplastic keratomileusis.

STERILE NONHEALING CORNEAL DEFECTS

An episode of a sterile nonhealing epithelial defect with subsequent stromal melting and perforation requiring penetrating keratoplasty has been reported after radial keratotomy.[27] This complication occurred in the area of intersecting incisions, which resulted in wound gape. For this and many other reasons, intersecting corneal incisions for refractive surgery have been abandoned.

Geggel[99] reported a case of sterile keratitis 34 months after radial keratotomy. This complication occurred in four adjacent incision sites; multiple biopsies failed to demonstrate a causative agent. This was associated with stromal edema and poor wound healing and required a penetrating keratoplasty for visual rehabilitation. Mackman[100] reported a case of recurrent sterile stromal keratitis requiring a conjunctival flap to achieve resolution.

Predisposing factors for sterile keratitis include delayed wound healing, epithelial edema, incisional epithelial plugs, dry eye, chronic steroids, and multiple surgeries. Every effort should be taken to avoid these risks.[100]

INFECTIOUS KERATITIS

Both bacterial and fungal infections of the cornea have been reported after radial keratotomy. Typically, these events have been categorized as early and late postoperative keratitis. Last postoperative keratitis has been reported as long as 40 months after surgery.

Early postoperative keratitis has been caused by multiple infectious agents. These include *Staphylococcus aureus, Staphylococcus epidermidis, Streptococcus pneumoniae,* diptheroids, *Pseudomonas* species, and *Mycobacterium chelonei.** These cases of keratitis occurred in the incision site and tend to spread quickly throughout the wound. Inflammation frequently involves the full depth of the wound and may increase the risk of crystalline keratopathy. The survey by Lewicky and Salz[3] of 24 refractive surgeons reported only five episodes of early postoperative keratitis; one required a corneal transplantation[3] (Figure 168-3).

*References 4, 10, 29, 51, 101-107.

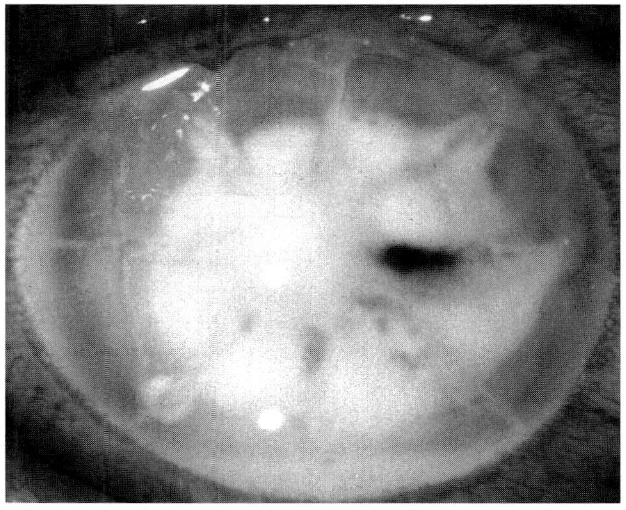

FIGURE 168-3 Delayed *Pseudomonas aeruginosa* keratitis in an eye that was undercorrected from original surgery and wearing a soft contact lens for best corrected vision. Cornea demonstrates a large infiltrative process with descemetocele formation in the 3 o'clock radial incision.

Late postoperative keratitis has been reported as late as 40 months after surgery.[105] Cottingham et al.[104] reported six episodes of late postoperative keratitis in 14,163 patients for an incidence of 1 in 2,400 cases.[104] The causative agents have included *Pseudomonas aeruginosa, S. epidermidis, Propionibacterium acnes, M. chelonei, Enterobacter gergoviae, Serratia liquefaciens,* and possibly *Moraxella.*[102,105,108] Most cases have been associated with attempted contact lens wear after radial keratotomy.

The cause of postoperative keratitis is probably multifactorial. The epithelial plug in the incision site often is extruded over time as the incision heals and scars, leading to epithelial irregularity and providing a portal of entry for bacteria. Additionally, epithelial irregularity over the incision site may predispose the cornea to infection. Transverse incisions may make the cornea locally anesthetic. All reported cases of delayed keratitis have occurred in the incision sites. The interpalpebral regions are the areas of the cornea that are most frequently involved in both early and late postoperative keratitis, indicating that exposure and drying are contributing factors.[102]

Fungal keratitis has been documented in the early postoperative period. Organisms involved have included *Candida parapsilosis.*[109] It is thus important to perform comprehensive cultures of all patients with resistant corneal ulcers and to consider fungal agents, especially if the ulcer does not respond to conventional therapy.

Other incisional keratotomies have been associated with late infections. Infectious crystalline keratopathy has been reported 3 months after relaxing incisions in an eye that had a history of steroid use and a previous penetrating keratoplasty for bullous keratopathy. The patient eventually required a repeat penetrating keratoplasty.[110]

All potential sources of infection such as blepharitis, conjunctivitis, and canaliculitis should be treated adequately before refractive surgery. All procedures should be performed in a sterile surgical field. Prophylactic antibiotics should be used in the immediate postoperative period until the epithelium is completely healed. Standard corneal ulcer protocols should be followed in the event of postoperative keratitis. All examinations of the patient should include slit lamp biomicroscopy of the anterior segment to search for evidence of keratitis or epithelial irregularities. Additionally, patients should be well informed of the signs and symptoms of keratitis.

ABNORMALITIES OF INCISION HEALING AND SCARRING

Early in the history of radial keratotomy, it was apparent that the healing of corneal incisions was crucial to the outcome of refractive keratotomy. Corneal incisions or corneal lacerations that are not tightly reapproximated heal by creation of an epithelial plug in the incision. This plug is apparent at the slit lamp as a lucid interval within the incision. This epithelial plug can persist in the incision for years after the original incision in the cornea.[50,111,112] Solid nests of epithelium, called epithelial inclusion cysts, can develop in the incisions. These inclusions were present in about 7% of scars at 1 year postoperatively in the PERK study. They may make the scar appear more dense and can be present as long as 79 months after radial keratotomy.[48] However, they are not clinically significant.[30]

Rowsey and Balyeat[31] reviewed epithelial ingrowth in corneal incisions with biomicroscopy. They found that epithelium in the incisions typically extrudes within the first 3 months. They discovered, however, that epithelium may be present in the wounds for as long as 1 year after surgery. Keratotomy incisions have now been evaluated histologically for their healing tendencies. Deg et al.[50] and Binder et al.[113] have found that wounds can show incomplete healing with epithelial plugs in the incisions for as long as 47 months after surgery. Some, but not all, of these patients received postoperative steroids.

It is now known that the epithelial plug may remain in the wound for years after radial keratotomy. Active fibroblasts also may remain in the wound for years. Therefore the wound healing response after radial keratotomy occurs over years. The wound may not regain its final tensile strength for years and even then may be weaker than in the original preoperative state.[114] Factors that have been proposed to cause delayed wound healing include use of topical corticosteroids, fluctuation of intraocular pressure, inherently weakening the cornea, and especially tangential incisions.

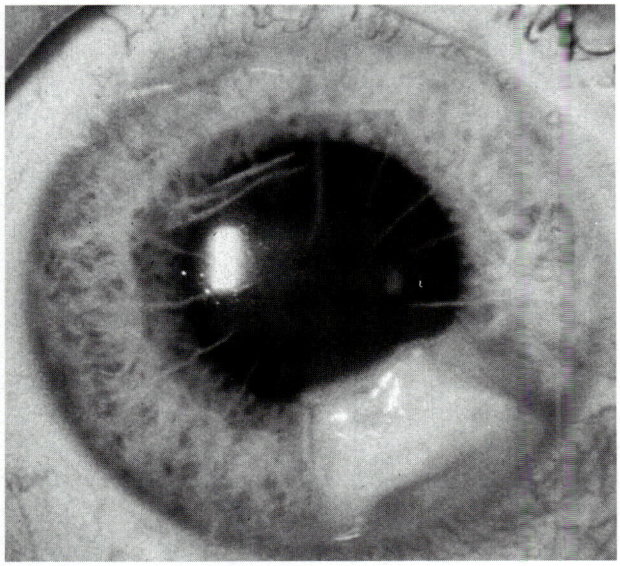

FIGURE 168-4 Intersecting radial and tangential incisions result in a lamellar dehiscence of the peripheral cornea.

Incomplete wound healing can become important during subsequent intraocular surgery. It is common for radial keratotomy wounds to open during trephination for penetrating keratoplasty. McNeill[115] reported a case of peripheral wound dehiscence 9 years after radial keratotomy when the patient was undergoing a penetrating keratoplasty. It is also common for radial keratotomy wounds to gape adjacent to a cataract wound. Progressive flattening of the central radial keratotomy cornea after cataract surgery suggests progressive wound dehiscence. Additionally, vascularization of scars, especially if stromal, may increase the chance of graft rejection.[24]

It is now well recognized that the intersection of incisions in refractive keratotomy creates excessive amounts of wound gape, increased and unpredictable scarring, delayed wound healing, and irregular astigmatism. Histopathologic examination of a representative specimen 6 months after surgery showed absence of scarring, retention of epithelium in the wound, and degeneration of adjacent keratocytes.[26] Therefore, these types of intersecting incisions, including the original Ruiz procedure, TL procedures, Flag incisions, and others[27,61,71,116-120] have been abandoned in refractive surgery. If a surgeon accidentally crosses incisions, he or she should consider surgical repair at the time (Figure 168-4).

A

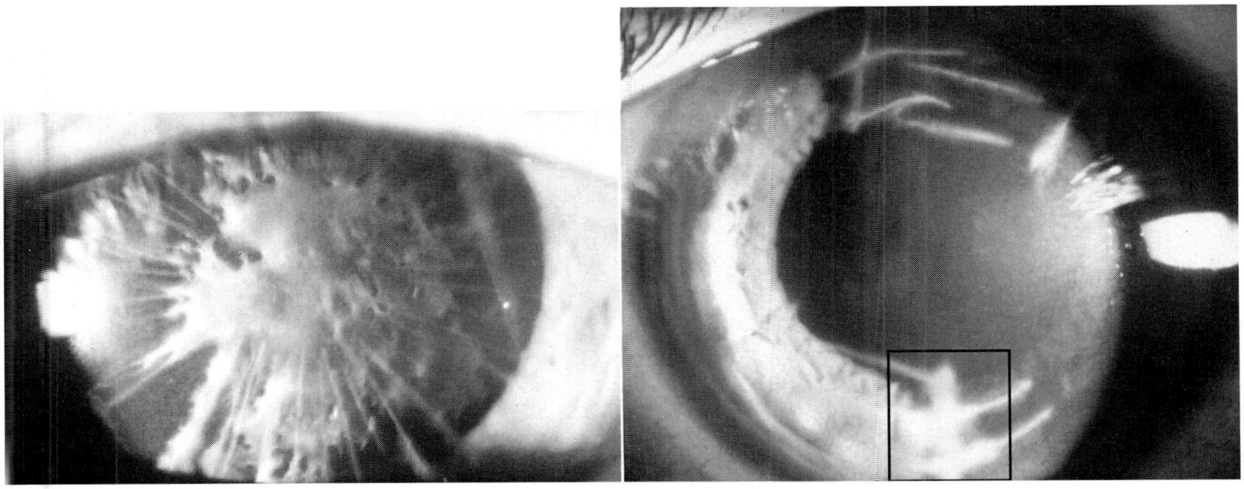

B

FIGURE 168-5 **A,** Multiple incisions and **B,** crossed incisions may result in hypertrophic scarring *(box)* of the cornea.

Many techniques are available for the enhancement of original refractive procedures. Making repeat incisions over original incisions is a common technique (deepening or lengthening), but it may lead to increased scarring in that location. There is no known relationship between individuals with keloid skin incisions and hypertrophic scars of the cornea. Additionally, normal skin healers can develop hypertrophic corneal scars after uncomplicated radial keratotomy[51] (Figure 168-5).

As with perforations caused by other traumatic injuries to the cornea, areas of perforation tend to create a plaque on the posterior corneal surface.[30] These tend to peak into the stroma as grayish areas of increased relucency.

Irregular or wavy incisions are often seen after radial keratotomy. However, these do not tend to affect the outcome. Waring[6] has discussed the possible mechanisms of irregular incisions including globe movement, surgeon inexperience, new or unfamiliar equipment, thin and flexible or double-edged knife blades, and stopping and restarting a centripetal incision.

Vascularization of the incision was a common occurrence when the incisions extended through the limbus. Rowsey and Balyeat[31] demonstrated that clear corneal incisions create a larger amount of myopic correction; current techniques avoid crossing the limbus. Vascularization of incisions is now infrequent. It occurs most commonly in the setting of contact lens wear, limbal cautery, and various inflammations of the scars.[61,116] In the PERK study, only 1.5% of incisions had more that 1 mm of vascularization at the 1-year report. At 3 years, 16 of 435 eyes in the PERK study had vascularization 5% to 50% of the incision length. Thirteen of these eyes had been wearing contact lenses. No complications from the vascularization could be identified.[30,51]

STRUCTURAL INTEGRITY OF THE CORNEA

Some worry that radial keratotomy may lead to structural weakness of the globe. Table 168-1 reviews several studies of structural integrity of the globe after radial keratotomy. The cornea may be weakened significantly if a microperforation occurs, or if the incisions are very deep. Most of the studies involve cadaveric eyes in which no healing occurs. Our studies with eye bank eyes demonstrated that with no incisions through Descemet's membrane, the post-radial keratotomy eye would tolerate 1,600 mm Hg infusion pressure with globe rupture at the optic nerve, not at the cornea.

Ruptured globe has been reported after radial keratotomy. Pearlstein et al.[126] have reported a patient who suffered blunt trauma to the eye 8 months after 8-incision radial keratotomy. The patient ruptured several incisions, with the laceration passing across the visual axis joining radial keratotomy incisions and extending to the limbus. Bloom et al.[127] have described a patient in which blunt trauma resulted in a full-thickness corneal laceration 22 months after the radial keratotomy involving two radial keratotomy wounds joined through the visual axis. Glasgow et al.[128] have also reported a case of blunt trauma, resulting in dehiscence of three radial keratotomy wounds, two of which joined across the visual axis. Additionally, pathologic evaluation confirmed that the rupture sites coincided with the radial keratotomy wounds.[26] Binder et al.[114] have reported three eyes that suffered wound rupture after blunt trauma one and two years after undergoing uneventful RK.

Table 168-1. Quantitated trauma in RK

Study	Eyes	Trauma	Procedure	Rupture pressure	Rupture site
Campos et al.[121]	Pig, cad	Lat comp	RK	240 mm Hg	RK incision
			Control	>280 mm Hg	ON or sclera
Lutterull et al.[122]	Pig, cad	Bench press	RK <70%*	N/A	Sclera
			RK >70%*		RK incision
Rylander et al.[123]	Pig, cad	Lat comp	RK	5 lb	75% incision for RK
			Control	6.8 lb	
		Axial comp	RK	5.8 lb	81% sclera for controls
			Control	7.6 lb	
Alcarez et al.[124]	Human, cad	Saline	RK	215 mm Hg	RK incision
		Infuse	PRK	1149 mm Hg	No corneal ruptures
Larson et al.[125]	Rabbit, live	Weighted ball	RK	50% of control	98% Incisional
			RK/microper	25% of control	2% ON

cad, cadaveric; ON, optic nerve; RK, radial keratotomy; PRK, photorefractive keratectomy; microper, microperforation; *, incision depth; N/A, not available; Lat comp, lateral compression; Axial comp, axial compression.

John and Schmitt,[129] however, report a patient with an 8-incision radial keratotomy 6 months before suffering trauma. The injury to the eye resulted in traumatic hyphema, traumatic iridoplegia, and angle recession. The corneal incisions remained intact and the refraction was stable. Spivack also described a patient who was in a plane crash after radial keratotomy and suffered severe facial trauma; however, the corneal incisions remained intact.[130] Forstot and Damiano[131] reported eight episodes of trauma after radial keratotomy. These episodes involved variable amounts of trauma to the orbital/globe area. In two of the episodes, rupture of one radial keratotomy wound was treated successfully with therapeutic contact lens without loss of visual acuity.

The possibility of structural weakness must be discussed with any patient considering radial keratotomy. This procedure should be avoided in some patients, such as contact sports participants, who are a high risk for trauma to their eyes. Unfortunately it is the active patient that often requests radial keratotomy.

ENDOTHELIAL CELL LOSS

Sato, in Japan, described the technique of posterior keratotomy for treatment of keratoconus in 1939; later he described its use to correct refractive errors.[132] His surgery involved the placement of incisions in the posterior aspect of the cornea. It is now well recognized that these patients developed bullous keratopathy 10 to 20 years after surgery.[132-134] Since this discovery, concern about the endothelium justifiably remains after anterior corneal incisions.

A study in rhesus monkeys revealed endothelial cell changes centrally in as many as 33% of eyes undergoing anterior radial keratotomy.[111] This study also revealed disruption in endothelial cells adjacent to the incisions. Histopathologic examination of human eyes has revealed that some incisions have linear endothelial abnormalities adjacent to the incision site.[111] Histopathologic evidence of endothelial cell migration, degeneration without inflammatory cells and areas of detachment of the endothelium are also seen along radial keratotomy incisions.[100]

The results of endothelial cell counts on humans are available in Table 168-2. These studies show mean endothelial cell count changes from +2% to −14.3%. The studies tend to show a cell loss related to the procedure but stable endothelial cell counts thereafter. Some data suggest that an optical zone less than 3.5 mm is related to a higher central endothelial cell loss. Additionally, enhancement procedures result in further endothelial cell loss.

The possible mechanisms of endothelial cell loss include mechanical or inflammatory damage and induced corneal instability.[27,135] Additionally contact lens wear can lead to endothelial cell morphologic changes that occur within 2 weeks of use and may be irreversible.[136] These changes make the interpretation of radial keratotomy data on the endothelium more difficult. Postoperative corneal edema has been reported.[27] The long-term clinical significance of these reports is uncertain. Clearly the long-term effects of radial keratotomy on the corneal endothelium need to be addressed. Any sign of progressive endothelial cell loss after radial keratotomy would warrant discontinuation of the procedure.

MISCELLANEOUS CORNEAL COMPLICATIONS

Several miscellaneous case reports of complications have been published. Nolan[140] reported a case of an army officer who was struck in the left eye with a tree branch 1 year after radial keratotomy. The patient had a piece of vegetable matter that perforated the eye through a prior incision. Durand et al.[94] reported the

Table 168-2. Endothelial cell loss studies in RK

Study	RK	Optical zone (mm)	Percentage of cell loss			Perforation
			1-3 months	6-12 months	>1 year	
Chiba et al.[137]	8	≥3.5		0.0%*		No
	8	<3.5		9.0%*		No
Chiba et al.[137]	8			1.6%*		No
	8			14.3%*		Yes
MacRae et al.[138]	8	3-5			3.3%	
	0	(control eye)			1.7%	
Rowsey et al.[21]	8		7.7%	8.3%	7.6%	No
	8		4.5%	2.8%	10%	Yes
Deitz et al.[12]	8		4.9%	1.6%		
Hoffer et al.[10]	16		9%		+2%	
	8			2.6%		
Rowsey and Balyeat[31]	8-16	3-5	5.6%	6.9%	4.5%	No
	8-16	3-5	4.6%	1%		Yes
Rowsey et al.[139]	2nd				14.6%	

*Statistically significant.

case of a patient with keratoconus who underwent radial keratotomy and experienced a microperforation. The patient subsequently developed an incisional abscess with a fistula and hypopyon. This abscess required treatment with intravenous antibiotics and subsequent penetrating keratoplasty. Deposits including fibers, metal fragments, fine particles, and possibly degenerated blood have been reported in the incision scars; but they do not appear to have clinical significance.[6] Epithelial downgrowth has been reported by Binder.[58] Heterophoria and ptosis have also been reported.[141,142]

Conclusion

The major complications of radial keratotomy are largely avoidable by meticulous attention to surgical detail. Patients should be informed of possible difficulties and of plans to follow, correct, or refer for consultation, if required. The most unhappy patients are not those with complications, but those who were not informed of a problem, ignored when complaining of a difficulty, or told that, "There is nothing that can be done." If patients believe that you are their primary advocate and informed consultant, they will remain an ally even in the face of corrected complications.

REFERENCES

1. Rapizzi A, Prosdocimo G, Gorla C, Martinuzzi A: Blood staining of the cornea following radial keratotomy, *J Refract Corneal Surg* 7:188-189, 1991.
2. Cross WD, Head WJ: Complications of radial keratotomy: an overview. In Sanders D, Hofmann RF, Salz J, editors: *Refractive corneal surgery,* Thorofare, NJ, 1986, Charles Slack.
3. Lewicky A, Salz JJ: Special Report: radial keratotomy survey, *J Refract Surg* 2:32-33, 1986.
4. O'Day DM, Femar SS, Elliott JH: Visual impairment following radial keratotomy: a cluster of cases, *Ophthalmology* 93:319-326, 1986.
5. Feldman RM, Crapotta JA, Feldman ST, Goldbaum MH: Retinal detachment following radial and astigmatic keratotomy, *J Refract Corneal Surg* 7:252-253, 1991.
6. Waring GO: *Refractive keratotomy for myopia and astigmatism,* St Louis, 1992, Mosby.
7. Hecht SD, Jamara RJ: Prospective evaluation of radial keratotomy using the Fyodorov formula: preliminary report, *Ann Ophthalmol* 14:319-330, 1982.
8. Leroux les Jardins S, Bertrand I, Massin M: Intraoperative and early postoperative complications in 466 radial keratotomies, *J Refract Corneal Surg* 8:215-216, 1992.
9. Nirankari VS et al: Ongoing prospective clinical study of radial keratotomy, *Ophthalmology* 90:637-641, 1983.
10. Hoffer KJ et al: Three years experience with radial keratotomy: the UCLA study, *Ophthalmology* 90:627-636, 1983.
11. Cowden JW, Bores LD: A clinical investigation of the surgical correction of myopia by the method of Fyodorov, *Ophthalmology* 88:737-41, 1981.
12. Deitz MR, Sanders DR, Marks RG: Radial keratotomy: an overview of the Kansas City Study, *Ophthalmology* 91:467-478, 1984
13. Cowden JW, Cichocki J: Radial keratotomy in monkeys: a one-year follow-up report, *Ophthalmology* 89:684-686, 1982.
14. Schachar RA: Indications, techniques, and complications of radial keratotomy, *Int Ophthalmol Clin* 23:119-128, 1983.
15. Arrowsmith PN et al: Visual, refractive, and keratometric results of radial keratotomy, *Arch Ophthalmol* 101:873-881, 1983.
16. Rowsey JJ, Balyeat HD: Radial keratotomy: preliminary report of complications, *Ophthalmic Surg* 13:27-35, 1982.
17. Rashid ER, Waring GO: Complications of radial and transverse keratotomy, *Surv Ophthalmol* 34:73-106, 1989.
18. Marmer RH: Radial keratotomy complications, *Ann Ophthalmol* 19:409-411, 1987.
19. Salz J et al: Radial keratotomy in fresh human cadaver eyes, *Ophthalmology* 88:742-746, 1981.
20. Gelender H, Gelber EC: Cataract following radial keratotomy, *Arch Ophthalmol* 101:1229-1231, 1983.

21. Rowsey JJ et al: *Complications of radial keratotomy. Acta: XXIV Int'l Congress of Ophthalmology,* Philadelphia, 1983, JB Lippincott.
22. Carter J et al: Cystoid macular edema following corneal-relaxing incisions, *Arch Ophthalmol* 105:70-72, 1987.
23. Baldone JA, Franklin RM: Cataract following radial keratotomy, *Ann Ophthalmol* 15:416-418, 1983.
24. Hersh PS, Kalevar V, Kenyon KR: Penetrating keratoplasty for severe complications of radial keratotomy, *Cornea* 10:170-174, 1991.
25. Ellis W: *Radial keratotomy and stigmatism surgery,* Irvine, Calif, 1986, Keith C. Terry and Associates.
26. Jester JV, Villasenor RA, Miyashiro J: Epithelial inclusion cysts following radial keratotomy, *Arch Ophthalmol* 101:611-615, 1983.
27. Karr DJ et al: Radial keratotomy complicated by sterile keratitis and corneal perforation: histopathologic case report and review of complications, *Ophthalmology* 92:1244-1248, 1985.
28. Uozato H, Guyton DL, Waring GO: Centering corneal surgical procedures, in Waring GO, editor: *Refractive keratotomy for myopia and astigmatism,* St Louis, 1992, Mosby.
29. Waring GO: The changing status of radial keratotomy for myopia, Part II, *J Refract Surg* 1:119-137, 1985.
30. Waring GO, Lynn MJ, Gelender H: Results of the evaluation of radial keratotomy (PERK) study one year after surgery, *Ophthalmology* 92:177-198, 1985.
31. Rowsey JJ, Balyeat HD: Preliminary results and complications of radial keratotomy, *Am J Ophthalmol* 93:433-455, 1982.
32. Wyzinski P: Why are refractive surgeons still wearing glasses? *Ophthalmic Surg* 18:349-351, 1987.
33. Sawelson H, Marks RG: Three year results of radial keratotomy, *Arch Ophthalmol* 105:81-85, 1987.
34. Sawelson H, Marks RG: Two year results of radial keratotomy, *Arch Ophthalmol* 103:505-510, 1985.
35. Schanzlin DJ et al: Diurnal change in refraction, corneal curvature, visual acuity, and intraocular pressure after radial keratotomy in the PERK study, *Ophthalmology* 93:167-175, 1986.
36. Neumann AC, Osher RH, Fenzl RE: Radial keratotomy: a comprehensive evaluation, *Ophthalmology* 56:275-301, 1984.
37. Bores LD, Myers W, Cowden J: Radial keratotomy: an analysis of the American experience, *Ann Ophthalmol* 13:941-948, 1981.
38. Gelender H, Flynn HW, Mandelbaum SH: Bacterial endophthalmitis resulting from radial keratotomy, *Am J Ophthalmol* 93:323-326, 1982.
39. Hoffer KJ et al: UCLA clinical trial of radial keratotomy: preliminary report, *Ophthalmology* 88:729-736, 1981.
40. Kremer FB, Marks RG: Radial keratotomy: prospective evaluation of safety and efficacy, *Ophthalmic Surg* 14:925-930, 1983.
41. Sarno EM, Smith RE, Schanzlin DJ: Comparison of clinical results following radial keratotomy, extended wear contact lenses, and myopic keratomileusis, *Int Ophthalmol Clin* 23: 167-192, 1983.
42. American Academy of Ophthalmology: Radial keratotomy for myopia, *Ophthalmology* 100:1103-1115, 1993.
43. Richmond RD: Special report: radial keratotomy as seen through operated eyes, *J Refract Surg* 3:22-27, 1987.
44. Wyzinski P: Diurnal cycle of refraction after radial keratotomy, *Ophthalmology* 94:120-124, 1987.
45. Wyzinski P, O'Dell L: Subjective and objective findings after radial keratotomy, *Ophthalmology* 96:1608-1614, 1989.
46. Bourque LB et al: Reported satisfaction, fluctuation of vision and glare among patients one year after surgery in the prospective evaluation of radial keratotomy (PERK) study, *Arch Ophthalmol* 104:356-363, 1986.
47. Waring GO, Steinberg EB, Wilson LA: Slit-lamp microscopic appearance of corneal wound healing after radial keratotomy, *Am J Ophthalmol* 100:218-224, 1985.
48. Jester JV et al: Variations in corneal wound healing after radial keratotomy: possible insights into mechanisms of clinical complications and refractive effects, *Cornea* 11:191-199, 1992.
49. Deg J, Binder PS: Wound healing after astigmatic keratotomy in human eyes, *Ophthalmology* 94:1291-1298, 1987.
50. Deg J, Zavala E, Binder PS: Delayed corneal wound healing following radial keratotomy, *Ophthalmology* 92:734-740, 1985.
51. Waring GO et al: Three year results of the prospective evaluation of radial keratotomy (PERK) study, *Ophthalmology* 94:1339-1354, 1987.
52. Busin M et al: Overcorrected visual acuity improved by antiglaucoma medication after radial keratotomy, *Am J Ophthalmol* 101:374-375, 1986.
53. Waring GO et al: Results of the prospective evaluation of the radial keratotomy (PERK) study five years after surgery, *Ophthalmology* 98:1164-1176, 1991.
54. Waring GO, Lynn MJ, McDonnell PJ, PERK Group: Results of the Prospective Evaluation of the Radial Keratotomy (PERK) study ten years after surgery, *Arch Ophthalmol* 112:1298-1308, 1994.
55. Arrowsmith PN, Marks RG: Visual, refractive, and keratometric results of radial keratotomy: one year follow-up, *Arch Ophthalmol* 102:1612-1617, 1984.
56. Foulks GN: Refractive keratoplasty: keratomileusis, keratophakia, and epikeratophakia, *Trans Pa Acad Ophthalmol Otolaryngol* 35;122-124, 1982.
57. Arrowsmith PN, Marks RG: Visual, refractive and keratometric results of radial keratotomy: five year follow-up, *Arch Ophthalmol* 197:506-511, 1989.
58. Binder PS: Resumed epithelial ingrowth following radial keratotomy, *CLAO J* 12:247-250, 1986.
59. Chen V, Lindstrom RL: Oblique orientation of incisions in four incision radial keratotomy, *Ophthalmic Surg* 23:359, 1992.
60. Binder PS, Charlton KH: Surgical procedures performed after refractive surgery, *Refract Corneal Surg* 8:61-74, 1992.
61. Sanders DR, Hofmann RF, Salz, JJ, editors: *Refractive corneal surgery,* Thorofare, NJ, 1986, Slack.
62. Milder B, Rubin M: *The fine art of prescribing glasses without making a spectacle of yourself,* Gainesville, Fla, 1978, Triad Scientific Publishers.
63. Arrowsmith PN et al: *Radial keratotomy: ARK Study Group,* Thorofare, NJ, 1984, Slack.
64. Salz JJ: Improving the results of radial keratotomy, *J Refract Surg* 1:167-171, 1985.
65. Deitz MR et al: Long term followup of metal blade radial keratotomy procedures, *Arch Ophthalmol* 112:614-620, 1994.
66. Starling J, Hofmann R: A new surgical technique for the correction of hyperopia after radial keratotomy: an experimental model, *J Refract Surg* 2:9-14, 1986.
67. Werblin TP, Stafford GM: The Casebeer system for predictable keratorefractive surgery, *Ophthalmology* 100:1095-1102, 1993.
68. Buzard KA: Deepening of incisions after radial keratotomy using the "tickle" technique, *Refract Corneal Surg* 7:348-355, 1991.
69. Busin M et al: The effect of changes in intraocular pressure on corneal curvature after radial keratotomy in the rabbit eye, *Ophthalmology* 93:331-334, 1986.
70. Andrade HA et al: Changes in contrast sensitivity and refraction after application of 0.5% pilocarpine solution in over- and under-corrected radial keratotomy patients with symptoms of glare and starbursts, *Invest Ophthalmol Vis Sci* 31(suppl):29, 1990.
71. Hofmann RF: Reoperations after radial keratotomy and astigmatic keratotomy, *J Refract Surg* 3:119-128, 1987.

72. Lyle WA, Jin JC: Circular and interrupted suture technique for correction of hyperopia following radial keratotomy, *Refract Corneal Surg* 8:80-83, 1992.
73. Damiano RE, Forstot SL, Duke DK: Surgical correction of hyperopia following radial keratotomy, *Refract Corneal Surg* 8:75-79, 1992.
74. Lindquist TD, William PA, Lindstrom RL: Surgical treatment of overcorrection following radial keratotomy: evaluation of clinical effectiveness, *Ophthalmic Surg* 22:12-15, 1991.
75. Rowsey JJ: Management of hyperopic shift after radial keratotomy, *Refract Corneal Surg* 8:325-330, 1992.
76. Jordan LT, Maxwell WA: Refractive surgery and informed consent, *J Cataract Refract Surg* 18:420-421, 1992.
77. Tamura M et al: Complications of hexagonal keratotomy following radial keratotomy, *Arch Ophthalmol* 109:1351, 1991.
78. Basuk WL et al: Complications of hexagonal keratotomy, *Am J Ophthalmol* 117:37-49, 1994.
79. Deitz MR, Sanders DR, Raanan MG: A consecutive series (1982-1985) of radial keratotomies performed with the diamond blade, *Am J Ophthalmol* 103:417-422, 1987.
80. Waring GO et al: Results of the Prospective Evaluation of Radial Keratotomy (PERK) study 4 years after surgery for myopia, *JAMA* 263:1083-1091, 1990.
81. Rowsey JJ et al: Predicting the results of radial keratotomy, *Ophthalmology* 90:642-654, 1983.
82. Fouraker BD et al: Results of four incision radial keratotomy at one year, *Invest Ophthalmol Vis Sci* 29(suppl): 7, 1988.
83. Cowden JW et al: Repeated radial keratotomy in the Prospective Evaluation of Radial Keratotomy study, *Am J Ophthalmol* 103:423-431, 1987.
84. Hofmann RF: Reoperations after radial and astigmatic keratotomy, *J Refract Surg* 3:119-128, 1987.
85. Franks S: Radial keratotomy undercorrections: a new approach, *J Refract Surg* 2:171-173, 1986.
86. Sawelson H, Marks RG: Two year results of reoperations for radial keratotomy, *Arch Ophthalmol* 106:497-501, 1988.
87. Villasenor RA, Cox KO: Radial keratotomy: reoperations, *J Refract Surg* 1:34-37, 1985.
88. Salz JJ et al: Four-incision radial keratotomy for low to moderate myopia, *Ophthalmology* 93:727-738, 1986.
89. Waring GO et al: Rationale for and design of the National Eye Institute Prospective Evaluation of Radial Keratotomy (PERK) study, *Ophthalmology* 90:40-58, 1983.
90. Moreira H et al: Multifocal corneal topographic changes after radial keratotomy, *Ophthalmic Surg* 23:85-89, 1992.
91. Maguire LJ, Bourne WM: A multifocal lens effect as a complication of radial keratotomy, *Refract Corneal Surg* 6:394-397, 1989.
92. Arffa RC, editor: *Grayson's diseases of the cornea,* ed 3, St Louis, 1991, Mosby.
93. Santos CI: Herpetic corneal ulcer following radial keratotomy, *Ann Ophthalmol* 15:82-85, 1983.
94. Durand L, Monnot JP, Burillon C, Assi A: Complications of radial keratotomy: eyes with keratoconus and late wound dehiscence, *Refract Corneal Surg* 8:311-314, 1992.
95. Steinberg EB et al: Stellate iron lines in the corneal epithelium after radial keratotomy, *Am J Ophthalmol* 98:416-421, 1984.
96. Nelson JD, Williams P, Lindstrom RL, Doughman DJ: Map-dot-fingerprint changes in the corneal epithelial basement membrane following radial keratotomy, *Ophthalmology* 92:199-205, 1985.
97. Gieser J, Sugar A: Radial keratotomy and corneal scarring, *Arch Ophthalmol* 110: 1527-1528, 1992.
98. Pelit F, Anwar M, Tabbara K, El-Maghraby A: Subepithelial reticular cicatrization following radial keratotomy in a patient with inactive trachoma, *Refract Corneal Surg* 8:240-241, 1992.
99. Geggel HS: Delayed sterile keratitis following radial keratotomy requiring corneal transplantation for visual rehabilitation, *Refract Corneal Surg* 6:55-58, 1990.
100. Mackman G: Delayed sterile keratitis following radial keratotomy successfully treated with conjunctival flap, *Refract Corneal Surg* 8:122-124, 1992.
101. Szerenyi K et al: Keratitis as a complication of bilateral, simultaneous radial keratotomy, *Am J Ophthalmol* 117:462-467, 1994.
102. Matoba AY et al: Bacterial keratitis after radial keratotomy, *Ophthalmology* 96:1171-1175, 1989.
103. Robin JB et al: *Mycobacterium chelonei* keratitis after radial keratotomy, *Am J Ophthalmol* 102:72-79, 1986.
104. Cottingham AJ et al: Bacterial corneal ulcers following keratorefractive surgery: a retrospective study of 14,163 procedures, Presented at the Ocular Microbiology and Immunology Meeting, San Francisco, September 28, 1986.
105. Mandelbaum S et al: Late development of ulcerative keratitis in radial keratotomy scars, *Arch Ophthalmol* 104:1156-1160, 1986.
106. Salz JJ: How safe is radial keratotomy? *J Refract Surg* 3:188-189, 1987.
107. Wilhelmus KR, Hamburg S: Bacterial keratitis following radial keratotomy, *Cornea* 2:143-146, 1983.
108. Shivitz IA, Arrowsmith PN: Delayed keratitis after radial keratotomy, *Arch Ophthalmol* 104:1153-1155, 1986.
109. Maskin SL, Alfonso E: Fungal keratitis after radial keratotomy, *Am J Ophthalmol* 114:369-370, 1992.
110. Kincaid MC, Fouraker BD, Schanzlin DJ: Infectious crystalline keratopathy after relaxing incisions, *Am J Ophthalmol* 111:374-375, 1991.
111. Ingraham HJ, Guber D, Green WR: Radial keratotomy: clinicopathologic case report, *Arch Ophthalmol* 103:683-688, 1985.
112. Yamaguchi T et al: Histologic study of a pair of human corneas after anterior radial keratotomy, *Am J Ophthalmol* 100:281-292, 1985.
113. Binder PS et al: An ultrastructural and histochemical study of long-term wound healing after radial keratotomy, *Am J Ophthalmol* 103:432-440, 1987.
114. Binder PS, Waring GO, Arrowsmith PN, Wang CL: Traumatic rupture of the cornea after radial keratotomy, *Arch Ophthalmol* 106:1584-1590, 1988.
115. McNeill JI: Corneal incision dehiscence during penetrating keratoplasty nine years after radial keratotomy, *J Cataract Refract Surg* 19:542-543, 1993.
116. Ellis W: *Radial keratotomy and astigmatism surgery,* Irvine Calif, 1986, Keith C. Terry and associates, pp. 117-130.
117. Franks JB, Binder PS: Keratotomy procedures for the correction of astigmatism, *J Refract Surg* 1:11-17, 1985.
118. Fyodorov SN: Surgical correction of myopia and astigmatism. In Schachar RA, Levy NS, Schachar L, editors: *Keratorefraction,* Denison, Texas, 1980, LAL.
119. Fyodorov SN, Durnev VV: Surgical correction of complicated myopic astigmatism by means of dissection of circular ligament of cornea, *Ann Ophthalmol* 13:115-118, 1981.
120. Gills JP: Trephination in combination with radial keratotomy for myopia. In Schachar RA, Levy NS, Schachar L, editors: *Keratorefraction,* Denison, Texas, 1980, LAL.
121. Campos M, Lee M, McDonnell PJ: Ocular integrity after refractive surgery: effects of photorefractive keratectomy, phototherapeutic keratectomy and radial keratotomy, *Ophthalmic Surg* 23:598-602, 1992.
122. Lutterull JK, Jester JV, Smith RE: The effect of radial keratotomy on ocular integrity in an animal model, *Arch Ophthalmol* 100:319-320, 1982.
123. Rylander HG, Welch AJ, Fremming B: The effect of radial

keratotomy in the rupture strength of pig eyes, *Ophthalmic Surg* 14:744-749, 1983.

124. Alcaraz LG et al: Comparative study of wound integrity after excimer laser photoablation and radial keratotomy, *Invest Ophthalmol Vis Sci* Suppl 33:999, 1992.
125. Larson BC, Kremer FB, Eller AW, Bernardina VB: Quantitated trauma following radial keratotomy in rabbits, *Ophthalmology* 90:660-667, 1983.
126. Pearlstein ES et al: Ruptured globe after radial keratotomy, *Am J Ophthalmol* 106:755-756, 1988.
127. Bloom HR, Sands J, Schneider D: Corneal rupture from blunt trauma 22 months after radial keratotomy, *Refract Corneal Surg* 6:197-199, 1990.
128. Glasgow BJ et al: Traumatic dehiscence on incisions seven years after radial keratotomy, *Am J Ophthalmol* 106:703-707, 1988.
129. John ME, Schmitt TE: Traumatic hyphema after radial keratotomy, *Ann Ophthalmol* 15:930-932, 1983.
130. Spivack L: Case report: radical keratotomy incisions remain intact despite facial trauma from plane crash, *J Refract Surg* 3:59-60, 1987.
131. Forstot SL, Damiano RE: Trauma after radial keratotomy, *Ophthalmology* 95:833-835, 1988.
132. Kanai A: Bullous keratopathy after anterior-posterior radial keratotomy for myopia and myopic astigmatism. *Am J Ophthalmol* 93:600-606, 1982.
133. Beatty RF, Smith RE: 30-year follow-up of posterior keratotomy, *Am J Ophthalmol* 103:330-331, 1987.
134. Yamaguchi T et al: Bullous keratopathy after anterior-posterior keratotomy for myopia and myopic astigmatism, *Am J Ophthalmol* 93:600-606, 1982.
135. Jester JV, Miyashiro JE, Rife L, Smith RE: Radial keratotomy in primate eyes: pathologic studies, *Invest Ophthalmol Vis Sci* 29(suppl): 69, 1982.
136. Holden BA et al: Effects of long-term extended contact lens wear on the human cornea, *Invest Ophthalmol Vis Sci* 26:1489-1501, 1985.
137. Chiba K et al: Morphometric analysis of corneal endothelium following radial keratotomy, *J Cataract Refract Surg* 13:263-267, 1987.
138. MacRae SM, Matsuda M, Rich LF: The effect of radial keratotomy on the corneal endothelium, *Am J Ophthalmol* 100:538-542, 1985.
139. Rowsey JJ et al: Endothelial cell loss after radial keratotomy, *Ophthalmology* 94(suppl):97, 1987.
140. Nolan BT: Clinical report: perforation by a foreign body through a pre-existing radial keratotomy wound, *Mil Med* 156:151-154, 1991.
141. Marmer RH: Ocular deviation induced by radial keratotomy, *Ann Ophthalmol* 20:451-452, 1988.
142. Linberg JV et al: Ptosis following radial keratotomy performed using a rigid eyelid speculum, *Ophthalmology* 93:1509-1512, 1986.

CHAPTER 169

RICHARD J. DUFFEY

Postoperative Complications of Radial Keratotomy

Expected Side Effects of Incisional Keratotomy

PAIN

Pain in the early postoperative period is to be expected for patients undergoing incisional keratotomy. This discomfort is secondary to breaks in epithelium and is worsened if large epithelial defects occur at the time of surgery. Several factors contribute to intraoperative stripping of epithelium, including excessive drying of the corneal epithelium, thicker diamond blades, unpolished footplates, dried epithelial debris on footplates and diamonds, and the shearing force of a front-cutting diamond, which tends to plow epithelium and lift it from its underlying basement membrane.

In the past, postoperative pain has been controlled with oral analgesics.[1] More recently, topical nonsteroidal antiinflammatory agents such as diclofenac have been used with success after refractive surgery to significantly reduce or eliminate this pain.[2-4] Repositioning epithelium that has been torn during surgery is helpful to speed the healing process. Use of cool compresses and ice is also recommended in the early postoperative period to minimize upper lid swelling. Patching the eye in the early postoperative period is practiced less often because it can actually increase postoperative pain.[5] Nonpreserved artificial tear drops are also helpful for lubrication to diminish discomfort and scratchiness in the early postoperative period.

GLARE AND STARBURST (SHORT TERM)

The term *photophobia* will be used to denote both glare and starburst that are commonly experienced by most patients after radial keratotomy. Before the use of nonsteroidal antiinflammatory agents, more than 90% of patients complained of photophobia in the early postoperative period in one study.[6] Most photophobia diminishes with time[7] and is less in patients that have fewer incisions and larger optical zones. Nonpreserved artificial tears, nonsteroidal antiinflammatory agents, and low concentrations of topical steroids all seem to diminish these symptoms.[2] Most patients will wear sunglasses in the first postoperative week, but the passage of time is most effective in decreasing photophobia.

DIURNAL FLUCTUATION IN VISION (SHORT TERM)

Corneal edema after radial keratotomy, particularly morning edema that causes increased gaping of wounds and increased central flattening of the cornea, leads to diurnal fluctuation of vision in the early postoperative period. This diurnal variation ranged from 1.00 to 3.50 diopters in 59% of eyes in one study[8] and between 0.50 and 4.25 diopters in 80% of eyes in the Prospective Evaluation of Radial Keratotomy (PERK) study.[9] Unhealed stromal incisions that increase stromal edema, eyelid swelling with pressure on the cornea, and the diurnal variation in intraocular pressure each contribute to this fluctuation in vision in the early postoperative period. The most effective treatment of this common side effect is the passage of time.

ANISOMETROPIA (TRANSIENT)

Most patients undergoing radial keratotomy in one eye at a time experience anisometropia in the interval period between the procedures on each eye. The higher the degree of preoperative myopia, the greater the anisometropia for the patient. Many surgeons and patients have chosen simultaneous bilateral radial keratotomy to significantly reduce this problem, but, not without additional risks such as simultaneous bilateral bacterial keratitis.[10-14] The anisometropia may be relieved by fitting the patient with a contact lens in the unoperated eye, but most patients tolerate this inconvenience by wearing no spectacles and depending on the operative eye or by wearing their previous spectacles sometimes with removal of the lens over the operative eye.

RAPID ONSET PRESBYOPIA IN OLDER PATIENTS

Patients older than 45 years of age will experience the rapid onset of symptomatic presbyopia after radial

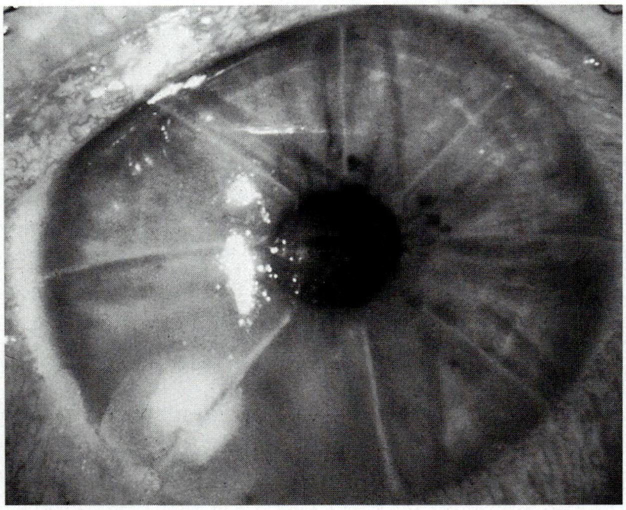

FIGURE 169-1 Acute onset bacterial keratitis involving one incision following radial keratotomy. (Courtesy Richard L. Lindstrom, MD.)

keratotomy. This problem is to be expected after surgery if no significant residual myopia remains. This fact must be explained preoperatively to patients in this age group. Temporary or permanent reading glasses are helpful in managing this problem. Morning edema in the early postoperative period may also cause a transient presbyopia in patients under the age of 40 years. This problem can be relieved with the use of temporary reading glasses.

Acute and Delayed, Potentially Severe, Sight-Threatening Complications

ULCERATIVE KERATITIS

Bacterial keratitis

As with all ophthalmic surgical procedures, incisional keratotomy runs the risk of bacterial invasion of the incisions and subsequent ulcerative keratitis (Figure 169-1). Early onset suppurative bacterial keratitis agents have included *Staphylococcus aureus* and *Staphylococcus epidermidis, Streptococcus pneumoniae, Pseudomonas,* and *Serratia marcescens.*[10-12,14-16] Delayed bacterial keratitis from *S. epidermidis, Pseudomonas aeruginosa, Moraxella, Propionibacterium acnes, Serratia liquefaciens,* and *Enterobacter gergoviae* has been documented.[15,17-19] Early onset bacterial keratitis is presumably secondary to the loss of the epithelial barrier to bacteria with direct invasion of the stroma with the infectious agent,

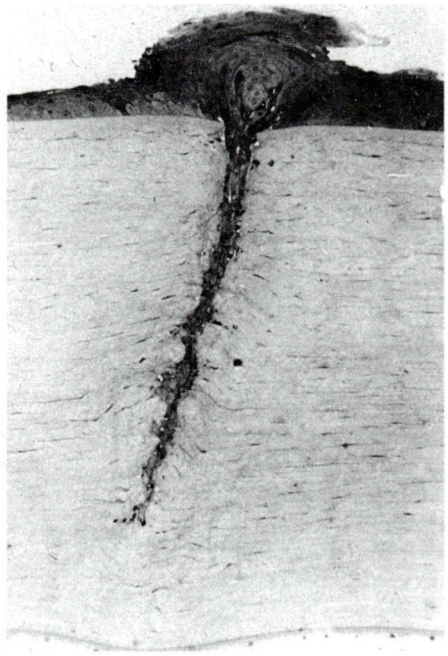

FIGURE 169-2 Radial keratotomy incision of 75% depth demonstrating intraincisional epithelial plugs and an elevated facet of epithelium overlying the incision. Such epithelial plugs can delay wound healing and predispose to recurrent erosion and bacterial adherence to the irregular epithelial surface overlying the incision. (From Binder PS et al: *Arch Ophthalmol* 106:1584-1590, 1988.)

most commonly gram-positive organisms.[15] Late onset keratitis may be secondary to an epithelial plug (Figure 169-2) within the keratotomy wound and irregular epithelium overlying the incision causing delayed wound healing and persistent subclinical recurrent erosions, thus predisposing the patient to invasion by bacteria at a later date, most commonly gram-negative organisms.[15]

Several reports of bilateral microbial keratitis occurring in patients who underwent radial keratotomy in both eyes within 24 hours[11] of one another or in both eyes simultaneously[10,12] have now been published. These cases involved acute onset bacterial keratitis within days of the procedures, with the same bacteria being present in both eyes. Treatment guidelines should include aggressive management of infectious keratitis in these patients because the infection can easily spread along the incision line to its base near Descemet's membrane, thus rapidly causing full-thickness ulcerative keratitis.[10] The infiltrates should be scraped and sent for Gram stain and culture with the initiation of fortified topical antibiotics immediately. If the infiltrate is deep in a corneal incision, the incision should be opened with a platinum spatula or Sinskey hook and appropriate Gram stains and cultures taken followed by irrigation of the incision with balanced salt solution in an attempt to debride the wound(s). Evidence suggests that topical povodone-iodine can be

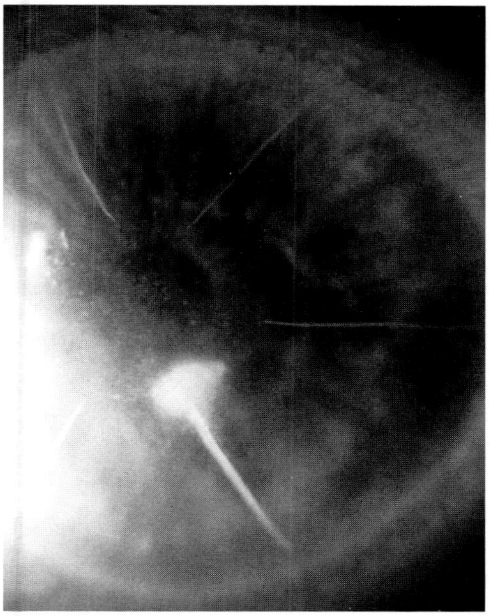

FIGURE 169-3 Stromal infiltrate at site of singular incision 3 months after radial keratotomy, culture-positive for *Candida parapsilosis.* (From Maskin SL, Alfonso E: *Am J Ophthalmol* 114:369-370, 1992.)

used safely after irrigation of these deep corneal abscesses to provide additional sterilizing effect.[10] Although the occurrence of simultaneous bilateral ulcerative keratitis is rare, it is possible; thus it is prudent to perform radial keratotomy on one eye at a time.

Fungal keratitis

Keratomycosis theoretically can occur in any patient after trauma to the cornea, including surgical trauma from radial keratotomy. A 24-year-old male patient developed a *Candida* abscess in one radial incision 1 month after uneventful 8-incision radial keratotomy.[20] He was also diagnosed at that time with cutaneous *Candida* involving the fingernail beds, the groin, the buttocks, and the feet. Presumably, the infection was inoculated into the cornea in the early postoperative period. He was successfully treated with ketoconazole systemically and topical fluconazole 0.5% and achieved a final visual acuity of 20/40 without correction and 20/30 with spectacle correction in the involved eye.

Candida parapsilosis fungal keratitis (Figure 169-3) has been described in a patient 3 months after radial keratotomy surgery.[21] This 35-year-old woman responded to topical amphotericin B and systemic ketoconazole, and best-corrected visual acuity returned to 20/20 in the affected eye.

Atypical *Mycobacterium* keratitis

Mycobacterium chelonei keratitis has been described in two patients from the same office following radial keratotomy.[22] One patient cleared with medical therapy alone of topical amikacin, but the second patient developed recurrent infiltrates, ultimately requiring penetrating keratoplasty.

Because atypical *Mycobacterium* species can survive and grow in some concentrations of standard cold disinfection solutions,[23] radial keratotomy instrumentation should be autoclaved between uses. This recommendation is further substantiated by similar clusters of mycobacterial keratitis cases occurring at other office and outpatient surgical facilities.[24,25]

Herpes simplex virus keratitis

Several cases of recurrent herpes simplex virus keratitis have been reported following radial keratotomy.[26-29] Whether the recurrence was caused by the topical corticosteroids used after radial keratotomy or the trauma of radial keratotomy surgery itself is unknown.[30] Nonetheless, it may be advisable that patients with a history of herpes simplex keratitis not undergo radial keratotomy because of this risk of recurrence.

Sterile keratitis

A case of sterile keratitis involving three adjacent incisions and the intervening stroma occurred in one patient several years after an 8-incision radial keratotomy.[31] Because it did not respond to antibiotics, lubricants and bandage contact lens placement, a conjunctival flap was required for cure. An anaerobic bacterial infection could not be ruled out despite negative cultures. A corneal melt also developed in a 35-year-old physician who underwent radial keratotomy combined with intersecting arcuate incisions.[32] The patient went on to develop keratolysis and subsequent perforation that required corneal transplantation (Figure 169-4). Final best corrected visual acuity was less than 20/200. This case emphasizes the importance of not allowing incisions to intersect during incisional keratotomy surgery (see Intersecting Incisions, Additional Corneal Complications).

A case of delayed sterile keratitis was documented 34 months after a 16-incision radial keratotomy procedure.[33] The keratitis was limited to the incisions, and the patient ultimately required a penetrating keratoplasty for restoration of vision. Histopathologic studies documented delayed corneal wound healing despite the lack of intersecting radial and transverse incisions; however, the patient did have dry eyes but no underlying rheumatoid disease.

From the foregoing cases of ulcerative keratitis following radial keratotomy, both early and late, as well as infectious and noninfectious, it is obvious that any patient who suffers persistent pain, redness, or decreased vision at any time after radial keratotomy

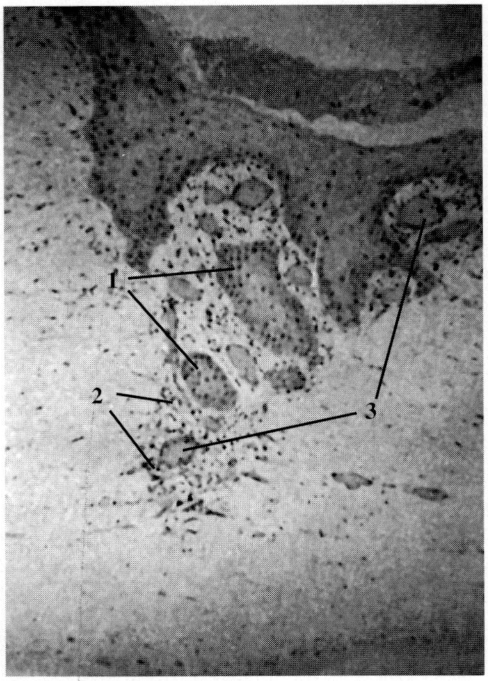

FIGURE 169-4 Recipient corneal button from 35-year-old physician who had previously undergone radial keratotomy complicated by corneal melt. Note 75% stromal thickness keratolysis with persistent epithelial plug (*1*) inflammatory cell infiltrates (*2*) with both superficial and deep vascularization (*3*) (Hematoxylin-eosin stain; ×10 original magnification). (From Karr DJ et al. *Ophthalmology* 92:1244-1248, 1985.)

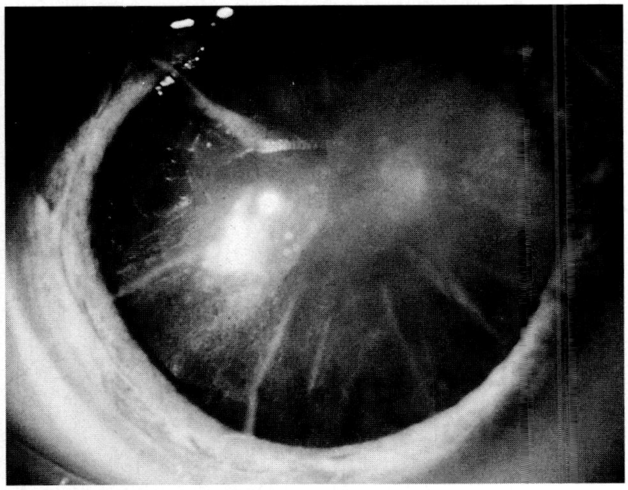

FIGURE 169-5 Cataract formation following macroperforation of the cornea and insult to the anterior lens capsule with the keratotomy knife blade. (Courtesy Walter Stark, MD.)

should consult the ophthalmologist as soon as possible.

ENDOPHTHALMITIS

Three case reports of endophthalmitis following incisional keratotomy have been published.[16,34,35] In each case there was a presumed microperforation at the time of surgery and the causative organism was *S. epidermidis,* which presented as pain, decreased visual acuity, and hypopyon formation between 8 and 10 days postoperatively. Cross and Head[36] identified an additional nine unpublished cases of endophthalmitis following radial keratotomy, including several cases with virulent gram-negative organisms. Microperforations in four large series have ranged from 2% to 11%, further emphasizing the importance of appropriate preoperative preparation of the eye, as with any intraocular procedure performed in a sterile operative environment with sterile instrumentation.[9,37-40] Close follow-up by the surgeon, particularly after a microperforation, and early intervention and treatment in suspected cases of endophthalmitis following radial keratotomy are essential for a successful outcome.

CATARACT FORMATION

Lens opacification can occur in a patient after radial keratotomy unrelated to the procedure simply as a result of the aging process as noted in six patients in the PERK study at 5-year follow-up.[9] Prolonged corticosteroid use can also lead to cataract formation.[34] Acute onset cataract formation has occurred in multiple patients following macroperforation of the cornea and direct insult to the anterior lens capsule (Figure 169-5) with the keratotomy knife.[34,41-44] This complication is avoidable with good surgical technique. A cooperative, well-stabilized patient and a surgeon who is well familiarized with the equipment and instrumentation and who follows a meticulous surgical technique, watching carefully for microperforations, especially during redeepening procedures, are essential for a successful incisional keratotomy. Treatment of clinically significant cataract formation after incisional keratotomy by modern techniques of cataract extraction and lens implantation is effective.[45] However, intraocular lens power calculations may be more difficult because of differences in true corneal power and measured keratometric power.[46]

EPITHELIAL DOWNGROWTH

Only one case of epithelial downgrowth has been reported following radial keratotomy.[47] A microperforation occurred at the time of surgery; however, the patient had an uneventful course for 4 months until a drop in visual acuity was noted (Figure 169-6). Despite the excellent outcome of 20/30 vision following full-thickness corneal cryotherapy, a drop in endothelial cell count would be expected. The degree of epithelial

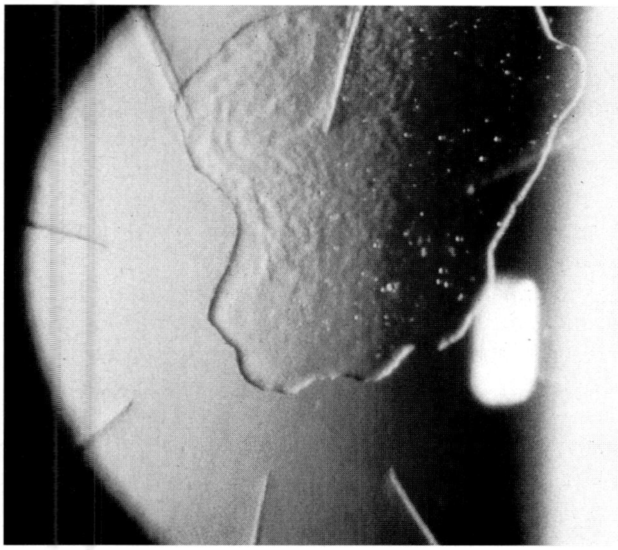

FIGURE 169-6 Retroillumination of cornea demonstrating epithelial ingrowth through microperforation site onto corneal endothelium 4 months after radial keratotomy. (Courtesy Perry S. Binder, MD.)

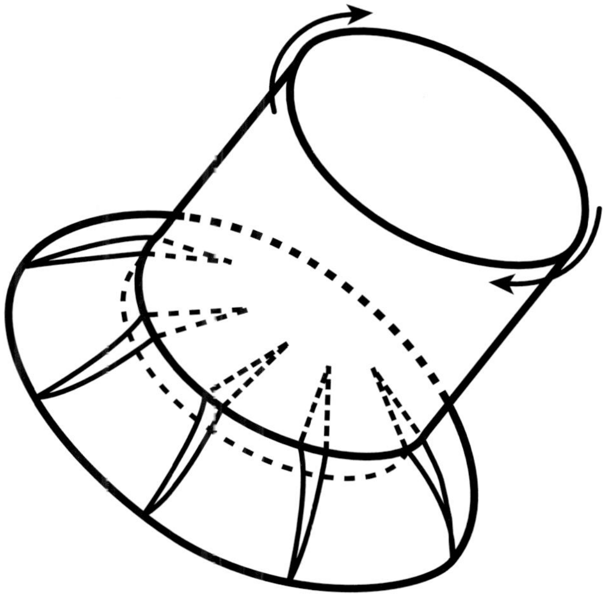

FIGURE 169-7 Schematic drawing of corneal trephine incising cornea that had previously undergone radial keratotomy. Delayed corneal wound healing can lead to separation of peripheral keratotomy wounds, making corneal transplantation difficult. (From Beatty RF et al: *J Refract Surg* 2:207-214, 1986.)

downgrowth at the time of diagnosis will determine prognosis, again emphasizing the importance of ophthalmic consultation for a patient who notices a significant drop in vision at any time after incisional keratotomy.

TRAUMATIC RUPTURE OF GLOBE AND WOUND HEALING

Animal studies have demonstrated that healed corneal incisions have a lesser tensile strength than the original nonincised cornea.[48-55] Full-thickness corneal wounds show little healing in the first week, approximately 30% of normal strength by 4 weeks, and no more than 50% of normal strength by 12 to 24 weeks.[54,55] Thus, the residual weakness of the cornea is not peculiar to incisional keratotomy, but is also true after corneal transplantation, cataract surgery with a clear corneal incision, or traumatic full-thickness perforating injury to the cornea.[48] One study noted that 3 months after radial keratotomy in rabbit eyes, the necessary force to rupture the incisions was less than half that required to rupture an unoperated cornea.[51] Microperforated corneas required even less blunt force to rupture.

McNeill[56] reported a 56-year-old man who had undergone radial keratotomy and 9 years later required a penetrating keratoplasty for visual distortion and monocular diplopia that had developed. During corneal transplantation surgery, one third of the peripheral radial keratotomy incisions spontaneously opened, making suturing difficult and demonstrating incomplete wound healing from the previous refractive surgical procedure (Figure 169-7). McNeill and Wilkins[57] have recommended that a purse-string suture be placed outside of the proposed donor/recipient interface intraoperatively before removal of the recipient donor button at the time of corneal transplantation in a patient who has previously undergone radial keratotomy. This technique can prevent separation of the peripheral radial keratotomy wounds at the time of trephination or corneal transplantation suturing.

Jester et al.[58] reported three histopathologic specimens 1 to 2 years after radial keratotomy. One eye had undergone penetrating keratoplasty and two eyes lamellar keratoplasty secondary to glare, severe astigmatism, overcorrection, or diplopia. All three corneas showed epithelial inclusion cysts into partially healed incisions with variable wound healing. These data support previous studies that showed delayed corneal wound healing as the most common histopathologic alteration after radial keratotomy and may explain to some degree the lack of predictability of refractive outcomes and subsequent refractive instability following radial keratotomy surgeries.

Binder and Charlton[59] examined some 132 histologic specimens following refractive procedures, 27 of which involved eyes following radial keratotomy and 11 following astigmatic keratotomy. These specimens demonstrated abnormalities in wound healing (Figure 169-2) associated with the clinical symptoms of loss of best corrected visual acuity, glare, under correction, and overcorrection. Because of this unpredictability in wound healing, they recommended extreme caution

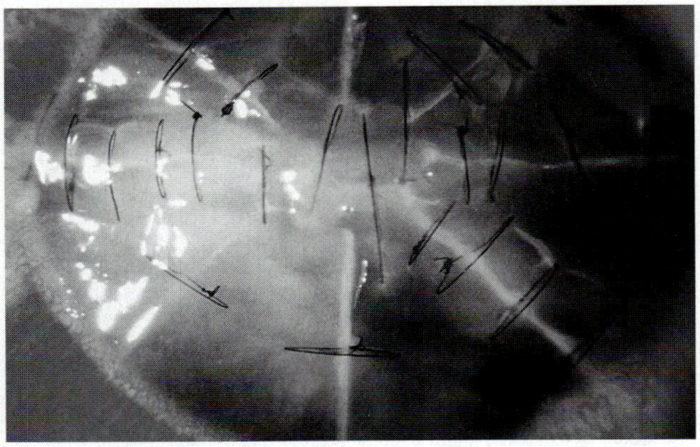

FIGURE 169-8 Traumatic rupture of all eight radial keratotomy incisions 8 months after original surgery secondary to severe blunt trauma to the globe, leading to the loss of the iris and lens and the subsequent need for penetrating keratoplasty. Note perforation through visual axis connecting 4:30 and 9 o'clock incisions. (From Pearlstein ES et al: *Am J Ophthalmol* 106:755-756, 1988.)

when combining different keratorefractive surgeries to the same eye.

Two patients with severe direct ocular trauma developed small perforations in radial incisions, leading to flat anterior chambers that were treated successfully with bandage contact lenses.[60] Severe ocular trauma 2 years after a 16-incision radial keratotomy in one patient[61] and 8 months after an 8-incision keratotomy in another[62] led to evulsion of the lens and iris and ultimately the need for penetrating keratoplasty (Figure 169-8). Blunt trauma from an elbow 24 days after radial keratotomy led to rupture of the cornea requiring repair and subsequent enucleation.[63] A more recent case of automobile airbag-associated corneal rupture 2 years after radial keratotomy has been reported, which required 31 sutures to close seven of eight incisions which ruptured.[64]

Ruptured incisions following hexagonal keratotomy have also been reported.[65] Likewise, surgical manipulations of corneas following incisional keratotomy have led to separation of incompletely healed wounds months to years after the original keratotomies were performed.[66-68] Campos et al.[69] compared the potential for rupture of pig globes after 4-incision radial keratotomy, photorefractive keratectomy with a 6 mm ablation zone, and phototherapeutic keratectomy at various depths. The eyes undergoing photorefractive keratectomy had the least risk of blunt trauma rupture. Intermediate risk was the phototherapeutic keratectomy eyes, whose risk of rupture increased significantly when greater than 40% of the anterior stroma was removed. The highest risk was in the radial keratotomy group.

Multiple cases of mild, moderate, and severe trauma to the orbit and globe have been reported in patients weeks to years after radial keratotomy without rupture of the incisions.[60] Similarly, one patient suffered severe blunt trauma to an eye 6 months after an 8-incision radial keratotomy leading to hyphema formation but without rupture of the incisions.[70] Another patient suffered facial and orbital fractures during a plane crash 4 months after 16-incision radial keratotomy and 2 months after astigmatic keratotomy to the same eye without rupture of the globe.[71]

Despite these latter cases of severe trauma to the globe and orbit without rupture of the keratotomy incisions, patients who undergo radial keratotomy should be made aware of their higher risk of damage to the eyes after blunt trauma. Safety goggles for sports such as racquetball, squash, and handball, as well as for contact sports such as basketball are an absolute requirement for these patients. Finally, boxers and others involved in severe contact/collision sports would be wisely directed away from incisional keratotomy surgery.[72] Corbe et al.[73] examined 273 eyes of previous radial keratotomy subjects applying for a flight crew position in the German armed forces and determined that because of alterations in corneal structure after surgery, only one in three applicants obtained a special dispensation to pursue the field applied for in that particular military branch. The United States military recommends that enlistees, particularly aviators, not be accepted if they have undergone radial keratotomy.[74,75]

Some authors have suggested that mini radial keratotomy performed with shorter incisions (e.g., from the 3.0 to 7.0 mm optical zone) might lessen the risk of traumatic rupture of the globe. Others dispute this possibility based on cadaver eye studies using mini radial keratotomy incisions.[76]

SIGHT-THREATENING COMPLICATIONS IN PERK AND OTHER STUDIES

Of the aforementioned severe sight-threatening complications of radial keratotomy, it is interesting to note that in the 793 PERK eyes followed closely for a decade and beyond, only two of these patients suffered a true sight-threatening complication attributable to the procedure.[5,9,77-79] Both of these complications were related to delayed bacterial keratitis, and both resolved with appropriate therapy, leading to a return of best corrected visual acuity of 20/20 in each.[18] One patient did develop a retinal detachment as reported in the 5-year PERK study results,[9] but it was thought to be unrelated to the previous radial keratotomy surgery. Eight other non-PERK cases of retinal detachment following radial keratotomy have been reported[80,81] (see Retinal Detachment section, Other Unusual Complications).

Similar results are reported by multiple non-PERK investigators with long-term follow-up.[37,53,82] This

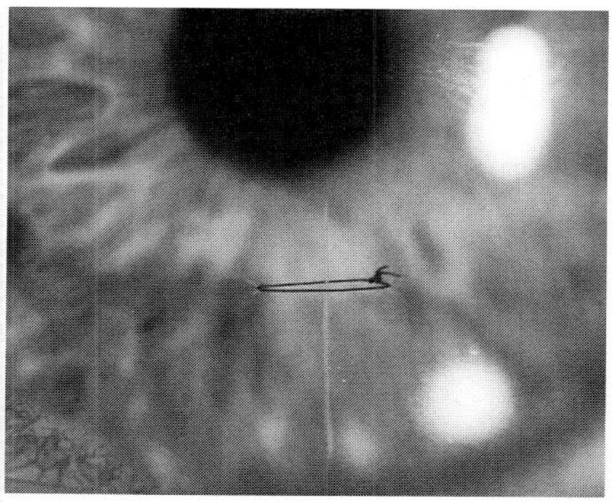

FIGURE 169-9 Macroperforation at the time of radial keratotomy requiring suturing for repair of persistent wound leak. Note that the perforation occurred in an inferior incision at its most central aspect where the cornea was thinnest.

finding might be expected because the surgery was performed in each of these studies by well-trained refractive surgeons using a specific reproducible technique and a relatively conservative approach to radial keratotomy. As the popularity of the procedure has spread, a higher number of complications might be expected. Overall, it is difficult to determine, either from published studies or anecdotally, the actual frequency in number of these specific complications listed previously. Nonetheless, when radial keratotomy has been performed conservatively, as in the PERK study and numerous other studies, the risk of severe sight-threatening complications has been acceptably low.

Bates et al.[83] reported 300 consecutive cases of radial keratotomy performed between 1985 and 1990 and found no sight-threatening complications and no loss of uncorrected visual acuity. Another report of 466 consecutive radial keratotomies listed seven eyes that suffered macroperforations (1.5%), all of which required suturing.[84] None of these eyes, however, developed bacterial keratitis or endophthalmitis as a consequence. Four patients in this study had incisions that extended 1 mm into the clear zone, but no case involved an incision through the visual axis. The errant incisions into the optical zone were made with front-cutting diamond knives and might have been prevented with a back-cutting blade. None of these patients suffered a loss of best corrected visual acuity. The authors concluded that macroperforations (Figure 169-9) were more common with centripetal incisions (limbus to central clear zone) than with centrifugal incisions (central optical zone mark to limbus).

Perhaps the worst reported cases of sight-threatening complications following radial keratotomy involved three patients who underwent the procedure in India and were subsequently evaluated in the United States for treatment.[69] No details of the original surgical technique are available, but they involved a

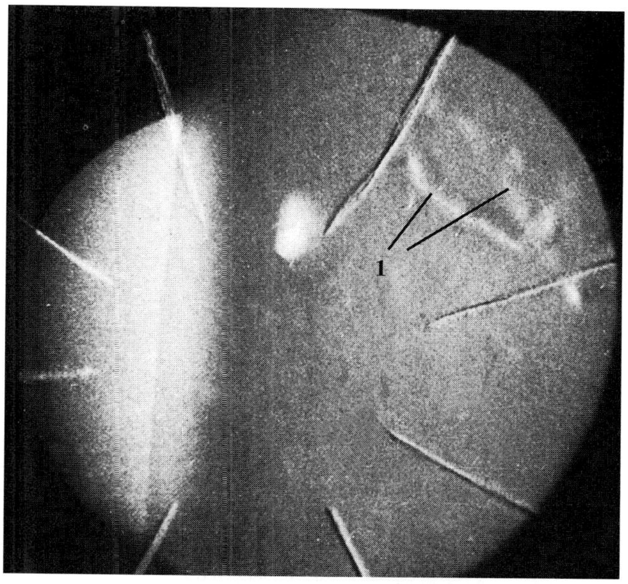

FIGURE 169-10 A maptype epithelial basement membrane change (*1*) following radial keratotomy, which may predispose a patient to recurrent epithelial erosions. (From Nelson JD et al: *Ophthalmology* 92:199-205, 1985.)

9-year-old, 27-year-old, and 37-year-old patient who had each undergone simultaneous bilateral radial keratotomy. Four of these six eyes ended up with light perception visual acuity following multiple surgical procedures to correct macroperforations and flat anterior chambers that resulted after the original radial keratotomy surgery. In one eye, the best-corrected visual acuity was 20/200 after similar multiple surgical procedures, and the final eye stabilized at a visual acuity of 20/40. Obviously, these severe complications are the exception to the rule, occurring when radial keratotomy is placed in the hands of an inadequately trained surgeon unable to provide appropriate post-operative follow-up and unable to deal with the rare complications associated with the procedure.

Additional Corneal Complications

EPITHELIAL/SURFACE PROBLEMS

Basement membrane/subepithelial changes

Incisions through epithelial basement membrane and Bowman's layer can lead to redundant new basement membrane in patients in the early postoperative period.[85] These epithelial changes appear similar to map-dot-fingerprint dystrophy and occur in as many as half of eyes undergoing radial keratotomy but persisting for less than 3 months in three fourths of those eyes (Figure 169-10). Recurrent epithelial erosions are rare after radial keratotomy as less than 1% of

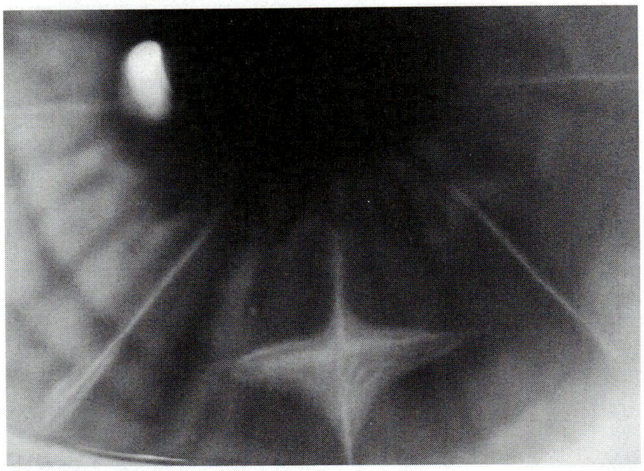

FIGURE 169-15 Intersecting tangential incision (T-cut) and radial incision causing hypertrophic thickened corneal scar at the intersection site.

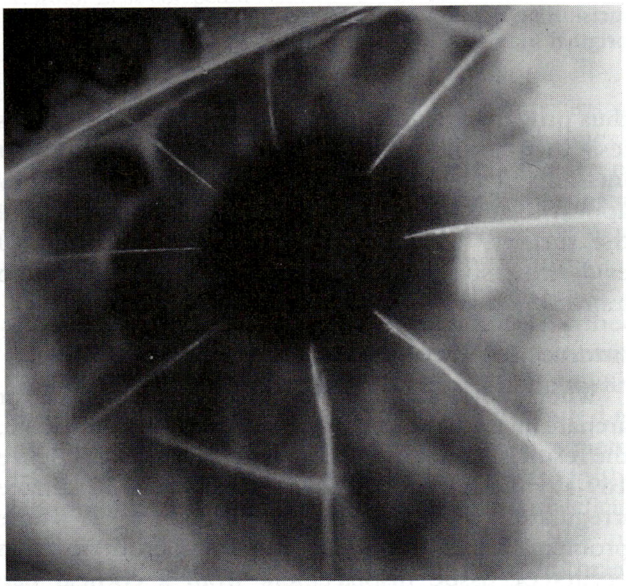

FIGURE 169-16 Ten-day postoperative slit lamp photograph of tangential incision inadvertently connected to radial incision causing a raised triangular facet of corneal tissue with its apex at the intersection point.

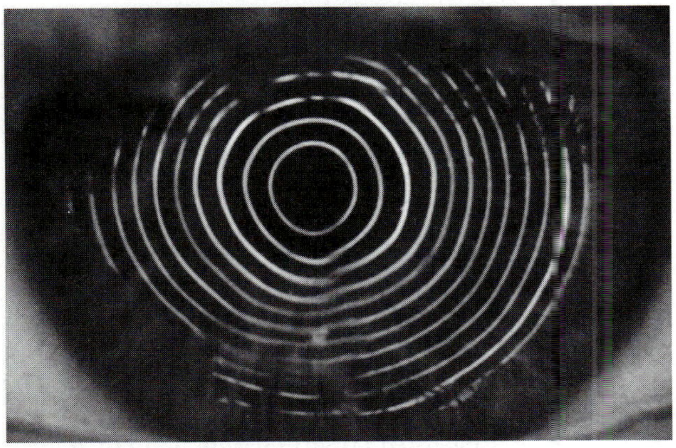

FIGURE 169-17 Photokeratoscope of same eye as in Figure 169-16 showing distorted mires secondary to corneal edema and irregular corneal surface overlying the facet of raised corneal tissue. Mild irregular astigmatism is noted extending into the central mires, and best corrected visual acuity is 20/25.

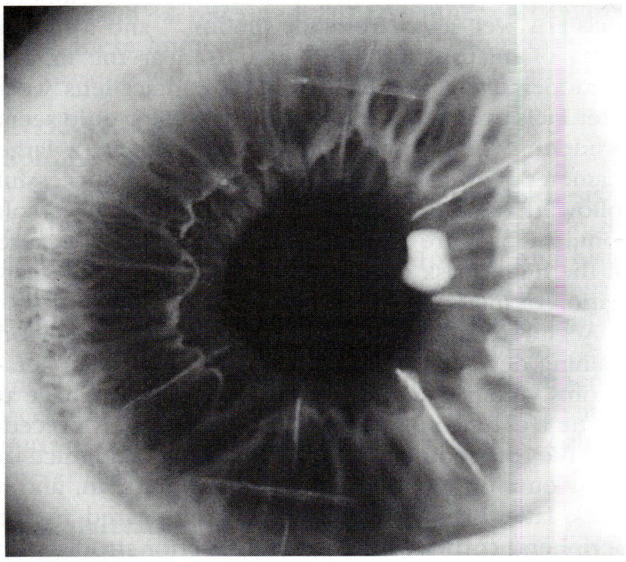

FIGURE 169-18 Slit lamp photograph of cornea demonstrating interrupted radial incisions, in the vertical meridian, which "jump" the transverse incisions. Note that there is no connection of radial and transverse incisions when jump radials are made.

When intersection does occur, hypertonic saline solutions are useful to decrease stromal edema at the intersection point. When a corneal facet develops at an intersection site because of edema, a bandage contact lens is effective in promoting reepithelialization and lessening the edema while at the same time decreasing the foreign body sensation experienced by the patient.

ENDOTHELIAL CHANGES

Microperforations and macroperforations through Descemet's membrane and endothelium directly injure endothelial cells and lead to thin scar formation visible at the perforation site by slit lamp examination. These corneas show a greater central endothelial cell loss than nonperforated corneas.[112] Most studies report less than a 10% endothelial cell loss adjacent to the incisions,[6,113,114] which does not appear to be progressive over time in animal[15,116] or human studies.[97,117] Overall, the extensive endothelial cell loss associated with Sato's technique of posterior radial keratotomy[117,118] performed in the 1940s and 1950s

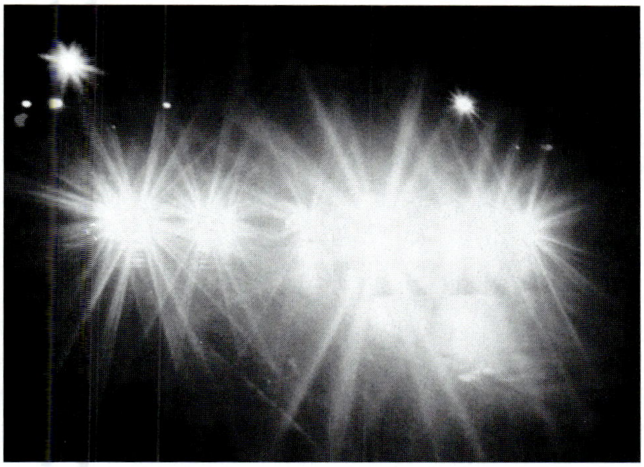

FIGURE 169-19 Photograph simulating severe disabling glare from oncoming headlights during nighttime driving in the rain with wet pavement. (Courtesy Michael R. Deitz, MD.)

has been seen only in a rare patient with extensive anterior incisional keratotomy.[119]

Vision Complications

GLARE AND STARBURST (LONG TERM)

Glare caused by the scattering of light rays can be broken down into a mild starburst effect, moderate glare that does not interfere with daily activities, and disabling glare that disrupts daily activities. Starbursting, such as the scattering of a point source of light (e.g., an automobile headlight) seldom interferes with a patient's ability to function and is commonly present in unoperated patients who use glasses and contact lenses.[120,121] Mild to moderate glare sometimes persists beyond the usual 3 to 6 months after radial keratotomy.[5,29,122,123] Disabling glare occurs rarely,[5,29,34] but when it does occur, it can cause some patients to curtail night driving (Figure 169-19) and even change their occupations.[34]

One study compared nine unoperated control eyes with ten radial keratotomy eyes an average of 5 years after surgery and determined that the number of incisions had no effect on glare.[124] However, the glare did increase with increasing pupillary size that occurs at dusk and with nighttime vision. Theoretically, a surgeon can decrease the risk of glare to the patient by increasing optical zone sizes and limiting irregular astigmatism from decentered optical zones and intersecting incisions.[125]

Sunglasses, particularly with a blue blocker, can be helpful for daytime glare; unfortunately, they cannot counter the increasing glare that develops from increasing pupil size at night.[98,125,126] If the disabling glare is primarily secondary to an irregular astigmatism, fitting with a rigid gas permeable lens can provide a new smooth optical surface to lessen this type of light scattering glare.

OPTICAL ABERRATION AND DECREASED CONTRAST SENSITIVITY

Optical aberration occurs in the center of the visual field when the cornea is not regular over the entrance pupil,[127] as is often the case after radial keratotomy, especially with smaller optical zones.[128] One measure of optical aberration is contrast sensitivity testing, which has been performed extensively after radial keratotomy.[129-134] The most important factor influencing contrast sensitivity as a measure of optical aberration in patients following radial keratotomy is pupil size.[135] Under photopic conditions with relatively small pupil sizes, contrast sensitivity thresholds are similar in eyes after radial keratotomy compared to unoperated control eyes.[127,136] However, under scotopic conditions when the pupil is often 5 mm in size or larger, studies have measured a clinically significant decrease in contrast sensitivity, especially with smaller optical zones,[129,136] possibly from light scattering at the central most aspect of the incisional scars. Contrast sensitivity under scotopic conditions has been noted to improve from between 6 months to 1 year after radial keratotomy.[127] Another study of 44 eyes showed a statistically significant decrease in contrast sensitivity in the first month after radial keratotomy, but by 4 months there was only a mild drop, and no difference existed at 1 year.[137]

A study of 32 corneas after radial keratotomy compared to 47 control, age-matched eyes demonstrated that surgical corneas showed a sharp inflection zone or "paracentral knee" 2.7 mm from the apex of the cornea.[138] Further, the mean range of dioptric power over the 4 mm entrance pupil was 3.80 ± 2.40 diopters in the radial keratotomy eyes compared to 2.00 ± 0.50 diopters in the normal control eyes. Although this corneal asphericity over the entrance pupil provides a multifocal lens effect, allowing better than expected uncorrected visual acuity in these patients, it simultaneously contributes to the optical aberration and decreased contrast sensitivity noted following radial keratotomy, particularly under scotopic conditions. Another study by Applegate[139] demonstrated that paracentral and peripheral corneal optics are degraded after radial keratotomy compared to both normal eyes of similarly low refractive errors and the same eye before surgery. These conclusions suggest that the use of as large a surgery-free zone as possible and meticulous centering of this surgery-free zone over the entrance pupil (Figure 169-20) are important to lessen the risk of optical aberration following radial keratotomy.

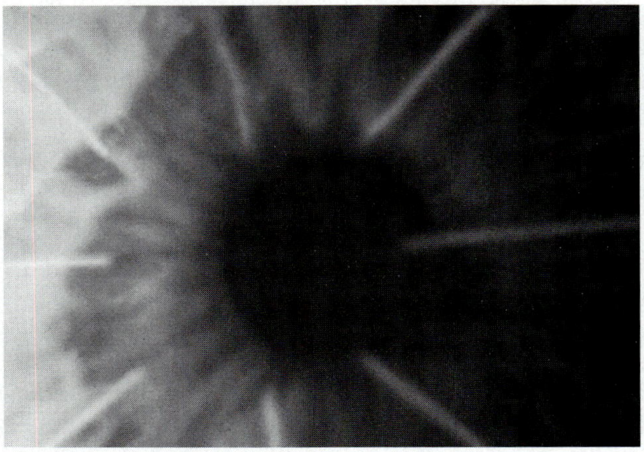

FIGURE 169-20 Cornea after 8-incision radial keratotomy demonstrating central optical clear zone eccentric to the entrance pupil.

DIMINISHED NIGHT (SCOTOPIC) VISION

Several factors contribute to the decreased nighttime vision well documented in some patients after radial keratotomy.[5,34,122,123] As is true of unoperated patients with simple myopia, patients with residual myopia following radial keratotomy have 0.33 to 0.50 diopters more myopia with a dilated pupil at night because of spherical aberration from the paracentral and peripheral cornea, which contributes to a loss of depth of focus.[140] This is particularly true when a more conservative approach is used in modern keratotomy following nomograms intended to keep a patient approximately 0.50 to 1.00 diopter myopic after surgery to lessen the risk of overcorrection, progressive hyperopia, and premature presbyopia.

A second cause of diminished night vision after radial keratotomy is the glare originating from irregularities over the entrance pupil from the most central aspect of the incision scars and the surface aberrations on the front surface of the cornea induced by these incisions. With a large pupil under scotopic conditions of decreased background luminance, Applegate[141] found that disabling glare increased when a point source of light was introduced to an eye following radial keratotomy, whereas such glare was minimal in the unoperated eye. This problem might account for the 3 of 435 patients studied 1 year after surgery in the PERK study who complained of disabling glare that reduced their ability to drive at night.[5] Prevention of this complication may be aided by using as large a central surgery-free zone as possible.

GHOSTING AND MONOCULAR DIPLOPIA

If the cornea is irregular over the entrance pupil, the retinal image generated loses edge definition and ghosting can occur.[126,142] This complication can be particularly disturbing under conditions of low illumination, and when severe can actually lead to monocular diplopia.[98,128] The best treatment plan is to prevent the problem by meticulous centering of the optical clear zone to keep incisions as distanced from the entrance pupil as possible.[36,90,98]

DIURNAL FLUCTUATION IN VISION (LONG TERM)

Diurnal fluctuation of visual acuity is secondary to changes in refraction at different times throughout the day. When diurnal fluctuation continues longer than 3 months, it can be arbitrarily recategorized from a side effect of radial keratotomy to a complication thereof. Its reported occurrence for up to several years after surgery varies from less than 5% to more than 50% of patients.[29,78,120,143,144]

Computerized corneal topography has been used to study eyes in patients who experienced diurnal variation in visual acuity.[144] Ninety-one percent of these patients had dumb-bell-shaped or split optical zones rather than the round concentric optical zones, which were found in 80% of the patients that demonstrated no diurnal fluctuation. Essentially, patients with large, round, central optical zones on corneal topography mapping proved to be free of diurnal fluctuation in vision. Kwitko et al.[145,146] studied central corneal topographic changes in 11 radial keratotomy and 12 penetrating keratoplasty patients comparing both the untreated and the surgically treated eyes of each patient. They determined that changes in corneal topography accounted for the diurnal fluctuation in refraction and visual acuity noted after radial keratotomy and penetrating keratoplasty.

One particularly interesting case was reported by White and Mader,[147] who documented a 1.00 diopter hyperopic fluctuation in refraction in a patient 1 year after radial keratotomy that occurred consistently as the patient traveled from sea level to 10,000 feet elevation in the mountains. The authors thought the acute relative corneal hypoxia at this elevation caused corneal expansion in the area of the keratotomy incisions, leading to additional flattening of the central cornea. They concluded that corneal scarring from healing wounds can lead to physiologic changes of the cornea and predispose such corneas to diurnal changes not otherwise present in normal corneas.

Diurnal fluctuation in vision when extreme can be debilitating to patients interfering with daily activities. In these rare patients, obtaining a refraction early in the day and a second one later in the afternoon or early evening is often adequate to provide the patient with two different spectacle corrections to carry out normal daily activities. Some surgeons have advocated fewer incisions or even mini radial keratotomy to produce an earlier stable refraction,[76] although no data have been published to support this claim.

RELATIONSHIP OF REFRACTION TO VISUAL ACUITY

After radial keratotomy, it is not uncommon for patients to have uncorrected visual acuities better than predicted based solely on cycloplegic refraction.[148,149] Computerized corneal topographic analysis of corneas after radial keratotomy often yields the appearance of a multifocal central cornea that provides greater asphericity. McDonnell et al.[148] used computerized corneal topographic mapping to identify distinct regions of differing central corneal curvature in 3 of 11 eyes after radial keratotomy. These regions of corneal curvature appeared to serve as multiple optical zones, allowing patients to experience excellent uncorrected visual acuity inconsistent with the postoperative spherical equivalent refractions in these patients. This effectively made the cornea a multifocal lens, giving patients better uncorrected visual acuity under photopic conditions, but not without the risk of degradation in contrast sensitivity or even possibly monocular diplopia at night. None of these three particular patients, however, expressed night vision complaints. Moreira et al.[149] found similar topographic changes following radial keratotomy. From a purely optical standpoint, the spherical aberration of the paracentral cornea with its aspheric shape following radial keratotomy may produce a larger blur circle on the retina and thus account for the surprisingly good uncorrected visual acuity in these patients.[150]

Fleming[151] measured corneal aspericity before and after radial keratotomy surgery in the central cornea 1.15 to 3.8 mm from the visual axis (keratoscope rings 2 through 9) with computerized topography. He found a statistically significant increase in corneal aspericity, particularly when smaller optical clear zones were used and concluded that it accounted for the better uncorrected visual acuity than expected after surgery relative to the residual refractive error.

Likewise, Moreira et al.[152] used corneal topography to demonstrate regional variability in corneal curvature, further demonstrating the multifocal lens effect of the aspheric cornea following radial keratotomy. This was perhaps even more strikingly noted in a study of cadaver eyes that underwent 4- and 8- incision radial keratotomy.[153] All eyes showed subregions of differing refractive powers within the clear central zone over the pupil, again giving a multifocal lens effect to the cornea. Pupil size will have a larger effect on refractive error following radial keratotomy, because a larger pupil allows a larger area of the cornea to affect refractive power.[154]

PSYCHOMETRIC CONSIDERATIONS

The patient's perception of visual function and subsequent restriction or freedom of activities play an important role in patient satisfaction after radial keratotomy. Despite the previously mentioned patients who experience glare, optical aberrations, and fluctuation in visual acuity, psychometric data from patients in the PERK study suggest that there is a threefold decrease in worry about eyesight and a 50% reduction in restriction of activities following radial keratotomy relative to unoperated control myopes.[9] Although overall patient satisfaction after radial keratotomy may not be the best measure of success of the procedure, "very satisfied" levels range from 48% to 71% in several studies.[130,155] Unfortunately, a later study that reported 99% of patients achieved 20/40 or better visual acuity after radial keratotomy, although with a greater than 33% reoperation rate, published no psychometric data to support patient satisfaction rates.[156] One would expect satisfaction to be high based on uncorrected visual acuity alone in this study population.

Many studies have used a visual acuity of 20/40 or better and a spherical equivalent refraction of +1.00 to −1.00 diopter as an indication of visual acuity and refractive success after radial keratotomy, respectively. However, a recent study suggests that if freedom from glasses and contact lens wear is the true measure of success after radial keratotomy, then this correlates much better with the visual acuity of greater than or equal to 20/20 in at least one eye and a spherical equivalent refraction of ± 0.50 diopters from emmetropia.[157]

Refractive Complications

PREDICTABILITY OF FINAL REFRACTION

Perhaps the major refractive complication of radial keratotomy is less than perfect predictability of final refractive error regardless of the incisional technique. When data from multiple studies are combined, the percentage of patients whose spherical equivalent refraction 1 year after surgery was outside the range of +1.00 diopters to −1.00 diopters varied from 5% to 16% in the low myopes (less than 3.00 diopters preoperative myopia) to 38% to 76% in the high myopes (greater than 6.00 diopters preoperative myopia).[5,9,37-39,158] Despite this less than perfect predictability, the 5-year PERK data demonstrate uncorrected visual acuity of 20/20 or better in 60% of eyes, 20/40 or better in 88% of eyes, and only 2% with less than 20/200.[9] Sixty-four percent of eyes had a final refraction between −1.00 and +1.00 diopters (see Table 169-1). Presented in a slightly different fashion, Salz et al.[38] reported 100% of eyes with 20/40 visual

Table 169-1. Series of radial keratotomy performed with a diamond knife

	PERK[5] (1 year)	PERK[9] (5 years)	PERK[159] (10 years)	Deitz et al.[37,160]	Salz et al.[38]	Spiegleman et al.[39]	Werblin and Stafford[156]
Demographics							
Number of consecutive eyes	435	793	793	972[37]	225	52	205
Surgery dates	1982-1983	1982-1983	1982-1983	1982-1985[37]	1980-1990	1986 and before	1990-1991
Percent of eyes follow-up	95%	95%	88%	68%[37]	100%	62%	100%
Follow-up time	1 yr	Up to 6.3 years	10 years	≥1 year[37]	≥1 year	≥1 year	≥1 year*
Reoperations included in data (%)	Yes 9%	Yes 12%	Yes 12%	No[37]	Yes 15%	No	Yes 33%†
Predictability							
Total % of eyes between +/−1.00 diopter	60%	64%	60%	76%[37]	73%	91%	NR
% Overcorrected >1.00 D	10%	17%	29%	13%[37]	3%	5%	NR
% Undercorrected >1.00 D	30%	19%	11%	12%[37]	NR	3%	NR
Total % of eyes with ≥20/40 visual acuity	78%	88%	85%	88%[37]	69%	88%	99%
Stability							
Number of eyes with follow-up data >1 yr	NA	757	693	77[160]	100	NR	NA§
Time interval	NA	3-6.3 yrs	6 mo-10 yr	1-2 yrs[160]	2-9 Yrs	NR	NA§
% of eyes with progressive effect of surgery ≥+1.00 D 6 mos. or more after surgery	4%‡	22%	43%	17%[190]	17%	20%	NA§
Complications							
Best corrected visual acuity loss of ≥2 Snellen lines	13%	3%	3%	0.3%[37]	2%	0%	NR
% Corneal perforations	2%	2%	2%	7-11%[37]	3.5%	6%	NR
Vision-threatening complications	0	2‖	2‖	1‖[37]	0	0	NR

NR, not reported; NA, not applicable.
* = 172 out of 205 eyes had ≥1 year follow up.
† = 23 out of 205 eyes had two or more reoperations (thus, three or ore total operations); 6 required suturing of previous incisions.
‡ = 4% of eyes developed between 0.62 to 1.25 diopters of progressive effect between 6 months and 1 year after surgery.
§ = Not enough time lapse for further follow-up studies.
‖ = Delayed bacterial keratitis.

acuity or better postoperatively when the preoperative refraction was less than −3.00 diopters, 73% when it was between −3.00 and −6.00 diopters, and 47% when the preoperative refraction was greater than −6.00 diopters.

Predictability can be affected by many factors, including inter-surgeon and intrasurgeon variability of technique, changes in instrumentation and equipment, and differences in wound healing among individuals. One study looked at the results of corneal fellows in training at UCLA from 1985 to 1991 who performed radial keratotomy in 79 eyes with at least 3 months follow-up.[161] Eighty-five percent of eyes were within 1.00 diopter of emmetropia, and 94% of eyes had an uncorrected visual acuity of 20/40 or better. No sight-threatening complications occurred in this group of patients, and no eyes lost greater than one line of best corrected visual acuity.

Despite increases in predictability with modern equipment, improved instrumentation, and better training of radial keratotomy surgeons, there is no consensus regarding the most effective surgical technique, suggesting that there is no one superior approach to radial keratotomy. In fact, in evaluating a study published in 1993[156] touting the most up-to-date technical improvements in instrumentation, equipment, and technique of radial keratotomy, the percentage of eyes with 20/40 visual acuity or better after one operation was slightly less than the original PERK data at 1 year follow-up with procedures performed in the early to mid 1980s.[5,162,163] Most would agree, however, that the initial use of one specific surgical technique used in a methodical, consistent, and reproducible fashion yields the best initial results.[164,165]

One improvement in technology that might heighten the predictability of radial keratotomy has been computerized corneal topography. Wilson and Klyce[166] screened 53 patients before radial keratotomy with the topographic modeling system and demonstrated that three patients (5.7%) had a forme fruste of keratoconus thus making these patients poor candidates for refractive surgery. Forty-two of these 43 patients were contact lens wearers (18 rigid and 24 soft lenses), and one third of these eyes demonstrated abnormal corneal topography including irregular astigmatism, corneal warpage, and the aforementioned occult ectatic disease of keratoconus. They concluded that appropriate preoperative detection and management, when possible, of these corneal topographic abnormalities are essential before undertaking any refractive surgical procedure; in some cases surgical intervention can be precluded altogether.

Many other studies have documented the unpredictability of radial keratotomy when it is performed on the unsuspecting keratoconus patient,[167-170] further stressing the value of performing preoperative corneal topography to rule out preexisting corneal ectatic disease and irregular astigmatism. Theoretically, this approach should improve the predictability of radial keratotomy by eliminating these patients from the operative pool.[170-172]

A newer concept in improving the predictability of radial keratotomy has been "enhancement" procedures or performing radial keratotomy as a titrated or staged procedure. Werblin and Stafford[156] reported on 205 eyes using a technique popularized by Casebeer (Table 169-1) and demonstrated that 99% of eyes following radial keratotomy and subsequent reoperation(s) had a visual acuity of 20/40 or better. Ninety percent of eyes demonstrated 20/25 visual acuity or better. Thirty-three percent of eyes had one or more reoperations. Additionally, six eyes required reopening and suturing of multiple incisions because of overcorrections or astigmatic shifts. Whether these newer techniques of radial keratotomy will make the procedure more predictable is unknown.[162,163,165,173]

The inherent variability in biologic systems, particularly pertaining to wound healing among individuals will forever limit the predictability of radial keratotomy until pharmacologic agents are developed that allow specific and precise modification of the wound healing process.[174] Epidermal growth factor is one such agent that may have a practical therapeutic use in modulating wound healing after radial keratotomy.[175]

UNDERCORRECTION

Undercorrection or residual myopia increases with successively larger degrees of preoperative myopia.[5,9,37-39,158] The PERK study demonstrated that 19% of eyes had greater than 1.00 diopter of myopia (Table 169-1) 5 years after surgery.[9] Undercorrection is preferable to overcorrection because (1) patients are accustomed to myopia, (2) reoperation might further decrease myopia, and (3) further progression of the effect of surgery may occur, bringing the patient closer to emmetropia in subsequent years.[90] Likewise, residual myopia slows the onset of presbyopia for the patient nearing or over the age of 40 to 45 years.

Some techniques of radial keratotomy use enhancements or reoperations routinely for treatment of undercorrections. In the series by Werblin and Stafford,[156] approximately one third of 205 consecutive eyes undergoing radial keratotomy required one or more enhancement procedures to further correct residual myopia. They found that in the preoperative myopia range of −2.00 to −3.12 diopters, 20% of eyes required one or more enhancement operations. In the preoperative range of −3.25 to −4.27 diopters, fully 51% required one or more enhancements. Finally, in the group of −4.50 to −8.00 diopters of preoperative myopia, 45% of eyes required one or more enhancements. Reoperations varied from redeepening and lengthening original incisions to adding incisions.

Treatment of undercorrection with spectacle and contact lenses is typically satisfactory if additional surgery will not correct residual myopia.[6,85,100,101,103] Most conservative surgeons intentionally plan for some small degree of residual myopia because of the well-documented continued progressive effect of radial keratotomy that occurs in many patients and the strong desire to prevent overcorrection.

A newer treatment approach to undercorrections has been the reduction of residual myopia with photorefractive keratectomy.[176-181] By combining these studies, a total of 114 eyes have been treated for undercorrection following radial keratotomy with the excimer laser. The largest of these series was reported by Durrie et al.[180] who studied 91 eyes and found that 1 year after photorefractive keratectomy, 89.7% of eyes had 20/40 visual acuity or better, and 75.9% were within 1.00 diopter of emmetropia. Mean residual myopia after radial keratotomy but before excimer laser treatment was −3.62 diopters. They concluded that in those eyes that had only a partial response to maximum safe refractive keratotomy, photorefractive keratectomy appeared to be a viable option for correcting residual myopia with acceptable safety and results. However, a 42-year-old man, who had undergone 16-incision radial keratotomy followed by photorefractive keratectomy for residual myopia, developed 3+ anterior stromal haze after the laser procedure.[181] Final best corrected visual acuity was 20/80 in this patient who represented a four line loss of best corrected visual acuity after the excimer laser procedure. Further studies are necessary to determine the ultimate safety of photorefractive keratectomy after radial keratotomy.

OVERCORRECTION

Overcorrection or secondary hyperopia is a more serious complication after radial keratotomy and can be broken down into three categories. Transient hyperopia in the first several weeks after surgery is secondary to corneal edema and resolves as the edema abates (see Diurnal Fluctuation in Vision, Expected Side Effects of Incisional Keratotomy). A second more serious type of overcorrection occurs from too much surgery and becomes a permanent overcorrection as measured several months after radial keratotomy. Finally, progressive hyperopia, as noted in the next section, can lead to a worsening of an original overcorrection or the development of overcorrection years following otherwise successful radial keratotomy surgery.

Using a hyperopic refraction of +1.00 diopters or more as a definition of overcorrection, 10% of the original 435 eyes in the PERK study were overcorrected at 1 year follow-up.[5] This number had increased to 17% of 793 eyes at 5-year and 29% at 10-year follow-up because of progressive hyperopia.[9,159] Deitz et al.[37] noted a 13% overcorrection rate at 1-year follow-up (Table 169-1). By using a more conservative nomogram, specifically to reduce the number of overcorrections, Salz et al.[38] performed 4-incision radial keratotomy in more than 50% of eyes and noted a 3% overcorrection rate in the 225 eyes followed for 1 year. Likewise, Spigelman et al.[39] performed an initial 4-incision radial keratotomy on 52 eyes and noted a 5% overcorrection rate at 1 year. In their series of 20[illegible] eyes with 1 year follow-up, Werblin and Stafford[156] did not report their overcorrection rate. However, in a subsequent authors' reply to a letter to the editor,[16[illegible]] they noted that at least six eyes had greater than 1.50 diopters of hyperopia on final follow-up, and six additional eyes required suturing, presumably some secondary to significant overcorrection.

Many surgeons have advocated 4-incision radial keratotomy to lessen the risk of overcorrection and progressive hyperopia, allowing additional incisions to be placed at a later time in the presence of residual myopia.[39,158,182] In its assessment of radial keratotomy, the American Academy of Ophthalmology has also suggested that the risk of overcorrection is lessened by initial placement of only four incisions whenever possible.[40] Despite this precaution, overcorrection has still been measured in 3% to 6% of eyes undergoing conservative 4-incision radial keratotomy.[39,158]

Mini radial keratotomy has been advocated by some surgeons to lessen the risk of immediate overcorrection and progressive hyperopia.[76] This variation of radial keratotomy involves shortening the incisions so that they spare the peripheral 2 to 2.5 mm of the cornea. No long-term follow-up data on this technique have been published, and some argue against its effectiveness.[76] Some have suggested that revision of previous radial keratotomy wounds by redeepening increases the risk of overcorrection because of the decreased predictability of effect from these deepened incisions.[183]

John[184] has suggested that prevention is the best mode of treatment of overcorrection. Avoiding microperforations and macroperforations intraoperatively and taking a conservative approach to surgical planning by using fewer incisions and larger optical zones are prudent approaches. Likewise, the patient can lessen the propensity for overcorrection in the postoperative period by avoiding eye rubbing and preventing direct pressure to the eyes during sleep.

Treatment of overcorrection in the early postoperative period includes hyperosmotic topical agents (5%

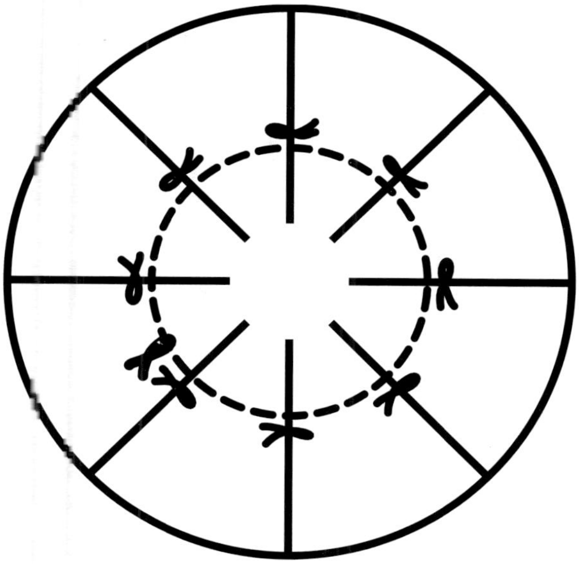

FIGURE 169-21 Schematic drawing of a purse-string suture through all 8 radial incisions at a 7 mm optical zone followed by interrupted sutures through each incision at an 8 mm optical zone used for correction of hyperopia after radial keratotomy. (From Lyle WA, Jin J: *Refract Corneal Surg* 3:80-83, 1992.)

sodium chloride), discontinuation of topical steroids, and use of antiglaucoma medication to decrease intraocular pressure.[36,90,185,186] Whether any of these treatments have a lasting effect is debatable. Conventional spectacle correction and contact lenses are excellent means for treating overcorrection when tolerated by the patient.[6,85,100,101,103] When these approaches are not an option or when they are unsuccessful, surgical intervention can be undertaken by opening the radial incisions with a Sinskey hook to remove the epithelial plug and suturing of the incision with a continuous purse-string suture and/or interrupted 10-0 nylon or mersilene sutures, which may be left in place permanently if a near emmetropic refraction results.[187,188]

Alio and Ismail[189] reported 13 patients who had their overcorrection treated with either purse-string suturing, interrupted sutures, or a combination of the two. The results suggested that neither purse-string nor radial suturing alone was enough to achieve a permanent effect on the cornea, and results were better when the two techniques were combined. Lyle and Jin[190] combined purse-string and interrupted sutures (Figure 169-21) in nine patients for treatment of overcorrection. Seventy-eight percent of the patients were able to be corrected within 1.00 diopter of emmetropia after suture placement, and all patients achieved an uncorrected visual acuity of 20/40 or better. The purse-string suture was placed at a 7 mm optical zone using 10-0 mersilene suture placed at a 60% depth, and the interrupted sutures were 10-0 mersilene at a 7.5 to 8 mm optical zone and 80% depth. Follow-up ranged from 3 to 10 months, with a mean of less than 6 months.

Damiano et al.[191] reported on 19 eyes of 18 patients that underwent double purse-string suturing for overcorrection after radial keratotomy, with an average follow-up of 24 months. This technique produced a significant steepening of the central cornea, which appeared stable for more than 1 year follow-up. Uncorrected visual acuity after suturing was 20/40 or better in 74% of eyes. No significant complications were reported, and no eyes lost any lines of refractive Snellen acuity.

PROGRESSIVE HYPEROPIA

Progressive hyperopia is defined as a continuation of the flattening process of the central cornea that leads to a greater than 1.00 diopter hyperopic direction shift in spectacle corrected visual acuity over time after radial keratotomy.[5] In assessing the stability of refraction between 6 months and 5 years postoperatively, a progressive effect greater than 1.00 diopters in the hyperopic direction has been measured in 22% of eyes in the PERK study[9] and 17% by Salz et al.[38] (Table 169-1). This result is comparable to the regressive effect of 1.00 diopter or more in the myopic direction in 2% and 6% of eyes, respectively, in these same studies. Progressive hyperopia has been noted in 20% of eyes by Spigelman et al.,[39] 17% by Deitz et al.,[160] 13% by Salz and Salz,[182] 22% by Arrowsmith and Marks,[82] and 26% by Waring[9] and further adds to the risk of overcorrection. In addition to the progressive hyperopia rates noted previously, Schneider et al.[192] noted a rate of 20% over 5 years in 350 radial keratotomy eyes operated on between 1985 and 1987. When looking at metal blade data where longer follow-up data are available, Deitz et al.[160] noted a 31% incidence of progressive hyperopia between 12 and 48 months after radial keratotomy. After an average of 8.5 years, this number had increased to a disturbing 54% of the original 225 eyes followed for at least 5 years.[193]

The PERK study group looked at stability of refraction 4 years after radial keratotomy in 341 eyes.[194] Between 2 weeks and 3 months postoperatively, 59% of eyes lost 1.00 diopter or more of initial effect. Between 3 and 6 months postoperatively, 95% of eyes showed less than 1.00 diopter of change in refraction. However, between 6 months and 4 years, 24% of eyes developed 1.00 diopter or more of progressive hyperopia, and 4% of eyes regressed 1.00 diopter or more. Seventy-two percent of eyes showed less than a 1.00 diopter change in either a myopic or hyperopic direction during this time frame. These authors noted that the average hyperopic shift over 4 years for this radial keratotomy study population was 0.40 diopter, roughly a 0.10 diopter hyperopic shift per year. The PERK study at 10 years with 88% follow-up on 793 eyes demonstrated a progressive hyperopic shift of 1.00 diopter or more in 43% of eyes,[159a] up from 22% noted at 5 years of follow-up[9] (Table 169-1). Patients with smaller optical zones tended to have more hyperopic shift compared to those with larger optical zones. As pointed out by Waring et al.[194] and MacRae,[195] further long-term follow-up and data analysis of the PERK study patients are necessary to determine the long-term stability of refractive error after radial keratotomy.

One particularly severe case of progressive hyperopia was reported by Waisberg[196] in a 27-year-old woman who initially had a spherical equivalent refraction of −3.00 diopters in both eyes before radial keratotomy. Over an 8-year period, her refraction had progressed from near plano after surgery to +9.00 diopters right eye and +8.75 diopters in the left eye, yielding best corrected visual acuities of 20/25 in both eyes. Damiano and Forstot[197] noted two patients with progressive flattening of the cornea after radial keratotomy over a 7- and 10-year period, respectively. The progressive hyperopia noted by cycloplegic refraction in these two patients was accounted for by further keratometric flattening of the central cornea with time.

As with initial overcorrection after radial keratotomy, prevention of progressive hyperopia is the best method of treatment. Minimizing enhancements or reoperations involving redeepening of previously made incisions, using larger optical zones and fewer incisions when possible, and not exceeding the limits of radial keratotomy are prudent recommendations to lessen this complication.[197] Perhaps mini radial keratotomy with shorter incisions will lessen the risk of progressive hyperopia over time.[76]

Treatment of progressive hyperopia is much like that of initial overcorrection after radial keratotomy. Spectacle correction is certainly the easiest, most reversible and least risky treatment option. Likewise, patients can be fitted with a contact lens.[6,85,100-102] Finally, opening of radial incisions with a Sinskey hook and curetting the epithelium followed by resuturing with either interrupted or a purse-string suture or combination thereof is an effective means of management.[187-191,198] Other useful surgical procedures include hyperopic epikeratoplasty, lamellar keratoplasty, and penetrating keratoplasty.[58,59,198]

ASTIGMATISM

Residual astigmatism

Like undercorrection of myopia, undercorrection of astigmatism or residual astigmatism can remain after radial keratotomy, with or without astigmatic keratotomy. Nomograms for astigmatic correction are less predictable than for myopia correction[199] and most surgeons do not use them unless the preoperative refractive astigmatism is 0.75 diopters or more. Tangential or arcuate incisions can be added, lengthened or redeepened following the initial radial/astigmatic keratotomy procedure if residual astigmatism is present. A potential major complication to avoid during astigmatic keratotomy is connection of radial incisions with tangential and arcuate incisions[36, 08-110] (see Intersecting Incisions, Additional Corneal Complications).

Induced astigmatism

Induced astigmatism can occur after radial keratotomy from radial incisions alone. In the PERK study, 15% of eyes had a greater than 1.00 diopter increase in astigmatism when no attempt was made to correct preexisting astigmatism.[9] Likewise, astigmatism can be induced at a new axis by overly aggressive tangential and arcuate incisions leading to a shift in astigmatism 90 degrees away from its original location. Increased or induced astigmatism ranging from 1.00 to 3.00 diopters has been noted in 2% to 11% of eyes after radial keratotomy.[5,34,82,200]

Treatment of induced astigmatism depends on its etiology. If there has been a 90 degree shift in astigmatism axis because excessive astigmatic incisions, these incisions can be resutured with 10-0 mersilene after being opened with a Sinskey hook and the epithelial plugs removed.[201] Likewise, additional tangential or arcuate incisions can be made in the new axis of the steep cylinder, making certain to avoid intersecting these new incisions with previously made radial incisions.

Computerized corneal topography has become an invaluable tool to assess both preoperative congenital astigmatism and postoperative residual or induced astigmatism. Using this information as a "road map" of the cornea allows the surgeon to design a specific surgical approach for correction of the preexisting or remaining astigmatism in an individual patient.

Irregular astigmatism

Irregular astigmatism is noted in all patients to some degree after radial keratotomy because of the less than perfectly smooth corneal surface that overlies the incisions.[90] However, when the incisions extend into a visual axis (Figure 169-22) or there is extensive hypertrophic scarring such as that caused by intersecting incisions, irregular astigmatism can be devastating and sight-threatening.[202,203] Poor surgical planning leading to excessive number and imprecise placement of incisions can also cause this disabling complication.[90] One patient underwent radial keratotomy

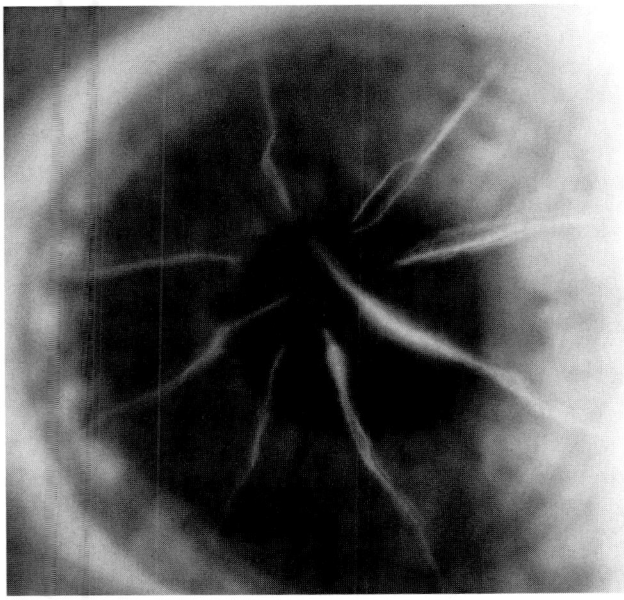

FIGURE 169-22 Twenty-seven-year-old patient who underwent 8-incision radial keratotomy followed by reoperation with redeepening of original incisions. Note how the second set of incisions extend outside of original incisions and how the 4 o'clock incision extends beyond the optical zone mark into the visual axis. Patient was left with irregular astigmatism, and best corrected visual acuity dropped from 20/20 preoperatively to 20/60 when last evaluated 4 months after reoperation.

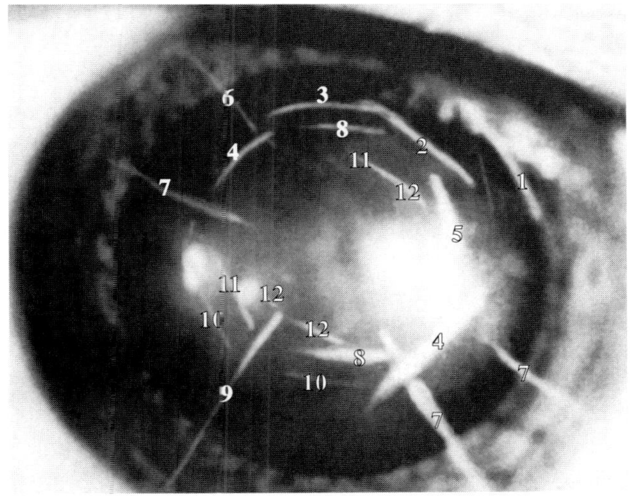

FIGURE 169-23 Cornea 6 weeks after the last of 12 keratotomy procedures. Multiple incisions are present in a double hexagonal pattern, leading to severe corneal ectasia. Keratometry readings after the twelfth operation were 60.5 axis 65 degrees by 46.5 axis 155 degrees. The numbers over the incisions refer to the operation in which the incision(s) was (were) made. The patient's refractive cylinder rotated clockwise with each procedure, causing the surgeon to "chase" the astigmatism with each successive procedure. (From Wellish KL et al: *J Refract Surg* 10:360-364, 1994.)

followed by 12 "enhancement" reoperations (Figure 169-23) for residual astigmatism, which ultimately led to corneal ectasia, similar to keratoconus, that required penetrating keratoplasty for restoration of vision.[106]

Computerized corneal topography and photokeratoscopy can be used to assess the presence and degree of irregular astigmatism in a cornea both before and after radial keratotomy. Maloney et al.[204] studied 29 corneas with topographic mapping following radial keratotomy and measured the degree of irregular astigmatism compared to 146 normal control eyes, 58 eyes with corneal transplantation, and 29 eyes with keratoconus. The topographic irregularity averaged 0.40 diopters in the normal eyes, 0.8 diopters in the radial keratotomy eyes, 2.00 diopters in the corneal transplantation eyes, and 3.00 diopters in the keratoconus eyes.

Treatment of irregular astigmatism depends on its etiology. If it exists preoperatively secondary to corneal warpage from rigid contact lens wear or a primary corneal diagnosis (e.g., keratoconus, pterygium, Salzmann nodules), radial keratotomy is best avoided,[166-172] either permanently or until the condition clears. Rigid contact lens fitting, although more difficult after radial keratotomy because of unusual topographic corneal changes[6,85] and neovascularization of incisions,[43,101,103] is a reversible, relatively safe, and effective treatment option for post radial keratotomy irregular astigmatism.[6,85,100] Fitting in this patient population can be difficult but may be aided by corneal topography.[205,206] If irregular astigmatism leads to severe visual disability and is untreatable by more conservative approaches, a patient may require lamellar or penetrating keratoplasty.[58,59,106]

PREMATURE PRESBYOPIA

Patients whose eyes are overcorrected in the early postoperative period secondary to edema can expect premature presbyopia if accommodative reserve is not adequate to compensate for the hyperopia. This is particularly true of patients over the age of 35 to 40 years. These patients must be extensively counseled regarding the need of reading glasses to treat normally occurring presbyopia following radial keratotomy if their final refraction is near emmetropia or hyperopic.[207] This counseling becomes particularly important if the patient's occupation requires extensive near work such as required of an accountant or secretary. If these patients spend much of their day without corrective lenses doing closeup work, they may be better advised against radial keratotomy. Another option for patients over 40 to 45 years of age includes keeping the nondominant eye mildly to moderately myopic for near vision while attempting to correct the dominant eye closer to emmetropia, as with a monovision contact lens technique.[90]

ANISOMETROPIA (PERMANENT)

A significant refractive difference exists between the two eyes in most patients who undergo radial keratotomy one eye at a time during the interval between operations. However, if a significant difference exists in final refraction between the two eyes after both eyes have undergone radial keratotomy, or if the patient elects not to have the second eye operated, this anisometropia can be permanent. In the PERK study, 385 of the original 435 patients chose to have second eye surgery. Of these, 88% had less than a 2.00 diopter spherical equivalent difference between the two eyes 5 years after surgery. However, 2% had greater than a 3.00 diopter difference after surgery. The mean difference was 0.62 diopters, with 65% of patients having a zero to one line difference in uncorrected vision between the two eyes, but 11% having a four line or more difference in uncorrected visual acuity.[9] Smaller degrees of anisometropia are common after bilateral radial keratotomy as noted in the 3-year follow-up of the PERK study, in which 41% of patients had asymmetry of 1.00 diopter or more between the two eyes.[78]

Greater degrees of anisometropia can persist when the patient chooses not to have the second eye operated, as did 50 patients of the original 435 in the PERK study.[9] Transient anisometropia can be minimized by shortening the time between surgery to the two eyes. Ninety-five percent of patients in the PERK study waited 1 year between surgery on the first and second eye.[78] Most surgeons today wait 1 to 6 weeks between surgeries from the first to the second eye; however, some surgeons practice simultaneous bilateral radial keratotomy, which eliminates this period of transient anisometropia.[10-12,208,209] This is not without additional risks for the patient, however, including simultaneous bilateral bacterial keratitis.[10-12]

Long-term treatment of permanent anisometropia can be managed with contact lens wear and special spectacle corrections as with any other patient suffering asthenopia from anisometropia.[140] Additional surgery may be performed on one or both eyes when appropriate to lessen or eliminate the anisometropia.

DECREASE IN BEST CORRECTED VISUAL ACUITY

A gain or loss of one Snellen line of vision is a normal variation in visual acuity from refraction to refraction; therefore, only a change of two lines or more of best corrected visual acuity is considered meaningful.[210] Twenty-five of 752 eyes (3%) lost two lines or more of best corrected visual acuity when considering 5-year

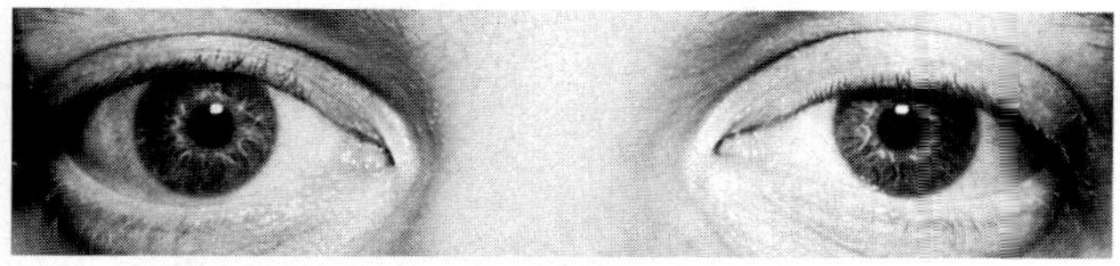

FIGURE 169-24 Acquired blepharoptosis of the left upper eyelid still present 6 months after radial keratotomy. (From Carroll RP, Lindstrom RL: *Am J Ophthalmol* 102: 800, 1986.)

data (see Table 169-1) from the PERK study.[9] Twenty-one eyes lost two lines, two eyes lost three lines, one eye lost four lines, and one eye lost seven lines. This seven line loss was from cataract formation noted on follow-up examination, but was thought to be unrelated to the previous radial keratotomy. Most of these eyes had better than 20/20 visual acuity preoperatively; thus only 10 eyes (1.3%) had a best spectacle correction visual acuity worse than 20/20. Six eyes corrected to 20/25, two eyes to 20/30, one eye to 20/40, and the eye with cataract formation to 20/80 visual acuity.

According to the American Academy of Ophthalmology Assessment of Radial Keratotomy,[79] a decrease in best corrected spectacle visual acuity of two lines or more may occur in about 1% of patients after radial keratotomy. Salz et al.[38] noted only one eye that had a best corrected visual acuity of less than 20/40 in his series of 225 consecutive eyes over 10 years. Three eyes lost two lines and one eye lost three lines of refractive visual acuity. The one eye with worse than 20/40 visual acuity had dropped to 20/60 from progression of myopic retinal degeneration thought to be unrelated to radial keratotomy. Marmer[121] noted an incidence of reduced best corrected visual acuity of 0.9% in a survey of over 63,000 cases of radial keratotomy. Treatment of this refractive complication is difficult because its etiology is often difficult to identify and when identifiable (e.g., irregular astigmatism), treatment options are limited.[106]

Other Unusual Complications

ESOTROPIA

Two cases of esotropia have been reported after radial keratotomy in patients whose preoperative myopia masked their reduced fusional amplitudes.[211] Both patients were less than 40 years of age and were overcorrected, leading to hyperopia in the postoperative period. This newly acquired need to accommodate for correction of the hyperopia combined with their reduced fusional divergence amplitudes led to a secondary esotropic strabismus. Keeping a patient intentionally undercorrected after surgery or at least avoiding overcorrection as much as possible is advisable in the presence of a preoperative large angle esophoria or intermittent esotropia.

BLEPHAROPTOSIS

As can occur with any eye surgery that requires a lid speculum, blepharoptosis (Figure 169-24) has been reported after radial keratotomy.[212,213] In one particular PERK study center that used a Knapp rigid lid speculum with a locking thumbscrew mechanism, seven of 68 patients developed ptosis in the first eye after radial keratotomy.[213] Five of these seven patients ultimately underwent radial keratotomy in the second eye, and four of five developed ptosis again in the second operative eye. The mechanism of development of blepharoptosis was thought to be secondary to a disinsertion of the levator aponeurosis as occurs after cataract surgery that involves a lid speculum with or without a superior rectus bridal suture.[214] The authors recommend that a flexible wire lid speculum might be less likely to induce ptosis than the rigid speculum.[212] Treatment of blepharoptosis after radial keratotomy would be the same as its repair after other forms of ocular surgery but should be delayed until both eyes have been operated and at least 6 months after the last surgery, because at least several patients have shown spontaneous resolution of ptosis following radial keratotomy.[36,213]

IRIDOCYCLITIS

A mild anterior chamber reaction is occasionally seen in the first week after radial keratotomy, especially if a large epithelial defect occurs at the time of surgery.[5] Several reports of moderately severe iridocyclitis (Figure 169-25), both associated with microperforations, have been noted.[215,216] A surgeon must follow these patients closely to rule out early endophthalmitis, with appropriate intervention depending on the severity of the case, the level of suspicion, and the patient's initial response to intensive antiinflammatory medication. As with all forms of iridocyclitis, use of a topical mydriatic will lessen discomfort and the associated photophobia.

GLAUCOMA

Glaucoma attributable to radial keratotomy has not been reported in a patient after surgery in the United States, however, shallowing or loss of the anterior chamber secondary to microperforation or macroperforation could narrow the angle and precipitate a secondary form of glaucoma. Hersh et al.[217] reported three patients who had been operated on in India, all of whom developed flat anterior chambers, secondary glaucomas, and corneal problems requiring multiple surgical interventions. Four of these six eyes ended up with light perception vision, one eye with 20/200 visual acuity, and one eye with 20/40 visual acuity.

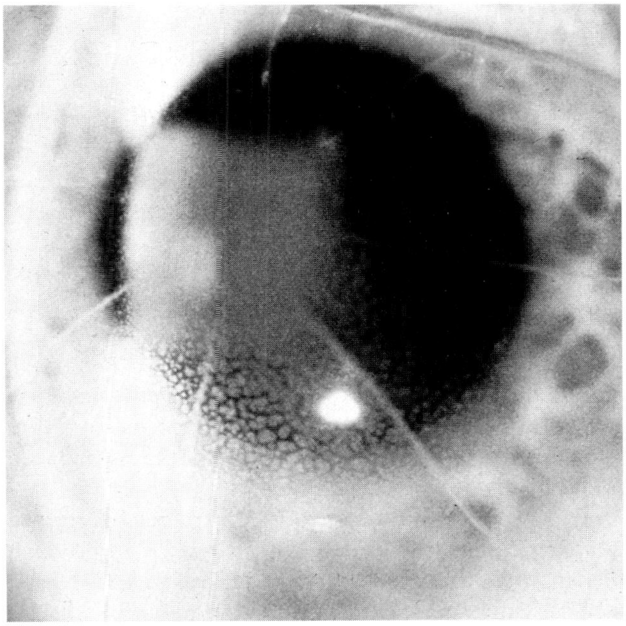

FIGURE 169-25 Moderately severe anterior uveitis with keratic precipitates in the early postoperative period following radial keratotomy complicated by a microperforation. (From Starling J, Hofmann R: *J Refract Surg* 2:96-98, 1986.)

Long-term topical steroid use can induce increased intraocular pressure and subsequent glaucoma after radial keratotomy. Published data suggest that long-term topical steroids do not increase the predictability or effectiveness of radial keratotomy and should be avoided for this reason alone, as well as for their increased risk of inducing glaucoma and cataract formation.[208]

Uncontrolled glaucoma is a contraindication to radial keratotomy because of the potential for increased flattening of the cornea induced by increased intraocular pressure.[186] Likewise, even controlled glaucoma is a relative contraindication because it may later become uncontrolled or even require surgical intervention. Despite some reports that the weakening of the peripheral cornea by radial keratotomy may lower intraocular pressure in patients and thus reduce their risk of glaucoma, Sastry et al.[218] reported on 134 eyes from the PERK study that showed no clinically significant difference in intraocular pressure from baseline between operated and unoperated eyes 1 year after surgery. There are no reported cases of glaucoma surgery in a patient who has previously undergone radial keratotomy. However, patients have undergone extracapsular cataract extraction and phacoemulsification after radial keratotomy with minimal technical difficulty, suggesting that other anterior segment surgery such as a filtering procedure would probably be well tolerated.[43,219]

RETINAL DETACHMENT

Only one patient in the original PERK study developed a retinal detachment,[9] but it occurred years after the procedure and was thought to be unrelated to the radial keratotomy procedure. Another case of retinal detachment occurred in a patient 1 month after a repeat radial keratotomy procedure complicated by microperforation.[81] The patient had preexisting lattice degeneration of the peripheral retina. Two possible mechanisms contributing to retinal tears in this patient may have been sudden decompression of the globe at the time of microperforation and possible ciliary spasm after the surgery. This second mechanism would be similar to that produced by miotic agents and their propensity to induce retinal detachments in high and moderate myopes.[34,220]

Several additional reported cases of retinal detachment have been associated with the use of miotics in the early postoperative period to lessen overcorrection[34,220]; another case was reported following double perforation of the globe and was associated with retrobulbar anesthesia at the time of radial keratotomy.[34] The latter case emphasizes the importance of avoiding retrobulbar and peribulbar anesthesia with radial keratotomy, as this type of anesthesia poses an unnecessary risk to the patient.

Rodriguez and Camacho[80] reported on the treatment of retinal detachment after refractive surgeries for myopia, including seven patients who underwent radial keratotomy. In each of the cases where scleral buckling was required to repair the retinal detachment, refractive changes were induced by an increase in the axial length of the eye, leading to recurrence of myopia and/or astigmatism. Refractive myopia increased a mean of -3.00 diopters after buckling. The authors thought that preexisting peripheral retinal degenerative changes were present in these patients preoperatively and recommended thorough examination of the peripheral retina to treat these abnormalities before radial keratotomy when appropriate.

REFERENCES

1. Ellis W: *Radial keratotomy and astigmatism surgery,* Irvine, Calif, 1986, Keith C Terry and Associates.
2. Sher NA et al: Topical diclofenac in the treatment of ocular pain after excimer photorefractive keratectomy, *Refract Corneal Surg* 9:425-436, 1993.
3. Arshinoff S et al: Use of topical nonsteroidal anti-inflammatory drugs in excimer laser photorefractive keratectomy, *J Cataract Refrac Surg* 20 (suppl):216-222, 1994.
4. Ferrari M: Use of topical nonsteroidal anti-inflammatory drugs after photorefractive keratectomy, *J Refract Corneal Surg* 10 (suppl):S287-289, 1994.
5. Waring GO et al: Results of the Prospective Evaluation of Radial Keratotomy (PERK) study one year after surgery, *Ophthalmology* 92:177-198, 1985.
6. Kremer FB, Marks RG: Radial keratotomy: prospective evaluation of safety and efficacy, *Ophthalmic Surg* 14:925-930, 1983.
7. Sawelson H, Marks RG: Three-year results of radial keratotomy, *Arch Ophthalmol* 105:81-85, 1987.
8. McDonnell PJ, Schanzlin DJ: Early changes in refractive error following radial keratotomy, *Arch Ophthalmol* 106:212-214, 1988.
9. Waring GO et al: Results of the Prospective Evaluation of Radial Keratotomy (PERK) study five years after surgery, *Ophthalmology* 98:1164-1176, 1991.
10. Duffey RJ: Bilateral *Serratia marcescens* keratitis following simultaneous bilateral radial keratotomy, *Am J Ophthalmol* 119:233-236, 1995.
11. Beldavs RA et al: Bilateral microbial keratitis after radial keratotomy, *Arch Ophthalmol* 111:440, 1993.
12. Szerenyi K et al: Keratitis as a complication of bilateral, simultaneous radial keratotomy, *Am J Ophthalmol* 117:462-467, 1994.
13. Kliger CH, Maloney RK: Keratitis as a complication of bilateral simultaneous radial keratotomy (letter), *Am J Ophthalmol* 118:680-681, 1994.
14. Grimmett MR, Holland EJ, Krachmer JH: Therapeutic keratoplasty after radial keratotomy, *Am J Ophthalmol* 118:108-109, 1994.
15. Matoba AY et al: Bacterial keratitis after radial keratotomy, *Ophthalmology* 96:1171-1175, 1989.
16. Gelender H, Flynn HW, Mandelbaum SH: Bacterial endophthalmitis resulting from radial keratotomy, *Am J Ophthalmol* 93:323-236, 1982.
17. McClellan KA et al: Suppurative keratitis: a late complication of radial keratotomy, *J Cataract Refract Surg* 14:317-325, 1988.
18. Mandelbaum S et al: Late development of ulcerative keratitis in radial keratotomy scars, *Arch Ophthalmol* 104:1156-1160, 1986.
19. Shivitz IA, Arrowsmith PN: Delayed keratitis after radial keratotomy, *Arch Ophthalmol* 104:1153-1155, 1986.
20. Holgado S, Luna JD, Juarez CP: Postoperative candida keratitis treated successfully with fluconazole, *Ophthalmic Surg* 24:132-134, 1993.
21. Maskin SL, Alfonso E: Fungal keratitis after radial keratotomy, *Am J Ophthalmol* 114:369-370, 1992.
22. Robin JB et al: *Mycobacterium chelonei* keratitis after radial keratotomy, *Am J Ophthalmol* 102:72-79, 1986.
23. Carson LA et al: Growth characteristics of atypical mycobacteria in water and their comparative resistance to disinfectants, *Appl Environ Microbiol* 36:839-842, 1978.
24. Lazar M et al: *Mycobacterium fortuitum* keratitis, *Am J Ophthalmol* 78:530, 1974.
25. Newman PE et al: A cluster of cases of mycobacterium chelonei keratitis associated with outpatient office procedures, *Am J Ophthalmol* 97:344-346, 1984.
26. Santos CI: Herpetic corneal ulcer following radial keratotomy, *Ann Ophthalmol* 15:82-85, 1983.
27. Santos CI: Herpes keratitis after radial keratotomy (letter reply), *Am J Ophthalmol* 93:806-807, 1982.
28. Santos CI: Herpes keratitis after radial keratotomy, *Am J Ophthalmol* 93:370, 1982.
29. Deitz MR, Sanders DR, Marks RG: Radial keratotomy: an overview of the Kansas City study, *Ophthalmology* 91:467-477, 1984.
30. Haruta Y et al: Recurrent herpes simplex virus type 1 corneal epithelial lesions after radial keratotomy in rabbit, *Arch Ophthalmol* 105:692-698, 1987.
31. Mackman G: Delayed sterile keratitis following radial keratotomy successfully treated with conjunctival flap, *Refract Corneal Surg* 8:122-124, 1992.
32. Karr DJ, Grutzmacher RD, Reeh MJ: Radial keratotomy complicated by sterile keratitis and corneal perforation, *Ophthalmology* 92:1244-1248, 1985.

33. Geggel HS: Delayed sterile keratitis following radial keratotomy requiring corneal transplantation for visual rehabilitation, *Refract Corneal Surg* 6:55-58, 1990.
34. O'Day DM, Feman SS, Elliott JH: Visual impairment following radial keratotomy: a cluster of cases, *Ophthalmology* 93:319-326, 1986.
35. Hanka RL, Gast TJ: Endophthalmitis following Ruiz procedure, *Arch Ophthalmol* 108:21-24, 1990.
36. Cross WD, Head WJ: Complications of radial keratotomy: an overview. In Sanders D, Hofmann RF, Salz J, editors: *Refractive Corneal Surgery,* Thorofare, NJ, 1986, Slack.
37. Deitz MR, Sanders DR, Raanan MG: A consecutive series (1982-1985) of radial keratotomies performed with the diamond blade, *Am J Ophthalmol* 103:417-422, 1987.
38. Salz JJ et al: Ten years experience with a conservative approach to radial keratotomy, *Refract Corneal Surg* 7:12-22, 1991.
39. Spigelman AV, Williams PA, Lindstrom RL: Further studies of four incision radial keratotomy, *Refract Corneal Surg* 5:292-295, 1989.
40. Waring GO: Ophthalmic procedures assessment—radial keratotomy for myopia, *Ophthalmology* 100:1103-1115, 1993.
41. Balcone JA, Franklin RM: Cataract following radial keratotomy, *Ann Ophthalmol* 15:416-418, 1983.
42. Gelender H, Gelber EC: Cataract following radial keratotomy, *Arch Ophthalmol* 101:1229-1231, 1983.
43. Sanders DR, Jofmann RF, Salz JJ, editors: *Refractive Corneal Surgery,* Thorofare NJ, 1986, Slack.
44. Stark WJ, Martin NF, Maumenee EA: Radial keratotomy: a risky procedure of unproven long-term success, *Surv Ophthalmol* 28:101, 106-111, 1983.
45. Casebeer JC et al: Phacoemulsification after T-Lex keratotomy, *J Cataract Refract Surg* 19:778-779, 1993.
46. Koch DD et al: Refractive complications of cataract surgery after radial keratotomy, *Am J Ophthalmol* 108:676-682, 1989.
47. Binder PS: Presumed epithelial ingrowth following radial keratotomy, *CLAO J* 12:247-250, 1986.
48. Maurice DM: The biology of wound healing in the corneal stroma: Castroviejo Lecture, *Cornea* 6:162-168, 1987.
49. Luttrull JK, Jester JV, Smith RE: The effect of radial keratotomy on occular integrity in an animal model, *Arch Ophthalmol* 100:319-320, 1982.
50. Rylander HG, Welch AJ, Fleming B: The effect of radial keratotomy in the rupture strength of pig eyes, *Ophthalmic Surg* 14:744-749, 1983.
51. Larson, BC et al: Quantitated trauma following radial keratotomy in rabbits, *Ophthalmology* 90:660-667, 1983.
52. McKnight SJ, Fitz J, Giangiacoma J: Corneal rupture following radial keratotomy in cats subjected to BB gun injury, *Ophthalmic Surg* 19:165-167, 1988.
53. Darakjian NE, Marchese A: Assessment of corneal strength post radial keratotomy in rabbit eye, *Invest Ophthalmol Vis Sci* 22(suppl):26, 1982.
54. Condon PI, Hill DW: The testing of experimental corneal wounds stitched with modern corneal scleral sutures: experimental corneal wound healing, *Ophthalmic Res* 5:137-150, 1973.
55. Gasset AR, Dohlman CH: The tensile strength of corneal wounds, *Arch Ophthalmol* 79:595-602, 1968.
56. McNeill JI: Corneal incision dehiscence during penetrating keratoplasty nine years after radial keratotomy, *J Cataract Refract Surg* 19:542-543, 1993.
57. McNeill JI, Wilkins DL: A purse-string suture for penetrating keratoplasty following radial keratotomy, *Refract Corneal Surg* 7:392-394, 1991.
58. Jester JV et al: Variations in corneal wound healing after radial keratotomy: possible insights into mechanisms of clinical complications and refractive effects, *Cornea* 11:191-199, 1992.
59. Binder PS, Charlton KH: Surgical procedures performed after refractive surgery, *Refract Corneal Surg* 8:61-74, 1992.
60. Forstot SL, Damiano RE: Trauma after radial keratotomy, *Ophthalmology* 95:833-835, 1988.
61. Binder PS et al: Histopathology of traumatic rupture of the cornea after radial keratotomy, *Arch Ophthalmol* 106:1584-1590, 1988.
62. Pearlstein ES et al: Ruptured globe after radial keratotomy, *Am J Ophthalmol* 755-756, 1988.
63. Simons KB, Linsalata RP, Zaragosa AM: Ruptured globe secondary to blunt trauma following radial keratotomy, *J Refract Surg* 4:132-135, 1988.
64. Goldberg MA et al: Airbag-associated corneal rupture two years after radial keratotomy. Presented at Castro Viejo Cornea Society Annual Meeting, San Francisco, California, October 1994.
65. McDonnell PJ, Lean JS, Schanzlin DJ: Globe rupture from blunt trauma after hexagonal keratotomy, *Am J Ophthalmol* 103:241-242, 1987.
66. Girard LJ et al: Delayed wound healing after radial keratotomy, *Am J Ophthalmol* 99:485-486, 1985.
67. Beatty RF, Robin JB, Schanzlin DJ: Penetrating keratoplasty after radial keratotomy, *J Refract Surg* 2:207-214, 1986.
68. Swinger CA, Barker BA: Myopic keratomileusis following radial keratotomy, *J Refract Surg* 1:53-55, 1985.
69. Campos M, Lee M, McDonnel PJ: Ocular integrity after refractive surgery: effects of photorefractive keratectomy, phototherapeutic keratectomy, and radial keratotomy, *Ophthalmic Surg* 23:598-602, 1992.
70. John ME, Schmitt TE: Traumatic hyphema after radial keratotomy, *Ann Ophthalmol* 15:930-932, 1983.
71. Spivak L: Case report: radial keratotomy incisions remain intact despite facial trauma from plane crash, *J Refract Surg* 3:59-60, 1987.
72. Vinger PF: Prescribing for contact sports, *Optom Clin* 3:129-143, 1993.
73. Corbe C et al: Aircrew fitness decisions and advances in refractive surgery techniques, *Ger J Ophthalmol* 2:146-149, 1993.
74. Enzenauer RW et al: Radial keratotomy in the soldier-aviator, *Mil Med* 158:521-528, 1993.
75. Nolan, BT: Perforation by a foreign body through a pre-existing radial keratotomy wound, *Mil Med* 156:39-42, 1991.
76. Thornton SP et al: Opinions on mini-radial keratotomy, *Refract Corneal Surg* 9:476-479, 1993.
77. Waring GO et al: Results of the Prospective Evaluation of Radial Keratotomy (PERK) study 4 years after surgery for myopia, *JAMA* 263:1083-1091, 1990.
78. Waring GO et al: Three-year results of the Prospective Evaluation of Radial Keratotomy (PERK) study, *Ophthalmology* 94:1339-1354, 1987.
79. Waring GO: Ophthalmic procedures assessment—radial keratotomy for myopia, *Ophthalmology* 95:671-687, 1988.
80. Rodriguez A, Camacho H: Retinal detachment after refractive surgery for myopia, *Retina* 12 (suppl):S46-S50, 1992.
81. Feldman RM et al: Retinal detachment following radial and astigmatic keratotomy, *Refract Corneal Surg* 7:252-253, 1991.
82. Arrowsmith PN, Marks RG: Four-year update on predictability of radial keratotomy, *J Refract Surg* 4:37-45, 1988.
83. Bates AK, Morgan SJ, Steele AD: Radial keratotomy: a review of 300 cases, *Br J Ophthalmol* 76:586-589, 1992.
84. Leroux les Jardins S, Bertrand I, Massin M: Intraoperative and early postoperative complications in 466 radial keratotomies, *Refract Corneal Surg* 8:215-216, 1992.
85. Nelson JD et al: Map-finger-dot changes in the corneal epithelial

basement membrane following radial keratotomy, *Ophthalmology* 92:199-205, 1985.

86. Gieser J, Sugar A: Radial keratotomy and corneal scarring, *Arch Ophthalmol* 110:1527-1528, 1992.
87. Bechara SJ, Grossniklaus HE, Waring GO: Subepithelial fibrosis after myopic epikeratoplasty, *Arch Ophthalmol* 110:228-232, 1992.
88. Davis RM et al: Corneal iron lines after radial keratotomy, *J Refract Surg* 2:174-178, 1988.
89. Steinberg EB et al: Stellate iron lines in the corneal epithelium after radial keratotomy, *Am J Ophthalmol* 98:416-421, 1984.
90. Rashid ER, Waring GO: Complications of radial and transverse keratotomy, *Surv Ophthalmol* 34:73-106, 1989.
91. Binder PS et al: An ultrastructural and histochemical study of long-term wound healing after radial keratotomy, *Am J Ophthalmol* 103:432-440, 1987.
92. Deg JK, Zavala EY, Binder PS: Delayed corneal wound healing following radial keratotomy, *Ophthalmology* 92:734-740, 1985.
93. Jester JV, Villasenor RA, Miyashiro J: Epithelial inclusion cysts following radial keratotomy, *Arch Ophthalmol* 101:611-615, 1983.
94. Yamaguchi T et al: Histologic study of a pair of human corneas after anterior radial keratotomy, *Am J Ophthalmol* 100:281-292, 1985.
95. Reed JW, Dohlman CH: Corneal cysts: a report of eight cases, *Arch Ophthalmol* 86:648-652, 1971.
96. Waring GO: Short-term results of the Prospective Evaluation of Radial Keratotomy (PERK) study. In Sanders D, Hofmann RF, Salz J, editors: *Refractive Corneal Surgery,* Thorofare NJ, 1986, Slack.
97. Rowsey JJ, Balyeat HD: Preliminary results and complications of radial keratotomy, *Am J Ophthalmol* 93:437-455, 1982.
98. Rowsey JJ, Balyeat HD: Radial keratotomy: preliminary report of complications, *Ophthalmic Surg* 13:27-35, 1982.
99. Salz JJ: Multiple complications following radial keratotomy in an elderly patient: a case report, *Ophthalmic Surg* 16:579-580, 1985.
100. Hofmann RF, Starling JC, Masler W: Contact fitting after radial keratotomy: one year results, *J Refract Surg* 2:155-162, 1986.
101. Shivitz IA, Russell BM, Arrowsmith PN: Contact lenses in the treatment of patients with overcorrected radial keratotomy, *Ophthalmology* 94:899-903, 1987.
102. Shivitz IA et al: Optical correction of postoperative radial keratotomy patients with contact lenses, *CLAO J* 12:59-62, 1986.
103. Wilhelmus KR, Hamburg S: Bacterial keratitis following radial keratotomy, *Cornea* 2:143-146, 1983.
104. Cottingham AJ et al: Bacterial corneal ulcers following keratorefractive surgery: a retrospective study of 14,163 procedures. Presented at the Ocular Microbiology and Immunology Group Meeting, San Francisco, September 28, 1986.
105. Rapizzi A et al: Blood staining of the cornea following radial keratotomy, *Refract Corneal Surg* 7:188-189, 1991.
106. Wellish KL et al: Corneal ectasia as a complication of repeated keratotomy surgery, *J Refract Corneal Surg* 10:360-364, 1994.
107. Waring GO, Steinberg EB, Wilson LA: Slit lamp microscopic appearance of corneal wound healing after radial keratotomy, *Am J Ophthalmol* 100:218-224, 1985.
108. Hofmann RF: Reoperations after radial keratotomy and astigmatic keratotomy, *J Refract Surg* 3:119-128, 1987.
109. Thornton SP: Graded non-intersecting transverse incisions for correction of idiopathic astigmatism. In Hofmann RF et al, editors: *Radial keratotomy: surgical techniques,* Thorofare NJ, 1986, Slack.
110. Lindstrom RL, Lavery GW: Correction of post-keratoplasty astigmatism. In Sanders DR, Hofmann RF, Salz JJ, editors: *Refractive Corneal Surgery,* Thorofare NJ, 1986, Slack.
111. Lipshitz I, Mayron Y, Loewenstein A: Combined transverse and interrupted radial keratotomy for compound myopic astigmatism, *Refract Corneal Surg* 8:280-285, 1992.
112. Chiba K et al: Morphometric analysis of corneal endothelium following radial keratotomy, *J Cataract Refract Surg* 13:263-267, 1987.
113. Hoffer KJ et al: Three years experience with radial keratotomy: the UCLA study, *Ophthalmology* 90:627-636, 1983
114. Rowsey JJ et al: Endothelial cell loss after radial keratotomy, *Ophthalmology* 94(suppl):97, 1987.
115. Dunn S et al: Endothelial cell loss following radial keratotomy in a primate model, *Arch Ophthalmol* 102:1666-1670, 1984.
116. Jester JV et al: Radial keratotomy in primate eyes: pathologic studies, *Invest Ophthalmol Vis Sci* 29 (suppl):69, 1982.
117. Aiello JP, MacRae SM, Rich LF: Radial keratotomy and the corneal endothelium: a morphometric analysis II, *Invest Ophthalmol Vis Sci* 29:280-285, 1988.
118. Akiyama K et al: Problems arising from Sato's radial keratotomy procedure in Japan, *CLAO J* 10:179-184, 1984.
119. Salz JJ: Progressive endothelial cell loss following repeat radial keratotomy—a case report, *Ophthalmic Surg* 13:997-999, 1982.
120. Arrowsmith PN, Marks RG: Visual, refractive, and keratometric results of radial keratotomy: one year follow-up, *Arch Ophthalmol* 102:1612-1617, 1984.
121. Marmer RH: Radial keratotomy complications, *Ann Ophthalmol* 19:409-411, 1987.
122. Bores LD: Historical review and clinical results of radial keratotomy. In Binder PS, editor: Refractive corneal surgery: the correction of aphakia, hyperopia and myopia, *Int Ophthalmol Clin* 23:93-118, 1983.
123. Waring GO et al: Changes in refraction, keratometry and visual acuity during the first year after radial keratotomy in the PERK study, *Invest Ophthalmol Vis Sci* 26(suppl):202, 1985.
124. Veraart HG et al: Stray light in radial keratotomy and the influence of pupil size and straylight angle, *Am J Ophthalmol* 114:424-428, 1992.
125. Swinger CA: Postoperative astigmatism, *Surv Ophthalmol* 31:219-248, 1987.
126. Maguire LJ: Keratorefractive surgery, success, and the public health, *Am J Ophthalmol* 117:394-398, 1994.
127. Ginsburg AP et al: Contrast sensitivity under photopic conditions in the Prospective Evaluation of Radial Keratotomy (PERK) study, *Refract Corneal Surg* 6:82-91, 1990.
128. Binder PS: Optical problems following refractive surgery, *Ophthalmology* 93:739-745, 1986.
129. Atkin A et al: Radial keratotomy and glare effects on contrast sensitivity, *Doc Ophthalmol* 62:129-148, 1986.
130. Bourque LB et al: Reported satisfaction, fluctuation of vision, and glare among patients one year after surgery in the Prospective Evaluation of Radial Keratotomy (PERK) study, *Arch Ophthalmol* 104:356-363, 1986.
131. McDonald MB, Haik M, Kaufman HE: Color vision and contrast sensitivity testing after radial keratotomy, *Am J Ophthalmol* 103:468-473, 1987.
132. Miller D, Miller R: Glare sensitivity in simulated radial keratotomy, *Arch Ophthalmol* 99:1961-1962, 1981.
133. Peyman GA, Spigelman AV: Reduction of glare after radial keratotomy: an experimental study, *Ophthalmic Surg* 12:727-730, 1981.
134. Trick LR, Hartstein J: Investigation of contrast sensitivity following radial keratotomy, *Ann Ophthalmol* 19:251-254, 1987.
135. Applegate RA, Gansel KA: The importance of pupil size in

optical quality measurements following radial keratotomy, *Refract Corneal Surg* 6:47-54, 1990.

136. Ginsburg AP et al: Effects of radial keratotomy on contrast sensitivity in the Prospective Evaluation of Radial Keratotomy (PERK) study, *Ophthalmology* (Suppl 2) 91:121, 1984.
137. Krasnov MM et al: The effect of radial keratotomy on contrast sensitivity, *Am J Ophthalmol* 150:651-654, 1988.
138. Bogan SJ et al: Computer-assisted videokeratography of corneal topography after radial keratotomy, *Arch Ophthalmol* 109:834-841, 1991.
139. Applegate RA: Acuities through annular and central pupils after radial keratotomy, *Optom Vis Sci* 68:584-590, 1991.
140. Milder B, Rubin M: *The fine art of prescribing glasses without making a spectacle of yourself,* Gainesville Fla, 1978, Triad Scientific.
141. Applegate RA et al: Radial keratotomy increases the effects of disability glare: initial results, *Ann Ophthalmol* 19:293-297, 1987.
142. Camp JJ et al: A computer model of the evaluation of the effect of corneal topography on optical performance, *Am J Ophthalmol* 109:379-383, 1990.
143. Schanzlin DJ et al: Diurnal change in refraction, corneal curvature, visual acuity, and intraocular pressure after radial keratotomy in the PERK study, *Ophthalmology* 93(Suppl 2):89, 1986.
144. McDonnell PJ, McClusky DJ, Garbus JJ: Corneal topography and fluctuating visual acuity after radial keratotomy, *Ophthalmology* 96:665-670, 1989.
145. Kwitko S et al: Computer-assisted study of diurnal variation in corneal topography after penetrating keratoplasty, *Ophthalmic Surg* 23:10-16, 1992.
146. Kwitko S et al: Diurnal variation of corneal topography after radial keratotomy, *Arch Ophthalmol* 110:351-356, 1992.
147. White LJ, Mader TH: Refractive changes with increasing altitude after radial keratotomy, *Am J Ophthalmol* 115:821-823, 1993.
148. McDonnell PJ, Garbus J, Lopez PF: Topographic analysis and visual acuity after radial keratotomy, *Am J Ophthalmol* 106:692-695, 1988.
149. Moreira H et al: Multifocal corneal topographic changes after radial keratotomy, *Ophthalmic Surg* 23:85-89, 1992.
150. Santos VR et al: Relationship between refractive error and visual acuity in the Prospective Evaluation of Radial Keratotomy (PERK) study, *Arch Ophthalmol* 105:86, 1987.
151. Fleming JF: Corneal asphericity and visual function after radial keratotomy, *Cornea* 12:233-240, 1993.
152. Moreira H et al: Corneal topographic changes over time after radial keratotomy, *Cornea* 11:465-470, 1992.
153. Lopez PF et al: Subregions of differing refractive power within the clear zone after experimental radial keratotomy, *Refract Corneal Surg* 7:360-367, 1991.
154. Holladay JT et al: The relationship of visual acuity, refractive error, and pupil size after radial keratotomy, *Arch Ophthalmol* 109:70-76, 1991.
155. Powers MK et al: Psychological findings in radial keratotomy patients two years after surgery, *Ophthalmology* 91:1193-1198, 1984.
156. Werblin TP, Stafford GM: The Casebeer system for predictable keratorefractive surgery, *Ophthalmology* 100:1095-1102, 1993.
157. Bourque LB et al: Spectacle and contact lens wearing six years after radial keratotomy in the Prospective Evaluation of Radial Keratotomy study, *Ophthalmology* 101:421-31, 1994.
158. Salz JJ et al: Four-incision radial keratotomy for low to moderate myopia, *Ophthalmology* 93:727-738, 1986.
159. Waring GO et al: Results of the prospective evaluation of radial keratotomy (PERK) study 10 years after surgery, *Arch Ophthalmol* 112:1298-1308, 1994.
160. Deitz MR, Sanders DR, Raanan MG: Progressive hyperopia in radial keratotomy, *Ophthalmology* 93:1284-1288, 1986.
161. Friedberg ML et al: Results of radial and astigmatic keratotomy by beginning refractive surgeons, *Ophthalmology* 100:746-751, 1993.
162. Bores LD: Radial keratotomy predictability, *Ophthalmology* 101:414-415, 1994.
163. Nordan LT, Maxwell WA: Radial keratotomy predictability, *Ophthalmology* 101:412-413, 1994.
164. Kremer F, Suscavage P: Radial keratotomy: improved predictability, *Ann Ophthalmol* 24:299-302, 1992.
165. Friedlander MH: Radial keratotomy predictability, *Ophthalmology* 101:411-412, 1994.
166. Wilson SE, Klyce SD: Screening for corneal topographic abnormalities before refractive surgery, *Ophthalmology* 101:147-152, 1994.
167. Durand L et al: Complications of radial keratotomy: eyes with keratoconus and late wound dehiscence, *Refract Corneal Surg* 8:311-314, 1992.
168. Ellis W: Radial keratotomy in a patient with keratoconus, *J Cataract Refract Surg* 18:406-409, 1992.
169. Mamalis N et al: Radial keratotomy in a patient with keratoconus, *Refract Corneal Surg* 7:374-376, 1991.
170. McDonnell PJ: Current applications of the corneal modeling system, *Refract Corneal Surg* 7:87-91, 1991.
171. Rowsey JJ et al: Corneal topography as a predictor of refractive change in the Prospective Evaluation of Radial Keratotomy (PERK) study, *Ophthalmic Surg* 22:370-380, 1991.
172. Wilson SE, Klyce SD: Advances in the analysis of corneal topography, *Surv Ophthalmol* 35:269-277, 1991.
173. Sugar A: Has radial keratotomy finally come of age? *Ophthalmology* 100:979-980, 1993.
174. Assil KK, Quantock AJ: Wound healing in response to keratorefractive surgery, *Surv Ophthalmol* 38:289-302, 1993.
175. Feldman ST: The effect of epidermal growth factor on corneal wound healing: practical considerations for therapeutic use, *Refract Corneal Surg* 7:232-239, 1991.
176. Hahn TW, Kim JH, Lee YC: Excimer laser photorefractive keratectomy to correct residual myopia after radial keratotomy, *Refract Corneal Surg* 9(suppl):S25-S29, 1993.
177. Frangie JP et al: Excimer laser keratectomy after radial keratotomy, *Am J Ophthalmol* 115:634-639, 1993.
178. Seiler T, Jean B: Photorefractive keratectomy as a second attempt to correct myopia after radial keratotomy, *Refract Corneal Surg* 8:211-214, 1992.
179. McDonnell PJ, Garbus JJ, Salz JJ: Excimer laser myopic photorefractive keratectomy after undercorrected radial keratotomy, *Refract Corneal Surg* 7:146-150, 1991.
180. Durrie DS, Schumer J, Cavanaugh TB: Photorefractive keratectomy for residual myopia after previous refractive keratotomy, *Refract Corneal Surg* 10(suppl):S235-S238, 1994.
181. Ribeiro JC, McDonald MB, Klyce SD: Photorefractive keratectomy after radial keratotomy in a patient with severe myopia, *Am J Ophthalmol* 118:106-108, 1994.
182. Salz JJ, Salz MS: Results of four- and eight-incision radial keratotomy for 6 to 11 diopters of myopia, *J Refract Surg* 4:46-50, 1988.
183. Olson RJ, Biddulph MC: Hyperopia, anisometropia, and irregular astigmatism in a patient following revisional radial keratotomy, *Ophthalmic Surg* 23:782-783, 1992.
184. John ME: High hyperopia after radial keratotomy, *J Cataract Refract Surg* 19:446-447, 1993.
185. Busin M et al: The effect of changes in intraocular pressure on corneal curvature after radial keratotomy in the rabbit eye, *Ophthalmology* 93:331-334, 1986.
186. Busin M et al: Overcorrected visual acuity improved by

antiglaucoma medication after radial keratotomy, *Am J Ophthalmol* 101:374-375, 1985.
187. Lindquist TD, Rubenstein JB, Lindstrom RL: Correction of hyperopia following radial keratotomy: quantification in human cadaver eyes, *Ophthalmic Surg* 18:432-437, 1987.
188. Lindquist TD, Williams PA, Lindstrom RL: Surgical treatment of overcorrection following radial keratotomy: evaluation of clinical effectiveness, *Ophthalmic Surg* 22:12-15, 1991.
189. Alio J, Ismail M: Management of radial keratotomy overcorrections by corneal sutures, *J Cataract Refract Surg* 19:595-599, 1993.
190. Lyle WA, Jin J: Circular and interrupted suture technique for correction of hyperopia following radial keratotomy, *Refract Corneal Surg* 8:80-83, 1992.
191. Damiano RE, Forstot SL, Dukes DK: Surgical correction of hyperopia following radial keratotomy, *Refract Corneal Surg* 8:75-79, 1992.
192. Schneider DM, Draghic T, Murthy RK: Combined myopia and astigmatism surgery: review of 350 cases, *J Cataract Refract Surg* 18:370-373, 1992.
193. Deitz MR et al: Long-term (5 to 12 year) follow-up of metal blade radial keratotomy procedures, *Arch Ophthalmol* 112: 614-620, 1994.
194. Waring GO et al: Stability of refraction during four years after radial keratotomy in the Prospective Evaluation of Radial Keratotomy study, *Am J Ophthalmol* 111:133-144, 1991.
195. MacRae S: Stability of refraction during four years after radial keratotomy in the Prospective Evaluation of Radial Keratotomy study, *Am J Ophthalmol* 113:111-112, 1992.
196. Waisberg Y: Bilateral high hyperopia after radial keratotomy, *J Cataract Refract Surg* 19:88-89, 1993.
197. Damiano RE, Forstot SL: Extreme corneal flattening after radial keratotomy, *Am J Ophthalmol* 112:738-741, 1991.
198. Thornton SP et al: Management of hyperopic shift after radial keratotomy, *Refract Corneal Surg* 8:325-330, 1992.
199. Franks JB, Binder PS: Keratotomy procedures for the correction of astigmatism, *J Refract Surg* 1:11-17, 1985.
200. Sawleson H, Marks RG: Two year results of radial keratotomy, *Arch Ophthalmol* 103:505-510, 1985.
201. Lindquist TD, Williams PA, Lindstrom RL: Management of overcorrection following astigmatic keratotomy, *J Refract Surg* 4:218-221, 1988.
202. Arciniegas A et al: Corneal astigmatism induced by the combination of arc and radial keratotomies: experimental research in rabbits, *J Refract Surg* 2:67-77, 1986.
203. Girard LJ et al: Case report: overcorrection of radial and arc keratotomies—two years postoperatively, *J Refract Surg* 2:232-235, 1985.
204. Maloney RK, Bogan SJ, Waring GO: Determination of corneal image-forming properties from corneal topography, *Am J Ophthalmol* 115:31-41, 1993.
205. McDonnell, PJ: Computerized analysis of corneal topography as an aid in fitting contact lenses after radial keratotomy, *Ophthalmic Surg* 23:55-59, 1992.
206. Astin CL: Keratoreformation by contact lenses after radial keratotomy, *Ophthalmic Physiol Opt* 11:156-162, 1991.
207. Waring GO: The changing status of radial keratotomy for myopia: Parts I & II, *J Refract Surg* 1:81-86, 119-137, 1985.
208. Haverbeke L: Assessing the efficacy of topical corticosteroids following radial keratotomy, *Refract Corneal Surg* 9:379-382, 1993.
209. Rashid ER, Waring GO: Complications of refractive keratotomy. In Waring GO, editor: *Refractive keratotomy for myopia and astigmatism,* St Louis, 1992, Mosby.
210. Nizam A et al: Stability of refraction and visual acuity during five years in eyes with simple myopia: the PERK Study Group, *Refract Corneal Surg* 8:439-847, 1992.
211. John ME, Howard C: Esotropia following radial keratotomy, *J Cataract Refract Surg* 17:246-247, 1991.
212. Carroll RP, Lindstrom RL: Blepharoptosis after radial keratotomy, *Am J Ophthalmol* 102:800-802, 1986.
213. Lindberg JV et al: Ptosis following radial keratotomy: performed using a rigid eyelid speculum, *Ophthalmology* 93:1509-1512, 1986.
214. Paris GL, Quickert MH: Disinsertion of the aponeurosis of the levator palpebrae superioris muscle after cataract extraction, *Am J Ophthalmol* 81:337-340, 1976.
215. Brodsky ME, Bauerberg JM, Sterzovsky A: Case report: probable fluorescein-induced uveitis following radial keratotomy, *J Refract Surg* 3:28-29, 1987.
216. Starling J, Hofmann R: Case report: anterior uveitis and transient hyperopia following radial keratotomy, *J Refract Surg* 2:96-98, 1986.
217. Hersh PS, Kalevar V, Kenyon KR: Penetrating keratoplasty for severe complications of radial keratotomy, *Cornea* 10:170-174, 1991.
218. Sastry SM et al: Radial keratotomy does not affect intraocular pressure, *Refract Corneal Surg* 9:459-464, 1993.
219. Markovits A: Extracapsular cataract extraction with posterior chamber intraocular lens implantation in a post radial keratotomy patient, *Arch Ophthalmol* 104:329, 331, 1986.
220. Hofmann RF, Starling JC, Hovland KR: Case report: retinal detachment after radial keratotomy surgery, *J Refract Surg* 1:226-230, 1985.

CHAPTER 170

R. BRUCE GRENE

Congenital Astigmatism

Over the last decade, several forces have converged to make the surgical reduction of astigmatism one of the most exciting applications of refractive surgery. Corneal transplantation surgeons have become active in refractive surgery, drawing on their extensive experience with postkeratoplasty astigmatism. Radial keratotomy specialists have contributed their incisional surgery skills and instrumentation for reduction of myopia. Computerized corneal topography work stations give expanded definition to the form, amount, and distribution of corneal astigmatism. The proliferation keratorefractive techniques (epikeratophakia, PRK, ALK, RK, AK, ALK-E, etc.) have given us ample clinical models to study congenital and postrefractive surgical astigmatism. This decade of fruitful activity has forged nothing less than a new paradigm for our understanding of astigmatism.

Refractive surgery is the art of altering corneal curvature without degrading its optical quality. The success of our surgical efforts depends largely on our understanding and management of three forms of astigmatism: regular, macroirregular, and microirregular astigmatism (Figure 170-1). The traditional model of astigmatism that worked well two decades ago is inadequate for today's state-of-the-art corneal and refractive surgeon. The three forms of astigmatism discussed here allow clinicians to understand the essential challenge of refractive surgery, which is the redistribution of corneal refractive power without degradation of the optical quality of the anterior corneal surface.

The clinical importance of astigmatism management cannot be overestimated. Refractive surgery is being performed on hundreds of thousands of men and women with refractive errors but otherwise healthy eyes. Subtle visual side effects that would be clinically acceptable postkeratoplasty become critical to the success of these elective keratorefractive surgeries.

Regular astigmatism describes astigmatism that is (1) corrected by a spheres lentical lens, (2) measured by manual and automated keratometry, and (3) targeted for reduction by astigmatic keratotomy. Regular refractive astigmatism is traditionally defined as the sum of corneal and lenticular astigmatism. In reality, the difference between corneal and refractive astigmatism includes both lenticular astigmatism and errors in measurement of corneal and refractive astigmatism. Regular astigmatism is a vector with direction (axis) and magnitude (diopters). The initially simple aspects of preoperative regular astigmatism quickly become complex when assessing the difference between preoperative and postoperative vectors. The determination of undercorrection versus overcorrection requires trigonometric analysis[1-3] This postoperative determination of regular astigmatism is further confounded by the coexistence of both forms of irregular astigmatism.

Macroirregular astigmatism is defined as the regional irregular distribution of corneal refracting power. These regional variations in corneal curvature are easily appreciated by noting the irregular distribution of various colors corresponding to corneal curvature on topographic maps. Macroirregular astigmatism can also be appreciated using manual keratometry to observe indentations or excrescences in the keratometric mire. Macroirregular astigmatism is seen with computerized topography when opposing hemimeridia lose their mirror image symmetry. The most common nonsurgical causes of macroirregular astigmatism are keratoconus and contact lens-induced corneal warpage. Macroirregular astigmatism is also quite common after astigmatic keratotomy. By examining the distribution corneal refractive power, the surgeon can identify regions of both undercorrection and overcorrection. This regional analysis is essential to guide enhancement procedures.

Whereas macroirregular astigmatism refers to larger regional areas of irregular corneal curvature, *microirregular astigmatism* refers to very small irregular variations in the corneal surface. Microirregular corneal astigmatism describes the optical smoothness of

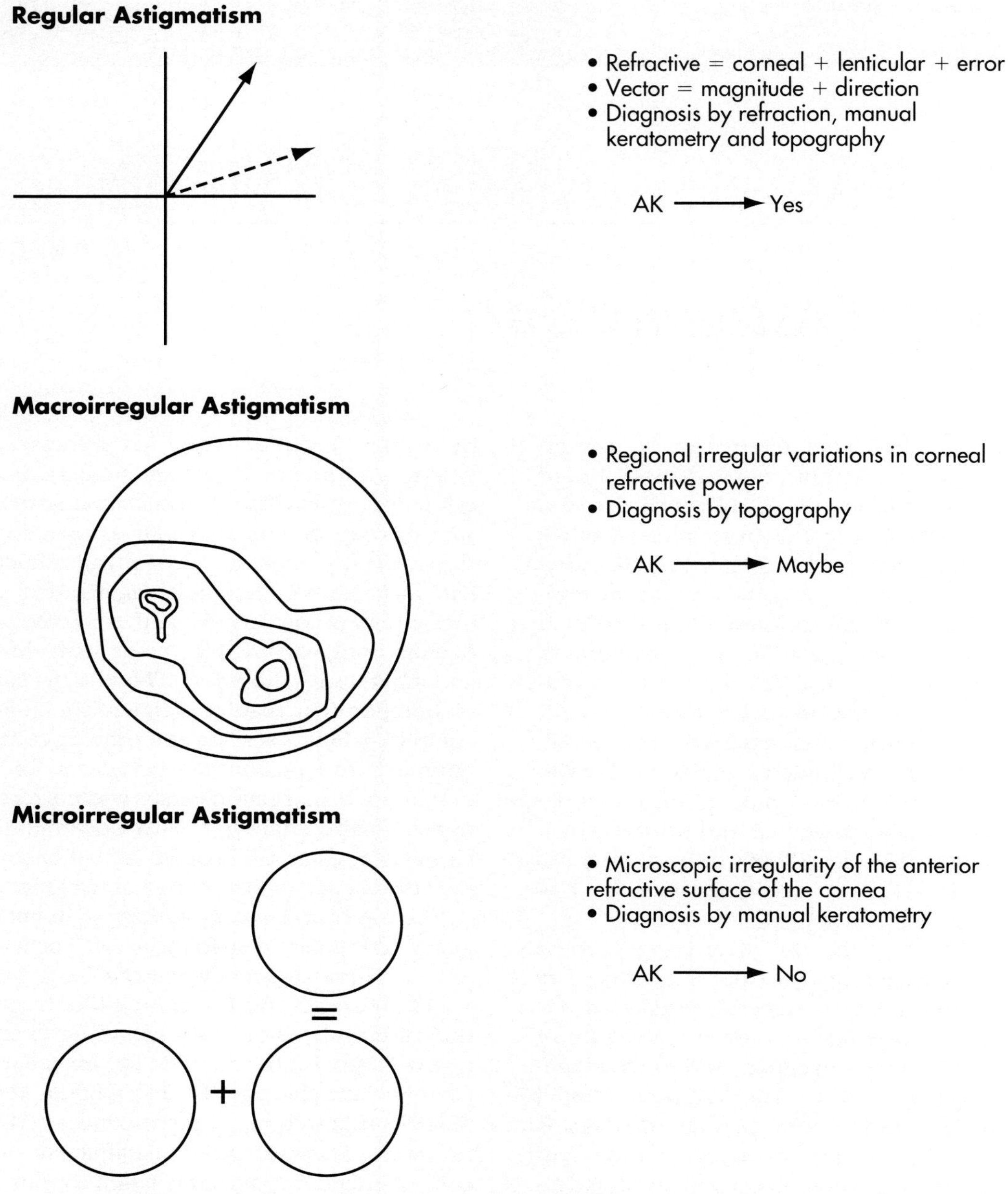

FIGURE 170-1 The three forms of astigmatism. (AK = Astigmatic keratotomy.)

the anterior corneal surface. Rippling resulting from postsurgical, posttraumatic, postinfectious scarring creates microirregularity. Tear film breakup and superficial punctate keratitis create irregularity of the anterior cornea. Virtually all keratorefractive procedures induce at least transient microirregular astigmatism. Because the degradation of image quality with symptoms of ghosting and decreased contrast sensitivity can be so bothersome to patients, microirregular astigmatism must be minimized. The risk of permanent microirregular astigmatism limits the upper range of both radial and astigmatic keratotomy. The diagnosis of microirregular astigmatism can be made to inspection of ring image on computerized topography systems or by inspection of the mires on manual keratometry. Inability to superimpose the mires crisply may range from mild (1+) to marked (4+). Regular, macroirregular, and microirregular astigmatism frequently coexist in patients who have undergone keratorefractive procedures.

The preoperative clinical importance of macroirregular and microirregular astigmatism stems from their ability to alert clinicians to various forms of corneal pathology. Postoperatively, macroirregular astigmatism may help identify areas of wound gape, inadequate incision depth, or errors in the placement of astigmatic keratotomy incisions. Postoperative microirregular astigmatism is important in understanding patients symptoms of decreased image quality. Clinically significant microirregular astigmatism can coexist with 20/20 Snellen acuity. Persistent microirregular astigmatism is a relative contraindication to additional incisional refractive surgery. Additional clinical significance is derived from Nordan's rule, which states that microirregular astigmatism exaggerates refractive hyperopia and regular astigmatism.

Patient Selection

Patient selection for astigmatic keratotomy begins with consideration of refractive data, but ultimately requires consideration of both nonclinical and clinical factors. Like radial keratotomy, astigmatic keratotomy has a fairly narrow range within which it is effective. Outside this range, astigmatic keratotomy may be associated with increased side effects and complications. The lower limit of astigmatism for which astigmatic keratotomy is indicated depends on the axis of astigmatism. For with-the-rule astigmatism, the lower limit for astigmatic keratotomy is 1.5 diopters. With-the-rule astigmatism is better tolerated than oblique and against-the-rule astigmatism because patients are able to blunt the optical effects of vertical astigmatism through squinting (stenopaic slit effect). The lower limit for correction of oblique and against-the-rule astigmatism is 1 diopter. When operating on 1 diopter or less of with-the-rule astigmatism, one risks the creation of new against-the-rule astigmatism, which patients tolerate poorly. Overcorrection of with-the-rule astigmatism should be avoided.

The upper limit of regular astigmatism that is consistently correctable through simple astigmatic keratotomy is 3.5 diopters. Experienced astigmatism surgeons disagree on the age effect for astigmatic keratotomy. The Astigmatism Reduction Clinical Trial (ARC-T) nomogram modified from Lindstrom's work has a significant age factor.[4] Nordan's nomogram has no age factor.[5] My own comparison of arcuate and straight transverse astigmatic keratotomy procedures shows a small increase in effect with increasing age.[6]

The patient's associated spherical refractive error must also be considered in patient selection for astigmatic keratotomy. Astigmatic keratotomy works well in conjunction with simultaneous radial keratotomy for those patients with low and moderate myopia. In patients with high myopia, astigmatic keratotomy is proven to be effective in conjunction with photorefractive keratectomy. Astigmatic keratotomy can be performed either before or after photorefractive keratectomy.

For hyperopic patients, astigmatic keratotomy offers one of few options available to reduce hyperopia. Astigmatic keratotomy flattens the cornea in the meridian of the incision and there is a compensatory steepening 90 degrees away. This effect, termed *coupling,* can be used to the patient's advantage. Although the exact ratio of flattening in the incised meridian to steepening in the unincised meridian is quite variable, on average it is 1:1. This means that the spherical component of a patient's minus cylinder refraction is made more myopic by astigmatic keratotomy. The net effect on the patient's spherical equivalent depends on the coupling ratio. With coupling of 1:2, the spherical equivalent remains unchanged: for 1:1, the spherical equivalent becomes more myopic; for 1:3 or greater, the spherical equivalent becomes more hyperopic.

After first determining that the candidate is in range for astigmatic keratotomy, attention turns to a second test: comparing the *current system of visual correction* to the likely outcome of refractive surgery. When comparing visual correction using glasses or contact lenses to the expected result from refractive keratotomy, it is important to stress to the patient the limits of refractive surgery. Refractive surgery provides good uncorrected vision but rarely perfect uncorrected vision. The patient will not likely see as well with uncorrected postoperative vision as with either spectacles or contact lenses. Estimates of the likely postoperative acuity must consider preoperative spherical refractive error and preoperative astigmatism. Particular attention should be placed on the patient's level of adaptation to contact lens wear. Generally speaking, astigmatic keratotomy should be reserved for patients who are experiencing problems with full-time contact lens wear or who are unhappy wearing spectacles.

It is useful to demonstrate to candidates the approximate level of acuity expected after refractive surgery. Myopes should be shown the level of uncorrected vision that is consistent with their spherical error. For low to moderate myopes, this is generally 20/40. For the purposes of demonstration, approximately two thirds of their refractive cylinder should be removed from the phoropter. For hyperopes, two thirds of their refractive astigmatism should be removed from their cylindrical correction and one half of this amount removed from their hyperopic spherical component. This simulates 2:1 coupling. The +2.00 to −3.00 diopter preoperative patient would be shown the eye chart with +1.00 to −1.00 diopter residual refractive error. For some patients, preoperative astigmatism limits contact lens use, and astigmatic keratotomy can improve contact lens adaptation.

The third aspect of patient selection evaluates the patient's overall lifestyle. The benefits of refractive surgery are greatest for men and women who lead an active lifestyle. People who farm, ranch, ride horses, or garden all benefit from decreased dependence on glasses or contact lenses. The obvious limitations of contact lenses and glasses for swimming, water skiing, snow skiing, and camping make patients who participate in these activities excellent candidates for refractive surgery. These tasks can generally be performed with the good, but not perfect, visual acuity achieved by astigmatic keratotomy.

The fourth consideration in patient selection deals with the patient's *expectations* for the benefits of surgery. The patient's expectations must be tempered by repeating the limitations of all refractive surgery procedures: refractive surgery will give *good but not perfect* uncorrected vision. Most patients are thrilled with the prospect of being able to do most activities without dependence on glasses or contact lenses. They generally accept the fact that they will need glasses to obtain perfect vision. Nonetheless, it is critical that this message be heard by patients before surgery.

In summary, patient selection depends on a four step test (Figure 170-2). After confirming that the patient is a potential candidate, attention turns to patient education and informed consent.

Patient Education and Informed Consent

For all elective surgical procedures, it is important to inform patients of the possible side effects and complications of astigmatic keratotomy. Patients must have time to evaluate both written and video education materials before signing informed consent documents.

Side effects associated with astigmatic keratotomy are minimal. The most common side effect is ghosting resulting from residual irregular astigmatism. This occurs most often when astigmatic keratotomy incisions are placed in optical zones smaller than 7 mm. Another potential cause of irregular astigmatism is postoperative wound gape caused by defective stromal healing. Fluctuation of vision is much less common in pure astigmatic keratotomy cases than with radial keratotomy procedures. Similarly, starburst is not generally associated with astigmatic keratotomy.

The complications most commonly associated with astigmatic keratotomy are similar to those for radial keratotomy. The risk of incisional keratitis with progression to endophthalmitis is small but real. Wound gape with associated overcorrection can occur with astigmatic keratotomy incisions as it does with radial keratotomy incisions. Indeed, because the cornea bends at right angles to transverse astigmatic keratotomy incisions, wound gape is significantly more frequent with astigmatic keratotomy than with radial keratotomy. This propensity for wound gape means that intraoperative perforations during astigmatic keratotomy are frequently associated with aqueous loss and shallowing of the anterior chamber. Not infrequently, this requires immediate suture closure. Few perforated astigmatic keratotomy incisions are "microperforations." Because of all of the preceding potential complications, astigmatic keratotomy candidates should be forewarned about the likelihood that they may require multiple procedures.

Preoperative Testing

Preoperative testing for astigmatic keratotomy candidates relies on screening for three forms of astigmatism (Figures 170-3,4,5). *Regular astigmatism* must be measured with manual refraction, either manifest or cycloplegic depending on the nomogram for correction of the patient's spherical error. Neither autorefraction nor autokeratometry readings should be used as the basis for refractive surgery procedures. Manual keratometry should also be performed to quantify the regular corneal astigmatism. Both the magnitude and axis of these readings should be compared. One should not assume that the variance between refractive and corneal regular astigmatism is due to lenticular astigmatism. Significant variation requires retesting or use of corneal topography instruments to help resolve the difference.

Macroirregular astigmatism is best detected using corneal topography power maps. *Microirregular astigmatism* is most easily diagnosed using manual keratometry, but inspection of ring images from corneal topography studies is also useful. Common causes of preoperative macroirregular and microirregular astigmatism include ocular surface disease with rapid tear break-up, superficial punctate keratitis, posttraumatic scarring, postinfectious scarring, keratoconus, and contact lens-induced corneal warpage.

Additional preoperative testing includes slit lamp examination to rule out corneal pathology, which might be a contraindication to astigmatic keratotomy. This includes significant ocular surface disease (keratoconjunctivitis sicca, meibomitis, exposure), Fuchs' dystrophy, intrastromal vessels, or significant corneal thinning.

Operative Methods

The operative technique for astigmatic keratotomy includes many approaches to achieve a common end

GRENE CORNEA
Cornea & Refractive Eye Surgery

FOUR STEP TEST

STEP 1

IS THE PATIENT IN RANGE?

For AK, I consider the lower limit indication for surgery to be 1.5 diopters refractive astigmatism. I perform AK for 1 diopter or more refractive astigmatism if simultaneous RK is being performed. The upper limit for AK is 3-1/2 to 4 diopters Above this level, modified full Ruiz procedures are utilized and strongly favored over AK.

STEP 2

RANK OPTIONS

Each patient is evaluated for the suitability of spectacle, contact lens, or surgical correction. Their grade (literally, a letter grade of A to F) is solicited for past or present success with contacts or glasses. Because the majority of refractive surgery patients will still require spectacles or contact lenses for their best vision postop, the specific advantages of decreased but continued dependency on corrective lenses must be discussed. This ranking process always puts the patient's interests first. The ethical refractive surgeon may direct patients to another doctor for contact lenses, and the ethical optometrist may refer contact lens wearers to a refractive surgeon.

STEP 3

EVALUATE PATIENT'S LIFESTYLE

Are there specific activities which will likely to aided by the surgery? This step examines a patient's work, hobbies and athletics. In general, activities for which glasses and contacts are poorly suited, but for which good (not perfect) vision is sufficient are the most compelling reasons to proceed with RK. Common examples are running, skiing, camping, farming, gardening, and swimming.

STEP 4

PATIENT'S EXPECTATIONS

It is essential that the surgeon and his staff accurately identify each patient's expectation of the benefits of surgery. This process involves a back and forth dialogue between the practice and the patient. The clear elucidation of the limits of refractive surgery begins in the seminar, is expanded during the consultation, and is reinforced during counseling for informed consent. Simply stated, RK makes the large majority of patients better and gives "perfect" results very rarely. We verbalize (repeatedly) the likely results of surgery, demonstrate a probable level of acuity in the phoropter or trial frame, and solicit the patient's comments as to the acceptability of this probable outcome. Finally, the patient is asked to recopy the following phrase in his or her own handwriting.

"I understand and am willing to accept the limitations of RK and/or AK surgery. I realize it is possible that I will need glasses or contact lenses to achieve my best possible level of vision following RK and/or AK surgery."

FIGURE 170-2 **Four step test. (AK = Astigmatic keratotomy; RK = radial keratotomy.)**

(corneal weakening). By using various combinations of incision length, incision depth, incision number, and optical zone diameter, the cornea is weakened in its steeper meridian. This creates a bowing forward of the cornea in the region of the "knee" with secondary central flattening. Various surgeons mix and match the four major variables of incision length, depth, number, and optical zone, depending on their specific nomogram. A fifth, minor factor, incision configuration, adds to the apparent complexity of competing schools of astigmatic keratotomy.

Like radial keratotomy, astigmatic keratotomy can be made more or less aggressive. Side effects and complications associated with astigmatic keratotomy

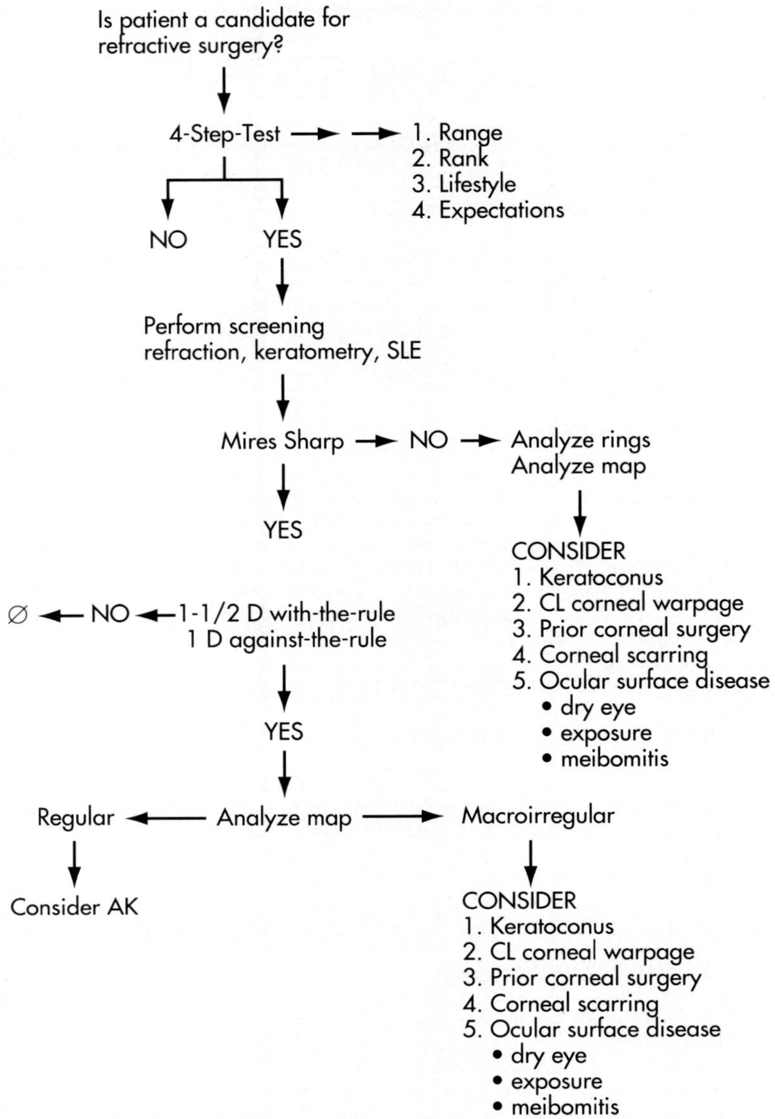

FIGURE 170-3 **Evaluation flow chart. (SLE = Slit lamp examination; CL = contact lens; D = diopter; AK = astigmatic keratotomy.)**

increase with more aggressive forms of surgery. The limiting factors for incision length include the risk of paradoxical coupling in which both the steeper and flatter meridia are flattened by surgery. Additional risks of excessive incision length include a higher propensity for wound gape. Incision depth is limited by the risk of perforation with wound leak, wound gape, and permanent irregular astigmatism. An increased number of incisions adds to the technical complexity of the procedure with an increased risk of bridged scarring between incisions. Smaller optical zones are associated with an increased risk of permanent irregular astigmatism.

Although much debate exists regarding the optical configuration of astigmatic keratotomy incisions, this is a more minor consideration than depth, length, number, and optical zone. There are three major schools of thought. Nordan favors a simple nomogram involving straight transverse incisions in three strengths. The ARC-T approach derived from Lindstrom's method involves arcuate transverse incisions at variable lengths. Both Nordan and ARC-T approaches use a 7 mm optical zone. Thornton involves multiple short incisions at various optical zones. Each configuration appears to work well when incisions are skillfully placed and conservative surgical parameters are respected (Figure 170-6).

RK PREOPERATIVE INFORMATION TECH: RR

NAME: DMA	AGE: 43	SEX: M	RACE: C	DATE: 10-5-94

ACTIVITIES/LIFESTYLE OD: Dr. T REF BY: Dr. T SEMINAR DATE: NA

CURRENT OCULAR MEDS:	SURGERIES:	INJURIES:	DISEASES:
NONE	NONE	NONE	NONE

WORK: cattle buyer

INTERESTS: coaching son's sport

CURRENT SYSTEM

CONTACTS Grade: ____

TOTAL YRS: ____
CURRENT TYPE: ____ YRS: ____
DAILY TIME: NONE
CURRENT AGE: ____
PROBLEMS: ____

GLASSES Grade: B−

DAILY TIME: Full-time
RX AGE: 3/93
PROBLEMS: in the way, get bumped
MEDICAL HISTORY: get dirty, get scratched
High Blood Pressure → minipress, → Propranolol

CURRENT NUMBERS UNCORRECTED DV OU 20/ UNCORRECTED NV OU 20/

	EXAM OD	EXAM OS
CURRENT SPECS:	−2.25 − 2.75 × 180 + ⁄ (ADD)	−2.00 − 2.75 × 180 + ⁄ (ADD)
D VA C: 20/	20	20
N VA C: 20/	20-2	20-2
D VA SC: 20/	400	400
N VA SC: 20/	20	20
KERATOMETRY:	41.50 @ 180 / 44.00 @ 090	40.87 @ 173 / 43.37 @ 083
IRR	(0) 1/4 2/4 3/4 4/4	0 1/4 2/4 3/4 4/4
CYLINDER +	2.50 @ 090	2.50 @ 083
TONOMETRY APPL	12	12
PUPIL SIZE	3 mm	3 mm
MANUAL REFRACTION BY:	−1.25 − 2.75 × 180 20/ 20-2 SE: −2.62	−1.00 − 2.75 × 180 20/ 20-2 SE: −2.37

EXAM

	OD	OS
LIDS/LASHES	(WNL)	WNL
CONJUNCTIVA	(WNL)	WNL
CORNEA	(WNL)	WNL
ANT CHAMBER	(WNL)	WNL
LENS	(WNL)	WNL
RETINA	(WNL)	WNL
CD:	.2	.2
MACULA:	MNL	MNL
EOMS:	WNL	WNL

DISCUSSION

Demod 20/40 thru −.50−.75×180 −.50−.75×180 Pt states "this would be wonderful!" Discussed monovision → pt declines. Wants maximum distance vision. Pt understands and accepts thin specs for perfection, also understands he will need specs for near tasks.

PLAN

RK/AK OU
goal −.50
Dr. R

RK PREOP01 01 10/94

FIGURE 170-4 Preoperative evaluation.

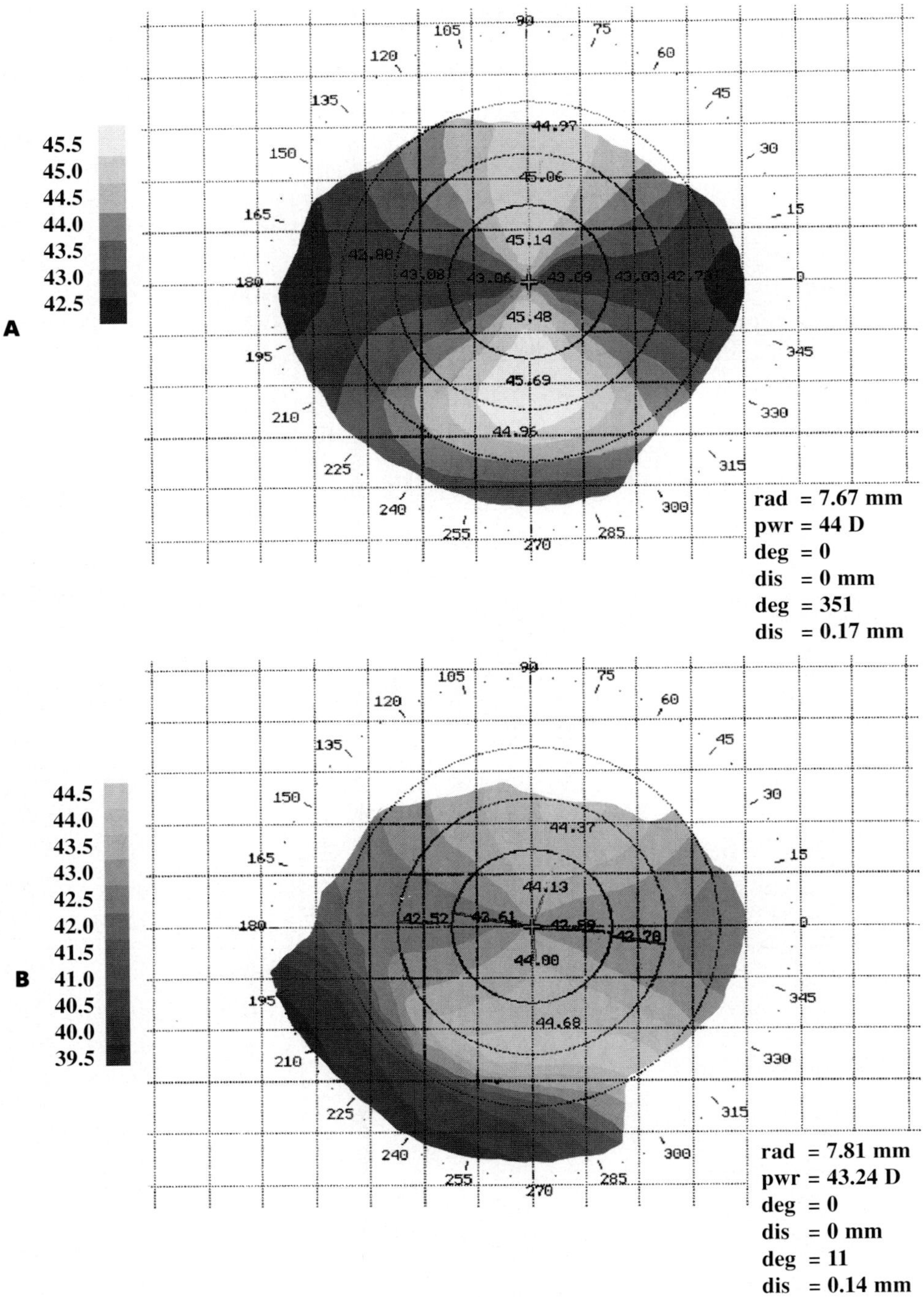

FIGURE 170-5 Topographic maps. **A,** With-the-rule regular corneal astigmatism before surgery. **B,** Six weeks after astigmatic keratotomy, a partial reduction in the patient's astigmatism is seen. This map shows the residual regular astigmatism. *Continued.*

Intraoperative Steps for Astigmatic Keratotomy

Before surgery, the patient receives three drops of broad-spectrum antibiotic. A single drop of 0.5% pilocarpine is administered. For enhancement procedures, the pilocarpine is omitted and a single drop of mydriacyl given so that preexisting incisions can be visualized against the red reflex. Ten milligrams of sublingual diazepam is administered.

The patient is brought to the operating suite and

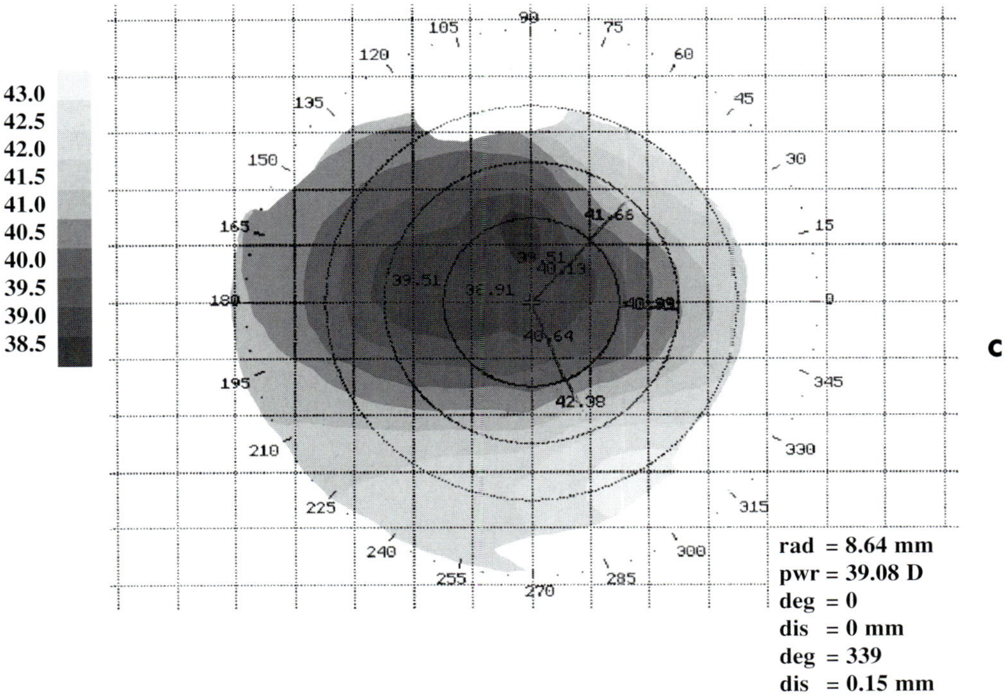

FIGURE 170-5, cont'd. Topographic maps. **C**, Two weeks later, the final map illustrates mild macroirregular astigmatism and no regular astigmatism following radial keratotomy enhancement after primary astigmatic keratotomy.

positioned comfortably in a reclining chair. The unoperated eye is covered, and the patient is asked to view the fixation light within the microscope. A visual axis marker is used to create a circular visual axis landmark. A 7 mm optical zone mark is made. Ultrasonic pachymetry is then used to determine corneal thickness at the intended astigmatic keratotomy site(s). The lid speculum has not yet been placed and the axis for pachymetry readings is estimated without the use of a Mendez ring. Actual readings are measured, and the diamond knife is set to 10% below this reading. The patient's lids are prepped while the diamond knife is set. The surgeon is gloved and a lid speculum placed. The vertical edge of a 45 degree double sharp diamond knife is used. A Mendez ring is used to determine the exact axis for surgery. Incisional markers 3.5 or 4.5 mm long are used to make an epithelial indentation. The patient is asked to look in the direction of gaze, which brings the intended astigmatic keratotomy site into a position of the surgeon's greatest advantage. The diamond then traces this mark. After surgery, analgesic and antibiotic drops are instilled. The patient is returned to recovery for postoperative counseling and dismissal.

Intraoperative Complications

The most serious intraoperative complications associated with astigmatic keratotomy are transection of another incision and corneal perforation. By the use of dilation during reoperation, previously placed radial and astigmatic keratotomy incisions can be easily visualized against the red reflex. This minimizes the risk of intersecting incisions. Intersected incisions generally require suture compression to alleviate the induced irregular astigmatism caused by edge elevation and wound gape. Similarly, patients who experience perforation during surgery generally require suture closure to prevent wound leak and subsequent wound gape with irregular astigmatism and overcorrection. Because these sutures induce significant corneal distortion, either soft lenses or rigid gas permeable lenses should be considered in the immediate postoperative period. This allows for more rapid visual rehabilitation because spectacles are of little benefit. Sutures should generally remain in place for 6 to 8 weeks. If contact lenses are required, the patient should be seen every 2 weeks to monitor possible corneal neovascularization.

Postoperative Management

The postoperative management of astigmatic keratotomy patients requires attention to issues of (1) infection, (2) inflammation, (3) pain, (4) ocular surface repair, (5) intraocular pressure, (6) visual rehabilitation, and (7) patient activities.

Infection is a rare but potentially serious complica-

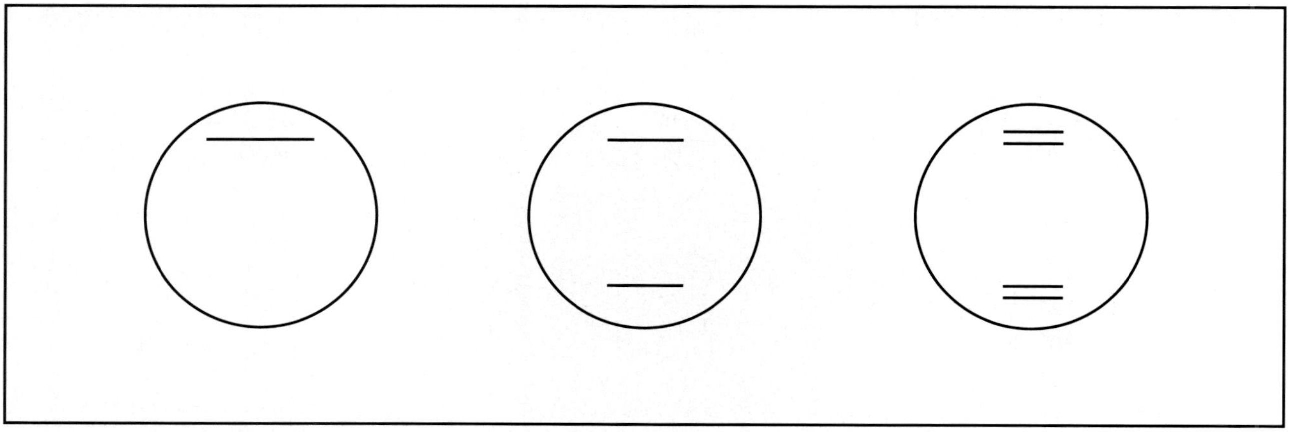

FIGURE 170-6 Three different surgical techniques of astigmatic keratotomy of equal strength.

tion of any incisional refractive procedure. Bacterial keratitis spreads rapidly along the incision and can quickly penetrate the thin barrier of remaining uncut stroma, progressing to frank endophthalmitis. Symptoms of bacterial infection must be clearly understood by all reception and technical staff. It is essential that the concerned patient's phone call not be passed off as the innocuous discomfort of a recently operated patient. Many patients experience discomfort after radial keratotomy or astigmatic keratotomy, but the increase in the severity of discomfort is unusual and should be considered a potential symptom of infection. The seriousness of acute bacterial keratitis justifies the use of powerful broad spectrum quinolone antibiotics for preoperative and postoperative prophylaxis.

Control of the inflammation can be divided into both acute and late phases. Acute phase inflammation primarily concerns reduction of the patient discomfort caused by lid edema, corneal edema, and ciliary spasm. The prolonged use of topical steroids has been advocated for modulation of wound repair. This approach is based on the belief that additional steroid use can decrease undercorrection by slowing stromal repair.

The control of pain has historically relied on the use of oral narcotics. New topical analgesic agents are a welcome addition to our armamentarium. Although astigmatic keratotomy is minimally painful, the goal of refractive surgery is to allow patients to return to work and play as quickly as possible. Every effort should be made to minimize the intensity and duration of pain.

Ocular surface repair is a critical element in reducing patient morbidity. Furthermore, rapid epithelialization mitigates against bacterial infection. Finally, the repair of the corneal epithelium is necessary for deturgescence of the cornea and reduction of irregular astigmatism caused by periincisional edema.

Although astigmatic keratotomy is less sensitive to variations of intraocular pressure than radial keratotomy, elevated IOP does lead to increase risk of wound gape and over correction.

The visual rehabilitation of astigmatic keratotomy patients is straightforward when pure astigmatism surgery is performed. Spherical loaner glasses can be provided immediately after surgery. For patients undergoing simultaneous reduction of myopia, postoperative acuity is generally adequate for most activities of daily living. Astigmatic keratotomy incisions that exhibit normal healing are associated with a stable refraction by 1 month. Although most patients prefer part-time spectacles following refractive surgery, contact lenses remain an option for patients who have undergone astigmatic keratotomy. Both soft and rigid gas-permeable lenses are acceptable. Lenses should be worn on a daily wear basis and examinations performed every few months during the first year to rule out erosion or neovascularization.

Patient activity following astigmatic keratotomy parallels guidelines for radial keratotomy patients. Patients are asked to avoid chlorinated water (pools or hot tubs) for 1 week and natural water (rivers, oceans, lakes) for 1 month. Any contact sport or racquet sport requires the use of protective eyewear. Patients are generally allowed to return to work on the second day after surgery.

Results of Astigmatic Keratotomy

There are limited descriptions of pure astigmatic keratotomy surgery in the literature. Merlin,[7] and Thorton[8] have described the basic principles of astigmatic keratotomy and published limited case reports. Thorton and Sanders[9] analyzed 106 procedures of astigmatic keratotomy. Unfortunately this analysis is confounded by the performance of simultaneous radial keratotomy. This same problem biases the results of the report of Newman et al.[10] of 154 astigmatic keratotomy procedures. The recently completed ARC-T is a multicenter prospective clinical trial reporting the work of nine experienced refractive surgeons. The study reports the findings of 159 eyes undergoing arcuate transverse keratotomy. All eyes had isolated astigmatic keratotomy as radial keratotomy was delayed for at least 1 month after the astigmatic keratotomy procedure.

Vector analysis was used to determine the net effect of astigmatic keratotomy in the ARC-T population. Patients reported in ARC-T had a mean age of 39.5 years (range 18 to 66). The population was 33% male, and 67% female. The mean preoperative refractive cylinder was 2.8 diopters. At 1 month, 43% of cases had residual refractive cylinder within 0.5 diopter of plano. Residual astigmatism of 1 diopter or less was present in 71% of cases. The rate of overcorrection of more than 1 diopter was only 6%, and complications were both infrequent and minimal in severity.

A more extensive comparision of 100 ARC-T and 100 straight-T astigmatic keratotomy procedures has been reported.[11] The ARC-T subgroup had preoperative astigmatism of 2.85 diopters ± 1.14 diopters refractive and 2.69 diopters ± 1.02 corneal astigmatism. The patient's postoperative astigmatism was 1.15 diopters ± 0.83 diopters refractive and 1.00 ± 0.84 diopters corneal astigmatism. The 100 straight-T astigmatic keratotomy patients had preoperative refractive astigmatism of 2.44 diopters + 0.80 diopters, and corneal astigmatism of 2.34 diopters + 0.76 diopters. Following their straight-transverse keratotomy, this population showed 1.06 diopters + 0.67 diopters refractive and 1.12 diopters + 0.62 diopters corneal astigmatism.

In summary, astigmatic keratotomy effectively eliminated two thirds of preoperative astigmatism in these patients. The majority of patients were left with 1 diopter or less in their life-long axis of astigmatism. There was no significant difference in the efficacy of arcuate versus straight-T incisions.

Future of Astigmatic Keratotomy

Incisional refractive procedures act through corneal weakening. This regional weakening with secondary flattening is both the strength and weakness of astigmatic keratotomy procedures. The advantage of astigmatic keratotomy is that a localized incision produces generalized flattening. This makes the procedure relatively forgiving with regard to axis identification. Conversely, excimer laser techniques require precise location of the axis of ablation.

The use of weakening keratotomy incisions limits the precision of astigmatic keratotomy. Different patients' corneas bend differently in response to similar incisions. In addition, wound healing is a major determinant of the ultimate effect of astigmatic keratotomy. The individual biologic response to weakening keratotomy incisions induces significant variability in the refractive response to surgery.

Future developments in astigmatism reduction must address accurate identification of the steeper corneal meridian. For astigmatic keratotomy techniques, improved methods of predicting corneal response to surgery must be developed. This includes better models of corneal mechanics and improved methods of predicting and controlling wound healing. Another essential requirement for more accurate astigmatism reduction is the ability of the surgeon to see what he or she is doing. Observing the alteration of corneal power with real time feedback allows for more precise surgical technique. The last decade has witnessed tremendous advancement in the understanding of astigmatism and the ability to reduce the patient's astigmatic error. The surgical reduction of astigmatism is a fertile area for clinical investigation.

REFERENCES

1. Holladay JT, Cravy TV, Koch DD: Calculating the surgically induced refractive change following ocular surgery, *J Cataract Refract Surg* 18:429-443, 1992.
2. Naylor EJ: Astigmatic difference in refractive errors, *Br J Ophthalmol* 52:422-425, 1968.
3. Alpins NA: A new method of analyzing vectors for change in astigmatism, *J Cataract Refract Surg* 19:524-533, 1993.
4. Lindstrom RL: Lans Distinguished Refractive Surgery Lecture: The surgical correction of astigmatism: a clinician's perspective, *Refract Corneal Surg.* 6:441-454, 1990.
5. Nordan LT, Grene RB: The importance of corneal asphericity and irregular astigmatism in refractive surgery, *Refract Corneal Surg* 6:200-204, 1990.
6. Grene RB, Lindstrom RL: Astigmatic keratotomy in the refractive patient: the ARC-T study. In Gills JP, Thornton SP, Martin RG, Sanders DR, ed *The surgical treatment of astigmatism,* Thorofare, NJ, 1994, Slack.
7. Merlin U: Curved keratotomy procedure for congenital astigmatism, *J Refract Surg* 3:92-97, 1987.
8. Thornton SP: Astigmatic keratotomy: a review of basic concepts with case reports, *J Cataract Refract Surg* 16:430-435, 1990.
9. Thorton SP, Sanders DR: Graded nonintersecting transverse incisions for correction of idiopathic astigmatism, *J Cataract Refract Surg* 13:27-31, 1987.
10. Newman AC, McCarty GR, Sanders DR, Raanan MG: Refractive evaluation of astigmatic keratotomy procedures, *J Cataract Refract Surg* 15:25-31, 1989.
11. Price FW et al: Astigmatism reduction clinical trial: a multicenter prospective evaluation of the predictability of arcuate keratotomy, *Arch Ophthal* 113:288-282, 1995.

CHAPTER 171

MICHAEL E. HETTINGER

Astigmatism and Cataract Surgery

Emphasis on postoperative astigmatism after cataract surgery has undergone a dramatic metamorphosis within the last 20 years. This developed in part because of rapid technologic advancements such as phacoemulsification, intraocular lenses, foldable intraocular lenses, and multifocal intraocular lenses. Twenty years ago, the intracapsular surgeon was more concerned with anatomical or structural integrity of the 11 to 12 mm cord length incision than the amount of induced postoperative astigmatism.[1] With the advent of aphakic contact lenses, some minimal residual postoperative with-the-rule (WTR) astigmatism was desirable, permitting the contact lens to be held in position by the upper lid or over the pupil. The development of phacoemulsification caused little alteration in astigmatism; however, because of the lengthy learning curve, complications, and the cataract incision being extended to 8 mm to accommodate intraocular lens insertion, planned extracapsular cataract extraction supplanted phacoemulsification as the procedure of choice for most cataract surgeons.

With extracapsular cataract surgery, the postoperative emphasis initially remained on incision security and not astigmatism. Many authors reported that nylon sutured extracapsular cataract incisions result in initial WTR astigmatism that decays with time to against-the-rule (ATR) astigmatism.[2-6] Narrow profiled intraocular lenses and foldable intraocular lenses, along with newer suturing techniques and posterior placement of cataract incisions, produced a revitalization of phacoemulsification for cataract surgery because these newer lenses could be inserted through smaller posterior incisions,[7-9] which permitted faster wound stability and earlier visual rehabilitation.

Variables in Producing Astigmatism after Cataract Surgery

INCISION LENGTH

The amount of surgically induced astigmatism after cataract surgery has been substantially decreased by reducing the length of the cataract incision.[3,8-14] Armeniades et al.[15] found that 12 mm incisions had a pronounced effect on tissue deformation, but 3 mm incisions did not. Extracapsular incisions of 10 to 11 mm in cord length all exhibit a drift towards ATR astigmatism. Smaller 6 to 7 mm tunnel incisions are reported to induce minimal astigmatic changes at 6 months.[15] Smaller incisions were documented to be beneficial in reducing postoperative astigmatism in the first 3 months, but no statistical difference in astigmatism existed between 4 mm, 6 mm, and 11 mm length incisions at 3 months.[17] These two studies do not address the long-term results of insidious drift to ATR astigmatism reported by others.[18,19] In his article on the structural analysis of cataract incision construction, Koch[20] introduces the concept of the incision funnel (Figure 171-1, *A*), which is an imaginary pair of curved lines approximately 3.0 mm apart at the limbus that diverge from the limbus, separating as the distance from the limbus increases. This concept of the external scleral incision was developed from mathematical analysis that demonstrated a curvilinear relationship between the length of the incision and amount of astigmatism that can develop[20] (Figure 171-1, *B*). Incisions constructed inside the incisional funnel will be astigmatically neutral. External incisions of various lengths can be fashioned to be astigmatically neutral; however, this can only be accomplished if the longer incisions are placed farther from the limbus (Figure 171-2, *A*). In phacoemulsification surgery, posterior incisions increase the length of the scleral tunnel that restricts lateral movement of the phacoemulsification tip and causes striations in the cornea limiting the surgeon's vision. This is referred to as "oar-locking."

EXTERNAL INCISIONS

Curvilinear scleral incisions following the limbus have significant potential for developing ATR astigmatism, because the inferior edge of the incision can sag away from the superior edge and it falls outside the incisional funnel[20] (Figure 171-2, *B*). Linear external scleral incisions have less potential for developing ATR astigmatism than curvilinear external scleral incisions because the ends of the linear incision are secured in the sclera and are farther away from the limbus than

scleral incision inside the incisional funnel or a 3.0 mm temporal self-sealing clear corneal incision and place arcuate corneal incision on the steep axis for the appropriate amount of surgery according to the desired nomogram. Alternatively, the surgeon may elect to operate on the steepest axis with a scleral incision that extends outside the incisional funnel with the length varying from 4.0 to 5.5 mm, depending on the amount of astigmatism—4.0 mm for 0.75 diopters, 4.5 mm for 1.00 diopters, 5.0 for 1.25 diopters, and 5.5 mm for 1.50 diopters. Surgeons should review their results and modify these numbers based on outcomes.

With-the-rule astigmatism > 1.50 diopters

The surgeon should perform astigmatic neutral surgery with an incision inside the incisional funnel or a 3.0 mm clear corneal incision. Arcuate incisions of the cornea should be made to correct the desired amount of astigmatism according to the nomogram the surgeon uses.

If astigmatic neutral surgery cannot be performed, the surgeon's usual surgery should be performed on-axis without sutures, if safe for the patient. If sutures are required, a snug, but not tight, horizontal anchor suture of 10-0 nylon should be used. If the resulting astigmatism is visually disabling for the patient, it can be corrected at a later, more appropriate time with incisional corneal surgery.

Against-the-rule astigmatism ≥0.75 diopters but <1.75 diopters

Two options exist for correcting this astigmatic problem. Using foldable intraocular lenses, a 3.0 mm temporal self-sealing clear corneal or a self-sealing scleral incision inside the scleral funnel is constructed and appropriate arcuate incisions from the surgeon's nomogram of choice are placed in the steep axis. The second option is for the surgeon to operate on the steep axis with a scleral incision that extends outside the incisional funnel with the length varying from 4.0 mm to 5.5 mm, depending on the amount of astigmatism—4.0 mm for 0.75 diopters, 4.5 mm for 1.00 diopters, 5.0 for 1.25 diopters, and 5.5 mm for 1.50 diopters.

Against-the-rule astigmatism >1.50 diopters

Astigmatic neutral surgery should be performed with an incision inside the incisional funnel or a 3.0 mm clear corneal incision along with arcuate incisions of the cornea to correct the desired amount of astigmatism. Surgeons who do not perform astigmatic neutral surgery should perform their usual surgery on axis without sutures, if safe for the patient. If the residual astigmatism causes visual dysfunction, it can be corrected at a later, more appropriate time with incisional corneal surgery.

OBLIQUE ASTIGMATISM

Oblique astigmatism is that astigmatism in which the steep axis lies between the 120 and 150 degrees meridian or between the 30 and 60 degrees meridian.

Oblique astigmatism ≥0.75 diopters but <1.75 diopters

Intraoperative correction of this quantity of oblique astigmatism depends on its location. With this degree of astigmatism located between the 120 and 150 degrees axis in the right eyes or between the 30 and 60 degree axis in the left eye, self-sealing astigmatically neutral cataract surgery can be performed at a site the surgeon chooses and appropriate corneal incisions can be placed in the steep axis. As an alternative, the surgeon may center the cataract incision on the steep axis and vary the length of the incision that extends beyond the incisional funnel, as described previously.

If this degree of astigmatism is located between 30 and 60 degrees in the right eye or between the 120 and 150 degree axis in the left eye, the surgeon will likely encounter difficulty operating on axis, superonasally for either eye. In these cases, I recommend performing self-sealing astigmatically neutral cataract surgery and performing the appropriate amount of arcuate incisional surgery to correct the oblique astigmatism. If the surgeon is unable to perform self-sealing astigmatically neutral cataract incisions and insert foldable intraocular lenses, the surgeon should perform the usual cataract operation and correct the astigmatism at the appropriate time with incisional corneal surgery.

Oblique astigmatism >1.50 diopters

It is possible to correct this astigmatic problem in the same manner as described previously for oblique astigmatism located between 30 and 60 degrees in the right eye and between 120 and 150 degrees in the left eye.

ASYMMETRIC ASTIGMATISM

This unusual type of astigmatism requires identification with computerized videokeratography (Figure 171-3), and, when present in patients undergoing cataract surgery, it can be corrected by performing astigmatism-neutral cataract surgery and asymmetric arcuate keratotomy in the steep axis.

NONORTHOGONAL ASTIGMATISM

This relatively rare type of astigmatism (Figure 171-4) also requires identification with computerized videokeratography. When present in patients undergoing cataract surgery, it can be corrected by astigmatism-neutral cataract surgery and by perform-

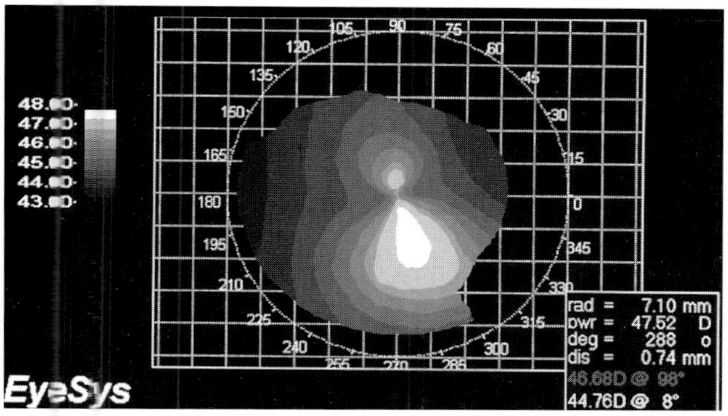

FIGURE 171-3 Asymmetric astigmatism.

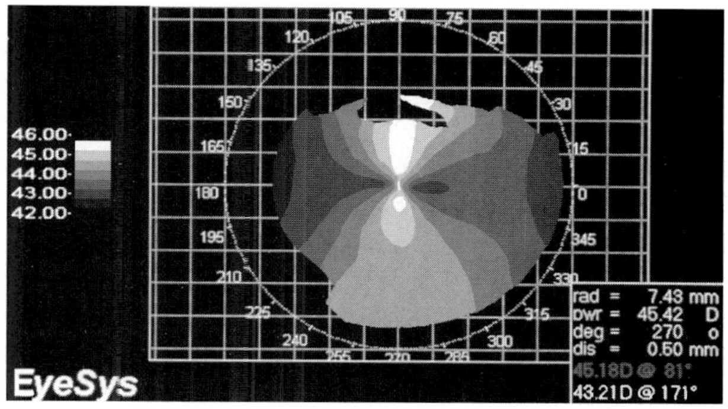

FIGURE 171-5 Preoperative videokeratography of −1.25 +2.50 ×90.

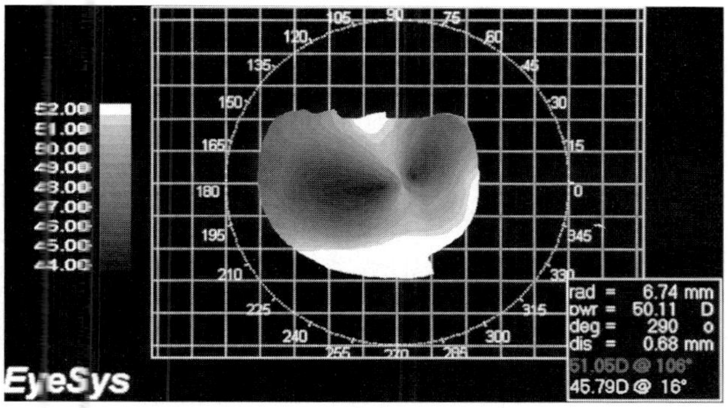

FIGURE 171-4 Nonorthogonal astigmatism.

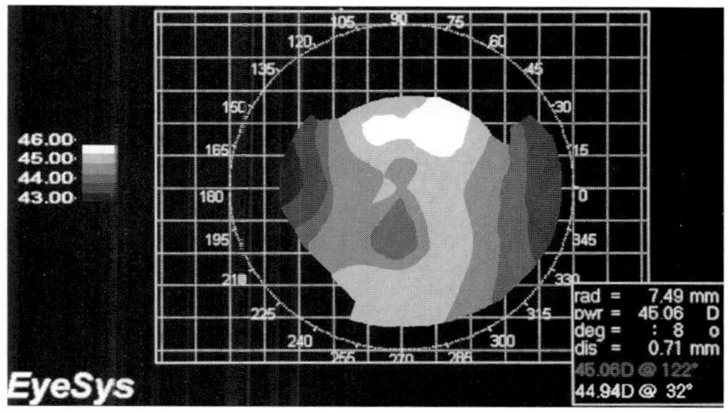

FIGURE 171-6 Postoperative videokeratography of Figure 171-5 after acruate keratotomy.

ing arcuate incisional corneal surgery in the steep axes, because, by definition, the cornea is steep in two separate axes.

RESIDUAL ASTIGMATISM AFTER CATARACT SURGERY

Postoperative cataract patients who desire surgical astigmatic correction should have a thorough understanding of what their postincisional astigmatic surgery refractive error will likely be if not plano. As an example, if a patient's refraction is −2.00 +2.00 × 180, and if the surgeon successfully eliminates the cylinder with arcuate transverse incisions, the patient's postoperative refraction will be −1.00 diopters. If the patient's refraction was −1.25 +2.50 × 90, and if one were to successfully eliminate the astigmatism with arcuate or transverse incisions, the postoperative refraction should be plano (Figure 171-5 and 171-6).

Patients desiring astigmatic incisional surgery must have a stable refraction and keratometry readings. Furthermore, videokeratography is strongly recommended. Lindstrom et al.[27] believe residual postoperative cataract astigmatism that causes functional visual impairment should not be corrected until 1 year after cataract surgery and when the eye has a stable refraction. Timing of this type of surgery depends on the cataract incision length, configuration, location, closure material, and technique. Smaller self-sealing incisions with frown or chevron configurations can be operated on much earlier than larger sutured curvilinear incisions. In a small series of patients with self-sealing 4 mm cataract incisions, the mean astigmatic decay was −0.28 diopters at 4 months and −0.45 diopter at 1 year.[32] It seems reasonable to use 6 months as an acceptable time for surgical intervention in postoperative cataract patients who have had small self-sealing incisions and desire incisional astigmatic surgery, provided their refraction and keratometry readings are stable.

The surgeon should select a nomogram with which he or she is comfortable. If the nomogram includes variables such as age, sex, intraocular pressure, or specific diamond knife, these must be considered.

Instruments Required for Incisional Astigmatic Surgery

Astigmatic refractive surgery should be carried out under an operating microscope with a rheostat to

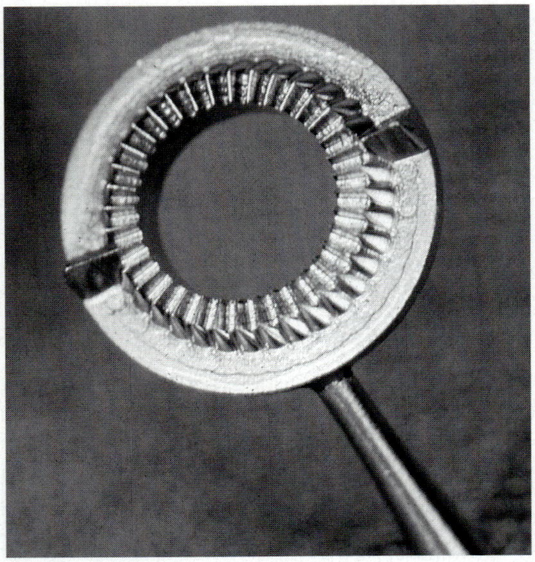

FIGURE 171-7 Thornton 360 arcuate corneal marker.

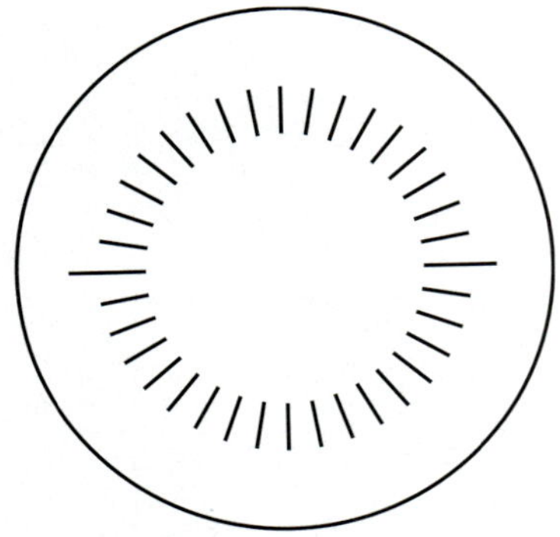

FIGURE 171-8 Impression the Thornton 360 arcuate marker leaves on the cornea. The divisions are 10° apart. The internal diameter of the marker is 6 mm. The outside diameter is 8 mm. (From Thornton SP: Inverse arcuate incision: a new approach to the correction of astigmatism, *Refract Corneal Surg* 10:27, 1994.)

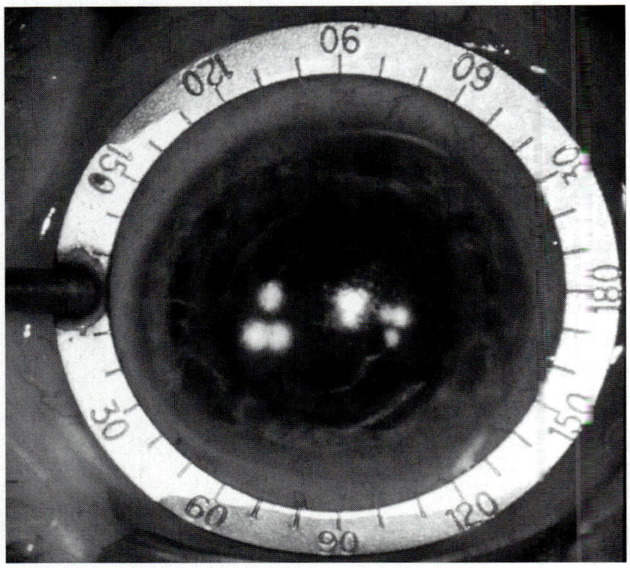

FIGURE 171-9 Mendez ruler on globe.

control light intensity. An ultrasonic pachymeter is required to measure corneal thickness over the area in which incisions are to be made. Optical zone markers of various diameters are needed to demarcate the appropriate optical zone or zones in which the surgeon plans to operate. Transverse markers of various lengths are needed if one prefers transverse over arcuate incisions. If one's preference is to perform arcuate keratotomy, Thornton has simplified the need for marking instruments by developing the 360 degree arcuate corneal marker (Figure 171-7). When the 36 blades of the marker are coated with a marking pen, it demarcates every 10 degrees for the entire 360 degrees with the inside diameter of the blades at 6 mm and the outside diameter at 8 mm, with the exception of two blades, which are oriented 180 degrees apart (Figure 171-8). A marking pen will assist in delineating the transverse or arcuate incisional area. The incision is made with a front-cutting diamond micrometer knife. Several companies make diamond knives specifically for arcuate keratotomy. The blade is set under a microscope with 100× magnification. A Mendez 360 degree ruler (Figure 171-9) will assist the surgeon in demarcating the steep axis intraoperatively.

Astigmatic Theory and Incisional Procedure

Many incisional astigmatism surgery nomograms are available for the beginning incisional refractive cataract surgeon. It is useful for the neophyte refractive cataract surgeon to discuss the benefits and problems of using certain nomograms with a colleague who is pleased with results using a particular nomogram. It is also extremely useful to observe that surgeon performing the procedure. It is important for the observer to watch several cases both through the oculars on the observer scope or on a monitor and without the assistance of the operating microscope. This approach provides a better view and understanding of the position of the surgeon's hands and arms during the operation.

This information helps the neophyte refractive surgeon decide whether to use straight or arcuate keratotomy. Straight incisions are easier to perform and require less skill. Arcuate incisions afford larger astigmatic corrections with incisions at the 6.0, 7.0, and 8.0 mm optical zones. With straight keratotomy inci-

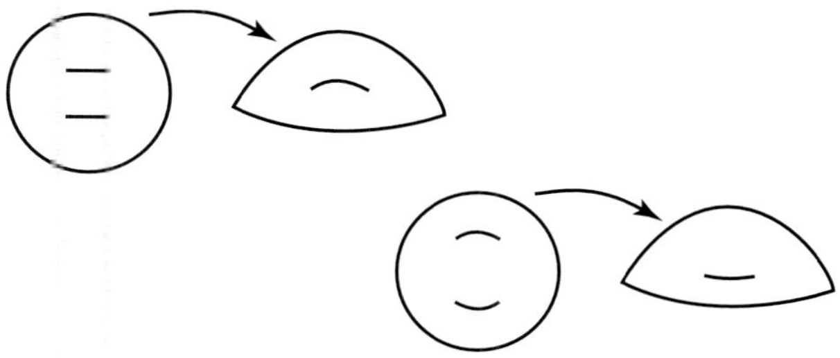

FIGURE 171-10 What appears to be a straight transverse line when viewed from above a spherical surface is actually an inverse arc. What appears to be a concentric arc from above is parallel to the equator and therefore transverse to the meridian. (From Thornton SP: *Radial and astigmatic keratotomy,* Thorofare, NJ, 1994, Slack.)

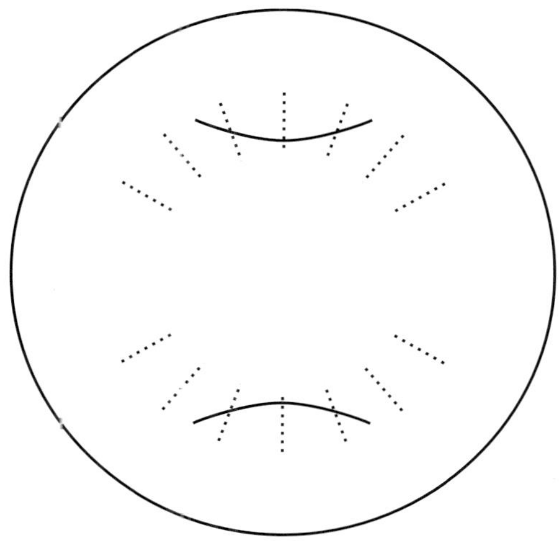

FIGURE 171-11 Inverse arcuate incision to correct astigmatism in the steep axis without coupling. (Modified from Thornton SP: *Radial and astigmatic keratotomy,* Thorofare, NJ, 1994, Slack).

sions, large corrections require an optical zone less than 6.0 mm, which can result in irregular astigmatism and glare.[27]

Properly placed transverse or arcuate incisions are of equal length on either side of the steep meridian and produce coupling when they do not increase the corneal circumference. With coupling, the steep meridian flattens and the flat meridian steepens. One can visualize coupling by graphically altering the two-dimensional shape of a football to that of a basketball without changing the circumference of the football.

Lavery and Linstrom[33] found that the relationship between corneal flattening and optical zone size of straight incisions was not linear, and the maximum effect was between 5.0 and 8.0 mm optical zone. Furthermore, Thornton[34] showed that straight incisions viewed from above a spherical surface are actually inverse arcs when viewed from the side, and arcuate incisions viewed from above are actually transverse incisions when viewed from the side. (Figure 171-10). Arcuate incisions result in 1:1 coupling, whereas straight incisions produce 2:1 coupling.[34] In 1:1 coupling, for every diopter of flattening in the steep meridian, the flat meridian steepens 1 diopter. With 2:1 coupling, for every diopter of flattening in the steep meridian, the flat meridian steepens only 0.5 diopter. Binder and Waring[35] found that the principal variable affecting coupling was incision length, with short incisions less than 2 mm yielding >1:1 coupling, with 2 mm to 5 mm length incisions yielding 1:1 coupling, and 5 mm to 6 mm length incisions yielding <1:1 coupling. Using cadaver eyes, Sabates et al.[36] studied paired transverse corneal incisions subtending a 45 degree arc at 5.0, 6.0, 7.0, and 8.0 mm optical zones and concluded that optical zones of 7.0 mm and 8.0 were less effective than 5.0 mm and 6.0 mm. Inverse arcuate incisions correct astigmatism in the steep axis of the cornea without steepening the flat axis; therefore, there is no coupling[34] (Figure 171-11). The nomogram for this procedure is available.[34]

ASTIGMATISM CORRECTION AT THE TIME OF CATARACT SURGERY

At the end of the astigmatically neutral cataract procedure, the globe is inflated through the small paracentesis incision to achieve an intraocular pressure that is slightly higher than normal. The appropriate optical zone marker is centered over the light reflex from the operating microscope, which is centered in the pupil. Patients who have retrobulbar or peribulbar anesthesia are unable to fixate on the operating microscope light at the time of the incisional astigmatic surgery. When topical anesthesia is used in cataract surgery, the patient should be able to fixate on the microscope light after the cataract procedure.

The Mendez ruler is placed on the globe, and the Thornton arcuate marker, inked with a marking pen, is placed on the carefully dried cornea, with the two longer blades oriented in the steep axis. If the blades are inked too much, or too much pressure is applied to the globe, the result will be thickened or smeared radial marks on the cornea. The ultrasonic pachymeter measures the corneal thickness over the arc of the cornea to be incised. The front cutting diamond blade is inspected and set under the microscope at 100% of the thinnest corneal reading. Because there is variation in corneal thickness from superior to inferior and from temporal to nasal, a reading is taken at each optical zone and over both areas of the cornea to be incised. This reading usually requires the diamond blade to be set twice for a pair of arcuate incisions and four times

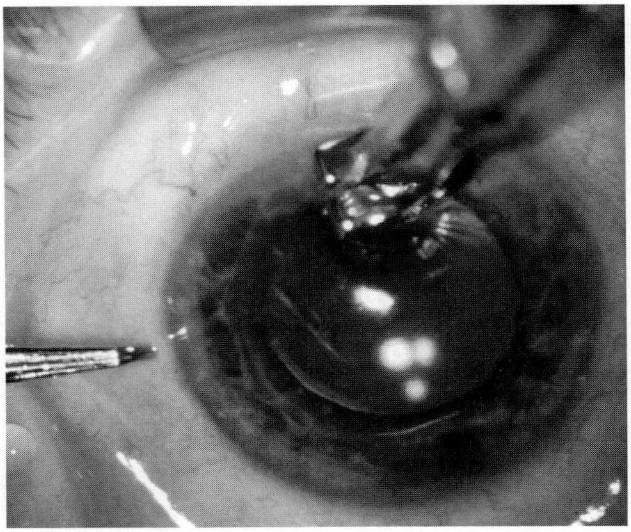

FIGURE 171-12 Diamond knife beginning arcuate incision toward fixation at the limbus.

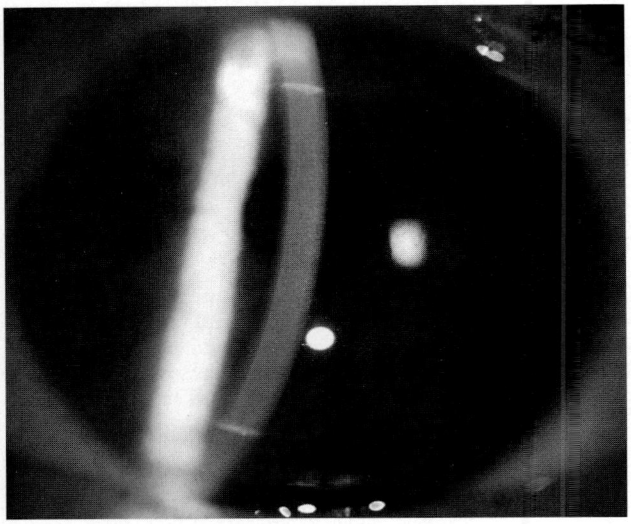

FIGURE 171-13 Slit lamp photograph of superior and inferior arcuate incisions.

for two pairs of arcuate incisions at two different optical zones.

Although the globe is immobilized with retrobulbar or peribulbar anesthesia, I fixate the globe with 0.25 double curved forceps at the limbus so that my incision moves toward fixation (Figure 171-12). The diamond blade is placed into the cornea, perpendicular to the globe, all the way to the footplates at the beginning of the arc. After waiting approximately 2 seconds, the blade is pushed along the arc to be incised. This cut is facilitated by slowly rotating the handle of the diamond knife between the ends of the thumb and first two fingers while applying constant downward pressure and slowly pushing the blade forward over the extent of the arc, keeping both footplates in contact with the cornea. The same procedure is repeated for each individual arc. (Figure 171-13) The astigmatism is checked with a quantitative surgical keratometer. At the end of the procedure, one drop of diclofenac (Voltaren) is applied to the cornea, which is then covered with a 12-hour collagen shield soaked in 0.5 ml of 1% prednisolone phosphate and 0.5 ml of tobramycin. Beginning on the first postoperative day, the patient medicates the operated eye with one drop of an antibiotic steroid combination for 5 days.

If transverse incisions are made, the appropriate optical zone marker or markers are centered over and applied to the cornea with gentle pressure. The Mendez ruler is placed on the globe, and the transverse marker is aligned tangential to the optical zone mark straddling the steep axis, creating parallel indentations 180 degrees apart. The ultrasonic pachymeter measures the cornea thickness over both areas to be incised, and the thinnest reading for each area is recorded. The diamond knife is inspected and set the same as for arcuate incisions. The globe is fixated and incisions made the same as for arcuate incisions; however, there is no need to rotate the knife between the thumb and fingers. Treatment at the end of the procedure is the same as for arcuate incisions.

RESIDUAL ASTIGMATISM CORRECTION AFTER CATARACT SURGERY

After an appropriate amount of time has elapsed from cataract surgery, residual astigmatism is corrected in the same manner as if it were to be corrected at the time of cataract surgery, except that the use of topical anesthesia allows for better localization of the visual axis over which to center the arcuate or transverse incisions. Proparacaine, 0.5%, is administered every 10 minutes for four doses, and one drop of diclofenac is given 30 minutes before surgery. Immediately after surgery, one drop of antibiotic and one drop of diclofenac are applied. No collagen shield or patch is used; otherwise, treatment is the same as for a procedure completed at the time of cataract surgery.

Complications

Several complications may occur with incisional surgery. The most serious is endophthalmitis, which requires a microperforation or macroperforation along with introduction of bacteria into the anterior chamber. Microperforation occurs as a result of inaccurate pachymetry readings, incorrect setting of the blade, or excessive pressure on the globe with the diamond knife. Most pachymeters will not measure the corneal thickness if the probe is not perpendicular to the surface. It is important to use the thinnest corneal reading to set the depth of the diamond blade. Microperforations are signaled by the presence of a bead of aqueous at the leading edge of the diamond blade. If a microperforation occurs, 20 μ should be taken off the diamond blade depth under the microscope before the procedure can be finished in that quadrant. If a second microperforation is located after decreasing the blade depth 20 μ, the procedure should be aborted. Microperforations are generally self-sealing. Patients with microperforations that are self-sealing on the operating table are started on topical ciprofloxacin, four times a day the day of surgery, and patients are examined the next day.

Macroperforations are unrecognized microperforations that are subsequently extended. They usually do not stop leaking aqueous, and the procedure should be aborted. If the chamber remains formed, these can be treated with one drop of diclofenac and a 12-hour collagen shield soaked in 0.5 ml of tobramycin. If the anterior chamber is flat, repair of the perforation with a butterfly 10-0 nylon suture is required. With reformation of the anterior chamber, one drop of diclofenac and a 12-hour collagen shield soaked in 0.5 ml of tobramycin are applied.

Corneal epithelial abrasions or flaps are not uncommon with a front-cutting diamond knife. The epithelial flap should be reapproximated to its original position. An antibiotic steroid combination drop is administered four times a day for 5 days.

IMMEDIATE TO INTERMEDIATE POSTOPERATIVE PERIOD

The most serious complication of astigmatic keratotomy is infectious keratitis, which occurs because bacteria have been given access to and colonized the corneal stroma. It should be treated aggressively like any other infectious keratitis. Pain, foreign body sensation, photophobia, and burning and stinging have been significantly reduced or eliminated with the use of diclofenac.[37]

INTERMEDIATE AND LONG-TERM POSTOPERATIVE PERIOD

Irregular astigmatism can occur immediately and last long after the surgery. It frequently develops in cases with smaller optical zones. Stabilization of irregular astigmatism can be aided with a bandage lens. Overcorrections should not be addressed surgically until there is stable videokeratography that correlates with the refraction.

Conclusions

Technologic improvements in phacoemulsification units, intraocular lenses, ultrasonic pachymeters, and diamond knives; a better understanding of how and why cataract incisions and wound closure techniques alter corneal stability and curvature; and new nomograms for astigmatic refractive surgery afford the cataract surgeon the opportunity to perform astigmatic neutral cataract surgery in patients without significant preoperative astigmatism and to correct preexisting astigmatism intraoperatively in cataract patients. In the future it is likely that second-generation exicmer lasers will be able to perform intraoperative correction of astigmatism. Finally, intraocular lenses containing cylindrical correction in given axis have received attention. For these to be effective, the surgeon must know how much postoperative astigmatism must be corrected, identify intraoperatively the axis of astigmatism, and ensure that the implant will not rotate away from the axis in which it is placed. As cataract surgeons, we have the ability to perform cataract surgery that provides rapid and stable visual rehabilitation. The future looks promising for patients to obtain excellent, rapid, and stable uncorrected visual acuity after cataract surgery.

REFERENCES

1. Swinger CA: Postoperative astigmatism, *Surv Ophthalmol* 31:219-248,1987.
2. Masket S: Keratorefractive aspects of the scleral pocket incision and closure method for cataract surgery, *J Cataract Refract Surg* 15:70-77,1989.
3. Shepherd JR: Induced astigmatism in small incision cataract surgery, *J Cataract Refract Surg* 15:85-88,1989.
4. Kondrot EC: Keratometric cylinder and visual recovery following phacoemulsification and intraocular lens implantation using a self-sealing cataract incision, *J Cataract Refract Surg* 17(suppl):731-733,1991.
5. Talamo JH et al: Natural history of corneal astigmatism after cataract surgery, *J Cataract Refract Surg* 17:313-318,1991.
6. Jampel HD et al: A computerized analysis of astigmatism after cataract surgery, *Ophthalmic Surg* 17:786-790,1986.
7. Werblin TP: Refractive stability after cataract extraction using a 6.5 millimeter scleral pocket incision with horizontal or radial sutures, *J Refract Corneal Surg* 10:339-342,1994.
8. Brint SF, Ostrick DM, Byran, JS: Keratometric cylinder and visual performance following phacoemulsification and implantation with silicone small incision or poly-(methyl methacrylate) intraocular lenses, *J Cataract Refract Surg* 17:32-36,1991.
9. Feil SH, Crandall AS, Olson RJ: Astigmatic decay following small incision, self-sealing cataract surgery, *J Cataract Refract Surg* 20:40-43,1994.
10. Newman AC et al: Small incisions to control astigmatism during cataract surgery, *J Cataract Refract Surg* 15:78-84,1989.
11. Gills JP, Sanders DR: Use of small incisions to control induced astigmatism and inflammation following cataract surgery, *J Cataract Refract Surg* 17(suppl):740-744,1991.

12. Grabow HB: Early results of 500 cases of no-stitch cataract surgery: *J Cataract Refract Surg* 17(suppl):726-730,1991.
13. Steinert RF et al: Astigmatism after small incision cataract surgery: a prospective randomized, multicenter comparison of 4- and 6.5- mm incisions, *Ophthalmology* 98:417-423,1991.
14. Martin RG et al: Effect of small incision intraocular lens surgery on postoperative inflammation and astigmatism: a study of the AMO SI-18 NB small incision lens, *J Cataract Refract Surg* 18:51-57,1992.
15. Armeniades CD et al: Effect of incision length, location, and shape on local corneal deformation during cataract surgery, *J Cataract Refract Surg* 16:83-87,1990.
16. Dam-Johansen M, Olsen T: Refractive results after phacoemulsification and ECCE A comparative study, *Acta Ophthalmol (Copenh)* 71:382-387,1993.
17. Leen MM, Ho CC, Yanoff M: Association between surgically induced astigmatism and cataract incision size in the early postoperative period, *Ophthalmic Surg* 24(9):586-592,1993.
18. Parker WT, Clorfeine GS: Long-term evaluation of astigmatism following planned extracapsular cataract extraction, *Arch Ophthalmol* 107:353-357,1989.
19. Richards SC et al: Long-term course of surgically induced astigmatism, *J Cataract Refract Surg* 14:270-276,1988.
20. Koch PS: Structural analysis of cataract incision construction, *J Cataract Refract Surg* 17(suppl):661-667,1991.
21. Singer JA: Frown incision for minimizing induced astigmatism after small incision cataract surgery with rigid optic intraocular lens implantation, *J Cataract Refract Surg* 17(suppl):677-688,1991.
22. Pallin SL: Chevron sutureless closure: a preliminary report, *J Cataract Refract Surg* 17(suppl):706-707,1991.
23. Siepser SB: Sutureless cataract surgery with radial transverse incision, *J Cataract Refract Surg* 17(suppl):716-718,1991.
24. Ernest PH: Corneal lip tunnel incision, *J Cataract Refract Surg* 20:154-157,1994.
25. Fine IH: Architecture and construction of a self-sealing incision for cataract surgery, *J Cataract Refract Surg* 17(suppl):672-676,1991.
26. Gimbel HV, Raanan MG, DeLuca M: Effect of suture material on postoperative astigmatism, *J Cataract Refract Surg* 18:42-50, 1992.
27. Lindstrom RL, Agapitos PJ, Koch DD: Cataract surgery and astigmatic keratotomy. In Dodick JM, Donnellfeld ED, editors: *Int Ophthalmol Clin* 34(2):145-164,1994.
28. Hayashi K, Nakao F, Hayashi F: Topographic analysis of early changes in corneal astigmatism after cataract surgery, *J Cataract Refract Surg* 19:43-47,1993.
29. Koch DD, Haff EA, Gay C: Computerized videokeratographic analysis of corneal topographic changes induced by sutured and unsutured 4 mm scleral pocket incisions, *J Cataract Refract Surg* 19(suppl):166-169,1993.
30. Fine HI: Infinity suture: modified horizontal suture for 6.5 mm incisions. In Gills JP, Sanders DR, editors: *Small incision cataract surgery; foldable lenses, one-stitch surgery, sutureless surgery, astigmatic keratotomy,* Thorofare, NJ, 1990, Slack.
31. Masket S: Horizontal anchor suture closure method for small incision cataract surgery, *J Cataract Refract Surg* 17(suppl):689-695,1991.
32. Masket S: One year postoperative astigmatic comparison of sutured and unsutured 4.0 mm scleral pocket incisions, *J Cataract Refract Surg* 19:453-456,1993.
33. Lavery GW, Lindstrom RL: Trapezoidal astigmatic keratotomy in human cadaver eyes, *J Refract Surg* 1:28-51,1985.
34. Thornton SP: *Radial and astigmatic keratotomy,* Thorofare, NJ, 1994, Slack.
35. Binder PS, Waring GO: Keratotomy for astigmatism. In Waring GO, editor: *Refractive keratotomy for myopia and astigmatism,* St Louis, 1991, Mosby.
36. Sabates MA et al: Induction of astigmatism by straight transverse corneal incisions, 45° long, at different clear zones in human cadaver eyes, *J Refract Corneal Surg* 10:327-332,1994.
37. Hettinger ME, Robin JB, Gill DJ: Diclofenac sodium (Voltaren) as an ocular analgesic—the RK experience. Paper presented at the 1995 CLAO meeting, Las Vegas, Nevada.

SECTION FIVE *Lamellar Refractive Procedures*

CHAPTER 172

WILLIAM E. WHITSON KEVIN C. CHANG
JULIAN A. PROCOPE FRANCIS W. PRICE, JR

Automated Lamellar Keratoplasty

Historical Perspectives

The concept of lamellar refractive keratoplasty was first introduced by Barraquer[1] in 1949. He later developed techniques for lamellar refractive surgery for correction of myopia and hyperopia in the early 1960s The techniques of keratomileusis and keratophakia were first performed on human subjects in the mid 1960s. The concept behind this procedure was to alter the refractive properties of the eye by changing the anterior curvature of the cornea. The original myopic keratomileusis procedure was a complex and technically demanding procedure. In this procedure, a corneal disk approximately 300 μm thick is removed with a keratome and then lathed into a concave shape while frozen using a cryolathe (Figure 172-1). After thawing, the tissue is replaced onto the stromal bed and sutured in place with a running eight-bite antitorque suture (Figure 172-2).

The first human keratophakia procedures for aphakia were performed by Barraquer in 1963 and 1964. The original microkeratome and those that have followed are based on a principle similar to that of a carpenter's plane in which an oscillating cutting blade in the keratome removes a lamellar section of corneal tissue when the keratome is passed across the cornea of an eye that is fixated by a suction ring. The first reported patient experienced acceptable visual results. However, recovery of visual acuity was slow, usually taking 6 to 8 months to achieve a stable level of vision postoperatively. This slow recovery was due to tissue damage from freezing of the cornea. With these techniques, extremely high degrees of myopia up to 34 diopters could be corrected.

Keratophakia and keratomileusis were first introduced into the United States in 1979 by Troutman and Swinger.[2] In 1980, Werblin et al[3] introduced the idea of epikeratoplasty. This procedure was first termed epikeratophakia but was later renamed epikeratoplasty. This procedure involved the removal of a disk of corneal tissue with a microkeratome from a donor globe. This disk was then frozen and lathed into a concave or convex lens and then lyophilized. This donor tissue was created in known dioptric powers. This donor cap was sutured onto the cornea to provide a new anterior refractive system. This was technically a much easier procedure to perform than myopic keratomileusis. In addition, it could be achieved at a significantly reduced cost to the surgeon because of the elimination of the microkeratome and cryolathe. However, epikeratoplasty did not gain widespread acceptance by surgeons or patients because of the unpredictability and instability of results. In addition, there was significant discomfort, delayed epithelial healing, and slow visual recovery in some patients.

In 1985, the keratomileusis procedure entered the next phase in its evolution. Krumeich and Swinger introduced the Barraquer-Krumeich-Swinger (BKS) system,[4] the first commercially available nonfreeze keratomileusis system. The procedure involved the use of an improved microkeratome to remove a lamellar section of tissue from the cornea of known diameter and thickness and inversion onto a suction dye that was preselected to set the cornea up for a myopic or hyperopic second resection on the stromal side of the disk. The primary advantage to this procedure was the elimination of freezing-related injury to the corneal tissue and the delay in recovery of useful vision. Visual recovery, however, was still slow.

Disadvantages included the need to create two microkeratome cuts with a manual microkeratome. The inherent lack of predictability of the refractive result using a manual microkeratome was heightened by the need for a second cut. Irregular astigmatism was a significant problem postoperatively in these patients.

By the early 1980s, the emergence of radial keratotomy and astigmatic keratotomy displaced keratomil-

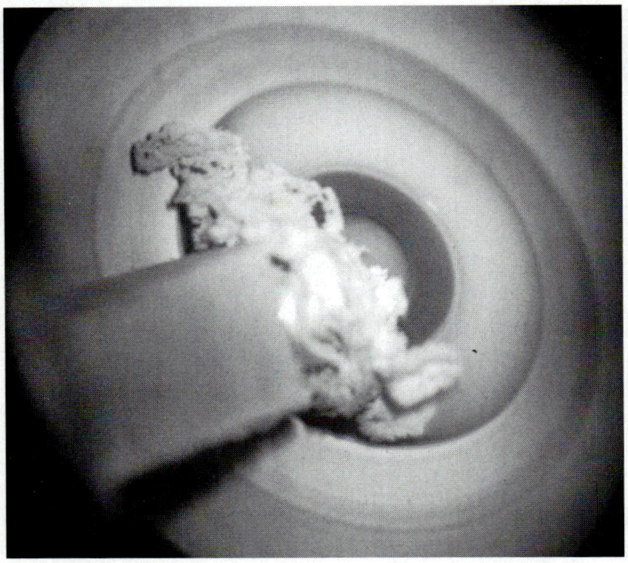

FIGURE 172-1 The resected lamellar cornea cap is placed on a cryolathe, frozen to rigidity, then lathed to create the desired dioptric power change. The tissue is dyed green to facilitate visualization.

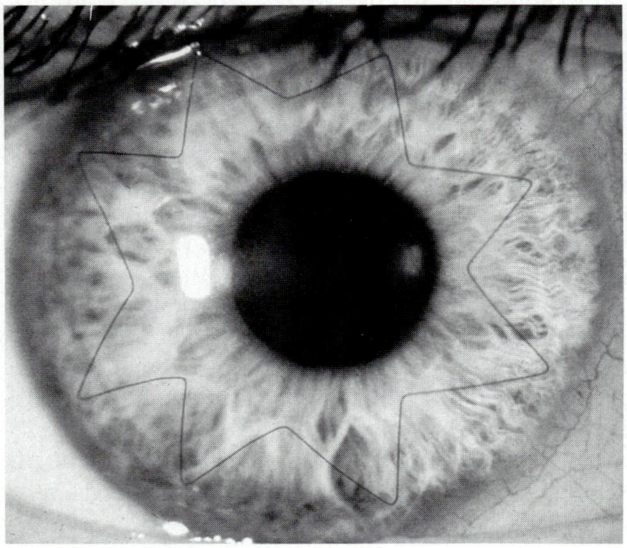

FIGURE 172-2 The lathed corneal button is held in place with an eight-bite antitorque suture.

eusis and keratophakia in the armamentarium of most refractive surgeons. The next major development in keratomileusis was that of keratomileusis in situ in which the refractive cut was made in the underlying stromal bed after the primary cap had been resected. Whereas the refractive resection was performed on the resected piece of tissue in myopic keratomileusis using the cryolathe, it is prepared in the stromal bed by the microkeratome in keratomileusis in situ. It was thought that resection of a lamellar disk from the bed would reduce the anterior corneal curvature by having the corneal cap "drape" into the resected bed underlying it, resulting in a larger optical zone than the diameter of the resected piece of stromal tissue.

Bas and Nano[5] reported their series of in situ keratomileusis. Seven percent of patients had 20/40 or better vision without correction. Twenty-seven percent of eyes were within ±1 diopter of the planned correction postoperatively. Undercorrection and irregular astigmatism were significant complications in their group. These authors concluded that keratomileusis in situ performed with the manual keratome was unsatisfactory in terms of accuracy, predictability, and the tendency to produce irregular astigmatism.

In the late 1980s, a new technique of keratomileusis in situ, later named *automated lamellar keratoplasty,* was introduced. The cornerstone of this new system was an automated, gear-driven keratome that controlled the speed with which the keratome passed across the cornea. This allowed for greater consistency and smoothness of the lamellar cut. Concurrent improvements and refinements in the pneumatic suction ring and related equipment reduced the technical difficulty of the procedure and have resulted in the ability to produce very smooth cuts. Ruiz's device is now called the automatic corneal shaper (Chiron Surgical Products, Irvine, California).

Originally, the corneal cap was sutured back into position. Guimaraes, et al later discovered that suturing of the lenticule was an unnecessary step because the lenticule would adhere to the underlying stromal bed within 24 hours. There is now a significantly reduced recovery time and less induced astigmatism resulting from elimination of the suturing step. Although irregular astigmatism rates have been lowered with this improved automated system, the microkeratome cuts are accurate to only ± 5 μm and the cuts are lamellar and not lenticular.

The argon fluoride 193 excimer laser is now being used in investigational studies to perform the refractive cut in in situ myopic keratomileusis via stromal ablation. Laser assisted in situ keratomileusis (LASIK) may be technically superior to conventional automated lamellar keratoplasty because the refractive cut in the stromal bed takes advantage of the excimer laser's greater precision and ability to create a lenticular resection of tissue. It is also thought that the LASIK procedure may be superior to excimer laser photorefractive keratectomy (PRK) in moderate to high degrees of myopia by eliminating the healing changes which occur when Bowman's layer is disrupted. In standard photorefractive keratectomy, this surface-healing process can induce stromal haze or collagen plaque formation, which can have major effects on regression,

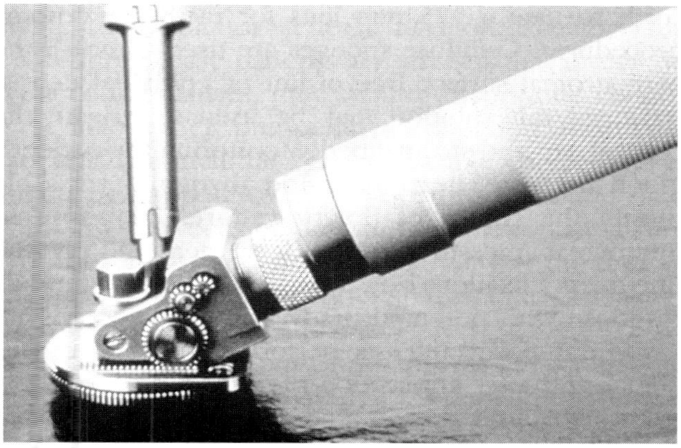

FIGURE 172-3 The automatic corneal shaper consists of gear-driven microkeratome with an electric motor drive attached to the grooved plate of the adjustable suction ring. (Courtesy Chiron Vision, Irvine, California.)

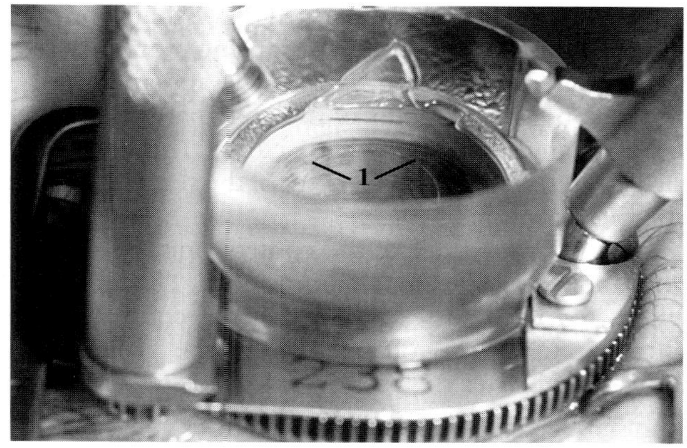

FIGURE 172-4 One of a set of acrylic applanation lenses that have specified diameter circles etched onto the posterior surface *(1)*. These lenses facilitate accurate resection diameter with the microkeratome.

corneal clarity, and rate of recovery of best corrected visual acuity.

The excimer laser with in situ keratomileusis was first reported by Pallikaris[6] and Burrato.[7] In these studies, laser ablation was applied to the undersurface of the resected corneal cap, and the corneal cap was sutured in place following photoablation. Burrato later performed direct excimer laser ablation of the stromal bed after removal of the keratectomy cap.[8]

New developments for future lamellar refractive surgery include intrastromal corneal rings, laser microkeratomes, and microkeratome diamond blades. Lamellar refractive techniques may allow us to avoid the usual wound healing responses that modify and reduce the predictability of refractive surgery results. With second- and third-generation excimer and solid state lasers in evolution, the precision and accuracy of today's keratomileusis procedures will continue to be refined.

Instrumentation

The centerpiece of the automated lamellar keratoplasty technique is the automatic corneal shaper (Figure 172-3). The automatic corneal shaper is a mechanical device that consists of the shaper head, a sharp oscillating blade, motor handle that may be driven by conventional electrical current, and a system of calibrated depth plates. The automated keratome has a reverse feature that allows the surgeon to construct a flap or hinge for the first keratectomy by bringing the keratome head to nearly traverse the cornea, hit a mechanical stop before complete resection of the corneal cap, and then reverse.

The next element of the system is a pneumatic fixation ring that is adjustable in height. This ring provides two separate features. The ring is able to fixate the patient's eye by means of suction created by a suction pump. The goal is to elevate the intraocular pressure to greater than 65 mm Hg using this suction system. This ensures a smooth and accurate lamellar cut. The second feature is a design of the pneumatic fixation ring that allows adjustment of the height of the microkeratome platform. Changing the height of the platform with relation to the cornea will alter the amount of corneal tissue projecting above the platform and thereby allow control of the diameter of the planned resection. The final function of the pneumatic fixation ring is to provide a grooved, geared track for passage of the motor-driven microkeratome across the cornea. The cutting blade reciprocates at 4,000 to 7,000 rpm. The cutting blade can be changed for each case because ultimate accuracy and smoothness of cuts depend on blades being extremely sharp. In the future, the use of a diamond blade instead of the current disposable metal blades may be feasible.

Applanation lenses are used during the procedure to delineate the area of cornea protruding above the suction ring platform. This lens system allows for the desired resection diameter to be set accurately by the surgeon. The applanation lens set is made of plastic, and each lens has a circular optical zone etched onto its applanation surface (Figure 172-4). The convex upper surface of the applanation lens acts as a magnifying glass for evaluation of the applanation. The underside of the lens has two levels, a more peripherally located level that rests on the fixation ring platform and a centrally located concave level that comes into contact with and applanates or flattens the corneal surface. A metal wrench is inserted and engages a gear on the ring, which can then adjust the height of the platform.

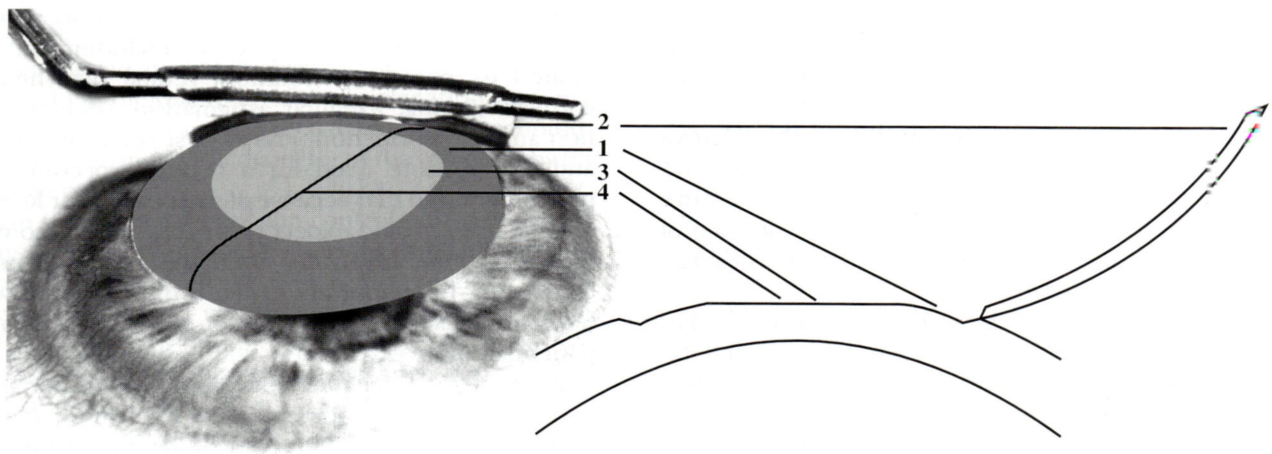

FIGURE 172-5 The microkeratome makes two passes. The first hinged cut is usually 7.2 mm in diameter *(1)* and is folded back *(2)* allowing the second cut of smaller diameter *(3)* to be made in the stromal bed. Removal of this second piece of stromal tissue causes the corneal cap to flatten when it is replaced over the flattened stromal bed *(4)* resulting in a reduction of dioptric refractive power of the cornea.

with the suction ring, we routinely use cardiac monitoring and a pulse oximeter during the procedure. The surgeon and assistants are properly gloved, the patient's eye prepped with povidone-iodine (Betadine), and the skin and lashes covered with a plastic drape. Linen is not recommended for this purpose because of increased chance of shedding fibers onto the operating field and possibly between the cap and stromal bed.

A speculum is inserted to hold the lids open. This is probably the most uncomfortable part of the procedure because the lids are not anesthetized and the palpebral fissure must be opened considerably to admit the adjustable suction ring. In eyes with small palpebral fissures such as those of Asians, a lateral canthotomy or even retrobulbar block may be necessary to achieve adequate lid relaxation. Preliminary experience in Taiwan showed that almost 10% of the cases have to be aborted because of inability to achieve good suction through a small palpebral fissure (personal communication from Hu, Department of Ophthalmology, National Taiwan University, 1994).

Instruments must be checked before initiation of the surgery. One should verify that adequate suction can be generated and that there is no kink or blockage in the suction line. The microkeratome must be inspected for its appropriate assembly and the presence of a depth plate (Figure 172-6). Failure to include a depth plate can cause the most dreaded complication of automated lamellar keratoplasty: perforation into the anterior chamber and damage to the anterior segment. One should make it a strict habit not to engage the microkeratome without a depth plate in position. The blade should be inspected to ensure that it is free of

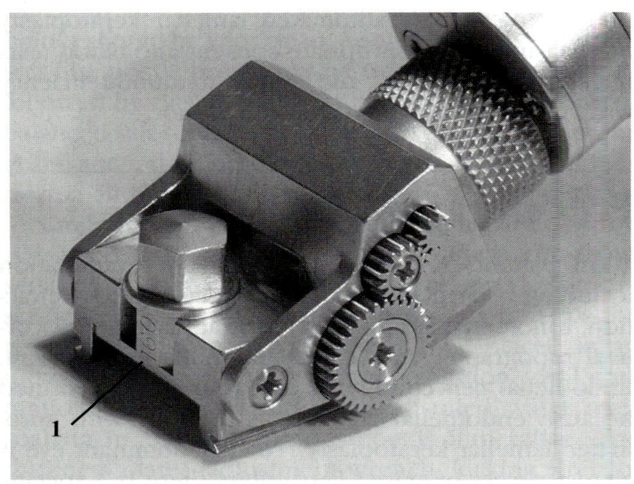

FIGURE 172-6 Close inspection of the assembled microkeratome head before each use is extremely important. The depth plate *(1)* should be properly seated and locked in place.

damage and oscillates smoothly. Finally, the ability of the microkeratome to pass along the suction ring smoothly, forward and backward, must be verified. Any hangup during the procedure increases the likelihood of irregular astigmatism and even permanent scarring in the visual axis.

The central corneal thickness is measured with a pachymeter. The visual axis is lightly marked with an indentation. The centration ring with the pararadial mark, which has been lightly touched with gentian violet, is used to mark the cornea. If the first cut creates a hinged cap, the pararadial line helps realign it

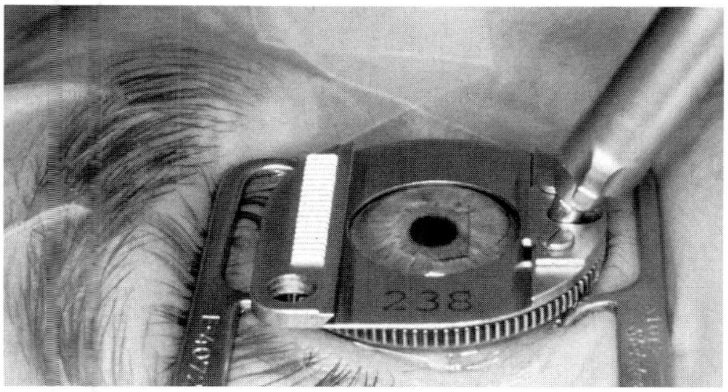

FIGURE 172-7 The suction ring is aligned over the visual axis and suction applied through the handle to raise the intraocular pressure to greater than 65 mm Hg.

properly. If the first resection leads to a completely excised cap, then the marks also ensure that the epithelial side would face up when the cap is replaced. The suction ring is then placed on the globe, using the marks as a guide for centration (Figure 172-7). Centration of the ring is critical; a decentered ring leads to decentered cuts and thus irregular astigmatism. If the ring is not centered satisfactorily, this should be corrected promptly, as prolonged suction leaves a groove on the sclera, making subsequent repositioning difficult.

After the suction is applied, an applanating tonometer is placed on the eye to ensure the intraocular pressure is greater than 65 mm Hg. The appropriate diameter applanation lens is placed on the ring and the wrench used to raise or lower the ring on the eye to achieve the correct diameter cut, which should be 7.2 mm or greater. One recalls that the first cut does not correct the myopia; therefore the diameter need not be exact. A few drops of balanced salt solution are placed to lubricate the corneal surface. The microkeratome is brought into the operating field and engaged onto the suction ring (Figure 172-8). The foot pedal is depressed to advance and then to reverse the microkeratome. In this automated lamellar keratoplasty system, a stop is placed on the microkeratome so that only a partial resection is made. In this case, the hinged flap is simply flipped backward (Figure 172-9). In cases in which a complete resection is made, the cap is placed in a special container and immersed in balanced salt solution for later retrieval.

The stromal bed is dried and the thickness of the cornea measured. The difference between this measurement and the pachymetry reading at the beginning of the case is the thickness of the cap. With the bed dry, a sizing tonometer of the appropriate size, which was predetermined from the nomogram, is placed on the cornea. The wrench is again used to adjust the ring height to the appropriate applanation diameter.

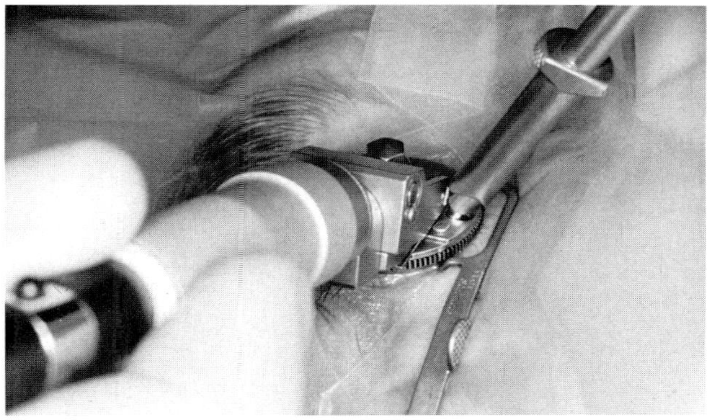

FIGURE 172-8 The microkeratome is engaged into the grooved track of the suction ring before actuating the electric motor, which drives both the forward motion gearing and the oscillating blade.

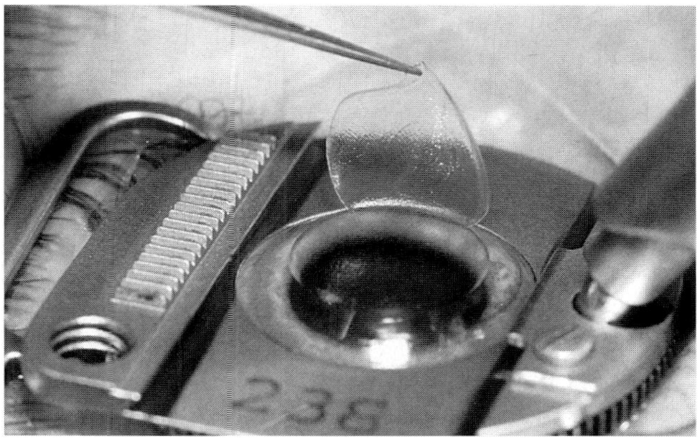

FIGURE 172-9 The microkeratome has been removed, revealing the 160 μm thick first lamellar cut. A small residual hinge of uncut tissue is evident.

The microkeratome, with the new appropriate depth plate for the refractive cut in proper, verified position is brought back to the operating field and the second cut made. Because the stop is still in place, the hinged cap is not resected. The lenticule created with the second cut will be discarded but should be saved until the end of the procedure. The central corneal thickness is measured again to determine the thickness of the lenticule, thus implying whether the desired correction will be achieved. The suction is discontinued and the ring removed, taking care not to damage the hinged cap. The stromal bed and the underside of the cap are lightly irrigated with balanced salt solution. Some surgeons use a sablehair brush to free up any epithelium or debris that might be present. The cap is then gently replaced, using previous marks for alignment (Figure 172-10). A Weck cell sponge is used to remove gently any excess fluid along the edge of the resection to promote adherence of the cap.

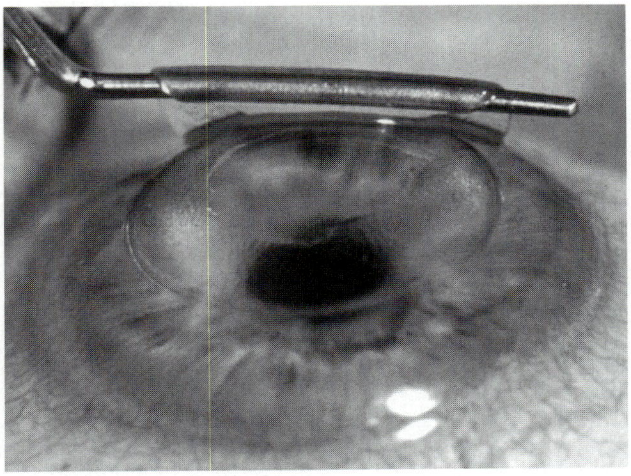

FIGURE 172-10 A spatula is used to replace the corneal cap back into position after the second cut is complete. Note the peripheral pararadial gentian violet mark, which aids in appropriate alignment of the cap.

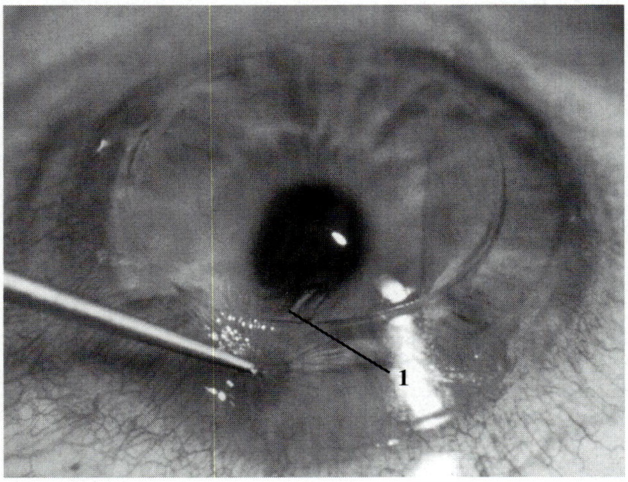

FIGURE 172-11 Stria *(1)* can be seen in the corneal cap adjacent to the area of peripheral indentation with a forceps. These striae indicate that the cap is adherent to the stromal bed and that the lid speculum can be safely removed.

A drop of balanced salt solution is placed in the center of the cornea to moisten the epithelium. At this point, we allow about 2 minutes and then check the adherence of the flap by gently indenting the cornea just beyond the resection to see if the resected flap develops stress stria from the indentation, thus indicating proper adhesion (Figure 172-11). The speculum is then carefully removed. The patient is asked to gently open and close the eye several times to make sure the cap is firmly adherent to the stromal bed. A few drops of topical antibiotic and ketoraloc are instilled and a clear plastic shield taped over the eye for protection. We no longer tape the eye shut or use eye patches. A bandage contact lens is not recommended because it may actually increase the possibility of displacing the cap. We do not use any topical medication until the follow-up examination the next day, when a steroid-antibiotic drop is given.

HYPEROPIC AUTOMATED LAMELLAR KERATOPLASTY

Performing hyperopic automated lamellar keratoplasty is similar to performing myopic automated lamellar keratoplasty, with the exception that only one pass of the microkeratome is made. Therefore the first cut is the refractive cut. The depth is set at about 70% of the total corneal thickness, leaving a much thinner residual stromal bed than the myopic procedure. Therein lies the fundamental concept of the hyperopic procedure; theoretically, it achieves the intended correction via a controlled ectatic effect. The diameter of the resection varies, depending on the amount of intended correction, and it can be determined from a nomogram. The range of correction varies with different manufacturers, but generally falls between −0.5 and +7.0 diopters. We have found that the predictability at the higher levels of hyperopia falls off considerably, and therefore we generally do not perform this procedure for corrections higher than about +5.5 diopters. Instead, we use keratophakia to correct higher hyperopia.

KERATOPHAKIA

With keratophakia, a piece of donor cornea is sandwiched within the stroma to increase the total refractive power of the recipient cornea. Similar to myopic automated lamellar keratoplasty, a cap is created with the keratome at a depth of 160 μm and a diameter of around 8 mm. A donor lenticule is placed on the stromal bed; it is centered over the visual axis and allowed to tightly adhere over 2 to 4 minutes. The flap is repositioned over the lenticule and again allowed to adhere tightly. If necessary, the flap can be gently sutured in place with three to five interrupted sutures to secure the lenticule. These sutures can be removed in 1 week. The diameter of the donor tissue is usually 4.2 mm, although 5.0 mm may be more effective. The lenticule can be carved from a donor globe, but it is more convenient and accurate if it is obtained from the refractive cut of a prior myopic automated lamellar keratoplasty procedure. The required thickness of the lenticule varies with the amount of hyperopic correction intended. A nomogram is not yet available, but in our experience, the dioptric shift achieved on the keratophakia eye is usually equal to or somewhat greater than the myopic resection from the donor eye. As in other procedures that involve donor tissue, appropriate laboratory tests and screening need to be performed. We require HIV and hepatitis B and

Table 172-1. Automatic corneal shaper

Myopic Shaping Calculations
First Cut (Disk) - Plate 160
Disk Diameter 7.0 to 8.0 mm

Diopters (sph. equiv.)	Optical zone (mm) 2nd cut lenticule	Requested resection (microns)	Plate number	Diopters (sph. equiv)	Optical zone (mm) 2nd cut lenticule	Requested resection (microns)	Plate number
2.5	5.0	33	30	16.5	4.0	108	105
3.0	5.0	39	35	17.0	4.0	111	110
3.5	4.7	40	40	17.5	4.0	113	110
4.0	4.5	41	40	18.0	4.0	116	115
4.5	4.5	46	45	18.5	4.0	118	115
5.0	4.2	43	40	19.0	4.0	121	120
5.5	4.2	47	45	19.5	4.0	123	120
6.0	4.2	51	50	20.0	4.0	125	125
6.5	4.2	55	55	20.5	3.7	109	105
7.0	4.2	59	55	21.0	3.7	111	110
7.5	4.2	63	60	21.5	3.7	112	110
8.0	4.2	66	65	22.0	3.7	114	110
8.5	4.2	69	65	22.5	3.7	116	115
9.0	4.2	73	70	23.0	3.7	118	115
9.5	4.2	77	75	23.5	3.7	120	120
10.0	4.2	80	80	24.0	3.7	122	120
10.5	4.2	83	80	24.5	3.7	123	120
11.0	4.2	87	85	25.0	3.7	125	125
11.5	4.2	90	90	25.5	3.7	127	125
12.0	4.2	93	90	26.0	3.7	129	125
12.5	4.2	96	95	26.5	3.7	130	130
13.0	4.2	100	100	27.0	3.7	132	130
13.5	4.2	102	100	27.5	3.7	134	130
14.0	4.2	106	105	28.0	3.5	121	120
14.5	4.2	108	105	28.5	3.5	122	120
15.0	4.2	112	110	29.0	3.5	124	120
15.5	4.2	114	110	29.5	3.5	125	125
16.0	4.2	117	115	30.0	3.5	126	125

The amount of myopia that can be corrected depends upon the thickness and diameter of the second cut resection as can be determined from the surgical nomogram.
If spherical equivalent is >15 diopters, or if corneal thickness is <0.530, use plate 130.

C testing. This testing increases the total cost to the patient.

Postoperative Care

We do not tape the lids closed or patch the eye. If this is done, the tape or patch needs to be removed with great care, making sure that the corneal cap is not dislocated and adherent to the tape or patches. In most cases, uncorrected vision is markedly improved by the next morning; the cornea is clear, the epithelium intact, and the lamellar cut barely visible. At this point, a combination steroid-antibiotic drop such as tobramycin and dexamethasone (Tobradex) is given, four times a day, for 7 days.

In most cases, the refraction stabilizes within a week to a month, but some fluctuation can occur for 3 to 6 months after surgery. This fluctuation may be more pronounced in higher myopic eyes. Topical steroid can be maintained for a longer period of time to retard healing, which tends to cause regression, if a myopic case is undercorrected. Precisely how much effect can be gained with topical steroids has not yet been quantitated.

Surgery can be performed on the second eye once the patient is functional with the first. If an enhancement procedure such as radial or astigmatic keratotomy is needed, it may be performed after the topography and refraction are stable, usually after 3 to 4 months.

Nomograms

MYOPIC AUTOMATED LAMELLAR KERATOPLASTY

Table 172-1 shows an example of the nomogram for myopic keratomileusis in situ. This particular example is used with the Chiron Automatic Corneal Shaper system originally developed by Ruiz. One notices immediately that the nomogram is not age-dependent, in stark contrast to that of radial keratotomy. The refractive results depend solely on the amount of tissue removed in the second cut as described earlier.

The first lamellar cut is set at a constant 160 μm depth in this nomogram for corrections up to 15 diopters. For higher corrections, which requires a deeper second cut, and/or thinner corneas (<0.530 mm), a shallower first cut is selected to leave a thicker stromal bed. We want at least 250 μm of residual stromal thickness after the second cut to avoid the possibility of inducing corneal ectasia. The diameter of the first resection should be at least 7.2 mm or greater.

The nomogram for the second refractive cut has three variables: intended correction, optical zone size (diameter of the resected lenticule), and thickness of intended resection. Smaller optical zone sizes or deeper cuts correct higher myopias; these two variables do not usually change simultaneously from one intended correction to the next. For example, between −5.0 to −16.0 diopters, the most commonly performed range of correction, the diameter of resection stays at 4.2 mm, and the depth increases. At 16.5 diopters, the optical zone decreases to 4.0 mm and the depth drops to 108 μm, less resected thickness than the cut for a 16.0 diopter correction. Notice that the cuts for 16 diopters and 18.5 diopters have similar depth (see Table 172-1), but the optical zone is 0.2 mm smaller for 18.5 diopters. Therefore sizing the refractive cut should be as precise as possible to avoid undercorrection or overcorrection.

The highest intended correction on this nomogram is 30 diopters. At this extreme, the results are not as predictable, and our data indicate a stronger trend toward regression.[9] Longer follow-up and larger patient population are needed to further evaluate this phenomenon.

HYPEROPIC AUTOMATED LAMELLAR KERATOPLASTY

Table 172-2 shows a hyperopia nomogram used with the automatic corneal shaper. Again, age is not a variable. This nomogram has two main features: (1) The disk diameter decreases as the intended correction gets higher, and (2) The depth of the first cut (refractive cut for hyperopic automated lamellar keratoplasty) is increased to generate a greater hyperopic effect.

Results

Recent automated lamellar keratoplasty results obtained by surgeons across the country have been quite good. Published data in the United States is as yet difficult to obtain, since the technique is still relatively new and most data that have been accepted are pending publication. One recent study by Dishler[10] reports an average preoperative myopia of −8.5 diopters, reduced to an average of to −0.94 diopters postoperatively. Sixty-five percent of patients were within 1.5 diopters of emmetropia, and 95% of patients had uncorrected visual acuity of 20/70 or better. Best corrected acuity was 20/30 or better in 95% of cases. A few patients, however, did lose two or more lines of best-corrected visual acuity. None of the patients in this study of 66 cases underwent any additional enhancement procedures such as radial or astigmatic keratotomy. Dishler also found that results in the higher myopes in the study were comparable to results in the lower myopes.

Automated lamellar keratoplasty appears to be a generally safe, effective, and reasonably predictable procedure. The percentage of patients realizing 20/40 or better vision uncorrected certainly does not rival that of radial keratotomy. However, most patients undergoing automated lamellar keratoplasty have such a high degree of refractive error that this outcome would not be realistic. As might be expected, patients with lower degrees of myopia tend to achieve better uncorrected visual acuity and greater predictability of final refraction. Most patients who undergo additional

Table 172-2. Automated lamellar keratoplasty hyperopic nomogram, Kerasys International

Diopters spherical equivalent	Optical zone mm	Calculation of desired cap resection
1.0	6.6	1. Measure apical pachometry
1.5	6.5	2. Multiply the apical pachometry × 0.7
2.0	6.4	3. Thickness plate = apical pachometry × 0.7 rounded to the nearest 0.25 mm plate
2.5	6.3	4. Select the thicker plate if result is exactly halfway between the nearest 0.25 mm plate
3.0	6.2	5. Add plates 425 μm and 0.450 μm to your ALK kit
3.5	6.1	Example: Apical pachometry = 580 μm
4.0	6.0	580 μm × .7 = 406 μm round to plate 400
4.5	5.8	
5.0-6.5	5.6	

The amount of hyperopic correction depends upon the depth of the cut (usually set at 70% of central corneal thickness) and the diameter of resection. The smaller the diameter, the higher the correction achieved.

enhancement surgery for undercorrection or regular astigmatism after automated lamellar keratoplasty will obtain a good visual result.

In a single center, a consecutive series of 174 eyes undergoing automated lamellar keratoplasty, Price and Whitson[9] found that at 6 or more months of follow-up, 75% of eyes achieved uncorrected visual acuity of 20/40 or better. The range of refractions in this group of patients was −5 to −23 diopters for myopes and +1.5 to −5.75 diopters for hyperopes. Because best achievable uncorrected visual acuity was the goal in the majority of these patients, additional enhancement procedures to correct residual myopia or astigmatism were performed in 53% of eyes. Six percent of eyes lost two or more lines of best corrected visual acuity. In this study, 1 to 2 diopters of undercorrection was the goal in most cases. Myopic eyes in the study had an average 5% loss of effect between 1 and 6 months postoperatively. However, the majority of eyes showed stable refraction postoperatively; 69% of hyperopic eyes had 20/40 or better uncorrected vision.

Automated lamellar keratoplasty is a powerful procedure for the correction of extreme degrees of myopia and hyperopia. Results are increasingly more predictable when compared with those realized in the original myopic keratomileusis procedures; however, there is still room for improvement. With continued refinement of the instrumentation and technique and with the advent of LASIK, automated lamellar keratoplasty promises to be a widely accepted technique for treating myopia of moderate to high degrees and hyperopia. Improved instrumentation and techniques should further reduce the complication rate.

Complications

Keratomileusis is a complex procedure. Advancement to automated in situ techniques has greatly reduced its complexity and enhanced its predictability. Nevertheless, a successful automated lamellar keratoplasty procedure consists of many steps, each of which must be performed accurately and precisely. There are delicate instruments made up of precision parts, which must be handled correctly and maintained rigorously. Before performing the first case, the surgeon should be thoroughly familiar with the instrumentation, the surgical steps, and the best ways to handle a complication.

We believe that automated lamellar keratoplasty should not be the surgeon's first experience with refractive procedures, not only because of its complexity, but also because patients may need future enhancement procedures such as radial keratotomy. There is a definite learning curve. Therefore we highly recommend taking a certifying course followed by multiple practice sessions on eye bank eyes or animal eyes before operating on a patient. Even in skilled hands, the procedure may lead to complications that cannot always be avoided. It is helpful to have access to a surgeon familiar with complicated anterior segment problems.

The best way to deal with complications is prevention. Before surgery, thorough examinations allow the surgeon to exclude those with contraindicated conditions such as keratoconus. Accurate manifest and cycloplegic refractions lower the incidence of undercorrection or overcorrection. Meticulous preparation, inspection, and testing of the instruments minimize intraoperative difficulties caused by equipment failure.

As with any surgery, many problems can occur during or after the automated lamellar keratoplasty. We briefly discuss some of the most common difficulties one may encounter intraoperatively and postoperatively.

INTRAOPERATIVE COMPLICATIONS

Inadequate suction/intraocular pressure

The suction ring serves two major purposes: it provides a stable platform for the microkeratome and it hardens the globe. If the globe is too soft, the blade cannot engage properly, resulting in an irregular cut. When suction is inadequate, immediately inspect the speculum, drape, and lashes to ensure they are not in the way. The suction line should be checked to ensure it is free of kinks or leaks. Chemotic or redundant conjunctiva may obstruct the suction port on the ring, especially if a retrobulbar block is given. In this situation, a smooth surfaced instrument can be used to milk away the subconjunctival fluid. In rare cases, a 360 degree peritomy followed by hemostasis may be needed to allow the ring direct contact with the sclera. Pressing on the globe or injecting retrobulbar fluid can increase the intraocular pressure to the required level. However, we do not recommend these methods because neither can be well controlled. It is best to abort the case if adequate suction or intraocular pressure cannot be achieved and the cause is not clear.

Thusfar there has been no report of retinal vascular conditions caused by the high intraocular pressure required in this procedure. This possibility is still a concern, however, especially in patients with systemic diseases known to compromise the circulation. Whenever a problem arises during the procedure that cannot be resolved quickly, the suction should be discontinued until the problem is solved.

Epithelial defects

If large corneal epithelial defects are noted before the first pass is made, the case should be rescheduled.

An irregular surface would cause the microkeratome to cut unevenly. If the epithelium sloughs off the cap after the first resection is made, the case can be completed. In this scenario, the cap should probably be sutured in place because epithelial integrity is crucial for the cap to adhere to the stromal bed. Without the epithelial barrier, fluid can seep into the interface and displace the flap.

No depth plate

Passing the microkeratome without a depth plate can create a full-thickness incision with dramatic entry into the anterior chamber in an eye pressurized to more than 65 mm Hg. Severe damage to the iris and lens most likely would ensue. This most dreaded complication is entirely avoidable. The importance of never engaging the microkeratome without checking the presence of a correctly positioned depth plate cannot be overemphasized.

Shaper head jams

If the keratome jams before completing the first pass, the procedure should be stopped and the keratome backed out slightly by reversing the foot pedal. The angle at which the motor unit is held must be appropriate to prevent binding. Care should be taken not to damage the cap resting on top of the blade. A forward cut should then be possible. If the unit still jams, the surgeon should back out entirely, reposition the partially resected cap, and abort the case. One should allow several weeks for the cornea to heal before returning to the operating room to proceed as if performing a first-time case.

Decentered or irregular cuts

Decentered or irregular cuts are made as a result of decentration of the suction ring or sudden eye or lid movements during the first pass. The surgeon should hold the instruments in a relaxed manner to avoid inadvertently torquing either the suction ring or the microkeratome.

If the irregularity or decentration occurs on the first cut, the case should be stopped and the flap repositioned properly and allowed to heal, as described earlier. If decentration happens on the second cut in a myopic case, it is important not to discard the lenticule. Doing so would result in healing on an irregular stromal bed and would induce irregular astigmatism. Instead, the surgeon should replace the second lenticule properly, wait a few minutes for it to adhere, and replace the cap. The cornea should be allowed to heal for several months and the procedure can be repeated with relative safety.

If the edge of an irregular first resection comes close to the visual axis, scarring may decrease vision permanently. A superficial keratectomy, excimer laser phototherapeutic keratectomy or a penetrating keratoplasty may be needed to restore vision.

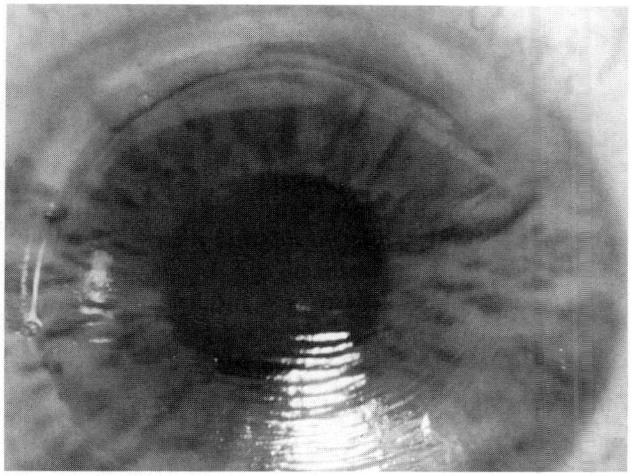

FIGURE 172-12 Poor adherence of the corneal cap has caused a partial displacement resulting in numerous anterior folds and irregular astigmatism. The cap was subsequently lifted, repositioned, and allowed to adhere appropriately.

Cuts at undesired depth

In a myopic case, the exact depth of the first resection is usually not problematic as long as there is enough residual depth for the second cut. If the cap is too shallow, it should be allowed to heal and the procedure attempted at a later date.

If the second cut (refractive cut) is too shallow, one can make up the difference with a third cut of appropriate residual thickness. If the second cut is too deep, the lenticule should be set aside; a third cut should be made at the desired depth for the original intended correction and the first lenticule replaced on the stromal bed and allowed to adhere before replacing the cap. When contemplating the need for additional or alternate lenticule resections, it is important to leave at least 250 μm of residual deep stroma to avoid the possibility of an inadvertent hyperopic automated lamellar keratoplasty response.

In a hyperopic case, a shallower resection results in undercorrection, which is undesirable because residual hyperopia is difficult to correct. One can repeat the procedure later with a deeper resection. However, the original cap may dehisce, leaving a free cap and a deeper hinged layer. It is quite a challenge to suture these together like a sandwich. On the other hand, the patient can sometimes be happy with diminished but residual hyperopia of 1 to 2 diopters. The glasses are thinner and lighter, and a bifocal may not always be needed. Overcorrecting a hyperopic patient is more desirable because the ensuing myopia can be corrected with radial keratotomy.

POSTOPERATIVE COMPLICATIONS

Dislocated cap

Partial (Figure 172-12) or complete dislocation of the lamellar cap can occur. A free, unhinged cap can be lost. This complication is certainly not desirable, but it may not always be disastrous. In a myopic case, the cornea should be allowed to reepithelialize and heal. The results can be satisfactory because this "capless automated lamellar keratoplasty" may create a situation similar to photorefractive keratectomy with the excimer laser. If inadequate vision results, an autologous lamellar keratoplasty is required. Purposeful creation of a capless automated lamellar keratoplasty is not advised.

A lost hyperopic cap will necessitate a lamellar corneal graft to preserve corneal integrity. If the dislocated cap is found either in the conjunctival sac or on the tape, it should be soaked in antibiotic solution and the stromal surfaces meticulously cleaned before being sutured in place.

Dislocation, a rare event, occurs more frequently after hyperopic automated lamellar keratoplasty and keratophakia procedures than with myopic automated lamellar keratoplasty. We use sutures to secure the dislocated cap in these cases. The sutures can be safely removed after 1 week. If dislocation occurs after a myopic procedure, we recommend irrigating and cleansing the stromal bed and the underside of the corneal cap before replacing it. One can simply allow the cap to adhere as with a standard procedure or secure the cap with sutures. We prefer interrupted sutures, but a number of antitorque suture techniques also work well. Regardless of the chosen technique, the cornea should be free of tension lines at completion.

Epithelial growth in the interface

A small amount of epithelium within 1 mm of the edge of the flap usually does not cause any problem (Figure 172-13). More centrally located epithelium can result in irregular astigmatism. Rarely, an entire sheet of epithelium can grow under the cap. It can cause necrosis of the overlying stroma or cap dislocation. Nd:YAG laser has been used successfully to treat small patches of centrally located epithelium, but can leave opacified spots in the stroma. Larger epithelial patches need to be removed. A preferred technique is to raise the flap and mechanically scrub and irrigate the bed. Irrigation alone does not work reliably.

Overcorrection and undercorrection

As mentioned earlier, the predictability of automated lamellar keratoplasty is reasonably good, but as with all refractive procedures, it is not 100% successful. Therefore it is always better to err on the myopic side (i.e., undercorrection for myopia and overcorrection for hyperopia). We generally aim for a postoperative refraction of -1.00 diopter. Enhancement with radial keratotomy can be performed safely after about 3 months. It is important to measure pachymetry at each of the keratotomy sites and to adjust the blade accordingly because corneal thickness can vary considerably after automated lamellar keratoplasty. A nomogram is not yet available for radial keratotomy after automated lamellar keratoplasty. We use the optical zone that would have corrected one third less than the intended correction on a virgin cornea.

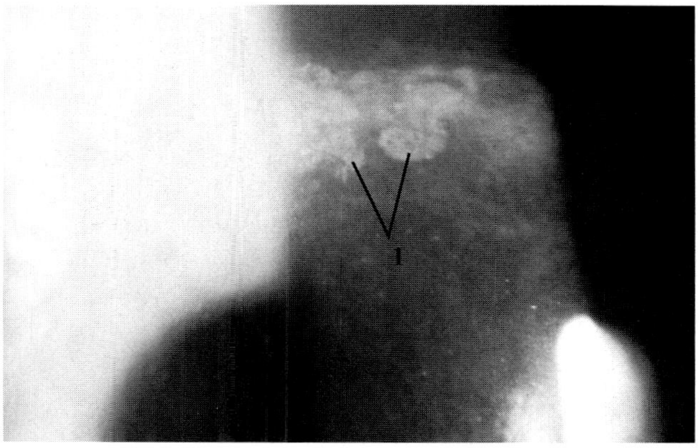

FIGURE 172-13 Whitish, opalescent debris in the peripheral interface represents sequestered nests of epithelial cells *(1)*. If these are more centrally located, they can result in visual disturbance from the opacity itself or from induced anterior corneal curvature changes.

Astigmatism

The astigmatic effect of automated lamellar keratoplasty is unpredictable. Using vector analysis, we have studied surgically induced astigmatism after this procedure. Our findings indicate that automated lamellar keratoplasty neither induces nor corrects astigmatism systematically. On the other hand, astigmatism, both in cylindrical value and axis, can change unpredictably in a significant number of patients (unpublished data). Small to moderate amounts of astigmatism are correctable with an astigmatic keratotomy. If an excessive amount of induced astigmatism is noted postoperatively, one should examine the site of the flat axis carefully for epithelial growth under the cap, which, if present, should be removed.

Irregular astigmatism is the most important cause of decreased visual acuity after automated lamellar keratoplasty (Figure 172-14). The incidence of irregular astigmatism is much smaller than what was seen in association with cryolathing keratomileusis. Frequently, the use of ocular lubricating drops and a

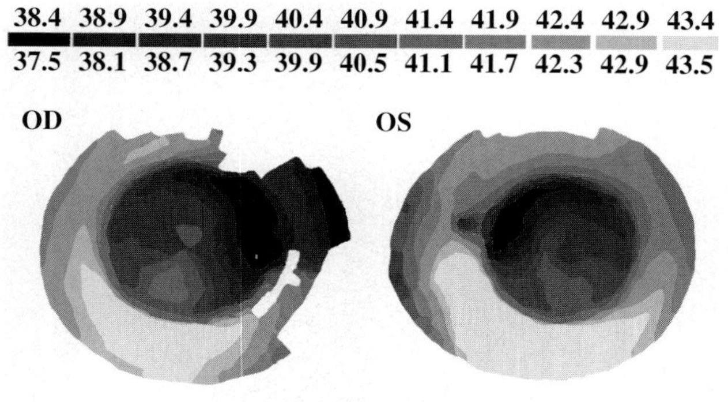

FIGURE 172-14 Topography of bilateral automated lamellar keratoplasty. Flattening in the central corneal is obvious. Variability of the topography in this area indicates subtle irregular astigmatism, which can result in some degree of visual degradation. **See color plate 172-14.**

wait-and-see approach will allow a reduction in irregular astigmatism over time. In some cases, the cap can be lifted and repositioned. Rigid contact lens may be needed in severe cases. An appropriately placed single T-cut can sometimes correct mild asymmetric astigmatism.

Enhancement

Overcorrections in myopic automated lamellar keratoplasty are quite uncommon, but can be treated with hyperopic automated lamellar keratoplasty or keratophakia, depending on the degree of overcorrection. Patients with significant residual myopia after myopic automated lamellar keratoplasty may be treated either with a repeat procedure, radial keratotomy, or excimer laser. Enhancement procedures should be delayed for 3 months after the original procedure.

For patients who are significantly undercorrected, a second myopic automated lamellar keratoplasty may be repeated within 1 or 2 weeks of the first procedure by lifting the cap and carefully positioning the suction ring to superimpose the new refractive cut over the initial second cut.

In our practice, for radial keratotomy correction of residual myopia following automated lamellar keratoplasty, we use the Casebeer or Arrowsmith radial keratotomy nomograms. A helpful modification is the use of larger optical zones for enhancement. In situations where a similar myopic correction may be achieved with an 8-cut rather than a 4-cut radial keratotomy, the 8-cut procedure is generally selected because of a larger optical zone. The larger optical zone seems to decrease potential problems with glare, halos, and night vision. We find that eyes that have had automated lamellar keratoplasty tend to respond more than predicted by the nomogram. Therefore, we aim to correct about one third less myopia than is present.

The surgical technique for radial keratotomy enhancement following myopic automated lamellar keratoplasty is similar to a standard radial keratotomy procedure. A DuoTrak knife is used, with the incision initiated at the optical zone mark and cut in a centrifugal fashion and then reversed back toward the optical zone. Incision length depends on the degree of correction required, but they are generally stopped 1.5 to 2 mm inside the limbus. Blade depth is set at 100% of the lowest paracentral pachymetry reading. Pachymetry is performed at 8 spots 1.5 mm from the corneal center. For correction of residual regular astigmatism, the ARC-T nomograms and incisions are preferred. We place the cuts at or just outside the first cap resection diameter (generally 7.2 mm).

Comparison with Other Refractive Surgery Procedures

Currently, surgical management of moderate to high degrees of myopia include (1) automated lamellar keratoplasty, (2) excimer laser PRK, (3) LASIK, (4) clear lens extraction and implantation of low power posterior chamber intraocular lens, and (5) radial keratotomy.

In terms of surgical management of low to moderate degrees of myopia, radial keratotomy has stood the test of time in terms of predictability, low complication rate, and widespread acceptance of the procedure by ophthalmic surgeons. The results of the recently published 10-year PERK study[11] showed that at 10 years, 53% of eyes obtained an uncorrected visual acuity of 20/20 or better, and 85% were 20/40 or better uncorrected. There was a 3% two- to three-line loss of best corrected visual acuity in this study. However, predictability was shown to be much better for lower levels of myopia as compared to higher levels. The incidence of regression, hyperopic shift, and other visual side effects such as ghost images and halos was greatest in the higher degrees of myopia. It appears therefore that as a means of correcting higher degrees of myopia, radial keratotomy demonstrates inferior accuracy and predictability when compared to automated lamellar keratoplasty.

In a recent study by Williams,[12] LASIK was compared directly with excimer laser PRK for severe myopia. Refractive errors ranged from −12 to −19.5 diopters in this group of patients. The study looked at 12 eyes from six extremely myopic patients. Patients had one eye treated with LASIK and the other eye with PRK. Results were similar between the two groups. Myopia was reduced an average of 66.7% by either procedure. Regression was similar between the two groups. However, in the PRK group there was a higher rate of postoperative corneal haze. In fact, none of the PRK corneas were entirely haze free throughout the postoperative follow-up period of 12 months. This study was in contrast to a similar study comparing PRK with LASIK reported by Pallikaris.[13] In that study, visual results were clearly superior with the LASIK procedure than with PRK. Both of these studies showed that persistent corneal haze was a feature of the PRK treatment. As yet, no prospective studies have directly compared automated lamellar keratoplasty with either PRK or LASIK.

Colin[14] reported the use of low-power intraocular lens implants and clear lens extractions for high myopes. He reported good visual results and predictability with few complications. This approach has not yet been widely embraced because of potentially more severe complications with an intraocular versus surface procedure. Durrie and Mack[15] reported results of the intrastromal corneal ring study group (ISCRS), which has found this procedure useful for correction of lower degrees of myopia; however, predictability and accuracy have thusfar been unsatisfactory.

A singular advantage of automated lamellar keratoplasty, at least at the present time, is the ability to correct both myopia and hyperopia with good results. Excimer laser may eventually be able to treat myopia, hyperopia, and astigmatism. At this time, laser treatment of astigmatism and hyperopia is being refined.

REFERENCES

1. Barraquer JI: Keratomileusis, *Int Surg,* 48:103-117, 1967.
2. Troutman RC, Swinger CA: Refractive keratoplasty: keratophakia and keratomileusis, *Trans Am Ophthalmol Soc* 76-329, 1978.
3. Werblin TP et al: Epikeratophakia—the surgical correction of aphakia: update 1981, *Ophthalmology* 89:916, 1982.
4. Krumeich JH, Swinger JA, Boyd B: The planar non-freeze lamellar refractive keratoplasty techniques. Non-freeze keratomileusis, non-freeze epikeratophakia. Edition of refractive surgery with the masters, *Highlights of ophthalmology* Coral Gables, Florida, 1987.
5. Bas AM, Nano HD: In situ myopic keratomileusis results in 30 eyes at 15 months, *Refract Corneal Surg* 7:223-231, 1991.
6. Pallikaris I: Laser in situ keratomileusis, *Lasers Surg Med* 10:463-468, 1994.
7. Buratto L: Excimer laser intrastromal keratomileusis: case reports, *J Cataract Refract Surg* 18:37-41, 1992.
8. Buratto L: Myopic keratomileusis with the excimer laser: one-year follow up, *Refract Corneal Surg* 9:12-19, 1993.
9. Price FW, Whitson WE: Automated lamellar keratomileusis in situ for myopia, *J Refract Surg* 12(1):29-35, 1996. (accepted for publication pending revision)
10. Dishler J: *Ocular Surgery News* 12:59,69, 1994.
11. Waring G, PERK Study Group: Results of the Prospective Evaluation of Radial Keratotomy (PERK) study 10 years after surgery, *Arch Ophthalmol* 112:1298-1308, 1994.
12. Williams J: *Ocular Surgery News* 12:52,71, 1994.
13. Pallikaris I: Excimer laser in-situ keratomileusis and photorefractive keratectomy for correction of high myopia, *Refract Corneal Surg* 10:498-510, 1994.
14. Colin J et al: The surgical treatment of high myopia: comparison of epikeratoplasty, keratomileusis and minus power anterior chamber lenses, *Refract Corneal Surg* 6:245-251, 1990.
15. Durrie DS, Mack R: Update on corneal rings, *Review of Ophthalmology* 1:80, 1994.

SECTION SIX *Laser Corneal Surgery*

CHAPTER 173

DANIEL S. DURRIE ROBERT J.S. MACK

Laser Refractive Keratoplasty: Instrumentation and Techniques

Instrumentation

This chapter attempts to simplify the complex technical aspects of laser photorefractive keratoplasty (PRK) and emphasize the importance of precise surgical technique in the performance of these procedures. Technical features of the various lasers currently manufactured are discussed, and the relevant surgical techniques are reviewed.

EFFECT OF THE LASER ON CORNEAL TISSUE

Interaction of the laser with corneal tissue

The argon fluoride excimer laser produces photochemical ablation of corneal tissue as opposed to thermal decomposition, which occurs with the absorption of other laser light.[1] The covalent intramolecular bonds of certain polymers and organic macromolecules are broken upon absorption of high energy photons of 193 nm light. The resultant fragments expand rapidly into a much larger volume and leave the surface at high velocities. Because thermal decomposition of tissue does not occur, the borders of the ablated tissue are well defined and correspond exactly to the pattern of light exposure.[2] Clinically important aspects of the beam include fluency, or laser energy density; frequency of the ablation pulses; beam size; and beam homogeneity. The various internationally available excimer lasers operate with the same argon fluoride gas and wavelength of 193 nm, but vary in many of the other parameters. These include beam shaping, homogenization, and alignment, as well as fluency, pulse rate, spot size, and transition zone from one area to another. The smoothness and uniformity of the beam ablation depend greatly on the homogeneity of the beam profile. This smoothness is thought to account for the clinical observation that the treated cornea can function quite well without Bowman's layer. Ensuring the homogeneity of the beam profile is the responsibility of the surgeon. This homogeneity should be rechecked frequently between treatments, because it may vary considerably. Similarly, alignment of the excimer beam must be verified with great regularity.

Maintenance of the excimer laser is expensive and can involve potential safety hazards. Most internationally available excimer lasers cost approximately $20,000 to $40,000 a year to maintain, which may or may not include a continual series of upgrades in both hardware and software. All involve some quantity of fluorine gas, which is highly toxic and may require special ventilation capabilities in the surgical suite.

The natural profile of the excimer laser beam leaving the cavity is rectangular with a gaussian distribution of laser intensity along one axis. In addition, focal areas within the beam of higher intensity can lead to uneven tissue ablation. Therefore several strategies for improving beam homogeneity have been attempted, including rotating prisms, slit beams, and absorbing cell systems.[3-7] The concave curvature of a myopic ablation pattern can be projected sequentially onto the cornea using (1) a mechanical iris aperture that opens during the procedure, thus ablating more centrally than peripherally, (2) several different circular apertures,[6,8] or (3) an ablatable mask.

A nonrefractive zone of transition between untreated cornea and treated cornea is created by some lasers to avoid a steep interface between these two areas. An ablatable mask of polymethylmethacrylate (PMMA) in the beam path has been used to transfer a new spherical or toric curvature to the cornea for the correction of myopia with astigmatism. This technology may prove promising as the algorithm develops in the future.

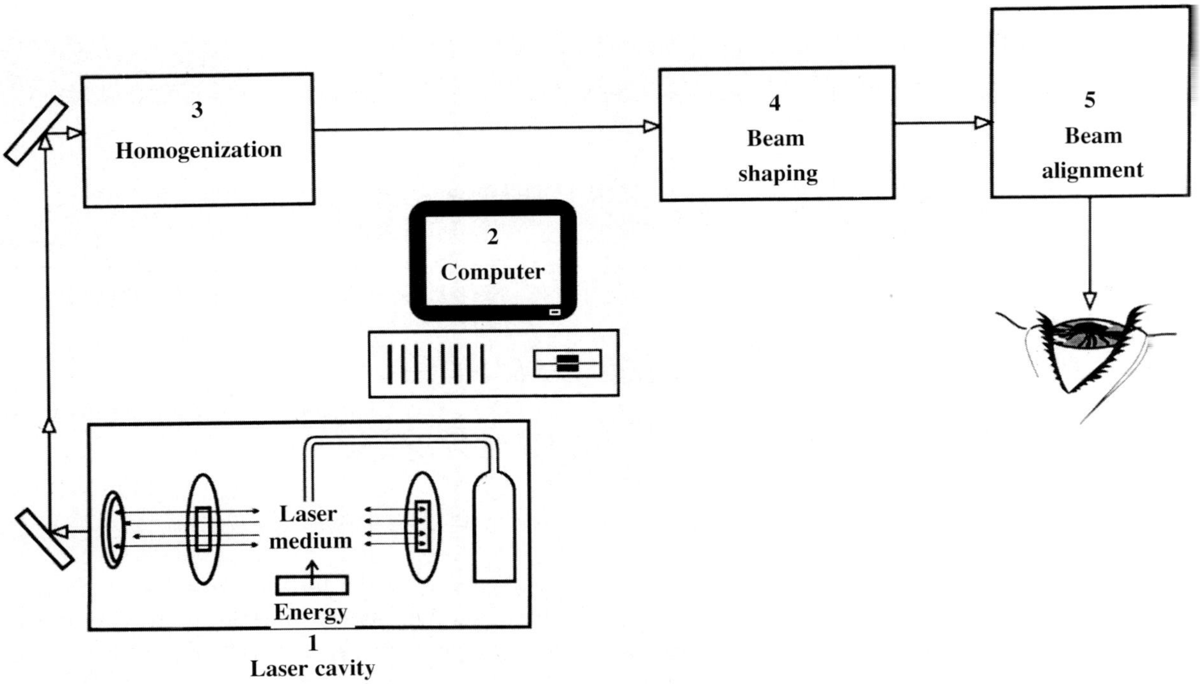

FIGURE 173-1 The five basic components of excimer lasers.

GENERAL FEATURES OF EXCIMER LASERS

Although excimer laser manufacturers emphasize the differences in the various components of each machine, each excimer laser is composed of the following five basic components (Figures 173-1 and 173-2).

Beam generation system

This system is a laser cavity that produces 193 nm wavelength light from the argon flouride gas. The light has a certain fluency, or laser energy density, when it leaves the tubes, which is then significantly reduced in some systems by the time the beam reaches the eye. The laser cavity may be made by the company selling the excimer laser system or purchased from another vendor. According to some manufacturers, the qualities of the laser tube itself can affect beam characteristics.

Beam control system

The beam control system is a computer that coordinates the various portions of the laser depicted in Figure 173-1. The computer provides a means to increase the power through the laser cavity as gases degrade in order to maintain a constant fluency of the beam. The computer also controls the repetition rate of the laser pulses and the treatment diameter in most systems. The computer controls the edge profile and other beam parameters such as multizone/multipass software and programs for astigmatism and phototherapeutic keratectomy (PTK).

Beam clean-up system

In general the excimer laser beam as produced by the laser cavity is nonhomogeneous and may have "hot spots" in the beam profile. Various systems exist for homogenizing the beam, such as prismatic spatial integrators or rotating prisms. Some manufacturers try to compensate for a nonhomogeneous excimer laser beam by projecting through a scanning slit, creating homogeneous ablation on the cornea, with no single area being consistently ablated more than surrounding tissue. Therefore, scanning systems tend not to include beam homogenizers. This may be advantageous because each optical element in the path of the beam degrades the energy density of the beam along the way.

Beam shaping system

The precise shape of the beam as it strikes the eye is controlled in various ways by the different laser manufacturers. There is commonly an optical diaphragm, which opens and closes in several possible patterns under computer control throughout the treatment. Other technologies such as the erodible mask and the fractile mask selectively block the excimer laser beam from certain areas of the cornea. As the mask ablates, the inverse contour of the mask is transferred to the cornea. Some lasers have scanning systems and progressively opening slits that move the beam back and forth across the cornea selectively to attain a certain contour. A laser's capacity to treat astigmatism or hyperopia is also determined by its beam shaping system.

A B C D E F G H

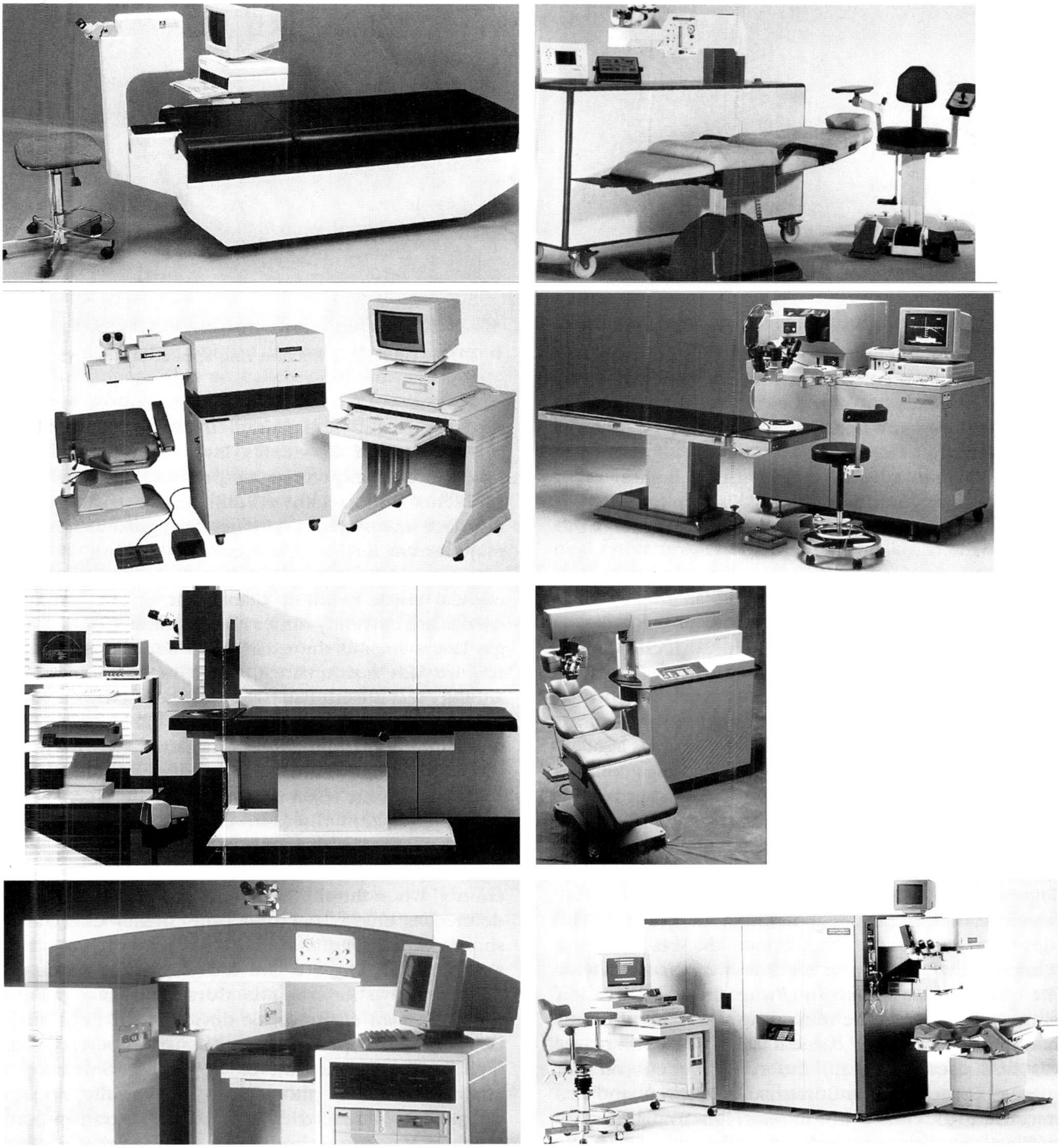

FIGURE 173-2 Excimer lasers manufactured by Autonomous **(A)**, Asculap-Meditec **(B)**, Lasersight **(C)**, Nidek **(D)**, Schwind **(E)**, Summit **(F)**, Technolas **(G)**, and Visx **(H)**.

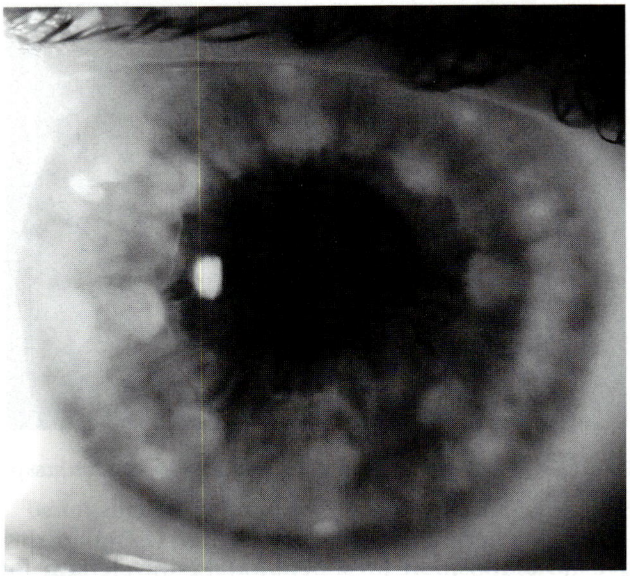

FIGURE 173-6 Holmium laser thermal keratoplasty immediately after surgery.

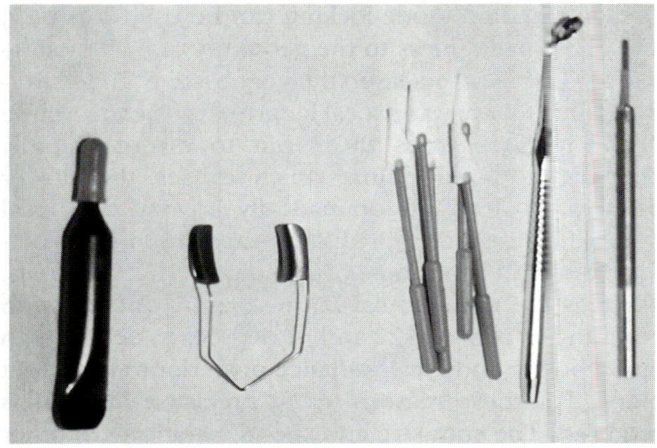

FIGURE 173-7 PRK equipment.

fixed configuration is used in the Sunrise Technology's Ho:YAG LTK device. This laser operates at a wavelength of 2.13 μm, has a 250 μsec pulse duration and a 5 Hz pulse repetition frequency.[13]

An ablatable mask of PMMA in the beam path has been used to transfer a new spherical or toric curvature to the cornea for the correction of myopia with astigmatism. In a study of 10 eyes of 10 patients with up to 6.00 diopters of spherical myopia and 2.75 diopters of astigmatism showed that 44% of these eyes improved by more than 0.5 diopter of cylindrical correction.[14] As noted above, this may prove to be a promising technology with correction of the algorithm in the future.

Surgical Technique

PREPARATION FOR SURGERY

The excimer laser is a complex device, and because the surgical procedure is dependent on a properly functioning laser, it is important to designate one individual as the laser technician. The laser technician should check the key laser parameters and make any necessary adjustments early in the morning on the day of surgery. It is valuable to be sure that the laser technician understands under what circumstances surgery should be cancelled. It is certainly better to inform patients before they leave home for the laser center that the surgery is either cancelled or delayed than to have them find this out once they have arrived. If a LASIK (laser assisted in situ keratomileusis) is to be performed, microkeratome equipment must be assembled and tested.

It is important to explain the procedure thoroughly to the patient before surgery. Explanation should include a basic description of the laser, photoablation, and the role of the patient in this surgical procedure. In general, the patient's job during surgery is to relax and look at the fixation light. The patient should be told that the light will blur during the procedure and that he or she should continue to maintain the same gaze because looking for a position where the light is clear again could decenter the ablation. Moreover, the patient should be told that a lid speculum and topical anesthesia are used. Also, it is important to explain what the surgeon will be doing during the procedure and the overall length of time of the individual steps. One should explain the medications that will be used preoperatively, intraoperatively, and postoperatively. It is also important to ask about allergies and other related medical conditions. Overall, the most important step is to reassure the patient so that he or she may be as relaxed as possible during the procedure. Sedation is rarely needed because patient fixation is better without it when good preoperative education has taken place.

The informed consent should be obtained by the surgeon. It should include a description of the goals of the procedure, as well as the potential risks, complications, and alternatives. As with all surgical procedures, all of the required forms must be properly filled out and reviewed before drops are given.

Patients have usually chosen excimer laser because of the precision that can be obtained with this computer-controlled device. Therefore it is important that the overall preoperative process be well organized. Poorly organized patient and paper flow during the preoperative period adds to apprehension and erodes confidence.

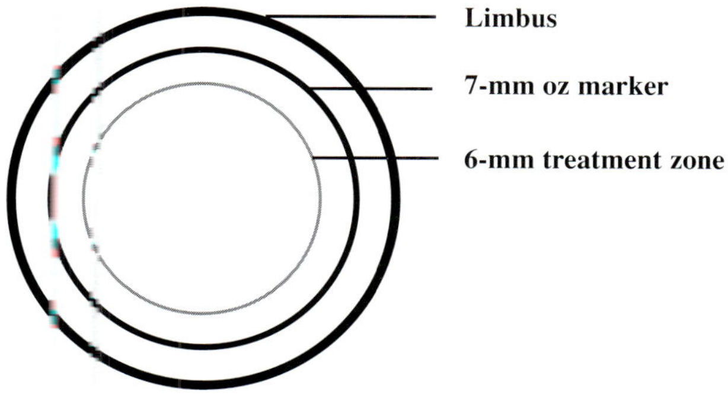

FIGURE 173-8 PRK epithelial debridement zones.

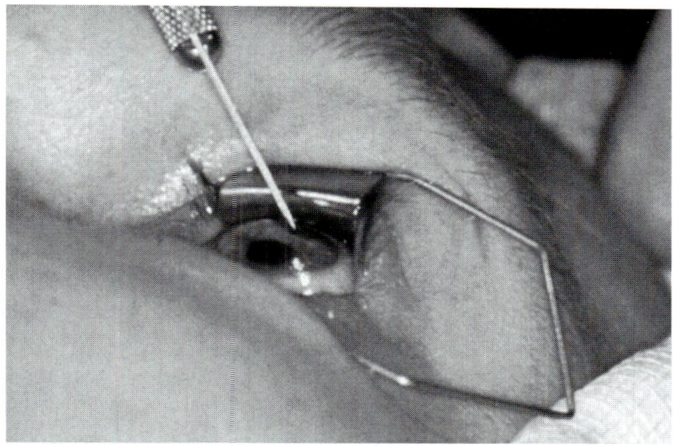

FIGURE 173-9 The 45-degree angle position for debridement. Debridement is performed in a "doughnut" shape, leaving removal of the central epithelium for last.

Topical anesthetics, topical antibiotics, and miotic agents are applied to the eye. Excessive anesthetic drops may be toxic to the epithelium and should be avoided. Nonsteroidal antiinflammatory drugs are sometimes applied preoperatively.

The handheld instruments required for excimer laser ablation are minimal (Figure 173-7) and should be well organized and available to the surgeon. These should include a sterile lid speculum, corneal markers, a spatula or blade for epithelial removal, and cellulose sponges.

PHOTOREFRACTIVE KERATECTOMY

In PRK, patient training is essential. One should describe to the patient the fixation system that is used, and he or she should be comfortably positioned under the operating microscope. It is usually valuable to fire a few pulses of the laser onto the patient's corneal epithelium to acquaint the patient with the sights, sounds, and odor of the laser as it ablates. Care should be taken not to fully ablate the epithelium and possibly damage the underlying stroma. Excessive ablation of epithelium also can make subsequent epithelial debridement difficult. It is beneficial to talk to the patient in a reassuring voice during the training period to relax the patient as much as possible. Long periods of silence are unnerving to the patient in this setting.

The next step is epithelial removal. It is important to control hydration during this step. Once epithelial removal is started, no further topical drops should be applied, and the epithelium should be removed quickly in a standard fashion. The area from which epithelium is to be removed should be marked with a marker that is at least 1 mm larger than the intended ablation diameter (Figure 173-8). A Paton or similar spatula or a sharper rounded blade, such as a 64 Beaver blade can be used to remove epithelium. The sharp cutting edge should be avoided, and the blade should be kept at a 45 degree angle to the surface and moved in only one direction (Figure 173-9). A peripheral "doughnut" of epithelium should be removed around the edges first, leaving the central epithelium intact. The laser should be armed and ready during this period before the central epithelium is removed. The surface must be cleaned thoroughly to remove any loose epithelium and prepare the surface for ablation. After all the epithelium is removed and the surface is cleaned with a dry cellulose sponge, the laser ablation procedure should proceed as quickly as possible.

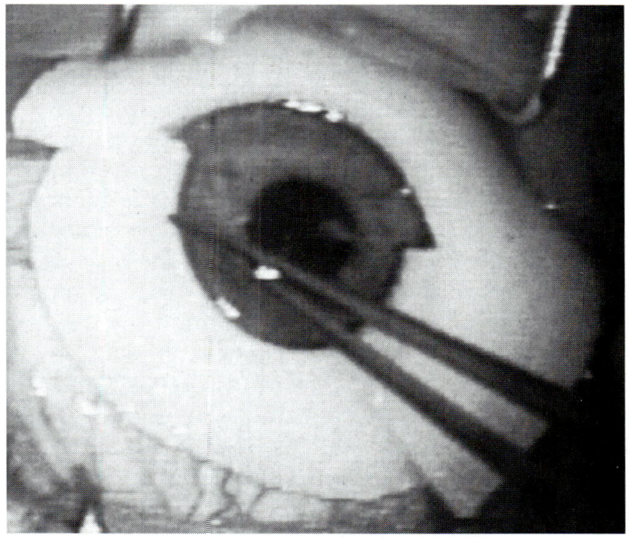

FIGURE 173-10 Instrument sponge saturated with tetracaine.

If a LASIK procedure is to be performed, both the cornea and the limbus must be anesthetized (Figure 173-10). A circular 14-mm sponge can be soaked in anesthetic and laid on the limbus to help anesthetize this area. The pupil center is marked with a blunt hook, and the optical zone and custom pararadial marks are applied. There must be good exposure, for which a

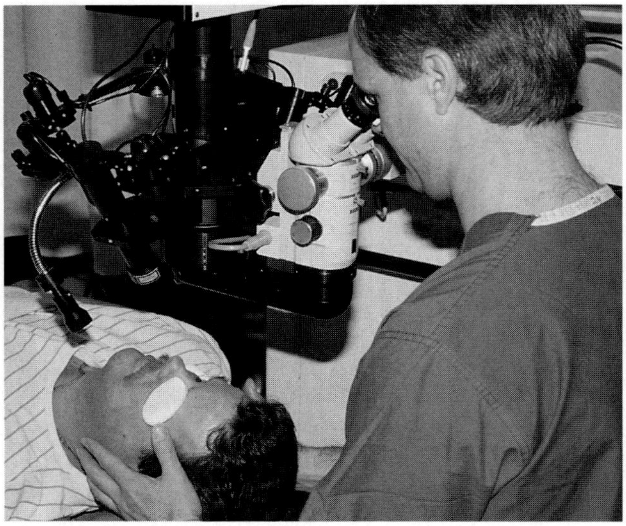

FIGURE 173-11 The surgeon's hands are positioned on the sides of the patient's head during PRK treatment.

lateral canthotomy is occasionally required. The microkeratome suction ring is then applied to the eye and applanation tension is checked. The intraocular pressure should be greater than 60 mm Hg to obtain an accurate microkeratome section. A 160 μm plate is used in most LASIK procedures, and the position and security of the plate must be checked. The resection is then performed, leaving a small hinge of tissue nasally, and the microkeratome is backed off. The patient is then positioned under the excimer laser, and the flap of tissue is carefully lifted with a forceps. The time between lifting the flap and the start of the ablation should be standardized. Because it usually takes approximately 10 seconds to align the laser, it is a good idea to leave a little extra time (such as 15 seconds) from the time the flap is elevated to the time of the ablation. This technique can help control hydration.

The laser procedure is then performed by careful realignment of the laser to the optical axis, and the laser firing is started. During the firing of the laser, the role of the surgeon is to hold the patient's head to monitor carefully that the laser starts and stays in the proper position and to press the pedal. Even though the laser is doing most of the work, there are saccades and fine movements caused by breathing and contraction of the patient's neck and head muscles, so one hand must be kept on the patient's head to keep the patient in position while the surgeon concentrates on the alignment of the laser beams with the cornea. This approach reassures the patient and ensures that the total ablation is delivered in the proper place (Figure 173-11). If there is significant movement during the procedure, the ablation should be stopped immediately. Excimer lasers have built-in memory of where the procedure is stopped, so that by repositioning and realigning the patient's eye, the procedure can be resumed and completed at any point. After the procedure, the patient should be reassured that the procedure is ended, and that things have gone well.

If a LASIK procedure is performed, the cap is moistened and then repositioned. It is important to wait 5 to 10 minutes in the LASIK procedure before removing the lid speculum. During this time, the "wrinkle test" is performed by placing the slight pressure on the peripheral cornea outside the area of the cap. If fine indentation wrinkles are transmitted into the cap, there is good adherence.

In the immediate postoperative period, the patient is instructed on the use of pain medications, antibiotic drops or ointment, and also topical nonsteroidal antiinflammatory drugs. The patient is given both a short-term and long-term follow-up schedule so that both patient and family understand the commitment to long-term care. The use of antibiotic drops or ointment is limited to the first few days until reepithelialization occurs. Pain medications after PRK usually consist of oral analgesics and topical nonsteroidal antiinflammatory agents. The LASIK procedure usually causes less pain, and strong analgesics are usually not needed. The use of postoperative steroids varies with the individual lasers, and it is important to follow a standardized system and carefully document records, including both the planned procedure and attempted correction. The patient should be informed about (1) discomfort after the procedure(s), (2) levels of vision to expect during the first 24 hours and the first weeks and months after the procedure, and (3) activities must be restricted in the immediate postoperative period.

Excimer laser instrumentation varies from one manufacturer to another, but all lasers are composed of five basic building blocks. Although the surgical technique may seem to be a simple "point and shoot" to the novice, there are many possibilities for a poor result, and meticulous attention to detail is required.

REFERENCES

1. Srinivasin R: Kinetics of the ablative photodecomposition or organic polymers in the far ultraviolet (193 nm), *J Vac Sci Technol Bull* 4:923-926, 1983.
2. Krauss JM, Puliafito CA, Steinert RF: Laser interaction with the cornea, *Surv Ophthalmol* 31:37-53, 1986.
3. Mendel ER, Kruegger RR, Puliafito et al: Excimer laser large area ablation of the cornea, *Invest Ophthalmol Vis Sci* 28 (suppl):275, 1987.
4. Munnerly CR, Koons SF, Marshall J: Photorefractive keratectomy: a technique for laser refractive surgery, *J Cataract Refract Surg* 14:46-52, 1988.
5. Hanna K, et al: A rotating slit delivery system for excimer laser refractive keratoplasty, *Am J Ophthalmol* 103:474, 1987.
6. Forster W, Beck R, Busse H: Design and development of a new

193-nanometer excimer laser surgical system, *Refract Corneal Surg* 9:293-299, 1993.

7. Fyodorov SN et al: PRK using an absorbing cell delivery system for correction of myopia from 4.00 to 26 diopters in 3,251 eyes, *Refract Corneal Surg* 9 (suppl):123-124, 1993.
8. L'Esperance FA et al: Excimer laser instrumentation and technique for human corneal surgery, *Arch Ophthalmol* 107:131-139, 1988.
9. Maxwell W, Nordan L: Myopic keratomileusis. In Thompson F, editor: *Myopia surgery,* New York, 1990, McMillan.
10. Price F: Keratomileusis. In Nordan L, Maxwell A, Davison J, editors: *The surgical rehabilitation of vision,* New York, 1992, Gower.
11. Buratto L, Ferarri M: Excimer laser intrastromal keratomileusis: case report, *J Cataract Refract Surg* 18:37-41, 1992.
12. Pallikaris I et al: Laser in situ keratomileusis, *Lasers Surg Med* 10:463-468, 1990.
13. Kruegger RR: Excimer laser: a step up in complexity and responsibility for the ophthalmic laser surgeon, *J Refract Corneal Surg* 10:83-89, 1994.
14. Maloney RK et al: A prototype erodible mask delivery system for the excimer laser, *Ophthalmology* 100:542-549, 1993.

CHAPTER 174

EZRA MAGUEN JEFFREY J. MACHAT JAMES J. SALZ

Results and Complications of Photorefractive Keratoplasty

Excimer laser photorefractive keratectomy (PRK) is establishing itself worldwide as a worthwhile set of refractive surgical procedures for the correction of myopia, myopic astigmatism, and hyperopia. Although in the United States, these surgical procedures have been limited by the U.S. Food and Drug Administration (FDA) restricting the number of procedures performed, the U.S. effort has contributed to a large multicenter controlled clinical study using three types of excimer lasers at a total of 30 clinical sites. Data from this study provides a fairly unbiased assessment of the performance of these procedures, their limitations, and their complications in the short- and medium-term periods after surgery.

The U.S. study may also provide a long-term outlook for the PRK procedures, even though the value of these data may be minimized by the emergence of better techniques and technologies for the performance of PRK; the conclusions derived from these studies may, therefore, be criticized as being antiquated.

There is a need to standardize data reporting in refractive surgery,[1] a need especially obvious in a report such as this in which data emanate from several sources that are not controlled by rigid protocols. An attempt will therefore be madè to report results obtained with comparable methods.

Complications will also be reported based on the U.S and international experiences. An attempt will be made to highlight the more frequent problems associated with PRK, and attempts at solving them will be discussed.

Results of PRK

PRK FOR THE CORRECTION OF LOW AND MODERATE MYOPIA

Under FDA-guided protocols three types of 193 nm excimer lasers have been evaluated since 1990 for the correction of myopia of up to 7.00 diopters with astigmatism not to exceed 1.50 diopter. The VISX models 2015 and 2020 lasers* and the Excimed model UV-200 LA† were evaluated. The VISX model 2015 laser was later discontinued, and the former two systems were evaluated during phase III of the FDA-guided protocols. Seven hundred patients were treated with each device. Five hundred eighty-five eyes for the Summit system and 521 for the VISX system were available for follow-up 1 year postoperatively.[2,3] Data from these two studies at the 1-year time gate will be used for reporting in this chapter. Data from other studies will be also used to allow better comparison between the two systems.

Patient selection was similar in both groups. In addition to the refractive criteria, best corrected visual acuity (BCVA) with spectacles of 20/40 or better and refractive stability for at least 1 year had to be demonstrated. Patients were required to be at least 18 years old and free of ocular disease and systemic autoimmune diseases. For contact lens wearers a washout period of no contact lens wear was mandatory.

The preoperative evaluation included a complete ophthalmic examination with pachymetry. Subsets of patients in each study underwent contrast sensitivity and glare testing, corneal topographic evaluations, specular microscopy, visual fields, and psychometric testing.

The surgical technique was specific to each system and is described elsewhere. The technique used with the Summit laser was consistent over the duration of the study. There was a major technical modification with the VISX 2020 laser when it became apparent that corneal haze could be improved by discontinuing nitrogen flow. Another change consisted of the discontinuation of the suction ring and reliance on patient fixation for globe stabilization. The impact of these changes will be discussed.

Postoperative management was similar with both systems and initially included patching with antibiotic-steroid ointment and cycloplegia along with various narcotic analgesics. With this initial regimen, patients

*VISX, Santa Clara, CA.

†Summit Technologies, Waltham, MA.

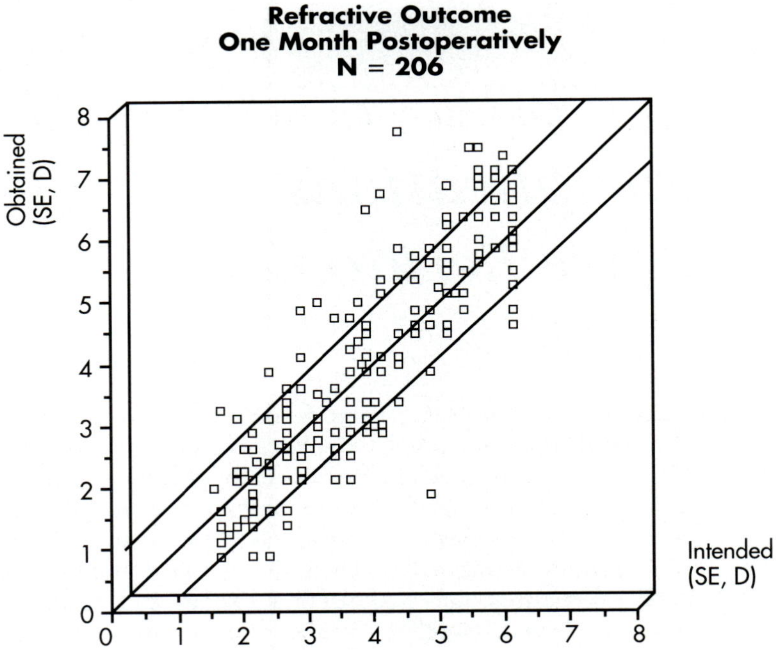

FIGURE 174-1 Scattergram, refractive outcome 1 month postoperatively.

endured severe pain for 24 to 48 hours. Sher described the combined use of topical nonsteroidal anti-inflamatory medication (NSAID) and a therapeutic soft contact lens for successful pain management,[4] and the short-term management of these patients was modified accordingly. Contact lenses and topical antibiotics were used until epithelialization was complete, usually within 72 hours of surgery. NSAID topically was used as necessary for pain control not exceeding four times daily. Once the epithelium has grown, Fluorometholone 0.25% eye drops were administered initially four times daily, slowly tapering over a 4-month period.

Refractive outcome

Figures 174-1 to 174-4 demonstrate the refractive outcome over time between 1 and 12 months postoperatively. These data were generated from a cohort of 250 eyes operated on at Cedars Sinai Medical Center, one of 10 VISX 2020 laser centers participating in phase III of the FDA-guided protocols.[5] These scattergrams represent achieved correction versus intended correction at different time gates. They reflect the following findings:

1. Results of eyes corrected for "low myopia," between 1.00 and 3.50 diopters, show less scatter, and data points are mostly confined to within ±1.00 diopter of emmetropia.
2. The eyes with preoperative myopia higher than 3.50 diopters show more scatter in the distribution of the data points throughout these figures.
3. There is a relatively high number of overcorrections 1 month postoperatively, primarily in eyes with preoperative myopia of more than 5.50 diopters.
4. Overcorrections are relatively rare thereafter, and outlying data points beyond ±1.00 diopter are mostly undercorrections. There was a slow progression toward emmetropia over the 12 months. Table 174-1 compares the percent of eyes within ±0.50 diopter and within ±1.00 diopter of emmetropia as obtained with the two systems.

Evaluation of the mean correction over time shows that the mean correction at 1 month is slightly hyperopic for VISX (+0.5 diopter) and significantly hyperopic for Summit (+1.6 diopters). Refraction stabilizes in both cases between 3 to 6 months. At 1 year the mean correction for Summit is +0.1 diopter and for VISX −0.5 diopter. Table 174-2 summarizes these data.

Uncorrected visual acuity

Table 174-3 summarizes the accuracy of postoperative uncorrected visual acuity (UCVA) 12 months postoperatively for the VISX and Summit systems. The Summit laser appears to fare better for vision of 20/20 or better, whereas no significant difference exists between the two systems for vision of 20/40 or better.

The Summit series provides data pertaining to the

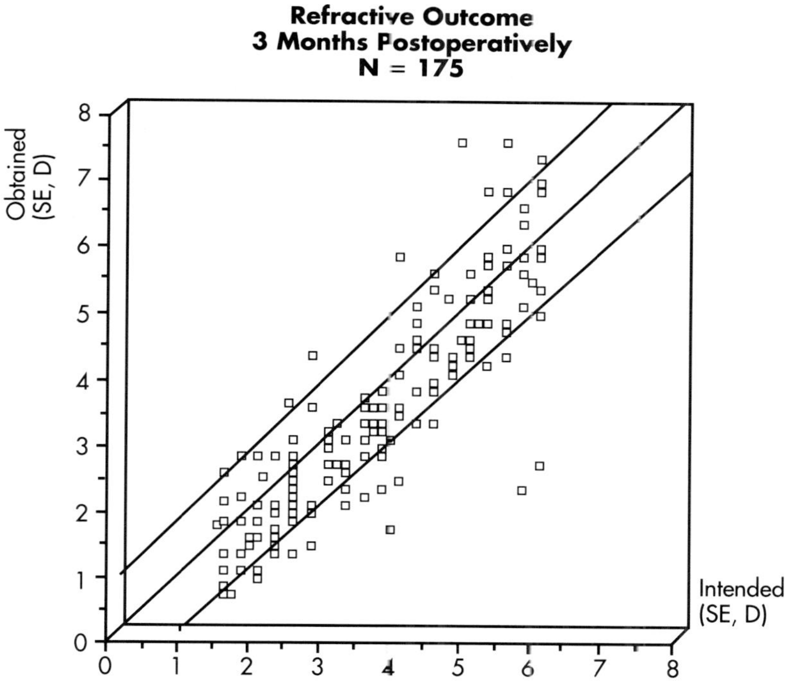

FIGURE 174-2 Scattergram, refractive outcome 3 months postoperatively.

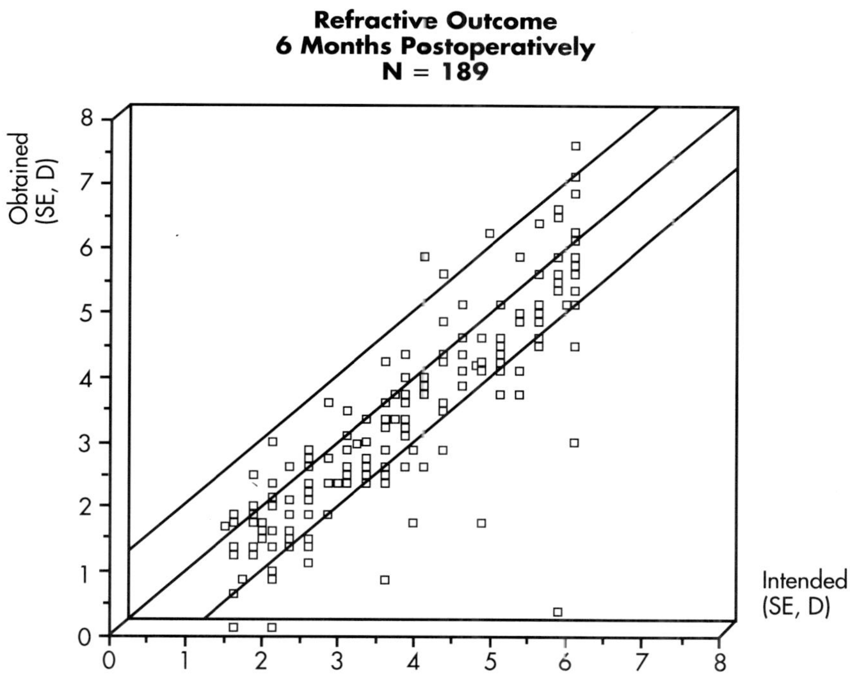

FIGURE 174-3 Scattergram, refractive outcome 6 months postoperatively.

predictability of attempted correction by comparing the percent of eyes seeing uncorrected 20/20 or better to the degree of preoperative myopia. From this comparison (Table 174-4), it is evident that predictability of attempted correction is better in lower preoperative myopia. VISX data (Table 174-5) evaluated the actual percentage of eyes seeing 20/20 or better in relation to preoperative myopia, and the same conclusion as for the Summit system could be drawn.

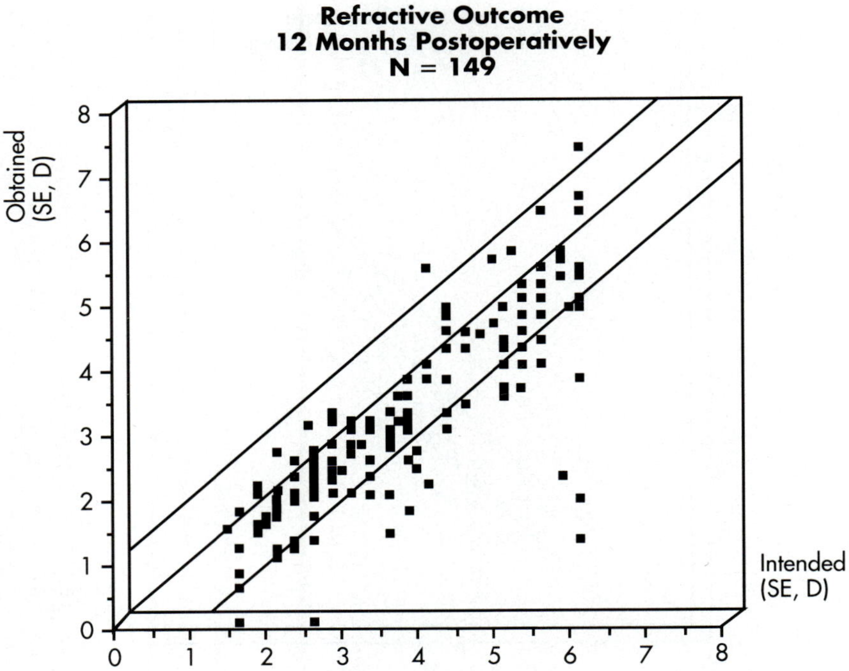

FIGURE 174-4 Scattergram, refractive outcome 12 months postoperatively.

Table 174-1. Refractive outcome at 12 months postoperatively

	VISX (% eyes)	Summit (% eyes)
±0.50 diopter	48.0	58.5
±1.00 diopter	78.0	77.7

Table 174-2. Mean spherical equivalent (SE) refraction over time

Time gate (months)	VISX (SE, diopter)	Summit (SE, diopter[s])
1	+0.50	+1.60
3	−0.20	+0.70
6	−0.30	+0.30
12	−0.50	+0.10

Table 174-3. UCVA 12 months postoperatively

UCVA	VISX (% eyes)	Summit (% eyes)
≥20/20	50	66.4
≥20/40	88	90.7

Table 174-4. Predictability of attempted correction compared to preoperative myopia for the Summit system

Preoperative myopia (diopters)	% of eyes with UCVA ≥20/20
1.5 to 2.9	80
3.0 to 3.9	68.4
4.0 to 4.9	69.2
5.0 to 5.9	58.9

Table 174-5. Deviation of intended correction compared to preoperative myopia (VISX)

Preoperative myopia (diopters)	% of eyes with UCVA ≥20/20
<2.0	65
2.0 to 4.0	57
>4.0	39

Spectacle BCVA

BCVA is an important indicator, since loss of such acuity as compared to preoperative values may indicate a corneal pathologic condition related to the refractive surgical procedure. The Summit series reported that 1 year postoperatively 96% of all eyes were seeing 20/20 or better and 99.8% of all eyes were seeing 20/40 or

Table 174-6. BCVA loss of 1.6 lines (VISX) or 2 lines (Summit) on the ETDRS chart 12 months postoperatively

Laser	No. of eyes/total eyes	% Eyes
Summit	18/585	3.07
VISX	8/519	1.5

better. VISX reported that 95% of all eyes had no change in their BCVA and 3.5% gained visual acuity at 1 year.

Another way of evaluating this issue is by assessing the number of eyes that lost two or more lines of BCVA on the ETDRS chart. VISX reported eyes that lost (or gained) ≥1.6 lines on the ETDRS visual acuity chart. The rationale for this type of reporting was that a lesser loss of BCVA has been shown to result from "noise." In addition, such a format allows comparison with data from the Prospective Evaluation of Radial Keratotomy (PERK) study.[6] Table 174-6 summarizes BCVA loss for the VISX and Summit systems.

Induced astigmatism

Induced refractive astigmatism is not uncommon after PRK; for the most part, induced astigmatism appears to decrease over time. It may result from surface irregularity secondary to the interaction between corneal collagen and the 193 nm laser beam. The VISX data reported 3.3% of eyes with induced astigmatism of 1.00 diopter or more 1 year postoperatively. Seiler, in his prospective study,[7] reported 5.6% of eyes with induced astigmatism of 0.75 to 1.5 diopters at the same time gate. The Cedars-Sinai study[5] reported that the change in the axis of astigmatism did not exceed 20°.

Postoperative superficial stromal corneal haze

The appearance of superficial stromal opacification of the cornea after PRK is extremely common and reflects a biologic healing response to PRK. Malley et al.[8] found in the monkey eye with immunofluorescence that the patterns produced during wound healing by excimer laser ablation and mechanical keratectomy were qualitatively identical. They concluded that corneal opacity associated with wound healing may result from the following factors: deposition of type III collagen, absence of sulfated keratan sulfate from the extracellular matrix, and the absence of Bowman's layer and an orderly array of collagen fibers. Fibronectin and laminin were also found in high quantities, associated with an increase in size and number of keratocytes adjacent to the treatment area.

Clinically, the development of reticulated corneal haze is a normal part of the healing process and appears during the first postoperative month. Its incidence peaks between 1 and 3 months postoperatively and gradually decreases over the first year. The haze scores obtained nationwide with the VISX and Summit lasers are described in Table 174-7. The density of the haze was scored in up to three subjective units whereby a 1+ score was deemed functionally significant. The hallmark of clinically significant haze is confluence. Confluent haze, whether focal or diffuse, arcuate or circular, is associated with a higher risk of (1) immediate and long-term regression and (2) loss of BCVA related to irregular astigmatism or abnormal topography. Corneal haze is not only related to depth of ablation but also to steep wound contours, intraoperative stromal hydration, and patient variability. Corneal haze appears to have decreased significantly with the discontinuation of nitrogen flow during surgery, and its scores are higher when the preoperative myopia is higher.

Table 174-7. Superficial stromal corneal haze, 1 year postoperatively

Type	Score	VISX (%)	Summit (%)
None	0.0	65.1	25.6
Trace	0.5	24.3	59.1
Mild	1 to 1.5	6.6	12.2
Moderate	2.0	0.4	2.6
Marked	≥3.0	0	0

Corneal haze may be observed with the slit lamp by sclerotic scatter. The opacities are located in the superficial stroma immediately beneath the epithelium covering the ablation zone. They may assume several appearances: thin granules, coarse clumps, or a confluent opacity involving part or all of the ablation zone. Over time, most opacities fade, and, in several cases, it is difficult to detect any opacification at all. Associated symptoms may include blurred vision with a decrease in uncorrected and BCVA, and symptoms related to light scattering such as a starburst effect when viewing oncoming lights in evening traffic.

Another school of thought associates night glare to spherical aberration alone and not to haze directly. Indeed a cornea may show dense haze with no glare, and clear corneas may be associated with severe glare. The method by which haze affects glare is by inducing myopia through steepening the corneal curvature and by affecting topography, reducing the effective optical zone. In the nationwide VISX data, glare testing with the BAT device in conjunction with the CSV 1000 contrast sensitivity device showed that 3.7% of 150 eyes had an abnormal response and 0.7% had such a response 12 months postoperatively. Seventeen per-

Table 174-9. Summary of three U.S. studies of PRK for high myopia 1 year postoperatively

Parameter	Summit	VISX 2015	VISX 2020
Range of preoperative myopia	8 to 15	8 to 19.5	6 to 10 diopters
Mean of preoperative myopia	10 ± 2.1 diopters	11.83 ± 2.92 diopters	7.10 diopters
% ±1 diopter of emmetropia	58	39	60
% ±2 diopter of emmetropia	79	74	100
% UCVA ³20/40	79	57	100
% Haze (score)	10 (≥2)(@ 6M)	30 (≥1.5)	NA
% Retreatments	6.1	13	NA
OZ (mm)	5 to 6.2 (s)	4/5/6 (m)	4.5 to 5 (s)
BCVA loss (≥2 lines) (%)	12	8.7	0

S, single; m, multiple zones; NA, not available.

studies. The same observations were made in a series of 14 eyes operated on at Cedars-Sinai Medical Center. There is no scientific explanation for the discrepancy between visual results and amount of astigmatism corrected. On the other hand, Dausch et al report their series[24] of myopic astigmatism correction with the MEL 60 laser.* In this series, the mean preoperative cylinder was −2.10 ± 0.93 diopters. Six months postoperatively the mean cylinder was −0.11 ± 0.37 diopters. UCVA was 20/40 or better in 54% of eyes 3 months postoperatively. This laser is capable of operating in the scanning mode of a slit beam. From these results, it appears that different delivery systems provide different final results, and further study is needed to better understand PARK.

PRK FOR THE CORRECTION OF HYPEROPIA

The correction of hyperopia by any refractive keratoplasty entails the steepening of the central cornea. This may be achieved by adding tissue to the central corneal stroma or by removing tissue from the peripheral cornea, thereby obtaining a centrally steepened profile. The excimer laser uses the latter principle to steepen the central cornea. The MEL 60 laser is capable of performing such an ablation in the scanning mode. An attempt is currently being made by VISX using a variable eccentric lens in connection with the existing delivery system to enable the 2020 model to perform hyperopic PRK.[25]

The only published series on hyperopic PRK is by Dausch et al.[24] using the MEL 60 laser. The study treats two groups: a low to moderate hyperopic group and an aphakic group. In general, the aphakic group fared less well because of more variability of the correction and larger amounts of corneal change postoperatively. The mild to moderate group featured 15 eyes of 15 patients. The preoperative hyperopia was +2.0 ± 7.5 diopters. The mean preoperative refraction was +4.7 ± 1.6 diopters, and the mean refraction was +0.53 ± 1.2 diopters 9 months postoperatively. The mean refractions at 1 month and 3 months postoperatively were −0.17 and +0.33 diopters, respectively, thereby demonstrating a tendency toward regression of the correction. Uncorrected visual acuity was 20/40 or better in 80% and 20/20 or better in 40% of eyes 1 year postoperatively. One eye lost two lines of BCVA because of a 1.3 mm decentration of the ablation. Peripheral corneal haze at the ablation site decreased significantly in all eyes 12 months after surgery. Haze was classified from grade 0 (none) to grade 3 (confluent). Table 174-12 shows the progression of mean haze scores over 12 months.

The recently developed hyperopia module for the VISX 2020 excimer laser was evaluated on eyes with subnormal vision at several centers in the United States, including Cedars-Sinai Medical Center. The study was designed to establish the safety of the procedure, which was achieved. Refractive and keratometric data are also available but cannot be properly interpreted because of the inability of the patients to be refracted or to properly fixate. The data suggest that a hyperopic ablation is feasible with the system and that there is some regression 3 months postoperatively.

*Aesculap-Meditec, Heroldsberg, Germany.

FACTORS AFFECTING RESULTS IN PRK

Nitrogen flow

As phase III of the FDA-guided study of PRK proceeded, VISX investigators became aware that discontinuation of nitrogen flow from the suction ring applied to the eye during surgery may reduce corneal haze and enhance the final surgical outcome. Maguen et al. evaluated the short-term outcome of such procedures and found significant improvement in results as compared to the same number of procedures performed with nitrogen flow.[26] Later it was found that with the same algorithm used for PRK with nitrogen flow, there were a significant number of undercorrections.[5] Figure 174-7 shows a comparison between series of PRK performed with and without nitrogen flow and demonstrates a mean spherical equivalent of −0.8 diopter 18 months postoperatively. This issue

Table 174-10. Summary of studies since 1992 of excimer PRK in high myopia

Study/year	No. of eyes	Refractive range (diopters)	Laser used	Ablation zone (mm)	No. of steps	% within 1 diopter	% within 2 diopters	% >2 lines lost	% haze	Haze scale
Sher 1992	16	−8.62 to −14.50	VISX 2015	5.5 to 6.0	1	NA	68.7	NA	25 (1.5+)	0-4
Ehlers and Hiortdal 1992	31	−6.35 to −16.77	Aesculap-Meditec	5.0	1	29	42	NA	29 (1+); 71.6% (2+)	0-3
Burrato and Ferrari 1993	40	6.00 to 10.000	Summit UV200	4 3 to 4 5	1	27.5	NA	40	77.5 (1+) 7.52 (2+)	0-4
Brancatto et al 1993	184	−6.00 to −25.00	Summit UV200	3.5 to 5.0	1 or 2	34.5 (<10) 28.2 (>10)	61.4 (<10) 46.1 (>10)	3.3	58 (1+) 14. (2+)	0-4
Cho et al 1993	19	−8.87 to 16.99	Summit UV200	4.5 to 5.0	2 or 3	16.7	22.2	NA	10.5 (1+)	0-4
Kim et al 1993	19	−8.00 to −13.50	Summit UV200	4.5 to 5.0	2	73.7	NA	NA	16 (1+)	0,TR, 1,2,3
Lavery 1993	33	−6.00 to −9.50	Summit UV200	5.0	2	45	84	NA	NA	0-4

No. of steps refers to multizone approach. Percentage of eyes within 1 or 2 diopters of attempted correction of emmetropia if not stated. Haze refers to various subjective scales that are listed in haze scale. NA, Not available.

Table 174-11. Mean preoperative and postoperative cylinder in three series using the VISX 2020 excimer laser

	Taylor et al 1993	Saedi et al 1994	Kim and McDonnell 1994
Mean preoperative cylinder	−1.39 ± 1.33 diopters	−2.1 ± 0.7 diopters	−1.51 ± 0.81 diopters
Mean postoperative cylinder	>0.61 ± 0.53 diopters	−1.0 to 0.5 diopters	−0.67 ± 0.6 diopters
Difference	43%	47%	44%

Table 174-12. Mean scores of corneal haze over 12 months

Month postoperatively	Mean haze score
1	1.25
2	1.4
12	0.8

Table 174-13. The effect of a larger optical zone and multizone treatments on the outcome of PRK

	VISX 2015 (%)	VISX 2020 (%)
No. of eyes	91	849
UCVA ≥20/40	98	96
UCVA ≥20/25	80	85
+1.00 diopter of attempted correction* or of emmetropia†	93*	92†

UCVA, Uncorrected visual acuity.

could be addressed by correcting the algorithm used for obtaining specific refractions. In our study, we have used the actual refraction rather than the spherical equivalent at the corneal plane to correct for this finding.

Optical zone size and multizone PRK

Two recent studies undertaken with the VISX 2015[27] and the VISX 2020[28] demonstrated improved results with the use of a larger optical zone than previously reported. An optical zone of 6 to 7 mm was used with the VISX 2015 laser. Ninety-one eyes underwent a single PRK to correct myopia. Lin reports 849 eyes that underwent a single procedure to correct myopia up to 6.00 diopters and astigmatism of up to a 3.50 diopter cylinder with the VISX 2020 laser. This series was performed with an optic zone of up to 6 mm, with several cases performed using various optical zones. Table 174-13 details the results of these two studies 1 year postoperatively and demonstrates that with the same hardware, improved results may be obtained by refining the surgical technique. Multizone PRK was previously discussed as an alternative for the correction of high myopia and as a means to obtain a more tapered transition zone, thereby improving on the tendency for regression in those with higher myopia.

Patient-related parameters

It appears that the most influential factor affecting the final outcome of PRK is the preoperative myopia. Additional factors were evaluated before designing the algorithm driving the laser as surgery proceeds. It was apparent that corneal thickness and keratometry do not significantly affect outcome even though mean keratometry is still a part of the VISX algorithm. Other factors, such as age and sex, have been evaluated. Srinivas et al[29] found in their series performed with the Summit excimer laser that a greater degree of hyperopia may occur in patients older than 40 years. Lipschitz (personal communication) also found in his series an influence of age on the final outcome of PRK using the Summit laser.

Complications of PRK

Many of the complications encountered in PRK patients such as undercorrections and overcorrections are similar to those experienced by patients who have undergone radial keratotomy. Other complications such as corneal haze and central islands, however, are specific to the excimer laser. It is extremely rare to obtain a final result that is the same or worse than the preoperative refraction, and no reports of lost vision or lost eyes have been published. Anecdotal reports of the need to perform corneal transplants after PRK have surfaced in Europe, yet no such occurrence has been reported in the United States under the FDA-guided long-term evaluation of PRK.

We will discuss complications of PRK from the following sources: A series of 240 procedures performed by five surgeons at Cedars-Sinai Medical Center in Los Angeles during the past 3 years,[5] the nationwide results of phase III of the FDA-guided VISX clinical trials 1 year postoperatively; a review of the literature and a series of over 1,000 procedures performed by Maguen at

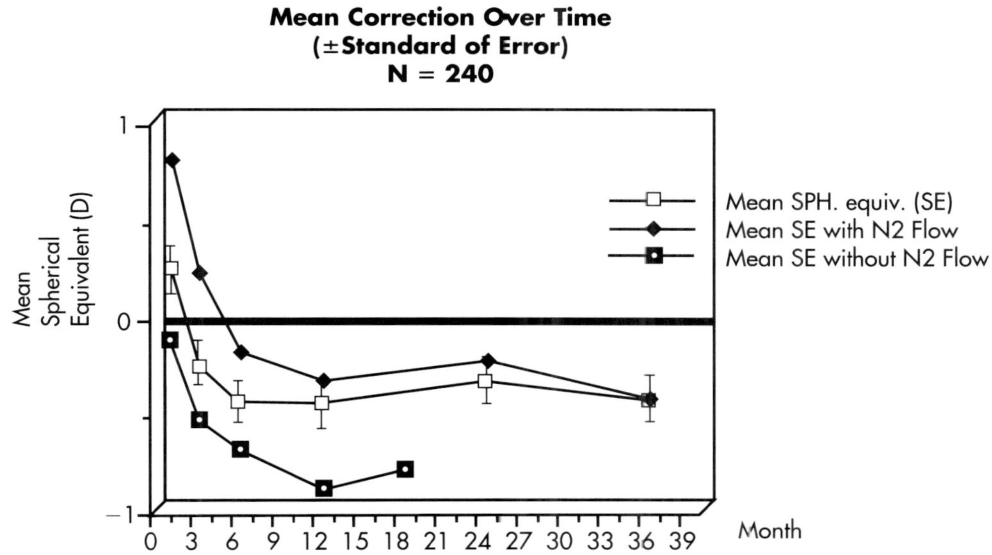

FIGURE 174-7 Mean correction over time, comparison between nitrogen (N_2) blow and no blow.

using the Summit, VISX, and Technolas excimer lasers.*

COMPLICATIONS RELATED TO UNPLANNED DEVIATIONS FROM INTENDED CORRECTION

Overcorrection, undercorrection, and induced astigmatism

The accepted standard of accuracy of the final optical correction in refractive surgery is a maximal deviation of ±1.00 diopter of the intended correction. In a series performed with the VISX model 20/20 excimer laser[5] at Cedars-Sinai Medical Center, the optical correction stabilized between 3 and 6 months postoperatively (Figure 174-7). Six months after surgery, 88% of a sample of 124 eyes were corrected within ±1.00 diopter of the intended correction. The amount of undercorrection was significantly larger than that of overcorrection, partly because of the discontinuation of nitrogen flow, which provided better short-term rehabilitation after PRK,[26] but induced a mean undercorrection of 0.8 diopter, 18 months postoperatively (Figure 174-7).[5]

A significant amount of overcorrection was reported by users of the Summit Technologies Excimed UV200 excimer laser. Gimbel[30] reported on the need to reduce the intended correction by 25% to neutralize the tendency toward overcorrection in his hands. Both the risk of overcorrection and the symptoms produced are substantially greater in patients over 40 years of age.

Undercorrections are more easily managed than overcorrections. Significant undercorrections can be managed by retreatment of the undercorrected eye with the excimer laser. Incisional keratotomy after PRK should be undertaken with caution because the nomograms available may not be accurate. At the present time there is no effective and safe treatment for overcorrection. If high doses of topical steroid are used on an overcorrected eye, the medication should be tapered down quickly, to be hopefully followed by decreased hyperopia. Overcorrected eyes not responsive to withdrawal of topical steroids may be fitted with an extended wear contact lens in an attempt to produce a hypoxic state of the cornea, thereby promoting regression.

Regular and irregular astigmatism may be induced after PRK. In the Cedars-Sinai series, 4% of 240 eyes showed induced regular astigmatism of 1.00 diopter or greater 12 months postoperatively.[5] Astigmatism increased more than 1.00 diopter in 6.1% of the 521 patients of the national VISX series. We have successfully treated three patients with peripheral arcuate incisions made peripheral to the ablation zone for regular astigmatism of 1.50 to 2.5 diopters after PRK.

Irregular astigmatism is often evident early in the healing period after excimer laser ablation reducing spectacle BCVA. Nitrogen flow produced a greater incidence of irregular astigmatism, which resolved over weeks to months with the smoothing of the epithelium.

Severe regression

Severe regression of most or all the correction obtained after PRK is rare. In our series, two of 240 patients showed severe regression. One case, previously

*The Laser Center, Inc., Windsor, Canada.

described (Figures 174-5 and 174-6), was associated with severe corneal haze, whereas the second case had a clear cornea. The possible etiologies of regression are unknown. Gartry found a correlation between corneal haze and regression.[31] The combined incidence of regression and haze was more frequent in patients with preoperative high myopia.[9] Wilson et al[32] found regression to be more common and more pronounced in eyes with intended correction of more than 5.00 diopters. Tengroth et al[33] reported the occurrence of regression after discontinuation of topical steroids and the ability to reverse regression after discontinuation of topical steroids and the abililty to reverse regression with the same medication. Carones[34] reported the same findings in six eyes. Several anecdotal reports note significant myopic regression after intense ultraviolet exposure during the first few months of healing. It is surmised that eyes which underwent PRK may be more sensitized to ultraviolet exposure and that further exposure can retrigger or accelerate the healing process. A series of six female patients who became pregnant in the immediate postoperative period after PRK were reported by Machat.[43] All eyes experienced myopic regression, two associated with severe haze. There appeared to be a definite correlation between hormonal imbalance and regression, with the most severe cases experiencing severe morning sickness. The least affected patient had the least problems with her pregnancy, and another non-pregnant patient being treated for a hormonal imbalance found her vision fluctuating dramatically. Her refraction changed by 1.00 diopter and vision fluctuated between 20/20 and 20/50 whenever her hormonal fluctuation peaked over her monthly cycle.

Because of the low incidence of severe regression in human eyes and the lack of an experimental model, it is impossible at this point to have a good understanding of this process and to prevent it. One may propose two possible mechanisms: (1) the overproduction of collagen and/or fibrous tissue and (2) epithelial hyperplasia filling the defect created by ablation. Treatment consists of starting or increasing the frequency or potency of topical steroids. Regression associated with haze can be retreated with the excimer laser in a transepithelial fashion along with stromal ablation in the amount necessary to correct the present myopia (PRK protocol). Caution should be exercised in treating clear corneas with the excimer laser, and one may consider transepithelial treatment with minimal stromal ablation (PTK protocol) if epithelial hyperplasia can be demonstrated with high power slit lamp observation. Clinically, multizone techniques using larger optical zones to blend in the new contour have reduced the risk of regression when correcting cases of high myopia.

COMPLICATIONS RELATED TO POSTOPERATIVE MEDICATIONS AND THERAPEUTIC CONTACT LENSES

Steroid-induced complications

Increase in intraocular pressure (steroid response). In the initial stages of the FDA-guided investigation of PRK, high doses of steroids were used such as prednisolone sodium acetate 1% (Pred Forte) eye drops four times daily to the operated eye.[35] Later, because of steroid response and other concerns, Fluorometholone 0.25% (FML) was used in an attempt to decrease the incidence of steroid-induced increase in intraocular pressure (IOP). The Cedars-Sinai series demonstrated an incidence of 1.7% of operated eyes in which an IOP equal to or higher than 25 mm Hg was measured at any time postoperatively. The same incidence was noted in the national VISX series. Other reports showed incidences ranging between 3.1% and 25.3%.[12] In series where higher incidences of steroid response were reported, higher potency topical steroids were used, such as dexamethasone 0.1%. Management of steroid response associated with PRK consists of the control of IOP with topical antiglaucoma medications while the topical steroid is continued. At times it may be necessary to reduce the potency of the topical steroid to achieve better IOP control. Fluorometholone 0.5% (FML Forte) eye drops may be an adequate substitute. In all cases, IOP reverted to normal values on discontinuation of topical steroids in our series, and no reports of persistent increased IOP exist in the literature.

Steroid-induced ocular herpes simplex keratitis. The use of topical steroids may induce ocular herpes simplex (HSV) keratitis. At the same time the immediate tissue response after PRK is an acute photokeratitis. This acute inflammatory response may in itself cause shedding of HSV, thereby inducing the viral keratitis. Indeed, such cases have been described,[36] and such a case was treated in our series of phototherapeutic keratectomy with success (Mannis, personal communication). Management consists of discontinuation of topical steroids and the use of trifluorothimidine eye drops every 2 hours initially, along with systemic acyclovir 200 mg one tablet five times daily. We screen all candidates for PRK for possible HSV dermatitis (cold sores or "fever blisters"), and treat these patients prophylactically with the same dose of acyclovir starting from 1 week preoperatively and continuing until the acute keratitis has subsided and the epithelium has regenerated over the treatment area. One might also consider a shorter term regimen of topical steroids, and while this medication is used, coverage by a topical antiviral agent should be considered.

Ptosis. Steroid-induced ptosis is more common in young females. It is minimal and measures usually 1 to

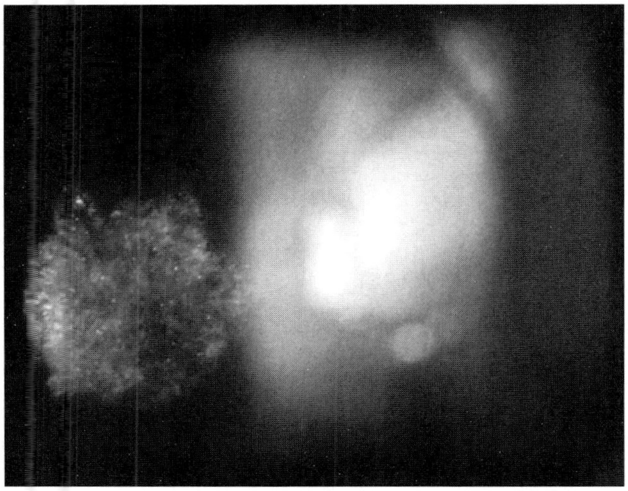

FIGURE 174-8 Posterior subcapsular cataract associated with PRK.

2 mm. It worsens as the day progresses, improves with decreasing frequency and potency of topical steroid used, usually resolves with discontinuation of topical steroids, but can be permanent. Ptosis may also occur as a result of stretching Müller's muscle with the use of a lid speculum. One case occurred in the Cedars-Sinai series and was corrected with a Müller muscle-conjunctival resection.

Posterior subcapsular cataracts. Three posterior subcapsular cataracts after the use of dexamethasone phosphate 0.1% were observed by Machat (Figure 174-8). All patients were treated by other surgeons. The duration and frequency of use varied from QID for 3 months to Q2H for 8 months to control regression. All cases underwent PRK with the Summit Excimed laser. No such cases were reported with the use of Fluorometholone.

Superficial keratopathy

A large variety of topical medications is used in conjunction with PRK. These include topical antibiotics, nonsteroidal anti-inflammatory drugs (NSAIDs), topical steroids, artificial tears, and, on occasion, antiglaucoma medications. It is therefore not surprising that on occasion we have encountered superficial keratopathy related to either the preservatives or to the topical medications themselves. Treatment consists of trying to identify the responsible medication and replacing it with an equivalent containing a different preservative. If this is not feasible, nonpreserved medication should be used. A nonspecific keratitis may develop in patients 1 week after excimer ablation lasting 1 to 3 weeks. The superficial punctate staining may be associated with an increase in clinical haze. These findings may reflect an ultraviolet photokeratitis related to underlying stromal inflammation. Treatment similarly consists of lubrication.

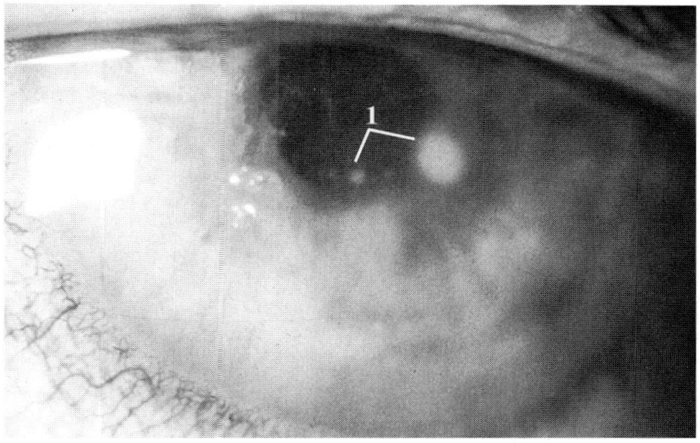

FIGURE 174-9 Corneal infiltrates (*1*) associated with PRK.

Complications related to therapeutic contact lenses

Sterile paracentral corneal infiltrate and infectious corneal ulcers. In the Cedars-Sinai series we encountered one episode of a paracentral sterile corneal infiltrate after PRK (Figure 174-9). Because of the lack of pathogens in the corneal scraping, it is unclear whether this was an infectious corneal ulcer or a corneal infiltrate associated with the use of disposable extended wear lenses as described by Serdahl et al.[37] One should always assume that such keratitis is infectious and treat it intensively. If the epithelium is intact, one may consider not scraping the cornea and follow the patient closely. Machat has treated six corneal ulcers out of a total of 3,000 patients evaluated in relation with PRK (Figure 174-10). The incidence of corneal ulcers in this series is 0.1%.[38] The annualized incidence of "contact lens–induced keratitis" in large Swedish population of disposable extended lens wearers is similar.[38] Therefore one may reasonably assume that corneal ulcers and infiltrates are mainly caused by contact lens wear rather than the surgical procedure itself. All eyes were treated with postoperative contact lenses. All resolved with fortified topical antibiotics. Two ulcers grew *Staphylococcus epidermidis* on cultures.

Other contact lens–related complications. Disposable extended wear contact lenses are now used in the majority of PRK procedures performed along with topical NSAIDs to control postoperative pain. At times, these lenses may dislocate, mostly because of loose fit. Our patients are instructed to patch the operated eye and not to reinsert the lens if such an event occurs in order to avoid infection. Systemic pain medication may then be used as needed, and a lens can be reinserted with sterile technique as soon as feasible.[39] Lenses that

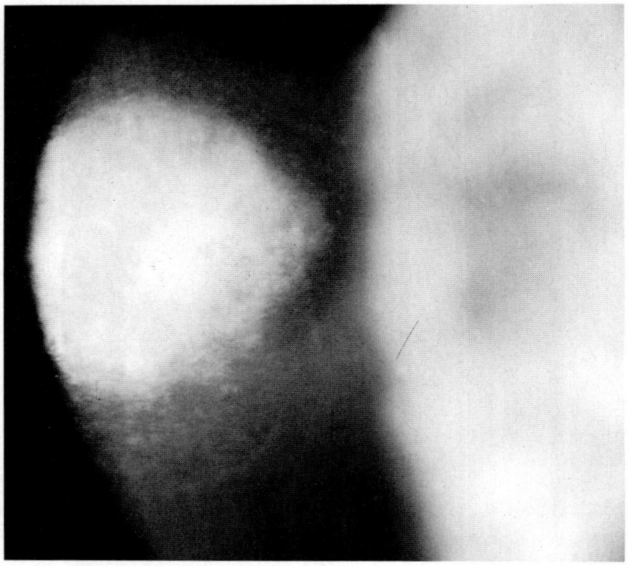

FIGURE 174-10 Corneal ulcer associated with PRK, after healing.

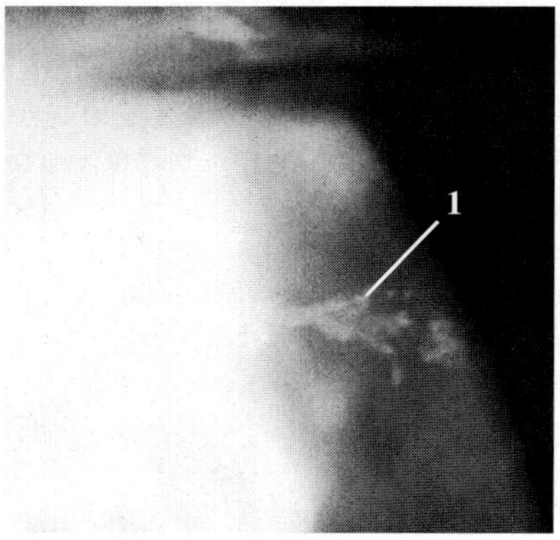

FIGURE 174-11 Recurrent corneal erosion (*1*) associated with PRK.

are fit too tightly may cause a variant of the "tight lens syndrome,"[40] which manifests itself by a red painful eye, chemosis, a tightly fitting lens, and, in the extreme, corneal edema. In most cases, replacing the lens with a flatter curve provides relief. Disposable lenses appear to undergo spoilage quickly and, in our experience, 72 hours postoperatively, patients complain of foreign body sensation and tearing that are relieved by the removal of the lens, if the epithelium is intact, or its replacement, if the epithelium needs further healing.

COMPLICATIONS RELATED TO CORNEAL WOUND HEALING

Plaque formation

Lindstrom (personal communication) described one case of epithelial plaque formation in an eye that previously underwent myopic epikeratoplasty to correct high myopia. The correction regressed, and PRK was performed. A dense epithelial plaque formed with a significant decrease in visual acuity. The plaque was debrided manually. The corneal cleared, but the correction obtained totally regressed. No similar findings were reported in normal corneas before surgery.

Table 174-14. Recurrent corneal erosions after PRK–surgical variables

Case #	Preoperative spherical equivalent (diopters)	Time (months) postoperatively	Nitrogen flow
1R	−6.00	9	F
1L	−6.00	14	NF
3	−1.75	1	F
4	−1.75	29	F
5	−5.62	5	NF

F, Nitrogen flow; NF, no nitrogen flow; R, right eye; L, left eye.

Recurrent corneal erosions

Four cases of recurrent corneal erosions (RCE) occurred after PRK in the Cedars-Sinai series. Several patients were also seen in The Laser Center's series (Figure 174-11). All patients were screened for ophthalmic diseases before surgery, and no evidence of corneal dystrophy was found. Two cases (one bilateral) display both the clinical signs and symptoms of RCE. One patient has intraepithelial cysts and is asymptomatic. One case demonstrated the symptoms of RCE but did not display the clinical signs of this syndrome.

Table 174-14 shows that there is no pattern in the following parameters that might explain the occurrence of RCE: preoperative refraction, time elapsed between surgery and onset of symptoms, and whether nitrogen flow was or was not used during surgery.

The incidence of RCE in the Cedars-Sinai series was 2.1%, a figure extremely close to the incidence reported in the general population.[41] In addition, the clinical features of this dystrophy may be absent even though the patient may develop them later. Also, the area of dystrophy was seen both within and away from the ablation zone. Therefore one cannot rule out the possibility that epithelial dystrophy was preexisting in these eyes. Only time and additional reports of this phenomenon will tell if this observation is of concern. The lack of pattern in several parameters suggests perhaps multiple causes for this finding: the frequent use of topical anesthetic and/or the physical force applied to the epithelial sheath during debridement with a blunt instrument could have an impact. It is a widely accepted observation among surgeons performing PRK that some epithelia can be debrided much easier than others. This may occur because the hemidesmosomal attachments are sometimes weaker, and the added trauma of frequent topical anesthetics, the debridement, and, perhaps, in some way, the photoablation contribute to the occurrence of this finding.

Treatment of recurrent corneal erosions under these circumstances is similar to that of RCE not associated with PRK. All symptomatic patients found relief with the use of hypertonic saline solution, and one patient was successfully treated with PTK in The Laser Center series.

COMPLICATIONS RELATED TO MECHANICAL FACTORS

Halos

Patients undergoing PRK complain sometimes of seeing halos around lights with or without a starburst effect. These two phenomena are related to light scattering, mostly caused by surface irregularity and corneal haze, or to spherical aberrations, as described earlier. In addition, the relation between the ablation zone diameter and the diameter of the pupil, especially in dim light is of importance. Gimbel reported 50% of surveyed patients described having rings or halos and 45.2% described a "haze effect" 8 months postoperatively with ablation zones between 4.5 and 5 mm.[30] Other studies reported an incidence between 10% and 78% of operated eyes, depending on the time interval between surgery and the report of the symptom.[31,42,43] The Laser Center series correlates this symptom mainly with the OZ size used. Incidences of 75% to 80% night glare were found with 4 mm OZ ablations, 35% to 40% night glare with 4.5 mm OZ ablations, 20% night glare with 5 mm OZ ablations, less than 5% night glare with 6 mm OZ ablations, and less than 0.5% night glare with 7 mm OZ ablations. The nationwide VISX data show that 30% of patients surveyed 1 year postoperatively complain of sensitivity to bright lights, compared to 17% who had the same complaint preoperatively.

Roberts and Koester[44] provide the theoretical framework to explain these symptoms by generating a ray tracing, defining the edge of the OZ for any given pupil size. They concluded that OZ diameters in PRK must be at least as large as the entrance pupil diameter to prevent foveal glare and larger than the entrance pupil diameter to prevent parafoveal glare. In addition, the postoperative corneal curvature also plays a role because it determines magnification of the pupil. Clinically a 7 mm OZ ablation seems to be adequate for 9 or 10 mm pupil dilation in dim light in The Laser Center series.

Indeed, measurement of the pupillary diameter in dim light before surgery is extremely important, and patients with very wide pupils should be advised preoperatively of this possible complication and, in extreme cases, discouraged from having refractive surgery.

Table 174-15. Decentration of the ablation zone in PRK

Amount of decentration (mm)	% of light rays falling on retinal that miss the OZ
0	0
0.5	16
1.0	31
2.0	61
3.0	86
4.0	100

Modified from Maloney RK: *Refract Corneal Surg* 6:363-371, 1990.

Management of halos and starburst effect should address the probable cause of the symptom. If corneal haze is the cause, treatment should be undertaken as described earlier. When OZs are less than 5.5 mm and there is a disparity between pupil size and the edge of the zone, one may attempt to enlarge the OZ in a transepithelial fashion with blending of the peripheral edge when residual myopia is present. If the symptomatic eye is emmetropic or hyperopic, peripheral retreatment should not be attempted. Low concentrations of pilocarpine were used anecdotally to remedy this symptom. We feel that the risks associated with chronic use of pilocarpine in myopic eyes preclude use of this medication as an alternative. Indeed, in our experience, this medication was not generally well tolerated, inducing in younger patients undergoing this surgery various symptoms, such as blurred vision, headaches, and dimming of light.

Decentration of ablation zone

Decentration of the ablation zone may occur because of inadequate fixation by the patient and because of an inadequate method of marking the optical center during PRK. Maloney[45] calculated the percentage of light rays falling on the retina that miss the OZ (Table 174-15), assuming a 4 mm optical zone and entrance pupil. Indeed, according to this author, a 1 mm decentration would result in a blurred ghost image and monocular diplopia. The Stiles-Crawford effect may reduce the intensity of this phenomenon. Several authors[22,30,46] clinically documented this finding and the presence of decreased uncorrected and BCVA in decentrations exceeding 1 mm. An extreme case is described in which uncorrected vision was 20/12 in bright light, whereas it was less than 20/200 in dim light because of decentration of the ablation zone. The amount of decentration was not documented.[22]

Treatment of significant decentration is difficult. If there is associated significant undercorrection, one may attempt retreatment after thoroughly evaluating

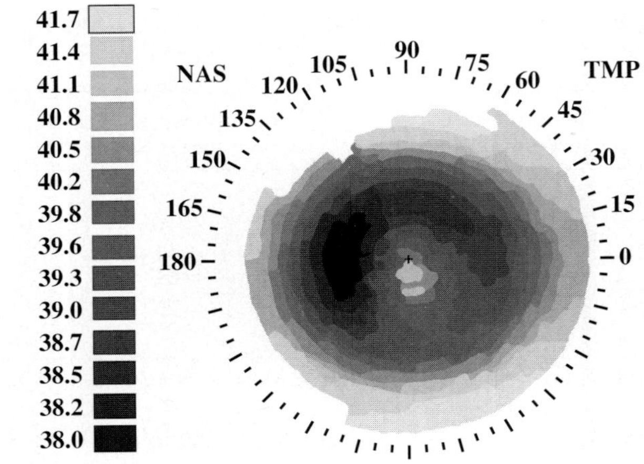

FIGURE 174-12 Topographic map of a central island.

the topography of the affected cornea. When residual myopia is present, one may attempt to treat it with a larger OZ to include the decentered area. At the same time, no reported cases of retreatment under these circumstances have been published. Small amounts of decentration should not be treated, since they rarely induce symptoms.

Central islands

Various topographic abnormalities have been described after excimer ablation. Lin et al identified four topographic patterns: (1) a uniform circular ablation (44% to 45%); (2) a central island of steepened cornea within the ablative zone (10% to 26%); (3) a keyhole ablative pattern (12%); and (4) a semicircular ablative pattern (18% to 33%).[47] Both the keyhole and the semicircular patterns demonstrated inadequate inferior ablations predominantly. Visual acuity was still excellent with BCVA often maintained.[47] The most significant topographic abnormality observed with respect to patient symptoms was the central island.

The definition of a central island is a central or pericentral steepening (1) of at least 1 to 3 diopters in height; (2) with a diameter of at least 1 to 3 mm; (3) measured at least 1 month postoperatively, and (4) associated with clinical symptoms of monocular diplopia, ghosting of images, or qualitative visual changes (Figure 174-12). Factors increasing central islands include (1) lasers with nonhomogeneous or flat energy beam profiles; (2) single zone techniques; (3) large OZs; (4) moderate or severe degrees of myopia; and (5) moist corneas intraoperatively.

There are four main theories as to the cause of central islands: (1) focal central epithelial hyperplasia; (2) vortex plume theory; (3) degradation of laser optics; and (4) acoustic shock wave theory. Central island formation is probably multifactorial.

Cases of focal epithelial hyperplasia have been documented in patients with central islands with corneal topography. However, these islands invariably are short lived and are clinically different. Patients do not have the classic ghosting of images commonly associated with central island formation. There is also no explanation as to why the epithelium would heal differently after myopic ablation with the Summit Excimed UV200 LA laser. The epithelium appears clinically normal in almost all cases of central islands. A diagnosis of central island formation is made from the association of clinical symptoms described by the patient and corneal topography, not by slit lamp examination.

The "vortex plume theory" proposed that the emitted plume of ablative debris forms a random vortex that centrally blocks successive pulses. This theory was advanced by Klyce based on his observation that central islands were detected once nitrogen blow was discontinued.[48] However, this theory fails to explain why central islands, although observed with the VISX, Taunton, and Technolas lasers, were essentially nonexistent with the Summit Excimed UV 200 unit. The Summit Excimed laser had no vacuum aspiration system, and the pulse repetition rate was twice that of the VISX, allowing half the time for plume dissipation before the next pulse, which, according to the vortex plume theory, should have resulted in a higher incidence of central islands.

Lin and other investigators have proposed that degradation of the beam optics centrally would result in a less ablative effect centrally.[47] Central islands, however, have been observed with normal calibration test plastics after replacement of optics as well as on new laser systems. In addition, nitrogen flow or the method of epithelial removal should have no effect on the incidence of central islands if the primary cause were a defect within the optical pathway, as clinically noted.

The theory that seems to have gained acceptance is that based on the acoustic shock wave model.[49] This model is based on clinical impressions while using both the Summit Excimed UV 200 and the VISX 20/20 excimer lasers. In over 1,500 cases, no central islands were seen with the Summit Excimed laser. However, a 17% incidence of central islands with the VISX 20/20 laser was noted.

In a study of 167 eyes of 97 consecutive patients, aged 20 to 58 years, of which 70% of participants were male, five operative techniques were studied prospectively for the incidence of central islands. Preoperative myopia ranged from −1.00 to −12.75 diopters, with up to −3.50 diopters of cylinder. The first three techniques were designed to look at the role of the VISX vacuum aspiration system on the incidence of central islands. The latter two techniques examined the

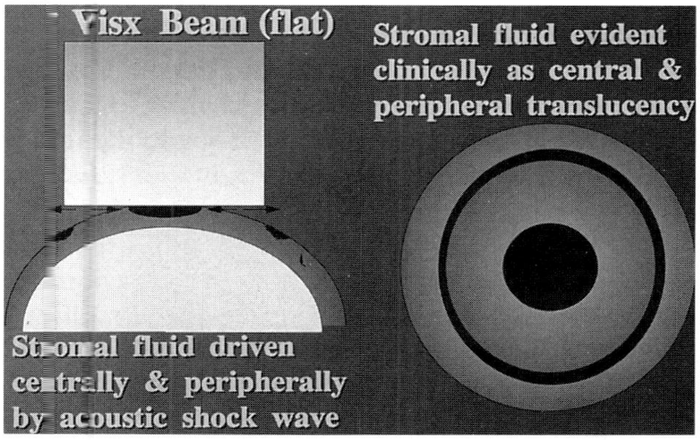

FIGURE 174-13 Fluid dynamics during ablation with the VISX laser as observed clinically, explaining the formation of a central island.

effect of central fluid accumulation. The basic technique involved blunt epithelial debridement followed by a no-blow PRK technique with patient self-fixation. A multizone technique was used for procedures above −6.00 diopters, and a 6 mm OZ was used for all single zone treatments.

The incidence of central islands in the first three subgroups ranged from 16.7% to 11.1%, as the vacuum aspiration system was turned off, then modified to have a wide nozzle, reducing air turbulance. The fourth subgroup was treated with a stall and wipe technique, whereby the central stromal fluid was wiped clear with a blunt spatula every few seconds intraoperatively or allowed to evaporate with the low vacuum aspiration. The incidence of central islands was reduced in group IV to 10.3% at 3 months.

Based on differences in the intraoperative hydration pattern observed while performing procedures with the Summit Excimed UV 200 and the VISX 20/20 systems, it was postulated that the altered hydration pattern was the cause of central islands. The corneal stroma in the Summit laser subgroup appeared uniformly moist intraoperatively. In contrast, the stroma in the VISX subgroup became moist centrally, appearing as an area of increased translucency, with the midperiphery remaining relatively dry intraoperatively. The periphery remained somewhat moist, thus creating a target pattern (Figure 174-13). It was estimated that half the pulses were being blocked by the stromal fluid centrally and, therefore, were being rendered ineffective, that is, the pulse energy centrally was removing fluid rather than stromal tissue, or the stroma became more hydrated and less compact centrally.

Based on these observations, a "pretreatment technique" was developed, treating the central 2 to 3 mm of the cornea before PRK. The pretreatment consists of an ablation of 1 μm per diopter of correction for single zone ablations of up to 6.00 diopters, and 0.6 μm per diopter of correction for multizone ablations above 6.00 diopters. There was a dramatic improvement in both the qualitative and quantitative visual results with the elimination of central islands in the final treatment group of 43 eyes. An additional 120 procedures were performed using Machat's modified formula with no occurrence of central islands. Data on uncorrected visual acuities demonstrate that 97.7% of eyes in the pretreatment study group achieved uncorrected vision of 20/40 or better 6 months postoperatively. These patients also noted qualitative subjective improvement in their vision often relative to their fellow eye, which was not pretreated but had no central island. Refractive predictability was improved, with three quarters of pretreated patients, being within 0.50 diopter of emmetropia. Leaving a moist cornea helped preserve corneal clarity, with three quarters of pretreated eyes graded as trace haze or clear, with no cases of clinically significant or confluent haze observed.

According to the model by Machat, each pulse produces an acoustic shock wave, the pattern of which is related to the energy beam profile of the laser. Intraoperative stromal hydration patterns are determined by the acoustic shock wave pattern. Flat or homogeneous energy beam profiles produce central fluid accumulation intraoperatively that result in reduced ablation centrally. Based on the acoustic shock wave model, blowing nitrogen would reduce islands by drying this central fluid pocket. Since excessive drying produces increased corneal haze, some investigators have used humidified gases with success.[50] Removal of the epithelium with alcohol was found to reduce the incidence of central islands by altering the stromal fluid dynamics. Larger optical zones would be at greater risk of inducing islands because of both the larger shock wave amplitude and the tendency of the beam energy to drop centrally as the diameter is increased. One can use the analogy of a tent to understand that as the tent poles are spread apart, the tent begins to sag centrally. This is why there is an increased beam edge effect creating circular shock waves. A recent series of PRK patients with the VISX 20/20 with a reduced fluence of 120 mj/cm^2 from the VISX standard of 160 mj/cm^2 resulted in an incidence of central islands greater than 90%. The effect of reduced fluence is to increase pulse-to-pulse variability, resulting in a less homogeneous beam profile and exacerbating the beam edge effect (Johnson, personal communication, ASCRS 1993 Summer Symposium). This dramatic increase in central island formation is best explained with this model. Single zone techniques for moderate myopia used the greatest number of successive pulses and therefore had the highest frequency of central islands in the study. Multizone techniques allow the stroma to dry between steps and, by starting each zone centrally, alter the

17. Buratto I, Ferrari M: Photorefractive keratectomy for myopia from 6.00 to 10.00D, *Refract Corneal Surg* 9(Suppl):34-36, 1993.
18. Lavery FL: Photorefractive keratectomy in 472 eyes, *Refract Corneal Surg* 9(Suppl):98-100, 1993.
19. Maloney RK et al: A prototype erodible mask delivery system for the excimer laser, *Ophthalmology* 100:542-549, 1993.
20. McDonnel PJ et al: Photorefractive keratectomy to create toric ablations for correction of astigmatism, *Arch Ophthalmol* 109: 710-713, 1991.
21. Saedi NF, Krueger RR, McDonnel PJ: Clinical analysis of excimer laser photorefractive keratectomy for compound myopic astigmatism, *Invest Ophthalmol Vis Sci* 35(Suppl):2022, 1994.
22. Taylor HR et al: Comparison of excimer laser treatment of astigmatism and myopia, *Arch Ophthalmol* 111:1621-1626, 1993.
23. Kim YJ, McDonnel PJ: Photorefractive keratectomy for astigmatism. In Salz JJ, editor: *Corneal laser surgery,* St Louis, 1994, Mosby.
24. Dausch D, Klein R, Schröder E: Excimer laser photorefractive keratectomy for hyperopia, *Refract Corneal Surg* 9:20-28, 1993.
25. Macy JI, Nesburn AB, Salz JJ: Laser correction of hyperopia, VISX blind eye study, United States results. In Salz JJ, editor: *Corneal laser surgery,* St Louis, 1994, Mosby.
26. Maguen E et al: Effect of nitrogen flow on recovery of vision after excimer laser photorefractive keratectomy without nitrogen flow, *J Refract Corneal Surg* 10:321-326, 1994.
27. Talley AR et al: Results one year after using the 193 excimer laser for photorefractive keratectomy in mild to moderate myopia, *Am J Ophthalmol* 118:304-311, 1994.
28. Lin D: *Ophthalmol Suppl* 1994.
29. Srinivas D et al: One year results of excimer laser photorefractive keratectomy for low to moderate myopia, *Arch Ophthalmol* 112:1427-1436, 1994.
30. Gimbel HV, Van Westenbrugge JA, Johnson WH: Visual, refractive, and patient satisfaction results following bilateral photorefractive keratectomy, *Refract Corneal Surg* (Suppl)9:S5-S10, 1993.
31. Gartry DS, Kerrmuir MG, Marshall J: Excimer laser photorefractive keratectomy. 18-month follow-up, *Ophthalmology* 99:1209-1219, 1992.
32. Wilson SE et al: Changes in corneal topography after excimer laser photorefractive keratectomy for myopia, *Ophthalmology* 90:1338-1347, 1991.
33. Tengroth B et al: Effects of corticosteroids in postoperative care following photorefractive keratectomies, *Refract Corneal Surg (Suppl)* 9:S61-S64, 1993.
34. Carones F, Brancato R, Venturi E: Efficacy of corticosteroids in reversing regression after myopic photorefractive keratectomy, *Refract Corneal Surg (Suppl)* 9(2):S52-S56, 1993.
35. McDonald MB et al: Central photorefractive keratectomy for myopia. Partially sighted and normally sighted eyes, *Ophthalmology* 98:1327-1337, 1991.
36. Pepose JS et al: Reactivation of latent herpes simplex virus by excimer laser photokeratectomy, *Am J Ophthalmol* 114:45-50, 1992.
37. Serdahl CL et al: Infiltrative keratitis associated with disposable soft contact lenses, *Arch Ophthalmol* 107:332-333, 1989.
38. Nilsson SEG, Montan PG: The annualized incidence of contact lens induced keratitis in Sweden and its relation to lens type and wear schedule: results of a 3-month prospective study, *CLAO J* 20:225-230, 1994.
39. Nesburn AB, Maguen E, Caroline PC: A method for sterile insertion of soft contact lenses, *Contact Lens Spectrum* p. 19, March 1992.
40. Wilson LA: Tight lens syndrome in contact lenses. In Dabezies O Jr, editor: *Contact lenses: the CLAO guide to basic and clinical practice,* New York, 1984, Grune & Stratton.
41. Waring GO, Rodrigues MM, Laibson PR: Corneal dystrophies. I. Dystrophies of the epithelium, Bowman's layer and stroma, *Surv Ophthalmol* 23:71-122, 1978.
42. Kim JH, Hahn TW, Lee YC: Photorefractive keratectomy in 202 myopic eyes, 1-year results, *Refract Corneal Surg (Suppl)* 9:S11-S15, 1993.
43. Machat JJ, Tayfour F: Photorefractive keratectomy for myopia, preliminary results in 147 eyes, *Refract Corneal Surg (Suppl)* 9:S16-S18, 1993.
44. Roberts CW, Koester CJ: Optical zone diameters for photorefractive corneal surgery, *Invest Ophthalmol Vis Sci* 34:2275-2281, 1993.
45. Maloney RK: Corneal topography and optical zone location in photorefractive keratectomy, *Refract Corneal Surg* 6:363-371, 1990.
46. Maguire LJ et al: Topography and raytracing analysis of patients with excellent visual acuity 3 months after excimer laser photorefractive keratectomy for myopia, *Refract Corneal Surg* 7:122-128, 1991.
47. Lin DTC, Sutton HF, Berman M: Corneal topography following excimer photorefractive keratectomy for myopia. *J Cataract Refract Surg Suppl* 19:149-154, 1993.
48. Parker PJ et al: Central topographic islands following photorefractive keratectomy, *Invest Ophthalmol Vis Sci Suppl* 34:803, 1993.
49. Maguen E, Machat JJ: Complications of photorefractive keratectomy, primarily with the VISX excimer laser. In Salz JJ editor: *Corneal laser surgery,* St Louis, 1994, Mosby.
50. Krueger RR et al: Corneal surface morphology following excimer laser ablation with humidified gases, *Arch Ophthalmol* 111: 1131-1137, 1993.
51. Seiler T, Wollensak J: Myopic photorefractive keratectomy with the excimer laser, *Ophthalmology* 98:1156-1163, 1991.
52. Pallikaris IG et al: Paraformaldehyde-induced keratitis after photorefractive keratectomy, *Am J Ophthalmol* 114:339-344, 1992.
53. Kim JH, Hahn TW, Lee YC: Clinical experience of two-step photorefractive keratectomy in 19 eyes with high myopia, *Refract Corneal Surg (Suppl)* 9:S44-S47, 1992.
54. Hersh PS, Jordan AJ, Mayers M: Corneal graft rejection episode after excimer laser phototherapeutic keratectomy, *Arch Ophthalmol* 111:735-736, 1993.

CHAPTER 175

DIMITRI T. AZAR SANDEEP JAIN WALTER STARK

Phototherapeutic Keratectomy

The excimer laser was introduced as a prospective tool in corneal surgery in 1983 and was later used in investigational protocols to treat patients with corneal pathologic conditions.[1] High energy ultraviolet light is emitted by the excimer laser to ablate corneal tissue with submicron precision without significant injury to nonablated tissue.[1-3] It can be used for reshaping the corneal curvature, for controlled removal of corneal tissue, or in reconstructive superficial keratectomy. In phototherapeutic keratectomy (PTK) the excimer laser is used to remove the anterior layers of the cornea. Excimer laser ablation has great potential to treat corneal opacities and to smooth corneal surface irregularities. The depth and shape of excimer laser ablative photodecomposition can be accurately controlled,[3-6] allowing for exact removal of the stroma and providing a relatively smooth base for better reepithelialization.[1,3,6]

Advantages of PTK over Mechanical Keratectomy Techniques

The excimer laser provides corneal surgeons with an excellent instrument for the management of anterior stromal opacities.[6] As opposed to nonlaser corneal surgery, there is a very clear boundary between the treated and untreated area at the ultrastructural level.[7] Reepithelialization and wound healing begin shortly after surgery and are associated with a relatively small degree of tissue reorganization.[7,8] Incisions made with diamond and steel blades produce irregular and more diffuse tissue damage as compared to the 193 nm argon fluoride excimer laser.[7] This is also in contrast to the 248 nm krypton excimer laser, which produces irregular and scattered areas of tissue damage.

The far ultraviolet (193 nm) laser radiation is thought to be within the limits of safety for the human eye. Adjacent tissues undergo minimal distortion and suffer no apparent thermal damage after 193 nm excimer laser PTK. The stromal lamellae show no evidence of distant disorganization.[1,3,4,6] There is evidence of endothelial cell loss when the remaining unablated stromal thickness is 40 μm or less.[6] It is not clear, however, whether similar endothelial loss would occur with equally deep mechanical lamellar dissection. Successfully treated patients can postpone or avoid more invasive surgical procedures, such as penetrating or lamellar keratoplasty.[1]

Indications for PTK

Opacities resulting from surgical or nonsurgical trauma, corneal inflammations, dystrophies, and degenerations limited to the anterior corneal layers have been successfully treated with PTK. Of 271 consecutive PTK cases at 17 VISX U.S. centers reviewed by Sanders, 55% of patients had corneal scars or leukomas, 39% had corneal dystrophies, and 5% had corneal surface irregularities.[9,10]

Surface irregularities resulting from epithelial dystrophies, Reis-Bücklers' dystrophy, band keratopathy, peripheral corneal degenerations, and corneal surgical procedures can be improved with PTK, especially if the surface irregularities are associated with significant visual impairment. PTK is less effective in treating deep scars, nodules, and band keratopathy. Calculated posttreatment corneal thickness should not be less than 250 μm. The use of PTK to treat microbial keratitis, including infectious crystalline keratopathy,[11-14] is very limited because of the risk of spreading microorganisms during treatment.[15]

Hyperopia may be a relative contraindication for PTK, because PTK results in further flattening of the cornea. Keratoconjunctivitis is a relative contradiction. Uncontrolled uveitis, severe blepharitis, lagophthalmos, and systemic immunosuppression are contraindications under many protocols.

Surgical Technique

PREOPERATIVE EVALUATION

Under most investigational protocols, preoperative evaluation includes visual acuity, visual potential (evaluated with pinhole, hard contact lens, and potential acuity meter), pupil size, slit lamp biomicroscopy,

Table 175-1. Typical laser parameters for PTK

Parameter	VISX Twenty/Twenty	Summit Excimed 200	Meditec LV 2000	Technolos Keracor 116
Fluency (mJ/cm²)	160 ± 10	180	250	120-200
Repetition rate (Hz)	5	10	20	10
Ablation rate (μm/pulse)	0.20 to 0.27	0.25	0.5	—
Ablation diameter (mm)	5.5 to 6, including 0.5 mm transition zone	6.5	7.0	7.0

Modified from Azar DT et al: Phototherapeutic keratectomy: the VISX experience. In Salz JJ, McDonnell PJ, McDonald MB, editors: *Corneal laser surgery,* St Louis, 1995, Mosby.

and dilated fundus examination. The depth of the intended treatment is measured using an optical pachometer.

PREOPERATIVE PREPARATION

The laser is calibrated before each treatment to ensure optimal performance. The overall operation of the laser is confirmed by ablating a standard treatment into a calibration plate made of polymethylmethacrylate (PMMA) or other material, depending on the laser used. The appropriate corneal ablation rate is determined using nomograms and is entered into the laser computer program.

Currently, most procedures are performed with the patient under topical anesthesia. Before treatment the plane of the corneal surface is determined by focusing the microscope at high magnification. Poor centration of laser treatment may result in a suboptimal outcome.

LASER TREATMENT

Table 175-1 summarizes the laser parameters that are ordinarily adopted for PTK. Nitrogen gas flow, used during the PMMA calibration in some lasers, is rarely used today. The decision whether to ablate using the laser or to remove the epithelium manually is based on the smoothness of the epithelium relative to the envisioned smoothness of Bowman's layer.

A transition zone is usually created during stromal ablation. It is intended to allow smooth and uniform reepithelialization over the ablation bed. This procedure is referred to as "standard taper" ablation. Sher et al used a "smoothing" technique in their early cases, wherein the eye was moved in a circular manner under the laser beam.[16] A similar "polish technique" was used in the Summit excimer laser clinical trials. The surgeon moved the patient's head in a brisk controlled circular manner under the laser beam to "polish" the corneal surface.[17,18] Stark et al later described a "modified taper" technique, wherein the surgeon attempts to decrease central flattening by moving the eye under the laser in a circular fashion and treating the circumference of the ablation zone with a 20 μm deep, 2 mm diameter spot size.[1] This edge modification creates a ring-shaped ablation pattern at the periphery of the PTK to reduce the hyperopic shift that is seen after PTK. When corneal opacities or irregularities are associated with myopic refractive errors, a combination of PTK and photorefractive keratotomy (PRK) should be considered. By allowing for approximately 1 diopter of hyperopic shift for every 20 μm of stromal ablation, the need for PRK to correct any myopic refractive error is reduced. Talamo et al have described clinical treatment strategies for optimizing the successful application of PTK to the treatment of superficial corneal pathology.[19] Table 175-2 summarizes this approach.

SURFACE IRREGULARITIES

After epithelial removal, whether manually or using the laser, a masking fluid (1% hydroxymethylcellulose, 0.5% tetracaine or Tears Naturale II) is usually applied to improve the smoothness of the stromal surface. The fluid in valleys prevents ablation of underlying tissue, leaving the exposed peaks to be ablated. A highly viscous fluid (2% hydroxymethylcellulose or Healon) does not cover an irregular surface uniformly and tends to partially cover peaks as well as valleys. A fluid of low viscosity tends to expose both peaks and valleys. In addition to creating a smooth corneal surface, masking agents may reduce the amount of induced hyperopia.

RECURRENT CORNEAL EROSIONS

Patients suffering from recalcitrant recurrent corneal erosions (map-dot-fingerprint dystrophy) may benefit from excimer PTK. The treatment depth is relatively minimal (5 to 10 μm) and is usually limited to Bowman's layer. Accordingly, significant postoperative hyperopic shift is not observed, and corneal wound healing is less prolonged. After epithelial debridement a Weck-Cel sponge can be used to sweep any residual deposits. In most cases of recurrent corneal erosions the use of surface modulators before laser ablation is not necessary.

CORNEAL DYSTROPHIES

Patients with recurrent granular or lattice dystrophy in a graft have relatively superficial lesions (Figures 175-1 and 175-2). The success rate in these cases is very

Table 175-2. Strategies for successful PTK

Pathologic lesion	Epithelial removal	Ablation technique	Masking fluid
Elevated, focal	No	Small spot size	Preoperatively, to adjacent normal epithelium
Extensive, evenly distributed	No	Large spot size "Smoothing" head rotation	Intraoperatively, if irregularities are increasing
Multiple, unevenly distributed	Yes	Varying spot size	Repeated focal application

From Azar DT et al: Phototherapeutic keratectomy: the VISX experience. In Salz JJ, McDonnell PJ, McDonald MB, editors: *Corneal laser surgery*, St Louis, 1995, Mosby.

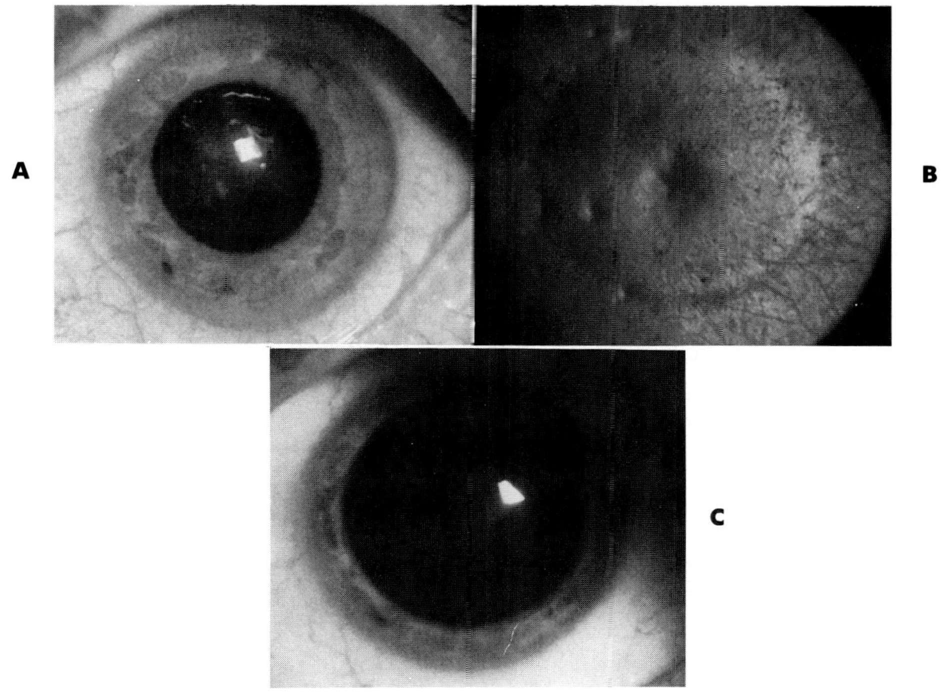

FIGURE 175-1 A 31-year-old man with a history of corneal lattice dystrophy underwent PTK. Preoperative best corrected visual acuity was 20/200. **A,** Note 75 μm stromal depth after epithelial ablation. **B,** Appearance of cornea 3 months after PTK by retroillumination. **C,** Marked improvement 24 months postoperatively. (From Azar DT et al: Phototherapeutic keratectomy: the VISX experience. In Salz JJ, McDonnell PJ, McDonald MB, editors: *Corneal laser surgery*, St Louis, 1995, Mosby.)

high and is similar to that for primary Reis-Bücklers' dystrophy, in which the deposits are limited to Bowman's layer[1] (Figure 175-3). Most patients achieve a relatively smooth ablation bed by treating through the epithelium. For patients with granular dystrophy involving the posterior stroma, the aim is to ablate most of the areas of diffuse haze between the granular deposits and not necessarily all the granular hyaline deposits (Figures 175-4 and 175-5).

CORNEAL SCARS

Treatment of corneal scars limited to the superficial stroma produces significant improvement in visual function.[1] Visual improvement with deeper postinfectious and posttraumatic scars is less likely to occur for several reasons.[15,20] The scar may ablate at rates different from that of the adjacent normal stroma, which may not benefit from laser ablation. This may result in postoperative irregular astigmatism. Peripheral elevated nodules may be treated with laser ablation after truncation with sharp blades. Central elevated nodules remain a major operative challenge.

POSTOPERATIVE MANAGEMENT

Postoperative medications include prophylactic antibiotics and anti-inflammatory agents. Sub-Tenon's

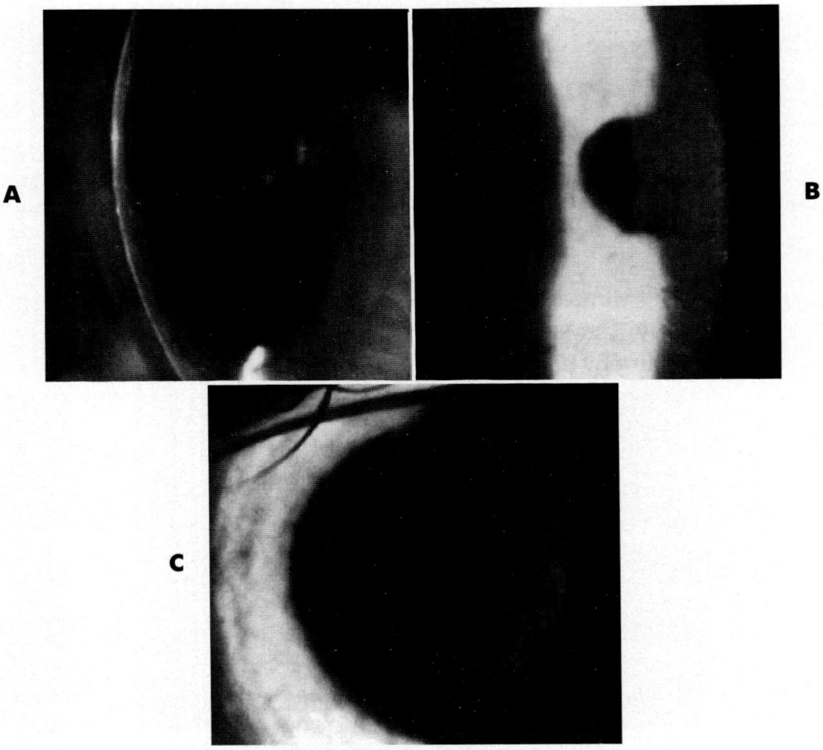

FIGURE 175-2 Lattice dystrophy. **A,** Preoperative appearance. **B,** Three months after phototherapeutic keratectomy. **C,** Nine months after PTK. (From Azar DT et al: Phototherapeutic keratectomy: the VISX experience. In Salz JJ, McDonnell PJ, McDonald MB, editors: *Corneal laser surgery,* St Louis, 1995, Mosby.)

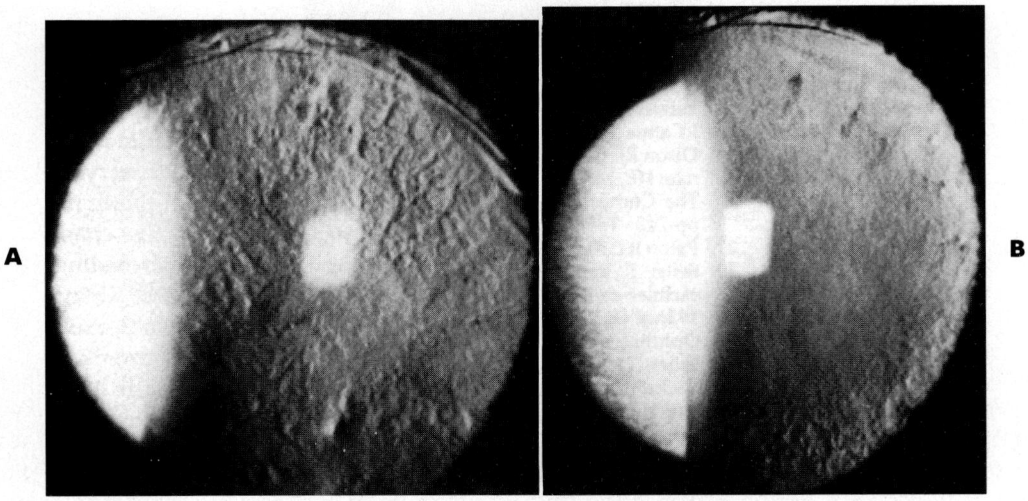

FIGURE 175-3 Reis-Bücklers' dystrophy. **A,** Pre-PTK and, **B,** 3 months postoperatively. (From Chamon W et al: *Ophthalmol Clin North Am* 6:399-413, 1993.)

injections of gentamicin and dexamethasone are given immediately postoperatively. After topical application of antibiotic ointment (bacitracin and erythromycin) and instillation of a cycloplegic agent (homatropine), the eye is patched. Alternatively, a therapeutic soft contact lens is applied with frequent application of comparable medications. Since the patient may experience severe pain in the first 24 hours, topical nonsteroidal anti-inflammatory agents and systemic sedative-analgesics may be needed for the first few

A 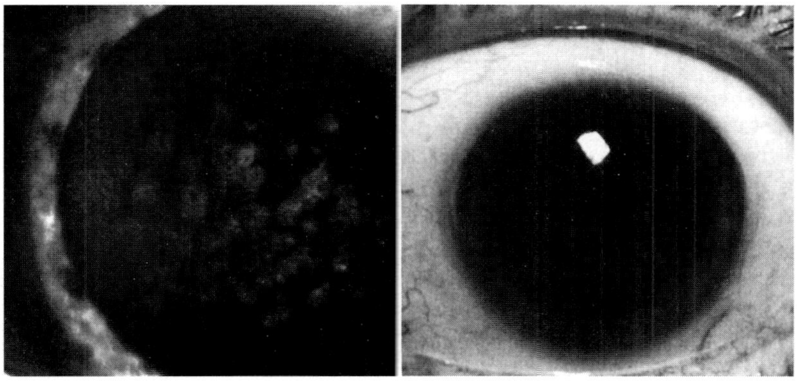 B

FIGURE 175-4 A 73-year-old woman with a history of granular dystrophy. The left eye was treated with 40 μm of stromal ablation combined with a modified tapering procedure. **A,** Preoperative clinical appearance of granular dystrophy and, **B,** 9 months postoperatively. (Reproduced from Azar DT et al: Phototherapeutic keratectomy: the VISX experience. In Salz JJ, McDonnell PJ, McDonald MB, editors: *Corneal laser surgery,* St Louis, 1995, Mosby.)

A 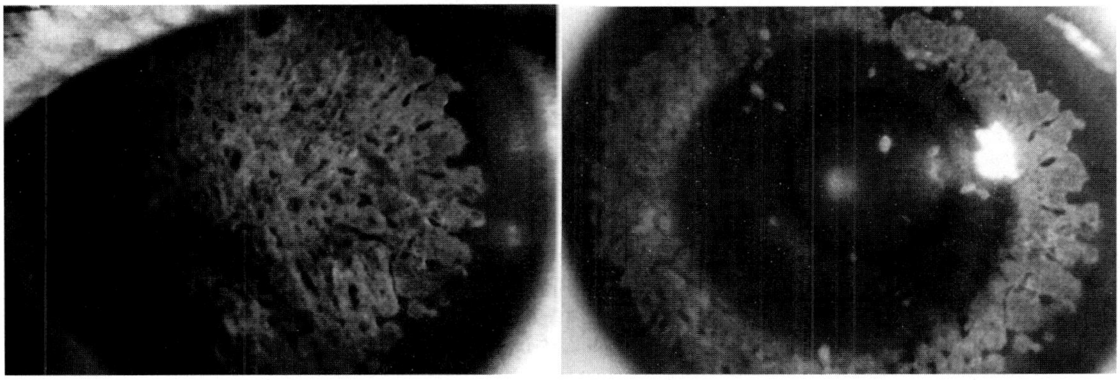 B

FIGURE 175-5 Preoperative, **A,** and 3 months' postoperative, **B,** appearance of a patient with granular dystrophy after 6 mm diameter, 195 μm deep PTK. The visual acuity improved from hand motion to 20/400. (From Azar DT et al: Phototherapeutic keratectomy: the VISX experience. In Salz JJ, McDonnell PJ, McDonald MB, editors: *Corneal laser surgery,* St Louis, 1995, Mosby.)

days. One percent prednisolone acetate or 0.1% fluorometholone drops are used four times daily for 1 week, then tapered to once daily by 1 month. The benefits of continued steroid drops may be outweighed by potential side effects, such as steroid-induced pressure elevation.

Most protocols require that patients be examined every 24 to 48 hours until reepithelialization, and then at 1 month, 3 months, 6 months, 12 months, and 24 months. Reepithelialization occurs within 1 week in most patients. After reepithelialization the postoperative examination at each visit includes symptomatic evaluation, a detailed anterior segment examination, and slit lamp biomicroscopy. In addition, all measurements (visual acuity, ocular pressure, etc.) taken during the preoperative evaluation are repeated.

Corneal haze is graded subjectively using slit lamp biomicroscopic examination as suggested by Fantes et al: 0 = clear; 0.5 = barely detectable; 1.0 = mild, not affecting refraction; 1.5 = mildly affecting refraction; 2.0 = moderate, refraction possible but difficult; 3.0 = opacity preventing refraction, anterior chamber easily viewed; 4.0 = impaired view of anterior chamber; and 5.0 = inability to see the anterior chamber. The cornea is divided into five hypothetical layers (superficial and deep epithelium, anterior and posterior stroma, and endothelium), and each layer is graded separately.

Subjective methods of grading corneal haze are not accurate and reproducible and suffer from interobserver variability and bias. Objective methods assess the magnitude of haze by measuring corneal light scattering. In collaboration with Dr. Russell McCally of the Applied Physics Laboratory at Johns Hopkins, we have developed an instrument for the objective measurement of haze. The "scatterometer" is a modified slit lamp microscope that measures backscattered light from a defined region of the cornea under standardized illumination conditions. Corneal light scattering is related to the degree of stromal scarring after excimer laser ablations. This instrument has been tested on laboratory animals and humans and found to yield reproducible results.[21] Both objective and subjective postoperative corneal clarity scores are usually lower than preoperative scores after PTK.[22]

Corneal Wound Healing After PTK

Reformation of basement membrane complexes and reestablishment of the basement membrane usually follow epithelial scrape wounds, resulting in a smooth epithelial surface with minimal stromal scarring.[1,6,10,23,24] Reepithelialization after excimer PTK usually occurs within the first week.[1-6,9,25,26] Anchorage of the epithelium to the stroma is achieved 1 to 3 months later, after adequate deposition of the adhesion structures (hemidesmosomes, basal lamina, and anchoring fibrils) of the new epithelium to the underlying stroma (Figures 175-6 and 175-7 and Table 175-3).[3,27]

Stromal wound healing occurs after formation of new corneal epithelium and while the adhesion structures are reforming. Some reports have noted that a pseudomembrane forms almost immediately after surgery. The pseudomembrane is thought to help hyperplastic migrating epithelial cells to fill in the wound and create a smooth epithelial surface.[3,25] Epithelial hyperplasia and stromal collagen deposition help restore the original corneal surface contour of shallow wounds.[1,5,25] Generally, hyperplasia takes place in deeper ablations and when there are apparent irregularities in the stromal bed.[10,24,26]

After reepithelialization a hypercellular zone of keratocytes is evident at the wound margins and within the anterior stroma.[3,26] A residual stromal depression persists after deep PTK despite the deposition of newly synthesized collagen by the keratocytes.[10,24]

After surgery the cornea may remain hazy for several months. Haze may result from the deposition of new irregular collagen fibers or from light scattering by "activated" keratocytes in the wound.[2,5,6,25] Postoperative treatment with steroids may reduce the thickness

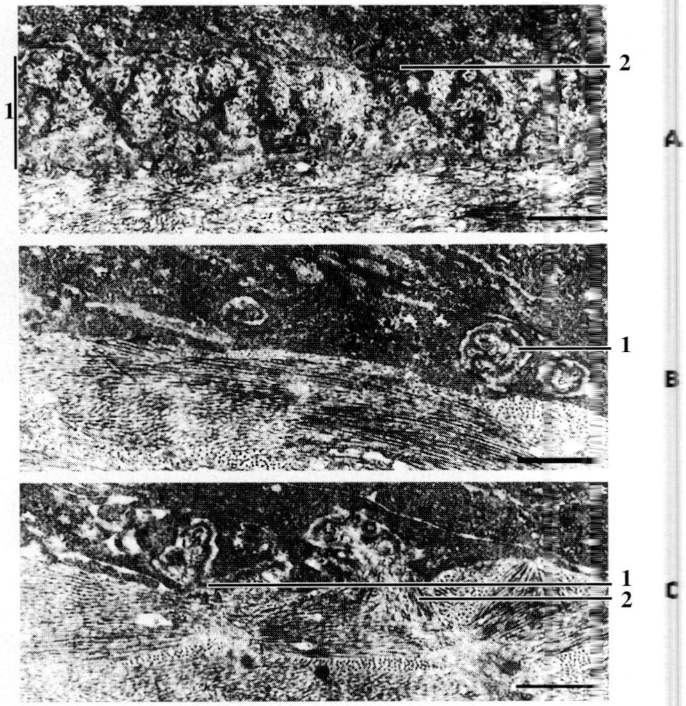

FIGURE 175-6 Electron microscopic findings 9 months after PTK for postkeratoplasty myopic astigmatism in a 43-year-old patient. **A**, Extensive duplication and multilamination of the basement membrane *(1)* and normal hemidesmosome reformation *(2)* at the sloping edge of treatment zone. **B**, Neighboring treated corneal regions showing areas of absent basement membrane and hemidesmosomes. Basal lamina can be seen in intracytoplasmic vacuoles *(1)* close to the basal cell membrane. **C**, Paracentral regions of the treated zone showing discontinuous basement membrane *(1)*. In this region, irregular collagen *(2)* is seen below the basal cell membrane. Bars indicate 1 μm. (From Fountain TR et al: *Arch Ophthalmol* 112:967-972, 1994.)

of the subepithelial layer of collagen and the density of subepithelial scarring.[5] Haze usually decreases after the 3- to 6-month period following surgery.[5,26]

When ablations are within 40 μm from Descemet's membrane, there is a loss of endothelial cells.[6-7] This may be related to acoustic or shock waves, and high pulse energy or resonance in the posterior cornea.[6,7,28] There is no evidence so far of endothelial cell loss or displacement if the ablations stay 40 μm above Descemet's membrane.[6,28,29]

Clinical Outcome

CLINICAL STUDY BACKGROUND

To date the clinical outcome of approximately 600 eyes, treated for various corneal diseases with excimer

A

B

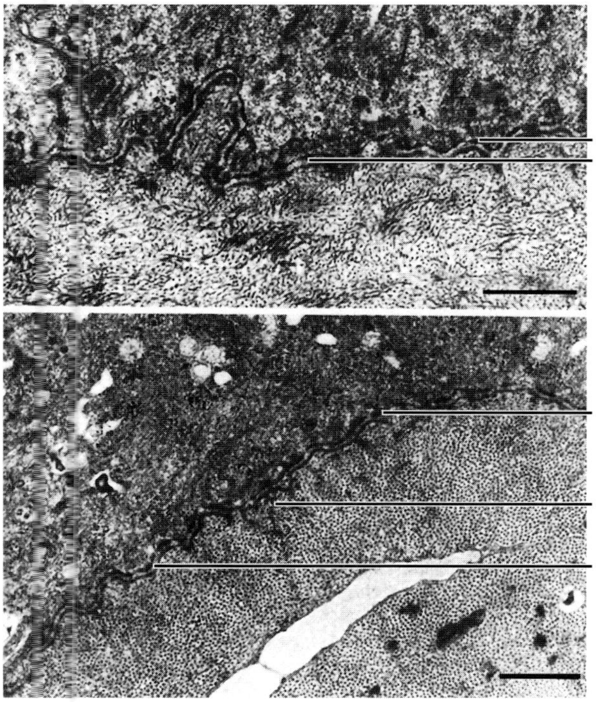

FIGURE 175-7 Epithelial basement membrane zones of two specimens obtained 11 months, **A**, and 15 months, **B**, after PTK in corneas with postinfectious scarring, **A**, and band keratopathy, **B**. Continuous unilamellar basement membrane *(1)* and abundant hemidesmosomes *(2)* are noted. Normal anchoring fibrils *(3)* are seen. Areas of abnormal basement membrane are not shown. Bars indicate 1 μm. (From Fountain TR et al: *Arch Ophthalmol* 112:967-972, 1994.)

Table 175-3. Reformation of hemidesmosomes and basal laminae after excimer laser PTK

Patient	Time after excimer laser (mo)	% of BCM occupied by HD	BL/100 μm^2 of BCM
1	6	37.7	18.0
2	9	36.1	49.6
3	11	35.2	19.0
4	15	36.2	24.4
Normal controls		24.5	32.0

From Fountain TR et al: *Arch Ophthalmol* 112:967-972, 1994.
*BCM, Basal cell membranes; HD, hemidesmosomes; BL, basal lamina.

laser PTK, has been reported in 26 published reports (Table 175-4). Four excimer lasers have been used: Twenty/Twenty,* LV 2000† (now VISX 20/15), Excimed 200,‡ and MEL 50.§ Thirty-six percent (203 eyes) were treated for recurrent corneal erosions, 20% (110 eyes) for corneal dystrophies, 16% (89 eyes) for corneal scars, 28% (157 eyes) for corneal irregularities, and one eye for recurrent corneal intraepithelial dysplasia.

RECURRENT EPITHELIAL EROSIONS AND CORNEAL DYSTROPHIES

Functional improvement was achieved in 77% of the 203 eyes after the initial treatment of recurrent epithelial erosions with PTK. In two studies the success rate improved to 95% (107/113) with retreatment. Corneal dystrophies and degenerations that have been treated with PTK to improve visual function or comfort include dystrophies of the epithelium and basement membrane (map-dot-fingerprint and Meesmann); dystrophies of Bowman's layer (Reis-Bücklers'); stromal dystrophies (granular, lattice, gelatinous droplike, macular, Schnyder), endothelial dystrophies (Fuchs'), and Salzmann nodular degeneration (Table 175-4). Greater success has been achieved in superficial corneal dystrophies like map-dot-fingerprint (100%), Meesmann (100%), and Reis-Bücklers' dystrophy (100%) than in stromal dystrophies like granular (67%), lattice (92%), and Schnyder dystrophy (67%).

CORNEAL SCARS

Corneal scars that have been successfully treated with PTK to improve visual function include postinfectious, posttraumatic, herpetic, trachomatous, and pterygium related. The success rate varies from 50% to 80%. Greater success has been achieved in superficial corneal scars such as those after pterygium surgery (80%) than in deeper postinfectious (50%) and posttraumatic scars (61%). One report has shown a high success rate in treating herpetic scars (80%). Despite the reported success, several investigators caution against using the excimer laser in herpetic disease because of the risk of recurrence.[1,10,20,45]

CORNEAL IRREGULARITIES

Corneal irregularities that have been successfully treated with PTK to improve visual function include band keratopathy (smooth and rough) and apical scars in keratoconus (proud nebulae). Of the 136 eyes treated for band keratopathy, 91% improved, while 81% of the 21 eyes treated for apical scars in keratoconus improved. As opposed to O'Bart's high success rate (113/122) in treating band keratopathy, other investigators have had little success.[16,20] The use of ethylene diamine tetraacetate (EDTA) remains the standard treatment for this condition.[1,10,16,20]

*VISX Inc., Santa Clara, CA.
†Taunton Technologies Co., Monroe, CT.
‡Summit Technologies Inc., Waltham, MA.
§Aesculap Meditec, Heroldsberg, Germany.

Table 175-4. PTK in corneal diseases

Pathology	Excimer laser used				Eyes	Follow-up (months)	Success (%)	References
	VISX	Summit	Meditec	Taunton				
Recurrent epithelial erosions	+	+	+	+	203	16.5	77%	30-37
Corneal dystrophies								
Reis-Bücklers'	+	+	−	+	32	6.2	100%	34,35,37-42
Lattice	+	+	−	−	25	11	92%	1,20,37,42
Granular	+	+	−	+	20	7.2	70%	1,16,20,34,35, 40,42
Salzmann's nodular	+	+	−	+	12	8.6	67%	1,16,34,35,37
Map-dot-fingerprint	+	+	−	−	10	5.2	100%	20,42
Schnyder	+	+	−	−	6	6	67%	34,35,42
Avellino	−	−	+	−	1	12	100%	43
Gelatinous droplike	−	+	−	−	1	4	100%	44
Meesmann's	+	+	−	−	2	9	100%	42
Fuchs' endothelial	+	+	−	−	1	9	100%	42
Corneal scars								
Postinfectious	+	+	−	+	12	8.5	50%	16,20,40
Posttraumatic	+	+	−	+	23	11.1	61%	16,20,32-35
Herpetic	+	+	−	+	24	15	71%	16,45,46
Trachomatous	−	+	−	−	3	6	67%	47
Pterygium	+	+	−	+	10	11.2	80%	16,32,34,35, 37,40
Stevens-Johnson syndrome	−	+	−	−	3	11.7	67%	32
Contact lens wear–related	+	+	−	−	2	3	50%	35,37
Unknown etiology	+	+	−	−	12	14.6	50%	1,35,37,48
Corneal irregularities								
Band keratopathy	+	+	−	+	136	12.3	91%	16,20,32, 37,49
Apical scars in keratoconus	+	+	−	−	21	9.7	81%	16,32,34,35, 50,51
Corneal intraepithelial dysplasia	−	−	+	−	1	26	100%	52

RESULTS OF MAJOR CLINICAL STUDIES

Representative postoperative results published in the five major reports are summarized in Table 175-5. The data comparing preoperative to postoperative best corrected visual acuity accumulated by Sanders from 271 consecutive PTK cases at 17 VISX U.S. centers are shown in Figures 175-8 to 175-11.[10] The average improvement in best corrected visual acuity was 1.8 lines ($p < 0.0001$). Ten percent (10%) of patients lost two or more lines of best corrected visual acuity, while 45% gained two or more lines. Seven percent (7%) of the patients lost three or more lines, while 36% gained that much. Analysis of the reasons for decreases in best corrected visual acuity showed corneal surface irregularity induced by PTK accounting for only 3% of cases. Two or more lines of improvement of uncorrected visual acuity were seen in 42% to 44% of patients, as opposed to reduction in 18% to 19% (Figure 175-8). Based on the dates of treatment, Sanders divided the 271 patients treated at U.S. VISX centers into quartiles.[10] He found that the first quartile had an average of 5.5 diopters of hyperopic effect and the last quartile had less than 2 diopters of hyperopia (Figure 175-9). The percentages of patients in Sanders' review who experienced moderate to severe levels of pain and tearing before treatment were 10% and 8%, respectively. Of these patients, only one experienced postoperative tearing; the rest were improved. Similarly, there was no significant worsening of photophobia, redness, or foreign body sensation. The effect of PTK on patients with moderate to severe epithelial corneal opacities shows that 86% to 88% of patients improved after treatment, and in only 1% did the condition worsen (Figure 175-10). From 60% to 62% of patients with anterior stromal opacities improved after treatment, and 2% worsened (Figure 175-11).[10]

Sher et al reported that 15% of patients lost two or more lines of spectacle-corrected visual acuity after PTK.[16] Chamon et al reported a 3% loss of one line of functional visual acuity, defined as the acuity achieved

Table 175-5. Results of major PTK

	Sher[16] (1991)	**Chamon[53] (1993)**	**Campos[20] (1993)**	**Sanders[10] (1995)**	**Durrie[18] (1995)**
Excimer laser	Taunton LV 2000	VISX Twenty/Twenty	VISX Twenty/Twenty	VISX Twenty/Twenty	Summit Excimed 200
Ablation technique	Myopic Combined Smoothing	Standard taper Modified taper	Uniform depth (disk ablation) Standard taper Modified taper	Uniform depth	Polish technique
Visual acuity (%)					
Better	48	74	61	80	67
Unchanged	36	16	28	10	28
Worse	15	10	11	10	11
Hyperopic shift (%)	50	Greater in standard taper	56	Greater in early treatments	20*
Best results (>75% success)	Keratoconus (apical scar)	Corneal dystrophies (lattice, granular, and Reis-Bückler's) Salzmann's degeneration	Corneal dystrophies (lattice, granular, and map-dot-fingerprint)	—	Corneal dystrophies (lattice, Schnyder's, Reis-Bückler's) Recurrent erosions Corneal scars
Moderate results (50%-75% success)	Corneal dystrophies Corneal scars Salzmann's nodule	Corneal scars Surgically induced myopia	—	—	
Poor results (<25% success)	Band keratopathy Recurrent erosions Herpetic scars	Band keratopathy Recurrent erosions	Band keratopathy Corneal scars		

Modified from Azar DT et al: Phototherapeutic keratectomy: the VISX experience. In Salz JJ, McDonnell PJ, McDonald MB, editors: *Corneal laser surgery,* St Louis, 1995, Mosby.
*Data calculated from scatterplot.

2. Salz JJ et al: One-year results of excimer laser photorefractive keratectomy for myopia, *Refract Corneal Surg* 8:270-273, 1992.
3. Gaster RN et al: Corneal surface ablation by 193 nm excimer laser and wound healing in rabbits, *Invest Ophthalmol Vis Sci* 30:90-97, 1989.
4. Trokel SL, Srinivasan R, Braren B: Excimer laser surgery of the cornea, *Am J Ophthalmol* 96:710-715, 1983.
5. Tuft SJ, Zabel RW, Marshall J: Corneal repair following keratectomy, *Invest Ophthalmol Vis Sci* 30:1769-1777, 1989.
6. Marshall J et al: Photoablative reprofiling of the cornea using an excimer laser: photorefractive keratectomy, *Lasers Ophthalmol* 1:23-44, 1986.
7. Marshall J et al: A comparative study of corneal incisions induced by diamond and steel knives and two ultraviolet radiations from an excimer laser, *Br J Ophthalmol* 70:482-500, 1986.
8. van Setten GB et al: Expression of tenascin and fibronectin in the rabbit cornea after excimer laser surgery, *Graefe's Arch Clin Exp Ophthalmol* 230:178-182, 1992.
9. Sanders D: Clinical evaluation of phototherapeutic keratectomy—VisX twenty/twenty excimer laser, FDA submission—written communication Feb, 1994.
10. Azar DT et al: Phototherapeutic keratectomy: the VISX experience. In Salz JJ, McDonnell PJ, McDonald MB, editors: *Corneal laser surgery,* St Louis, 1995, Mosby.
11. Keates RH, Drago PC, Rothchild EJ: Effect of excimer laser on microbiological organisms, *Ophthalmic Surg* 19:715-718, 1988.
12. Gottsch JD et al: Excimer laser ablative treatment of microbial keratitis, *Ophthalmology* 98:146-149, 1991.
13. Serdarevic O et al: Excimer laser therapy for experimental *Candida* keratitis, *Am J Ophthalmol* 99:534-538, 1985.
14. Eiferman RA, Forgey DR, Cook YD: Excimer laser ablation of infectious crystalline keratopathy, *Arch Ophthalmol* 110:18, 1992.
15. Pepose JS et al: Reactivation of latent herpes simplex virus by excimer laser photokeratectomy, *Am J Ophthalmol* 114:45-50, 1992.
16. Sher NA et al: Clinical use of 193-nm excimer laser in the treatment of corneal scars, *Arch Ophthalmol* 109:491-498, 1991.
17. Thompson V, Durrie DS, Cavanaugh TB: Philosophy and technique for excimer laser phototherapeutic keratectomy (review), *Refract Corneal Surg* 9:81-85, 1993.
18. Durrie DS, Schumer JD, Cavanaugh T: Phototherapeutic keratectomy: the VISX experience. In Salz JJ, McDonnell PJ, McDonald MB, editors: *Corneal laser surgery,* St Louis, 1995, Mosby.
19. Talamo JH, Steinert RF, Puliafito CA: Clinical strategies for excimer laser therapeutic keratectomy, *Refract Corneal Surg* 8:319-324, 1992.
20. Campos M et al: Clinical follow-up of phototherapeutic keratectomy for treatment of corneal opacities, *Am J Ophthalmol* 115:433-440, 1993.
21. McCally RL et al: A simple device for objective measurement of haze following excimer ablation of cornea, *SPIE* 1877:20-25, 1993.
22. Braunstein RE et al: Objective measurement of corneal haze in human corneas following excimer laser keratectomy, *Invest Ophthalmol Vis Sci* 34(Suppl):2013, 1994.
23. Azar DT, Chamon W, Stark WJ: Phototherapeutic keratectomy. In: Stenson S, editor: *Surgical management in external diseases of the eye,* Tokyo, Igaku-Shoin (in preparation).
24. Azar DT: Epithelial and stromal wound healing following excimer laser keratectomy, *Semin Ophthalmol* 9:102-105, 1994.
25. Courant D et al: Corneal wound healing after photokeratomileusis treatment on the primate eye, *Laser Light Ophthalmol* 3:189-195, 1990.
26. Hanna KD et al: Corneal stromal wound healing in rabbits after 193-nm excimer laser surface ablation, *Arch Ophthalmol* 107:899-900, 1989.
27. Fountain TR et al: Reassembly of corneal epithelial adhesion structures after excimer laser keratectomy in humans, *Arch Ophthalmol* 112:967-972, 1994.
28. Bende T, Seiler T, Wollensak J: Side effects in excimer corneal surgery: corneal thermal gradients, *Graefe's Arch Clin Exp Ophthalmol* 226:277-280, 1988.
29. Ozler SA et al: Acute ultrastructural changes of cornea afer excimer laser ablation, *Invest Ophthalmol Vis Sci* 33:540, 1992.
30. Ohman L, Fagerholm P, Tengroth B: Treatment of recurrent corneal erosions with the excimer laser, *Acta Ophthalmol* 72:461-463, 1994.
31. Dausch D et al: Phototherapeutic keratectomy in recurrent corneal epithelial erosion, *Refract Corneal Surg* 9:419-424, 1993.
32. Fagerholm P et al: Phototherapeutic keratectomy: long-term results in 166 eyes, *Refract Corneal Surg* 9(Suppl):76-81, 1993.
33. Forster W et al: Phototherapeutic keratectomy in corneal diseases, *Refract Corneal Surg* 9(Suppl):85-90, 1993.
34. Rapuano CJ, Laibson PR: Excimer laser phototherapeutic keratectomy, *CLAO J* 19:235-240, 1993.
35. Rapuano CJ, Laibson PR: Excimer laser phototherapeutic keratectomy for anterior corneal pathology, *CLAO J* 20:253-257, 1994.
36. John ME et al: Excimer laser phototherapeutic keratectomy for treatment of recurrent corneal erosion, *J Cataract Refract Surg* 20:179-181, 1994.
37. Hersh PS et al: Phototherapeutic keratectomy: strategies and results in 12 eyes, *Refract Corneal Surg* 9(Suppl):90-95, 1993.
38. Rogers C, Cohen P, Lawless M: Phototherapeutic keratectomy for Reis Bucklers' corneal dystrophy, *Aust NZ J Ophthalmol* 21:247-250, 1993.
39. Lawless MA, Cohen PR, Rogers CM: Retreatment of undercorrected photorefractive keratectomy for myopia, *J Refract Corneal Surg* 10(Suppl):174-177, 1994.
40. Hahn TW, Sah WJ, Kim JH: Phototherapeutic keratectomy in nine eyes with superficial corneal disease, *Refract Corneal Surg* 9(Suppl):115-118, 1993.
41. McDonnell PJ, Seiler T: Phototherapeutic keratectomy with excimer laser for Reis-Buckler's corneal dystrophy, *Refract Corneal Surg* 8:306-310, 1992.
42. Orndahl M et al: Treatment of corneal dystrophies with excimer laser, *Acta Ophthalmol* 72:235-240, 1994.
43. Cennamo G et al: Phototherapeutic keratectomy in the treatment of avellino dystrophy, *Ophthalmologica* 208:198-200, 1994.
44. John ME et al: Excimer laser photoablation of primary familial amyloidosis of the cornea, *Refract Corneal Surg* 9(Suppl):138-141, 1993.
45. Vrabec MP et al: Electron microscopic findings in a cornea with recurrence of herpes simplex keratitis after excimer laser phototherapeutic keratectomy, *CLAO J* 20:41-44, 1994.
46. Fagerholm P, Ohman L, Orndahl M: Phototherapeutic keratectomy in herpes simplex keratitis: clinical results in 20 patients, *Acta Ophthalmol* 72:457-460, 1994.
47. Goldstein M et al: Phototherapeutic keratectomy in the treatment of corneal scarring from trachoma, *J Refract Corneal Surg* 10(Suppl):290-292, 1994.
48. McDonnell JM, Garbus JJ, McDonnell PJ: Unsuccessful excimer laser phototherapeutic keratectomy. Clinicopathologic correlation, *Arch Ophthalmol* 110:977-979, 1992.
49. O'Brart DP et al: Treatment of band keratopathy by excimer laser phototherapeutic keratectomy: surgical techniques and long term follow up, *Br J Ophthalmol* 77:702-708, 1993.

50. Steinert RF, Puliafito CA: Excimer laser phototherapeutic keratectomy for a corneal nodule, *Refract Corneal Surg* 6:352, 1990.
51. Moodaley L et al: Excimer laser superficial keratectomy for proud nebulae in keratoconus, *Br J Ophthalmol* 78:454-457, 1994.
52. Dausch D, Landesz M, Schroder E: Phototherapeutic keratectomy in recurrent corneal intraepithelial dysplasia, *Arch Ophthalmol* 112:22-23, 1994.
53. Chamon W et al: Phototherapeutic keratectomy, *Ophthalmol Clin North Am* 6:399-413, 1993.
54. Gartry D, Muir MK, Marshall J: Excimer laser treatment of corneal surface pathology: a laboratory and clinical study, *Br J Ophthalmol* 75:258-269, 1991.
55. Seiler T et al: Side effects in excimer corneal surgery: DNA damage as a result of 193 nm excimer laser radiation, *Graefe's Arch Clin Exp Ophthalmol* 226:276, 1988.
56. Krueger RR, Sliney DH, Trokel SL: Photokeratitus from subablative 193-nanometer excimer laser radiation, *Refract Corneal Surg* 8:274-279, 1992.

Table 176-1. Basic refractive mechanisms of intrastromal devices

Alloplastic device type	Refractive index dependent	Modify central corneal curvature
Central*—lenticular		
Pocket incision	+	−
Lamellar incision	−	+
Peripheral—ring/toroid	−	+

*Combinations of mechanisms possible.

Intrastromal implant types

Centrally placed: lenticular shaped
- Refractive index similar to cornea: modifies central corneal curvature; requires lamellar keratectomy; keratotomy
- Dissimilar refractive index: modifies effective corneal index of refraction; can use pocket dissections

Peripherally placed: ring-shaped, toroid, or arcuate
- Modifies central corneal curvature

Implant materials:
- Rigid or semi-rigid:
  - Homoplastic (human donor)
  - Xenogenic (e.g., porcine)
  - Synthetic or alloplastic
    - Nutrient impermeable to semipermeable—polymethylmethacrylate (PMMA), silicone, polysulfone
    - Relatively nutrient permeable—hydrogels, fenestrated materials
- Viscous or injectable
  - Gels, polymers

the cornea is considered in cross section with the anterior surface a fixed arc length, the addition of bulk in the corneal periphery pushes out the peripheral anterior and posterior corneal surfaces minutely, requiring compensatory central corneal flattening.[14-16] The stresses required to effect central corneal flattening are quite small and should be tolerated physiologically. Ring-shaped implants may also be suited to take advantage of the mechanical principles of circumferential centrifugal expansion or centripetal constriction (purse-string) to flatten or steepen central corneal curvature.[15,17]

Implants designed to be placed in mid to deep central stromal pockets routinely use material(s) with an index of refraction different from that of corneal stroma (n = 1.376).[18-21] These implants can directly modulate the cornea's refractive properties without necessarily altering anterior corneal curvature. They generally displace stroma and Descemet's membrane posterior to the lamellar dissection, since anterior stroma and Bowman's layer are relatively inelastic and resist curvature changes.

Physiologic Considerations of Intrastromal Devices

The corneal stroma and epithelium receive their nutrition by diffusion of essential chemicals from the aqueous humor and the limbal blood supply.[20-23] Intrastromal devices have the potential to block the diffusion of essential nutrients such as glucose to the stromal layers and epithelium anterior to the implant, resulting in stromal and epithelial atrophy, ulceration, and neovascularization.[1,24-26] Maurice postulated that extrusion of large nutrient-impermeable implants may occur because of nutritional deprivation.[22] He calculated that a disk 4 mm in diameter, impermeable to solute placed at full-thickness depth in the stroma, would completely block glucose diffusion to the central basal epithelium; placing the same disk closer to the epithelium or using a larger disk would result in a broader zone of glucose depletion.

Animal data support tolerance of relatively nonpermeable lenses such as polysulfone no larger than 5 mm in diameter.[27,28] Choyce implanted 5 to 6 mm polysulfone lenticular lenses into the posterior stroma of patients to correct aphakia and myopia and found some of these to be remarkably well tolerated, whereas others were not.[18,26]

To further predict the effect of stromal implants on nutrition of the anterior corneal layers, McCarey and Schmidt developed an electrical analog model of the cornea that predicts the availability of glucose to these corneal layers.[29] The model allows variation of the diameter, depth, permeability, and thickness of the stromal implant. The authors found that the most important physical characteristic for corneal tolerance of a 4 mm or larger intracorneal lens is its permeability to glucose. A water-impermeable midstromal lens of diameter 4 to 7 mm demonstrated a severe reduction in available epithelial glucose at the corneal apex for a constant thickness implant. In comparison, 70% hydrogel lenticules of equal diameters and thickness showed only a small reduction in available glucose. Decreasing the hydrogel implant thickness (e.g., as noted in the central portion of a myopic lenticule) allows an incremental improvement in central corneal glucose availability. Placing the lenticule more deeply in the stroma allows for an additional improvement in glucose availability because of improved lateral glucose diffusion across anterior stroma.

Figure 176-1 demonstrates calculations obtained for 5 mm midstromal −9 diopter lenticules of donor stroma and of 70% water hydrogel, +3 diopter 38.6% hydrogel, −9 diopter PMMA, and 1 mm wide PMMA stromal corneal ring. The data predict good apical stromal and epithelial glucose availability for the myopic stromal lenticules, the hyperopic hydrogel lenticules, and the intrastromal corneal ring. A severe reduction of central anterior stromal and epithelial glucose levels is noted for the PMMA lenticule.

Clinical and Histopathologic Observations

Tolerance of alloplastic intrastromal implants in animal models has been reviewed.[20,30-32] This tolerance noted in animal models has frequently not carried over to human studies. Polysulfone lenticules were initially reported as reasonably well tolerated in humans,[18,25,26] but no long-term reports of safety have been generated. Nutritional considerations are believed to be responsible for changes seen in stroma anterior to the implants, causing opacification and necrosis.[33] There are few reports of hydrogel lenses in humans, but these lenses still appear promising,[32-35] particularly with the adoption of smaller diameter inlays. ICRs composed of PMMA have been well tolerated up to 3 years postoperatively in blind eyes and for 2 years in sighted eyes.[5,36-38]

Complications associated with surgical implantation of intrastromal devices in patient eyes have been frequently reported, including problems related to faulty pocket or lamellar dissections and implantation of foreign bodies, such as lint and epithelial inclusions. Neovascularization originating from the limbus to the edges of some implants has been reported; this may be associated with faulty surface wound healing or as a reaction to stromal necrosis related to large impermeable implants.

Side effects and complications directly related to devices used in clinical study have been noted in some cases and are backed by histologic findings.* No significant inflammation has been seen in tissues surrounding the implants. Lenticular implants may have significant epithelial thinning and visually significant calcification, or other opacification formation in anterior stroma and Bowman's layer, as well as a reduction in adjacent stromal keratocyte population. Clinically significant fibrosis at the stromal interface surrounding hydrogel material has been observed in some cases, but not reported with polysulfone or PMMA implants. Amorphous or lipidlike deposits may be seen at the implant/stromal interface; when seen with the ICR, these tend to be an early finding and typically dissipate several months after implantation.

ICR may show collagen/proteoglycan deposits in the PMMA ring suture holes, suggesting a localized stromal space filling phenomenon. Deposits seen with other implants have also been imputed to represent a similar space-occupying, wound-healing mechanism.[30] Polysulfone, hydrogel, and PMMA implant surgeries have been associated with the formation of tiny refractile deposits in the vicinity of the implant/lamellar dissection interfaces. These deposits are nonprogressive and are not visually significant. At the time of this writing, no human studies have been performed with gel injection techniques to assess the clinical and histopathologic response; polyethylene oxide gel has been well tolerated in cats with up to 3 years follow-up.[6]

Removal of intrastromal implants has the potential for restoring the normal histology of the cornea, and in some cases the central cornea can return to its preoperative curvature. Reversibility has been demonstrated after explantation of hydrogel inlays and the ICR.[32,36,41]

*References 18, 25, 26, 32, 34, 37-40.

Current Device Investigations

Devices currently being investigated for long-term safety and efficacy in clinical trials conducted under FDA guidelines include the ICR and the small diameter corneal inlay (SDCI).†

ICR

Preliminary Studies

The ICR was introduced into the literature in 1987 by Fleming et al.[4] The prototype device was a relatively large-diameter, open-ended PMMA ring that used Reynolds' concept of mechanical ICR expansion and constriction to correct, respectively, myopia and hyperopia. The ring was inserted via a small peripheral corneal incision into a midstromal 360-degree lamellar channel created by an annular-shaped dissector. The dissector was novel in that it did not invade the central visual region of the cornea and could create an arcuate dissection via a small peripheral corneal incision. The early rabbit studies demonstrated excellent tolerance of the ring and the

†Chiron, Inc., Irvine, CA.

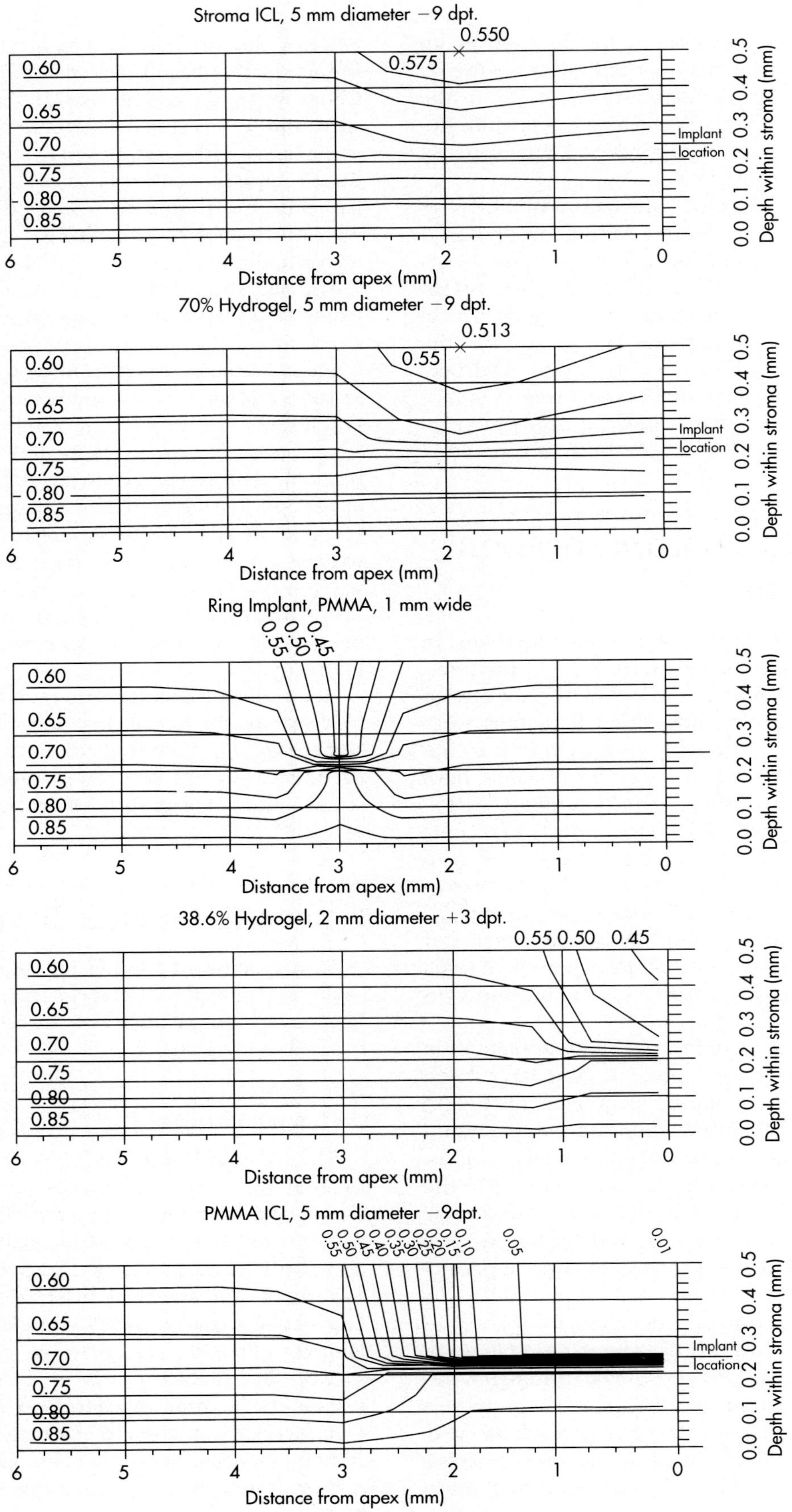

FIGURE 176-1 **Glucose availability curves for five different intrastromal devices placed at midperipheral depth. (Courtesy BE McCarey.)**

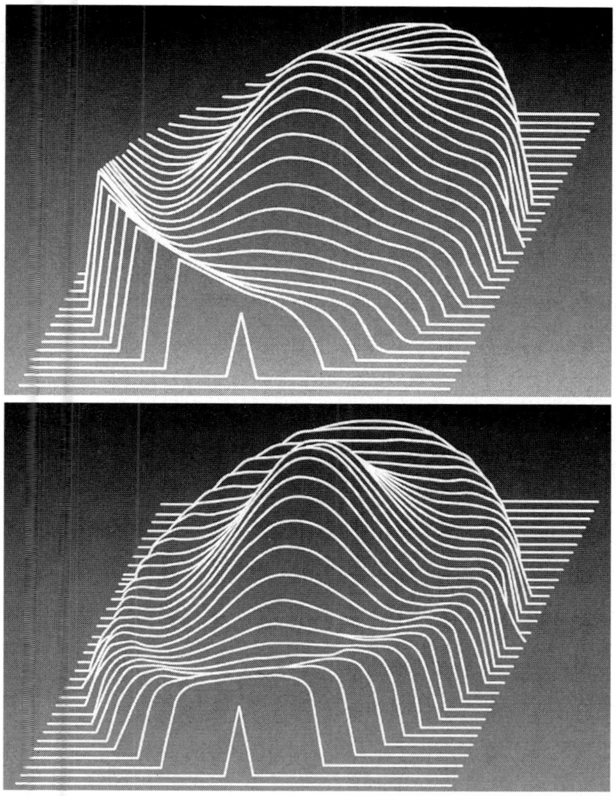

FIGURE 176-2 Laser holographic interferometry (wave unit map) of a cornea before *(top)*and after *(bottom)*implantation with a 0.3 mm ICR. Physiologic corneal positive asphericity remains intact postoperatively. (Courtesy KeraVision, Inc., Fremont, CA.)

capability of flattening and steepening the cornea keratographically.

Early eye bank eye studies in 1987 showed the preliminary ICR design to be too large for many human eyes; thus its dimensions were modified. Subsequent eye bank eye studies confirmed the efficacy of expansion for flattening the central cornea,[15] but, of importance for current ICR designs, approximately 3.5 diopters of central corneal flattening could be obtained simply from the 0.3 mm thickness of the ICR itself. Subsequent eye bank eye and patient studies have used the thickness principle alone for the correction of low to moderate myopia.[14,15] A performance curve has been generated with videokeratography and laser holographic interferometry in eye bank eyes, which suggests between 7 and 10 diopters of myopic correction can be obtained from the thickest ICR tested.

Eye bank eye studies have also demonstrated that the ICR can maintain the natural positive asphericity that is routinely present in the normal central cornea.[42] A laser holographic interferometer study of a cornea preoperatively and after implantation with a 0.30 mm ICR is shown in Figure 176-2. The cornea is positively

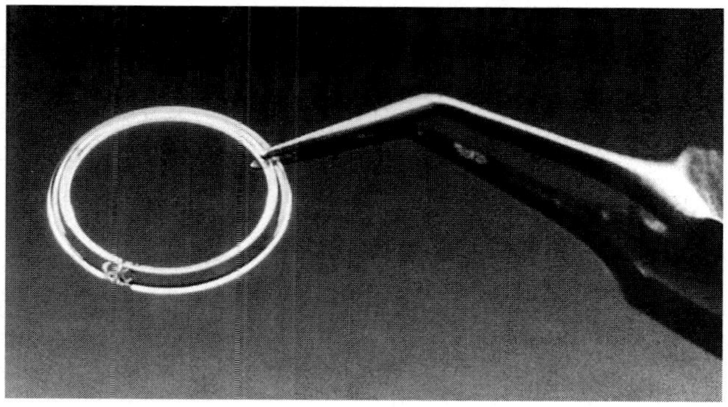

FIGURE 176-3 ICR. (Courtesy KeraVision, Inc., Fremont, CA.)

aspheric in both examinations. This would provide a theoretical contrast sensitivity advantage over most other refractive surgical techniques, which can induce negative corneal asphericity and attendant increased spherical aberration. This concept must be investigated in comparative clinical trials using sensitive measures of central corneal curvature, such as laser holographic interferometry and clinical tools that discern subtle losses of visual function, for example, contrast sensitivity testing.

Operative procedure

The ICR procedure may be performed under topical anesthesia for cooperative patients. The visual axis is marked, and the peripheral corneal thickness is measured by pachymetry over the incision site, typically at 12 o'clock.[15] A diamond knife is set to 66% of the peripheral corneal thickness and is used to create a small incision allowing introduction of the channeling tool. A Suarez spreader is used to initiate the lamellar dissection. The intrastromal channel is created with a proprietary set of instruments.* A vacuum centering guide is applied to the globe, and the stromal dissector is introduced through the incision and rotated to create the midperipheral circular channel. The dissector is rotated out of the channel, and the vacuum centering guide is removed. One end of the open-ended ICR (Figure 176-3) is inserted into the channel, and the ring is dialed into place. The leading and trailing ends of the ICR may then be attached to each other, and the corneal incision is closed with 10-0 nylon sutures. A bandage contact lens or eye patch may be placed for the immediate postoperative period.

Clinical trials

The first ICRs in human nonfunctional eyes were placed by Walton Nosé et al, Sao Paulo, Brazil,[5] in 1991, and followed later that year in a U.S. phase I clinical trial by Schanzlin et al.[43] The ICR was well tolerated in both

*KeraVision, Inc., Fremont, CA.

studies beyond 1 year. Stromal channel haze present the first day postoperatively decreased to nearly undetectable levels by the twelfth month. Lamellar channel deposits were sometimes observed in the first months postoperatively, and, if the incision was placed too close to the limbus, mild pannus or single vessel stromal neovascularization in the incision area could be seen. Clinical parameters, including intraocular pressure, corneal pachymetry, and endothelial cell counts, remained stable. Five patients developed an arcuate epithelial iron line concentric with the inner margin of the ICR.[44] At the 12-month follow-up period, mean keratometric and retinoscopic central corneal flattening for the one size (0.3 mm thick) ICR was approximately 2.5 diopters.

Potential reversibility of the ICR procedure was demonstrated by planned removal of the rings from five of the patients 1 year after implantation. The explant procedures were easily performed and were uncomplicated, and, 3 months after ICR removal, average retinoscopic and keratometric values had returned to their preoperative state and remained stable through 1 year of postexplant follow-up.[45]

The first sighted eye ICR study was performed by Nosé et al.[40] Ten eyes of 10 patients with preoperative myopic refractive errors ranging from −2.63 to −4.25 diopters underwent implantation of a 0.3 mm thick ICR. One case was complicated by a small tear in Descemet's membrane made at the time of the channel dissection. Persistent focal edema necessitated explantation of the ICR after 6 months of follow-up, and the patient's best corrected visual acuity returned to 20/20. Two patients developed corneal infiltrate at the incision site during the early postoperative period; both resolved with topical antibiotic therapy. Slit lamp findings showed peripheral corneal haze in the lamellar channel that gradually diminished and lamellar channel deposits (Figure 176-4). There were no instances of implant extrusion or migration. For the nine patients retaining ICRs at 1 year, uncorrected visual acuity of 20/40 or better was achieved, with a stable, average reduction of myopia of −2.25 ±0.5 D 12 months postoperatively. Results at 24 months postoperatively demonstrated no new complications and a mean refractive correction of −2.51 ±0.43 diopters. Best corrected visual acuities remained 20/20 or better.

A U.S. phase II multicenter clinical trial of the ICR was initiated in 1993, with enrollment of 90 patients completed in 1994. The study incorporates a range of ICR thicknesses[37] and tests their effect on a wider range of myopia. The most common postoperative observations to date include peripheral corneal haze, lamellar channel deposits, ICR suture hole deposits, and late fluorescein staining at the incision site.

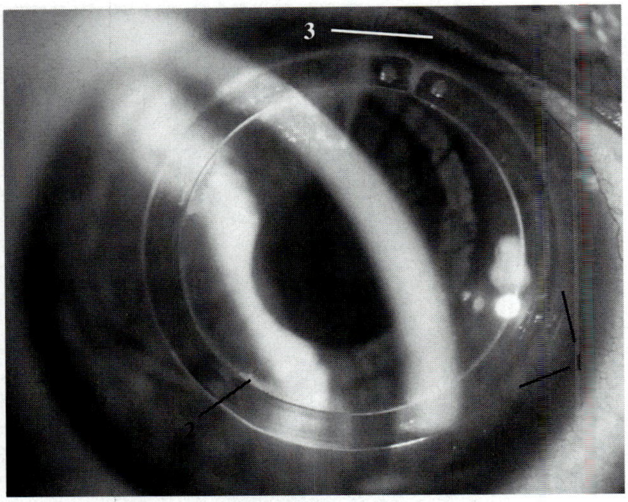

FIGURE 176-4 ICR clinical appearance in a subject 9 months postoperatively. Note the peripheral channel haze (*1*), lamellar channel deposits (*2*), and vascularization of incision site too close to limbus (*3*). (Courtesy KeraVision, Inc., Fremont, CA.)

SDCI

Preliminary studies

The SDCI concept is that of a biocompatible lenticular implant measuring approximately 2 mm, which has a diameter less than that of the optical zone in bright light conditions (Figure 176-5). Its composition relative to that of the surrounding tissues produces a multifocal system suitable for correction of presbyopia and possibly other refractive error.[38,46] A related ring-shaped device has also been proposed but is not yet in clinical trials.[47]

Animal safety studies have shown the SDCI is biocompatible and well tolerated.[48] A study of 18 hydrogel inlays in 14 rabbits demonstrated a total of 14 inlays remained in the eyes, while four extruded from the eyes at various times postoperatively. Of the 14 eyes with retained implants, all eyes had a very slight haze in the tunnel at the 6-month follow-up examination. Histologic examination of two eyes 7 months after implantation revealed normal histology of the corneal tissue surrounding the implanted lenticule.

Feline safety studies of +2.5-diopter biconvex and meniscus-shaped hydrogel inlays were performed. The biconvex design was associated with minimal haze and/or small scattered deposits, with normal histopathology. The meniscus design showed no evidence of haze or deposits in a preliminary study and in a second study showed only faint, light-reflecting specks on or near both inlays implanted in the eyes of one cat In one cat the inlay was successfully explanted at 7 months to prove reversibility.

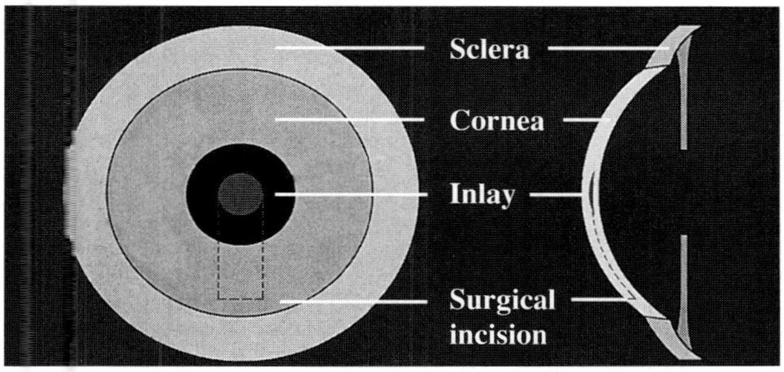

FIGURE 176-5 Concept of the SDCI measuring smaller than the effective optical zone in bright light conditions. (Courtesy Chiron, Inc., Irvine, CA.)

Operative procedure

The SDCI may be performed under topical anesthesia for cooperative patients. The optical zone is marked with a 2 mm marker. A peripheral 2 mm clear corneal stromal incision is made parallel to the limbus to approximately 75% depth. A Suarez spreader is used to initiate a lamellar pocket dissection, and the dissection is continued with a blunt spatula to incorporate the 2 mm central optical zone. The SDCI is then placed on a spatula and is inserted into the most central portion of the pocket. The incision site may be sutured if incision gape is present.

Clinical trials

The current SDCI is a 1.9 mm, 45% water hydrogel lens, refractive index 1.425, 30 to 60 μm thick, and is available in powers up to +4 diopters.[45] The first seven SDCIs were placed in nonfunctional human eyes by Eduardo Martines at Sao Paulo University, Sao Paulo, Brazil (personal communication).* One inlay was inadvertently inserted into the anterior chamber. Each subject had slight small particles in the tunnel during the first postoperative week that remained unchanged through at least 6 months postoperatively. No deposits formed on the inlays (Figure 176-6). Three inlays were explanted to demonstrate reversibility at 2, 9, and 13 months after implantation. No difficulties were encountered, and the tunnels in all three cases remained clear after removal, with the exception of the small particles present since the beginning of the surgery.

The first sighted eye SDCI study was performed by Martines in Brazil. Five inlays were successfully implanted in five presbyopic eyes (uncorrected near vision of J5 or worse) under topical anesthesia, and the subjects were followed for 12 months. By 1 week postoperatively, all five eyes were quiet, and four eyes had small particles in the tunnel. After 12 months the particles were visible only in one eye. At the 3-month

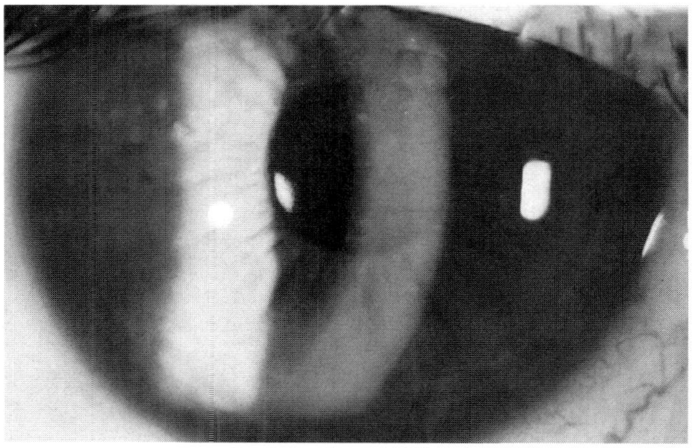

FIGURE 176-6 SDCI clinical appearance. Implant is barely detectable. (Courtesy Chiron, Inc., Irvine, CA.)

examination, three of the subjects had J1-J2 uncorrected near vision, and the remaining two subjects had J3 uncorrected near vision. At the 4-month examination, inlay exchanges were performed on two patients because of insufficient near reading vision. From 4 to 12 months postoperatively, near vision remained good in all but one subject (an inlay exchange subject), but variable decreases in uncorrected and best corrected distance visual acuity occurred. Four of the five subjects reported no visual complaints of glare, halos, haze, double vision, multiple images, or blurred and distorted images at any visit. One subject reported slight diplopia with near vision at 3 and 12 months.

Phase II multicenter clinical studies of the SDCI are in progress in the United States and involve 24 presbyopic and 24 pseudophakic patients.

*Chiron, Inc., Irvine, CA.

REFERENCES

1. Barraquer JI: Modification of refraction by means of intracorneal inclusions, *Int Ophthalmol Clin* 6:53-78, 1966.
2. Komai Y, Ushiki T: The three-dimensional organization of collagen fibrils in the human cornea and sclera, *Invest Ophthalmol Vis Sci* 32:2244-2258, 1991.
3. Barraquer JI: Keratomileusis for myopia and aphakia, *Ophthalmology* 88:701-708, 1981.
4. Fleming JF et al: The intrastromal corneal ring: two cases in rabbits, *J Refract Surg* 3:227-232, 1987.
5. Nosé W et al: Intrastromal corneal ring—one-year results of first implants in humans: a preliminary nonfunctional eye study, *Refract Corneal Surg* 9:452-458, 1993.
6. Takesue Y et al: Long-term clinical and histological results of gel injection adjustable keratoplasty (GIAK) in the cat, *Invest Ophthalmol Vis Sci* 4:2024, 1994.
7. Rowsey JJ: Ten caveats in keratorefractive surgery, *Ophthalmology* 90:148-155, 1983.
8. Buzard KA: Keratophakia. In Schwab IR, editor: *Refractive keratoplasty,* New York, 1987, Churchill Livingstone.
9. Binder PS et al: Hydrogel keratophakia in non-human primates, *Curr Eye Res* 1:535-542, 1981/2.
10. Binder PS et al: Refractive keratoplasty: microkeratome evaluation, *Arch Ophthalmol* 100:802-806, 1982.

11. Werblin TP et al: Stability of hydrogel intracorneal implants in non-human primates, *CLAO J* 9:157-161, 1983.
12. McCarey BE, Andrews DM: Refractive keratoplasty with intrastromal hydrogel lenticular implants, *Invest Ophthalmol Vis Sci* 21:107-115, 1981.
13. Koenig SB et al: Refractive keratoplasty with hydrogel implants in primates, *Ophthalmic Surg* 15:225-229, 1984.
14. Silvestrini T et al: A geometric model to predict the change in corneal curvature from the intrastromal corneal ring (ICR), *Invest Ophthalmol Vis Sci* 35:2023, 1994.
15. Burris TE et al: Effects of intrastromal corneal ring size and thickness on corneal flattening in human eyes, *Refract Corneal Surg* 7:46-50, 1991.
16. Parel J-M, Comander J: Mathematical model of gel injection adjustable keratoplasty (GIAK), *Invest Ophthalmol Vis Sci* 35: 2024, 1994.
17. Fleming JF, Wan WL, Schanzlin DJ: The theory of corneal curvature change with the Intrastromal Corneal Ring, *CLAO J* 15:146-150, 1989.
18. Choyce DP: The correction of refractive errors with polysulfone corneal inlays, *Trans Ophthalmol Soc UK* 104:332-342, 1985.
19. Watsky MA, McCarey BE, Beekhius WH: Predicting refractive alterations with hydrogel keratophakia, *Invest Ophthalmol Vis Sci* 26:240-243, 1985.
20. McCarey BE, Lane SS, Lindstrom RL: Alloplastic corneal lenses, *Int Ophthalmol Clin* 28:155-164, 1988.
21. McCarey BE et al: Refractive predictability of myopic hydrogel intracorneal lenses in nonhuman primate eyes, *Arch Ophthalmol* 108:1310-1315, 1990.
22. Maurice DM: Nutritional aspects of corneal grafts and prostheses. In Raycroft PV, editor: *Corneo-plastic surgery. Proceedings of the Second International Corneo-Plastic Conference, 1967,* London, 1969, Pergamon.
23. Maurice DM: The cornea and sclera. In Davson H, editor: *The eye.* vol 1b. *Vegetative physiology and biochemistry,* Orlando, 1984, Academic Press.
24. Bock R, Maumenee AE: Corneal fluid metabolism, experiments and observations, *Arch Ophthalmol* 50:262, 1953.
25. Kirkness CM, McG. Steele AD, Garner A: Polysulfone corneal inlays. Adverse reactions: a preliminary report, *Trans Ophthalmol Soc UK* 104:343-350, 1985.
26. Lane SS et al: Polysulfone intracorneal lenses, *J Refract Surg* 1:208-216, 1985.
27. Lane SS, McCarey BE, Lindstrom RL: Alloplastic corneal lenses. In Schwab IR, editor: *Refractive keratoplasty,* New York, 1987, Churchill Livingstone.
28. Kobayashi H et al: Tissue reactions induced by modified poly(vinyl alcohol) hydrogels in rabbit cornea, *J Biomed Mat Res* 26:1583-1598, 1992.
29. McCarey BE, Schmidt FH: Modeling glucose distribution in the cornea, *Curr Eye Res* 9:1025-1039, 1990.
30. McDonald MB et al: Assessment of the long-term corneal response to hydrogel intrastromal lenses implanted in monkey eyes for up to five years, *J Cataract Refract Surg* 19:213-222, 1993.
31. Assil KK, Quantock AJ: Wound healing in response to keratorefractive surgery. *Surv Ophthalmol* 38:289-302, 1993.
32. Werblin TP, Patel AS, Barraquer JI: Initial human experience with Permalens myopic hydrogel intracorneal lens implants, *Refract Corneal Surg* 8:23-26, 1992.
33. Werblin TP: Lamellar refractive surgery: where have we been and where are we going? *Refract Corneal Surg* 5:167-175, 1989.
34. Werblin TP, Barraquer J: Intracorneal lenses, *inFocus,* 2:14, 1994.
35. Barrett GD, Durrie DS, Lindstrom RL: *Use of a small diameter corneal inlay to create a multifocal cornea in presbyopia and pseudophakia,* International Society of Refractive Keratoplasty pre AAO meeting, abstracts, Oct 29, 1994.
36. Nosé W, Neves R, Belfort R: *The ICR (Intrastromal Corneal Ring): long term followup from the Brazilian clinical studies,* International Society of Refractive Keratoplasty pre AAO meeting, abstracts, Oct 28, 1994.
37. Durrie DS, Schanzlin DJ, Asbell PA: *The ICR (Intrastromal Corneal Ring): phase II update,* International Society of Refractive Keratoplasty pre-AAO meeting, abstracts, Oct 28, 1994
38. Durrie, DS, et al: *The ICR (Intrastromal Corneal Ring): theory and surgical technique,* International Society of Refractive Keratoplasty pre-AAO meeting, abstracts, Oct 28, 1994.
39. Quantock AJ, Assil KK, Schanzlin DJ: Electron microscopic evaluation of intrastromal corneal rings explanted from nonfunctional human eyes, *J Refract Corneal Surg* 10:142-148, 1994.
40. Nosé W et al: The intrastromal corneal ring: twelve month sighted eye study (submitted for publication).
41. Binder PS et al: Alloplastic implants for the correction of refractive errors, *Ophthalmology* 91:806-814, 1984.
42. Burris TE et al: Flattening of central corneal curvature with intrastromal corneal rings of increasing thickness: an eye-bank eye study, *J Cataract Refract Surg* 19(Suppl):182-187, 1993.
43. Schanzlin DJ et al and ICR study group: One year results of the intrastromal corneal ring in nonfunctional human eyes, *Arch Ophthalmol* (In press).
44. Assil KK, et al: Corneal iron lines associated with the intrastromal corneal ring, *Am J Ophthalmol* 116:350-356, 1993.
45. Barrett, AM, Schanzlin, DJ, and the ICR study group: Corneal curvature analysis following explantation of the intrastromal corneal ring, *Invest Ophthalmol Vis Sci* 34(Suppl):1240, 1993.
46. Barrett GD, Link WJ, Reich CJ: *Corneal inlay lenses.* United States patent number 5,336,261, Aug 9, 1994.
47. Barrett GD, Link WJ, Reich CJ: *Method of implanting corneal inlay lenses smaller than the optic zone,* United States patent number 5,196,026, Mar 23, 1993.
48. Reich CJ: *Small-diameter corneal inlay lens for the correction of presbyopia, proceedings of the American Chemical Society Division of Polymeric Materials:* Science and Engineering, vol 69, 1993.

CHAPTER 177

KEITH P. THOMPSON JAN DANIEL

Synthetic Epikeratoplasty

Synthetic epikeratoplasty is an investigational procedure in which a biocompatible synthetic lenticule is attached to the anterior surface of a deepithelialized host cornea. Epithelialization of the lenticule restores the ocular surface. Thus the radius of the anterior corneal surface can be changed and the optical power of the host cornea modified, allowing treatment of myopia, hyperopia, and astigmatism.

Background

Epikeratoplasty (originally termed epikeratophakia), using human donor tissue, was first described by Werblin and Kaufman in the early 1980s,[1,2] and extensive efforts to refine this technique were made by McDonald.[3,4] This technique employs lenticules harvested from lyophilized corneal tissue or fresh cadaver eyes with a microkeratome. The lenticule is shaped using the cryolathe invented by Barraquer, the Barraquer-Krumeich-Swinger nonfreezing lathe, or, more recently, the excimer laser. After shaping, the graft lenticule containing an intact Bowman's layer and anterior corneal stroma is sutured to the deepithelialized recipient cornea within a circular keratotomy.[5-7] The patient's epithelium usually re-covers the lenticule within 1 week.

Compared with classic keratomileusis or keratophakia, epikeratoplasty avoids the need for an intrastromal cut with the microkeratome, decreasing the risk of severe complications. The procedure is less technically demanding and easier to learn. The use of suitable methods of tissue preservation allows for manufacture of the graft lenticule by an off-site commercial firm with reproducible quality standards, thus improving the uniformity and quality of the lenticules because of the standardized procedures. In addition, it eliminated the need for lathing procedures at the time of surgery. Epikeratoplasty is a partially reversible procedure, since the lenticule can be removed.

Epikeratoplasty suffers from several unsolved problems that have prevented its widespread acceptance. Epikeratoplasty depends on a limited supply of human donor lenticules. Widespread commercial use of human donor tissue has raised ethical problems, and there is some risk for transmission of infectious agents. Visual recovery after epikeratoplasty is prolonged; many patients require up to 1 year to achieve their best corrected visual acuity. Because of possible distortions occurring with shaping and suturing the lenticule, irregular astigmatism is common and many patients have lost best corrected visual acuity after the procedure.[8] Postoperative cellular remodeling[9] can render the refractive outcome of epikeratoplasty unpredictable. After extensive clinical trials during the 1980s that revealed the deficiencies of epikeratoplasty and failure of the procedure to gain Food and Drug Administration (FDA) approval in the United States, the procedure is no longer used for the routine treatment of ametropia and is rarely used in the management of aphakic patients in whom an intraocular lens is contraindicated. In the United States, epikeratoplasty is still monitored by the FDA and is performed on an investigational device exemption at only two clinical centers.

Many of the deficiencies of epikeratoplasty have been associated with the use of tissue lenticules and might be avoided by using a suitable synthetic material.[10,11] This would eliminate problems with tissue availability and the risk for transmission of infectious diseases. A synthetic lenticule, not containing keratocytes, would avoid postoperative synthesis of collagen fibers, resulting in scarring and changes in the shape of the lenticule as a result of tissue remodeling. Synthetic materials could also potentially provide superior optical properties compared to tissue lenticules and could be shaped more precisely.

A synthetic lenticule attached to the cornea could be ablated with an excimer laser system for refining its curvature and adjusting the refractive result of the procedure.[12] Since this ablation would be performed on an acellular lenticule, Bowman's layer would not be violated, and the postoperative haze in the ablation area and regression of the refractive effect that occur frequently after excimer laser photorefractive keratectomy might be avoided. This adjustment could be performed immediately after the attachment to correct for inaccuracies in the optical power of the lenticule or

Table 177-1. Potential biomaterials for synthetic epikeratoplasty

Materials	Examples	Advantages	Disadvantages
Pure collagen	Cross-linked human type IV collagen	Clear	Susceptible to proteolysis
	Cross-linked bovine type I or III collagen (fibrillar)	Strong epithelium affinity	Fibrillar collagen less transparent
Collagen synthetic copolymers	HEMA-collagen composites	Good optical properties, potentially more stable	Susceptible to proteolysis, brittle
Coated synthetics	Laminin-, fibrin-, or fibronectin-coated HEMA	Proven biocompatibility of hydrogels, not susceptible to proteolysis	Dependent on attached coating, difficult to achieve stable epithelial attachment
Bioactive synthetics	Blown synthetic microfibers	Resistant to proteolysis	Difficult to achieve stable epithelial attachment

Requirements for biomaterials used for synthetic epikeratoplasty

- Optically clear
- Support epithelial spreading and attachment
- Permeable to nutrients and metabolites
- Biocompatible
- Stable

later to correct for changes in the refraction of the eye.

If a synthetic lenticule could be attached directly to Bowman's layer, maintenance of an intact Bowman's layer might permit the whole procedure to be completely reversible and preserve the structural integrity of the cornea. This procedure would allow the refractive outcome of synthetic epikeratoplasty to be independent of corneal stromal wound healing, considered to be a major factor in limiting the predictability of all the corneal refractive procedures currently in use.[13]

Potential Biomaterials for Synthetic Epikeratoplasty

The requirements that a synthetic material suitable for epikeratoplasty should meet are summarized in the box above. Based on these criteria, several potential biomaterials for investigation were selected and listed in Table 177-1.

Since type I and III collagens are the primary components of Bowman's layer,[14] collagen-containing or collagen-derived materials are good candidates for biomaterials for epikeratoplasty. Collagen supports the migration and attachment of corneal epithelial cells. Successful synthesis of copolymers consisting of 2-hydroxyethyl methacrylate (HEMA) and collagen have been reported.[15] Those copolymers may combine the advantages of both components, such as the biologic activity of collagen and the superior optical performance of HEMA. Collagen synthetic copolymers may be a suitable material for synthetic epikeratoplasty. However, the use of collagen-containing biomaterials increases the vulnerability of the lenticule to breakdown by proteinolytic enzymes released by corneal and immunologic cells.

Extensive use of HEMA for lens implants in cataract surgery has shown this material to be stable and well tolerated,[16] making hydrogel biomaterials potentially suitable for synthetic epikeratoplasty. Hydrogels are not susceptible to enzymatic degradation. However, to ensure sufficient spreading and stable attachment of the corneal epithelium, the HEMA lenticule must be coated with a suitable biomaterial to support cell attachment. Successful epithelialization of a polyvinyl alcohol copolymer lens coated in this manner has been achieved in vitro and in an animal model.[17] However, long-term epithelial adhesion to coated hydrogel polymers in vivo has not been demonstrated.

Recently a blown mixture of polypropylene and polybutylene microfibers has been employed to imitate the structure of the extracellular matrix.[18] Although this material does not contain collagen, its surface charge may support epithelial migration and attachment to its surface.

In Vitro Trials for Evaluation of Potential Biomaterials

Before initiating animal studies, potential biomaterials for epikeratoplasty should be evaluated by in vitro analysis of their physical and physiologic properties.

OPTICAL CHARACTERISTICS

Excellent optical performance is a prerequisite for an appropriate biomaterial that covers the central corneal surface. Therefore the transmission of light in the visible spectrum must be measured by spectroscopy in potential biomaterials. In contrast to donor tissue lenticules, synthetic materials do not require keratocytes to maintain optical clarity.

SUPPORT OF EPITHELIAL MIGRATION

The ability to support epithelial migration and cell attachment is one of the most important characteristics of a potential biomaterial for synthetic epikeratoplasty. Presumably, to ensure stable long-term adhesion, the epithelium will need to form normal attachment complexes to the synthetic lenticule. These subcellular components have been described previously and include hemidesmosomes, basement membrane, and anchoring fibrils.[19] To screen a potential biomaterial for its ability to support cell migration and attachment, rabbit corneal epithelium was removed from the cornea by dispase method. The cells are cultured at the surface of potential biomaterial in cell culture medium for an appropriate period. Then the cell sheet is examined by shaking. If the epithelium remains attached to the synthetic surface, the cell-lenticule sheet may be examined by transmission electron microscopy and immunohistochemistry for epithelial attachment structures.

PERMEABILITY

Since the corneal epithelium derives its nutrition from the aqueous humor, a suitable lenticule for epikeratoplasty must be permeable to nutrients and metabolites. In vivo studies with intracorneal lenses have shown that impairment of intracorneal diffusion caused by impermeable implants may lead to epithelial thinning or even aseptic necrosis. Glucose has been used to determine the diffusion rate in potential synthetic materials. However, glucose is a small molecule and does not necessarily represent the diffusion rate of more complex proteins such as neurotrophic factors released from intracorneal nerves or cytokines produced by keratocytes that may be necessary for long-term epithelial viability.

Kim et al have investigated the permeability of the cornea to radiolabeled inulin (molecular weight [MW] about 7,000 daltons [D]) and dextran (MW about 50,000 D).[20] This method was deemed a suitable approach for testing the permeability of potential synthetic materials. Data obtained from native rat corneas served as a control. The results of a preliminary study are shown in Table 177-2.

Table 177-2. Coefficients of permeability in potential biomaterials (mm/sec × 10^{-5})

	Inulin	Dextran
Corneal stroma (rat model)	7.0 ± 0.2	5.0 ± 0.1
Collagen type IV	8.3 ± 0.5	4.0 ± 0.4
Collagen type I	8.7 ± 0.3	15.0 ± 0.2
HEMA-type IV collagen	33.1 ± 15.1	19.8 ± 14.7

STABILITY

To ensure long-term refractive stability the synthetic lenticule must be capable of withstanding erosion and breakdown caused by naturally occurring corneal enzymes. Two major types of proteolytic enzymes are present in the cornea: (1) collagenases released by keratocytes that are capable of breaking down native interstitial collagen molecules and (2) neutral proteases secreted by both keratocytes and epithelial cells that break down denatured collagen, which is characterized by a loss of its typical helical structure. Consequently, epithelial cells exposed to denaturated collagen have the ability to remodel it.

Like avascular hyaline cartilage the cornea has a low turnover rate of collagen, and there is no collagenase detectable in the normal cornea.[21] Bowman's layer, which separates the corneal epithelium from the stroma, is probably synthesized by the epithelium during embryogenesis. This layer remains the same thickness throughout life unless it is destroyed or damaged by disease or injury. With respect to a stable refractive effect, a potential biomaterial for synthetic epikeratoplasty will be required to provide stability similar to that of Bowman's layer. A synthetic lenticule composed of a material that is susceptible to breakdown may induce intracorneal pathologic processes such as proteolysis, resulting in the breakdown of Bowman's layer and remodeling of stromal collagen.

To test the stability of potential materials, an in vitro approach was used in which these materials were exposed to corneal enzymes (collagenases and proteases) for a defined period. The stability of human type IV collagen copolymer can be compared with native rabbit stroma after 20 hours of exposure to different enzymes. The data suggest that type IV collagen is much more susceptible to trypsin, a neutral protease, than is the native rabbit stroma.

EXCIMER LASER ABLATION CHARACTERISTICS

Appreciating past experience with refractive surgery, it seems unlikely that these procedures will be capable of correcting refractive errors as accurately and predictably as glasses or contact lenses that provide a best corrected visual acuity of 20/20 in the otherwise healthy eye. Furthermore, the refractive status of the eye may change after surgery. For these reasons, it may be desirable to reshape the lenticule surface either immediately after the epikeratoplasty procedure to

Table 177-3. Summary of the postoperative outcome

Animal	Complete epithelization of the lenticule	Use of hand restraints	Postoperative outcome	Animal status
1	*	No	Lenticule expulsed day 1	Removed from study
2†	*	No	Lenticule expulsed day 3	Removed from study
3	No	No	Erosion of lenticule, 4 weeks	Sacrificed 4 weeks postoperatively
4†	Partial	No	Erosion of lenticule, 6 weeks	Sacrificed 6 weeks postoperatively
5	Yes	Yes	Peripheral focal erosion of lenticule, 4 months	Sacrificed 4 months postoperatively
6	Yes	Yes	Peripheral focal erosion of lenticule, 4 months	Sacrificed 4 months postoperatively
7	Yes	Yes	Lenticule stable over 42 months	Sacrificed 42 months postoperatively

*Extensive eye rubbing.
†Anterior surface of the lenticule was ablated with an excimer laser before the attachment.

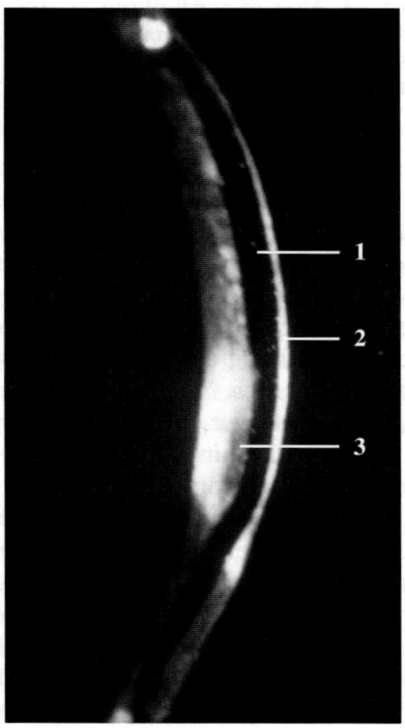

FIGURE 177-2 Slit lamp photomicrograph of a human-derived type IV collagen lenticule *(1)* in a primate 42 months after epikeratoplasty. The epithelium *(2)* covers the synthetic lenticule completely, and there is no evidence of epithelial erosions. The lenticule remains stable with respect to its thickness. Note the clarity of the synthetic material compared to the underlying native host cornea *(3)*.

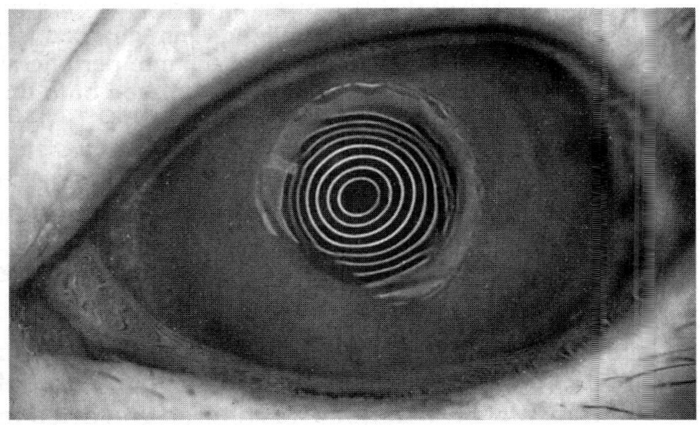

FIGURE 177-3 Keratoscope photograph after synthetic epikeratoplasty in a primate 21 months postoperatively. Astigmatism is present, but the regular mires indicate that the lenticule permits a smooth ocular surface.

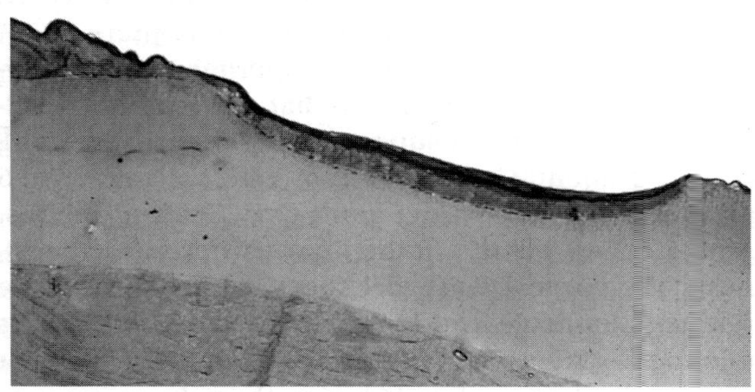

FIGURE 177-4 Light micrograph of section of synthetic epikeratoplasty lenticule at erosion site. Erosion sites typically occur adjacent to the stromal pocket and are characterized by cellular infiltration into the lenticule. Note the thickened epithelium in the erosion. Underlying stroma is normal.

epithelium to be about three cell layers thick. Bowman's layer underlying the synthetic lenticule was normal. There was no evidence for activated keratocytes except close to the intrastromal pocket, where keratocytes were found in increased size and number (Figure 177-4). Few specimens revealed invasion of keratocytes into the lenticule. The middle and posterior stromal portion as well as Descemet's membrane and the endothelium were found to be normal. Basal epithelial cells were found with hemidesmosomes and focal segments of basement membrane were apparent.

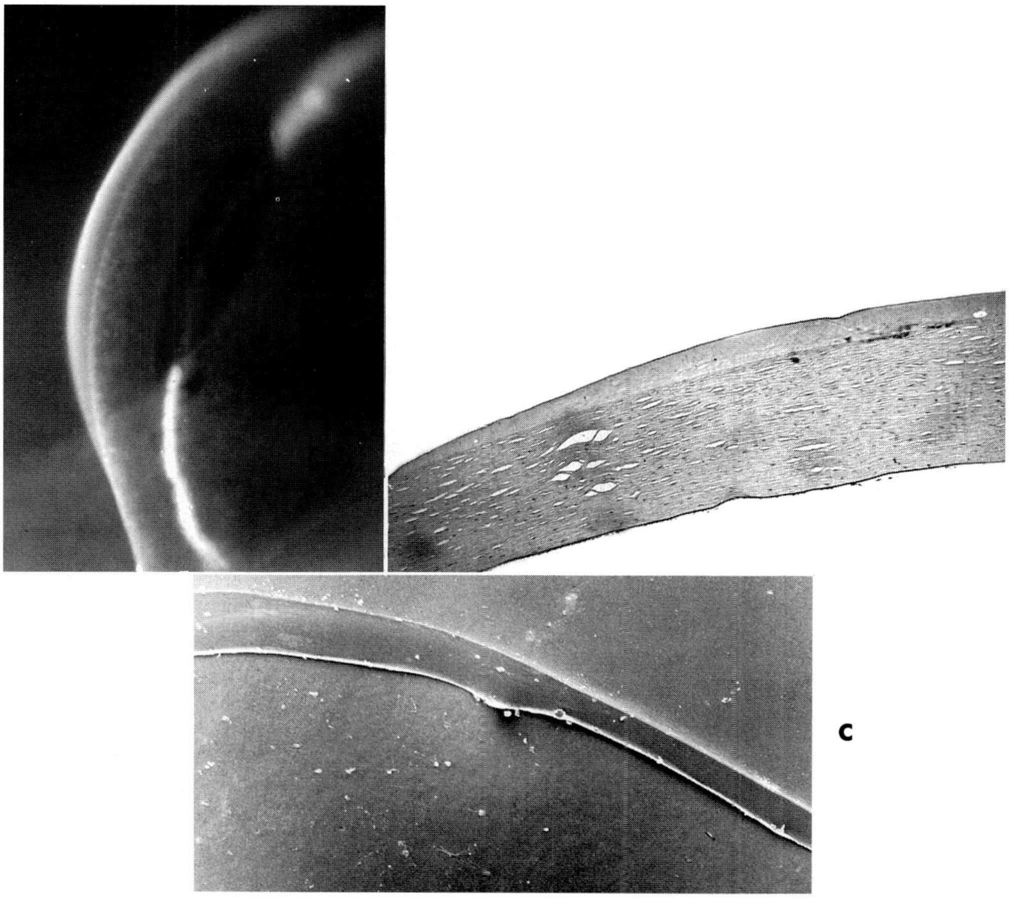

FIGURE 177-5 **A,** Using a type I collagen with a polymerizing agent, a lenticule of collagen can be polymerized in situ onto the deepithelialized cornea while leaving Bowman's layer intact. **B,** The collagen is tightly adherent to Bowman's layer, as shown in this light micrograph. **C,** By nicking the surface and creating a surgical plane, it can be peeled from the surface without damaging Bowman's layer (scanning electron micrograph). Using this technique, it may be possible to bond collagen lenticules to the cornea in a reversible fashion without damaging the underlying cornea.

All physiologic components of the epithelial adhesion complex were localized immunohistochemically at the epithelial lenticule interface.

The results of preliminary studies in nonhuman primates suggest that synthetic epikeratoplasty is feasible. However, further efforts are needed to optimize the properties of the material and to refine the attachment procedure. Synthetic type IV collagen lenticules were found to support attachment and migration of the corneal epithelium in vitro as well as in vivo. The appearance of hemidesmosomes, anchoring fibril components, and basement membrane is promising because the production of normal attachment complexes is considered a prerequisite for stable long-term attachment of the corneal epithelium to the lenticule surface. There was no evidence of epithelial toxicity, recurrent epithelial erosions, infiltration, neovascularization, or other adverse complications. Additionally, the type IV collagen lenticules were clearer than the corneal stroma, probably because the cross-linked matrix does not contain continuous helical collagen fibers. We found no difference in results between ablated and nonablated lenticules. Therefore it may be possible to adjust the anterior curvature or surface characteristics of the synthetic lenticule by means of an excimer laser.

However, type IV collagen lenticules were found to thin gradually in most of our animals. Frequently these thinning areas were located close to the intrastromal pocket, suggesting that activated keratocytes released proteolytic enzymes that degraded the type IV collagen molecules of the synthetic lenticule.[32,33] Other possible sources of the proteolytic enzymes are epithelial cells and leukocytes. Biochemical examination of the specimen harvested from animal 6 revealed that at least four neutral proteases with activity for gelatin (and for type IV collagen)[34] were present in the lenticule, two of which were found in the active form.[35] The exact nature of these enzymes is unknown, although the measured molecular weights referred to different type IV collagenases. These proteases degrade type IV collagen but do not break down type I collagen, which is a major component of the native human cornea. Type I collagen is uniquely degraded enzymatically by interstitial and polymorphonuclear collagenases.[34] Since we did not find these enzymes either in the thinned lenticule or in the host cornea, synthetic lenticules consisting of type I collagen may have acceptable stability (Figure 177-5).

Past experience with synthetic intracorneal implants to change the refractive status of the eye has shown that considerable attention must be given to avoid any impairment in intracorneal diffusion of nutrients and metabolites resulting in epithelial thinning or even aseptic necrosis. We found that the epithelium overlying the synthetic lenticule was thinned generally to three cell layers. Whether this change was caused by diminished diffusion or insufficient reinnervation of the epithelium covering the lenticule remains to be determined. Corneal nerves or neurotrophic agents have been shown to support normal epithelial morphology and physiology[36]; nevertheless, stable epithelialization has been observed over completely or partially denervated corneal grafts and human epikeratoplasty lenticules. Furthermore, synthetic collagen matrices have demonstrated the potential for allowing epithelial reinnervation.[37]

Synthetic epikeratoplasty is not expected to offer correction of ametropia in humans in a safe and predictable manner in the near future. However, the shortcomings of all refractive procedures in current use and the potential advantages of this new approach support further research. Increasing the stability of synthetic biomaterials while maintaining the support for epithelial spreading and attachment as well as refining the lenticule attachment method will be the primary objective of further experimental studies.

Acknowledgment

This study was supported in part by NIH grant No. EY007388-02, Yerkes Primate Research Center Core grant No. RR-00165, Research to Prevent Blindness, Inc., by P30 EY06360 (an NIH Departmental Core Grant), a research grant from G.E. Medical Systems, Milwaukee, Wisconsin, and Domilens, Inc., Lyon, France.

REFERENCES

1. Werblin TP, Klyce SD: Epikeratophakia: the surgical correction of aphakia. I. Lathing of corneal tissue, *Curr Eye Res* 1:123-129, 1981.
2. Werblin TP, Kaufman HE: Epikeratophakia: the surgical correction of aphakia. II. Preliminary studies in a non-human primate model, *Curr Eye Res* 1:131-137, 1981.
3. McDonald MB et al: Epikeratophakia for myopia correction, *Ophthalmology* 92:1417-1422, 1985.
4. McDonald MB et al: The nationwide study of epikeratophakia for aphakia for adults, *Am J Ophthalmol* 103:358-365, 1987.
5. Grabner G: Myopic epikeratophakia. Results, complications, and new techniques. In Schachar RA, Le NS, Schachar L, editors: *Keratorefractive surgery,* Denison, TX, 1990, LAL.
6. Keates RH et al: Carbon dioxide laser use in wound sealing and epikeratophakia, *J Cataract Refract Surg* 13:290-295, 1987.
7. Rostron CK: Epikeratophakia grafts glued with autologous cryoprecipitate, *Eur J Implant Refract Surg* 1:105, 1989.
8. Barrett G, Moore MB: A new method of lathing corneal lenticules for keratorefractive procedures, *J Re Surg* 4:142-147, 1988.
9. Grabner G: Complications of epikeratophakia for the correction of aphakia, myopia, hyperopia, and keratoconus (German), *Fortschr Ophthalmol* 8:4-11, 1991.
10. McDonald MB: The future direction of refractive surgery, *Refract Corneal Surg* 4:158-167, 1988.
11. Thompson KP, Hanna K, Waring GO III: Emerging technologies for refractive surgery: laser adjustable synthetic epikeratoplasty, *Refract Corneal Surg* 5:46-48, 1989.
12. Thompson KP et al: Current status of synthetic epikeratoplasty (review), *Refract Corneal Surg* 7:240, 1991.
13. Thompson KP: Will the excimer laser resolve the unsolved problems with refractive surgery? *Refract Corneal Surg* 6:315-317, 1990.
14. Nimni ME, Harkness RD: *Molecular structures and functions of collagen.* In Nimni ME, editor: *Collagen* vol. 1, Boca Raton, FL, 1988, CRC Press, Inc.
15. Rao KP, Joseph KT: *Collagen graft copolymers and their biomedical applications.* In Nimni ME, editor: *Collagen,* vol. III, *Biotechnology,* Boca Raton, FL, 1988, CRC Press, Inc.
16. McCarey BE et al: Refractive predictability of myopic hydrogel intracorneal lenses in nonhuman primate eyes, *Arch Ophthalmol* 108:1310-1315, 1990.
17. Trinkaus-Randall V et al: Development of a biopolymeric keratoprosthetic material. Evaluation *in vitro* and *in vivo, Invest Ophthalmol Vis Sci* 29:393-400, 1988.
18. Trinkaus-Randall V et al: *In vitro* evaluation of fibroplasia in a porous polymer, *Invest Ophthalmol Vis Sci* 31:1321-1326, 1990.
19. Gipson IK et al: Reassembly of the anchoring structures of the corneal epithelium during wound repair in the rabbit, *Invest Ophthalmol Vis Sci* 30:425-434, 1989.
20. Kim JH et al: Solute permeability of the corneal endothelium and Descemet's membrane, *Exp Eye Res* 12:231-238, 1971.
21. Brown SI, Weller CA: Cell origin of collagenase in normal and wounded corneas, *Arch Ophthalmol* 83:77, 1970.
22. Hanna KD et al: Interaction of type IV collagen with a 193 nm excimer laser (abstract), *Invest Ophthalmol Vis Sci* 30(ARVO Suppl):189, 1989.
23. Albinet P et al: Epikeratoplastie sans susture ava lentille de Collagene IV chez le singe: description de la technique chirurgicale [Epikeratoplasty without sutures using collagen IV lens in monkeys: description of the surgical techniques] (French), *Fr Ophthalmol* 13:109-114, 1990.
24. Waring GO III, Hanna KD: The Hanna suction punch block and trephine system for penetrating keratophakia, *Arch Ophthalmol* 107:1536-1539, 1989.
25. Bailes JE et al: Review of tissue welding applications in neurosurgery (review), *Microsurgery* 8:242-1987.
26. Flemming AFS et al: Laser assisted microvascular anastomosis of arteries and veins: Laser tissue welding, *Br J Plast Surg* 41: 378-388, 1988.

27. Gailitis RP et al: Laser welding of synthetic epikeratoplasty lenticules to the cornea, *Refract Corneal* 6:430-436, 1990.
28. Robin JB et al: Preliminary evaluation of the use of mussel adhesive protein in experimental epikeratoplasty, *Arch Ophthalmol* 106:973-977, 1988.
29. Rostron CK et al: Experimental epikeratophakia with biological adhesive, *Arch Ophthalmol* 106:1103, 1988.
30. De Toledo AR et al: Preliminary evaluation of a new collagen-derived bioadhesive (abstract #1556), *Invest Ophthalmol Vis Sci* 31(ARVO Suppl):317, 1990.
31. Gipson IK, Spurr-Michaud SJ, Tisdale AS: Hemidesmosomes and anchoring fibril collagen appear synchronously during development and wound healing, *Dev Biol* 16:253-262, 1988.
32. Johnson-Muller B, Gross J: Regulation of corneal collagenase production: epithelial-stromal cell interaction, *Proc Natl Acad Sci USA* 75:4417-4421, 1978.
33. Johnson-Wint B, Gross J: Regulation of connective tissue collagenase production: stimulators from adult and fetal epidermal cells, *J Cell Biol* 98:90-96, 1984.
34. Matrisian LM: Metalloproteinases and their inhibitors in matrix remodeling, (review), *Trends Genet* 6:5, 1990.
35. Emonard H, Grimaud JA: Matrix metalloproteinases: a review, *Cell Molecular Biol* 36:131-153, 1990.
36. Beuerman RW, Tanelian DL, Schimmelpfennig B: *Nerve tissue interactions in the cornea.* In Cavanagh H, editor: *The cornea: Transactions of the World Congress on the Cornea III,* New York, 1988, Raven Press.
37. Akelman E et al: *Regeneration of a peripheral nerve through a bioresorbable nerve guide in primate: A preliminary study.* Proceedings of 34th Annual Meeting of the Orthopedic Research Society, 1988.

CHAPTER 178

GEORGE O. WARING, III

The Future of Refractive Surgery: Searching for the Ideal Procedure and Method of Delivery

Predicting the Future

Writing about the future of refractive keratoplasty has two attractive elements: It can be written about from a personal point of view, and one does not have to adhere to proven data.

Refractive surgery has been developing for over 100 years. Surely those prescient 19th century clinicians and investigators could not have anticipated the rate and direction of growth in refractive surgery over the past decade. Indeed, even the originators of modern techniques (Sato for refractive keratotomy, José Barraquer for keratomileusis, and Strampelli and Joaquin Barraquer for phakic intraocular lenses) could not have anticipated the advent of excimer laser corneal surgery.[1-3] Thus our ability to predict the future is inextricably constrained by our present fund of knowledge.

Criteria for Judging Refractive Surgical Procedures

Since we can anticipate neither the improvements in current techniques nor the uniquely new methods that will emerge, we are left with another alternative: to design criteria by which we can judge both present and future procedures. With such a checklist in mind, coping with rapid and unexpected change becomes easier.

Elsewhere I have proposed standard criteria for reporting refractive surgical procedures.[4] Here I propose 13 practical qualitative clinical criteria by which one can judge a refractive surgical procedure to estimate its acceptability for general clinical use (Table 178-1).

The author is a consultant for Summit Technology in excimer laser photorefractive keratectomy, for Chiron Corporation in refractive keratotomy, and for Tomey, Inc. in videokeratography.

EFFICACY

The cautious refractive surgeon who seeks to create realistic expectations on the part of patients will state that a given procedure can reduce *or* eliminate ametropia and dependence on optical correction. Thus the criteria for efficacy from the patient's point of view are functional ones: can the patient function without spectacles or contact lenses, or can the use of these optical devices be reduced to a minimal level that is acceptable to the patient? I am proposing these functional criteria for efficacy instead of a quantitative level of refractive error or visual acuity because these are the standards by which patients judge the outcome. They really do not care about residual numbers—only about their ability to see adequately without optical correction.

Thus reports of refractive surgery should contain information about the spectacle and contact lens–wearing status of the population studied, with clear distinctions between use of corrective eye wear for distance vision and for near vision. There are no established, agreed on criteria, but a reasonable goal for practical clinical purposes might be that 90% of the surgical population be free of distance corrective eye wear at least 90% of the time. Such criteria, allowing for the use of near correction, would render patients free of spectacles for all but a small amount of time for specific situations, such as night driving or attending the theater, where the best possible vision is needed and would deem a procedure effective if 90% of patients wore no corrective eye wear for routine daily activities. If we wished to be stricter, we could simply increase these levels to 95%—the usual cutoff for "significance."

What level of uncorrected visual acuity can we use to judge efficacy? The answer is simple—the same level that we use to judge efficacy of spectacles and contact lenses: 20/20 (6/6, 1.0, LogMar 0.0), remembering that the resolving power of the normal human eye can often do much better: 20/16, 20/12, or even 20/10. What level

Table 178-1. Thirteen criteria for assessing refractive surgical procedures

Criteria	Definition of success	Mnemonic
1. Efficacy	Reduction or elimination of need for corrective lenses	Every
2. Versatility	Treatment of myopia, hyperopia and astigmatism (and ideally presbyopia)	Viable
3. Predictability	Refractive outcome same as desired outcome	Procedure
4. Safety	Preservation of best spectacle-corrected preoperative visual acuity	Should
5. Quality of vision	Preservation of preoperative levels of contrast sensitivity, absence of glare, and patient's subjective judgment of sharp, clear vision day and night.	Qualify
6. Stability	Refraction changes minimally after surgery	Surely
7. Adjustability	Ability to surgically modify the refraction after the initial operation	As A
8. Reversibility	Ability to return the eye to its baseline state	Really
9. Complexity	Technique mastered by average, well-trained cataract surgeon	Completely
10. Corneal Contours	Minimal optical aberration from postoperative shape of cornea	Clear
11. Cost	As affordable as spectacles or contact lenses	Choice
12. Satisfaction	High rate of acceptance by patients and eye care professionals	Sans
13. Reports	Results published in peer reviewed ophthalmic literature	Reservations

of residual refractive error can we use to judge efficacy? The answer is simple—the same level we use to judge spectacles and contact lenses: ±0.50 diopter (or being stricter, ±0.25 diopter). Not only has the 20/20, ±0.50 diopter level of success been established by long-standing custom, but it also has been demonstrated in the Prospective Evaluation of Radial Keratotomy (PERK) Study[5] to be necessary for the majority of refractive surgery patients to be rid of their glasses or contact lenses and for them to judge refractive surgical procedures as highly successful (see box).

Attempts to alter the 20/20 standard by quoting good results at the levels of 20/25, 20/30, and 20/40 or by clinging to ±1.00 diopter as success only obfuscate the real clinical condition and appear to be efforts to make the results appear better than they are. Such information can be valuable and can help readers compare levels of success in different studies, but they do not form adequate criteria for efficacy.

Criteria for effective refractive surgery (PERK study—6 years, 328 patients)

Determinants of highly satisfied patients (regression analysis)

1. No spectacles or contact lenses for distance vision
2. Uncorrected visual acuity of 20/20 or better in at least one eye

Determinants of freedom from distance optical correction

	Percent of patients without optical correction
1. Visual acuity in best eye	
20/10 to 20/20	77
20/25 to 20/40	34
2. Refraction in both eyes	
±0.50 diopter	85
±1.00 diopter	33

VERSATILITY

The ideal refractive surgical procedure should be able to treat myopia, hyperopia, astigmatism—and even presbyopia. Such versatility would enable the surgeon to master one technique, with some variations for the different types of refractive correction, rather than investing the time, energy, and money to master many. Of course, this assumes that our ideal technique can meet the other 12 criteria equally well for all types of refractive correction—a tall order for the operation that treats everything.

PREDICTABILITY

Predictability is the ability of a refractive surgical procedure to achieve the desired refractive outcome. Predictability is affected by variability in the skill of the surgeon, variability among instruments, and variability in the biologic response of each eye. The surgical procedure that controls each of these best will have the most predictable outcomes.

Most of the time this is a refraction of plano or more commonly mild residual myopia of −0.50 diopter spherical equivalent refraction with less than 0.50 diopters of astigmatism. Of course, if the patient and surgeon desire a different outcome, such as a residual refraction of −1.50 diopters in the nondominant eye to achieve monovision for preservation of uncorrected reading vision, then the predictability of the procedure would be its ability to approximate −1.50 diopters. In fact, monovision is a commonly sought refractive state because approximately half the patients in most refractive surgery studies are over the age of 35 years. If the monovision does not work, a repeat operation on the undercorrected eye can usually be carried out to approximate emmetropia. Therefore it is erroneous to think of the endpoint of refractive surgery as emmetropia. It is rather the desired refractive outcome for each individual eye.

Predictability can be measured by calculating the prediction interval or confidence interval for the change in refraction, as described elsewhere.[6] For example, calculating the 90% prediction interval for the PERK surgical technique (which is now outdated) demonstrated that the surgeon could have 90% confidence that the refractive change would be between 1.50 and 5.32 diopters. This means that a patient with −4.00 diopters of myopia preoperatively could have a 90% chance at 1 year of having a refraction of between −2.50 and +1.32 diopters. Clearly, the predictability of the PERK technique of refractive keratotomy is far below that of fitting spectacles and contact lenses, where the 90% prediction interval should approximate 1.00 to 0.50 diopter.

Surgeons reporting results of refractive surgical procedures should report a 90% or 95% confidence or prediction interval. The computations are simple when the number of eyes is greater than 30. The 90% prediction interval equals the mean refractive change plus or minus the standard deviation times 1.645.[6] Although we commonly estimate predictability in terms of a symmetrical range around the desired outcome (e.g., ±0.50 diopters), an asymmetrical range is preferable because undercorrections in treating myopia are almost always more desirable than overcorrections. Management of an undercorrection usually involves repeating the original operation (an enhancement procedure), whereas management of an overcorrection often involves a different procedure that is more difficult to control and quantify.

SAFETY

The simple criterion of spectacle-corrected visual acuity after the procedure being the same as or within one line of baseline spectacle visual acuity is a useful standard for safety. A difference of one line (three letters) has been shown to be within the bounds of normal biologic variation.[7]

Loss of spectacle-corrected visual acuity can occur from small problems such as mild irregular astigmatism with a subtle loss of vision from 20/10 to 20/20. Although this is a loss of three Snellen lines, most patients would not notice the loss because they now see well without optical correction. Rare problems such as full thickness laceration of the cornea with an improperly set microkeratome, loss of a keratomileusis disk, laceration of the lens during refractive keratotomy, endothelial damage from a minus power phakic intraocular lens, and microbial keratitis or endopthalmitis can be devastating for the affected patient. The relative risk of such vision-threatening complications must be compared among procedures.

QUALITY OF VISION

The subjective quality of the patient's vision should be the same after surgery as it was before surgery with spectacle or contact-lens correction. Presently, there are no accurate and precise clinical tests to objectively verify the quality of a patient's vision. Contrast sensitivity function can be measured using sine wave gradings or letters of graded contrast, and although there is disagreement about the meaning of changes in contrast at different spatial frequencies, this test gives a more realistic estimate of the patient's visual functioning under the graded contrasts of daily living than does high contrast Snellen visual acuity. Similarly, glare tests need improvement and refinement. One of the most commonly used is the brightness acuity test (BAT), which measures Snellen visual acuity under proximal glare conditions, but which is not sensitive enough to pick up subtle changes in glare—particularly those specific patterns such as starburst after refractive keratotomy and halos after photorefractive keratectomy. Subjective questionnaires can help assess the patient's own perceptions, but the same questions must be asked preoperatively and postoperatively. Asking a patient, "Is the quality of your vision as good after surgery as it was before surgery?" is a very difficult question for patients to answer, because most of them conceive of this as the quality of vision preoperatively without correction compared to postoperaatively without correction, and in the vast majority of cases it is better postoperatively. Such questions must clearly specify the conditions as with spectacle correction or with contact lens correction before surgery, and questions should be designed to that the same question can be asked exactly before surgery as after surgery: e.g., "The quality of my vision now with spectacle (or contact lens) correction is ______.", and the patient grades it on analog scale from excellent to poor. The postoperative question would then be the same, specifying the quality without optical correction, using the same analog scale for response.

Commonly, in talking with patients, a clinican will find that the patient is generally pleased with the outcome and if asked, would have the surgery again; however, a more in-depth conversation frequently reveals a cautionary, "But . . . ", the patient expressing a desire to see more sharply, with less glare, or better at night. Clearly, ophthalmic clinical science faces a big challenge in accurately measuring the quality of a patient's vision after refractive surgery.

STABILITY

Stability of refraction, of vision, and of the cornea or the material used to effect the refractive change is a requisite for success. Concerning short-term stability, the earlier it can be achieved after surgery, the better. Patients desire rapid recovery of vision and do not want to wait around for a few weeks or months to achieve their final correction. Concerning long-term stability, neither surgeons nor patients want a procedure that might be unstable over many years, such as the hyperopic shift after radial keratotomy, even if the shift is small, gradual, and can be offset by an initial small undercorrection. It takes 3 to 5 years to document the long-term stability of a corneal refractive surgical procedure—even if the procedures involve synthetic materials. The proportion of eyes changing refraction by 1.00 diopter or more during the time interval is a good measure of stability.

ADJUSTABILITY

One advantage of spectacles and contact lenses is adjustability. All patients expect to buy a new pair of glasses every couple of years, realizing that their refraction (or the styles of spectacles) change somewhat over time. The ideal refractive surgical procedure is also adjustable. Adjustability is particularly important in procedures that have less predictability.

The first type of adjustability concerns adjusting the outcome of the surgery within the first few weeks to months after surgery. Intentional undercorrection has become part of surgical planning for the correction of myopia because procedures such as refractive keratotomy and laser in situ keratomileusis (LASIK) can be repeated to treat residual myopia. Intentional undercorrection with early adjustment (enhancement) helps avoid overcorrection. Adjustment of sutures after penetrating keratoplasty helps reduce astigmatism.

Although the ideal refractive surgical procedure would create a completely perfect correction in one operation, staged or titrated surgery in which multiple procedures are done to adjust the outcome to the specific biologic response and visual needs of an individual patient are accepted by both surgeons and patients. Nevertheless, procedures that have a more accurate result with only a single operation will surely be judged superior.

The second type of adjustability is more theoretical. It responds to changes in the eye over years—changes induced either by the surgery itself or by normal biologic processes, including a progression of axial myopia or the appearance of presbyopia. This type of adjustability may require a repeat of the initial operation or the use of a different technique. For example, LASIK could theoretically accommodate two types of long-term adjustment. If the myopia progressed, the flap could be lifted and a second myopic ablation done in the bed. When this patient became presbyopic the flap could again be lifted and a small diameter plus power intracorneal lens could be implanted in at least one eye to provide near vision. Alternatively, a hyperopic excimer laser ablation might be performed.

REVERSIBILITY

If a procedure does not work properly, can it be undone? Contact lenses, if they become uncomfortable or inconvenient, are often exchanged by patients for spectacles. In general, refractive procedures that employ synthetic materials in the eye, such as phakic intraocular lenses or an intracorneal lens or rings are reversible, whereas procedures that alter corneal structure are not. An operation that can be reversed easily and safely will have considerable advantage.

CORNEAL SHAPE AND CONTOURS

The normal cornea is radially asymmetric and aspheric; refractive surgical procedures must provide corneal contours that are within physiologic bounds and that induce minimal optical aberrations. For example, excimer laser photorefractive keratectomy may create inflection zones at the edge of the ablation. If these overlay the pupil, they produce optical aberrations and cause symptoms of glare and halos. Increasing the diameter of the ablation from 4.5 to 6.5 or 7.0 mm will place the inflection zone outside the normal pupil and will decrease symptoms. Similarly, increasing the diameter of an intraocular lens from 4.5 to 6.0 mm will decrease edge glare at night.

Videokeratography provides a method of measuring corneal contours; indices of surface regularity are being developed to quantify the results of refractive surgery beyond the simple measurement of corneal radius of curvature, refracting power, and regular astigmatism. For example, the central elevation-depression magnitude index developed by Klyce[8] can quantify central steep islands after photorefractive keratectomy.

The criteria for acceptable corneal contours are not yet defined. Clearly, they are different from normal contours, which are prolate (steeper centrally and flatter peripherally), whereas after most surgical procedures to correct myopia, the cornea becomes oblate (flatter centrally and steeper paracentrally or peripherally). Psychophysical testing and laboratory ray tracing will be required to define the limits of acceptable corneal contours.

COMPLEXITY OF INSTRUMENTS AND SURGERY

Judging the risks and benefits of complex instruments and procedures is difficult. In general, we might think that simpler instruments and less complex techniques are better, but of course only if they give equal or superior results. For example, few would challenge the premise that after cataract extraction the implantation of an intraocular lens makes the procedure more complex, but the complexity can be mastered by the average ophthalmic surgeon and provides a quality of vision for the patient vastly superior to that of the aphakic state. Complexity of instruments is important, particularly when instruments such as an excimer laser are used, because the surgeon becomes dependent on technical support for proper functioning. Although the surgeon remains the captain of the ship in terms of medical responsibility, he does not have the knowledge to actually adjust and control the instrument that creates the refractive effect—the excimer laser and delivery system. Refractive surgical procedures involve instrumentation that renders the surgeon dependent on manufacturers, whether it be intraocular lenses, intracorneal lenses, diamond knives, or lasers. On the other hand, complex instruments and procedures that can be mastered by only a handful of experts after time-consuming and costly training of surgeons will not serve the general needs of the profession or patients because of lack of accessibility. Cryolathe keratomileusis is probably the best example of highly complex equipment and an extremely demanding set of manual skills—both of which blocked the popular adoption of this technique by surgeons. On the other hand, excimer laser photorefractive keratectomy is seen by many individuals as being so simple that it could be done by nonophthalmic surgeons.

When trying to evaluate the complexity of a particular technique we can ask how easy a procedure is to learn, how complex the equipment is to maintain, and how consistently a procedure can be performed.

COST

There are two types of costs associated with refractive surgical procedures: the actual cost to the surgeon of performing the procedure and the cost to the patient to receive the procedure.

In terms of actual cost, the extremes are represented by phakic intraocular lenses and the LASIK procedure. To implant a phakic intraocular lens the surgeon needs only a few additional hand instruments and can work in a standard operating environment where standard equipment is already available; the cost of the lens itself is usually borne by the patient. By contrast, to do the LASIK procedure, the surgeon needs a microkeratome and excimer laser that cost approximately $500,000 in the United States with ongoing costs of at least $50,000 per year for disposables and maintenance in addition to the periodic expense of upgrades and technology. The surgeon can charge approximately the same price for implanting a phakic intraocular lens and doing a LASIK procedure, so the differential cost to the surgeon or facility is enormous, whereas the differential cost to the patient is minimal. Market forces will play a role and will drive the price of equipment and procedures up or down, depending on competitive pressures.

Thus, in evaluating refractive surgical procedures, the surgeon must consider the overall profitability of a specific technique, factoring in requirements for ongoing training.

SATISFACTION OF THE PATIENT

Refractive surgery is a patient-driven subspecialty because the surgery is elective and the patients naturally compare the results with their already familiar spectacles and contact lenses. Thus a high level of patient satisfaction is required for a given procedure to remain popular. Satisfied patients are those who have an effective, predictable, safe procedure that gives good quality vision with optimal corneal contours, is adjustable, and can be purchased at reasonable cost. But it is difficult to measure a patient's satisfaction, which is often determined by important subtleties and nuances of the patient's visual and psychologic experience.

Most refractive surgery patients are pleased with the overall outcome, and they are happy about the fact they do not have to wear spectacles as much as they used to, but the results are frequently not as good as they desire. Similarly, asking patients to grade their level of satisfaction on a 0 to 100 scale gives only relative values. A patient may grade his or her satisfaction high, because he or she has no other procedure for comparison. If he or she had received a more effective procedure, the grade would be lower for the first, less effective procedure and higher for the second, more effective one. Thus we must develop more probing, exquisitely sensitive psychometric tests to measure patient satisfaction and use these tests more uniformly in evaluating refractive surgical procedures.

REPORTED RESULTS

Adequate data must be available to surgeons and patients for them to make adequate judgments about individual procedures. Unfortunately, many operations that have been developed have had periods of popularity based on statements from ophthalmologists who proffer their wares with the label "In my experience" and with vigorous commercial marketing, but with a paucity of reported results. This phenomenon occurred, for example, with hexagonal keratotomy, epikeratoplasty, automated lamellar keratoplasty, and deep lamellar keratotomy for hyperopia. In the first 1 or 2 years of their development, these procedures were propagated through weekend courses, industry adver-

KERATOMILEUSIS

Keratomileusis is the surgical technique that creates a plano anterior corneal disk or flap with parallel surfaces using a microkeratome (or, in the future, some other instrument such as a laser or water jet). The refractive change is then created either on the back of the disk or flap (keratomileusis) or in the stromal bed of the cornea (keratomileusis in situ). The current preferred technique is excimer laser in situ keratomileusis (LASIK). In this regard, the future is present because the LASIK procedure is becoming increasingly popular outside of the United States and is under FDA investigation in the United States.

A few reports have appeared in the peer reviewed literature, and more are required to meet the 13 criteria. The procedure is effective and reasonably predictable. It is safe when done properly, but misuse of the microkeratome, decentration of the excimer laser, or loss of the disc flap can cause permanent corneal damage. The quality of vision and corneal contours depends on the refinements of the microkeratome cut and the contours created by the excimer laser ablation. Optical aberrations occur at the edge of the ablation and central steep islands occur in some cases. Because wound healing is minimal, the procedure is expected to be stable, but this remains to be documented; 30 years of human experience with keratomileusis have shown no large long-term shifts in corneal contour. It is adjustable because repeated operations can be done for residual myopia and astigmatism, and when the techniques of hyperopic correction with an excimer laser are refined, it might be possible to adjust an overcorrection, although ablation of an already flattened surface may require different algorithms. The procedure is not reversible. Both the microkeratome and the excimer laser are complex, expensive instruments, but the surgery itself is no more complex than phacoemulsification. Early patient satisfaction is high because there is minimal pain and rapid recovery of vision; of course, overall patient satisfaction will depend on the accuracy and stability of the results.

INTRASTROMAL PHOTOREFRACTIVE KERATECTOMY

Another type of intrastromal surgery involves the use of a picosecond Nd:YAG laser or a Nd:YSGG laser to produce photodisruption within the stroma, creating vacuoles that, if present superficially enough, will cause the central cornea to collapse and flatten.[10] How predictably this can be done depends on the accuracy of the size and location of the vacuoles. The quality of vision and corneal contours depends on the pattern of the photodisruption. It is likely that the procedure will remain stable because it is confined to the stroma. Whether it can be adjusted and repeated remains to be seen. It is not reversible.

The instrumentation is complex, but the technique of surgery is simple. The lasers are costly. Patients have not yet been treated, and we must await reported results.

LASER PHOTOREFRACTIVE KERATECTOMY

Surgeons use excimer lasers to perform photorefractive keratectomy to sculpt or reshape the corneal surface. Solid state lasers emitting at wavelengths close to 193 nm will probably be used in the future because they are cheaper to make and easier to maintain.

The big question is whether photorefractive keratectomy on the surface of the cornea will find continued widespread use or whether it will be replaced by intrastromal surgery, such as the LASIK procedure. My opinion is that the LASIK technique will replace photorefractive keratectomy in the same way that small incision, corneal valve, phacomulsification cataract extraction is replacing extracapsular cataract extraction. Photorefractive keratectomy will be used by many surgeons for some years because of regulatory restrictions on other procedures, because the technique is simpler than LASIK, because the intrastromal procedures must be proven before surgeons will adopt them, because photorefractive keratectomy has considerable momentum among ophthalmic laser manufacturers, and because refractive surgery services companies wish to capitalize on its technical simplicity.

Using the 13 criteria outlined, we can contrast photorefractive keratectomy and LASIK. Both are effective, and since similar algorithms are used both on the surface and in the bed, the versatility and effectiveness will probably remain comparable. Predictability should be better for LASIK because corneal stromal wound healing plays less of a role, but improved algorithms and contours for surface photoablation might make the two procedures similar in their predictability. Photorefractive keratectomy is safer because LASIK requires the use of a microkeratome. Quality of vision might be better after LASIK because Bowman's layer and the epithelium remain intact. LASIK is more quickly adjustable because recovery from the procedure is generally within days, whereas recovery from photorefractive keratectomy takes weeks to months. Neither procedure is reversible. LASIK should be more stable over time because there is less stromal wound healing. Corneal contours should be similar in the two procedures, since the same laser and algorithms are used, but stromal wound healing after PRK can create irregular areas of steepening and flattening. Patient satisfaction should be higher after LASIK because the procedure is less painful, recovery of vision is faster and postoperative topical medication is minimal. Far more reports are presently available on photorefractive keratectomy than on LASIK.

REFRACTIVE KERATOTOMY

Discussing refractive keratotomy (radial keratotomy for myopia and transverse keratotomy for astigmatism) sounds more like a glance toward the past than a look into the future. Will refractive keratotomy be part of refractive surgery in the future? I think so for the following reasons:

1. It is a time-honored procedure that has been done for over 100 years and improved continuously for the past 50 years.
2. The surgical techniques are refined and well established and have been taught to thousands of ophthalmologists around the world.
3. Many ophthalmologists will not have access to an excimer laser and/or a microkeratome and therefore will use refractive keratotomy.
4. Arcuate transverse keratotomy is an accurate and simple way to correct residual astigmatism after other procedures, including photorefractive keratectomy, LASIK, and intraocular lenses.
5. Refractive keratotomy might find a role in underdeveloped and developing countries, where the majority of individuals with myopia do not have spectacles and therefore are less productive citizens throughout their working years. If refractive keratotomy could be performed on these people effectively and cheaply, it is likely that their economic productivity and social contributions would increase.

Radial keratotomy can effectively eliminate myopia, achieving a refractive outcome within 0.50 diopter in 60% of eyes and within 1.00 diopter in 80% with reasonable predictability. The procedure is adjustable in one direction because repeated operations can reduce residual myopia or astigmatism. Approximately 30% of eyes will require one or more repeated operations to adjust the outcome nearer to the stated goal. Vision-threatening complications and severe glare are extremely rare after refractive keratotomy, making it a reasonably safe procedure. The quality of vision is good as shown by psychometric tests. However, corneal contours are severely altered by refractive keratotomy, with a polygonal topographic pattern and subtle optical aberrations perceived as halos and starbursts (from the scars) when the pupil is dilated. The procedure is not reversible. The operation requires good clinical skill but is not unduly complex. Special instruments must be purchased at a cost of approximately $25,000. Patient satisfaction is high, and there are hundreds of articles now reporting results of refractive keratotomy. Stability of the procedure is good in the short term, but a shift of refraction in the hyperopic direction of 1 diopter or more occurs in approximately half of the eyes over 10 years.[11]

THERMAL KERATOPLASTY

Ophthalmic surgeons have known for more than 100 years that heating the cornea causes contraction of the stroma and flattening in the area heated with a compensatory steepening in the unheated area. The secret of success for thermal keratoplasty, which is usually used to treat hyperopia and hyperopic astigmatism, seems to be in the accurate delivery of enough thermal energy to the stromal collagen to cause it to shrink the exact amount to predictably change the corneal power and then retain that shape indefinitely. This seems to require a permanent change in the molecular structure of the collagen, so that there is not a gradual loss of the initial effect.

The holmium:YAG infrared laser is the instrument under evaluation for future use. The efficacy and predictability depend on the stability of the outcome, which is currently not very good, because a large percentage of the initial effect is lost in the weeks to months after surgery. When the burns are applied outside a 6 mm diameter zone, the procedure seems to be reasonably safe with minimal reduction in the quality of vision. The procedure can be repeated, making it adjustable in the direction of a fuller reduction or a repeated reduction in far-sightedness. This adjustability might be useful. If the procedure is found to lose its effect after 1 or 2 years, it potentially could be repeated periodically, rather like buying a new pair of reading glasses. It is not reversible. Use of the solid-state holmium:YAG laser is not complex, although the surgeon must depend on the expensive and technologically complex functioning of the laser. Corneal contours resulting from the thermal keratoplasty remain to be defined, but some unusual shapes may result. Patient satisfaction depends on the outcomes. Few reports are now appearing in the literature.

Delivery of Refractive Surgical Services

The delivery of medical care is becoming dominated by economics, government control, and business influences throughout the world. In the United States the change from individual or small group private practice to domination by governments and large health care corporations is accelerating. Refractive surgery is not immune to these events.

HIGH PROFITS, HIGH COST

Two features of refractive surgery distinguish it from routine ophthalmic care:

1. The surgery is elective and is usually paid for by the patient.
2. The cost of purchasing and maintaining equipment—especially an excimer laser—is high.

The self-pay aspect means that there will be minimal third party price cutting and the cost of the procedure can remain between $1,000 and 2,000 per eye in the United States, unless surgeons get into a price war. If 10% of the 0.7 billion people with myopia in the United States have refractive surgery at $1,000 per eye, a $1.4 billion industry exists. The high cost of equipment means that individual surgeons and small groups cannot provide these services, unless they are able to secure a high volume of surgery to offset the costs. These two motivating factors—high profits and high cost—have spawned a new medical entity: the refractive surgery service or management company. As of this writing, there are approximately 20 such companies in various stages of development. Most of them promise high profit at minimal cost to the refractive surgeon, based on the following:

1. Large numbers of patients will seek refractive surgery.
2. There will be an initial surge in surgical volume when the excimer laser is approved for clinical use in the United States.
3. The company that can capitalize on this initial surge will be successful.
4. Excimer laser photorefractive keratectomy will be the cornerstone of refractive surgery for many years, making it easy to train large numbers of ophthalmologists to do the procedure and manage the patients according to simple formulas.
5. Volume purchasing of lasers and supplies will bring down the overall cost.
6. Optometrists wish to participate in refractive surgery networks and will refer patients to surgeons if they can receive acceptable comanagement fees or equity participation in the company.
7. Ophthalmic surgeons are willing to join networks that offer a "turnkey" approach, where the surgeon simply must perform the surgery with minimal financial or personal investment.
8. Successful companies can be taken public or sold to larger health care entities at a handsome profit.

Critical readers will spot the strengths and weaknesses of these premises, any of which can be challenged; only the test of the marketplace will prove whether these premises are valid.

MODELS FOR REFRACTIVE SURGERY COMPANIES

There is a full spectrum of business models for these companies, ranging from simple ambulatory refractive surgery centers where each surgeon pays a fee to use the center and its equipment, to a fully integrated refractive surgery provider system.

Most companies fall into one of the following categories based on the type of group and philosophy behind the company. There is considerable overlap and most are founded on common premises. These include business-driven, optometric-driven, corporation-driven, and ophthalmic-driven models.

1. Business driven
2. Optometric driven
3. Health care corporation driven
4. Ophthalmic driven

BUSINESS AND REFRACTIVE SURGERY

For better or worse, the future of refractive surgery will be shaped strongly by business interests. Manufacturers of refractive surgery instruments, such as excimer lasers, and supplies, such as intraocular lenses, play a major role in determining the surgical techniques available to surgeons and patients. Government entities, such as the FDA, have strong regulatory control in some countries over the manufacture and distribution of refractive surgery instruments and products, whereas in other countries, government regulation is almost nonexistent.

Business interests are strong because of the high potential profits and businessmen—including those who manufacture refractive surgery instruments and sell them to ophthalmic surgeons—will attempt to control the delivery of refractive surgery services. Refractive surgeons should not abrogate their authority and responsibility by yielding control to nonophthalmic interests; rather they should take the leadership in this arena in the best interests of fulfilling the social contract with their most important partners—their patients.

REFERENCES

1. Schimmelpfennig BH, Waring GO: Development of refractive keratotomy in the nineteenth century. In Waring GO: *Refractive keratotomy for myopia and astigmatism,* St Louis, 1992, Mosby.
2. Akiyama K et al: Development of radial keratotomy in Japan, 1939-1960. In Waring GO: *Refractive keratotomy for myopia and astigmatism,* St Louis, 1992, Mosby.
3. Waring GO: Development of refractive keratotomy in the Soviet Union, 1960-1990. In Waring GO: *Refractive keratotomy for myopia and astigmatism,* St Louis, 1992, Mosby.
4. Waring GO: Standardized data collection and reporting for refractive surgery, *Refract Corneal Surg* 8(Suppl):1-42, 1992.
5. Bourque LB et al, PERK Study Group: Spectacle and contact lens wearing six years after radial keratotomy in the Prospective

Evaluation of Radial Keratotomy Study, *Ophthalmology* 101:421-431, 1994.

6. Lynn MJ, Waring GO, Kutner MH: Predictability of refractive keratotomy. In Waring GO: *Refractive keratotomy for myopia and astigmatism,* St Louis, 1992, Mosby.
7. Lynn MJ et al, PERK Study Group: Symmetry of refractive and visual acuity outcome in the Prospective Evaluation of Radial Keratotomy (PERK) Study, *Refract Corneal Surg* 5:75-81, 1989.
8. Klyce SD et al: Evaluating refractive surgery with corneal topography, *Invest Ophthalmol Vis Sci* 36:S1, 1995.
9. Thompson KP, Hanna KD, Waring GO: Emerging technologies for refractive surgery: laser adjustable synthetic epikeratoplasty, *Refract Corneal Surg* 5:46-48, 1989.
10. Habib MS et al: Wound healing following intrastromal photorefractive keratectomy with the Nd:YLF picosecond laser in the cat, *J Refract Surg* 1995;11:442-447, 1995.
11. Waring GO, Lynn MJ, McDonnell PJ, and the PERK Study Group: Results of the Prospective Evaluation of Radial Keratotomy (PERK) Study 10 years after surgery, *Arch Ophthalmol* 112: 1298-1308, 1995.

Index

Note: Numbers in italics and preceded by *A* refer to terms mentioned in the *Cornea Color Atlas.*

A

Aberrant epithelial resurfacing, 205
Ablation
  intrastromal, 2000, 2001
  lacrimal, 675
  plasma-mediated, 2185
  in synthetic epikeratoplasty, 2235-2236
  in trichiasis, 569
Ablepharon, 872, 873
ABMD; *see* Anterior basement membrane dystrophy
ABO blood group matching, 1764
Abrasion, 1404-1407, *A227*
  Acanthamoeba keratitis and, 1267
  in astigmatic keratotomy, 2163
  from blunt trauma, 1930
  dust trail linear, *A262*
  epithelial, 1404-1406
  stromal, 1407
Abscess
  conjunctival, *A54*
  eyelid, *A28*
  suture, 1700-1701, *A279*
Acanthamoeba keratitis, 1267-1273, 1311-1312, *A199-202*
  clinical findings, 1268-1270
  confocal microscopy in, 344-345
  contact lens-induced, 1466-1467
  corneal ulcer in, 405
  differential diagnosis, 1271
  laboratory diagnosis, 1270-1271
  penetrating keratoplasty in, 1553
  prevention, 1273
  pseudodendrites in, 431
  risk factors, 1267-1268
  therapeutic keratoplasty for, 1845
  treatment, 1271-1273
Acanthosis nigricans, 999
Acarina, 655-656
Accreditation by Eye Bank Association of America, 470-471
Acetazolamide, 1823
Acetic acid, 1437
N-Acetylcysteine, *A32, A209*
  in ligneous conjunctivitis, 867
  in superior limbic keratoconjunctivitis, 860
Acid, 1437
Acid-fast stain, 306
Acid injury, 676, 1437-1442, *A259*
Acidic fibroblast growth factor, 185-188
Acne, 458
Acquired immunodeficiency syndrome
  after penetrating keratoplasty, 1706
  bacterial keratitis in, 1142
  conjunctivitis in, 769-770
  corneal infections in, 1017-1022
  disorders related to, *A111*
  erythema multiforme in, 839
  herpes zoster in, 1233
  Kaposi's sarcoma in, *A45*
  molluscum contagiosum in, *A26*
  Reiter's syndrome in, 785, 1518
Acquired lacrimal gland deficiency, 674
Acquired melanosis, *A41*
Acridine-orange stain, 305-306, 1159-1160
Acrochordon, 583
Acrodermatitis enteropathica, 994
Acrospiroma, eccrine, 593
Actinic keratosis, 585, 606, *A11-12*
Actinomyces, 802, *A35*
  in bacterial conjunctivitis, 768
  in canaliculitis, 692
  in dacryoadenitis, 687
  eyelid and, 653, 654
Acular; *see* Ketorolac
Acute anterior uveitis 1516-1517
Acute bacterial keratitis, *A177*
Acute conjunctivitis, 764-766, 767
Acute follicular conjunctivitis, 750-752
Acute hemorrhagic conjunctivitis, 1245-1246
Acute lymphocytic leukemia, 970
Acute membranous conjunctivitis, 752
Acute myeloid leukemia, 969-970
Acute papillary conjunctivitis, 750
Acute perivasculitis, 1532
Acute retinal necrosis, 1232
Acute spastic entropion, 561
Acyclovir, *A280*
  following keratoplasty, 1805
  in herpes simplex blepharoconjunctivitis, 643
  in herpes simplex keratitis, 1214, 1218-1219
  in neonatal conjunctivitis, 794
  in postherpetic neuralgia, 1238
  postoperative, 1767-1768
  therapeutic keratoplasty with, 1846
  in varicella zoster virus infection, 645, 1236-1237
Addressins, 86
Adellen, 392
Adenine arabinoside
  corneal effects, 1023
  in herpes simplex virus keratitis, 1214
  in infectious epithelial keratitis, 1215
  in neonatal conjunctivitis, 794
  in neonatal herpes simplex virus kerato-conjunctivitis, 794
  toxicity of, 849-850
Adenitis, 642
Adenoma
  pleomorphic, 593
  sebaceous, 596
Adenosine triphosphate, 3
Adenovirus
  in conjunctivitis, 750-751, 773-775
  laboratory investigation of, 309
Adhesins, 133, 1144, 1146
Adhesion complex, 199-200
Adhesion molecules, 85-86, 87
  in allograft rejection, 95
  in interior segment, 100
Adhesion receptor families, 87
Adhesives
  in acid injury, 1441
  in anterior segment surgery, 1932-1933
  in corneal perforation, 1818-1825
  in progressive stromal keratolysis, 1180
  in surgery for corneal thinning disorders, 1795
  in synthetic epikeratoplasty, 2236
Adjunctive therapy
  in bacterial keratitis, 1179-1181
  in pterygium, 1880-1883
Adjustability of refractive surgery, 2246
Adrenochrome deposits, 420, *A113*
Adult inclusion conjunctivitis, 783-785, *A58-59*
Advanced lattice dystrophy type I, *A129*
Advancement conjunctival flap, 1904, 1905
Afipia felis, 799
African eye worm, 658
Against-the-rule astigmatism, 876, 2158
Agar, *A196*
Age
  anterior uveitis and, 1494
  Bitot's spot and, 957
  corneal arcus and, 1119-1120
  corneal edema and, 410
  donor-recipient issues, 489
  penetrating keratoplasty and, 1581
  postkeratoplasty astigmatism and, 1681
Agenesis, corneal, 872
Agglutination, 1162
Aggrecan, 34
AIDS; *see* Acquired immunodeficiency syndrome
Air bubble indentations, *A263*
Alcaine; *see* Proparacaine
Alcian blue stain, *A93, A124*
Aldose reductase, 979
Alkali injury, 1443-1451, *A259-260*
  corneal perforation in, 1815-1816
  corneal ulcer after, *A292*
  dry eye following, 676
  emergency treatment, 1445-1447
  epidemiology and natural history, 1443
  graft failure and, 1762
  new research initiatives, 1450
  repair, 1443-1445, 1446-1447
  transitional stage treatment, 1447-1448
  visual rehabilitation, 1440-1450
Alkaline protease
  corneal infection and, 1147

- Alkaline protease—cont'd
  - in ocular wound healing, 186
  - pseudomonal, 133
- Alkaptonuria, 912, *A91*
- Alkylating agents, 1511
- Allergic ocular disease, 106-110
  - conjunctivitis, 805-810, *A65*
  - epiphora in, 696
  - eyelid, *A28*
  - immunopathology of, 108-109
  - rhinoconjunctivitis, 806-808
  - toxicity ***versus***, 847-849
- Allergic shiner, 807
- Allograft rejection, 90-96, 1687-1696
  - afferent immune response in, 91-94
  - animal models, 90-91
  - clinical features, 1689-1692
  - differential diagnosis, 1692-1693
  - efferent immune response in, 94-96
  - herpes simplex disease and, 1800, 1806-1808
  - historical perspective, 1687
  - immunology of, 1757-1761
  - immunomodulation, 96
  - induced after phototherapeutic keratoplasty, 2209
  - management strategy, 1695
  - methods for improving graft survival, 1764-1769
  - in pediatric penetrating keratoplasty, 1732-1734, 1751-1752
  - penetrating keratoplasty in, 1555
  - prevention, 1694
  - recognition of risk factors, 1687-1689
  - treatment, 1693-1694, 1769
- Allograft tolerance, 96
- Alomide; ***see*** Lodoxamide
- Alpha-5 β-1 integrin receptor, 206
- Alpha-chymotrypsin, 867
- Alpha toxin, 133
- Alpha$_6$β$_4$ integrin heterodimer, 200
- Alport's syndrome, 1073
- Alternate pathway of complement, 81-85, 144
- Amantadine, 1028
- Amaurosis, Leber's congenital, *A154*
- Amblyopia, 1735, 1748-1750
- American incision, 2016
- Amikacin, 1169, 1178
- Amino acid metabolism disorders, 910-915
  - alkaptonuria, 912
  - amyloidosis, 912-913, 914
  - cystinosis, 910-912
  - gout, 913-914
  - porphyria, 915
  - tyrosinemia II, 912
  - xeroderma pigmentosa, 914-915
- Amino acids deprivation, 964
- Amino penicillins, 1167
- Aminocaproic acid, 1931
- Aminoglycosides, 1168-1169, 1177-1178
  - in acute bacterial conjunctivitis, 766
  - preoperative, 2060
  - in staphylococcal blepharitis, 634
  - toxicity of, 850
- Amiodarone, 907, 908, *A115*
- Amitriptyline, 646, 1238
- Ammonia burn, *A259*
- Ammoniated mercury ophthalmic ointment, 657
- Amodiaquine, 1026
- Amorphous stromal dystrophy, *A141*
- Amoxicillin, 1006
- Amphotericin B
  - in fungal keratitis, 1258, 1259, 1260
  - toxicity of, 850-851
- Amyloidosis, 420, *A7, A103*
  - conjunctival, 731-732, 733
  - corneal, 912-913, 914, 1123-1125
  - in lattice dystrophy, 1048
  - in syphilitic interstitial keratopathy, 1294
- Analgesics, 1238
- Analyzed Area, 2047
- Androgenic steroids, 681
- Anemia, iron deficiency, 968
- Anesthesia
  - in anterior segment surgery, 1934-1935
  - in automated lamellar keratoplasty, 2169
  - complications in radial keratotomy, 2101
  - in conjunctival limbal autograft, 1948
  - in penetrating keratoplasty, 1582
    - in herpes simplex disease, 1803
    - with intraocular lens exchange, 1605
  - in radial keratotomy, 2060-2061, 2062
  - in Schirmer test, 667
  - for scleral perforation, 1965-1966
  - in therapeutic keratoplasty, 1848-1849
  - topical, *A215*
    - abuse of, 1354-1356
    - corneal effects, 1023, 1024
    - toxicity of, 851
- Anesthesimeter, 2023
- Angiogenesis, 151-153
- Angiogenin, 152
- Angiography, 1476
- Angiolymphoid hyperplasia with eosinophilia, 591
- Angiotensin converting enzyme, 1526
- Angle closure glaucoma, 1076
- Angular artery, 65-66
- Angular blepharitis, 634-635, *A24*
- Anhidrotic ectodermal dysplasia, 994
- Anhydrous ammonia burn, *A259*
- Animal studies
  - of diabetic cornea, 979
  - in interstitial keratitis, 1296
- Aniridia, 894, *A176*
- Anisocoria, 2209
- Anisometropia
  - after incisional refractive surgery, 2117
  - after radial keratotomy, 2107, 2136
- Ankyloblepharon, 829, 830
- Ankylosing spondylitis, 1519
- Anterior basement membrane, 2108
- Anterior basement membrane dystrophy, 200
- Anterior chamber
  - anterior segment surgery and, 1927-1928, 1929
  - corneal perforation and, 1816
  - epithelialization of, 329-330, 1709-1713
  - examination in anterior uveitis, 1498-1499, 1500
  - Fuchs' heterochromic iridocyclitis and, 1537
  - intraoperative hemorrhage, 1641-1642
  - ocular immune response, 104-105
  - viscoelastic placement in penetrating keratoplasty, 1586
- Anterior chamber angle
  - development of, 885-887
  - examination in anterior uveitis, 1498-1499, 1500
  - reconstructive procedures after anterior segment trauma, 1953
- Anterior chamber-associated immune deviation, 93-94, 104-105
- Anterior chamber cleavage syndromes 885-896, *A83-86*
  - corneal abnormalities
    - central, 888-889
    - peripheral, 889-893
  - development of angle, 885-887
  - differential diagnosis, 894
  - examination, 893-894
  - treatment, 894-895
- Anterior chamber epithelial inclusion cyst, *A258*
- Anterior chamber flare, 1498
  - in acute anterior uveitis, 1516-1517
  - corneal allograft rejection and, 168[illegible]
- Anterior chamber intraocular lens 15[illegible]8
  - evaluation, 1622
  - technique, 1612-1613
- Anterior chamber paracentesis, 1501-1502
- Anterior conjunctival plexus, 30-31, 3[illegible]
- Anterior corneal dystrophy, 1033-1042, *A119-124*
  - Bowman's layer, 1039-1042
  - epithelial basement membrane dystrophy, 1034-1039
  - Meesmann's juvenile epithelial dystrophy, 1033-1034
  - minimal visual loss in, 452
- Anterior embryotoxon, 1119
- Anterior episcleral arterial circle, 30-3[illegible], 36
- Anterior infraciliary approach, 56[illegible]
- Anterior segment
  - acid burns, 1437-1442
  - alkali injury
    - emergency treatment, 1445-1447
    - epidemiology and natural history, 1443
    - new research initiatives, 145[illegible]
    - repair, 1443-1445, 1446-1447
    - transitional stage treatment, 1447-1448
    - visual rehabilitation, 1440-1450
  - corneal edema and, 412
  - dermoids and, 377
  - examination before penetrating keratoplasty, 1567
  - high resolution ultrasound, 35[illegible]
  - hypersensitivity reactions and, 106-116
    - type I, 106-110
    - type II, 110-112
    - type III, 112-114
    - type IV, 114-116
  - ischemia, *A258*
  - ocular immune response, 96-106
    - anterior chamber, 104-105
    - conjunctiva, 98-101
    - cornea, 101-104
    - sclera, 105-106
    - tear film and lacrimal gland, 96-9[illegible]
  - skeletal and connective tissue disorders, 925-942
    - classification of, 925-926, 927-928
    - craniofacial malformation syndromes, 926-929
    - dermo-chondro-corneal dystrophy of Francois, 938
    - Ehlers-Danlos syndrome, 930-934, 935
    - Goldenhar syndrome, 929-930
    - Hallermann-Streiff syndrome, 930
    - hypophosphatasia, 939
    - Kniest syndrome, 935-936
    - Marfan syndrome, 936-937

skeletal and connective tissue disorders—cont'd
oculo-dento-osseous dysplasia, 937-938
osteogenesis imperfecta, 934-935
Sotos syndrome, 938
Stickler syndrome, 935
syndrome of acromegaly, 939
Treacher Collins syndrome, 930
treatment of, 939-940
Werner syndrome, 938-939
viral infections and, 1248
Wegener's granulomatosis and, 948
Anterior segment surgery
cyclectomy, 1957-1964
complications, 1963-1964
indications, 1957-1958
postoperative care, 1963
procedure, 1958-1963
results, 1964
surgical anatomy, 1958
rehabilitation after trauma, 1947-1955, *A293-294*
conjunctiva, 1949, 1948
cornea, 1949-1952
estimating visual potential, 1947-1948
graft failure and, 1763
iris and angle, 1953
in penetrating keratoplasty with intraocular lens implantation, 1609-1610, 1611, 1620
temporary keratoprosthesis, 1953-1954
vitreous and lens, 1952-1953
scleral perforation, 1965-1973
anesthesia for, 1965-1966
with fixation sutures, 1639, 1640
surgical repair, 1966-1972
for trauma, 1925-1945
anesthesia, 1934-1935
antibiotics, 1933-1934
blunt trauma, 1929-1930
corneal laceration repair, 1935-1938
corneoscleral lacerations, 1938-1939
external examination, 1926-1929, 1930
foreign bodies, 1932, 1942
hyphema, 1930-1932
iridodialysis, 1939-1940
iris trauma, 1939
lens trauma, 1940-1941
management of tissue loss, 1938
patient evaluation, 1925-1926
postoperative care, 1942-1943
postoperative complications, 1943-1944
prevention of endophthalmitis, 1933
suture removal, 1943
tissue adhesive, 1932-1933
visual rehabilitation, 1943
vitreous presentation, 1941-1942
Anterior segment trauma
reconstruction after, 1947-1955
conjunctiva, 1949, 1948
cornea, 1949-1952
estimating visual potential, 1947-1948
iris and angle, 1953
temporary keratoprosthesis, 1953-1954
vitreous and lens, 1952-1953
surgical management, 1925-1945
anesthesia, 1934-1935
antibiotics, 1933-1934
blunt trauma, 1929-1930
corneal laceration repair, 1935-1938
corneoscleral lacerations, 1938-1939
external examination, 1926-1929, 1930
foreign bodies, 1932, 1942
hyphema, 1930-1932
iridodialysis, 1939-1940
iris trauma, 1939
lens trauma, 1940-1941
management of tissue loss, 1938
patient evaluation, 1925-1926
postoperative care, 1942-1943
postoperative complications, 1943-1944
prevention of endophthalmitis, 1933
suture removal, 1943
tissue adhesive, 1932-1933
visual rehabilitation, 1943
vitreous presentation, 1941-1942
Anterior stromal cautery, 414
Anterior stromal keratectomy, 1868
Anterior stromal puncture, 203-204
in ocular surface disease, 1868-1869, 1870
in recurrent erosion syndrome, 1321-1324, 1325
Anterior uveitis, 1493-1503, *A269-272*
Behçet's disease, 1529-1535, *A271*
classification, 1500-1501
demography, 1494-1495
diagnostic evaluation, 1501-1502
Fuchs' heterochromic iridocyclitis, 1537-1540
HLA-B27 related, 1515-1521
idiopathic, 1505-1513
classification and previous occurrence, 1505, 1506
consultation in, 1508
laboratory evaluation, 1507-1508
physical examination in, 1506-1507
treatment of, 1508-1513
in juvenile rheumatoid arthritis, 1370-1371, 1541-1548, *A272*
patient history, 1493-1494
physical examination in, 1495-1500
in sarcoidosis, 1524-1525
symptoms, 1493
syphilitic interstitial keratitis and, 1282, 1283
treatment, 1502-1503
Anterior vitrectomy, 1558, 1745-1746
Anterior vitreous, 1499-1500
Anthrax, eyelid, 638
Antibiotics, 1165-1177
in acute bacterial conjunctivitis, 766
aminoglycosides, 1168-1169
in anterior segment surgery, 1933-1934
in anterior segment trauma, 1934
in bacterial keratitis, 1177-1179
in blepharitis, 623-624
cephalosporins, 167-1168
chloramphenicol, 1173-1174
in corneal abrasion, 1404-1405, *A227*
in corneal erosion, *A262*
in corneal perforation, 1818
in corneal ulcer, *A266*
in dacryoadenitis, 687
in dacryocystis, 689
in eyelid necrosis, 637-638
fluoroquinolones, 1169-1171
in foreign body injuries, *A244*
glycopeptides, 1168
in gonococcal conjunctivitis, *A62*
in hordeolum, 635
impairment of epithelial wound healing, 189-190
in infectious crystalline keratopathy, 1702
in interstitial keratitis, 1299, 1300
macrolides and lincosamides, 1171-1172
in marginal staphylococcus keratitis, 1394
in meibomian gland dysfunction, 630-631
in necrotizing scleritis, 1369
in neurotrophic ulcer, *A193*
penicillins, 1166-1167
peptide, 1175
in phlyctenulosis, 1392
in postkeratoplasty keratitis, 1699
in postoperative endophthalmitis, 1704
for postoperative epithelial defects, 1663
preoperative, 1582
before radial keratotomy, 2060
in recurrent corneal erosion, 202
rifampin, 1174
routes of administration, 1175-1177
spectinomycin, 1174-1175
in staphylococcal blepharitis, 634
in stromal infiltrate, *A266*
sulfonamides, 1174
for suspected sterile infiltrates, 432
tetracyclines, 1173
toxicity of, 850-851
in trachoma, 783
trimethoprim, 1174
in Whipple's disease, 946
Antibody
allograft rejection and, 94
in herpes simplex virus keratitis, 1213
in juvenile rheumatoid arthritis, 1544
in Mooren's ulcer, 1398
response to antigen, 81
Antibody-mediated immune response, 89
Anticardiolipin, 1377
Anticollagenases, 209
Anticonvulsants, 840
Antifungals
in fungal keratitis, 1258-1261
toxicity of, 850-851
Antigen
in allograft rejection, 91-93
antibody response to, 81
B-cell presentation of, 90
cytotoxic hypersensitivity response to, 110-112
in phlyctenular keratoconjunctivitis, 1389
processing of, 88-89
Antigen modulation, 1765
Antigen presenting cell, 74, 76, 77, 88
Antiglaucoma medications, 1025-1026
Antihistamines, 109-110
in allergic conjunctivitis, 808
in atopic keratoconjunctivitis, 816
to improve graft survival, 1785
in vernal keratoconjunctivitis, 813
Antiinflammatory agents, 209
Antimalarial agents, 1026
Antimetabolites, 1512
Antimicrobial removal device, 307
Antimicrobials
in anterior segment trauma, 1934
erythema multiforme and, 840
susceptibility testing, 1163, 1166

Antimicrobials—cont'd
therapeutic keratoplasty with, 1849
Antineutrophil cytoplasmic antibody, 1381
Antinuclear antibody
in relapsing polychondritis, 1380
in systemic lupus erythematosus, 1377
Antipseudomonal penicillins, 1167
Antitorque suture, 1589, 1630
Antiviral agents, *A280*
following keratoplasty, 1805
in herpes simplex blepharoconjunctivitis, 643
in herpes simplex keratitis, 1213-1214
in infectious epithelial keratitis, 1215-1216
toxicity of, 849-850
Aphakia, 1720-1721
Aphakic bullous keratopathy, 1423-1435, *A256*
Brown-McLean syndrome and, 1426
etiology of, 1426-1430, 1431
histopathology of, 1425
incidence of, 1423-1425
optic section and, 250
pathogenesis of, 1425-1426
slit beam of, 290, 291
treatment of, 1431-1432
Aphakic corneal edema, 1554
Apo-retinol-binding protein, 955
Apocrine hidrocystoma, 593
Applanation lenses, 2167-2168
Apraclonidine hydrochloride, 850
Aqueous drainage for postkeratoplasty glaucoma, 1727
Aqueous humor
immune recognition and, 93
immunoregulatory factors in, 95
tear film and, 49
Aqueous layer, 50-52, 666, *A29*
Aqueous leak, *A296*
Aqueous tear deficiency, 673-679
non-Sjögren's, 673-676
Sjögren's syndrome, 676-679
Ara-A; *see* Adenine arabinoside
Arachnida
in canaliculitis, 692
in eyelid infection, 655-656
Arcuate keratotomy, 1682
Arcus juvenilis, *A164*
Arcus senilis, 389-390, 423, 1119-1120, *A164*
Argon laser ablation, 569
Argon laser photocoagulation
in corneal injury, *A241*
in epithelial ingrowth, *A258*
Argon laser trabeculoplasty, 1725-1726
Argyrol, *A112*
Argyrosis, 917, 1027, *A112*
Arlt's line, 443, 749
Arne study, 2084-2086, 2094
Arsphenamine, 1276
Arteriovenous malformation, eyelid, 590
Arthritis
external eye diseases and, 457-458
Lyme disease and, 1004
in Reiter's syndrome, 1517
rheumatoid, 1359-1375, *A217-220*
articular manifestations, 1360
extra-articular manifestations, 1360-1361
juvenile, 1370-1371, 1541-1548, *A272*
keratitis in, 1364-1365, 1366, 1367
keratoconjunctivitis sicca in, 1361-1362
macroulcerative peripheral keratitis and, 396-397
ocular chrysiasis and, 425
pathogenesis, 1359-1360
scleritis in, 1362-1364, 1365, 1366
treatment, 1367-1370
Arthus reaction, 113
Artificial tears
in cicatricial pemphigoid, 831
in macroulcerative peripheral keratitis, 397
in neurotrophic keratopathy, 1216
in rheumatoid arthritis-associated keratoconjunctivitis sicca, 1368
toxic ulcerative keratopathy secondary to, 848
Ascorbic acid, 1440-1441
Asculap-Meditec excimer laser, 2183
Aspergillus, 407, 1254, *A195, A196*
Aspirin
in juvenile rheumatoid arthritis, 1544
in Kawasaki disease, 951
in postherpetic neuralgia, 1238
in vernal keratoconjunctivitis, 813
Astemizole
in atopic keratoconjunctivitis, 816
to improve graft survival, 1785
Astigmatic dial, 218
Astigmatic keratotomy, 2143-2153
cataract, 2155-2164
complications, 2162-2163
incision variables, 2155-2156
instruments for incisional astigmatic surgery, 2159-2160
preoperative evaluation, 2156-2157
surgical decisions, 2157-2159
theory and incisional procedure, 2160-2162
informed consent, 2146
instrumentation, 2018, 2020
intraoperative complications, 2151
operative methods, 2146-2148, 2152
patient selection, 2145-2146, 2147
postoperative management, 2151-2152
preoperative testing, 2146, 2148, 2149, 2150-2151
results, 2152-2153
Astigmatism, 875-876
after automated lamellar keratoplasty, 2177-2178
after cataract surgery, 2155-2164
complications, 2162-2163
incision variables, 2155-2156
instruments for incisional astigmatic surgery, 2159-2160
preoperative evaluation, 2156-2157
surgical decisions, 2157-2159
theory and incisional procedure, 2160-2162
after photorefractive keratoplasty, 2195
after radial keratotomy, 2107, 2134-2135
astigmatic keratotomy in, 2143-2153
informed consent, 2146
intraoperative complications, 2151
operative methods, 2146-2148, 2152
patient selection, 2145-2146, 2147
postoperative management, 2151-2152
preoperative testing, 2146, 2148, 2149, 2150-2151
results, 2152-2153
birth injury and, 1410
contact lens for, 1458-1460
corneal dermoid and, 377
corneal laceration and, 1936
correction at time of cataract surgery, 2161-2162
eccentric lamellar graft for, 1832
following anterior segment trauma, 1944
high, *A288*
irregular, 448
after astigmatic keratotomy, 2163
after automated lamellar keratoplasty, 2177
after radial keratotomy, 2134-2135
videokeratopathy in, 2053
photoastigmatic refractive keratectomy for, 2197-2198, 2200
photorefractive keratoplasty results, 2197-2198, 2200
in posterior keratoconus, 878
postkeratoplasty, 1651-1652, 1675-1685
intraoperative factors, 1677-1679
postoperative factors, 1679-1684
preoperative factors, 1675-1677
radial keratotomy incisions and, 2079-2082
refractive properties and responses, 219
regular, 875-876, 2143, 2144, 2146
suture adjustment for, 1632-1637
Terrien's degeneration and, 1126
Asymmetric astigmatism, 2158, 2159
Atopic disease, 1092
Atopic keratoconjunctivitis, 109, 753, 813-816, *A67-68*
Atopy, 106-110, 457
Atrophy, iris, *A160, A161-162*
in anterior uveitis, 1498
essential, 1107-1110
in herpes simplex keratouveitis, *A188*
in herpes zoster, *A194*
in leprosy, 1008
in postsyphilitic keratopathy, 1286
sectoral, *A194*
specular microscopy of, 325
Atropine, 1025
Auspitz sign, 989
Australian eye banking, 482-483
Auto refractor, 2019
Autoantibody
in cicatricial pemphigoid, 828
in rheumatoid arthritis, 1359
in systemic lupus erythematosus, 1377
Autoimmunity, 89-90
cicatricial pemphigoid and, 827-833
Fuchs' heterochromic iridocyclitis and, 1538
Automated lamellar keratoplasty, 1991, 2165-2179
comparison with other refractive procedures, 2178-2179
complications, 2175-2178
corneal topographic analysis in, 2052
enhancement, 2178
historical perspectives, 2165-2167
instrumentation, 2167-2168
nomograms, 2173-2174
operative procedure, 2169-2173
patient selection, 2168-2169
postoperative care, 2173
predictive formulas for, 2027-2028, 2029
preoperative evaluation, 2169
results, 2174-2175
Automatic corneal shaper, 2167, 2173
Autonomous excimer laser, 2183
Avascular keratitis, 1008
Avascular retrocorneal membrane, *A287*
Avellino dystrophy, 1051-1053, *A134*
Avulsion, pterygium, 1876-1877

Axenfeld-Rieger syndrome, 885, 889-891, 1115, 1116, *A84*
  50-degree mirror photography of, 301
  corneal opacity in, 370-371
Axial power, 227-229
Azar 91Z lens, 1424
Azathioprine
  in Behçet disease, 1533
  in cicatricial pemphigoid, 832
  for idiopathic uveitis, 1512
  in Mooren's ulcer, 1400
  in rheumatoid arthritis, 1367
  in systemic lupus erythematosus, 1378
Azithromycin, 1172
  in chlamydial infection, 785, 793
  in inclusion conjunctivitis, 751
  in trachoma, 783
Azoles, 1258
Azotobacter, 1141
Aztreonam, 1168

B

B cell, 70-72
  inflammation and, 143
  in rheumatoid arthritis, 1359
  in Sjögren's syndrome, 677-678
BacLight, 1161
Bacillus anthracis, 638
Bacillus cereus
  in keratitis, 1140-1141
  in peripheral corneal ulcer, 399
Bacitracin, 1175
  in bacterial conjunctivitis, 767
  eye drops, 1176
  impairment of epithelial wound healing, 189-190
  in staphylococcal blepharitis, 634
  toxicity of, 850
Bacterial corneal ulcer, 398-399
Bacterial infection, 1139-1189, *A177, A178*
  in acquired immunodeficiency syndrome, 1019-1020
  after astigmatic keratotomy, 2152
  after radial keratotomy, 2118-2119
  antimicrobial susceptibility testing in, 1163
  causes, 1139-1141
  chronic granulomatous disease, 947
  clinical features, 1147-1152, 1153
  conjunctivitis, 759-772, *A53-54; see also* conjunctivitis
    acute, 764-766, 767
    chronic, 766-769
    hyperacute, 761-763
    manifestations of, 760-761
    natural defenses, 759-760
    neonatal, 790-791
    syndromes, 769-770
    unusual causes, 769
  contact lens-induced, 1465-1466
  corneal; *see* Keratitis
  diagnosis, 1155
  eyelid, 621-624, 633-640, *A25*
    angular blepharitis, 634-635
    anthrax, 638
    chalazion, 635
    chancroid, 638
    classification, 621-623
    differential diagnosis, 623
    hordeolum, 635
    management, 623-624
    mycobacterial, 639
    preseptal cellulitis, 635-638
    staphylococcal blepharitis, 633-634
    syphilis, 638
  histopathology, 1152-1155
  laboratory investigation, 1155-1163
    culture, 1155-1158
    culture media, 1160-1163
    stain, 1158-1160, 1161
  lacrimal gland, 687-689
  Lyme disease, 1311
  mycobacterial, 1310-1311
  of nasolacrimal sac, 689-691
  pathogenesis, 1144-1147
  risk factors, 1141-1144, 1145
  therapeutic keratoplasty for, 1843-1844
  treatment, 1165-1181
    adjunctive, 1179-1181
    aminoglycosides, 1168-1169
    cephalosporins, 167-1168
    chloramphenicol, 1173-1174
    fluoroquinolones, 1169-1171
    glycopeptides, 1168
    macrolides and lincosamides, 1171-1172
    penicillins, 1166-1167
    peptide antibiotics, 1175
    rifampin, 1174
    routes of administration, 1175-1177
    spectinomycin, 1174-1175
    sulfonamides, 1174
    tetracyclines, 1173
    trimethoprim, 1174
  ulceration in, *A266*
Bacteroides, 636
Band keratopathy, 390
  anterior uveitis and, 1497
  calcific, 420, *A171, A172*
  corneal degeneration in, 1127-1129, 1130
  in juvenile rheumatoid arthritis, 1543, *A272*
  phototherapeutic keratectomy in, 2217
  pigmented, 418
  in posterior polymorphous dystrophy, 1063, 1065, 1066
  in sarcoidosis, 1524
  silicone oil and, 1029
Bandage soft contact lens, 1457
  in acid injury, 1441
  in corneal abrasion, 1405-1406
  in corneal perforation, 1823, 1830
  in corneal ulceration after keratoplasty, 1697
  in macroulcerative peripheral keratitis, 397
  for postoperative epithelial defects, 1662-1663
  in recurrent corneal erosion, 203 1319
Bard-Parker blade, 1157, 1158
Barraquer-Krumeich-Swinger system, 2165
Barraquer needle holder, 1572
Barron corneal donor button punch, 1575, 1576
Barron radial vacuum trephine, 1574
Bartonella henselae, 799, *A63*
Basal cell, 6-8
Basal cell carcinoma, *A14*
  conjunctival, 735
  eyelid, 601-605
Basal cell nevus syndrome, 614, 994
Basal lamina, 152-153
Basement membrane, 8-9, 2123-2124
Basement membrane collagenases, 147
Basic fibroblast growth factor
  in corneal wound healing, 21, 185-188
  inflammatory response and, 145
Basophil, 77
  in giant papillary conjunctivitis, 822
  inflammation and, 141-142
Bassen-Kornzweig disease, 904
Bauerberg study, 2084-2086, 2094
Beam alignment system of excimer laser, 2184
Beam clean-up system of excimer laser, 2182
Beam control system of excimer laser, 2182
Beam generation system of excimer laser, 2182
Beam shaping system of excimer laser, 2182
Beam splitter, 284
Bee sting, 1419-1420
Behçet's disease, 1529-1535, *A271*
Bell's palsy, 679
  lagophthalmos and, 574, 577
  in Lyme disease, 1005
Bell's phenomenon, 575, 576
Benign hereditary intraepithelial dyskeratosis, 701, 702
Benign lymphoid hyperplasia, *A44*
Benign monoclonal gammopathy, 976-977, *A105*
Benign mucoepidermoid papilloma of conjunctiva, 702-703
Benign pigmented lesion, 596-598
Benign tumor
  conjunctival, 701-704
    benign hereditary intraepithelial dyskeratosis, 701, 702
    dacryoadenoma, 703-704
    inverted papilloma, 702-703
    pseudoepitheliomatous hyperplasia and keratoacanthoma, 701-702, 703
    pterygia and pinguecula, 704
    squamous papilloma, 702, 703
  eyelid, 581-600, *A7-13*
    adnexal, 592-596
    approach to diagnosis and management, 582
    dermal, 586-592
    epidermal, 582-586
    histology of eyelid skin, 581-582
    pigmented lesions, 596-598
Benoxinate, 1023
Benzalkonium chloride
  impairment of epithelial wound healing, 189
  toxicity of, 851
Best corrected visual acuity
  after photorefractive keratoplasty, 2191, 2194-2195
  after radial keratotomy, 2136
Beta-blockers
  in corneal perforation, 1823
  in postkeratoplasty glaucoma, 1725
  postoperative, 1942
Beta-lactam antibiotics, 1168
Betaxolol, 895
Biber-Haab-Dimmer dystrophy, 913, 1050-1051
Bietti's crystalline dystrophy, 424, *A141*
Bietti's nodular corneal degeneration, 1122
Bilirubin deposits, 422, *A96*
Biochemistry
  of diabetic cornea, 979
  scleral, 31-35, 36, 37, 38
Biologic adhesives in synthetic epikeratoplasty, 2236

Chlamydial infection, 779-788, *A58-61*
  in acquired immunodeficiency syndrome, 1020
  biologic features, 779
  Chlamydia psittaci, 787
  in chronic follicular conjunctivitis, 756
  Cogan's syndrome *versus,* 1309
  corneal opacity in, 379-380
  in inclusion conjunctivitis, 751
    adult, 783-785
    neonatal, 786-787, 791-792
  laboratory investigation of, 307-308
  in lymphogranuloma venereum, 787
  in neonatal conjunctivitis, 789-790
  pathogenesis, 779-780
  phlyctenulosis, 1389
  in Reiter's syndrome, 785-786
  in trachoma, 780-783
Chlorambucil
  in Behçet disease, 1533
  for idiopathic uveitis, 1511
  in systemic lupus erythematosus, 1378
Chloramphenicol, 1173-1174
  in bacterial conjunctivitis, 767
  in corneal abrasion, 1406
  in dacryocystis, 689
  in gonococcal conjunctivitis, 763
  impairment of epithelial wound healing, 189-190
  toxicity of, 850
  in Whipple's disease, 946
Chloroacetophenone, 853-854
Chlorobutanol, 851-852
Chloroquine
  corneal deposits, *A115*
  corneal effects, 1026
  drug-induced lipidosis, 907
Chlorpromazine, 1026
Chocolate agar, 306, 1161
Cholesterol, 1055
Cholesterol esters, 629
Chondroitin, 11, 32
Chorioretinal scar, 1537-1538
Choristoma, 376, 723-725, 1921-1922
Choroidal detachment, 1668-1669
Choroidal hemorrhage
  after penetrating keratoplasty, 1668-1669
  expulsive, 1642-1643
Christoffel-Blinden Mission and Sightsavers, 483, 484
Chronic actinic keratopathy, 1122
Chronic bullous disease of childhood, 993
Chronic granulomatous disease, 947-948
Chronic lymphocytic leukemia, 970-971
Chronic myeloid leukemia, 970
Chronic progressive external ophthalmoplegia, *A214*
Chronic renal failure, *A106*
Chrysiasis, 425, 916, *A116*
Churg-Strauss syndrome, 1384
Cicatricial ectropion, 565, *A1*
Cicatricial entropion, 562, 565, *A3*
Cicatricial pemphigoid, 827-833, 993, *A69-70*
  drug-induced, 853
  keratoprosthesis for, 1857
  poor prognosis for penetrating keratoplasty, 1763
Cicatrization
  in conjunctivitis, 749
  in trachoma, 781
Cicatrizing conjunctivitis, 757, 827
Ciliary body tumor, 1957
Cimetidine, 1238
CIN; *see* Corneal intraepithelial neoplasia
Ciprofloxacin, 1169-1171
  in bacterial conjunctivitis, 767
  corneal deposits, 420, *A112*
  corneal effects, 1023
  in corneal perforation, 1824
  in gonococcal conjunctivitis, 763
  in microbial keratitis, 433
  minimal inhibitory concentration, 1178
  in neonatal conjunctivitis, 793, 794
  postoperative, 1645-1646
  in staphylococcal blepharitis, 634
  toxicity of, 850
Circumcorneal flush, 1689
Circumscribed posterior keratoconus, *A81*
Citrobacter, 1704
Clarithromycin, 1172
Class I antigen, 1759
Class II antigen, 1759
Classic pathway of complement, 81-85, 144
Climatic droplet keratopathy, 1121, 1122
Climatotherapy, 813
Clindamycin, 1172
  in dacryoadenitis, 687
  in dacryocystis, 689
  in meibomian gland dysfunction, 631
Clinical Laboratories Improvement Act, 525-527
Clinoril, 1272-1273
Clock dial, 218
Clofazimine, 1009
Clonal anergy, 88, 89
Clostridial infection
  in eyelid necrosis, 637
  in keratitis, 1141
Clotrimazole
  in *Acanthamoeba* keratitis, 1271-1272
  in fungal keratitis, 1259
Cloxacillin
  in dacryoadenitis, 687
  in dacryocystis, 689
Clutton's joints, 1289
CMV; *see* Cytomegalovirus
Coalescence, specular microscopy of, 323
Coalition on Donation, 550
Coat's white ring, 420, 1131, *A246*
Coaxial light source, 2063-2064
Cocaine, 1023
Coccidioides immitis, 802
  in eyelid infection, 653-654
  phlyctenulosis in, 1389
Cochet-Bonnet esthesiometer, 280
Coefficient of variation of corneal powers, 2054
Cogan-Reese syndrome, 325, 1108, 1110-1111, 1307-1310, *A160, A162, A204*
Colchicine, 1533
Colibri-style forceps, 1576, 1577
Collagen
  in Bowman's layer, 9
  corneal reaction to injury, 166
  in corneal stroma, 10-11
  in Descemet's membrane, 14
  response to infection, 145
  scleral, 31-32, 36, 37, 38
  for synthetic epikeratoplasty, 2234
  for synthetic lenticule, 2237-2240
Collagen shield, 1177
  in corneal perforation, 1823
  in fungal keratitis, 1261
  for postoperative epithelial defects, 1662
Collagen vascular disease, 1377-1387, *A221-224*
  Churg-Strauss syndrome, 1384
  giant cell arteritis, 1384
  mixed connective tissue disease, 1379
  polyarteritis nodosa, 1383-1384
  polymyositis and dermatomyositis, 1379-1380
  relapsing polychondritis, 1380-1381
  systemic lupus erythematosus, 1377-1378
  systemic sclerosis, 1378-1379
  Wegener's granulomatosis, 1381-1382
Collagenase, 147, 207
Collarette, 239, 633, 634, 755
Collimating keratoscope, 225
Colony-forming-unit-granulocyte-erythroid-macrophage-megakaryocyte, 967
Combined continuous and interrupted suture
  adjustment for astigmatism, 1633-1634
  technique, 1630
Combined incision, 2071-2077, 2078, 2079, 2080
Combined nevus, conjunctival, 715
Combined posterior transconjunctival approach, 566
Comedone, 585
Complement, 81-85
  corneal infection and, 1146
  inflammatory response and, 144-145
Compound 606, 1276
Compound microscope, 2069
Compound nevus, 596-597, 719, *A8*
Compress
  in chalazion, 635
  in cicatricial pemphigoid, 831
  in meibomian gland dysfunction, 630
Computed tomography
  in anterior segment trauma, 1929
  in ciliary body tumor, 1957
  radial keratotomy and, 2097
  before refractive surgery, 2009
Computerized videokeratography, 2020, *A148*
  in asymmetric astigmatism, 2158, 2159
  incisional refractive surgery and, 2157
  in minimal visual loss, 450-451
  in nonorthogonal astigmatism, 2158-2159
Concretion, conjunctival, 1135
Confocal microscopy, 335-350, 2023
  in *Acanthamoeba* keratitis, 344-345
  current in vivo imaging systems, 336-337
  digital image acquisition and processing, 338-339, 340
  of endothelium, 342-343
  of epithelium, 339-342
  in excimer laser photorefractive keratectomy, 345-347
  in fungal keratitis, 1255
  in herpetic keratitis, 347
  history of, 335-336
  in infectious keratitis, 1164-1165
  methodology, 337-338
  normal corneal structures, 339
  surface toxicity and incisional wound healing, 347-348
  in wound healing, 343, 344, 345
Congenital alacrima, 673-674
Congenital amaurosis, *A154*
Congenital anterior staphyloma, 374, 8[illegible]0
Congenital astigmatism surgery, 2143-2153
  informed consent, 2146
  intraoperative complications, 2151
  operative methods, 2146-2148, 2152

patient selection, 2145-2146, 2147
postoperative management, 2151-2152
preoperative testing, 2146, 2148, 2149, 2150-2151
results, 2152-2153
Congenital conjunctival lesions, 723-727
choristoma, 723-725
cysts, 727
hamartoma, 725-726
Congenital corneal anesthesia, 1352
Congenital corneal opacity, 367-386
bacterial and chlamydial diseases and, 379-380
birth trauma and, 369-370
cerebro-oculo-skeletal syndrome and, 383
corneal dystrophies and, 374-378
developmental abnormalities and, 370-374
fetal alcohol syndrome and, 382
Fryns syndrome and, 382-383
glaucoma and, 368-369
history and physical examination, 367-368, 369
infectious diseases and, 378-379
metabolic diseases and, 380-382
penetrating keratoplasty, 383-384
penetrating keratoplasty in, 1554
Congenital dermoid, 376-377
Congenital ectropion, 565, 567, *A2*
Congenital entropion, 561, 563
Congenital glaucoma, *A82*
congenital corneal opacity and, 368-369
keratoglobus *versus,* 1103
megalocornea *versus,* 873-874
retroillumination from fundus, 300
Congenital hereditary endothelial dystrophy, 1084-1088, *A147*
clinical characteristics of, 1064
corneal edema in, 410
corneal opacity in, 374-375
Congenital hereditary stromal dystrophy, 375, 1058
Congenital herpes simplex keratitis, 1194-1195
Congenital ichthyosiform erythroderma, 996-997
Congenital nevus, 597, 598
Congenital oculodermal melanocytosis, *A9*
Congenital porphyria, *A91*
Congenital rubella, 1246-1247
Congenital spherocytosis, 967-968
Congenital syphilis
Cogan's syndrome *versus,* 1309
disseminated, 1291, 1293
nonocular manifestations, 1288-1291, 1292
pathogenesis of, 1294-1295
syphilitic interstitial keratitis and, 1278-1282, 1283
Congo red stain, *A129*
Conjunctiva, 41-47
abscess of, *A54*
acid injury and, 1439
amyloidosis and, 1125
anatomy of, 41-42
atopic keratoconjunctivitis and, 814
bacterial flora of, 759
benign lymphoid hyperplasia of, *A44*
burn of, *A259*
cicatricial pemphigoid and, 827
contact lens complications, 1461-1463
Cryptococcus neoformans infection, 1020
cyclectomy and, 1959
degeneration, 1133-1135
concretions, 1135, *A52*
pinguecula, 1133-1134
pterygium, 1134-1135
dry eye and, *A30*
embryology, 41
examination
in anterior uveitis, 1495-1497
before penetrating keratoplasty, 1566
tear film, 272
foreign body in, 1932, *A233, A242, A243*
groove in, *A263*
hemangioma, *A46*
herpes simplex ulcer, *A182*
herpes zoster ophthalmicus and, 1227-1228
histology, 42-44
inflammation of, *A52*
ischemia of, *A259*
Kaposi's sarcoma of, *A45*
keratinization of, *A6*
keratoacanthoma of, *A37*
lesions of, *A40-42, A45*
lymphangioma of, *A44*
lymphatic drainage, 45
lymphoma of, *A44, A45*
management of neoplasia, 1911-1924
limbal dermoid, 1921-1922
lymphoid proliferations, 1920-1921
melanocytic neoplasms, 1912-1916
squamous neoplasms, 1916-1920
ocular immune response, 98-101
palpebral, 42
acute bacterial conjunctivitis and, 764
anterior uveitis and, 1495
arterial blood supply, 44-45
capillary hemangioma, 738-739
cyst on, *A50*
follicles in, *A51*
histology, 43
lymphoma of, *A45*
primary acquired melanosis, 717
red eye and, 442-443
superior limbic keratoconjunctivitis and, 857
phlyctenule of, 1390, *A183, A225*
physiology of, 46
pyogenic granuloma of, *A47*
reconstructive procedures after anterior segment trauma, 1949, 1948
Reiter's syndrome and, *A74*
response to infection, 130-131
sarcoidosis and, 1523-1524
scarring of, *A216*
scleral perforation surgery and, 1967
Stevens-Johnson syndrome and, *A73*
vascular supply of, 44-45
vernal keratoconjunctivitis and, 811
Conjunctival associated lymphoid tissue, 98, 99
Conjunctival autograft
after anterior segment trauma, 1948
indications for, 1888
in pterygium, 1877-1879, 1880
Conjunctival basement membrane zone, 43
Conjunctival biopsy
in chronic conjunctivitis, 753
in metabolic disease, 917-918
Conjunctival epithelium
development of, 41
giant papillary conjunctivitis and, 821
ocular surface replacement and, 1887-1888
vernal keratoconjunctivitis and, 812
Conjunctival flap, 1903-1909, *A289-290*
in acid injury, 1441
advancement, 1904, 1905
bipedicle, 1904, 1906
complications, 1905-1909
in corneal edema, 414
in corneal perforation, 1830
in corneal thinning, 1794
in *Fusarium* keratitis, 1261
high resolution ultrasound of, 358
indications, 1903-1904, 1905
keratoprosthesis and, 1859
in neurotrophic keratopathy, 1216
postoperative care, 1905
in pterygium, 1877-1879, 1880
single-pedicle, 1904, 1907
surgical technique, 1904, 1908
Conjunctival neoplasms, *A37-50*
melanocytic, 715-722, *A40-42*
malignant melanoma, 719-722
management of, 1912-1916
melanosis, 715-719
nevi, 715, 716
squamous, 701-714, *A37-39*
benign hereditary intraepithelial dyskeratosis, 701, 702
conjunctival intraepithelial neoplasia, 704-707
corneal epithelial dysmaturation and epithelial dysplasia, 707-710
dacryoadenoma, 703-704
inverted conjunctival papilloma, 702-703
management of, 1916-1920
mucoepidermoid carcinoma, 710
papilloma, 702, 703
pseudoepitheliomatous hyperplasia and keratoacanthoma, 701-702, 703
pterygia and pinguecula, 704
sebaceous cell carcinoma, 710-712
spindle cell carcinoma, 710
squamous cell carcinoma, 707, 708
subepithelial, 723-743, *A43-50*
amyloid, 731-732, 733
basal cell carcinoma, 735
choristoma, 723-725
conjunctival cyst, 727
elastofibroma oculi, 729
fibrous histiocytoma, 733, 734
granulomatous and histiocytic lesions, 729-730, 731
hamartoma, 725-726
hematic cyst, 732
Kaposi's sarcoma, 733-734, 735
keloid, 730-731
lymphoid lesions, 736-738
malignant melanoma, 735-736
nodular fasciitis, 729
oncocytoma, 734-735
pinguecula and pterygium, 728-729
pyogenic granuloma and capillary hemangioma, 727-728
Conjunctival scraping
in allergic conjunctivitis, 807-808
in chronic conjunctivitis, 753
in Parinaud's oculoglandular syndrome, 797
Conjunctival squamous dysplasia, 705
Conjunctival surgery
for corneal thinning disorders, 1794-1795
flaps, 1903-1909
in acid injury, 1441

Conjunctival surgery—cont'd
  flaps—cont'd
    advancement, 1904, 1905
    bipedicle, 1904, 1906
    complications, 1905-1909
    in corneal edema, 414
    in *Fusarium* keratitis, 1261
    high resolution ultrasound of, 358
    indications, 1903-1904, 1905
    in neurotrophic keratopathy, 1216
    postoperative care, 1905
    in pterygium, 1877-1879, 1880
    single-pedicle, 1904, 1907
    surgical technique, 1904, 1908
  neoplasia, 1911-1924
    limbal dermoid, 1921-1922
    lymphoid proliferations, 1920-1921
    melanocytic neoplasms, 1912-1916
    squamous neoplasms, 1916-1920
  ocular surface transplantation, 1887-1902
    conjunctival, 1889-1892
    limbal, 1892-1898, 1899
    mucous membrane, 1898-1901
    principles of, 1887-1889
  in pterygium, 1873-1885
    chemotherapy, 1880-1882
    conjunctival flaps and autografts, 1877-1879, 1880
    excision and avulsion, 1876-1877
    histopathology, 1874-1875
    lamellar and penetrating keratoplasty, 1879
    medical approaches, 1875-1876
    mucous membrane and skin graft, 1879-1880
    pathogenesis, 1874
    prevalence, 1873
    radiation therapy, 1822-1883
    transplantation of pterygium head, 1877
  in superior limbic keratoconjunctivitis, 859
  transplantation, 1889-1892
Conjunctival xerosis, 957-958
Conjunctivitis, *A51-76*
  acute, 750-752
  acute hemorrhagic, 1245-1246
  allergic, 805-810, *A65*
  anatomic localization, 749-750
  atopic, 109, 753, 813-816, *A67-68*
  bacterial, 759-772, *A53-54*
    acute, 764-766, 767
    chlamydial, *A58-61*
    chronic, 766-769
    hyperacute, 761-763
    manifestations of, 760-761
    natural defenses, 759-760
    syndromes, 769-770
    unusual causes, 769
  chlamydial, 779-788, *A58-61*
    adult inclusion conjunctivitis, 783-785
    biologic features, 779
    Chlamydia psittaci, 787
    chronic follicular, 756
    Cogan's syndrome *versus,* 1309
    lymphogranuloma venereum, 787
    neonatal, 786-787, 791-792
    pathogenesis, 779-780
    phlyctenulosis, 1389
    Reiter's syndrome, 785-786
    trachoma, 780-783
  chronic, 752-757, *A54*
  cicatricial pemphigoid, 827-833, 993, *A69-70*
    drug-induced, 853
    keratoprosthesis for, 1857
    poor prognosis for penetrating keratoplasty, 1763
  cicatrizing, 757
  clinical features of, *A51-52*
  conjunctival injection, 745
  erythema multiforme
    drug-induced, 1028
    dry eye in, 675
  exudate in, 749
  factitious, *A76*
  follicular, *A51*
    chronic, 756-757
    related to topical medications, 852
    in sarcoidosis, 1524
    toxic, 757, *A74*
  giant papillary, 753, 819-825, *A52, A68*
    from contact lens, 1461-1462, *A261*
    differential diagnosis, 823
    histopathology and pathogenesis, 821-823
    immunopathology of, 109
    meibomian gland dysfunction and, 629
    prognosis, 824-825
    symptoms and signs, 819-821, 822
    treatment, 823-824
  gonococcal, *A54, A62*
  granulomatous, 757
  inclusion
    adult, 783-785, *A58-59*
    Chlamydia trachomatis in, 751
    neonatal, 786-787, *A62*
    peripheral corneal and, 399-400
  in Kawasaki disease, 950
  lid imbrication syndrome and, 573
  ligneous, 756, 863-868, *A76*
  linear immunoglobulin A disease in, *A70*
  membranous, 752, 757
  in molluscum contagiosum, 775-776
  morphologic responses, 746-749
  in mumps, 776
  neonatal, 789-795
  in Newcastle disease, 776
  in onchocerciasis, 1011
  ophthalmia neonatorum, 789-795, *A62*
  papillary, *A6*
    adenovirus in, 775
    chronic, 753-756
    giant, *A52, A68, A261*
  parasitic, *A64*
  Parinaud's oculoglandular syndrome, 797-803, *A63*
    cat-scratch disease in, 797-799, 800
    granulomatous conjunctivitis secondary to, 749
    lymphogranuloma venereum in, 802
    sporotrichosis in, 801
    syphilis in, 801-802
    tuberculosis in, 801
    tularemia in, 799-801
  in psoriasis, 989
  in Reiter's syndrome, 1517, *A74*
  in rubella, 776
  in rubeola, 776-777
  severe, *A52*
  Stevens-Johnson syndrome, 836, 1028, *A71-73*
    bilateral pseudomembranous conjunctivitis in, 748
    dry eye in, 675-676
    intracorneal keratoprosthesis for, *A295*
    keratoprosthesis for, 1857
    in type III ocular hypersensitivity, 113-114
  superior limbic keratoconjunctivitis, 393, 754-755, 857-862, *A75*
    contact lens-induced, 1462-1463, *A265*
  toxic, 847-856, *A74*
    cosmetics and skin care products, 853
    follicular, 757
    hair care products, 853, 854
    papillary, 756
    related to topical medications, 849-853
    tear gas weapons and lacrimating agents, 853-854
    therapeutic considerations, 854-855
    toxicity *versus* allergy, 847-849
  trachoma in, *A60-61*
  vaccinia, 649
  in varicella, 777
  vernal keratoconjunctivitis, 393, 750, 753, 811-813, *A66*
    giant papillary conjunctivitis *versus* 823
    immunopathology of, 108-109
  viral, 773-777, *A55-57*
    cytomegalovirus in, 775
    Epstein-Barr virus in, 775
    herpes simplex virus in, 775, 1196, *A179, A180*
  in Wegener's granulomatosis, 948, 1382
Conjunctivitis-otitis media syndrome, 769
Connective tissue, keratoconus and, 1093
Connective tissue disorders, 925-942
  classification of, 925-926, 927-928
  craniofacial malformation syndromes, 926-929
  dermo-chondro-corneal dystrophy of Francois, 938
  Ehlers-Danlos syndrome, 930-931, 935
  Goldenhar syndrome, 929-930
  Hallermann-Streiff syndrome, 930
  hypophosphatasia, 939
  Kniest syndrome, 935-936
  Marfan syndrome, 936-937
  oculo-dento-osseous dysplasia, 937-938
  osteogenesis imperfecta, 934-935
  Sotos syndrome, 938
  Stickler syndrome, 935
  syndrome of acromegaly, 939
  Treacher Collins syndrome, 930
  treatment of, 939-940
  Werner syndrome, 938-939
Consent, 487
  for donor tissue removal, 494
  in pediatric penetrating keratoplasty, 1740-1741
  before refractive surgery, 2011
  in tissue procurement, 531-532
Contact allergy, 808-809, 1461
Contact burn, 1416
Contact dermatitis, 991, *A28*
Contact lens
  after corneal trauma, 1947-1948
  after keratoplasty, 1654, 1749-1750
  after radial keratotomy, 2106
  complications from, 1461-1470, *A261-266*
    Acanthamoeba keratitis, 1267
    conjunctival, 1461-1463
    corneal infiltrates, 429-435
    corneal warpage, 454
    endothelial, 1469
    epithelial, 1463-1465

evaporative dry eye, 690
fungal keratitis, 1254
giant papillary conjunctivitis, 819, 1461-1462
induced warpage, 2044-2045, 2046
keratoconjunctivitis, 861
lids and orbit, 1461, 1462
meibomian gland dysfunction, 629
microbial keratitis, 1142-1143
Pseudomonas keratitis, *A178*
red eye, 440
stromal, 1465-1469
fitting abnormal cornea, 220-221, 1457-1460
following anterior segment trauma, 1943
indications for, 1453-1456
for keratoconus, 1094, 1099
in minimal visual loss, 448
specular microscopy of, 330
therapeutic, 1455
in corneal edema, 414
in macroulcerative peripheral keratitis, 397
in minimal visual loss, 448
in neurotrophic keratopathy, 1216
in recurrent corneal erosion, 203
in sterile corneal ulceration, 208
in superior limbic keratoconjunctivitis, 859
in ulcerative keratitis, 1179
ultraviolet chromophores in, 1414
Continuing technical education, 472-473
Continuous lavage of antibiotics, 1176-1177
Contractile proteins, 166
Contrast acuity, 2023
Contrast sensitivity
evaluation before refractive surgery, 2009
in minimal visual loss, 447-448
problems after radial keratotomy, 2127-2128
Contusion injury, 1408
Copper
corneal deposits and, 425
foreign body, *A253*
metabolic disorders, 915-916
Corn husk foreign body, *A242, A244*
Cornea
abnormal; *see* Corneal abnormalities
abrasion, 1404-1407, *A227*
Acanthamoeba keratitis and, 1267
in astigmatic keratotomy, 2163
from blunt trauma, 1930
dust trail linear, *A262*
epithelial, 1404-1406
stromal, 1407
absence of, 871-872, 873
acquired immunodeficiency syndrome and
bacterial keratitis and, 1142
conjunctivitis in, 769-770
corneal infections in, 1017-1022
disorders related to, *A111*
erythema multiforme in, 839
herpes zoster in, 1233
Kaposi's sarcoma in, *A45*
molluscum contagiosum lesions with, *A26*
Reiter's syndrome in, 785, 1518
anatomy and physiology, 1-25
Bowman's layer, 9
Descemet's membrane, 14-15
endothelium, 15-17
epithelium, 4-9
innervation, 3
optical properties, 1-3
stroma, 10-14
tear fluid, 4
vascular system, 3
blood in, *A235*
chrysiasis in, *A116*
contusion from blunt trauma, 1930
cyan mottling of, *A263*
dermatologic disorders, 989-1002, *A107-108*
genetic, 994-999
immunobullous, 992-993
inflammatory and papulosquamous, 989-992
dermoid of, *A80*
development abnormalities of; *see* Developmental corneal abnormalities
ectasia of, *A159*
edema of; *see* Corneal edema
effects of local and systemic therapies, 1023-1031
drug deposition, 1026-1027
ophthalmic surgical solutions, 1028-1030
topical ophthalmic medications, 1023-1026
toxic effects, 1027-1028
endocrine disease and, 979-988
diabetes mellitus, 979-981
hyperparathyroidism, 981-983
hypoparathyroidism, 981
multiple endocrine neoplasia, 984-985
thyroid disease, 983-984
foreign body in; *see* Foreign body
gout and, *A96*
hematologic disorders and, 967-978, *A102-105*
Bruton's hypogammaglobulinemia, 972-973
crystalline keratopathy and, 977
erythroid line, 967-969
hematopoiesis and, 967
leukemia, 969-972
lymphoma, 972
plasma cell dyscrasia, 973-977
herpes zoster ophthalmicus and, 1228-1231
high resolution ultrasound, 353-354, 355
immunologic disorders and, *A217-226*; *see also* Immunologic disorders
collagen vascular disease, 1377-1387, *A221-224*
Mooren's ulcer, 398, 399, 1397-1401, *A226*
phlyctenulosis, 1389-1395
rheumatoid arthritis, 1359-1375, *A217-220*
staphylococcal disease, 1392-1394, *A225*
infections of; *see* Corneal infection
infectious disease and, 1003-1016
brucellosis, 1012-1013
leprosy, 1006-1009
Lyme disease, 1003-1106
onchocerciasis, 1010-1012
tuberculosis, 1009-1010
inflammatory disease and
chronic granulomatous disease, 947-948
corneal, 393-398, 399
dermatologic, 989-992
inflammatory bowel disease, 943-945
Kawasaki disease, 949-951
scleral, 1479-1491
Wegener's granulomatosis, 948-949
Whipple's disease, 945-946
iridocorneal endothelial syndrome, 1107-1118, *A160-162*
Axenfeld-Rieger syndrome *versus*, 894
clinical course, 1112, 1115
clinical features, 1107-1111, 1112
differential diagnosis, 1112-1115, 1116
etiology, 1111-1112, 1113-1114
history and background, 1107, 1108
management, 1115
minimal visual loss in, 453
posterior polymorphous dystrophy *versus*, 1066
specular microscopy in, 325
laceration, *A229, A231*
anterior segment surgery in, 1935-1938
penetrating keratoplasty in, *A294*
laser effect on, 2181
local effects of topical anesthetic, 1354-1355
maintenance of normal integrity, 17-21
metabolic diseases and, 897-924
alkaptonuria, 912
amyloidosis, 912-913, 914
calcium, 916
conjunctival biopsy in, 917-918
copper, 915-916
cystinosis, 910-912
diabetes mellitus, 897-899
drug-induced lipidoses, 907-909
dyslipoproteinemias, 903-905
galactosialidodis, 910
glycogenosis type I, 903
gold, 916-917
gout, 913-914
lipidoses, 905-906
macular corneal dystrophy, 902
mannosidosis and fucosidosis, 902-903
mucolipidoses, 909-910
porphyria, 915
silver, 917
systemic mucopolysaccharidoses, 899-902
tear enzyme analysis, 918
tyrosinemia II, 912
xeroderma pigmentosa, 914-915
nerves of, *A167*
noninflammatory ectatic disorders, 1091-1106, *A148-155*
keratoconus, 1091-1100, *A148-155*
keratoglobus, 1102-1103, *A158*
pellucid marginal degeneration, 1100-1101, *A156-157*
posterior keratoconus, 1103-1104
nutritional disorders and, 955-966, *A100-101*
amino acids deprivation, 964
discrete colliquative keratopathy, 964
vitamin A deficiency, 955-963
vitamin B deficiency, 963
vitamin C deficiency, 963-964
ocular immune response, 101-104
phlyctenule of, *A225*
photo slit lamp biomicrography, 284-304
biomicroscope, 284-285
direct illumination, 288-291, 292, 293, 294-296
indirect illumination, 291-293, 296-298
preparation for, 285-288

Cornea—cont'd
  photo slit lamp biomicrography—cont'd
    special techniques, 301-304
  reaction to injury, 163-182
    cell death, 163, 165
    cell migration, 166, 167
    collagen and, 166
    endothelial, 174
    epithelial, 168-171
    excimer photoablation, 178-179
    granulation tissue, 166
    inflammation, 163-165
    mechanisms of injury, 167-168
    penetrating and perforating injuries, 174-177, 178
    protein mediators of cell activity, 166
    stromal, 171-174
    variations in wound healing, 177-178
  recurrent keloid of, *A48*
  as refractive medium, 215-216
  residual interstitial keratopathy and, 1284-1285, 1286, 1287
  response to infection, 129-162
    fibrosis, 149-151
    inflammation and loss of function, 129, 130
    intrinsic barriers and immune response, 130-131
    mechanisms of microbial invasion, 131-133
    recruited cells, 141-144
    resident cells and surface receptors, 134-141
    soluble mediators, 144-145
    ulceration, 145-149
  sarcoidosis and, 1524, 1525
  scar; *see* Corneal scar
  skeletal disorders and, 925-942, *A97-98*
    classification of, 925-926, 927-928
    craniofacial malformation syndromes, 926-929
    dermo-chondro-corneal dystrophy of Francois, 938
    Ehlers-Danlos syndrome, 930-934, 935
    Goldenhar syndrome, 929-930
    Hallermann-Streiff syndrome, 930
    hypophosphatasia, 939
    Kniest syndrome, 935-936
    Marfan syndrome, 936-937
    oculo-dento-osseous dysplasia, 937-938
    osteogenesis imperfecta, 934-935
    Sotos syndrome, 938
    Stickler syndrome, 935
    syndrome of acromegaly, 939
    Treacher Collins syndrome, 930
    treatment of, 939-940
    Werner syndrome, 938-939
Cornea farinata, 425-426, 1132-1133, *A165*
Cornea plana, 876-877
Cornea verticillata, 417, 418, *A87, A115*
Corneal abnormalities, *A77-86*
  after radial keratotomy, 2111-2112
  anterior chamber cleavage syndromes, 885-896, *A83-86*
    central, 888-889
    development of angle, 885-887
    differential diagnosis, 894
    examination, 893-894
    peripheral, 889-893
    treatment, 894-895
  contact lens fitting in, 1457-1460
  corneal opacity and, 370-374, *A77-82*
  in floppy eyelid syndrome, 571
  minimal visual loss, 447-455
    conditions causing, 451-454
    examination techniques, 447-451
    patient history in, 447, 448
  phototherapeutic keratectomy for, 2217
  refraction of abnormal cornea, 215-221
  size and shape, 871-883
    absence of cornea, 871-872, 873
    astigmatism, 875-876
    congenital anterior staphyloma and keratectasia, 880
    keratoglobus, 878-880
    megalocornea, 872-874, 875
    microcornea, 874, 875
    oval cornea, 874-875
    posterior keratoconus, 877-878
    sclerocornea, 876-877
  in syphilitic interstitial keratitis, 1288, 1290, 1291
Corneal arcus, 1119-1120
Corneal biopsy
  in bacterial keratitis, 1163-1165
  in corneal ulcer, 405, 408
  in fungal keratitis, 1256-1257
  using slit lamp, 305
Corneal blood staining, 421-422
Corneal color map, 229-234
Corneal degeneration, 1119-1133
  amyloid, 1123-1125
  arcus senilis, 1119-1120
  band keratopathy, 1127-1129, 1130
  calcareous degeneration, 1129-1130
  climatic droplet keratopathy, 1121, 1122
  Coats' white ring, 1131
  cornea farinata, 1132-1133
  crocodile shagreen, 1131-1132
  dellen, 1133
  Hassall-Henle bodies, 1131
  high resolution ultrasound in, 355, 356
  iron lines, 1130-1131
  keloids, 1126
  limbal girdle of Vogt, 1127, 1128
  lipid, 1120-1121
  minimal visual loss in, 453-454
  neurotrophic keratitis, 1339-1347
    biochemical basis, 1340-1341
    clinical causes, 1339-1340
    clinical findings, 1341-1342, 1343
    evaluation of, 1343-1344
    histopathology, 1342-1343
    management, 1344-1345
  penetrating keratoplasty in, 1555
  polymorphic amyloid, 426-427
  recurrent corneal erosion in, 202
  reticular degeneration of Koby, 1130
  Salzmann's nodular degeneration, 1125-1126
  senile furrow, 1132, 1133
  spheroidal, 418-420
  Terrien's marginal corneal degeneration, 1126-1127
Corneal deposits, 417-428
  amyloid, *A7*
  in benign monoclonal gammopathy, 976
  brown, *A251, A252*
  chloroquine, *A115*
  deep stromal pigmented, 425
  deep stromal refractile/crystalline, 426-427
  mercury, *A112*
  in multiple myeloma, 974
  nonpigmented deep stromal, 425-426
  silver, *A112*
  stelazine, *A117*
  stromal nonpigmented, 422-423
  stromal pigmented, 421-422
  stromal refractile/crystalline, 423-425
  superficial nonpigmented, 420
  superficial pigmented, 417-420
  superficial refractile/crystalline, 420-421
  in Waldenstrom's macroglobulinemia, 975
  xanthogranuloma, *A7, A49*
Corneal devices
  intrastromal, 2225-2232
    clinical and histopathologic observations, 2227
    intrastromal corneal ring, 2227-2229
    physiologic considerations, 2226-2227, 2228
    refractive mechanisms, 2225-2226
    small diameter corneal inlay, 2230-2231
  synthetic epikeratoplasty, 2233-2241
    attachment of lenticule to cornea, 2236
    background, 2233-2234
    in vitro trials, 2234-2236
    potential biomaterials, 2234
    type IV collagen lenticules, 2237-2240
Corneal diagnostic techniques, 275-281
  corneal sensation, 279-280
    Acanthamoeba keratitis and, 1268
    decreased, 54
    in diabetes mellitus, 980
    in lagophthalmos, 575, 577
    preoperative, 1802
  corneal staining, 275-277, 278
  pachymetry, 277-279
    in automated lamellar keratoplasty, 2168
    in corneal edema, 412-413, 453, 1403
    for determining allograft rejection, 1691
    in keratoconus, 1097
    before keratoplasty, 1566
    during radial keratotomy, 2065-2067
    before refractive surgery, 2010
Corneal disease
  in dermatomyositis, 1379-1380
  high resolution ultrasound in, 354-355, 357
  in leprosy, 1007-1008
  in mixed connective tissue disease, 1379
  noninflammatory ectatic, 1091-1106, *A148-155*
    keratoconus, 1091-1100
    keratoglobus, 1102-1103
    pellucid marginal degeneration, 1100-1101
    posterior keratoconus, 1103-1104
  peripheral, 387-401
    anatomic and physiologic considerations, 387
    degenerative, 389-392
    infectious, 398-400
    inflammatory, 393-398, 399
    neoplastic, 387-389
    secondary to disease of contiguous structures, 392-393
  in polymyositis, 1379-1380
  in relapsing polychondritis, 1380-1381
  in rheumatoid arthritis, 1359-1375
    articular manifestations, 1360
    extra-articular manifestations, 1360-1361
    juvenile, 1370-1371
    keratitis in, 1364-1365, 1366, 1367

keratoconjunctivitis sicca in, 1361-1362
pathogenesis, 1359-1360
scleritis in, 1362-1364, 1365, 1366
treatment, 1367-1370
in systemic sclerosis, 1377-1378, 1378-1379
Corneal dystrophy
anterior, 1033-1042
Bowman's layer, 1039-1042
epithelial basement membrane dystrophy, 1034-1039
Meesmann's juvenile epithelial dystrophy, 1033-1034
corneal opacity in, 374-378
dermatochondral corneal dystrophy of Francois, 994
high resolution ultrasound in, 355, 356
minimal visual loss in, 452-453
phototherapeutic keratectomy for, 2212-2213, 2214, 2215, 2217
posterior, 1063-1090
congenital hereditary endothelial dystrophy, 1084-1088
Fuchs' endothelial dystrophy, 1073-1084; *see also* Fuchs' dystrophy
polymorphous, 1063-1073; *see also* Posterior polymorphous dystrophy
pre-Descemet's, 426
stromal, 1043-1062, *A125-141*
Avellino dystrophy, 1051-1053, *A134*
Bietti's crystalline corneal-retinal dystrophy, *A141*
central cloudy dystrophy, 1056-1057
congenital hereditary, 1058
fleck dystrophy, 1055-1056, *A140*
gelatinous droplike dystrophy, 1053
granular dystrophy, 1043-1045, *A131-133*
lattice dystrophy, 1048-1051, 1052, 1053, *A125-130*
macular dystrophy, 1045-1048, *A135-136*
minimal visual loss in, 452-453
posterior amorphous stromal dystrophy, 1058-1059, *A141*
pre-Descemet's dystrophy, 1047-1058, *A140*
Schnyder's crystalline dystrophy, 1054-1055, *A137*
subepithelial mucinous, 420
Corneal edema
after cataract extraction, 409-415, *A257*
after radial keratotomy, 2103, 2117
alkali burn with, *A259*
in allergic inflammation, 806, 807
birth injury and, 1410
from blunt trauma, 1930
in Chandler's syndrome, 1110
clinical causes, 409, 410
corneal allograft rejection and, 1691
cystoid macular, *A281*
endothelial rejection with, *A287*
epithelial or fibrous ingrowth *versus*, 1715
evaluation of, 409-413
from forceps injury, *A236-237, A239*
in Fuchs' dystrophy, 1075, *A145*
in herpes zoster ophthalmicus, 1227, 1230-1231
high resolution ultrasound in, 354-355
infrared radiation and, 1414
from lint foreign body, *A255*
in posterior polymorphous dystrophy, 376, 1064, *A142-144*
postoperative causes, 1429-1430, 1431
pseudophakic and aphakic, 1423-1435, *A256*
Brown-McLean syndrome and, 1426
etiology of, 1426-1430, 1431
histopathology of, 1425
incidence of, 1423-1425
pathogenesis of, 1425-1426
treatment of, 1431-1432
from retained intraocular foreign body, *A250*
specular microscopy of, 329
in syphilitic interstitial keratitis, 1280
treatment, 413-415
Corneal elastosis, 1122
Corneal endothelium, 15-17
adhesion molecules on, 137-138
blunt trauma to, 1408
contact lens complications, 1469
corneal edema and, 411-412
in donor tissue evaluation, 505, 506
immune response and, 91-92, 102
postsyphilitic keratopathy and, 1284-1285
reaction to injury, 174
specular microscopy of, 314, 317-318
ultraviolet irradiation and, 1412
wound healing, 193-195
Corneal epithelial dysmaturation, 707-710
Corneal epithelium, *A169*
abrasion of, 1404-1406
adhesion molecules on, 137-138
contact lens complications, 1463-1465
corneal edema and, 411
as defense barrier, 1142
degeneration of; *see* Corneal degeneration
in donor tissue evaluation, 503
epidermal growth factor in, 21
immune responses and, 101
ingrowth of, 1709-1713
maintenance of normal corneal integrity, 17
ocular surface replacement and, 1888-1889
posterior membrane dystrophies and, 1068
reaction to injury, 168-171
specular microscopy of, 318, 505-507
ultraviolet irradiation and, 1412
variable in photorefractive keratoplasty outcome, 2036
wound healing, 183-190, 205
Corneal erosion, *A262*
in contact allergy, 809
in donor tissue evaluation, 503
in epithelial basement membrane dystrophy, 1036-1037
recurrent, 200-202, 203, 1317-1326, *A205-208*
after corneal abrasion, 1406
anterior stromal puncture for, 1321-1324, 1325
debridement and superficial keratectomy for, 1320-1321
diagnosis, 1318-1319
in epithelial basement membrane dystrophy, 1036
excimer phototherapeutic keratectomy for, 1325-1326
in lattice dystrophy, 1048, 1049
medical treatment, 1319
pathophysiology, 1317
phototherapeutic keratectomy for, 2212, 2217
surgery in, 1865-1866, *A293*
YAG laser procedures in, 1324-1325
in vernal keratoconjunctivitis, 811
Corneal hypesthesia, 1339-1347
biochemical basis, 1340-1341
clinical causes, 1339-1340
clinical findings, 1341-1342, 1343
evaluation of, 1343-1344
histopathology, 1342-1343
management, 1344-1345
in ocular leprosy, 1007
Corneal immunologic disorders, *A217-226*
collagen vascular disease, 1377-1387, *A221-224*
Churg-Strauss syndrome, 1384
giant cell arteritis, 1384
mixed connective tissue disease, 1379
polyarteritis nodosa, 1383-1384
polymyositis and dermatomyositis, 1379-1380
relapsing polychondritis, 1380-1381
systemic lupus erythematosus, 1377-1378
systemic sclerosis, 1378-1379
Wegener's granulomatosis, 1381-1383
marginal staphylococcal keratitis, 1392-1394, *A225*
Mooren's ulcer, 398, 399, 1397-1401, *A226*
conjunctival resection in, 1794
deep lamellar keratoplasty for, 1775
immune response in, 114
marginal staphylococcus keratitis *versus*, 1393
pellucid marginal degeneration *versus*, 1101
penetrating keratoplasty in, *A277*
nonrheumatoid collagen vascular disease in, *A221-224*
phlyctenulosis, 1389-1395
rheumatoid arthritis, 1359-1375, *A217-220*
articular manifestations, 1360
extra-articular manifestations, 1360-1361
juvenile, 1370-1371, 1541-1548, *A272*
keratitis in, 1364-1365, 1366, 1367
keratoconjunctivitis sicca in, 1361-1362
macroulcerative peripheral keratitis and, 396-397
ocular chrysiasis and, 425
pathogenesis, 1359-1360
scleritis in, 1362-1364, 1365, 1366
treatment, 1367-1370
Corneal infection, *A177-202*
Acanthamoeba keratitis, 1267-1273, 1311-1312, *A199-202*
clinical findings, 1268-1270
confocal microscopy in, 344-345
contact lens-induced, 1466-1467
corneal ulcer in, 405
differential diagnosis, 1271
laboratory diagnosis, 1270-1271
penetrating keratoplasty in, 1553
prevention, 1273
pseudodendrites in, 431
risk factors, 1267-1268
therapeutic keratoplasty for, 1845
treatment, 1271-1273

Corneal infection—cont'd
  in acquired immunodeficiency syndrome, 1017-1022
  bacterial keratitis, 1139-1189, *A177-178*
    in acquired immunodeficiency syndrome, 1019-1020
    adjunctive treatment, 1179-1181
    after astigmatic keratotomy, 2152
    after radial keratotomy, 2118-2119
    aminoglycosides, 1168-1169
    antimicrobial susceptibility testing in, 1163
    causes, 1139-1141
    cephalosporins, 1167-1168
    chloramphenicol, 1173-1174
    clinical features, 1147-1152, 1153
    contact lens-induced, 1465-1466
    corneal biopsy, 1163-1165
    corneal opacity in, 379-380
    in corneal perforation, 1815-1816
    culture, 1155-1158
    culture media, 1160-1163
    diagnosis, 1155
    fluoroquinolones, 1169-1171
    glycopeptides, 1168
    histopathology, 1152-1155
    macrolides and lincosamides, 1171-1172
    pathogenesis, 1144-1147
    penicillins, 1166-1167
    peptide antibiotics, 1175
    rifampin, 1174
    risk factors, 1141-1144, 1145
    routes of administration, 1175-1177
    spectinomycin, 1174-1175
    stain, 1158-1160, 1161
    sulfonamides, 1174
    tetracyclines, 1173
    trimethoprim, 1174
    ulceration in, *A266*
  fungal keratitis, 1253-1265, *A195-198*
    after radial keratotomy, 2119
    clinical features, 1255, 1256, 1257
    epidemiology, 1253-1254
    laboratory diagnosis, 1255-1258
    medical therapy, 1258-1261
    pathogenesis, 1253
    peripheral corneal and, 399
    risk factors, 1254-1255
    surgical therapy, 1261-1263
    therapeutic keratoplasty for, 1844-1845, 1846
  Fusarium, A195
  herpes simplex, 1191-1223, *A179-188, A280*
    Acanthamoeba keratitis *versus,* 1271
    in acquired immunodeficiency syndrome, 1019
    after keratoplasty, 1705
    after radial keratotomy, 2108, 2119
    in atopic keratoconjunctivitis, 814
    chronic, *A188*
    confocal microscopy in, 347
    congenital and neonatal, 1194-1195
    with conjunctivitis, *A180*
    with corneal perforation, *A184*
    diagnosis, 1212-1213
    disciform, *A185*
    epidemiology, 1191-1193
    epithelial, *A181*
    inflammatory response in, 104
    laboratory investigation of, 308
    management, 1213-1219
    marginal staphylococcus keratitis *versus,* 1393
    necrotizing, *A187*
    neurotrophic ulcer in, *A184*
    pathogenesis, 1193-1194
    penetrating keratoplasty in, 1799-1811
    peripheral, 399, *A187*
    phlyctenular lesion *versus,* 1391
    recurrent, 1195-1212, 1213
    steroid-induced, 2202
    stromal scars in, *A183*
    therapeutic keratoplasty for, 1845-1846, 1847, 1848
    with ulcers, 290, A182
    viral structure and classification, 1191
    vitamin A deficiency and, 961
  herpes zoster ophthalmicus, 644, 1226-1233
    corneal allograft rejection *versus,* 1692
    corneal scarring from, *A192*
    corticosteroids in, 1237
    diagnosis, 1235-1236
    with indolent corneal ulcer, *A193*
    medical therapy, 1236-1237
    neuralgia in, 1237-1238
    with neurotrophic ulcer, *A193*
    ophthalmic complications, 1227-1232
    pathogenesis, 1234
    pathology, 1234-1235
    signs and symptoms, 1226-1227
    subepithelial infiltrates in, *A190*
  viral
    flavivirus and bunyavirus, 1247
    herpesvirus, 1244-1245
    opacity in, 378-379
    orthomyxovirus, 1249
    papovavirus, 1245
    paramyxovirus, 1247-1248
    picornavirus, 1245-1246
    poxvirus, 1243-1244
    togavirus, 1246-1247
Corneal injury; *see* Corneal trauma
Corneal intraepithelial neoplasia, 388-389, 1917
Corneal keloid, 377-378
Corneal leukoma of Rosenthal and Kloepfer, 939
Corneal media contamination, 514-515
Corneal mucous plaque, 1228-1229
Corneal nerve
  leprosy and, 1007-1008
  photo slit lamp biomicrography of, 292
Corneal opacity, 448, *A77-82*
  acid injury and, 1439
  after photorefractive keratoplasty, 2195-2196
  after phototherapeutic keratectomy, 2215-2216
  congenital, 367-386
    bacterial and chlamydial diseases and, 379-380
    birth trauma and, 369-370
    cerebro-oculo-skeletal syndrome and, 383
    corneal dystrophies and, 374-378
    developmental abnormalities and, 370-374
    fetal alcohol syndrome and, 382
    Fryns syndrome and, 382-383
    glaucoma and, 368-369
    history and physical examination, 367-368, 369
    infectious diseases and, 378-379
    metabolic diseases and, 380-382
    penetrating keratoplasty in infant, 383-384
  degeneration characterized by, 389-391
  in donor tissue evaluation, 504
  high resolution ultrasound of, 385
  in infant, 1739
  keratoprosthesis for, 1855-1863
  in lattice dystrophy, 1048
  in leprosy, 1007
  in macular corneal dystrophy, 1045-1046
  penetrating keratoplasty in, 1555
  in posterior keratoconus, 878
  in posterior polymorphous dystrophy, 1063-1064, 1067
  in sarcoidosis, 1525
  in syphilitic interstitial keratitis, 1281
  in trachoma, 782
Corneal perforation, 1815-1832
  during astigmatic keratotomy, 2151
  etiology, 1815-1816
  herpes simplex keratitis with, *A184*
  necrotic, *A230*
  prevention, 1830-1831
  signs and symptoms, 1816-1818
  terminology, 1816, 1817
  therapeutic keratoplasty in, 1845
  tissue glue for, 1932-1933
Corneal scar
  after radial keratotomy, 2110-2111, 2125
  from chemicals, *A216*
  conjunctival intraepithelial neoplasia with, *A38*
  in erythema multiforme, 836, 837
  from herpes zoster ophthalmicus, *A192*
  with inactive trachoma, *A61*
  from lightning, *A240*
  minimal visual loss in, 451
  in neurotrophic keratopathy, *A2[illegible]1*
  with pellucid marginal degeneration, *A157*
  phototherapeutic keratectomy for, 2213, 2217
  from radiation keratopathy, *A214*
  residual interstitial keratopathy and, 1293
  in rheumatoid arthritis, *A220*
  secondary to trauma, *A274*
  in syphilitic interstitial keratitis, 1281, *A203*
  from varicella infection, *A273*
Corneal scraping
  in *Acanthamoeba* keratitis, 1270
  in bacterial keratitis, 1156-1158
  in fungal keratitis, 1256
  in itching and burning eye, 458-459
  in marginal staphylococcus keratitis, 1394
  in microbial keratitis after keratoplasty, 1698-1699
Corneal sensation, 279-280
  Acanthamoeba keratitis and, 1268
  decreased, 54
  in diabetes mellitus, 980
  in lagophthalmos, 575, 577
  preoperative, 1802
Corneal shape evaluation, 223-235
  keratometry, 224-225
  keratoscopy, 225-226, 227
  refractive surgery and, 2246
  videokeratoscopy, 226-234
Corneal storage media, 512

Corneal surgery
  automated lamellar keratoplasty, 2165-2179
    comparison with other refractive procedures, 2178-2179
    complications, 2175-2178
    enhancement, 2178
    historical perspectives, 2165-2167
    instrumentation, 2167-2168
    nomograms, 2173-2174
    operative procedure, 2169-2173
    patient selection, 2168-2169
    postoperative care, 2173
    preoperative evaluation, 2169
    results, 2174-2175
  in corneal perforation, 1815-1832
    etiology, 1815-1816
    patch graft, 1827-1829
    penetrating keratoplasty, 1825-1826
    postoperative care, 1823-1824
    postoperative complications, 1824-1825
    preoperative evaluation, 1818
    prevention, 1830-1831
    signs and symptoms, 1816-1818
    terminology, 1816, 1817
    tissue adhesives, 1818-1825
  in corneal thinning disorders, 1789-1798
    alternative approaches, 1795-1797
    conjunctival, 1794-1795
    eyelid, 1794
    pellucid marginal corneal degeneration, 1789-1790, 1791
    Terrien's marginal degeneration, 1790-1793
    tissue adhesive, 1795
  high resolution ultrasound in, 356-358
  keratoprosthesis, 1855-1863, *A295-296*
    after anterior segment trauma, 1953-1954
    complications, 1859-1861
    design and materials, 1856
    historical background, 1855-1856
    indications, 1857, 1858
    surgical procedure, 1857-1859, 1860
  lamellar keratoplasty, 1773, 1833-1842, *A293*
    after anterior segment trauma, 1949-1951
    complications, 1840, 1841
    free band, *A245*
    high resolution ultrasound of, 356, 357
    indications, 1833, 1834, 1835
    in pellucid marginal corneal degeneration, 1789-1790
    penetrating *versus,* 1833-1834, 1835
    preoperative evaluation, 1834-1836
    in pterygium, 1879
    surgical technique, 1836-1841
    in Terrien's marginal degeneration, 1791
  for ocular surface disease, 1865-1872
    anterior stromal puncture, 1868-1869, 1870
    cauterization, 1866
    phototherapeutic keratectomy, 1869-1870
    superficial keratectomy, 1866-1868
    treatment options, 1865, 1866
  therapeutic keratoplasty, 1843-1854
    for *Acanthamoeba* keratitis, 1845
    antimicrobial therapy, 1849
    for bacterial infection, 1843-1844
    donor material, 1849
    for fungal keratitis, 1844-1845, 1846
    for herpetic keratitis, 1845-1846, 1847, 1848
    for persistent epithelial defects, 1846-1847, 1849
    postoperative management, 1851-1852
    presurgical evaluation, 1847-1849
    surgical technique, 1849-1851
    visual prognosis, 1852
Corneal thinning
  degeneration in, 391-392
  lamellar keratoplasty for, 1833
  minimal visual loss in, 451-452
  in noninflammatory ectatic diseases, 1091
  surgery for, 1789-1798
    alternative approaches, 1795-1797
    conjunctival, 1794-1795
    eyelid, 1794
    pellucid marginal corneal degeneration, 1789-1790, 1791
    Terrien's marginal degeneration, 1790-1793
    tissue adhesive, 1795
Corneal topography, 216, 223-235, 2039-2058
  in assessment of surgical result, 2048-2055, 2056
  before astigmatic keratotomy, 2150, 2151
  in bilateral automated lamellar keratoplasty, 2178
  challenges for future, 2055-2056
  in diurnal variation in visual acuity, 2128
  in keratoconus, 1096-1097, *A148*
  keratometry, 224-225
  keratoscopy, 225-226, 227
  of pellucid marginal degeneration, *A157*
  preoperative screening, 2042-2048
  videokeratoscopy, 226-234, 2039-2042
Corneal transplantation, 1581-1592, *A273-296*
  Acanthamoeba keratitis and, 1272
  in acid injury, 1441
  after anterior segment trauma, 1951-1952
  allograft rejection, 90-96, 1687-1696
    afferent immune response in, 91-94
    animal models, 90-91
    clinical features, 1689-1692
    differential diagnosis, 1692-1693
    efferent immune response in, 94-96
    historical perspective, 1687
    immunology of, 1757-1761
    immunomodulation, 96
    management strategy, 1695
    methods for improving graft survival, 1764-1769
    in pediatric penetrating keratoplasty, 1732-1734, 1751-1752
    penetrating keratoplasty in, 1555
    prevention, 1694
    recognition of risk factors, 1687-1689
    treatment, 1693-1694, 1769
  in aphakic bullous keratopathy, 1431
  astigmatism following, 1675-1685
    intraoperative factors, 1677-1679
    postoperative factors, 1679-1684
    preoperative factors, 1675-1677
  cataract extraction and, 1593-1601
    extracapsular cataract extraction, 1596-1600
    extraction techniques, 1594-1595
    phacoemulsification, 1595-1596
  complications, 1659-1673
    anterior synechia formation, 1668
    choroidal detachment and hemorrhage, 1668-1669
    elevated intraocular pressure, 1666-1667
    filamentary keratitis, 1663-1664
    fixed dilated pupil, 1669
    hyphema, 1669
    infection, 1669-1670
    inflammation, 1667
    intraoperative, 1639-1644, *A274-278*
    late, *A279-282*
    persistent epithelial defects, 1661-1663
    primary donor failure, 1670-1671
    pupillary block, 1668
    suture exposure and related infection, 1664-1665
    wound leaks and wound displacement, 1659-1661
  in congenital hereditary endothelial dystrophy, 1086
  contact lens fitting after, 1459
  in corneal edema, 414-415
  in corneal laceration, *A294*
  in corneal perforation, 1825-1826
  for corneal thinning disorders, 1789-1798
    alternative approaches, 1795-1797
    conjunctival, 1794-1795
    eyelid, 1794
    pellucid marginal corneal degeneration, 1789-1790, 1791
    Terrien's marginal degeneration, 1790-1793
    tissue adhesive, 1795
  donor tissue evaluation, 501-508
    penlight examination, 501
    slit lamp examination, 501-505, 506
    specular microscopy, 505-507
  donor tissue removal for, 493-500
    consent for, 494
    corneoscleral rim excision, 497-498, 499-500
    donor maintenance and identification, 494
    enucleation procedure, 495-497
    in situ corneal scleral rim excision, 498-500
    public and professional education, 493-494
  donor tissue storage, 509-517
    media contamination, 514-515
    methods of, 510-514
    principles of corneal preservation, 509-510
  epithelial ingrowth and, 1709
  expected outcomes, 1559-1560
  in Fuchs' dystrophy, 1077
  in fungal keratitis, 1261, 1262
  glaucoma after, 1719-1730
    clinical presentation, 1722
    incidence, 1719-1720
    management, 1724-1728
    mechanisms, 1722-1724
    risk factors, 1720-1722
  in herpes simplex disease, 1219, 1799-1811
    anesthesia, 1803
    complications, 1806-1810
    donor tissue requirements, 1802

Cytology—cont'd
  Epstein-Barr virus, 309-310
  herpes simplex virus, 308
  in microbial keratitis, 305-307
  varicella zoster virus, 308-309
Cytomegalovirus
  in acquired immunodeficiency syndrome, 1017-1018
  in conjunctivitis, 775
  cornea and, 1244
  retinitis, *A111*
Cytosine arabinoside, 1027
Cytotoxic agents
  in Behçet's disease, 1533
  in relapsing polychondritis, 1381
  in systemic lupus erythematosus, 1378
  in Wegener's granulomatosis, 1383
Cytotoxic hypersensitivity response, 110-112
Cytotoxic T cell, 73, 92, 143

D

Dacron mesh, *A296*
Dacryoadenitis, 687-689, 1247, *A36*
Dacryoadenoma, 703-704
Dacryocystitis, 689-691, *A36*
  chronic, 754
  in sarcoidosis, 1523
  in sporotrichosis, 655
Dacryocystography, 699
Dacryocystorhinostomy, 699-700
Dacryostenosis, 1523
Daily wear contact lenses, 1453-1454
Dapsone
  in cicatricial pemphigoid, 832
  in leprosy, 1009
  in relapsing polychondritis, 1381
Darier's disease, 994
Data tracking software, 2021-2023
Debridement
  in *Acanthamoeba* keratitis, 1272
  in epithelial basement membrane dystrophy, 1037-1038
  in eyelid necrosis, 637
  in fungal keratitis, 1258, 1261
  in ligneous conjunctivitis, 867
  in ocular surface disease, 1866-1868
  in photorefractive keratectomy, 2187
  in recurrent erosion syndrome, 1320-1321
Debris on contact lens, *A261*
Decay accelerating factor, 85
Decorin, 34
Deep episcleral plexus, 30-31, 36
Deer fly, 658
Deficient aqueous production, 673-679
Degeneration
  conjunctival, 727-733, 1133-1135
    amyloid, 731-732, 733
    concretions, 1135
    elastofibroma oculi, 729
    granulomatous and histiocytic lesions, 729-730, 731
    hematic cyst, 732
    keloid, 730-731
    nodular fasciitis, 729
    pinguecula, 728-729, 1133-1134
    pterygium, 728-729, 1134-1135
    pyogenic granuloma and capillary hemangioma, 727-728
  corneal, 389-392, 1119-1133
    amyloid, 426-427, 1123-1125
    arcus senilis, 1119-1120
    band keratopathy, 1127-1129, 1130
    calcareous, 1129-1130
    climatic droplet keratopathy, 1121, 1122
    Coats' white ring, 1131
    cornea farinata, 1132-1133
    crocodile shagreen, 1131-1132
    dellen, 1133
    Hassall-Henle bodies, 1131
    high resolution ultrasound in, 355, 356
    iron lines, 1130-1131
    keloids, 1126
    limbal girdle of Vogt, 1127, 1128
    lipid, 1120-1121
    neurotrophic keratitis, 1339-1347
    reticular degeneration of Koby, 1130
    Salzmann's nodular, 1125-1126
    senile furrow, 1132, 1133
    spheroidal, 418-420
    Terrien's marginal, 1126-1127
Degos' syndrome, 1000
Dehydration in erythema multiforme, 841
Deitz study, 2086-2088, 2095
Delayed-type hypersensitivity, 114-116
Dellen, 1133, *A212*
Demodicosis, 655-656
Demulcents, 56-57
Dendrites
  epithelial keratitis with, *A181*
  herpes simplex keratitis with, *A182*
  herpes zoster, 189
Dendritic cell, 4-5, 76, 77, 104
Dendritic keratitis
  after keratoplasty, 1806
  rose bengal stains in, 268
Dendritic ulcer, 1197-1199
Deoxyribonucleic acid probe assay, 1162-1163
Deoxyribonucleic acid virus, 1243-1245
Deposition, 417-428
  amyloid, *A7*
  in benign monoclonal gammopathy, 976
  brown, *A251-252*
  chloroquine, *A115*
  deep stromal pigmented, 425
  deep stromal refractile/crystalline, 426-427
  mercury, *A112*
  in multiple myeloma, 974
  nonpigmented deep stromal, 425-426
  silver, *A112*
  stelazine, *A117*
  stromal nonpigmented, 422-423
  stromal pigmented, 421-422
  stromal refractile/crystalline, 423-425
  superficial nonpigmented, 420
  superficial pigmented, 417-420
  superficial refractile/crystalline, 420-421
  in Waldenstrom's macroglobulinemia, 975
  xanthogranuloma, *A7*, *A49*
Dermatan sulfate, 11, 32
Dermatitis
  contact, 991, *A28*
  exfoliative, 990
  herpetiformis, 993
  from operating room equipment, *A228*
  seborrheic, 989-990
Dermatochondral corneal dystrophy of Francois, 994
Dermatofibroma, 592
Dermatologic disorders, 989-1002, *A107-108*
  genetic, 994-999
  immunobullous, 992-993
  inflammatory and papulosquamous disorders, 989-992
Dermatologic examination of eyelid, 2[illegible]7
Dermatomyositis, 1379-1380, *A224*
Dermatonecrotoxin, 133
Dermatophytosis, 654-655
Dermis
  benign tumors of, 586-592
  eyelid, 61
Dermo-chondro-corneal dystrophy of Francois, 938
Dermoid, 387-388, 723-724, 725, *A80*
  corneal opacity in, 376-377
  eyelid, 585-586
  transformation, 872
Dermolipoma, 723-724, 725
Descemetocele
  patch graft in, 1827
  signs and symptoms, 1816-1818
Descemet's membrane, 14-15, 190
  birth injury to, 1410
  cataract extraction from, *A257*
  congenital hereditary endothelial dystrophy and, 1086-1087
  corneal arcus and, 1119
  corneal edema and, 411-412
  detachment of, *A275*
  in donor tissue evaluation, 505
  forceps injury, *A238-239*
  Fuchs' dystrophy and, 1075, 1077-1078
  green-yellow discoloration in, *A253*
  Hassall-Henle bodies, 1131
  herpes simplex and, *A186*
  intraocular lens and, 1429
  iris atrophy and, 1109
  keratoconus and, 1094
  keratoglobus and, 879
  lamellar keratoplasty and, 1835, 1840, 1841
  macular dystrophy and, 1047
  posterior membrane dystrophies and, 1068, 1069-1070
  postkeratoplasty retained host, 1640-1641
  primary congenital glaucoma and, 36[illegible]
  residual interstitial keratopathy and, 1293-1294
  sclerocornea and, 876
  syphilitic interstitial keratitis and, *A263*
  syphilitic interstitial keratopathy and, 1285, 1286
  wrinkles in, 262
Descemet's warts, 1131
Desert fever, 654
Desipramine, 1238
Desmosome, 6
Detergent injury, *A227*
Developmental corneal abnormalities, *A77-86*
  anterior chamber cleavage syndromes, 885-896, *A83-86*
    central, 888-889
    development of angle, 885-887
    differential diagnosis, 894
    examination, 893-894
    peripheral, 889-893
    treatment, 894-895
  corneal opacity and, 370-374, *A77-82*
  size and shape, 871-883
    absence of cornea, 871-872, 873
    astigmatism, 875-876
    congenital anterior staphyloma and keratectasia, 880

keratoglobus, 878-880
megalocornea, 872-874, 875
microcornea, 874, 875
oval cornea, 874-875
posterior keratoconus, 877-878
sclerocornea, 876-877
in syphilitic interstitial keratitis, 1288, 1290, 1291
Dexamethasone
in Behçet disease, 1533
following keratoprosthesis, 1859
impairment of stromal wound healing, 193
in penetrating keratoplasty, 1589
in vernal keratoconjunctivitis, 813
Dexsol, 512
Diabetes mellitus, 979-981
corneal erosion in, 201-202
corneal manifestations, 897-899
fungal keratitis and, 1255
specular microscopy in, 330
Diamidine, 1271
Diamond calibration microscope, 2020, 2022
Diamond knife
calibration and adjustment, 2067-2070
design for combined incision technique, 2073
foot plates, 2017-2018
holding, 2075
Diathermy, 1961
Dibromopropamidine, 1271
Diclofenac
for idiopathic uveitis, 1508
preoperative, 2060
Dietary history, 1495
Diethylcarbamazine
in loiasis, 658
in onchocerciasis, 1012
Differential Sector Index, 2047
Diffuse endotheliitis, 1209, 1210
Diffuse endotheliopathy, 1408, 1409
Diffuse illumination
in photo slit lamp biomicrography, 288, 289
in slit lamp examination, 244-246
Diphtheroids, 46
Dipivefrin, 850
Diplopia
after photorefractive keratoplasty, 2209
after radial keratotomy, 2128
Direct fluorescent antibody test, 307, 309
Direct illumination
in donor tissue evaluation, 502
in photo slit lamp biomicrography, 288-291, 292, 293, 294-296
in slit lamp examination, 244-254, 255, 256
Direct mail fundraising, 545
Direct retroillumination from iris, 293, 298
Dirofilariasis, 659
Discharge
in bacterial conjunctivitis, 760
in red eye, 438-439
Disciform edema, 1205, 1207
Disciform endotheliitis, 1207-1209
Disciform keratitis, 1205, 1207, 1229, *A185*
Discoid lupus erythematosus, *A222*
Discrete colliquative keratopathy, 964
Disease modifying antirheumatic drugs
in juvenile rheumatoid arthritis, 1544, 1545
in rheumatoid arthritis, 1367
Dismorphic sialidosi, 909
Dissection of pterygium, 1876
Distichiasis, 568-569, *A4*
Diurnal variation
after incisional refractive surgery, 2117, 2128-2129
in corneal edema, 410
Dohlman-Doane keratoprosthesis, 1857, 1858, *A295*
Donor tissue
distribution of, 519-524
ethics in, 533-534
eye banking systems for, 475-476
vision research and, 556
evaluation of, 501-508
in herpes simplex disease, 1802
penlight examination, 501
slit lamp examination, 501-505, 506
specular microscopy, 505-507
failure of, 1670-1671
lamellar, 1838
management in penetrating keratoplasty, 1583
in pediatric penetrating keratoplasty, 1741-1742
preparation for transplantation, 1573-1576
procurement of
death to preservation time, 488-489
ethics in, 531-532
screening in, 487-488
public relations and education, 547-551
removal of, 493-500
consent for, 494
corneoscleral rim excision, 497-498, 499-500
donor maintenance and identification, 494
enucleation procedure, 495-497
in situ corneal scleral rim excision, 498-500
public and professional education, 493-494
role in vision research, 553-558
for sclera grafting, 1969
storage of, 509-517
media contamination, 514-515
methods of, 510-514
principles of corneal preservation, 509-510
syphilis and, 1299-1301
for therapeutic keratoplasty, 1849
Double continuous suture
adjustment for astigmatism, 1637
technique, 1632
Down's syndrome, 1092
Doxycycline, 1173
in brucellosis, 1013
in chlamydial infection, 785
in chronic conjunctivitis, 769
in cicatricial pemphigoid, 831
in inclusion conjunctivitis, 751
in Lyme disease, 1006
in meibomian gland dysfunction, 631
in ophthalmia neonatorum, 793
in rosacea, 396
in syphilitic corneal disease, 1299
Dracunculiasis, 659
Drainage for postkeratoplasty glaucoma, 1727
Draping, 2061-2063
Drug delivery, contact lens for, 1455-1456
Drug deposits, 1026-1027
Drug-induced disorders
cicatricial pemphigoid, 853
erythema multiforme, 836
lipidoses, 907-909
ocular pemphigoid, 993
toxic conjunctivitis, 849-853
Dry eye, 663-686, *A29-35*
classification, 663, 664
diagnosis, 663-672
character of ocular irritation, 664
dye staining, 668-669, 670
fluorophotometry, 668
impression cytology, 671-672
meibomian gland evaluation, 669-670
ocular ferning test, 671
serum autoantibodies, 669
tear evaporation, 670
tear film evaluation, 269-273, 664-667
tear film osmolarity, 668
tear protein analysis, 670-671
tear turnover and aqueous tear production, 667-668
evaporative, 679-680
increased tear film evaporation, 54
lacrimal gland disease and, 53
non-Sjögren's aqueous tear deficiency, 673-676
Sjögren syndrome aqueous tear deficiency, 676-679
therapeutic keratoplasty in, 1847
therapy, 680-682
Dubroff lens, 1424
Dural-cavernous fistula, *A102-103*
Duration of photographic exposure, 288
Dust trail linear abrasion, *A262*
Dye test
in dry eye, 668-669, 670
in epiphora, 698-699
Dysautonomia, *A35*
Dyskeratosis, 705, 994
Dyslipoproteinemia, 903-905
Dysplasia
ectodermal, 994-995
epithelial, *A265*
oculoauriculovertebral, *A97*
Dystonia, 250
Dystrophy
anterior corneal, 1033-1042, *A119-124*
Bowman's layer, 1039-1042
epithelial basement membrane dystrophy, 1034-1039
Meesmann's, 1033-1034, *A122*
congenital hereditary endothelial, 374-375, 1084-1088
dermatochondral corneal dystrophy of Francois, 994
Fleck, 423, 1055-1056, *A140*
Fuchs,' 1073-1084, *A145-146*
clinical presentation and course, 1073-1076
differential diagnosis, 1076
electron microscopy, 1078-1081, 1082, 1083
epithelial layer, 1083
histopathology, 1077-1078
pathogenesis, 1083-1084
penetrating keratoplasty in, *A274*
prognosis and management, 1077
specular microscopy in, 323, 324
stroma and Bowman's membrane, 1081-1083
lattice, 1048-1051, 1052, 1053, *A125-130*
corneal deposits in, 423
direct and indirect retroillumination from iris, 261, 299
keratoprosthesis in, 1858

Excimer laser ablation
  characteristics in synthetic epikeratoplasty, 2235-2236
  wound healing response to, 179
Excimer laser in situ keratomileusis, 2250
Excimer laser photorefractive keratectomy, *A300*
  complications, 2200-2209
    central islands, 2206-2208
    decentration of ablation zone, 2205-2206
    halos, 2205
    plaque formation, 2204-2205
    recurrent corneal erosions, 2203-2205
    steroid-induced, 2202-2203
    therapeutic contact lenses-induced, 2203-2204
    unplanned deviations from intended correction, 2201-2202
  confocal microscopy in, 345-347
  future of, 2250-2251
  high resolution ultrasound in, 358
  laser assisted in situ keratomileusis *versus,* 2166-2167
  in recurrent corneal erosion, 204
  results, 2191-2200
    in high myopia, 2197, 2198, 2199
    in hyperopia, 2198, 2200
    in low and moderate myopia, 2191-2197
    in myopic astigmatism, 2197-2198, 2200
    nitrogen flow and, 2198-2200, 2201
    optical zone size and, 2200
Excimer laser phototherapeutic keratectomy, 2211-2223
  advantages and indications, 2211
  in band keratopathy, 1129
  clinical outcome, 2216-2221
  in lattice dystrophy, 1051
  in recurrent erosion syndrome, 1325-1326
  side effects and complications, 2221
  surgical technique, 2211-2216
  wound healing after, 2216, 2217
Excision
  in conjunctival intraepithelial neoplasia, 1917
  in malignant melanoma of conjunctiva, 1915-1916
  in Mooren's ulcer, 1400
  pterygium, 1876-1877
  in squamous cell papilloma, 1917
Excisional biopsy, 866-867
Exclusion criteria, 2043
Exfoliative dermatitis, 990
Exoenzyme-S, 1147
Exophthalmos, 696
Exotoxin, 1146-1147
Explosion injury, 1407-1408
  corneal foreign body from, *A247*
  intracorneal keratoprosthesis after, *A295*
Exposure
  in donor tissue evaluation, 503
  evaporative dry eye, 679
Exposure keratitis, 1846-1847
Exposure keratopathy, *A214*
  in corneal perforation, 1815-1816
  in herpes zoster ophthalmicus, 1230
Expulsive choroidal hemorrhage, 1642-1643
Extended wear contact lens, 1454
External eye diseases, 457-459
External photography, 283-284
Extracapsular cataract extraction, 1594-1595, 1596-1600
Extracellular matrix
  angiogenesis and, 152-153
  maintenance of normal corneal integrity, 18-20
  response to infection, 145-146
  sterile corneal ulceration and, 205-206
Extracellular matrix proteins, 188-189
Extraocular muscles
  anterior segment surgery and, 1927
  examination in anterior uveitis, 1495
  herpes zoster ophthalmicus and, 1231
Exudate, 760
Eye area sensitivity syndrome, 853
Eye Bank Association of America, 481-482, 539
  annual statistics, 476
  Clinical Laboratories Improvement Act, 526
  on corneal tissue distribution, 519
  on donor tissue removal, 493
  ethics in procurement, 534
  Interim Final Rule, 528
  Medical Standards, 463-464
  purpose, organization, medical standards, and certification, 469-473
  reported penetrating keratoplasties, 1551, 1552
  on tissue banking, 527-528
  on vision research, 553
Eye Bank Association of India, 484
Eye Bank for Sight Restoration, 477-478, 537
Eye banking, 485-558
  ethics in, 531-535
  evolution, structure, and function, 475-480
  Eye Bank Association of America, 469-473
  governmental relations, 525-529
  international, 481-484
  medical legal issues, 537-541
  medical standards, 485-492
    consent, 487
    death to preservation time, 488-489
    donor screening, 487-488
    fees, 486-487
    government regulations, 486
    historical development, 485-486
  public relations and education, 547-551
  role in vision research, 553-558
  structure and function, 463-467
  syphilis and, 1299-1301
  tissue distribution in, 519-524
  tissue evaluation, 501-508
    penlight examination, 501
    slit lamp examination, 501-505, 506
    specular microscopy, 505-507
  tissue removal, 493-500
    consent for, 494
    corneoscleral rim excision, 497-498, 499-500
    donor maintenance and identification, 494
    enucleation procedure, 495-497
    in situ corneal scleral rim excision, 498-500
    public and professional education, 493-494
  tissue storage, 509-517
    media contamination, 514-515
    methods of, 510-514
    principles of corneal preservation, 509-510
Eye Banks for Responsible Regulation, 528
Eye examination, 213-364
  in anterior segment trauma, 1926-1929, 1930
  in anterior uveitis, 1497-1498
  in chronic conjunctivitis, 752-753
  confocal microscopy, 335-350
    in *Acanthamoeba* keratitis, 344-345
    current in vivo imaging systems, 336-337
    digital image acquisition and processing, 338-339, 340
    of endothelium, 342-343
    of epithelium, 339-342
    in excimer laser photorefractive keratectomy, 345-347
    in herpetic keratitis, 347
    history of, 335-336
    methodology, 337-338
    normal corneal structures, 339
    surface toxicity and incisional wound healing, 347-348
    in wound healing, 343, 344, 345
  corneal diagnostic techniques, 275-281
    corneal sensation, 279-280
    corneal staining, 275-277, 278
    pachymetry, 277-279
  in corneal injury, 1403-1404
  eyelid, 237-242
  high resolution ultrasound, 351-359
    in corneal disease, 354-356, 357
    in corneal surgery, 356-358
    examination techniques, 352-353, 354
    instrumentation, 351-352, 353, 354
    of normal cornea, 353-354, 355
  in itching and burning eye, 458
  laboratory investigation, 305-311
    adenovirus, 309
    Chlamydia trachomatis, 307-308
    Epstein-Barr virus, 309-310
    herpes simplex virus, 308
    in microbial keratitis, 305-307
    varicella zoster virus, 308-309
  before penetrating keratoplasty, 1564-1569
  in penetrating keratoplasty with intraocular lens implantation, 1504
  photo slit lamp biomicrography, 284-304
    biomicroscope, 284-285
    direct illumination, 288-291, 292, 293, 294-296
    indirect illumination, 291-293, 296-298
    preparation for, 285-288
    special techniques, 301-304
  points of emphasis, 361-364
  refraction of abnormal cornea, 215-221
  before refractive surgery, 2008
  slit lamp examination, 243-268
    before anterior segment surgery, 1927, 1928
    approach to, 263-268
    before astigmatic keratotomy, 2145
    in congenital corneal opacification, 367
    in corneal abrasion, 1404
    in corneal edema, 410-412
    in corneal infiltrates in contact lens patient, 429-430
    in corneal perforation, 1819
    in corneal trauma, 1403-1404
    direct illumination in, 244-254, 255, 256
    in donor tissue evaluation, 501-505, 506

in foreign body injury, 1417
in granular dystrophy, 1043, 1044
indirect illumination, 254-260
instrumentation, 243, 244
in itching and burning eye, 458
in keratoconus, 1094
before keratoplasty, 1567
in macular dystrophy, 1046
in minimal visual loss, 449
before penetrating keratoplasty, 1565-1569
in penetrating keratoplasty and intraocular lens exchange, 1604
of peripheral cornea, 260-261, 266
postoperative, 1647
in red eye, 442
before refractive surgery, 2010
in uveitis, 1506
vital dyes, 261-263, 266, 267, 268
specular microscopy, 313-334, 2023
in Chandler's syndrome, 1110
in corneal edema, 413
of diabetic cornea, 980
of donor tissue, 490, 505-507
epithelial, 317-318
in epithelial ingrowth, 1711
in Fuchs' dystrophy, 1076
improvements in instrumentation and methods, 316-317
in vivo findings, 323-330
in iris atrophy, 1110
optical principles, 313
in posterior polymorphous dystrophy, 1063, 1065, 1066
in pseudophakic corneal edema, 1603
qualitative morphometric analysis, 319-321
quantitative morphometric analysis, 321-323
tear film, 269-273
topographic analysis, 216, 223-235
keratometry, 224-225
keratoscopy, 225-226, 227
videokeratoscopy, 226-234
Eye poking, 1354
Eye pressing, 1354
Eye rubbing, 1094, 1354
Eyeglasses
after anterior segment trauma reconstruction, 1947-1948
after radial keratotomy, 2106
following anterior segment trauma, 1943
for keratoconus, 1099
for keratoglobus, 1102-1103
Eyelash
biomicroscopic examination of, 238-239
examination before penetrating keratoplasty, 1565-1566
ptosis in floppy eyelid syndrome, 571
Eyelid, 61-67, *A1-6*
anatomy, 563
atopic keratoconjunctivitis and, 814
capillary hemangioma, *A10*
contact dermatitis, 991
contact lens complications, 1461, 1462
epithelium of, 61-62, 63
examination before penetrating keratoplasty, 1565-1566
examination of, 237-242
herpes zoster ophthalmicus and, 1227
inflammation of, *A19-28*
allergic, *A28*
bacterial infection in, *A25*
blepharitis in, *A19-24*
parasitic infection in, *A27*
viral infection in, *A26*
Kaposi's sarcoma, *A18, A45*
lid margin, 62
molluscum contagiosum lesions, *A26*
nevus, 258
nodular malignant melanoma, *A17*
orbicularis oculi muscle, 62
physiology and biomechanics, 66-67
sarcoidosis and, 1523
scarring of, *A216*
sebaceous cell carcinoma, *A16*
sensory innervation, 65
surgery for corneal thinning disorders, 1794
tarsal plates, 62-64
varix, *A13*
Eyelid abnormalities
corneal infection and, 1142
distichiasis, 568-569
ectropion, 565-568 695, *A1-2*
entropion, 561-565, 566, *A3*
in cicatricial pemphigoid, 829
classification and pathophysiology, 561-562
differential diagnosis, 562
epiphora and, 696
management, 562-565, 566
in Stevens-Johnson syndrome, 842
in trachoma, 783
eyelid retraction, 578-579
floppy eyelid syndrome, 238, 571-573, *A6*
lagophthalmos, 574-578, 1007, *A5*
lid imbrication syndrome, 573-574, *A6*
trichiasis, 568-569, *A4*
biomicroscopic examination in, 240
in cicatricial pemphigoid, 829
in Stevens-Johnson syndrome, 842
in trachoma, 783
Eyelid infection
bacterial, 633-640
angular blepharitis, 634-635
anthrax, 638
chalazion, 635
chancroid, 638
hordeolum, 635
mycobacterial, 639
preseptal cellulitis, 635-638
staphylococcal blepharitis, 633-634
syphilis, 638
blepharitis, *A19-24*
angular, 634-635
in chronic granulomatous disease, 947-948
classification, 621-623
differential diagnosis, 623
herpes, *A180*
herpetic, 642
management, 623-624
meibomian gland dysfunction in, 625-632
microulcerative peripheral keratitis and, 394
psoriasis and, 939
in recurrent ocular herpes, 1195-1196
in rosacea, 990
staphylococcal, 633-634
fungal, 653-655
meibomian gland dysfunction, 625-632, 755
associated conditions, 628-629
classification, 627
diagnosis, 627-628
evaporative dry eye, 679
histopathology, 629
increased tear film evaporation, 54-55
lipid composition of meibomian secretion, 629-630
meibomian gland anatomy, 625, 626
physiology, 625-627
role of microorganisms, 630
in rosacea, 990
terminology, 625
treatment, 630-631
parasitic, 655-660
seborrhea, 625-632
associated conditions, 628-629
classification, 627
diagnosis, 627-628
histopathology, 629
lipid composition of meibomian secretion, 629-630
meibomian gland anatomy, 625, 626
physiology, 625-627
role of microorganisms, 630
terminology, 625
treatment, 630-631
viral, 641-651
herpes simplex virus, 641-643
molluscum contagiosum, 646-647
smallpox, 648-649
varicella zoster virus, 643-646
verruca vulgaris, 647-648
Eyelid retraction, 578-579
Eyelid retractors, 64-65
Eyelid speculum, 2015
Eyelid tumor, *A7-18*
benign, 581-600, *A7-13*
adnexal, 592-596
approach to diagnosis and management, 582
dermal, 586-592
epidermal, 582-586
histology of eyelid skin, 581-582
pigmented lesions, 596-598
malignant, 601-619, *A14-18*
basal cell carcinoma, 601-605
basal cell nevus syndrome, 614
Kaposi's sarcoma, 613-614
malignant melanoma, 612-613
Merkel cell carcinoma, 610-611
Muir-Torre syndrome, 616
premalignant lesions, 606-607
sebaceous cell carcinoma, 608-610
squamous cell carcinoma, 605-606, 607-608
xeroderma pigmentosum, 615-616
Eyeline, 477, 478, 523
EYENET, 477, 478

F

Fab fragment, 80
Fabry's disease, 905, 906, *A87-89*
corneal opacity in, 382
corneal verticillata in, 298, 417
sclerotic scatter of, 260
Facial artery, 65-66
Facial nerve palsy, 1005
Facial skin herpes simplex infection, *A179*
Factitious disorders, 1349-1358, *A215-216*
conjunctivitis, *A76*
keratoconjunctivitis, 1349-1350, 1351
Munchausen syndrome, 1350-1351
Munchausen syndrome by proxy, 1351
self-induced trauma, 1352-1354
topical anesthetic abuse, 1354-1356

Familial amyloidotic polyneuropathy type IV, 913
Familial dysautonomia, *A35*
Familial dysbetalipoproteinemia, 904
Familial high density lipoprotein deficiency, 904
Familial lecithin-cholesterol acyltransferase deficiency, 904
Family history, 1495
Fascia lata graft for scleral perforation, 1971
Fat, prolapsed orbital, *A50*
Favre-Racouchot syndrome, 585
Fc fragment, 80
Federal government regulation of tissue banking, 525-529, 540-541
Fees in eye banking, 486-487
Fenestration of conjunctival capillary, 45
Ferrous foreign body, 1418
Ferry line, *A169*
Fetal alcohol syndrome, 382
Fever
  in brucellosis, 1012-1013
  pharyngoconjunctival, 774
  vitamin A deficiency and, 960
Fibrin
  in anterior uveitis, 1498
  in epithelial wound healing, 205
Fibrinogen, 205
Fibrinolytic system, 145
Fibroblast, 150, 1713
Fibroblast collagenase, 186
Fibroblast growth factor, 152
Fibronectin, 86, 166
  in epithelial wound healing, 18, 184, 188-189
  functions of, 205-206
  to improve graft survival, 1785
  for postoperative epithelial defects, 1663
  scleral, 34-35, 38
  in sterile corneal ulceration, 208
Fibrosis
  after radial keratotomy, 2108-2109
  corneal response to infection, 149-151
Fibrous histiocytoma, 733, 734
Fibrous ingrowth, 1713-1715
Fibrous tissue tumor, 592
Filamentary keratitis, 1327-1332, 1663-1664, *A209*
Fill light, 284-285
Film color balance and sensitivity, 287
Fimbriae, 1144
First-In-First-Out inventory control, 521
Fish eye disease, 423, 904, *A90*
Fisherman's keratitis, 1122
Fistula, dural-cavernous, *A102-103*
Fixed dilated pupil after penetrating keratoplasty, 1669
Fixed frame analysis of cell size, 321
FK506, 1513
Flagella, 1144-1145
Flame burn, 1415-1416
Flap
  conjunctival, 1903-1909, *A289-290*
    in acid injury, 1441
    advancement, 1904, 1905
    bipedicle, 1904, 1906
    complications, 1905-1909
    in corneal edema, 414
    in corneal perforation, 1830
    in corneal thinning, 1794
    in *Fusarium* keratitis, 1261
    high resolution ultrasound of, 358
    indications, 1903-1904, 1905
    keratoprosthesis and, 1859
    in neurotrophic keratopathy, 1216
    postoperative care, 1905
    in pterygium, 1877-1879, 1880
    single-pedicle, 1904, 1907
    surgical technique, 1904, 1908
Flavivirus, 1247
Flavobacterium, 1704
Fleck dystrophy, 1055-1056, *A140*
  congenital corneal opacity in, 376
  corneal deposits in, 423
Fleischer ring, *A150, A152, A169*
  keratoconus and, 1094-1095, 1096
  photo slit lamp biomicrography of, 303
Flieringa rings, 1571, 1572
Floppy eyelid syndrome, 238, 571-573, 755, *A6*
Fluconazole, 1259
Fluctuation of vision after photorefractive keratoplasty, 2209
Flucytosine
  in fungal keratitis, 1258
  in neonatal conjunctivitis, 794
Fluorescein, 275-277, 278
  in contact lens fit, 261, 266
  in dry eye diagnosis, 669
  in foreign body injury, 1417
  for minimal visual loss evaluation, 449
  photography of, 301-302
  pooling in contact lens, *A263*
  staining characteristics of, 670
  in tear-break-up time, 664-665
Fluorescein angiography
  in episcleritis, 1476
  in penetrating keratoplasty and intraocular lens exchange, 1604
Fluorescein clearance test, 668
Fluorescein stain
  of dendritic epithelial patterns, *A262*
  in dry eye syndrome, *A33-34*
  of herpes zoster dendrites, *A189*
  in punctate keratitis, *A210*
  in superficial punctate keratopathy, *A30*
  in tear film evaluation, 271
  in thermal corneal injury, *A241*
Fluorocytosine, 1259
Fluorophotometry, 668
Fluoroquinolones, 1169-1171, 1178
  postoperative, 1646
  preoperative, 2060
  in staphylococcal blepharitis, 634
  toxicity of, 850
5-Fluorouracil, 1027, 1029
Flurbiprofen, 1508
Fluress; *see* Benoxinate
FN receptor, 206
Focal dermal hypoplasia, 995-996
Focal illumination in slit lamp examination, 246-254, 255, 256
  broad-beam illumination, 246-247, 248
  optic section, 247-252, 253
  specular reflection, 252-254, 255, 256
  Tyndall's phenomenon, 252, 253
Follicle
  conjunctival, *A51*
  in conjunctivitis, 746-748
    adult inclusion, 783-784
    bacterial, 760-761
  in trachoma, 781
Follicular blepharitis, 622
Follicular conjunctivitis, *A51*
  in acquired immunodeficiency syndrome, 1020
  acute, 750-752
  chronic, 756-757
  herpes simplex virus, 1196
  in Lyme disease, 1004
  related to topical medications, 852
  in sarcoidosis, 1524
  toxic, 757, *A74*
Folliculitis, 1530
Food and Drug Administration, [illegible]32
  Interim Final Rule, 528
  on refractive surgery, 2248
  on tissue banking, 527-528, 540-541
Forceps, 2015-2016
  injury, 369-370, *A236-239*
  large toothed, 1572
  used in securing donor to recipient cornea, 1576-1577
Foreign body, 1416-1419, *A227-254*
  abrasions in, *A227*
  after blast injury, *A233*
  in anterior segment, 1925-192[illegible], 19[illegible]2
  anterior segment surgery for, 1932
  conjunctival, *A233*
  copper, *A253*
  corn husk, *A242, A244*
  direct focal illumination of, 295
  direct retroillumination from iris, 2[illegible]8, 299
  elastic cord in, *A228*
  from explosion injury, *A247*
  of eyelid, *A28*
  glass, *A247, A250*
  glue in, *A232*
  grasshopper leg, *A242*
  hair, *A248*
  iron, *A244-246, A251-252*
  lacerations in, *A229-231*
  lint, *A255*
  metallic, *A243, A278*
  optic section of, 251
  perforated staphyloma from, *A246*
  photo slit lamp biomicrography of, [illegible]94
  retained, *A250*
  sclerotic scatter of, 260
  ultraviolet light in, *A228*
  vegetable, *A249*
Foreign body sensation
  after radial keratotomy, 2103
  in corneal abrasion, 1404
Forniceal conjunctiva, 42, 43
Fornix
  geography of, 41, 42
  reconstruction, 1891
4° C moist chamber storage, 510-511
Fracture, stromal, 1409
Franceschetti syndrome, 930
Francois dyscephalic syndrome, 9[illegible]0
Freckle
  conjunctival, 716
  eyelid, 598
Free-band lamellar keratoplasty, *A245*
Friedberg study, 2084-2086, 2094
Fright reflex, 66
Frozen section control, 604
Fryns syndrome, 382-383
Fuchs' dimples, 1133
Fuchs' dystrophy, 1073-1084, *A14[illegible]-14[illegible]*
  cataract in, 1593, 1594
  clinical characteristics of, 1064
  clinical presentation and course, 10[illegible]3-1076
  differential diagnosis, 1076
  electron microscopy, 1078-1081, 1082, 1083
  epithelial layer, 1083

- histopathology, 1077-1078
- minimal visual loss in, 453
- optic section of, 251
- pathogenesis, 1083-1084
- penetrating keratoplasty in, *A274*
- prognosis and management, 1077
- specular microscopy in, 323, 324
- specular reflection of, 256
- stroma and Bowman's membrane, 1081-1083

Fuchs' heterochromic iridocyclitis, 1537-1540
Fucosidosis, 902-903
Fudge factors, 225
Fund-raising in eye banking, 543-546
Fundus
- examination before refractive surgery, 2010
- retroillumination from, 259-260, 264, 265

Fungal infection
- after radial keratotomy, 2109
- chronic granulomatous disease, 947
- corneal
  - in acquired immunodeficiency syndrome, 1019-1020
  - ulceration in, 405
- eyelid, 621, 653-655
- lacrimal gland, 687-689
- in neonatal conjunctivitis, 792
- phlyctenulosis in, 1389
- in postoperative endophthalmitis, 1704

Fungal keratitis, 1253-1265, *A195-198*
- after radial keratotomy, 2119
- clinical features, 1255, 1256, 1257
- epidemiology, 1253-1254
- laboratory diagnosis, 1255-1258
- medical therapy, 1258-1261
- pathogenesis, 1253
- peripheral corneal and, 399
- risk factors, 1254-1255
- surgical therapy, 1261-1263
- therapeutic keratoplasty for, 1844-1845, 1846

Furrow degeneration, 391, 1101, *A167*
Fusarium, 1254, *A195-196*
Fusobacterium
- in acute bacterial conjunctivitis, 765
- in canaliculitis, 692

Fyodorov silicon, 2003
Fyodorov technique, 2102

G

Galactosialidodis, 910
Galardin, 192, 193
Gamma-benzene hexachloride, 657
Gammopathy, benign monoclonal, *A105*
Gangliosidosis type I, 382
GasPak Pouch system, 1161
Gaucher's disease, 1134
Gel injection adjustable keratoplasty, 2225
Gelatinase, 147
- in ocular wound healing, 186
- in sterile corneal ulceration, 207

Gelatinous droplike dystrophy, 420, 1053
General sedation, 2061
Generalized gangliosidoses, 906
Genesis incision, 2018
Genetic disorders, dermatologic, 994-999
Gentamicin
- in bacterial conjunctivitis, 767
- in corneal abrasion, 1406
- corneal effects, 1024
- in corneal perforation, 1818
- drug-induced lipidosis, 909
- eye drops, 1176
- impairment of epithelial wound healing, 189-190
- in microbial keratitis, 433
- in penetrating keratoplasty, 1589
- toxic keratoconjunctivitis secondary to, 848
- in tularemia, 800-801

Geographic ulcer, 1199
German measles
- conjunctivitis in, 776
- cornea and, 1246-1247

Gerontoxon, 1119
Ghost vessel, 1284, 1285
Ghosting, after radial keratotomy, 2128
Giant cell arteritis, corneal disease in, 1384
Giant papillary conjunctivitis, 753, 819-825, *A52, A68*
- from contact lens, 1461-1462, *A261*
- differential diagnosis, 823
- histopathology and pathogenesis, 821-823
- immunopathology of, 109
- meibomian gland dysfunction and, 629
- prognosis, 824-825
- symptoms and signs, 819-821, 822
- treatment, 823-824

Giemsa stain
- in bacterial keratitis, 1158, 1159
- in *Chlamydia trachomatis* infection, 307
- in fungal keratitis, 1255
- in herpetic blepharitis, 642
- in postoperative endophthalmitis, 1704
- in trachoma, 782
- in varicella zoster virus infection, 645

Gilles de la Tourette syndrome, 1353
Glands of Krause, 42, 50-51
Glands of Moll, 62, 63, *A13*
Glands of Wolfring, 42, 50
Glare
- after incisional refractive surgery, 2117
- after photorefractive keratoplasty, 2195-2196
- after radial keratotomy, 2103-2104, 2127-2129

Glare tester, 2019
Glass foreign body, *A247, A250*
Glass striae, *A165*
Glasses
- after anterior segment trauma reconstruction, 1947-1948
- after radial keratotomy, 2106
- following anterior segment trauma, 1943
- for keratoconus, 1099
- for keratoglobus, 1102-1103

Glaucoma, *A82*
- after cyclectomy, 1963
- after keratoplasty in herpes simplex, 1808
- after keratoprosthesis, 1860, 1861
- after penetrating keratoplasty, 1568-1569, 1719-1730
  - clinical presentation, 1722
  - incidence, 1719-1720
  - management, 1724-1728
  - mechanisms, 1722-1724
  - pediatric, 1753
  - risk factors, 1720-1722
- after radial keratotomy, 2136
- after therapeutic keratoplasty, 1851-1852
- in Axenfeld-Rieger syndrome, 893
- congenital corneal opacity and, 368-369
- donor tissue research in, 554, 556
- epithelial ingrowth and, 1712
- in Fuchs' heterochromic iridocyclitis, 1537, 1539
- in human leukocyte antigen-B27-positive patient, 1517
- in iridocorneal endothelial syndrome, 1112
- in juvenile rheumatoid arthritis, 1543
- postoperative, 372
- in postsyphilitic keratopathy, 1286-1287, 1288
- specular microscopy in, 326

Globe
- fixation in radial keratotomy, 2069, 2081
- fixation with forceps, 2016
- perforation during radial keratotomy, 2101-2102
- rupture of, 1926, 2121-2122

Globe supporting rings, 1571, 1572
Glomus tumor of eyelid, 590-591
Glucocorticoids, 681
Glucose availability curves, 2228
Glucuronic acid, 34
Glue injury, *A232*
Glycocalyx, 6, 43, 49, 1145
Glycogenosis type I, 903
Glycopeptides, 1168
Glycosaminoglycan metabolism disorders, 897-903
- diabetes mellitus, 897-899
- glycogenosis type I, 903
- macular corneal dystrophy, 902
- mannosidosis and fucosidosis, 902-903
- mucolipidoses, 909-910
- systemic mucopolysaccharidoses, 899-902

Glycosaminoglycans
- in corneal stroma, 10-11
- macular dystrophy and, 1047
- scleral, 32

Glycosylation-dependent cell adhesion molecule 1, 135
GM_1 gangliosidosis type I, 906
Goblet cell
- conjunctival, 44
- epithelial ingrowth and, 1711
- giant papillary conjunctivitis and, 821
- impression cytology and, 671-672
- in mucous layer, 49-50

Gold compounds
- corneal effects, 1026-1027
- deposits, 425, *A116*
- in juvenile rheumatoid arthritis, 1544-1545
- metabolic disorders, 916-917
- in rheumatoid arthritis, 1367

Gold weight implantation, 578
Goldenhar's syndrome, 929-930, *A97*
- epibulbar dermoids in, 377
- limbal dermoids and, 1922

Goldmann three-mirror lens, 301
Gonioplasty, 1609
Gonioscopy, 260-261, 266
- in anterior chamber cleavage syndromes, 893-894
- in corneal injury, *A249-251*
- in Fuchs' heterochromic iridocyclitis, *A270*
- in iris-nevus syndrome, *A162*
- before keratoplasty, 1567
- in penetrating keratoplasty and intraocular lens exchange, 1604
- in posterior embryotoxon, 889-891

Goniotomy, 895
Gonococcal conjunctivitis, 750, *A54, A62*
Gorlin's syndrome, 614-615
Gottron's sign, 1379, 1380
Gout, *A96*
  corneal crystals in, 421
  corneal manifestations, 913-914
  pigmented band keratopathy in, 418
Government
  impact on medical standards, 486
  regulation of tissue banking, 525-529, 540-541
GPC; *see* Giant papillary conjunctivitis
Graft
  in anterior segment trauma, 1938
  diameter as prognostic factor, 1762
  failure of, *A282, A287*
  granular dystrophy in, *A133*
  large diameter, 1773-1779
  macular dystrophy in, *A136*
  methods for improving survival, 1764-1769
  in scleral perforation surgery, 1967-1971
  in Terrien's marginal degeneration, 1791-1793
Graft-*versus*-host disease, 674-675, *A35*
Gram-negative bacteria
  in keratitis, 1140, 1141
  penicillin and, 1167
Gram-positive bacteria
  cephalosporins and, 1167-1168
  in keratitis, 1139
  penicillin and, 1167
Gram stain
  in bacterial keratitis, 1156, 1158-1159
  in fungal keratitis, 1255
  in microbial keratitis, 305-306
  in postoperative endophthalmitis, 1704
  therapy selection and, 1165
Gramicidin, 1175
Granular cell tumor, 587
Granular dystrophy, 1043-1045, *A131-133*
  corneal deposits in, 422
  minimal visual loss in, 452
  phototherapeutic keratectomy for, 2212-2213, 2214, 2215
Granulation tissue, 166
Granulocyte, 141-142
Granuloma
  in conjunctivitis, 749
  eosinophilic, *A105*
  pyogenic, *A47*
  in sarcoidosis, 1523-1524
Granulomatosis, *A222-224*
Granulomatous conjunctival lesion, 729-730, 731
Granulomatous conjunctivitis, 757
Grasshopper leg in conjunctivitis, *A242*
Graves' disease, 696, 983-984
Gray line, 239
Green-yellow discoloration, *A253*
Groenouw type II macular dystrophy, 902
Growth factors
  in endothelial wound healing, 195
  in epithelial wound healing, 185-188
  to improve graft survival, 1785
  maintenance of normal corneal integrity, 21
  in sterile corneal ulceration, 206, 208-209
  in stromal wound healing, 191
Gut-associated lymphoid tissue, 87-88
Guttae, *A145-146*
  aphakic bullous keratopathy and, 1427
  corneal edema and, 412
  in donor tissue evaluation, 505
  in Fuchs' dystrophy, 1073-1075
  in macular corneal dystrophy, 1045
  specular microscopy of, 323, 324

H

Haab's striae, 369, *A82*
Haemophilus aegyptius, 765
Haemophilus ducreyi, 638
Haemophilus influenzae
  in acute bacterial conjunctivitis, 764-765
  Bruton's hypogammaglobulinemia and, 972-973
  in conjunctivitis-otitis media syndrome, 769
  in dacryoadenitis, 689
  in eyelid necrosis, 637
  in nonsuppurative preseptal cellulitis, 636
Hair care products, 853, 854
Hair follicle tumor, 594-596
Hair groom gel, 853, 854
Hairs in cornea, *A248*
Hallermann-Streiff syndrome, 930
Hamartoma, 725-726
Hand dominance and incisions, 2079
Hand-Schüller-Christian disease, 904-905, *A105*
Hanna artificial anterior chamber, 1574, 1575
Hanna trephine system, 1573, 1574
Haptotaxis, 166, 167
Hassall-Henle bodies, 1131
Haze; *see* Corneal opacity
Head lice, 656
Health Care Financing Administration
  Clinical Laboratories Improvement Act and, 526
  organ procurement and, 537
Hearing loss
  in Cogan's syndrome, 1307
  in syphilis, 1288-1289, 1292
  in syphilitic interstitial keratitis, 1288-1289, 1292
Heat cauterization, 1866
Heavy chain, 80
Heerfordt's syndrome, 1525
Helmholtz's fudge factor, 225
Helper T cell, 73
Hemangioma
  capillary, *A10*
  in conjunctivitis, *A46*
Hematic cyst, conjunctival, 732
Hematologic disorders, 967-978, *A102-105*
  Bruton's hypogammaglobulinemia, 972-973
  crystalline keratopathy and, 977
  erythroid line, 967-969
  hematopoiesis and, 967
  leukemia, 969-972
  lymphoma, 972
  plasma cell dyscrasia, 973-977
Hematopoiesis, 967
Hematopoietic system, 71
Hemidesmosome, 8, 184, 199-200
Hemochromatosis, 968-969
Hemorrhage
  after cyclectomy, 1963
  after penetrating keratoplasty, 1668-1669
  anterior chamber, 1641-1642
  in Behçet disease, 1532
  from blunt trauma, 1930
  expulsive choroidal, 1642-1643
  intraocular use of tissue plasminogen activator and, 1667
  in soft contact lens wearer, *A264*
  subconjunctival, *A234*
  suprachoroidal, 1583, *A274*
Hemorrhagic conjunctivitis, 776
Hemorrhagic lymphangiectasia, 726
Henderson-Patterson body, 647
Heparin, 142
Hepatitis B virus infection, 1706
Hepatitis C virus infection, 1397-1398
Hepatocyte growth factor, 187
Herbert's pits, 400, 749, 781, 782, *A60-61*
Hereditary endothelial dystrophy, 374-375, *A147*
Hereditary hemorrhagic telangiectasia, 726
Hereditary progressive arthro-ophthalmopathy, 935
Hereditary stromal dystrophy, 375
Herniated orbital fat, 725
Herpchek test, 1212-1213
Herpes gestationis, 993
Herpes simplex infection, 1191-1223, *A179-188, A280*
  Acanthamoeba keratitis *versus*, 1271
  in acquired immunodeficiency syndrome, 1019
  after corneal transplantation, 1597
  after penetrating keratoplasty, 1705
  after radial keratotomy, 2108, 2119
  in atopic keratoconjunctivitis, 814
  blepharitis, *A180*
  chronic, *A188*
  confocal microscopy in, 347
  congenital and neonatal ocular herpes, 1194-1195
  conjunctival flaps in, 1903
  in conjunctivitis, 751-752, 775, *A186*
  corneal opacity in, 378-379
  with corneal perforation, *A184*
  with dendrites, *A182*
  diagnosis, 1212-1213
  disciform, *A185*
  epidemiology, 1191-1193
  epithelial, *A181*
  eyelid, 641-643
  of facial skin, *A179*
  in follicular conjunctivitis, 751
  graft failure and, 1762, 1767-1768
  inflammatory response in, 104
  from insect bite, *A254*
  interstitial, *A186*
  keratouveitis, 1692, *A186-188*
  laboratory investigation of, 308
  management, 1213-1219
  marginal staphylococcus keratitis *versus,* 1393
  of mouth, *A179*
  necrotizing, *A187*
  in neonatal conjunctivitis, 790, 792
  in Parinaud's oculoglandular syndrome, 802
  pathogenesis, 1193-1194
  penetrating keratoplasty in, 1799-1811
    anesthesia, 1803
    complications, 1806-1810
    donor tissue requirements, 1802
    indications, 1799-1800
    preoperative evaluation, 1801-1802
    preoperative medications, 1802
    prognosis, 1800
    surgical technique, 1803-1805
    timing of surgery, 1800-1801
  peripheral corneal and, 399

with peripheral inflammatory disease, *A187*
phlyctenular lesion *versus,* 1391
phlyctenulosis in, 1389
postoperative epithelial defects and, 1663
primary ocular herpes, 1195
recurrent ocular herpes, 1195-1212, 1213
blepharitis in, 1195-1196
conjunctivitis in, 1196
endotheliitis, 1205-1211
infectious epithelial keratitis, 1196-1201
iridocyclitis, 1211-1212, 1213
neurotrophic keratopathy, 1201-1202
stromal disease, 1202-1205
scars from, *A183*
scleritis, *A188*
stain of dendrite, 276
steroid-induced, 2202
therapeutic keratoplasty for, 1845-1846, 1847, 1848
ulcer in, *A182, A184, A290*
vesicle, *A179*
viral structure and classification, 1191
vitamin A deficiency and, 961
Herpes zoster, 1225-1242, *A189-194*
corticosteroids in, 1237
definition, epidemiology, and prevalence, 1225
dendrites, *A189*
herpes zoster ophthalmicus, 1226-1233, 1234-1236
in immunocompromised patient, 1233-1234
in interstitial keratitis, 1313
medical therapy, 1236-1237
neurotrophic ulcer after, *A193-194*
postherpetic neuralgia, 1237-1238
prevention, 1238-1239
in scleritis, 1487, *A194*
sectoral iris atrophy in, *A194*
therapeutic keratoplasty in, 1846
uveitis, *A191*
varicella, 1226
Herpes zoster ophthalmicus, 644, 1226-1233
in acquired immunodeficiency syndrome, 1018
corneal allograft rejection *versus,* 1692
corneal scarring from, *A192*
corticosteroids in, 1237
diagnosis, 1235-1236
with indolent corneal ulcer, *A193*
medical therapy, 1236-1237
neuralgia in, 1237-1238
ophthalmic complications, 1227-1232
pathogenesis, 1234
pathology, 1234-1235
signs and symptoms, 1226-1227
subepithelial infiltrates in, *A190*
Hesburg-Barron vacuum trephine, 1572-1573
Hesburg lens, 1424
Heterochromia
in Fuchs' heterochromic iridocyclitis, 1537, 1538, *A270*
with intraocular iron foreign body, *A251*
Hexagonal keratotomy, 2097, *A298*
historical background, 1986-1987
recurrent corneal erosion and, 202, 203
Hexosamine, 32
Hidrocystoma, apocrine, 593
Hidrotic ectodermal dysplasia, 994
High astigmatism, 1458-1460, *A288*
High magnification techniques
confocal microscopy, 335-350, 2023
in *Acanthamoeba* keratitis, 344-345
current in vivo imaging systems, 336-337
digital image acquisition and processing, 338-339, 340
of endothelium, 342-343
of epithelium, 339-342
in excimer laser photorefractive keratectomy, 345-347
in fungal keratitis, 1255
in herpetic keratitis, 347
history of, 335-336
in infectious keratitis, 1164-1165
methodology, 337-338
normal corneal structures, 339
surface toxicity and incisional wound healing, 347-348
in wound healing, 343, 344, 345
high resolution ultrasound, 351-359
in corneal disease, 354-356, 357
in corneal surgery, 356-358
examination techniques, 352-353, 354
instrumentation, 351-352, 353, 354
of normal cornea, 353-354, 355
specular microscopy, 313-334, 2023
in Chandler's syndrome, 1110
in corneal edema, 413
of diabetic cornea, 980
of donor tissue, 490, 505-507
epithelial, 317-318
in epithelial ingrowth, 1711
in Fuchs' dystrophy, 1076
improvements in instrumentation and methods, 316-317
in vivo findings, 323-330
in iris atrophy, 1110
optical principles, 313
in posterior polymorphous dystrophy, 1063, 1065, 1066
in pseudophakic corneal edema, 1603
qualitative morphometric analysis, 319-321
quantitative morphometric analysis, 321-323
High resolution ultrasound, 351-359
in corneal disease, 354-356, 357
in corneal surgery, 356-358
examination techniques, 352-353, 354
instrumentation, 351-352, 353, 354
of normal cornea, 353-354, 355
HIPO syndrome, 377
Hirschman iris hook, 1577
Histamine, 144
Histiocyte tumor, 591-592
Histiocytic conjunctival lesion, 729-730, 731
Histiocytosis X, 904-905
Histoacryl blau D-3508, 1819
Histocompatibility antigen, 1759
Histocompatibility matching, 1694
Histoplasma, 687
Hoffer study, 2088-2091, 2095
Holmium laser, 2185
Holmium:YAG laser, 1980, 2251
Holographic topography map, 2023
Homatropine
in acute anterior uveitis, 1516
for idiopathic uveitis, 1508
in ulcerative keratitis, 1179
Honan balloon, 1582-1583
Hook, 1577-1578
Hordeolum, 635, *A20*
Horizontal oval cornea, 874-875
Hormones, meibomian glands and, 627
Horner-Trantas dots, *A66*
in giant papillary conjunctivitis, 820
in vernal keratoconjunctivitis, 811
Host sensitization, 91
Hot wire thermokeratoplasty technique, 1989
Hudson-Stähli line, 1130, *A169*
Human immunodeficiency virus infection, 1017
after penetrating keratoplasty, 1706
bacterial keratitis in, 1142
conjunctivitis in, 769-770
corneal infections in, 1017-1022
disorders related to, *A111*
erythema multiforme in, 839
herpes zoster in, 1233
Kaposi's sarcoma in, *A45*
molluscum contagiosum in, *A26*
Reiter's syndrome in, 785, 1518
Human leukocyte antigen, 91-93
in Behçet disease, 1529
in juvenile rheumatoid arthritis, 1544
major, 91-93
minor, 93
pathogenesis of disease, 1515-1516
in rheumatoid arthritis, 1359
in Sjögren's syndrome, 679
Human leukocyte antigen-B27
in Reiter' syndrome, 785
in uveitis, 1515-1521, *A272*
Human leukocyte antigen marker, 839-841
Human mucosal lymphocyte antigen, 99
Human papillomavirus
in benign conjunctival epithelial growths, 705
in corneal infection, 1245
in verruca vulgaris, 647-648
Human recombinant epidermal growth factor, 208
Humoral immune response, 806
Hunter syndrome, 381, 901
Hurler-Scheie syndrome, 901
Hurler syndrome, 381, 899-901, *A92*
Hurricane keratitis, 852-853
Hutchinson's melanotic freckle, 598
Hutchinson's sign, 1226, *A189*
Hutchinson's teeth, 1288, 1289
Hyaline
in granular dystrophy, 1043-1045
in ligneous conjunctivitis, 864
Hyaluronan, 12, 19-20
Hyaluronic acid, 19-20, 32
Hyaluronidase, 867, 1147
Hydroa vacciniforme, 999
Hydrochloric acid, 1437
Hydrocystoma, eccrine, 593
Hydrofluoric acid, 1438
Hydrogen peroxide, 1273
Hydrops, *A157-158*
Hydroxychloroquine
corneal effects, 1026
in rheumatoid arthritis, 1367
in systemic lupus erythematosus, 1378
2-Hydroxyethyl methacrylate, 2234
Hydroxyl radical, 141-142
Hydroxyzine, 1238
Hymenolepis nana, 1389
Hyperacute bacterial conjunctivitis, 761-763, *A53*
Hyperbaric oxygen, 1765

Hyperbetalipoproteinemia, 904
Hypercalcemia
  calcific band keratopathy and, 420
  hyperparathyroidism and, 982
Hypercholesterolemia, *A96*
Hyperchylomicronemia, 904
Hyperemia
  in *Acanthamoeba* keratitis, 1268
  in giant papillary conjunctivitis, 819
Hyperlipoproteinemia, 903-904
Hyperopia
  after phototherapeutic keratectomy, 2221
  after radial keratotomy, 2049, 2105, 2132, 2133-2134
  excimer photorefractive keratectomy for, 2198, 2200
Hyperopic automated lamellar keratoplasty, 2172, 2174
Hyperosmotic lubricants, 1319
Hyperparathyroidism, 981-983
Hyperplasia
  conjunctival, *A44*
  sebaceous gland, 596
Hyperprebetalipoproteinemia, 904
Hyperproteinemia, 904
Hypersensitivity reaction, 106-116
  of conjunctiva, *A65*
  of eyelids, *A28*
  type I, 106-110
  type II, 110-112
  type III, 112-114
  type IV, 114-116
Hypertonic solutions
  in corneal edema, 413-414
  in recurrent corneal erosion, 202-203
Hypertrophy after radial keratotomy, 2125
Hyperuricemia, 913
Hyphema, 422, *A235*
  after penetrating keratoplasty, 1669
  anterior segment surgery for, 1930-1932
  in anterior uveitis, 1498
Hypolipoproteinemia, 904
Hypoparathyroidism, 981
Hypophosphatasia, 939
Hypophosphatemia, 982
Hypopyon
  in anterior uveitis, 1498, 1499
  in bacterial keratitis, 1148
Hypoxia, *A264*
  contact lens complication, 1464
  in corneal infiltrates in contact lens patient, 430

I

Ibuprofen, 1368
ICE syndrome; *see* Iridocorneal endothelial syndrome
Ichthyosis, 996-997, *A107*
ICR; *see* Intrastromal corneal ring
Idiopathic corneal endotheliopathy, 1210
Idiopathic uveitis, 1505-1513
  classification and previous occurrence, 1505, 1506
  consultation in, 1508
  laboratory evaluation, 1507-1508
  physical examination, 1506-1507
  treatment, 1508-1513
Idoxuridine
  corneal effects, 1023
  in herpes simplex virus keratitis, 1213-1214
  toxicity of, 849-850
IDU; *see* Idoxuridine
Iduronic acid, 34
Illumination intensity, 287-288
Imaging studies
  before anterior segment surgery, 1928-1929, 1930
  meibomian gland, 240-241
Imbibition pressure, 11
Imidazoles
  in fungal keratitis, 1258
  toxicity of, 850
Imipenem, 1168
Immune complex, 113-114
Immune-mediated scleritis, 1479-1485
Immune privilege, 90-96
Immune response, 68-127
  in allograft rejection, 1757-1761
  antigen processing, 88-89
  in Behçet disease, 1530
  components of immune system, 69-88
    cellular, 69-74, 75
    dendritic cell, 76, 77
    Langerhans cell, 76
    null lymphocyte, 74-76
    soluble mediators, 78-85
    tissue, 85-88
  contact lens-induced, 1464-1465
  corneal response to infection, 130-131
  in herpes simplex keratitis, 1193, 1194
  hypersensitivity reactions, 106-116
    type I, 106-110
    type II, 110-112
    type III, 112-114
    type IV, 114-116
  immune privilege and corneal transplantation, 90-96
  immunologic tolerance and autoimmunity, 89-90
  in Mooren's ulcer, 1398-1399
  overview, 68-69
  regulatory components of anterior segment, 96-106
    anterior chamber, 104-105
    conjunctiva, 98-101
    cornea, 101-104
    sclera, 105-106
    tear film and lacrimal gland, 96-98
Immune ring, 1204, 1205
Immune stromal keratitis
  herpes simplex virus keratitis and, 1202-1205, 1206, 1207
  treatment, 1217
Immune system, 69-88
  cellular components, 69-74, 75
  dendritic cell, 76, 77
  Langerhans cell, 76
  null lymphocyte, 74-76
  soluble mediators, 78-85
  tissue components, 85-88
Immunobullous disorders, 992-993
Immunocompromised patient
  conjunctivitis and, 769-770
  herpes zoster in, 1233-1234
  Parinaud's oculoglandular syndrome in, 799
  varicella zoster virus infection in, 645
Immunofluorescent assay, 1005
Immunoglobulin A, 52, 81
Immunoglobulin A disease, *A70*
Immunoglobulin E, 81
  atopic keratoconjunctivitis and, 815
  in giant papillary conjunctivitis, 822
  regulation of, 108
Immunoglobulin G, 310
Immunoglobulin M, 81
  B cells and, 70
  Epstein-Barr virus infection and, 310
Immunoglobulins, 73, 80-85
  characteristics of, 80-81
  distribution on ocular surface, [illegible]38
  in tear film, 52, 97-98
  in tears, 759
Immunologic disorders, *A217-226*
  collagen vascular disease, 1377-1387, *A221-224*
    Churg-Strauss syndrome, 138[illegible]
    giant cell arteritis, 1384
    mixed connective tissue disease, 1379
    polyarteritis nodosa, 1383-13[illegible]4
    polymyositis and dermatomyositis 1379-1380
    relapsing polychondritis, 138[illegible]-1381
    systemic lupus erythematosus, 1377-1378
    systemic sclerosis, 1378-1379
    Wegener's granulomatosis, 1[illegible]81-1383
  marginal staphyloccocal keratitis, 13[illegible]2-1394
  Mooren's ulcer, 398, 399, 1397-1401, *A226*
    conjunctival resection in, 179[illegible]
    deep lamellar keratoplasty for, 17[illegible]5
    immune response in, 114
    marginal staphylococcus keratitis *versus,* 1393
    pellucid marginal degeneration *versus,* 1101
    penetrating keratoplasty in, *A[illegible]77*
  nonrheumatoid collagen vascular disease in, *A221-224*
  phlyctenulosis, 1389-1395
  rheumatoid arthritis, 1359-1375, *A2[illegible]7-220*
    articular manifestations, 1360
    extra-articular manifestations, 136[illegible]-1361
    juvenile, 1370-1371, 1541-15[illegible]8, *A[illegible]72*
    keratitis in, 1364-1365, 1366, 136[illegible]
    keratoconjunctivitis sicca in, 1361-1362
    macroulcerative peripheral keratitis and, 396-397
    ocular chrysiasis and, 425
    pathogenesis, 1359-1360
    scleritis in, 1362-1364, 1365, 1366
    treatment, 1367-1370
  staphylococcal disease in, *A225*
Immunologic tolerance, 89-90
Immunomodulation
  in allograft rejection, 96
  through anterior chamber associated immune deviation, 105
Immunosuppressive agents
  for acute corneal allograft rejection, 1694
  in Cogan's syndrome, 1310
  in idiopathic uveitis, 1510-1513
  for improving graft survival, 1765-17[illegible]6
  in necrotizing scleritis, 1369
Impending perforation, 1816
Impetigo, 637, 992
Import dependent/net importer eye bank network, 475, 476
Importer/export eye bank network, 47[illegible], 476
Impression cytology
  in bacterial keratitis, 1158
  in conjunctival xerosis, 961
  in dry eye, 56, 671-672

In situ corneal scleral rim excision, 498-500
In vivo confocal imaging, 337-339
Incipient trachoma, 781
Incision
  American, 2016
  centripetal, 2016
  confocal microscopy of, 347-348
  genesis, 2018
  hand dominance and, 2079
  in phacoemulsification with penetrating keratoplasty, 1595, 1596
  radial keratotomy, 2070-2077, 2078, 2079, 2080
    abnormal healing after, 2110-2111
    marking location, 2065
    problems after, 2124-2126
  relaxing, 1681-1682
  variables in producing astigmatism after cataract surgery, 2155-2156
Incisional keratitis, 2146
Incisional refractive surgery, 1979-1987, *A291-299*
  astigmatic theory and incisional procedure, 2160-2162
  expected side effects, 2117-2118
  hexagonal keratotomy, 1986-1987
  instruments for, 2159-2160
  postoperative complications, 2162-2163
  radial keratotomy, 1979-1986; *see also* Radial keratotomy
Inclusion blennorrhea, *A62*
Inclusion cell disease, 909
Inclusion conjunctivitis
  adult, 783-785, *A58-59*
  Chlamydia trachomatis in, 751
  chronic follicular, 756
  neonatal, 786-787, *A62*
  peripheral corneal and, 399-400
Inclusion cyst, 585, *A258*
Incontinentia pigmenti, 998
India, eye banking in, 484
Indirect illumination
  in donor tissue evaluation, 502-503
  in photo slit lamp biomicrography, 291-293, 296-298
Indirect retroillumination from iris, 293, 299
Individual cell analysis, 322-323
Indomethacin
  in dacryoadenitis, 688-689
  for idiopathic uveitis, 1508
  in rheumatoid arthritis-associated scleritis, 1368
Infant
  congenital corneal opacity, 367-386
    bacterial and chlamydial diseases and, 379-380
    birth trauma and, 369-370
    cerebro-oculo-skeletal syndrome and, 383
    corneal dystrophies and, 374-378
    developmental abnormalities and, 370-374
    fetal alcohol syndrome and, 382
    Fryns syndrome and, 382-383
    glaucoma and, 368-369
    history and physical examination, 367-368, 369
    infectious diseases and, 378-379
    metabolic diseases and, 380-382
    penetrating keratoplasty in, 383-384
  penetrating keratoplasty in, 1731-1756
    complications, 1735
    future studies, 1735-1736
    graft survival, 1732-1734
    indications, 1732
    postoperative care, 1655-1656, 1746-1753
    preoperative evaluation, 1736-1742
    prognosis, 1763
    special considerations, 1766-1767
    surgical management, 1742-1746
    visual outcome, 1734-1735
Infection
  after astigmatic keratotomy, 2151-2152
  after keratoprosthesis, 1860, 1861
  after penetrating keratoplasty, 1669-1670, 1697-1707
    Creutzfeldt-Jakob disease, 1706
    endophthalmitis, 1703-1705
    hepatitis B virus, 1706
    human immunodeficiency virus, 1706
    infectious crystalline keratopathy, 1701-1703
    microbial keratitis, 1697-1700
    rabies, 1705-1706
    recurrent herpetic keratitis, 1705
    suture abscess, 1700-1701
  bacterial; *see* Bacterial infection
  chlamydial, *A58-59*
  in corneal perforation, 1815-1816
  corneal responses to, 129-162
    angiogenesis, 151-153
    fibrosis, 149-151
    inflammation and loss of function, 129, 130
    intrinsic barriers and immune response, 130-131
    mechanisms of microbial invasion, 131-133
    recruited cells, 141-144
    resident cells and surface receptors, 134-141
    soluble mediators, 144-145
    ulceration, 145-149
  Epstein-Barr virus, *A110*
  herpes simplex; *see* Herpes simplex infection
  herpes zoster; *see* Herpes zoster
  Proteus, A280
  suture-related, 1664-1665
  varicella, *A109, A273*
  viral; *see* Viral infection
Infection control in penetrating keratoplasty, 1582
Infectious crystalline keratopathy, 1701-1703, *A177, A280*
Infectious disease, 1003-1016, *A109-110*
  aqueous tear deficiency in, 674
  brucellosis, 1012-1013
  corneal, 398-400
  corneal opacity in, 378-379
  leprosy, 1006-1009
  Lyme disease, 1003-1006
  onchocerciasis, 1010-1012
  tuberculosis, 1009-1010
Infectious keratitis
  after radial keratotomy, 2109-2110
  in astigmatic keratotomy, 2163
  contact lens-induced, 1465-1467
  herpes simplex virus, 1196-1201
  therapeutic keratoplasty in, 1848
  treatment, 1215-1216
Infectious scleritis, 1485-1489, *A178*
Inferior marginal tear strip, 270-271
Inferior rectus muscle, 65
Infiltrates
  in *Acanthamoeba* keratitis, 1268-1269
  after penetrating keratoplasty, *A284, A286*
  allograft rejection and, 1689-1690, 1758
  associated with photorefractive keratoplasty, 2203
  in contact lens patient, 429-435, 1467-1468
  in donor tissue evaluation, 504
  endothelial rejection and, 1807
  in fungal keratitis, 1256
  in herpes zoster ophthalmicus, 1228, *A190*
  in marginal staphylococcus keratitis, 1392, 1393
  in Mooren's ulcer, 1397
  stromal, *A265-266*
  suture-related, 1665
  in syphilitic interstitial keratitis, 1280
Inflammation
  during active interstitial keratitis, 1282, 1283
  after astigmatic keratotomy, 2152
  after penetrating keratoplasty, 1667
  allergic, *A28*
  in anesthetic abuse, 1355
  in anterior uveitis, 1498, 1501, 1506
  in Cogan's syndrome, 1308-1309
  conjunctival, *A52*
  corneal allograft rejection and, 1689
  corneal reaction to injury, 163-165
  corneal response to infection, 129, 130
  eyelid, *A19-28*
    allergic, *A28*
    bacterial infection in, *A25*
    blepharitis in, *A19-24*
    parasitic infection in, *A27*
    physical examination in, 240
    viral infection in, *A26*
  in Fuchs' heterochromic iridocyclitis, 1539
  in giant papillary conjunctivitis, 819
  herpes simplex keratitis with, *A187*
  in juvenile rheumatoid arthritis, 1543
  mechanisms of microbial invasion, 131-133
  in syphilitic interstitial keratitis, 1280
  therapeutic keratoplasty and, 1852
  in trachoma, 781
Inflammatory bowel disease, 943-945, 1518-1519, *A99*
Inflammatory conjunctival lesion, 727-733
  amyloid, 731-732, 733
  elastofibroma oculi, 729
  granulomatous and histiocytic, 729-730, 731
  hematic cyst, 732
  keloid, 730-731
  nodular fasciitis, 729
  pinguecula and pterygium, 728-729
  pyogenic granuloma and capillary hemangioma, 727-728
Inflammatory disease
  chronic granulomatous disease, 947-948
  corneal, 393-398, 399
  dermatologic, 989-992
  inflammatory bowel disease, 943-945
  Kawasaki disease, 949-951
  scleral, 1479-1491
    immune-mediated, 1479-1485
    infectious, 1485-1489
  Wegener's granulomatosis, 948-949
  Whipple's disease, 945-946
Inflammatory ectropion, 567

Influenza, 1249
Informed consent
  in astigmatic keratotomy, 2146
  in laser surgery, 2186
  in pediatric penetrating keratoplasty, 1740-1741
  before refractive surgery, 2011
Infraorbital artery, 66
Infrared radiation injury, 1414
Infratrochlear artery, 66
Initial body, 779
Injury; *see* Trauma
Innervation
  conjunctival, 45
  corneal, 3
  eyelid, 65
  lacrimal gland, 51
Insect bite, *A254*
Insect corneal foreign body, 1418-1419
Instantaneous curvature, 229
Instrumentation
  automated lamellar keratoplasty, 2167-2168
  complexity of, 2246-2247
  corneal transplantation, 1571-1579
    preparation of donor cornea, 1573-1576
    preparation of recipient bed, 1572-1573, 1574, 1575
    preparation of recipient globe, 1571-1572
    used in securing donor to recipient cornea, 1576-1579
  high resolution ultrasound, 351-352, 353, 354
  laser refractive keratoplasty, 2181-2186
  refractive surgery, 2013-2024
    additional technology, 2019-2023
    astigmatic keratotomy instrumentation, 2018, 2020
    future advances, 2022, 2023, 2024
    investigative aids, 2023
    operating room equipment, 2013-2014
    primary procedure instrumentation, 2015-2018, 2019
    secondary procedure instrumentation, 2018-2019, 2020
    surgical supplies and medications, 2014-2015
Insulin-like growth factor-1, 191
Integrins, 86, 135, 136
  in corneal epithelium, 8
  distribution on ocular surface, 137, 138
  in epithelial wound healing, 18-19, 205
Intercellular adhesion molecule-1, 86, 103, 136-139
Interferon, 79-80
  Chlamydia trachomatis and, 781
  in Mooren's ulcer, 1400
Interferon-α, 83
Interferon-β, 83, 103
Interferon-γ, 134
Interim Final Rule, 528
Interleukin, 78-79
Interleukin-1, 78-79, 82, 139
Interleukin-1α, 150
Interleukin-2, 79, 82, 816
Interleukin-3, 82
Interleukin-4, 79, 82
Interleukin-5, 82
Interleukin-6, 18-19, 79, 82
Interleukin-7, 82
Interleukin-8, 79, 82, 139
Interleukin-9, 82
Interleukin-10, 79, 82
Interleukin-11, 83
Interleukin-12, 79, 83
International eye banking, 481-484
International Federation of Eye Banks, 483-484
Interrupted suture, 1628-1629, 1630
Interstitial collagenases, 147
Interstitial keratitis, *A203-204*
  herpes simplex, 1202-1205, 1206, 1207, *A186*
  in herpes zoster ophthalmicus, 1230
  nonsyphilitic, 1307-1315
    Acanthamoeba infection, 1311-1312
    Cogan's syndrome, 1307-1310
    herpes virus, 1312-1313
    leishmaniasis, 1312
    Lyme disease, 1311
    microsporidial infection, 1312
    mycobacterial infection, 1310-1311
    onchocerciasis, 1312
    trypanosomiasis, 1312
  syphilitic, 1275-1306, *A274*
    acquired syphilis and, 1282-1284
    congenital syphilis and, 1278-1282, 1283
    developmental stigmata in, 1288, 1290, 1291
    differential diagnosis, 1297
    epidemiology, 1277-1278
    hearing loss in, 1288-1289, 1292
    history of, 1275-1277
    joints and, 1289-1291
    laboratory investigation, 1297-1299
    pathogenesis, 1294-1297, 1298
    pathology, 1291-1294
    residual interstitial keratopathy and, 1284-1287, 1288
    treatment, 1299-1301
  in tuberculosis, 1010
Intestinal lipodystrophy, 945-946
Intracapsular cataract extraction, *A256*
Intracellular signal transduction, 21
Intracorneal lenses and rings, 2249
Intradermal nevus, 597, *A8*
Intradermal skin test, 848
Intraepithelial epithelioma, 705
Intraepithelial neoplasia, 754, *A38*
Intraepithelial ointment, 421
Intraocular blood, *A235*
Intraocular inflammation, 326
Intraocular lens implantation
  comparison of fixation techniques, 1623
  complications of, 1423-1425
  penetrating keratoplasty with, 1558, 1603-1626
    anterior segment reconstruction, 1609-1610, 1611
    evaluation, 1619-1623
    explantation, 1606-1608
    implantation technique, 1610-1617, 1618, 1619, 1620
    indications and goals of surgery, 1603-1604
    open-sky subtotal vitrectomy, 1608-1609
    patient preparation, 1605
    postoperative care, 1618-1619
    preoperative assessment, 1604-1605
    suturing of donor cornea, 1617-1618
    trephination of recipient cornea, 1605-1606
  specular microscopy following, 327
Intraocular pressure, 11
  after automated lamellar keratoplasty, 2175
  after photorefractive keratoplasty, 2202
  anterior segment surgery and, 1928
  in anterior uveitis examination, 150[illegible]
  corneal allograft rejection and, 1691
  in corneal edema, 414
  in epithelial ingrowth, 1712
  etiology of uveitis and, 1506-1507
  penetrating keratoplasty
    control during, 1582-1583
    elevated after, 1666-1667
    examination before, 1568-1569
  syphilitic interstitial keratitis and, 1286-1287
  therapeutic keratoplasty and, 1348
Intraocular refractive procedures, 200[illegible]-2003
Intraocular surgery, 1979
Intraoperative ultrasonic pachymetry, 2065-2067
Intrastromal ablation, 2000, 2001
Intrastromal corneal ring, 1993, 2225, 2227-2229
Intrastromal devices, 2225-2232
  clinical and histopathologic observations, 2227
  intrastromal corneal ring, 2227-2229
  physiologic considerations, 2226-2227, 2228
  refractive mechanisms, 2225-2226
  small diameter corneal inlay, 2230-2231
Intrastromal photoablation, 1982
Intrastromal photorefractive keratectomy, 2250
Intrastromal pocket, 2236
Intravascular papillary endothelial hyperplasia, 591
Intravenous immunoglobulin, 951
Intrinsic barriers to infection, 130-131
Inverted conjunctival papilloma, 702-703
Inverted follicular keratosis, 584-585
Investigative aids, 2023
Involutional ectropion, 565, 567, *A1*
Involutional entropion, 561-562, 563-564, *A3*
Ion transport system, 17
Iowa corneal punch, 1574, 1575
Iridectomy, 372
Iridocorneal adhesion, 892
Iridocorneal endothelial syndrome, 1117-1118, *A160-162*
  Axenfeld-Rieger syndrome *versus*, 894
  clinical course, 1112, 1115
  clinical features, 1107-1111, 1112
  differential diagnosis, 1112-1113, 1116
  etiology, 1111-1112, 1113-1114
  history and background, 1107, 1108
  management, 1115
  minimal visual loss in, 453
  posterior polymorphous dystrophy *versus*, 1066
  specular microscopy in, 325
Iridocyclectomy, 1957-1964
  complications, 1963-1964
  indications, 1957-1958
  postoperative care, 1963
  procedure, 1958-1963
  results, 1964
  surgical anatomy, 1958
Iridocyclitis, 1211-1212, 1213, *A269-270*
  after radial keratotomy, 2136
  in Behçet disease, 1531-1532

Fuchs' heterochromic, 1537-1540
herpes simplex virus, 1218
in juvenile rheumatoid arthritis, 1541, 1542, 1543
in sarcoidosis, 1524-1525
Iridodialysis
in anterior segment trauma, 1928
traumatic, 1939-1940
Iridoplasty
in anterior segment reconstruction, 1609-1610, 1611
in postkeratoplasty glaucoma, 1725
Iridoschisis, *A254*
Iris
anterior segment surgery and, 1928, 1929, 1939
bicolored irides, 1538
cyclectomy and iridocyclectomy, 1957-1964
complications, 1963-1964
indications, 1957-1958
postoperative care, 1963
procedure, 1958-1963
results, 1964
surgical anatomy, 1958
direct and indirect retroillumination from, 256-259, 261, 262, 263
examination in anterior uveitis, 1498-1499, 1500
foreign body attached to, 1942
iridocorneal endothelial syndrome, 1107-1118
clinical course, 1112, 1115
clinical features, 1107-1111, 1112
differential diagnosis, 1112-1115, 1116
etiology, 1111-1112, 1113-1114
history and background, 1107, 1108
management, 1115
iron deposits in, 422
nevus, 325, 1108, 1111, 1112, *A160, A162*
penetrating keratoplasty and
examination before, 1567
intraoperative damage, 1640-1641
pediatric, 1745
photo slit lamp biomicrography of, 292
posterior membrane dystrophies and, 1068
reconstructive procedures after anterior segment trauma, 1953
sarcoidosis and, 1524
transillumination of, 260, 265
xanthogranuloma on, *A7*
Iris atrophy, *A160-162*
in anterior uveitis, 1498
essential, 1107-1110, *A160-162*
in herpes simplex keratouveitis, *A188*
in herpes zoster, *A194*
in leprosy, 1008
in postsyphilitic keratopathy, 1286
sectoral, *A194*
specular microscopy of, 325
Iris-claw, 1982
Iris nodule syndrome, 1111
Iris-sutured posterior chamber intraocular lenses
evaluation, 1622
technique, 1613-1614
Iritis
in *Acanthamoeba* keratitis, 1269
after photorefractive keratoplasty, 2209
in Cogan's syndrome, 1307
Iron deficiency anemia, 968
Iron foreign body
in cornea, *A244-246, A251*
intraocular, *A251-252*
in iris, *A252*
Iron lines, 417-418, 419, 1130-1131, *A169*
after radial keratotomy, 2108, 2124
Iron overload, 968-969
Irregular astigmatism
after astigmatic keratotomy, 2163
after automated lamellar keratoplasty, 2177
after radial keratotomy, 2134-2135
contact lens for, 1458-1460
videokeratopathy in, 2053
Irregular Astigmatism Index, 2047
Irrigating cannula, 2018
Irrigating solutions
corneal effects, 1028
endothelial toxicity, 1427-1428
specular microscopy following induction, 329
Irrigation
of acid injury, 1438-1440
of wound, 2080
Irritation from contact lens, *A262*
Ischemia, *A258-260*
Isobutyl-2-cyanoacrylate, 1819
Isotretinoin
corneal effects, 1027-1028
meibomian gland dysfunction and, 629
meibomian gland expression and, 241
Itching, 457-459
in atopic keratoconjunctivitis, 814
in onchocerciasis, 1011
in vernal keratoconjunctivitis, 811
Ivermectin, 1012
Ixodes dammini tick, 1003

J

Jackson cross cylinder procedure, 218-220
Japanese eye banking, 483
Jarisch-Herxheimer reaction, 1299
Jellyfish sting, 1420
Jo-1 antibody, 1379
Joint
congenital syphilis and, 1289-1291
juvenile rheumatoid arthritis and, 1541
rheumatoid arthritis and, 1360
Junctional nevus, 596
Juvenile rheumatoid arthritis, 1370-1371, 1541-1548, *A272*
Juvenile xanthogranuloma, 591-592, 730, 904-905, 1000

K

K-Sol, 512
Kala-azar, 657
Kallikrein, 145
Kaposi's sarcoma, 1000, *A18, A45*
conjunctival, 733-734, 735
eyelid, 613-614
Kassowitz's law, 1295
Katzin corneal scissors, 1578
Kawasaki disease, 949-951
Kaye dots, 1665
Kayser-Fleischer ring, 390-391, 425, 915-916, *A95-96*
Kelman-McPherson forceps, 1576
Keloid
conjunctival, 730-731
corneal, 377-378, 1126, *A48*
Keratan sulfate, 11, 32
Keratectasia, 880
Keratectomy, phototherapeutic, 2211-2223, *A300*
advantages and indications, 2211
clinical outcome, 2216-2221
side effects and complications, 2221
surgical technique, 2211-2216
wound healing after, 2216, 2217
Keratic precipitates
in anterior uveitis, 1497
broad-beam illumination of, 247
corneal edema and, 412
in donor tissue evaluation, 505
endothelial rejection and, 1758
formation of, 136
in Fuchs' heterochromic iridocyclitis, 1537, 1538
in uveitis, 1506, *A191*
Keratinization
in erythema multiforme, 836, 837
of upper palpebral conjunctiva, *A6*
Keratinocyte growth factor, 187
Keratinoid corneal degeneration, 1122
Keratitis
Acanthamoeba, 1267-1273, 1311-1312, *A199-202*
clinical findings, 1268-1270
confocal microscopy in, 344-345
contact lens-induced, 1466-1467
corneal ulcer in, 405
differential diagnosis, 1271
laboratory diagnosis, 1270-1271
penetrating keratoplasty in, 1553
prevention, 1273
pseudodendrites in, 431
risk factors, 1267-1268
therapeutic keratoplasty for, 1845
treatment, 1271-1273
anterior uveitis and, 1497
avascular, 1008
bacterial, 1139-1189, *A177-178*
in acquired immunodeficiency syndrome, 1019-1020
adjunctive therapy in, 1179-1181
aminoglycosides in, 1168-1169
antimicrobial susceptibility testing in, 1163
causes, 1139-1141
cephalosporins in, 167-1168
chloramphenicol in, 1173-1174
clinical features, 1147-1152, 1153
contact lens-induced, 1465-1466
corneal biopsy, 1163-1165
culture in, 1155-1158
culture media for, 1160-1163
diagnosis, 1155
drug therapy routes, 1175-1177
fluoroquinolones in, 1169-1171
glycopeptides in, 1168
histopathology, 1152-1155
macrolides and lincosamides in, 1171-1172
Mycobacterium fortuitum, A178
pathogenesis, 1144-1147
penicillins in, 1166-1167
peptide antibiotics in, 1175
Pseudomonas, A178
rifampin in, 1174
risk factors, 1141-1144, 1145
spectinomycin in, 1174-1175
staining in, 1158-1160, 1161
Streptococcus pneumoniae, A299
sulfonamides in, 1174
tetracyclines in, 1173
trimethoprim in, 1174

Lamellar keratoplasty—cont'd
  indications, 1833, 1834, 1835
  in pellucid marginal corneal degeneration, 1789-1790
  penetrating *versus*, 1833-1834, 1835
  preoperative evaluation, 1834-1836
  in pterygium, 1879
  surgical technique, 1836-1841
  in Terrien's marginal degeneration, 1791
Lamellar stroma, 190
Lamellar surgery, 1990-2001
  epikeratoplasty, 1994-1996
  keratomileusis, 1991-1992
  keratophakia, 1992-1993
  photorefractive keratectomy, 1996-2001
  synthetic keratophakia, 1993-1994, 1995
Lamina fusca, 30
Laminin, 14, 86, 149-150
Landers-Foulks keratoprosthesis, 1953, 1954
Langerhans cell, 4-5
  antigen processing by, 92, 99, 1142
  in corneal graft rejection, 1688
  histiocytosis, 904-905
  immune response and, 76, 139-141
Large diameter corneal graft, 1773-1779
Large diameter therapeutic sclerokeratoplasty, 1776
Laser-assisted in situ keratomileusis, 1991, 2166, 2178-2179
  adjustability, 2246
  corneal topographic analysis in, 2052
  costs, 2247
  instrumentation for, 2184-2186
  procedure, 2187-2188
Laser confocal microscope, 336
Laser flare photometer, 1516-1517
Laser holographic interferometry, 2229
Laser photocoagulation
  in corneal injury, *A241*
  in epithelial ingrowth, *A258*
  to improve graft survival, 1785
Laser photorefractive keratectomy, *A300*
  future of, 2250-2251
  historical background, 1996-2001
Laser refractive keratoplasty, 2181-2189
  instrumentation, 2181-2186
  surgical technique, 2186-2188
Laser surgery
  in anterior chamber cleavage syndromes, 895
  in band keratopathy, 1129
  instrumentation in, 2184-2186
  laser-assisted in situ keratomileusis, 1991, 2166, 2178-2179
    adjustability, 2246
    corneal topographic analysis in, 2052
    costs, 2247
    instrumentation for, 2184-2186
    procedure, 2187-2188
  laser refractive keratoplasty, 2181-2189
    instrumentation, 2181-2186
    surgical technique, 2186-2188
  photocoagulation
    in corneal injury, *A241*
    in epithelial ingrowth, *A258*
    to improve graft survival, 1785
  photorefractive keratoplasty
    complications, 2200-2209
    historical background, 1997-1998
    predictability, 2030-2037
    results, 2191-2200
  phototherapeutic keratectomy, 2211-2223
    advantages and indications, 2211
    clinical outcome, 2216-2221
    in ocular surface disease, 1869-1870
    side effects and complications, 2221
    surgical technique, 2211-2216
    wound healing after, 2216, 2217
  refractive keratoplasty, 2181-2189
    instrumentation, 2181-2186
    surgical technique, 2186-2188
  in trichiasis, 569
Lasersight excimer laser, 2183
LASIK; *see* Laser-assisted in situ keratomileusis
Latency-associated transcripts, 1193
Lateral perpendicularity, 2076
Lateral rectus tendon, 41
Lateral tarsal strip, 565
Laterality
  in anterior uveitis, 1501
  in corneal edema, 409-410
Lattice dystrophy, 1048-1051, 1052, 1053, *A125-130*
  corneal deposits in, 423
  direct and indirect retroillumination from iris, 261, 299
  keratoprosthesis in, 1858
  minimal visual loss in, 452
  phototherapeutic keratectomy for, 2212-2213, 2214, 2215
  phototherapeutic keratectomy in, 2214
  specular microscopy in, 325
Lattice theory of transparency, 215-216
Lavery study, 2091-2093, 2095
Lax eyelid syndrome, 572
Laxity of eyelid, 238
LCAT deficiency; *see* Lecithin-cholesterol acyltransferase deficiency
Leaking descemetocele, 1816
Leber's congenital amaurosis, *A154*
Lecithin-cholesterol acyltransferase deficiency, 423, 1120, *A90*
Legal issues in eye banking, 537-541
Legislation in eye banking, 525-529
Legislative consent, 537-539
Leiomyoma, 587
Leishmania, 657-658, 1312, 1389
Leishmanin skin test, 658
Lens
  anterior segment surgery and, 1928, 1940-1941
  anterior segment trauma and, 1952-1953
  contact; *see* Contact lens
  dislocation, 1941
  examination in anterior uveitis, 1499-1500
  foreign body attached to, 1942
  intraocular, *A256*
  penetrating keratoplasty and
    examination before, 1567-1568
    intraoperative damage, 1640-1641
    management in, 1583
  syphilitic interstitial keratitis and, 1286
Lensectomy, 1745-1746
Lentigo maligna melanoma, 598
  conjunctival, 717
  eyelid, 612
Lentigo senilis, 598
Lentigo simplex, 598
Lepromatous leprosy, 1006
Leprosy, 1006-1009
  eyelid and, 639
  ocular lesions of, 1141
Lesch-Nyhan syndrome, 1353
Lester hook, 1577
Letterer-Siwe disease, 904-905
Leukemia, 969-972
Leukocyte
  angiogenesis and, 151
  trafficking, 85-86, 87, 136
Leukocyte adhesion deficiency, 135
Leukocyte selectin, 135-136
Levator aponeurosis, 65
Levator palpebrae superiorus muscle, 65
Levocabastine, 808, 816
Lice, crab, *A27*
Lid; *see* Eyelid
Lid edema
  in *Acanthamoeba* keratitis, 126[illegible]
  in bacterial keratitis, 1148
  in corneal birth injury, 1410
  in dermatomyositis, 1380
  in herpes zoster ophthalmicus, 1227
Lid hygiene
  in blepharitis, 623-624
  in cicatricial pemphigoid, 831
  in meibomian gland dysfunction, 63[illegible]
  in staphylococcal blepharitis, 6[illegible]4
Lid imbrication syndrome, 573-574, *A*[illegible]
Lid margin, 62
  atopic keratoconjunctivitis and, 814
  biomicroscopic examination of, 239
  ectropion, 565-568
  entropion, 561-565, 566
  meibomian gland dysfunction and, [illegible]28
Lid massage, 630
Lid scrub, 630
Lid telangiectasia, 1379
Lidocaine, *A215*
  in penetrating keratoplasty, 18[illegible]3
  in postherpetic neuralgia, 1238
  preoperative, 2060
Lieberman gravity-action corneal donor punch, 1575
Lieberman system, 1573, 1574
Ligase chain reaction, 307-308
Light chain, 80
Light filament reflex centration, 2063
Light microscopy
  in macular dystrophy, 1046-1047
  in phlyctenulosis, 1394
Lightning injury, *A240*
Ligneous conjunctivitis, 756, 863-868, *A76*
Limbal arcades, 30-31, 36
Limbal autograft, 1888
Limbal conjunctival resection, 1[illegible]94
Limbal dermoid, 387, 1921-1922, *A8*[illegible]
Limbal girdle degeneration, *A16*[illegible]
Limbal girdle of Vogt, 1127, 1128
Limbal guttering, 1364, 1366
Limbal ischemia, 1439
Limbal perforation, *A254*
Limbal sarcoid nodule, *A46*
Limbal stem cell, 17-18
Limbal transplantation, 1892-1898, 1[illegible]99
Limbal vascular keratitis, 1228
Limbal vernal keratoconjunctivitis, *A*[illegible]*6*
Limbus
  histology, 43-44
  immune response and, 131
  phlyctenulosis of, 1390
  vascular supply and regulation of corneal neovascularization, [illegible]03
Limulus lysate assay, 1164
Lincomycin, 1172
Lincosamides, 1171-1172
Lindane; *see* Gamma-benzene hexachloride

Linear endotheliitis, 1209-1211, 1212
Linear epidermal nevus, 585
Linear immunoglobulin A disease, 993, *A70*
Linear scleroderma, 1378
Link protein, 34
Lint foreign body, *A255*
Lions Club, 463, 483, 545, 546
Lipid degeneration, 1120-1121
Lipid keratopathy, 1230
Lipid layer, 52, 625-627, 666, *A29*
Lipid mediators, 144
Lipid metabolism disorders, 903-909
  drug-induced lipidoses, 906-909
  dyslipoproteinemias, 903-905
  lipidoses, 905-906
  mucolipidoses, 909-910
Lipidosis, 905-906, 907-909
Lipids
  corneal arcus and, 1119
  deposition, 423
  in meibomian secretion, 629-630
  secreted by macrophages, 143
Lipodermoid, *A80*
Lipoma, pleomorphic, 739
Lipopolysaccharide-binding protein, 131
Lipopolysaccharides
  of endotoxins, 1147
  mechanism of microbial invasion, 131-132
Lipoprotein metabolism disorders, 903-909
  drug-induced lipidoses, 907-909
  dyslipoproteinemias, 903-905
  lipidoses, 905-906
Lisch nodule, *A13*
Lissamine green B, 670
Listeria monocytogenes, 1141
Living Bank, 531
Livostin; *see* Levocabastine
Loa loa worm, *A64*
Local therapy, corneal effects, 1023-1031
  drug deposition, 1026-1027
  ophthalmic surgical solutions, 1028-1030
  topical ophthalmic medications, 1023-1026
  toxic effects, 1027-1028
Lodoxamide, 808, 1785
Lofgren's syndrome, 1525
Loiasis, 658, *A64*
Looped anterior chamber intraocular lens, *A256*
Loratadine
  in atopic keratoconjunctivitis, 816
  to improve graft survival, 1785
Louis-Bar syndrome, 726
Louse infestation, 656-657
Lowe syndrome, *A48*
Lowenstein-Jensen agar, 306
Lower eyelid imbrication, *A6*
Lubricating ointments
  in cicatricial pemphigoid, 831
  in dry eye, 680
  for epithelial basement membrane corneal dystrophy, 1037
  in rheumatoid arthritis-associated keratoconjunctivitis sicca, 1368
Lupus erythematosus
  discoid, *A222*
  systemic, 1377-1378, *A221*
Lyme disease, 757, 1003-1006, 1311, *A110*
Lymph nodes, 85
Lymphangiectasis, *A43*
Lymphangioma, *A44*
  conjunctival, 738
  eyelid, 589-590
Lymphatics
  conjunctival, 45
  eyelid, 65-66
  immune recognition and, 93
  malignant melanoma and, 721
Lymphocyte
  inflammation and, 143-144
  ocular immune response and, 70-74
  recirculation and homing, 86
Lymphocyte function-associated antigen-1, 136, 138
Lymphogranuloma venereum, 787
  in acquired immunodeficiency syndrome, 1020
  in Parinaud's oculoglandular syndrome, 802
Lymphoid conjunctival lesion, 736-738, 1920-1921
Lymphoid hyperplasia of conjunctiva, *A44*
Lymphoid organs, 85-88
Lymphoid stem cell, 71
Lymphokines, 78-80
Lymphoma, 972
  conjunctival, *A44-45*
  subconjunctival, 737
Lysozyme, 670-671, 1526

M

M cell, 88
M-K medium, 511
MacCallan classification and staging of trachoma, 781
Mace, 853-854
Macro lens, 283
Macroglobulinemia, *A104*
Macroirregular astigmatism, 2143-2145, 2146
Macrolides, 1171-1172
Macroperforation, 2163
Macrophage, 75-76
  allograft rejection and, 94
  inflammation and, 143
  in tears, 759
Macroulcerative peripheral keratitis, 396-398, 399
Macular dystrophy, 1045-1048, *A135-136*
  corneal deposits in, 422-423
  glycosaminoglycan metabolism in, 902
  minimal visual loss in, 453
Macular edema, 1653-1654
Maculopapular rash
  in herpes zoster ophthalmicus, 1227
  in varicella, 1226
Madarosis
  in ocular leprosy, 1007
  in staphylococcal blepharitis, 633
Magnetic resonance imaging
  in anterior segment trauma, 1929, 1930
  in ciliary body tumor, 1957
Major histocompatibility class II antigen, 72
Major histocompatibility complex, 88, 134, 1515
Malakoplakia, 769-770
Malbran procedure, 1774
Malignant atrophic papulosis, 1000
Malignant melanoma
  conjunctival, 719-722, 735-736, 754, 1914-1916, *A41*
  eyelid, 612-613, *A17*
Malignant tumor
  conjunctival, 704-712
    conjunctival intraepithelial neoplasia, 704-707
    corneal epithelial dysmaturation and epithelial dysplasia, 707-710
    mucoepidermoid carcinoma, 710
    sebaceous cell carcinoma, 710-712
    spindle cell carcinoma, 710
    squamous cell carcinoma, 707, 708
  eyelid, 601-619, *A14-18*
    basal cell carcinoma, 601-605
    basal cell nevus syndrome, 614
    Kaposi's sarcoma, 613-614
    malignant melanoma, 612-613
    Merkel cell carcinoma, 610-611
    Muir-Torre syndrome, 616
    premalignant lesions, 606-607
    sebaceous cell carcinoma, 608-610
    squamous cell carcinoma, 605-606, 607-608
    xeroderma pigmentosum, 615-616
Malingering, 1349, 1352
Maloney intraoperative qualitative keratometer, 1578
MALT; *see* Mucosa-associated lymphoid tissue
Mandel intraoperative keratometer, 1579
Mandibulofacial dysotosis, 930
Mannosidosis, 902-903
Map-dot-fingerprint corneal dystrophy, 452, 1035, *A119-121*
Marfan syndrome, 936-937
Marginal furrow, 397-398
Marginal infiltrates, 113
Marginal staphyloccocal keratitis, 1392-1394
Marginal ulcer, 1199-1200
Markers for allograft rejection, 95-96
Maroteaux-Lamy syndrome, 381-382, 900, 901-902, *A93*
Masquerade syndrome, 754
Mast cell, 77-78
  in atopic keratoconjunctivitis, 815
  in conjunctiva and limbus, 99
  in giant papillary conjunctivitis, 822
  inflammation and, 142
  in type I hypersensitivity reaction, 106-108
  vernal keratoconjunctivitis and, 812
Mast cell mediators, 106-108
Matrix metalloproteases, 166
Matrix metalloproteinases
  in ocular wound healing, 186
  response to infection, 146-148
  in sterile corneal ulceration, 207
  in stromal wound healing, 191-192
  in ulcerative keratitis, 1179
Matrix metalloproteinases inhibitors, 209
Maumenee-Park speculum, 1571, 1572
Mayo stand, 2014
McAdam classification, 1380
McCoy cell culture, 793
McGuire lens, 1459
McNeill-Goldmann blepharostat ring, 1571
McPherson-type forceps, 1576
Measles, 752
  conjunctivitis in, 776-777
  cornea and, 1247
  interstitial keratitis in, 1313
  vitamin A deficiency and, 961
Mechanical ectropion, 567
Mechanical trauma, 1555, *A227-254*
Mechanoreceptors, 29-30
Medial canthal ligament laxity, 564
Medial rectus tendon, 41
Mediators, soluble, 144-145
Medical Examiners Law, 494, 538

- Medical legal issues in eye banking, 537-541
- Medical standards in eye banking, 485-492
  - consent, 487
  - death to preservation time, 488-489
  - donor screening, 487-488
  - Eye Bank Association of America, 469-470, 485
  - fees, 486-487
  - government regulations, 486
  - historical development, 485-486
- Medicare, 545
- Medication history, 457
- Medroxyprogesterone, 1785
- Meesmann's dystrophy, 1033-1034, *A122*
  - corneal deposits in, 420
  - fluorescein staining of, 302
  - indirect transillumination from iris, 263
  - minimal visual loss in, 452
- Megalocornea, 872-874, 875, 1103, *A78*
- Meibography, 625, 626, 628
- Meibometry, 626
- Meibomian gland, 42
  - anatomy of, 625, 626
  - chalazion and, 635
  - evaluation in dry eye, 669-670
  - examination of meibomian expression, 240, 241
  - imagery of, 240-241
  - tear film evaluation and, 272
- Meibomian gland dysfunction, 625-632, 755
  - associated conditions, 628-629
  - classification, 627
  - diagnosis, 627-628
  - evaporative dry eye, 679
  - histopathology, 629
  - increased tear film evaporation, 54-55
  - lipid composition of meibomian secretion, 629-630
  - meibomian gland anatomy, 625, 626
  - physiology, 625-627
  - role of microorganisms, 630
  - in rosacea, 990
  - terminology, 625
  - treatment, 630-631
- Meibomian seborrhea, 623
- Meibomianitis, 625
- Meibomitis, 54, 625, *A21*
- Melanocytic conjunctival neoplasm, 715-722, *A40-42*
  - malignant melanoma, 719-722
  - management of, 1912-1916
  - melanosis, 715-719
  - nevi, 715, 716
- Melanocytosis, *A9*
- Melanoma
  - conjunctival, *A41*
  - eyelid, 597, *A17*
- Melanosis, 715-719, *A9, A41-42*
- Melkersson-Rosenthal syndrome, 998
- Membrane
  - in conjunctivitis, 748, 760, 761
  - Descemet's, 14-15, 190
    - birth injury to, 1410
    - cataract extraction from, *A257*
    - congenital hereditary endothelial dystrophy and, 1086-1087
    - corneal arcus and, 1119
    - corneal edema and, 411-412
    - detachment of, *A275*
    - in donor tissue evaluation, 505
    - forceps injury, *A238-239*
    - Fuchs' dystrophy and, 1075, 1077-1078
    - green-yellow discoloration in, *A253*
    - Hassall-Henle bodies, 1131
    - herpes simplex and, *A186*
    - intraocular lens and, 1429
    - iris atrophy and, 1109
    - keratoconus and, 1094
    - keratoglobus and, 879
    - lamellar keratoplasty and, 1835, 1840, 1841
    - macular dystrophy and, 1047
    - posterior membrane dystrophies and, 1068, 1069-1070
    - postkeratoplasty retained host, 1640-1641
    - primary congenital glaucoma and, 369
    - residual interstitial keratopathy and, 1293-1294
    - sclerocornea and, 876
    - syphilitic interstitial keratitis and, *A203*
    - syphilitic interstitial keratopathy and, 1285, 1286
    - wrinkles in, 262
  - in neonatal inclusion conjunctivitis, 792
  - retrocorneal, 1709-1717, *A281*
    - differential diagnosis, 1715
    - epithelial ingrowth, 1709-1713
    - fibrous ingrowth, 1713-1715
- Membrane attack complex-1, 136
  - distribution on ocular surface, 138
  - inflammatory response and, 144-145
- Membrane cofactor protein, 85
- Membranous conjunctivitis, 752, 757
- Memory cell, 89
- Mendez ruler, 2160
- Mercuric oxide
  - in pediculosis, 657
  - in staphylococcal blepharitis, 634
- Mercury deposits, 425, *A112*
- Meretoja syndrome, 913, 1050, *A128*
- Merkel cell carcinoma, 610-611
- Mesodermal dysgenesis syndrome, 885
- Metabolic diseases, 897-924, *A87-96*
  - alkaptonuria, 912, *A91*
  - amyloidosis, 912-913, 914
  - calcium, 916
  - congenital porphyria, *A91*
  - conjunctival biopsy in, 917-918
  - copper, 915-916
  - corneal opacity in, 380-382
  - cystinosis, 910-912, *A94*
  - diabetes mellitus, 897-899
  - drug-induced lipidoses, 907-909
  - dyslipoproteinemias, 903-905
  - Fabry's disease, *A87-89*
  - fish eye disease, *A90*
  - galactosialidodis, 910
  - glycogenosis type I, 903
  - gold, 916-917
  - gout, 913-914, *A96*
  - Hurler's syndrome, *A92*
  - hypercholesterolemia, *A96*
  - lecithin-cholesterol acyltransferase deficiency, *A90*
  - lipidoses, 905-906
  - macular corneal dystrophy, 902
  - mannosidosis and fucosidosis, 902-903
  - Maroteaux-Lamy syndrome, *A93*
  - Morquio's syndrome, *A93*
  - mucolipidoses, 909-910
  - porphyria, 915
  - Sheie's syndrome, *A92-93*
  - silver, 917
  - systemic mucopolysaccharidoses, 899-902
  - Tangier disease, *A91*
  - tear enzyme analysis, 918
  - tyrosinemia II, 912
  - Wilson's disease, *A95-96*
  - xeroderma pigmentosa, 914-915
- Metaherpetic ulcer, *A184*
- Metallic foreign body, *A243, A278*
- Methazolamide, 1823
- Methicillin, 769
- Methotrexate
  - in cicatricial pemphigoid, 832
  - corneal effects, 1027
  - in Mooren's ulcer, 1400
  - in necrotizing scleritis, 1369
  - in rheumatoid arthritis, 1367
- Methyl-2-cyanoacrylate, 1819
- Methylprednisolone
  - for allograft rejection, 1694, 1759
  - in Behçet disease, 1533
  - in Wegener's granulomatosis, 1583
- Metronidazole
  - to improve graft survival, 1785
  - in meibomian gland dysfunction, 631
- Miconazole
  - in *Acanthamoeba* keratitis, 1271
  - in fungal keratitis, 1259, 1260
- Microbes, mechanisms of invasion, 132-133
- Microbial keratitis
  - after penetrating keratoplasty, 1697-1700
  - bacteria in, 1140
  - corneal infiltrates *versus*, 430-432
  - laboratory investigation, 305-307
  - penetrating keratoplasty in, 1554
- Microbiologic testing, 305-311
  - adenovirus, 309
  - *Chlamydia trachomatis*, 307-308
  - of donor tissue, 489
  - Epstein-Barr virus, 309-310
  - herpes simplex virus, 308
  - in microbial keratitis, 305-307
  - varicella zoster virus, 308-309
- Microcornea, 373, 874, 875, *A78*
- Microcyst, 1033, 1034
- Microirregular astigmatism, 2143-2145, 2146
- Microkeratome, 2184
- Microperforation, 2162-2163
- Microphthalmos, *A77*
- Microscope
  - compound, 2069
  - diamond calibration, 2020, 2022
  - manipulation in radial keratotomy, 2063
  - selection of, 2013
- Microscopy
  - confocal, 335-350
    - in *Acanthamoeba* keratitis, 344-345
    - current in vivo imaging systems, 336-337
    - digital image acquisition and processing, 338-339, 340
    - of endothelium, 342-343
    - of epithelium, 339-342
    - in excimer laser photorefractive keratectomy, 345-347
    - in herpetic keratitis, 347
    - history of, 335-336
    - methodology, 337-338
    - normal corneal structures, 339
    - surface toxicity and incisional wound healing, 347-348
    - in wound healing, 343, 344, 345
  - electron
    - for adenovirus, 309
    - of epithelial ingrowth, 1711-1712
    - for herpes simplex virus, 308

light
in macular dystrophy, 1046-1047
in phlyctenulosis, 1394
specular, 313-334
in Chandler's syndrome, 1110
in corneal edema, 413
of diabetic cornea, 980
of donor tissue, 490, 505-507
epithelial, 317-318
in epithelial ingrowth, 1711
in Fuchs' dystrophy, 1076
improvements in instrumentation and methods, 316-317
in vivo findings, 323-330
in iris atrophy, 1110
optical principles, 313
in posterior polymorphous dystrophy, 1063, 1065, 1066
in pseudophakic corneal edema, 1603
qualitative morphometric analysis, 319-321
quantitative morphometric analysis, 321-323
Microsporidial infection, *A111*
in acquired immunodeficiency syndrome, 1020-1021
eyelid, 654-655
in interstitial keratitis, 1312
MicroTrak Direct Specimen Test, 782
Microtremor, 2082
Microulcerative peripheral keratitis, 394-396
Middlebrook agar, 306, 1162
Migration in epithelial wound healing, 184
Milia, 583
Mineral acids, 1437
Mineral metabolism disorders, 915-917
Mini-radial keratotomy, 2097
Minimal bactericidal concentration, 1163
Minimal inhibitory concentration, 1163
Minimal visual loss, 447-455
conditions causing, 451-454
examination techniques, 447-451
patient history in, 447, 448
Minimum antibacterial concentration, 1163
Minocycline, 1173
corneal effects, 1027
in meibomian gland dysfunction, 631
Minus power anterior chamber lens, 1982, 2002
Miotic pupil centering, 2063
Miotics
corneal effects, 1029
in postkeratoplasty glaucoma, 1725
Mite infection, 655-656
Mitomycin
in anterior chamber cleavage syndromes, 895
in canalicular obstructions, 699
in cervical intraepithelial neoplasia, 1918
conjunctival autograft *versus,* 1890-1891
corneal effects, 1029
in pterygium, 1881-1882
pterygium excision with, *A291*
Mitosis
in endothelial wound healing, 194
specular microscopy of, 323
Mixed connective tissue disease, 1379
MMPs; *see* Matrix metalloproteinases
Mohs surgery, 604
Molecular linking in synthetic epikeratoplasty, 2236
Moll's gland cyst, *A13*
Molluscum contagiosum, *A26*
in acquired immunodeficiency syndrome, 1020
conjunctivitis in, 756-757, 775-776, 852
cornea and, 1243-1244
eyelid and, 646-647
Molteno implant, 1727
Monoclonal antibody, 81, 1694
Monoclonal gammopathy, 976-977, *A105*
Monocular diplopia, 2104
Monocyte
inflammation and, 143
matrix-degrading proteinases of, 148
migration of, 86
Monokines, 76, 78-80
Mononuclear phagocytic system, 75-76
Montenegro test, 653
Moon's molar, 1288, 1289
Mooren's ulcer, 398, 399, 1397-1401, *A226*
conjunctival resection in, 1794
deep lamellar keratoplasty for, 1775
immune response in, 114
marginal staphylococcus keratitis *versus,* 1393
pellucid marginal degeneration *versus,* 1101
penetrating keratoplasty in, *A277*
Moraxella, A24
in angular blepharitis, 634-635
in conjunctivitis, 756, 764, 765, 766-769
in corneal ulcer, *A188*
in keratitis, 1139, 1150-1151
in peripheral corneal ulcer, 399
Morphea, 1378
Morphology of diabetic cornea, 980
Morquio syndrome, 381, 901, *A93*
Mouse-derived epidermal growth factor, 208
Mouth
capillary hemangioma, *A10*
herpes simplex vesicles, *A179*
oral aphthous ulcer, 1530, 1531
Sjögren's syndrome and, 678-679
Mucinous dystrophy, *A124*
Mucocutaneous junction, 42
Mucocutaneous lymph node syndrome, 949-951
Mucoepidermoid carcinoma, 710, 1920
Mucolipidoses, 380-381, 909-910
Mucomyst; *see* Acetylcysteine
Mucopolysaccharidoses
corneal deposits in, 423
corneal opacity in, 381-382
systemic, 899-902
Mucosa-associated lymphoid tissue, 86-88
Mucosal addressin cell adhesion molecule-1, 135
Mucosulfatidoses, 906
Mucous fishing syndrome, 755, 1352
Mucous layer of tear film, 49-50, *A29*
Mucous membrane
graft, 1879-1880
Stevens-Johnson syndrome and, 837
transplantation, 1888, 1898-1901
Muir-Torre syndrome, 616
Muller's muscle, 65
Multifocal cornea, 2108
Multiple endocrine neoplasia, 984-985
Multiple mucosal neuroma syndrome, 984-985
Multiple myeloma, 973-975, *A104*
Multiple sulfatase deficiency, 906
Mumps, 752, 802
conjunctivitis in, 776
cornea and, 1247
interstitial keratitis in, 1313
Munchausen syndrome, 1350-1351
Munnerlyn's model, 2032-2033, 2034, 2036, 2208
Munson's sign, 303-304, 1094, *A149*
Mutton-fat keratic precipitates, 1497-1498
Mycobacterial infection
after radial keratotomy, 2119
corneal ulcer in, 405
eyelid, 639
keratitis, 1141, 1151-1152
nonsyphilitic interstitial keratitis, 1310-1311
phlyctenulosis in, 1389
Mycobacterium fortuitum keratitis, *A178*
Mycobacterium leprae, 1006
in eyelid infection, 639
in keratitis, 1141
in nonsyphilitic interstitial keratitis, 1311
in scleritis, 1487-1488
Mycobacterium tuberculosis, 801, 1009
in conjunctivitis, 769
in interstitial keratitis, 1310-1311
phlyctenulosis and, 395
in scleritis, 1487
Mycosis fungoides, *A18*
Mydriatics, 1371
Myelitis, 1233
Myeloid stem cell, 71
Myeloid system, 75-77
Myopia, *A300*
after radial keratotomy, 2105
photorefractive keratoplasty results, 2191-2197, 2198, 2199
sclera and, 35-39
Myopic automated lamellar keratoplasty
nomogram, 2173-2174
procedure, 2169-2172
Myopic epikeratoplasty, 1981
Myopic keratomileusis, 1980, 1991-1992, 2025-2028, 2029
Myxoma, pleomorphic, 739

N

Nails, Reiter's syndrome and, 1518
Nalidixic acid, 1169
Nanophthalmos, *A78*
Naphazoline hydrochloride, 816
Naproxen, 688-689
Nasal-lacrimal reflex, 668
Nasolacrimal canal, 697, 698
Nasolacrimal sac, 689
Natamycin
in fungal keratitis, 1258, 1259, 1260
in neonatal conjunctivitis, 794
toxicity of, 850
National Association of Medical Examiners, 494
National Disease Research Interchange, 480
National Organ Transplant Act, 525, 537
Natural killer cell, 74-75
NCR Project, 478
Necrosis
around keratoprosthesis, 1860
in bacterial keratitis, 1152
in corneal perforating wound, *A230*
in erythema multiforme, 841
eyelid, 637-638
in herpes zoster ophthalmicus, 1232
stromal, *A260*
in syphilitic interstitial keratitis, 1280
Necrotizing cellulitis, 637-638

- Necrotizing herpes simplex keratitis, *A187*
- Necrotizing keratitis, 1202, 1203, 1773
- Necrotizing scleritis, *A268*
  - after beta irradiation for pterygium, 1883
  - in rheumatoid arthritis, 1363, 1364, 1369-1370, *A217*
  - in Wegener's granulomatosis, 1382, *A223*
- Needle holder, 1571-1572, 1577, 2018
- Negative staining, 276, 278
- *Neisseria gonorrhoeae, A53*
  - in conjunctivitis, 750, 761-763
  - in keratitis, 1141
  - in neonatal bacterial keratitis, 379
  - in neonatal conjunctivitis, 790-791
  - in peripheral corneal ulcer, 399
  - phlyctenulosis in, 1389
- *Neisseria meningitidis, A53*
  - in conjunctivitis, 750, 761-763
  - in keratitis, 1141
- Neodymium:yttrium-aluminum garnet laser, 2184-2186
- Neodymium:yttrium-lithium fluoride laser, 2184-2186
- Neomycin, 1169
  - contact allergy from, 809
  - eye drops, 1176
  - impairment of epithelial wound healing, 189-190
  - in staphylococcal blepharitis, 634
  - toxicity of, 850
- Neonate
  - congenital corneal opacity, 367-386
    - bacterial and chlamydial diseases and, 379-380
    - birth trauma and, 369-370
    - cerebro-oculo-skeletal syndrome and, 383
    - corneal dystrophies and, 374-378
    - developmental abnormalities and, 370-374
    - fetal alcohol syndrome and, 382
    - Fryns syndrome and, 382-383
    - glaucoma and, 368-369
    - history and physical examination, 367-368, 369
    - infectious diseases and, 378-379
    - metabolic diseases and, 380-382
    - penetrating keratoplasty in, 383-384
  - conjunctivitis, 786-787, 789-795, *A62*
  - herpes simplex keratitis, 1194-1195
- Neoplasm
  - benign eyelid, 581-600, *A7-13*
    - adnexal, 592-596
    - approach to diagnosis and management, 582
    - dermal, 586-592
    - epidermal, 582-586
    - histology of eyelid skin, 581-582
    - pigmented lesions, 596-598
  - ciliary body, 1957
  - cyclectomy and iridocyclectomy in, 1957-1964
    - complications, 1963-1964
    - indications, 1957-1958
    - postoperative care, 1963
    - procedure, 1958-1963
    - results, 1964
    - surgical anatomy, 1958
  - lacrimal gland, *A31*
  - malignant eyelid, 601-619, *A14-18*
    - basal cell carcinoma, 601-605
    - basal cell nevus syndrome, 614
    - Kaposi's sarcoma, 613-614
    - malignant melanoma, 612-613
    - Merkel cell carcinoma, 610-611
    - Muir-Torre syndrome, 616
    - premalignant lesions, 606-607
    - sebaceous cell carcinoma, 608-610
    - squamous cell carcinoma, 605-606, 607-608
    - xeroderma pigmentosum, 615-616
  - melanocytic conjunctival, 715-722, *A40-42*
    - malignant melanoma, 719-722
    - melanosis, 715-719
    - nevi, 715, 716
  - squamous conjunctival, 701-714, *A37-39*
    - benign hereditary intraepithelial dyskeratosis, 701, 702
    - conjunctival intraepithelial neoplasia, 704-707
    - corneal epithelial dysmaturation and epithelial dysplasia, 707-710
    - dacryoadenoma, 703-704
    - inverted conjunctival papilloma, 702-703
    - mucoepidermoid carcinoma, 710
    - papilloma, 702, 703
    - pseudoepitheliomatous hyperplasia and keratoacanthoma, 701-702, 703
    - pterygia and pinguecula, 704
    - sebaceous cell carcinoma, 710-712
    - spindle cell carcinoma, 710
    - squamous cell carcinoma, 707, 708
  - subepithelial conjunctival, 723-743, *A43-50*
    - amyloid, 731-732, 733
    - basal cell carcinoma, 735
    - choristoma, 723-725
    - conjunctival cyst, 727
    - elastofibroma oculi, 729
    - fibrous histiocytoma, 733, 734
    - granulomatous and histiocytic lesions, 729-730, 731
    - hamartoma, 725-726
    - hematic cyst, 732
    - Kaposi's sarcoma, 733-734, 735
    - keloid, 730-731
    - lymphoid lesions, 736-738
    - malignant melanoma, 735-736
    - nodular fasciitis, 729
    - oncocytoma, 734-735
    - pinguecula and pterygium, 728-729
    - pyogenic granuloma and capillary hemangioma, 727-728
- Neoplastic disease, peripheral corneal, 387-389
- Neosporin
  - in *Acanthamoeba* keratitis, 1272
  - preoperative, 2060
- Neovascularization
  - in Cogan's syndrome, 1308-1309
  - in erythema multiforme, 836, 837
  - limbal vascular supply and, 103
  - secondary lipid degeneration and, 1120-1121
  - in syphilitic interstitial keratitis, 1280-1281
  - in trachoma, 782
- Nerve supply
  - conjunctival, 45
  - corneal, *A167*
- Net exporter/self-sufficient eye bank network, 475, 476
- Neural tissue tumor, 587
- Neuralgia
  - herpes zoster ophthalmicus and, 1232, 1237-1238
  - postherpetic, 646
- Neurilemmoma, 587
- Neuritis, radial, *A201*
- Neurocrestopathies, 885
- Neuroendocrine carcinoma of eyelid, 610-611
- Neurofibroma, 587, *A13*
- Neurogenic keratopathy, *A213*
- Neuroglial choristoma, 724-725
- Neurologic complications
  - in herpes zoster ophthalmicus, 1232-1233
  - in Whipple's disease, 945
- Neurologic disorders, self-induced trauma in, 1353
- Neuroma, 587
- Neuroparalytic keratitis, 1903
- Neurosyphilis, 1287-1288
- Neurotrophic keratitis, 1339-1347
  - biochemical basis, 1340-1341
  - clinical causes, 1339-1340
  - clinical findings, 1341-1342, 1343
  - evaluation of, 1343-1344
  - histopathology, 1342-1343
  - management, 1344-1345
- Neurotrophic keratopathy, *A211-212*
  - in corneal perforation, 1815-1816
  - in herpes simplex virus keratitis, 1201-1202
  - in herpes zoster ophthalmicus, 1229
  - infectious epithelial keratitis *versus*, 1203
  - treatment, 1216
- Neurotrophic ulcer, *A184, A290*
  - corneal perforation from, *A194*
  - ophthalmicus with, *A193*
- Neutrophil, 76-77
  - in chronic granulomatous disease, 947
  - corneal infection and, 1145-1146
  - matrix-degrading proteinases of, 148
  - migration of, 86
  - response to infection, 130, 141-142
- Neutrophil collagenase, 186
- Neutrophil elastase, 186
- Nevocellular nevus, 596-597
- Nevus
  - blue, 597-598
  - congenital, 597, 598
  - conjunctival, 715, 716, *A40*
  - eyelid, *A8*
  - flammeus, 588
  - linear epidermal, 585
  - management of, 1913
  - nevocellular, 596-597
  - of Ota, 598, 716, *A9*
- New World leishmaniasis, 657
- Newborn; *see* Neonate
- Newcastle disease, 752
  - conjunctivitis in, 776
  - cornea and, 1247-1248
- Nidek excimer laser, 2183
- Night blindness, 957
- Night vision after radial keratotomy, 2128
- Nihon Eye Bank Association, 483
- Nikolsky's sign, 838
- Nirankari study, 2091-2093, 2095
- Nitric oxide, 142
- Nitrogen flow, 2198-2200, 2201
- Nits, *A27*

Nocardia
in dacryoadenitis, 687
in keratitis, 1141
in scleritis, *A268*
Nodular degeneration, *A169*
Nodular elastosis with cysts and comedones, 585
Nodular fasciitis, 729, *A48*
Nodular melanoma of eyelid, 612-613, *A17*
Nodular scleritis, 1363, 1364, *A267*
Nodule
Lisch, *A13*
Salzmann's, *A174*
Nomogram
automated lamellar keratoplasty, 2173-2174
radial keratotomy, 2031, 2032
Non B, non T lymphocyte, 74-76
Non Sjögren's aqueous tear deficiency, 673-676
Noninfectious keratopathy, *A205-216*
dellen in, *A212*
exposure, *A214*
factitious disorders, 1349-1358, *A215-216*
conjunctivitis, *A76*
keratoconjunctivitis, 1349-1350, 1351
Munchausen syndrome, 1350-1351
Munchausen syndrome by proxy, 1351
self-induced trauma, 1352-1354
topical anesthetic abuse, 1354-1356
filamentary keratitis, 1327-1332, 1663-1664, *A209*
neurogenic, *A213*
neurotrophic keratitis, 1339-1347, *A211-212*
biochemical basis, 1340-1341
clinical causes, 1339-1340
clinical findings, 1341-1342, 1343
evaluation of, 1343-1344
histopathology, 1342-1343
management, 1344-1345
recurrent corneal erosion, 200-202, 203, 1317-1326, *A205-208*
after corneal abrasion, 1406
anterior stromal puncture, 1321-1324, 1325
debridement and superficial keratectomy, 1320-1321
diagnosis, 1318-1319
in epithelial basement membrane dystrophy, 1036
excimer phototherapeutic keratectomy, 1325-1326
in lattice dystrophy, 1048, 1049
medical treatment, 1319
pathophysiology, 1317
phototherapeutic keratectomy for, 2212, 2217
surgery in, 1865-1866, *A293*
YAG laser procedures, 1324-1325
superficial punctate keratitis of Thygeson, 1333-1337, *A210*
disease course, 1334-1336
history of, 1333-1334
pathogenesis, 1336
toxicity in, *A215*
Noninfectious peripheral infiltrative keratitis, 394
Noninfectious ulcerative keratitis, 1555
Noninflammatory ectatic disorders, 1091-1106, *A148-155*
keratoconus, 1091-1100, *A148-155*
keratoglobus, 1102-1103, *A158*
pellucid marginal degeneration, 1100-1101, *A156-157*
posterior keratoconus, 1103-1104
Noninvasive break-up time, 665-667
Nonorthogonal astigmatism, 2158-2159
Nonpigmented deposits, 417, 418, 425-426
Nonrheumatoid collagen vascular disease, *A221-224*
Nonsteroidal antiinflammatory drugs
erythema multiforme and, 840
in idiopathic uveitis, 1508-1509
to improve graft survival, 1785
in juvenile rheumatoid arthritis, 1544
in rheumatoid arthritis, 1367
in rheumatoid arthritis-associated scleritis, 1368-1369
Nonsuppurative preseptal cellulitis, 636-637
Nonsyphilitic interstitial keratitis, 1307-1315, *A204*
Acanthamoeba infection, 1311-1312
Cogan's syndrome, 1307-1310
herpes virus, 1312-1313
leishmaniasis, 1312
Lyme disease, 1311
microsporidial infection, 1312
mycobacterial infection, 1310-1311
onchocerciasis, 1312
trypanosomiasis, 1312
Nontuberculous mycobacterial keratitis, 1152
Norfloxacin, 1170, 1171
postoperative, 1645-1646
in staphylococcal blepharitis, 634
toxicity of, 850
Normal flora of conjunctiva, 45-46
Nosema
in acquired immunodeficiency syndrome, 1020
in interstitial keratitis, 1312
Novatec laser, 2185
Nuclear factor of activated T cell, 89
Nucleic acid metabolism disorders, 910-915
alkaptonuria, 912
amyloidosis, 912-913, 914
cystinosis, 910-912
gout, 913-914
porphyria, 915
tyrosinemia II, 912
xeroderma pigmentosa, 914-915
Null cell, 74-76, 143
Nummular keratitis
in brucellosis, 1013
in sarcoidosis, 1524
Nut-and-bolt keratoprosthesis, *A296*
Nutrient supply to cornea, 3
Nutritional disorders, 955-966, *A100-101*
amino acids deprivation, 964
discrete colliquative keratopathy, 964
vitamin A deficiency, 955-963
vitamin B deficiency, 963
vitamin C deficiency, 963-964
Nylon suture, *A68*

O

O antigen polysaccharide, 131
Oblique astigmatism, 876, 2158
Obstetric injury, 1409-1411
Obstructive lacrimal disease, 675-676
Obstructive sleep apnea, 572
Occupation
anterior uveitis and, 1495
red eye and, 440
OCP; *see* Ocular cicatricial pemphigoid
Ocular argyrosis, 426
Ocular chrysiasis, 425
Ocular cicatricial pemphigoid, 675, *A69-70*
Ocular cicatrization, drug-induced, 1025-1026
Ocular dominance determination, 2010-2011
Ocular ferning test, 671
Ocular immune response, 68-127
in allergic conjunctivitis, 805-806
antigen processing, 88-89
components of immune system, 69-88
cellular, 69-74, 75
dendritic cell, 76, 77
Langerhans cell, 76
null lymphocyte, 74-76
soluble mediators, 78-85
tissue, 85-88
in herpes simplex keratitis, 1194
hypersensitivity reactions, 106-116
type I, 106-110
type II, 110-112
type III, 112-114
type IV, 114-116
immune privilege and corneal transplantation, 90-96
immunologic tolerance and autoimmunity, 89-90
overview, 68-69
regulatory components of anterior segment, 96-106
anterior chamber, 104-105
conjunctiva, 98-101
cornea, 101-104
sclera, 105-106
tear film and lacrimal gland, 96-98
Ocular melanocytosis, 716
Ocular surface, 49, 50
assessment of, 216
moistening in radial keratotomy, 2077-2079
phototherapeutic keratectomy and, 2212
problems after radial keratotomy, 2123-2124
Ocular surface disease
corneal surgery in, 1865-1872
anterior stromal puncture, 1868-1869, 1870
cauterization, 1866
phototherapeutic keratectomy, 1869-1870
superficial keratectomy, 1866-1868
treatment options, 1865, 1866
penetrating keratoplasty for, 1781-1788
Ocular surface transplantation, 1887-1902
conjunctival, 1889-1892
limbal, 1892-1898, 1899
mucous membrane, 1898-1901
principles of, 1887-1889
Oculo-dento-osseous dysplasia, 937-938
Oculoauriculovertebral dysplasia, *A97*
Oculodermal melanocytosis, 716, *A9*
Oculomandibulodyscephaly, 930
Odd Fellows, 463
Ofloxacin, 1170, 1171
in bacterial conjunctivitis, 767
in gonococcal conjunctivitis, 763
in microbial keratitis, 433
minimal inhibitory concentration, 1178
postoperative, 1645-1646
toxicity of, 850
Old World leishmaniasis, 657
Oligosaccharidoses, 902-903

- *Onchocerca volvulus,* 1010-1011
- Onchocerciasis, 658-659, 1010-1012, 1312
- Oncocytoma
  - conjunctival, 734-735
  - eyelid, 586
- Opacity, corneal; *see* Corneal opacity
- Open angle glaucoma, 1075-1076
- Open-sky subtotal vitrectomy
  - evaluation, 1620
  - technique, 1608-1609
- Operating room
  - equipment, 2013-2014
  - preparation, 2061-2063
- Operative planning sheet, 2062
- Ophthalmia neonatorum, 762, 789-795, *A62*
- Ophthalmic artery, 45, 66
- Ophthalmic dye, 670
- Ophthalmic ointments, 421, *A114*
- Ophthalmic vein, 66
- Ophthalmoplegia, *A214*
- Ophthetic; *see* Proparacaine
- Opposite Sector Index, 2047
- Optic nerve
  - herpes zoster ophthalmicus and, 1232
  - sarcoidosis and, 1526
- Optic section, 247-252, 253, 288-289, 290
- Optical aberration after radial keratotomy, 2127-2128
- Optical clear zone, 2075
- Optical cylinder, *A296*
- Optical zone markers, 2015, 2064
- Optisol, 512-513
- Oral aphthous ulcer, 1530, 1531
- Oral disease in Sjögren's syndrome, 678-679
- Orbicularis ligament, 238
- Orbicularis oculi muscle, 62
- Orbicularis oculi paralysis, 577
- Orbit
  - contact lens complications, 1461, 1462
  - preoperative evaluation, 1565
  - sarcoidosis and, 1523
- Orbital apex syndrome, 1231
- Orbital cellulitis, *A25*
- Orbital decompression, 579
- Orbital fat, 725, *A50*
- ORC stableflex lens, 1424
- Organ culture, 513-514
- Organ Procurement and Transplantation Network, 537
- Organ Procurement Organizations, 520, 537
- Organic acids, 1437
- Oriel 18011 Encoder Mike Controller, 338
- Oriental sore, 657
- Orthomyxovirus, 752, 1249
- Osmolarity of normal tear film, 51
- Osseous choristoma, 724-725
- Osteogenesis imperfecta, 934-935, *A98*
- Ota, nevus of, *A9*
- Outcome analysis, 2053-2055, 2056
- Outer zone markers, 2015
- Oval cornea, 874-875
- Overcorrection
  - in automated lamellar keratoplasty, 2177
  - in radial keratotomy, 2104-2105, 2106, 2132-2133
- Oxacillin, 1176
- Oxygen supply to corneal, 3
- Oxyphilic adenoma, 734-735

P

- P-selectin, 135-136
- Pachymetry, 277-279
  - in automated lamellar keratoplasty, 2168
  - in corneal edema, 412-413, 453, 1603
  - for determining allograft rejection, 1691
  - in keratoconus, 1097
  - before keratoplasty, 1566
  - during radial keratotomy, 2065-2067
  - before refractive surgery, 2010
- Pachyonychia congenita, 998
- PAF; *see* Platelet activating factor
- Pain
  - in *Acanthamoeba* keratitis, 1268, 1272-1273
  - after photorefractive keratoplasty, 2209
  - after phototherapeutic keratectomy, 2221
  - after radial keratotomy, 2102
  - in anterior uveitis, 1493
  - in bacterial keratitis, 1147-1148
  - in corneal abrasion, 1404
  - in corneal edema, 410
  - in corneal infiltrates in contact lens patient, 429
  - in corneal perforation, 1816
  - in epithelial ingrowth, 1710
  - in incisional refractive surgery, 2117
  - in red eye, 439
- Palisades of Vogt, 42
- Palpebral conjunctiva, 42
  - acute bacterial conjunctivitis and, 764
  - anterior uveitis and, 1495
  - arterial blood supply, 44-45
  - capillary hemangioma, 738-739
  - cyst on, *A50*
  - follicles in, *A51*
  - histology, 43
  - lymphoma of, *A45*
  - primary acquired melanosis, 717
  - red eye and, 442-443
  - superior limbic keratoconjunctivitis and, 857
- Palpebral fissure width, 54
- PAM; *see* Primary acquired melanosis
- Pan-American Association of Eye Banks, 482
- Pan T-cell marker, 138
- Pannus, 1008
- Panophthalmitis, 1486
- Papilla, 746, 748
  - in bacterial conjunctivitis, 760-761
  - in giant papillary conjunctivitis, 819-820
  - in vernal keratoconjunctivitis, 811, 812
- Papillary conjunctivitis, 761, *A6*
  - acute, 750
  - chronic, 753-756, 775
  - in floppy eyelid syndrome, 571
  - giant, 753, 819-820, *A52, A68, A261*
  - toxic, 756
- Papillary hypertrophy, 781
- Papilloma
  - conjunctival, 702, 703, *A37*
  - eyelid, *A26*
- Papovavirus, 1245
- Papulosquamous disorders, 989-992
- Paralysis of seventh nerve, *A214*
- Paralytic ectropion, 567, *A2*
- Paramyxovirus, 752, 776, 1247-1248
- Paraneoplastic pemphigus, 992
- Parasitic infection, 1312, *A27*
  - *Acanthamoeba* keratitis, 1311-1312
  - conjunctivitis, *A64*
  - eyelid, 621-622, 655-660
- Parathyroid disease, 981-983
- Parenteral antibiotics, 1177
- Parinaud's oculoglandular syndrome, 797-803, *A63*
  - cat-scratch disease in, 797-799, 800
  - granulomatous conjunctivitis secondary to, 749
  - lymphogranuloma venereum in, 802
  - sporotrichosis in, 801
  - syphilis in, 801-802
  - tuberculosis in, 801
  - tularemia in, 799-801
- Patch graft, 1889-1892
  - in bacterial keratitis, 1180-1181
  - in corneal abrasion, 1404-1405
  - in corneal perforation, 1823, 1827-1829
- Patch test, 848-849
- Patching
  - in acid injury, 1441
  - in corneal abrasion, 1405
  - for epithelial basement membrane corneal dystrophy, 1037
  - for postoperative epithelial defects, 1662
  - in recurrent corneal erosion, 202, 1219
  - in superior limbic keratoconjunctivitis, 859
  - in ulcerative keratitis, 1179
- Pathologic responses
  - corneal responses to infection, 129-162
    - angiogenesis, 151-153
    - fibrosis, 149-151
    - inflammation and loss of function, 129, 130
    - intrinsic barriers and immune response, 130-131
    - mechanisms of microbial invasion, 131-133
    - recruited cells, 141-144
    - resident cells and surface receptors, 134-141
    - soluble mediators, 144-145
    - ulceration, 145-149
  - ocular immune response, 68-127
    - in allergic conjunctivitis, 805-806
    - anterior chamber, 104-105
    - antigen processing, 88-89
    - cellular components, 69-74, 75
    - conjunctiva, 98-101
    - cornea, 101-104
    - dendritic cell, 76, 77
    - in herpes simplex keratitis, 1194
    - hypersensitivity reactions, 105-116
    - immune privilege and corneal transplantation, 90-96
    - immunologic tolerance and autoimmunity, 89-90
    - Langerhans cell, 76
    - null lymphocyte, 74-76
    - overview, 68-69
    - sclera, 105-106
    - soluble mediators, 78-85
    - tear film and lacrimal gland, 96-98
    - tissue, 85-88
  - persistent epithelial defects and sterile ulceration, 204-209
  - sterile corneal erosions, 199-203
  - wound healing, 183-198
    - in abrasion, 1406
    - after infection, 149-151
    - after phototherapeutic keratectomy, 2216, 2217
    - after radial keratotomy, 2121-2122
    - in child, 1767
    - endothelial, 193-195

epithelial, 183-190
excimer photoablation and, 179
extracellular matrix and, 18-20
in vivo four-dimensional analysis, 343, 344, 345
migration in, 17
specular microscopy of, 318, 323
steroid delay of, 1024
stromal, 190-193
in ulceration, 205
variations in, 177-178
Patient education, 1582
Patient history
in anterior uveitis, 1493-1494
in atopic keratoconjunctivitis, 815-816
in chronic conjunctivitis, 752
in congenital corneal opacity, 367-368, 369
in corneal edema, 409-410
in corneal infiltrates in contact lens patient, 429
in corneal injury, 1403
in corneal ulcer, 403
in donor tissue removal, 495
in dry eye, 269
in eyelid examination, 237
in minimal visual loss, 447, 448
in ocular trauma, 1925-1926
in penetrating keratoplasty, 1563
with intraocular lens implantation, 1604
for ocular surface disease, 1781-1784
pediatric, 1736
in red eye, 437-440
before refractive surgery, 2008
Patient positioning, 2061
Patient preparation
in anterior segment surgery, 1934-1935
in penetrating keratoplasty with intraocular lens implantation, 1605
Patient satisfaction in refractive surgery, 2247
Patient selection
in astigmatic keratotomy, 2145-2146, 2147
in automated lamellar keratoplasty, 2168-2169
in penetrating keratoplasty, 1581-1582
in refractive surgery, 2007-2008
Paton, R. Townley, 463
Paton spoon/spatula, 1578
Pediatric patient; *see* Child
Pediculosis, 656-657
Pellucid marginal degeneration, 391, 1100-1101, *A156-157*
minimal visual loss in, 452
surgery for, 1789-1790, 1791
Pelvic inflammatory disease, 785
Pemphigoid, 992-993
cicatricial, *A69-70*
keratoprosthesis for, 1857
Pemphigus, 992
Pemphigus foliaceus, 992
Pemphigus vulgaris, 992
Penetrating keratoplasty, 1581-1592, *A273-296*
Acanthamoeba keratitis and, 1272
in acid injury, 1441
after anterior segment trauma, 1951-1952
allograft rejection, 90-96, 1687-1696
afferent immune response in, 91-94
animal models, 90-91
clinical features, 1689-1692
differential diagnosis, 1692-1693
efferent immune response in, 94-96
historical perspective, 1687
immunology of, 1757-1761
immunomodulation, 96
management strategy, 1695
methods for improving graft survival, 1764-1769
in pediatric penetrating keratoplasty, 1732-1734, 1751-1752
prevention, 1694
recognition of risk factors, 1687-1689
treatment, 1693-1694, 1769
in aphakic bullous keratopathy, 1431
astigmatism following, 1675-1685
intraoperative factors, 1677-1679
postoperative factors, 1679-1684
preoperative factors, 1675-1677
cataract extraction and, 1593-1601
extracapsular cataract extraction, 1596-1600
extraction techniques, 1594-1595
phacoemulsification, 1595-1596
complications, 1659-1673
anterior synechia formation, 1668
choroidal detachment and hemorrhage, 1668-1669
elevated intraocular pressure, 1666-1667
filamentary keratitis, 1663-1664
fixed dilated pupil, 1669
hyphema, 1669
infection, 1669-1670
inflammation, 1667
intraoperative, 1639-1644, *A274-278*
late, *A279-282*
persistent epithelial defects, 1661-1663
primary donor failure, 1670-1671
pupillary block, 1668
suture exposure and related infection, 1664-1665
wound leaks and wound displacement, 1659-1661
in corneal edema, 414-415
in corneal laceration, *A294*
in corneal perforation, 1825-1826
for corneal thinning disorders, 1789-1798
alternative approaches, 1795-1797
conjunctival, 1794-1795
eyelid, 1794
pellucid marginal corneal degeneration, 1789-1790, 1791
Terrien's marginal degeneration, 1790-1793
tissue adhesive, 1795
epithelial ingrowth and, 1709
expected outcomes, 1559-1560
in Fuchs' dystrophy, 1077
in fungal keratitis, 1261, 1262
glaucoma after, 1719-1730
clinical presentation, 1722
incidence, 1719-1720
management, 1724-1728
mechanisms, 1722-1724
risk factors, 1720-1722
in herpes simplex disease, 1219, 1799-1811
anesthesia, 1803
complications, 1806-1810
donor tissue requirements, 1802
indications, 1799-1800
preoperative evaluation, 1801-1802
preoperative medications, 1802
prognosis, 1800
surgical technique, 1803-1806
timing of surgery, 1800-1801
high astigmatism in, *A288*
high resolution ultrasound of, 356, 357
high-risk, 1757-1772
immunology of rejection, 1757-1761
methods for improving graft survival, 1764-1769
risk factors, 1761-1763
history of, 1581, 1582
indications for, 1551-1561
anatomic, 1552-1553
associated procedures, 1556-1558
clinical, 1553-1556
functional, 1553
general considerations, 1551-1552
number of cases, 1551, 1552
trends, 1556, 1557
infections after, 1697-1707
Creutzfeldt-Jakob disease, 1706
endophthalmitis, 1703-1705
hepatitis B virus, 1706
human immunodeficiency virus, 1706
infectious crystalline keratopathy, 1701-1703
microbial keratitis, 1697-1700
rabies, 1705-1706
recurrent herpetic keratitis, 1705
suture abscess, 1700-1701
instrumentation, 1571-1579
preparation of donor cornea, 1573-1576
preparation of recipient bed, 1572-1573, 1574, 1575
preparation of recipient globe, 1571-1572
used in securing donor to recipient cornea, 1576-1579
intraocular lens exchange with, 1603-1626
anterior segment reconstruction, 1609-1610, 1611
evaluation, 1619-1623
explantation, 1606-1608
implantation, 1610-1617, 1618, 1619, 1620
indications and goals of surgery, 1603-1604
open-sky subtotal vitrectomy, 1608-1609
patient preparation, 1605
postoperative care, 1618-1619
preoperative assessment, 1604-1605
suturing of donor cornea, 1617-1618
trephination of recipient cornea, 1605-1606
keratitis after, 1143, 1145
lamellar *versus*, 1833-1834, 1835
with large diameter corneal graft, 1773-1779
in Mooren's ulcer, 1794
in ocular surface disease, 1781-1788
patient education, 1582
patient selection, 1581-1582
pediatric, 383-384, 1731-1756
complications, 1735
future studies, 1735-1736
graft survival, 1732-1734
indications, 1732
postoperative care, 1746-1753
preoperative evaluation, 1736-1742
prognosis, 1763

Postoperative care—cont'd
  for child, 1767
  in conjunctival flap, 1905
  in corneal perforation, 1823-1824
  in cyclectomy and iridocyclectomy, 1963
  in keratoprosthesis, 1857-1859, 1860
  in penetrating keratoplasty
    care after three months, 1654-1655
    early, 1646-1648
    immediate, 1645-1646
    in infants and children, 1655-1656, 1746-1753
    with intraocular lens implantation, 1618-1619
    with large diameter corneal graft, 1774-1775
    for ocular surface disease, 1786
    one to twelve weeks, 1648-1654
  in phototherapeutic keratectomy, 2213-2216
  in radial keratotomy, 2077
  in therapeutic keratoplasty, 1851-1852
Postoperative complications, 1659-1673
  in anterior segment surgery, 1943-1944
  anterior synechia formation, 1668
  in automated lamellar keratoplasty, 2175-2178
  choroidal detachment and hemorrhage, 1668-1669
  in conjunctival flap, 1905-1909
  in corneal perforation, 1824-1825
  elevated intraocular pressure, 1666-1667
  in excimer photorefractive keratectomy, 2200-2209
  filamentary keratitis, 1663-1664
  fixed dilated pupil, 1669
  hyphema, 1669
  in incisional refractive surgery, 2162-2163
  infection, 1669-1670
  inflammation, 1667
  in keratoprosthesis, 1859-1861
  in lamellar keratoplasty, 1840, 1841
  persistent epithelial defects, 1661-1663
  in photorefractive keratoplasty, 2195-2196
  in phototherapeutic keratectomy, 2221
  primary donor failure, 1670-1671
  pupillary block, 1668
  in radial keratotomy, 2102-2104, 2117-2142
    blepharoptosis, 2136, 2137
    cataract formation, 2120
    endophthalmitis, 2120
    endothelial changes, 2126-2127
    epithelial and surface problems, 2123-2124
    epithelial downgrowth, 2120-2121
    esotropia, 2136-2137
    expected side effects, 2117-2118
    glaucoma, 2137
    intrastromal changes, 2124-2126
    iridocyclitis, 2137
    refractive, 2129-2136
    retinal detachment, 2138
    sight-threatening, 2122-2123
    traumatic rupture of globe and wound healing, 2121-2122
    ulcerative keratitis, 2118-2120
    vision, 2127-2129
  suture exposure and related infection, 1664-1665
  wound leaks and wound displacement, 1659-1661
Postsyphilitic keratopathy, 1284-1285
Posttraumatic recurrent erosion, *A205-207*
Posttraumatic suppurative preseptal cellulitis, 636
Potassium iodide, 801
Potential acuity meter, 448-449
Povidone-iodine, 787
Poxvirus, *A26*
  in conjunctivitis, 752
  in corneal infection, 1243-1244
PPMD; *see* Posterior polymorphous dystrophy
Prausnitz-Kustner reaction, 847
Pre-Descemet's dystrophy, 426, 1047-1058, *A140*
Predictability, 2025-2037
  keratomileusis, 2025-2028, 2029
  photorefractive keratoplasty, 2030-2037
  radial keratotomy, 2028-2030, 2031, 2032, 2095-2096, 2129-2131
  refractive surgery, 2244-2245
Prednisolone
  after phototherapeutic keratectomy, 2215
  for allograft rejection, 1694, 1769
  in anterior uveitis, 1502-1503
  in atopic keratoconjunctivitis, 816
  in Behçet disease, 1533
  for idiopathic uveitis, 1508, 1509
  in juvenile rheumatoid arthritis, 1371
  in Mooren's ulcer, 1400
  in phlyctenulosis, 1391
  in vernal keratoconjunctivitis, 813
Prednisone
  in acute anterior uveitis, 1516
  in cicatricial pemphigoid, 831
  in dacryoadenitis, 688
  following keratoprosthesis, 1859
  for hyphema, 1931
  in ligneous conjunctivitis, 867
  in Mooren's ulcer, 1400
  in necrotizing scleritis, 1369
  in Wegener's granulomatosis, 1383
Premalignant lesion of eyelid, 606-607
Preoperative evaluation
  in anterior segment surgery, 1925-1926
  in astigmatic keratotomy, 2146, 2148, 2149, 2150-2151
  in automated lamellar keratoplasty, 2169
  of cataract patient with astigmatism, 2156-2157
  in corneal perforation, 1818
  corneal topography in, 2042-2048
  in lamellar keratoplasty, 1834-1836
  in penetrating keratoplasty, 1563-1569
    for herpes simplex disease, 1801-1802
    with intraocular lens implantation, 1604-1605
    for ocular surface disease, 1781-1784
    pediatric, 1736-1742
  in phototherapeutic keratectomy, 2211-2212
  in refractive surgery, 2007-2012
  in scleral perforation, 1966-1967
  therapeutic keratoplasty, 1847-1849
Preoperative preparation
  in laser surgery, 2186-2187
  in penetrating keratoplasty, 1582-1583
    in herpes simplex disease, 1802
    pediatric, 1741
  in phototherapeutic keratectomy, 2212
  in radial keratotomy, 2060-2061, 2062
Prereduced anaerobically sterilized media, 1161
Presbyopia
  after incisional refractive surgery, 2117-2118
  after radial keratotomy, 2108, 2135-2136
  contact lens correction, 1454
Preseptal cellulitis, 635-638, *A25*
Preservatives
  impairment of epithelial wound healing, 189
  toxicity of, 851-852
Pressure patch
  for postoperative epithelial defects, 1562
  in recurrent corneal erosion, 20[illegible]
  in superior limbic keratoconjunctivitis, 859
Presumed autoimmune corneal endotheliopathy, 1210
Prilocaine, 1238
Primary acquired melanosis, 1913-1914, 1915, *A41*
Primary acquired nasolacrimal duct obstruction, 689
Primary corneal amyloidosis, 912-913, 914, *A103*
Primary corneal dysplasia, 705
Primary corneal endotheliopathy, 1554
Primary corneal epithelial dysmaturation, 705
Primary dystrophic disorders, 200
Primary ocular herpes, 1195
PRK; *see* Photorefractive keratoplasty
Procaine penicillin G, 1299
Procurement fees, 534
Progelatinase, 1146
Progressive external ophthalmoplegia, *A214*
Progressive herpetic corneal endotheliitis, 1210
Progressive outer retinal necrosis, 1232
Propamidine isethionate, 1271
Proparacaine, 1023
Properdin system, 81-85
Prophylaxis
  in anterior segment trauma, 1934
  in neonatal conjunctivitis, 794
Propionibacterium, 630, 1140
Proptosis, 575, 1381-1382
Prostaglandins, 144
Protease inhibitors
  in *Pseudomonas aeruginosa* infection, 192-193
  in stromal wound healing, 191-192
Proteases
  bacterial, 133, 1146-1147
  in epithelial cell migration, 184-185
Protein energy malnutrition, 960
Protein kinase C, 21
Protein mediators of cell activity, 166
Protein metabolism disorders, 910-915
  alkaptonuria, 912
  amyloidosis, 912-913, 914
  cystinosis, 910-912
  gout, 913-914
  porphyria, 915
  tyrosinemia II, 912
  xeroderma pigmentosa, 914-915
Proteinases, degradative, 148-149
Proteins
  secreted by macrophages, 143
  in tear fluid, 51-52
Proteoglycanases, 147
Proteoglycans, scleral, 32-34
Proteolytic enzymes, 20
Proteus, 1141, *A280*

Proteus syndrome, 725
Proximal illumination
in photo slit lamp biomicrography, 291-292, 297
in slit lamp examination, 254-255, 257-258
Pruritus, 457-459
in atopic keratoconjunctivitis, 814
in onchocerciasis, 1011
in vernal keratoconjunctivitis, 811
Prussian blue stain
in keratoconus, *A155*
in pterygium, *A169*
Pseudo-Hurler polydystrophy, 909
Pseudocryptophthalmos, 872
Pseudocyst, 1100
Pseudodendrite
in herpes zoster ophthalmicus, 1228
in soft contact lens wearers, 431
Pseudoelastosis, 729
Pseudoepitheliomatous hyperplasia, 701-702, 703
Pseudoguttae, 506-507, *A145*
Pseudomembranes
in bacterial conjunctivitis, 760, 761
in neonatal inclusion conjunctivitis, 792
Pseudomembranous conjunctivitis, 761
Pseudomonas, A54
in acquired immunodeficiency syndrome, 1019
in acute bacterial conjunctivitis, 765
after radial keratotomy, 2109
in corneal infiltrates in contact lens patient, 430
in corneal ulcer, 399, *A266*
epithelial ulceration and, 1150
in eyelid necrosis, 637
in keratitis, 1139, *A178*
in neonatal conjunctivitis, 790
in postoperative endophthalmitis, 1704
protease inhibitors for, 192-193
in scleritis, *A268*
stromal extracellular matrix and, 145-146
therapeutic keratoplasty for, 1843-1844
virulence factors, 1144-1145
Pseudopemphigoid, 993
Pseudophakic bullous keratopathy, 1423-1435
Brown-McLean syndrome and, 1426
etiology of, 1426-1430, 1431
histopathology of, 1425
incidence of, 1423-1425
optic section of, 251
pathogenesis of, 1425-1426
treatment of, 1431-1432
Pseudophakic corneal edema, 1554, *A256*
Pseudophakodonesis, 1430
Pseudopterygium, 1135
Psoriasis, 989, 990, *A108*
Psychologic evaluation before refractive surgery, 2011
Psychometric considerations in radial keratotomy, 2129
Psychosis, self-induced trauma and, 1353
Pterygium, 728-729, 1134-1135, *A168-169, A291*
conjunctival transplantation in, 1889-1891
management of, 1873-1885
chemotherapy, 1880-1882
conjunctival flaps and autografts, 1877-1879, 1880
excision and avulsion, 1876-1877
histopathology, 1874-1875
lamellar and penetrating keratoplasty, 1879
medical approaches, 1875-1876
mucous membrane and skin graft, 1879-1880
pathogenesis, 1874
prevalence, 1873
radiation therapy, 1822-1883
scleritis after surgery, 1487
transplantation of pterygium head, 1877
minimal visual loss and, 453-454
peripheral cornea and, 392-393
with pseudoepitheliomatous hyperplasia, 703
squamous conjunctival, 704
PTK; *see* Phototherapeutic keratectomy
Ptosis, *A5*
after conjunctival flap procedure, 1909
steroid-induced, 2202-2203
Pubic crab, 656-657
Pubic louse, 656-657
Public relations in eye banking, 547-551
Punctal disease, 696-697, 699
Punctal ectropion, *A2*
Punctal occlusion
in dry eye, 680-681
at time of penetrating keratoplasty, 1768
Punctal plug, *A34*
Punctal reapposition procedure, 568
Punctate epithelial erosion, 276, 278
Punctate epithelial keratitis, *A30, A210*
in atopic keratoconjunctivitis, 814
corneal staining, 276
in floppy eyelid syndrome, 571
in herpes zoster ophthalmicus, 1228
in leprosy, 1008
minimal visual loss in, 451
in onchocerciasis, 1011
in Reiter's syndrome, 1518
in rosacea, 990
superficial Thygeson, 1333-1337
disease course, 1334-1336
history of, 1333-1334
pathogenesis, 1336
Punctate marginal keratitis, 394
Punctum examination, 238
Pupil
anterior segment surgery and, 1927
examination in anterior uveitis, 1495
fixed after penetrating keratoplasty, 1669
Pupillary block
after penetrating keratoplasty, 1668
in epithelial ingrowth, 1712
Pupillary miosis, 2060
Purse-string suture, 2133
Pyogenic granuloma, *A47*
conjunctival, 727-728
eyelid, 590
Pyrethrin ointment, 657
Pyrimidines
in fungal keratitis, 1259
toxicity of, 850
Pyrinate, 657

Q

Qualitative keratometer, 1578-1579
Qualitative morphometric analysis of specular images, 319-321
Quality of vision in refractive surgery, 2245
Quantitative morphometric analysis of specular images, 321-323
Quickert-Rathburn suture, 563, 564
Quinacrine, 1026

R

Rabies, 1705-1706
Racial melanosis, *A42*
Racquet flap, 1904
Radial keratotomy, *A297-299*
complications, 2101-2116, 2117-2142
blepharoptosis, 2136, 2137
cataract formation, 2120
corneal, 2108-2113
early postoperative, 2102-2104
endophthalmitis, 2120
endothelial changes, 2126-2127
epithelial and surface problems, 2123-2124
epithelial downgrowth, 2120-2121
esotropia, 2136-2137
expected side effects, 2117-2118
glaucoma, 2137
intraoperative, 2101-2102
intrastromal changes, 2124-2126
iridocyclitis, 2137
refractive, 2104-2108, 2129-2136
retinal detachment, 2138
sight-threatening, 2122-2123
traumatic rupture of globe and wound healing, 2121-2122
ulcerative keratitis, 2118-2120
vision, 2127-2129
contact lens fitting after, 1459-1460
correction of residual myopia, 2178
fungal keratitis following, 1255
high resolution ultrasound in, 356-358
historical background, 1979-1986
incisions surviving trauma, 1409
keratitis after, 1143, 1145
minimal visual loss following, 454
penetrating keratoplasty after, 1589-1590
peripheral incisions, 1979
predictability, 2028-2030, 2031, 2032
published studies, 2084-2096
results of, 2083-2093
surgical techniques, 2059-2082
astigmatism, 2079-2082
diamond knife calibration and adjustment, 2067-2070
globe fixation, 2069, 2081
incision, 2070-2077, 2078, 2079, 2080
intraoperative ultrasonic pachymetry, 2065-2067
marking central clear zone, 2064
microtremors, 2082
moistening ocular surface, 2077-2079
postoperative considerations, 2077
preoperative preparation, 2060-2061, 2062
radial marking, 2064-2065
visual axis determination and marking, 2063-2064
Radial keratotomy knives, 2016-2017
Radial marking, 2064-2065
Radial neuritis, *A201*
Radial wing marker, 2015
Radiant energy injury, 1411-1414
Radiation keratopathy, *A214*
Radiation therapy, *A114*
in basal cell carcinoma of eyelid, 604-605
of conjunctival lymphoid tumor, 1921
in pterygium, 1882-1883
Radiation trauma, *A227-254*
Radionuclide scan, 699
Ramsay Hunt syndrome, 1233
Rapid diagnostic tests, 307-308
Rapid plasma reagin test, 1298

Rash, 837-838
Raynaud's phenomenon, 1378
Reactive arthritis, 785
Reactive conjunctival lesion, 727-733
  amyloid, 731-732, 733
  elastofibroma oculi, 729
  granulomatous and histiocytic lesions, 729-730, 731
  hematic cyst, 732
  keloid, 730-731
  nodular fasciitis, 729
  pinguecula and pterygium, 728-729
  pyogenic granuloma and capillary hemangioma, 727-728
Reactive oxygen intermediates, 132
Real-time corneal topographic analysis, 2056
Recombinant human epidermal growth factor, 185-188
Reconstructive penetrating keratoplasty, 1553
Reconstructive procedures, *A289-296*
  after anterior segment trauma, 1947-1955
    conjunctiva, 1949, 1948
    cornea, 1949-1952
    estimating visual potential, 1947-1948
    iris and angle, 1953
    temporary keratoprosthesis, 1953-1954
    vitreous and lens, 1952-1953
  automated lamellar keratoplasty, 2165-2179
    comparison with other refractive procedures, 2178-2179
    complications, 2175-2178
    enhancement, 2178
    historical perspectives, 2165-2167
    instrumentation, 2167-2168
    nomograms, 2173-2174
    operative procedure, 2169-2173
    patient selection, 2168-2169
    postoperative care, 2173
    preoperative evaluation, 2169
    results, 2174-2175
  conjunctival flaps, 1903-1909
    in acid injury, 1441
    advancement, 1904, 1905
    bipedicle, 1904, 1906
    complications, 1905-1909
    in corneal edema, 414
    in *Fusarium* keratitis, 1261
    high resolution ultrasound of, 358
    indications, 1903-1904, 1905
    in neurotrophic keratopathy, 1216
    postoperative care, 1905
    in pterygium, 1877-1879, 1880
    single-pedicle, 1904, 1907
    surgical technique, 1904, 1908
  conjunctival transplantation, 1889-1892
  in corneal and conjunctival neoplasia, 1911-1924
    limbal dermoid, 1921-1922
    lymphoid proliferations, 1920-1921
    melanocytic neoplasms, 1912-1916
    squamous neoplasms, 1916-1920
  in corneal perforation, 1815-1832
    etiology, 1815-1816
    patch graft, 1827-1829
    penetrating keratoplasty, 1825-1826
    postoperative care, 1823-1824
    postoperative complications, 1824-1825
    preoperative evaluation, 1818
    prevention, 1830-1831
    signs and symptoms, 1816-1818
    terminology, 1816, 1817
    tissue adhesives, 1818-1825
  for corneal thinning disorders, 1794-1795
  cyclectomy, 1957-1964
    complications, 1963-1964
    indications, 1957-1958
    postoperative care, 1963
    procedure, 1958-1963
    results, 1964
    surgical anatomy, 1958
  high resolution ultrasound in, 356-358
  keratoprosthesis, 1855-1863, *A295-296*
    after anterior segment trauma, 1953-1954
    complications, 1859-1861
    design and materials, 1856
    historical background, 1855-1856
    indications, 1857, 1858
    surgical procedure, 1857-1859, 1860
  lamellar keratoplasty, 1773, 1833-1842, *A293*
    after anterior segment trauma, 1949-1951
    complications, 1840, 1841
    free band, *A245*
    high resolution ultrasound of, 356, 357
    indications, 1833, 1834, 1835
    in pellucid marginal corneal degeneration, 1789-1790
    penetrating *versus*, 1833-1834, 1835
    preoperative evaluation, 1834-1836
    in pterygium, 1879
    surgical technique, 1836-1841
    in Terrien's marginal degeneration, 1791
  for ocular surface disease, 1865-1872
    anterior stromal puncture, 1868-1869, 1870
    cauterization, 1866
    phototherapeutic keratectomy, 1869-1870
    superficial keratectomy, 1866-1868
    treatment options, 1865, 1866
  ocular surface transplantation, 1887-1902
    conjunctival, 1889-1892
    limbal, 1892-1898, 1899
    mucous membrane, 1898-1901
    principles of, 1887-1889
  in pterygium, 1873-1885
    chemotherapy, 1880-1882
    conjunctival flaps and autografts, 1877-1879, 1880
    excision and avulsion, 1876-1877
    histopathology, 1874-1875
    lamellar and penetrating keratoplasty, 1879
    medical approaches, 1875-1876
    mucous membrane and skin graft, 1879-1880
    pathogenesis, 1874
    prevalence, 1873
    radiation therapy, 1822-1883
    transplantation of pterygium head, 1877
  scleral perforation, 1965-1973
    anesthesia for, 1965-1966
    with fixation sutures, 1639, 1640
    surgical repair, 1966-1972
  therapeutic keratoplasty, 1843-1854
    for *Acanthamoeba* keratitis, 1845
    antimicrobial therapy, 1849
    for bacterial infection, 1843-1844
    donor material, 1849
    for fungal keratitis, 1844-1845, 1846
    for herpetic keratitis, 1845-1846, 1847, 1848
    for persistent epithelial defects, 1846-1847, 1849
    postoperative management, 1851-1852
    presurgical evaluation, 1847-1849
    surgical technique, 1849-1851
    visual prognosis, 1852
Rectus muscle surgery, *A258*
Recurrent conjunctivitis, 775
Recurrent corneal erosion, 200-202, 203, 1317-1326, *A205-208*
  after corneal abrasion, 1406
  anterior stromal puncture, 1321-1324, 1325
  debridement and superficial keratectomy, 1320-1321
  diagnosis, 1318-1319
  in epithelial basement membrane dystrophy, 1036
  excimer phototherapeutic keratectomy, 1325-1326
  in lattice dystrophy, 1048, 1049
  medical treatment, 1319
  pathophysiology, 1317
  phototherapeutic keratectomy for, 2212, 2217
  surgery for, 1865-1866, *A293*
  YAG laser procedures, 1324-1325
Recurrent herpes simplex infection, *A280*
  after penetrating keratoplasty, 1705
  keratitis, 1195-1212, 1213
    blepharitis in, 1195-1196
    conjunctivitis in, 1196
    endotheliitis, 1205-1211
    infectious epithelial keratitis, 1196-1201
    iridocyclitis, 1211-1212, 1213
    neurotrophic keratopathy, 1201-1202
    stromal disease, 1202-1205
  keratouveitis, *A188*
  vesicles in, *A179*
Recurrent interstitial keratitis, 1282
Recurrent keloid, *A48*
Red eye, 437-445
  in anterior uveitis, 1493
  contact lens-induced, 1468
  patient history in, 437-440
  physical examination in, 440-444, 445
Red pulp, 85
Red reflex, 1095, 1097
Reflex view
  of Fuchs' dystrophy, *A146*
  of Haab's striae, *A82*
Refractile/crystalline deposits, 417, 418
  deep stromal, 426-427
  stromal, 423-425
  superficial, 420-421
Refraction
  of abnormal cornea, 215-221
  after photorefractive keratoplasty, 2192, 2193, 2194
  evaluation before refractive surgery, 2008-2009
  intrastromal corneal device and, 2225-2226
  radial keratotomy
    complications, 2104-2108, 2129-2136
    visual acuity after, 2129

variable in photorefractive keratoplasty outcome, 2035
Refractive index, 3
Refractive surgery, *A297-300*
assistive technology and instrumentation, 2013-2024
additional technology, 2019-2023
astigmatic keratotomy instrumentation, 2018, 2020
future advances, 2022, 2023, 2024
investigative aids, 2023
operating room equipment, 2013-2014
primary procedure instrumentation, 2015-2018, 2019
secondary procedure instrumentation, 2018-2019, 2020
surgical supplies and medications, 2014-2015
astigmatic keratotomy, 2143-2153
cataract surgery with, 2155-2164
informed consent, 2146
instrumentation, 2018, 2020
intraoperative complications, 2151
operative methods, 2146-2148, 2152
patient selection, 2145-2146, 2147
postoperative management, 2151-2152
preoperative testing, 2146, 2148, 2149, 2150-2151
results, 2152-2153
automated lamellar keratoplasty, 1991, 2165-2179
comparison with other refractive procedures, 2178-2179
complications, 2175-2178
corneal topographic analysis in, 2052
enhancement, 2178
historical perspectives, 2165-2167
instrumentation, 2167-2168
nomograms, 2173-2174
operative procedure, 2169-2173
patient selection, 2168-2169
postoperative care, 2173
predictive formulas for, 2027-2028, 2029
preoperative evaluation, 2169
results, 2174-2175
contact lens fitting after, 1459-1460
corneal topography, 2039-2058
in assessment of surgical result, 2048-2055, 2056
challenges for future, 2055-2056
preoperative screening, 2042-2048
videokeratoscope, 2039-2042
evaluation of surgical outcomes, 1977-1978
future of, 2243-2253, 2251
criteria for judging procedures, 2243-2248
delivery of refractive surgical services, 2251-2252
intrastromal photorefractive keratectomy, 2250
keratomileusis, 2250
laser photorefractive keratectomy, 2250-2251
refractive keratotomy, 2251
surgery confined to corneal stroma, 2249
synthetic devices, 2248-2249
thermal keratoplasty, 2251
high resolution ultrasound in, 356-358
historical emergence, 1977
incisional, 1979-1987
hexagonal keratotomy, 1986-1987
radial keratotomy, 1979-1986
intraocular procedures, 2001-2003
intrastromal devices, 2225-2232
clinical and histopathologic observations, 2227
intrastromal corneal ring, 2227-2229
physiologic considerations, 2226-2227, 2228
refractive mechanisms, 2225-2226
small diameter corneal inlay, 2230-2231
lamellar, 1990-2001
epikeratoplasty, 1994-1996
keratomileusis, 1991-1992
keratophakia, 1992-1993
photorefractive keratectomy, 1996-2001
synthetic keratophakia, 1993-1994, 1995
laser refractive keratoplasty, 2181-2189
instrumentation, 2181-2186
surgical technique, 2186-2188
minimal visual loss following, 454
patient selection
in astigmatic keratotomy, 2145-2146, 2147
in automated lamellar keratoplasty, 2168-2169
in penetrating keratoplasty, 1581-1582
in refractive surgery, 2007-2008
photorefractive keratectomy, 1981
automated lamellar keratoplasty *versus,* 2178-2179
corneal topographic analysis, 2050
historical background, 1996-2001
intrastromal, 2250
results, 2097-2098
surgical technique, 2187-2188
photorefractive keratoplasty
complications, 2200-2209
historical background, 1997-1998
predictability, 2030-2037
results, 2191-2200
phototherapeutic keratectomy, 2211-2223
advantages and indications, 2211
clinical outcome, 2216-2221
in ocular surface disease, 1869-1870
side effects and complications, 2221
surgical technique, 2211-2216
wound healing after, 2216, 2217
predictive formulas, 2025-2037
keratomileusis, 2025-2028, 2029
photorefractive keratoplasty, 2030-2037
radial keratotomy, 2028-2030, 2031, 2032
principles of, 1978-1979, 1980-1982
radial keratotomy, *A297-299; see also* Radial keratotomy
complications, 2101-2116, 2117-2142
contact lens fitting after, 1459-1460
correction of residual myopia, 2178
fungal keratitis following, 1255
high resolution ultrasound in, 356-358
historical background, 1979-1986
incisions surviving trauma, 1409
keratitis after, 1143, 1145
minimal visual loss following, 454
penetrating keratoplasty after, 1589-1590
peripheral incisions, 1979
predictability, 2028-2030, 2031, 2032
published studies, 2084-2096
results of, 2083-2093
surgical techniques, 2059-2082
synthetic epikeratoplasty, 2233-2241
attachment of lenticule to cornea, 2236
background, 2233-2234
in vitro trials, 2234-2236
potential biomaterials, 2234
type IV collagen lenticules, 2237-2240
thermal keratoplasty, 1987-1990
future of, 2251
historical background, 1987-1990
Holmium laser, 2185-2186
Regression analysis, 2029
Regular astigmatism, 875-876, 2143, 2144, 2146
Reis-Bücklers' dystrophy, 1039-1042, *A123*
minimal visual loss in, 452
phototherapeutic keratectomy in, 2214
Reiter's syndrome, 785-786, *A74*
in acquired immunodeficiency syndrome, *A111*
Behçet disease *versus,* 1532-1533
HLA-B27 related uveitis in, 1517-1518
Rejection reactions to penetrating keratoplasty, *A283-287*
Relapsing polychondritis, 1380-1381
Relaxing incision, 1681-1682
Religious outreach program, 548
Renal failure, *A106*
Reoperation with photorefractive keratoplasty, 2196, 2197
Required request law, 531
Research
in alkali injury, 1450
donor tissue for, 553-558
Resection
in Mooren's ulcer, 1794
in pellucid marginal corneal degeneration, 1790
wedge, 1681
Residual horizontal laxity, 564-565
Residual interstitial keratopathy
pathology of, 1293-1294
syphilitic interstitial keratitis and, 1284-1287, 1288
Reticular degeneration of Koby, 1130
Reticulate body, 779
Reticulohistiocytoma, 730
Retina
anterior segment surgery and, 1928
Behçet syndrome, 1530, 1532
herpes zoster ophthalmicus and, 1232
iron deposits in, 422
penetrating keratoplasty and examination before, 1569
pediatric, 1746
Retinal detachment
after cyclectomy, 1964
after keratoprosthesis, 1861
after radial keratotomy, 2138
Retinitis, *A111*
Retinoic acid, 963
Retinoids, 831
Retinol, 955
Retinopathy, 1246-1247
Retinoscopy
in minimal visual loss, 449
in refraction of abnormal cornea, 216-217
Retraction of eyelid, 578-579
Retractor complex, 562

Soft contact lens
  bandage, 1457
    in acid injury, 1441
    in corneal abrasion, 1405-1406
    in corneal perforation, 1823, 1830
    in corneal ulceration after keratoplasty, 1697
    in macroulcerative peripheral keratitis, 397
    for postoperative epithelial defects, 1662-1663
    in recurrent corneal erosion, 203, 1319
  complications, *A261-266*
  therapeutic
    in corneal edema, 414
    in sterile corneal ulceration, 208
    in superior limbic keratoconjunctivitis, 859
  ulcerative keratitis and, 1143
  for visual rehabilitation following keratoplasty, 1654-1655
Solar keratosis, 585
Solid organ distribution system, 519
Soluble mediators, 78-85, 144-145
Somatoform disorders, 1349
Soper Cone lens, 1458
Sorbitol, 979
Sotos syndrome, 938
South America, eye banking in, 482
Soybean casein digest broth, 1162
Sparganosis, 660
Spastic entropion, *A4*
Spatula, 1577-1578
Spectacles
  after anterior segment trauma reconstruction, 1947-1948
  after radial keratotomy, 2106
  following anterior segment trauma, 1943
  for keratoconus, 1099
  for keratoglobus, 1102-1103
Spectinomycin, 763, 1174-1175
Specular microscopy, 313-334, 2023, *A161*
  in Chandler's syndrome, 1110
  in corneal edema, 413
  of diabetic cornea, 980
  of donor tissue, 490, 505-507
  epithelial, 317-318
  in epithelial ingrowth, 1711
  in Fuchs' dystrophy, 1076
  improvements in instrumentation and methods, 316-317
  in vivo findings, 323-330
  in iris atrophy, 1110
  optical principles, 313
  in posterior polymorphous dystrophy, 1063, 1065, 1066
  in pseudophakic corneal edema, 1603
  qualitative morphometric analysis, 319-321
  quantitative morphometric analysis, 321-323
Specular photomicrograph
  of corneal vesicles, *A81*
  of polymorphous dystrophy, *A143-144*
Specular reflection, 252-254, 255, 256
  of normal cornea, 295
  in photo slit lamp biomicrography, 290-291, 295, 296
Speculum, 1571, 1572, 1583
Spherocylindrical lens, 224
Spherocytosis, congenital, 967-968
Spheroidal degeneration, 390, 418-420, 1121, 1122, 1124-1125, *A173*
Spigelman study, 2086-2088, 2094
Spindle cell carcinoma, 710
Spiradenoma, eccrine, 592
Spirochete-associated keratitis, 1554
Spirometra, 660
Spitz nevus, 715
Spleen, 85
Split-thickness dermal graft for scleral perforation, 1972
Spondyloepiphysial dysplasia tarda, *A98*
Sporotrichosis
  eyelid and, 655
  in Parinaud's oculoglandular syndrome, 801
Sporotrichum, 687
Squames, 183
Squamous cell carcinoma, *A15, A39*
  conjunctival, 707, 708
  eyelid, 605-606, 607-608
  management of, 1918-1920
Squamous cell papilloma, 1917
Squamous conjunctival neoplasm, 701-714, *A37-39*
  benign hereditary intraepithelial dyskeratosis, 701, 702
  conjunctival intraepithelial neoplasia, 704-707
  corneal epithelial dysmaturation and epithelial dysplasia, 707-710
  dacryoadenoma, 703-704
  inverted conjunctival papilloma, 702-703
  management of, 1916-1920
  mucoepidermoid carcinoma, 710
  papilloma, 702, 703
  pseudoepitheliomatous hyperplasia and keratoacanthoma, 701-702, 703
  pterygia and pinguecula, 704
  sebaceous cell carcinoma, 710-712
  spindle cell carcinoma, 710
  squamous cell carcinoma, 707, 708
Squamous metaplasia, 671-672
Sri Lanka, eye banking in, 484
Stability
  of refractive surgery, 2246
  of synthetic epikeratoplasty, 2235
Stableflex-semiflexible closed loop, 1606-1608
Stain
  acid-fast, 306
  acridine-orange, 305-306, 1159-1160
  alcian blue, *A93, A124*
  in bacterial infection, 1158-1160, 1161
  carbol-fuchsin, 1159
  congo red, *A129*
  corneal, 275-277, 278
  corneal blood, 421-422
  in dry eye, 668-669, 670
  fluorescein
    of dendritic epithelial patterns, *A262*
    in dry eye syndrome, *A33-34*
    of herpes zoster dendrites, *A189*
    in punctate keratitis, *A210*
    in superficial punctate keratopathy, *A30*
    in tear film evaluation, 271
    in thermal corneal injury, *A241*
  Giemsa
    in bacterial keratitis, 1158, 1159
    in *Chlamydia trachomatis* infection, 307
    in fungal keratitis, 1255
    in herpetic blepharitis, 642
    in postoperative endophthalmitis, 1704
    in trachoma, 782
    in varicella zoster virus infection, 645
  Gram
    in bacterial keratitis, 1156, 1158-1159
    in fungal keratitis, 1255
    in microbial keratitis, 305-306
    in postoperative endophthalmitis, 1704
    therapy selection and, 1165
  lactophenol cotton blue, *A196*
  in microbial keratitis, 305-306
  Prussian blue
    in keratoconus, *A155*
    in pterygium, *A169*
  rose bengal, 261-263, 267, 275-277, 278, *A30-31*
    in dry eye, 56, 668-669
    in herpes zoster, *A189*
    in lid imbrication syndrome, 573-574
    photography of, 301, 302
    staining characteristics of, 67[illegible]
    in superior limbic keratoconjunctivitis, 858
    in tear film evaluation, 273
  Wright-Giemsa, 1159
  Ziehl-Neelsen
    in bacterial keratitis, 1159
    in microbial keratitis, 306
Staphyloccocal marginal infiltrate, 1201
Staphyloccocal marginal keratitis, 1392-1394
Staphylococcal blepharoconjunctivitis, 755
Staphylococcal keratoconjunctivitis, 24[illegible]
Staphylococcus, A24, A225
  in acquired immunodeficiency syndrome, 1019
  in blepharitis, 633-634, *A19*
  normal ocular flora, 1149
Staphylococcus aureus, A177
  in blepharitis, 622, 633
  in conjunctivitis, 764, 766-769
  in corneal ulcer, 405
  in dacryoadenitis, 687
  in erysipelas, 637
  in impetigo contagiosa, 637
  in keratitis, 1139, 1392, 1698
  in meibomian gland dysfunction, 63[illegible]
  normal conjunctival flora, 46
  in phlyctenular keratoconjunctivitis, 1389
  in posttraumatic suppurative preseptal cellulitis, 636
  in suture abscess, 1700, *A279*
Staphylococcus aureus enterotoxin, 1[illegible]2
Staphylococcus epidermidis
  in blepharitis, 622, 633
  in keratitis, 1140, 1392, 1698
  in meibomian gland dysfunction, 63[illegible]
  normal conjunctival flora, 46
  in postoperative endophthalmitis, 1703
  in suture abscess formation, 1700
Staphyloma
  corneal opacity in, 374
  perforated, *A246*
Starburst after incisional refractive surgery, 2117, 2127-2129
Stelazine deposits, *A117*
Stellate laceration, 1937-1938
Stem cell, 71, 1888-1889
Sterile corneal defect, 2109
Sterile corneal erosion, 199-204
Sterile corneal ulcer, 191-192, 204-20[illegible]
Sterile infiltrates, 1467-1468
Sterile keratitis, 2119-2120

Steroids
in acid injury, 1441
in atopic keratoconjunctivitis, 816
delayed epithelial wound healing, 1024
in erythema multiforme, 841-842
in juvenile rheumatoid arthritis, 1371
in meibomian gland dysfunction, 631
in rheumatoid arthritis, 1367
side effects of, 1511
in vernal keratoconjunctivitis, 813
Stevens-Johnson syndrome, 1028, *A71-73*
bilateral pseudomembranous conjunctivitis in, 748
dry eye in, 675-676
keratoprosthesis for, 1857, *A295*
in type III ocular hypersensitivity, 113-114
Stickler syndrome, 935
Sting, 1419-1420
Strabismus, 1735
Streptococcal toxin, 1147
Streptococcus faecalis, A177
Streptococcus pneumoniae, A278, A280
in acute bacterial conjunctivitis, 764
in dacryoadenitis, 687, 689
in keratitis, 1139, 1149-1150, 1698, *A299*
in nonsuppurative preseptal cellulitis, 636
in suture abscess formation, 1700
Streptococcus pyogenes
in acute bacterial conjunctivitis, 764
in erysipelas, 637
in posttraumatic suppurative preseptal cellulitis, 636
Streptococcus pyogenes erythrogenic toxin, 132
Streptococcus viridans, A177
in infectious crystalline keratopathy, 1702, *A280*
normal conjunctival flora, 46
Streptodornase, 1147
Streptokinase, 1147
Streptolysin O, 1147
Streptomycin, 800
Stress line, 505, 506
Stress testing, 413
Striate melanokeratosis, 417, *A42*
Stroma, 10-14
abrasion of, 1407
adhesion molecules on, 137-138
adhesion of epithelium to, 199-200
congenital hereditary endothelial dystrophy and, 1086
contact lens complications, 1465-1469
corneal edema and, 411, 412
corneal transparency and, 3
deposits in
nonpigmented, 422-423, 425-426
pigmented, 421-422
in donor tissue evaluation, 504-505
dystrophy of; *see* Stromal dystrophy
edema of, 411, 412
in acid injury, 1440
endothelial rejection with, *A287*
Fuchs' dystrophy with, *A145*
fungal keratitis and, 1253
glass foreign body in, *A247*
herpes simplex virus disease and, 1202
immune responses and, 101-102
infiltrates, 1256, *A265-266*
infrared radiation and, 1414
injuries and fractures, 1409
intrastromal corneal devices, 2225-2232
clinical and histopathologic observations, 2227
intrastromal corneal ring, 2227-2229
physiologic considerations, 2226-2227, 2228
refractive mechanisms, 2225-2226
small diameter corneal inlay, 2230-2231
keratoconus and, 1094, 1095
necrosis, 1690
necrosis and perforation of, *A260*
nonsyphilitic interstitial keratitis, 1307-1315, *A204*
Acanthamoeba infection, 1311-1312
Cogan's syndrome, 1307-1310
herpes virus, 1312-1313
leishmaniasis, 1312
Lyme disease, 1311
microsporidial infection, 1312
mycobacterial infection, 1310-1311
onchocerciasis, 1312
trypanosomiasis, 1312
posterior membrane dystrophies and, 1068
reaction to injury, 171-174
repair after infection, 149
response to infection, 145
scarring of, *A183-184, A300*
spheroidal degeneration and, 1122
surgery confined to, 2249
vascularization of, *A264*
vegetable foreign matter in, *A249*
wound healing, 190-193
Stromal dystrophy, 1043-1062, *A125-141*
Avellino dystrophy, 1051-1053, *A134*
Bietti's crystalline corneal-retinal dystrophy, *A141*
central cloudy dystrophy, 1056-1057
congenital hereditary, 375, 1058
Fleck dystrophy, 1055-1056, *A140*
gelatinous droplike dystrophy, 1053
granular dystrophy, 1043-1045, *A131-133*
lattice dystrophy, 1048-1051, 1052, 1053, *A125-130*
macular dystrophy, 1045-1048, *A135-136*
minimal visual loss in, 452-453
penetrating keratoplasty in, 1554
posterior amorphous stromal dystrophy, 1058-1059, *A141*
pre-Descemet's dystrophy, 1047-1058, *A140*
Schnyder's crystalline dystrophy, 1054-1055, *A137*
subepithelial mucinous, 420
Stromal keratitis, 1278
Stromelysin-1, 147, 186
Stye, 635, 698, *A20*
Sub-Tenon's injection, 1510, 1512
Subconjunctival hemorrhage, 1307, *A234*
Subconjunctival injection of antibiotics, 1176
Subconjunctival lymphoma, 737
Subconjunctival plasmacytoma, 738
Subepithelial congenital melanosis, 716-717
Subepithelial conjunctival neoplasm, 723-743, *A43-50*
amyloid, 731-732, 733
basal cell carcinoma, 735
choristoma, 723-725
conjunctival cyst, 727
elastofibroma oculi, 729
fibrous histiocytoma, 733, 734
granulomatous and histiocytic lesions, 729-730, 731
hamartoma, 725-726
hematic cyst, 732
Kaposi's sarcoma, 733-734, 735
keloid, 730-731
lymphoid lesions, 736-738
malignant melanoma, 735-736
nodular fasciitis, 729
oncocytoma, 734-735
pinguecula and pterygium, 728-729
pyogenic granuloma and capillary hemangioma, 727-728
Subepithelial fibrosis, 829, 830
Subepithelial haze, 179
Subepithelial infiltrates, 773-774
after penetrating keratoplasty, *A284, A286*
corneal staining, 276
in herpes zoster ophthalmicus, *A190*
in trachoma, 781
Subepithelial mucinous dystrophy, 420, *A124*
Subject reflectivity, 288
Subluxated lens, 265
Substance P, 20
Substantia propria
anatomy of, 44
atopic keratoconjunctivitis and, 815
neoplasms of, 723-743, *A43-50*
amyloid, 731-732, 733
basal cell carcinoma, 735
choristoma, 723-725
conjunctival cyst, 727
elastofibroma oculi, 729
fibrous histiocytoma, 733, 734
granulomatous and histiocytic lesions, 729-730, 731
hamartoma, 725-726
hematic cyst, 732
Kaposi's sarcoma, 733-734, 735
keloid, 730-731
lymphoid lesions, 736-738
malignant melanoma, 735-736
nodular fasciitis, 729
oncocytoma, 734-735
pinguecula and pterygium, 728-729
pyogenic granuloma and capillary hemangioma, 727-728
vernal keratoconjunctivitis and, 812
Sulfacetamide
in bacterial conjunctivitis, 767
in dacryocystis, 689
Sulfamethoxazole, *A268*
Sulfisoxazole, 794
Sulfonamides, 1174
erythema multiforme and, 839
toxicity of, 850
Sulforhodamine B, 670
Sulfur granule, 653
Sulfuric acid, 1437
Sulindac; *see* Clinoril
Summit excimer laser, 2183
Sunflower cataract, *A253*
Superficial cell, 5-6
Superficial episcleral plexus, 30-31, 36
Superficial keratectomy, 1320-1321
in ocular surface disease, 1866-1868
in recurrent corneal erosion, 203
Superficial nonpigmented deposits, 420
Superficial pigmented deposits, 417-420
Superficial punctate keratitis of Thygeson, 1333-1337, *A210*
disease course, 1334-1336

Superficial punctate keratitis of Thygeson—cont'd
  history of, 1333-1334
  pathogenesis, 1336
Superficial punctate keratopathy, *A30*
Superficial refractile/crystalline deposits, 420-421
Superficial spreading melanoma of eyelid, 612, 613
Superior forniceal conjunctiva, 41
Superior limbic keratoconjunctivitis, 393, 857-862, *A75*
  conjunctivitis in, 754-755
  contact lens-induced, 1462-1463, *A265*
Superior rectus muscle, 65
Suppressor T cell, 73
Suprachoroidal hemorrhage, 1583, *A274*
Supraorbital artery, 66
Supraorbital nerve, 65
Suprofen, 824
Surface Asymmetry Index, 2047
Surface markers, 72
Surface proteins, 100
Surface receptors, 134-141
Surface Regularity Index, 2040, 2053-2054
Surgeon preparation, 2061, 2062
Surgery; *see also* Corneal surgery
  in corneal edema, 414-415
  for corneal thinning disorders, 1789-1798
    alternative approaches, 1795-1797
    conjunctival, 1794-1795
    eyelid, 1794
    pellucid marginal corneal degeneration, 1789-1790, 1791
    Terrien's marginal degeneration, 1790-1793
    tissue adhesive, 1795
  in ectropion, 567-568
  in entropion, 563-565, 566
  in epithelial ingrowth, 1712-1713
  in fungal keratitis, 1261-1263
  for glaucoma after penetrating keratoplasty, 1725-1728
  in herpes simplex keratitis, 1219
  for hyphema, 1931-1932
  for keratoconus, 1099
  large diameter corneal graft, 1773-1774
  in ocular surface disease, 1785-1786
  before pediatric penetrating keratoplasty, 1742-1746
  in pellucid marginal degeneration, 1101
  in posterior polymorphous dystrophy, 1067
  in pterygia, *A291*
  in recurrent erosion syndrome, 1319-1326
  refractive; *see* Refractive surgery
  in rheumatoid arthritis-associated ocular disease, 1370
  for scleral perforation, 1966-1972
  scleritis after, 1487
  supplies and medications, 2014-2015
  technique development from eye bank material, 556
  trauma in, *A255-258*
Surgical trauma, 1423-1435
  Brown-McLean syndrome, 1426
  etiology of, 1426-1430, 1431
  histopathology of, 1425
  incidence of, 1423-1425
  pathogenesis, 1425-1426
  treatment of, 1431-1432
Suryidev style 10 lens, 1424
Suture, 1627-1638
  adjustment of, 1652-1653
  in anterior segment trauma, 1932
  combined continuous and interrupted
    adjustment for astigmatism, 1633-1634
    technique, 1630
  in conjunctival autografting, 1878
  in corneal laceration repair, 1935-1936
  double continuous
    adjustment for astigmatism, 1637
    technique, 1632
  in entropion treatment, 563, 564
  erosion of, *A279*
  in herpetic eye, 1804, 1805
  nylon, *A68*
  in penetrating keratoplasty, 1586-1589
    astigmatism following, 1679-1681
    complications after, 1664-1665
    with intraocular lens implantation, 1617-1618
    pediatric, 1744-1745, 1750-1751
  perforation of sclera, 1639, 1640
  removal of, 1633, 1943
  for scleral fixation ring, 1583-1584
  sealing a suture track leak, 1660-1661
  single continuous
    adjustment for astigmatism, 1634-1637
    techniques, 1630-1632
  single interrupted
    adjustment for astigmatism, 1633
    technique, 1628-1629, 1630
  of stellate laceration, 1937-1938
  in synthetic epikeratoplasty, 2236
  for treatment of overcorrection, 2133
  variables in producing astigmatism after cataract surgery, 2156
  of zig-zag incision, 1937
Suture abscess, 1664, 1700-1701
Suture granuloma, *A47*
Sweat gland tumor, 592-594
Swelling pressure, 11
Symblepharon
  in cicatricial pemphigoid, 829, 830
  in erythema multiforme, 836, 837
Symmetrel; *see* Amantadine
Syndrome of acromegaly, 939
Synechia, *A272*
  after keratoplasty in herpes simplex, 1808-1809
  formation after penetrating keratoplasty, 1668
  graft failure and, 1763
Synechiolysis, 1558
Synthetic devices, 2248-2249
Synthetic epikeratoplasty, 2233-2241
  attachment of lenticule to cornea, 2236
  background, 2233-2234
  in vitro trials, 2234-2236
  potential biomaterials, 2234
  type IV collagen lenticules, 2237-2240
Synthetic keratophakia, 1993-1994, 1995
Syphilis, *A203*
  corneal opacity in, 380
  eyelid and, 638
  Lyme disease *versus,* 1005
  in Parinaud's oculoglandular syndrome, 801-802
  syphilitic interstitial keratitis and, 1278-1284
Syphilitic interstitial keratitis, 1275-1306, *A203*
  acquired syphilis and, 1282-1284
  congenital syphilis and, 1278-1282, 1283
  developmental stigmata in, 128[illegible], 1290, 1291
  differential diagnosis, 1297
  epidemiology, 1277-1278
  hearing loss in, 1288-1289, 129[illegible]
  history of, 1275-1277
  joints and, 1289-1291
  laboratory investigation, 1297-1299
  pathogenesis, 1294-1297, 1298
  pathology, 1291-1294
  penetrating keratoplasty in, *A274*
  residual interstitial keratopathy and, 1284-1287, 1288
  treatment, 1299-1301
Syphilitic posterior uveitis, 1282
Syphilitic scleritis, 1487
Syphilitic uveitis, *A272*
Syringocystadenoma papilliferum, 594
Syringoma, 592
Systemic lupus erythematosus, 1377-1378, *A221*
Systemic mucopolysaccharidoses, [illegible]99-[illegible]02
Systemic sclerosis, 1378-1379
Systemic therapy, corneal effects, 1023-1031
  drug deposition, 1026-1027
  ophthalmic surgical solutions, 1028-1030
  topical ophthalmic medications, 102[illegible]-1026
  toxic effects, 1027-1028

T

T cell, 72-74
  antigen presentation and, 88-89
  erythema multiforme and, 839
  in immune response, 1759-176[illegible]
  immunoglobulin E response and, 1[illegible]
  inflammation and, 143
  in ligneous conjunctivitis, 864
  in Mooren's ulcer, 1398
  in phlyctenulosis, 1394
  in rheumatoid arthritis, 1359
  in Sjögren's syndrome, 677
  vernal keratoconjunctivitis and, 812
T cell receptor, 73, 88, 111
T cell superantigen, 132-133
T cut, 1683
Tacrolimus, 1694
Taenia solium, 659
Tandem scanning confocal microscopy, 336-337
  in *Acanthamoeba* keratitis, 344-345, 1270-1271
  digital image acquisition and processing, 338-339, 340
  in excimer laser photorefractive keratectomy, 345-347
  in herpetic keratitis, 347
  in vivo imaging methodology, 337-338
  normal corneal structures, 339, 340
  research applications, 339-343, 344, 345
  surface toxicity and incisional wound healing and, 347-348
  of tear film, 347
Tangier disease, 423, 904, 1120, *A91*
Tape tarsorrhaphy, 1216
Tarantula hair, 1418-1419, *A248*
Tarsal conjunctiva, 42
Tarsal gland, 625
Tarsal plates, 62-64
Tarsoconjunctival flap, 1967, 1968
Tarsorrhaphy, 1589, 1794
  in corneal perforation, 1830
  in neurotrophic keratopathy, 1216

for postoperative epithelial defects, 1662
in rheumatoid arthritis-associated keratoconjunctivitis sicca, 1368
at time of penetrating keratoplasty, 1768
Tear enzyme analysis, 918
Tear evaporation, 670
Tear film, 49-60
anatomy and physiology, 49-52
confocal microscopy of, 347
disorders of, 52-57
decreased tear secretion, 53-54
diagnostic tests, 55-56
dry eye, 55, 56, 663
increased tear film evaporation, 54-55
pharmaceutical progress, 56-57
evaluation of, 269-273, 664-667
meibomian gland and, 625-627
ocular immune response, 96-98
optic section and, 250
osmolarity, 668
red eye and, 442
response to infection, 130
specular reflection of, 254, 255
Tear film break-up time, 271
in dry eye, 56, 664-665
in meibomian gland dysfunction, 627
Tear fluid, 4
Tear function index, 668
Tear gas weapons, 853-854
Tear meniscus, 238
Tear production disorders, *A29-36*
canaliculitis, 691-693, *A36*
in actinomycosis, 653
chronic, 754
epiphora in, 697
in sporotrichosis, 655
dacryoadenitis, 687-689, 1247, *A36*
dacryocystitis, 689-691, *A36*
chronic, 754
in sarcoidosis, 1523
in sporotrichosis, 655
dry eye, 663-686, *A29-35*
character of ocular irritation, 664
classification, 663, 664
dye staining, 668-669, 670
evaporative, 679-680
fluorophotometry, 668
impression cytology, 671-672
increased tear film evaporation, 54
lacrimal gland disease and, 53
meibomian gland evaluation, 669-670
non-Sjögren's aqueous tear deficiency, 673-676
ocular ferning test, 671
serum autoantibodies, 669
Sjögren syndrome aqueous tear deficiency, 676-679
tear evaporation, 670
tear film evaluation in, 269-273, 664-667
tear film osmolarity, 668
tear protein analysis, 670-671
tear turnover and aqueous tear production, 667-668
therapeutic keratoplasty in, 1847
therapy, 680-682
epiphora, 374, 695-700
Tear protein analysis, 670-671
Tears
decreased, 53-54
epiphora and, 695-700
evaluation of production, 667-668
as infection barrier, 129-130
Technicians practical performance test, 472
Technolas excimer laser, 2183
Tectonic keratoplasty, 1553, 1833
Teflon cutting block, 1574, 1575
Temafloxacin, 850
Temperature reversal, 17
Temporal artery, 66
Temporal skin hemangioma, *A10*
Tenon's capsule, 1967
Tenon's fascia, 29, 30, 31
Tenotomy scissors, 1577
Terfenadine
in atopic keratoconjunctivitis, 816
to improve graft survival, 1785
Terrien's marginal degeneration, 1126-1127, *A175*
minimal visual loss in, 452
Mooren's ulcer *versus,* 1399
pellucid marginal degeneration *versus,* 1101
perforation in, 1816
peripheral cornea and, 391-392
surgery for, 1790-1793
Territorial rights in tissue procurement, 534
Testosterone undecenoate, 681
Tetracaine
corneal effects, 1023, 1354
preoperative, 2060
Tetracycline, 1173
in blepharitis, 623-624
in chlamydial infection, 785
corneal effects, 1027
to improve graft survival, 1785
in Lyme disease, 1006
in lymphogranuloma venereum, 787
in meibomian gland dysfunction, 630-631
in neonatal conjunctivitis, 793, 794
in phlyctenulosis, 1392
in rosacea, 396
in staphylococcal blepharitis, 634
in syphilis, 802
in trachoma, 783
Thayer-Martin agar, 306, 1161
Thelaziasis, 660
Theodore's superior limbic keratoconjunctivitis, 861, *A75*
Therapeutic contact lens, 1455
in corneal edema, 414
in macroulcerative peripheral keratitis, 397
in neurotrophic keratopathy, 1216
in recurrent corneal erosion, 203
in sterile corneal ulceration, 208
in superior limbic keratoconjunctivitis, 859
in ulcerative keratitis, 1179
Therapeutic keratoplasty, 1843-1854
for *Acanthamoeba* keratitis, 1845
antimicrobial therapy, 1849
for bacterial infection, 1843-1844
donor material, 1849
for fungal keratitis, 1844-1845, 1846
for herpetic keratitis, 1845-1846, 1847, 1848
for persistent epithelial defects, 1846-1847, 1849
postoperative management, 1851-1852
presurgical evaluation, 1847-1849
surgical technique, 1849-1851
visual prognosis, 1852
Therapeutic procedures, *A289-296*
anterior segment reconstruction, 1947-1955, *A293-294*
conjunctiva, 1949, 1948
cornea, 1949-1952
estimating visual potential, 1947-1948
graft failure and, 1763
iris and angle, 1953
in penetrating keratoplasty with intraocular lens implantation, 1609-1610, 1611, 1620
temporary keratoprosthesis, 1953-1954
vitreous and lens, 1952-1953
automated lamellar keratoplasty, 2165-2179
comparison with other refractive procedures, 2178-2179
complications, 2175-2178
enhancement, 2178
historical perspectives, 2165-2167
instrumentation, 2167-2168
nomograms, 2173-2174
operative procedure, 2169-2173
patient selection, 2168-2169
postoperative care, 2173
preoperative evaluation, 2169
results, 2174-2175
conjunctival flaps, 1903-1909, *A289-290*
in acid injury, 1441
advancement, 1904, 1905
bipedicle, 1904, 1906
complications, 1905-1909
in corneal edema, 414
in *Fusarium* keratitis, 1261
high resolution ultrasound of, 358
indications, 1903-1904, 1905
in neurotrophic keratopathy, 1216
postoperative care, 1905
in pterygium, 1877-1879, 1880
single-pedicle, 1904, 1907
surgical technique, 1904, 1908
conjunctival transplantation, 1889-1892
in corneal and conjunctival neoplasia, 1911-1924
limbal dermoid, 1921-1922
lymphoid proliferations, 1920-1921
melanocytic neoplasms, 1912-1916
squamous neoplasms, 1916-1920
in corneal perforation, 1815-1832
etiology, 1815-1816
patch graft, 1827-1829
penetrating keratoplasty, 1825-1826
postoperative care, 1823-1824
postoperative complications, 1824-1825
preoperative evaluation, 1818
prevention, 1830-1831
signs and symptoms, 1816-1818
terminology, 1816, 1817
tissue adhesives, 1818-1825
for corneal thinning disorders, 1794-1795
cyclectomy, 1957-1964
complications, 1963-1964
indications, 1957-1958
postoperative care, 1963
procedure, 1958-1963
results, 1964
surgical anatomy, 1958
high resolution ultrasound in, 356-358
keratoepithelialplasty, *A292*

Therapeutic procedures—cont'd
keratoprosthesis, 1855-1863, *A295-296*
after anterior segment trauma, 1953-1954
complications, 1859-1861
design and materials, 1856
historical background, 1855-1856
indications, 1857, 1858
surgical procedure, 1857-1859, 1860
lamellar keratoplasty, 1773, 1833-1842, *A293*
after anterior segment trauma, 1949-1951
complications, 1840, 1841
free band, *A245*
high resolution ultrasound, 356, 357
indications, 1833, 1834, 1835
in pellucid marginal corneal degeneration, 1789-1790
penetrating *versus*, 1833-1834, 1835
preoperative evaluation, 1834-1836
in pterygium, 1879
surgical technique, 1836-1841
in Terrien's marginal degeneration, 1791
for ocular surface disease, 1865-1872
anterior stromal puncture, 1868-1869, 1870
cauterization, 1866
phototherapeutic keratectomy, 1869-1870
superficial keratectomy, 1866-1868
treatment options, 1865, 1866
ocular surface transplantation, 1887-1902
conjunctival, 1889-1892
limbal, 1892-1898, 1899
mucous membrane, 1898-1901
principles of, 1887-1889
in pterygium, 1873-1885, *A291*
chemotherapy, 1880-1882
conjunctival flaps and autografts, 1877-1879, 1880
excision and avulsion, 1876-1877
histopathology, 1874-1875
lamellar and penetrating keratoplasty, 1879
medical approaches, 1875-1876
mucous membrane and skin graft, 1879-1880
pathogenesis, 1874
prevalence, 1873
radiation therapy, 1822-1883
transplantation of pterygium head, 1877
in recurrent erosions, *A293*
scleral perforation, 1965-1973
anesthesia for, 1965-1966
with fixation sutures, 1639, 1640
surgical repair, 1966-1972
therapeutic keratoplasty, 1843-1854
for *Acanthamoeba* keratitis, 1845
antimicrobial therapy, 1849
for bacterial infection, 1843-1844
donor material, 1849
for fungal keratitis, 1844-1845, 1846
for herpetic keratitis, 1845-1846, 1847, 1848
for persistent epithelial defects, 1846-1847, 1849
postoperative management, 1851-1852
presurgical evaluation, 1847-1849
surgical technique, 1849-1851
visual prognosis, 1852
Thermal-based refractive surgery, 1978
Thermal cautery, 859-860
Thermal keratoplasty
future of, 2251
historical background, 1987-1990
Holmium laser, 2185-2186
Thermal trauma, 1414-1416, 1891-1892, *A227-254*
Thermokeratoplasty, 202, 203
Thiel-Behnke corneal dystrophy, 1039-1042
Thimerosal, 852, *A28*
Thioglycolate broth, 306, 1161
Thiol broth, 1161
Thiols, 209
Thiotepa, 1880-1881
34° C organ culture, 513-514
Thoft technique, 1895
Thorazine deposits, *A117*
Thornton 360 arcuate corneal marker, 2160
Thygeson's superficial punctate keratitis, *A210*
Thymus, 85
Thyroid eye disease, 859, 983-984, *A106, A214*
Tick, 1003
Tight junctional complex, 6
Tight lens syndrome, 1468
Timolol
corneal effects, 1025
in corneal perforation, 1823
in penetrating keratoplasty, 1589
toxicity of, 850
Tinea palpebrum, 654-655
Tissue adhesive
in acid injury, 1441
in anterior segment surgery, 1932-1933
in corneal perforation, 1818-1825
in corneal thinning disorders, 1795
in progressive stromal keratolysis, 1180
Tissue banking
distribution of donor tissue, 519-524
federal regulation of, 527-528, 540-541
storage in, 509-517
media contamination, 514-515
methods of, 510-514
principles of corneal preservation, 509-510
true costs of, 544-545
Tissue Banks International, 478, 539
Tissue culture
from eye bank eyes, 555
for herpes simplex virus, 308
Tissue Distribution and Information Center, 478
Tissue Distribution Center, 478
Tissue evaluation, 501-508
penlight examination, 501
slit lamp examination, 501-505, 506
specular microscopy, 505-507
Tissue inhibitors of metalloproteinases, 147, 148
in sterile corneal ulceration, 207
in stromal wound healing, 192
Tissue matching, 1764-1765
Tissue plasminogen activator
in ocular wound healing, 186
in postvitrectomy fibrin formation, 1667
in sterile corneal ulceration, 206-207
Tissue procurement
ethics in, 531-532
legislation in, 527-528
processing fees, 544
Tissue removal, 493-500, 532
consent for, 494
corneoscleral rim excision, 497-498, 499-500
donor maintenance and identification, 494
enucleation procedure, 495-497
in situ corneal scleral rim excision, 498-500
preparation and processing, 532
public and professional education, 493-494
Tissue storage, 509-517
media contamination, 514-515
methods of, 510-514
principles of corneal preservation, 509-510
Tobramycin, 1169
in conjunctivitis, 767, 793, 794
in corneal abrasion, 1406
corneal effects, 1024
in corneal perforation, 1824
eye drops, 1176
in microbial keratitis, 433
in postkeratoplasty keratitis, 1699
toxicity of, 850
Togavirus, 752, 1246-1247
Tonometry
in anterior chamber cleavage syndrome, 894
before refractive surgery, 2010
Topical anesthetics
abuse of, 1354-1356
corneal effects, 1023, 1024
before radial keratotomy, 2060-2061 2062
toxicity of, 851
Topical antibiotics, 1023-1025, 20[illegible]0
Topical ophthalmic medications
corneal effects, 1023-1026
related to toxic keratoconjunctivitis, 849-853
Topographic analysis, 216, 223-23[illegible]
in bilateral automated lamellar keratoplasty, 2178
in keratoconus, 1096-1097, *A14[illegible]*
keratometry, 224-225
keratoscopy, 225-226, 227
of pellucid marginal degeneration, *A157*
videokeratoscopy, 226-234
Total ankyloblepharon, 872
Touton giant cell, 730
Toxic conjunctivitis, 847-856, *A74*
cosmetics and skin care products, 853
hair care products, 853, 854
related to topical medications, 849-853
tear gas weapons and lacrimating agents, 853-854
therapeutic considerations, 854-855
toxicity *versus* allergy, 847-849
Toxic follicular conjunctivitis, 757
Toxic papillary keratoconjunctivitis, 75[illegible]
Toxin, 1146
Toxin-A, 1146, 1147
Toxoplasmosis, 1538
Trabecular carcinoma of eyelid, 610-611
Trabeculectomy, 895
Trabeculitis, 1218
Trabeculum, 1068
Trachoma, 756, 780-783, *A60-61*
diffuse illumination of, 246
dry eye in, 675
peripheral corneal and, 399-400

phlyctenular lesion *versus,* 1391
scarring from, 749
Transforming growth factor-α
in corneal wound healing, 187
in epithelial wound healing, 184
in sterile corneal ulceration, 206
Transforming growth factor-β, 79, 83
angiogenesis and, 152
in corneal wound healing, 187
in epithelial wound healing, 184
in sterile corneal ulceration, 206
in stromal wound healing, 191
Transillumination
cyclectomy and, 1959-1960
meibomian gland, 241
Transplantation
corneal; *see* Corneal transplantation
ocular surface, 1887-1902
conjunctival, 1889-1892
limbal, 1892-1898, 1899
mucous membrane, 1898-1901
principles of, 1887-1889
of pterygium head, 1877
tissue distribution for, 519
Transretinoic acid, 843
Transscleral Nd:YAG cyclophotocoagulation, 1726-1727
Transsclerally fixated posterior chamber intraocular lenses
evaluation, 1622-1623
technique, 1614-1617, 1618, 1619, 1620
Transverse keratotomy, 1683
Trap-door scleral flap, 1969
Trapezoidal keratotomy, 1682-1683
Trauma, 1403-1422, *A227-260*
abrasions, 1404-1407, *A227*
acid burns, 1437-1442, *A259*
alkali burns, *A259-260*
blast, *A233*
blunt, 1407-1411, 1926, *A228*
after penetrating keratoplasty, *A282*
after radial keratotomy, 2111-2112
anterior segment surgery for, 1929-1930
limbal perforation after, *A254*
specular microscopy of, 330
from contact lens, *A264*
in corneal perforation, 1815-1816
dermatitis in, *A228*
epoxy glue, *A232*
explosion
corneal foreign body from, *A247*
intracorneal keratoprosthesis after, *A295*
forceps, *A236-239*
foreign body in, 1416-1419
fungal keratitis and, 1254
hemorrhage in, *A234-235*
herpetic keratitis in, *A254*
infrared radiation, 1414
keratoconjunctivitis in, *A228*
lacerations, *A229-231*
lightning, *A240*
in ligneous conjunctivitis, 865
mechanisms of, 167-168
patient approach, 1403-1404
penetrating, *A229, A231*
reaction to, 163-182
cell death, 163, 165
cell migration, 166, 167
collagen and, 166
endothelial, 174
epithelial, 168-171
excimer photoablation, 178-179
granulation tissue, 166
inflammation, 163-165
mechanisms of injury, 167-168
penetrating and perforating injuries, 174-177, 178
protein mediators of cell activity, 166
stromal, 171-174
variations in wound healing, 177-178
scar secondary to, *A274*
self-induced, 1352-1354
specular microscopy of, 330
stings, 1419-1420
surgical, *A255-258*
thermal, 1414-1416, *A241*
ultraviolet radiation, 1411-1414
Traumatic hyphema, *A235*
Treacher Collins syndrome, 930
Trephination
in corneal perforation, 1826
of donor cornea, 1585
of host cornea, 1585-1596
improper, 1605-1606
in penetrating keratoplasty with intraocular lens implantation, 1605-1606
in lamellar keratoplasty, 1836
to reduce wound leaks, 1660
in therapeutic keratoplasty, 1850
Trephine, 1572-1573, 1574, 1575
Treponema pallidum, 801, 1276
in conjunctivitis, 769
in eyelid infection, 638
in keratitis, 1141
Treponemal test, 1298
Tretinoin
in cicatricial pemphigoid, 831
in Sjögren's syndrome, 681-682
Triamcinolone
in Behçet disease, 1533
following keratoprosthesis, 1859
Trichiasis, 568-569, *A4*
biomicroscopic examination in, 240
in cicatricial pemphigoid, 829
in Stevens-Johnson syndrome, 842
in trachoma, 783
Trichilemmoma, 595
Trichoepithelioma, 594-595
Trichofolliculoma, 595
Trichophyton, 654-655
Trifluridine
in epidemic keratoconjunctivitis, 774
in herpes simplex blepharoconjunctivitis, 643
in herpes simplex virus keratitis, 1214
in infectious epithelial keratitis, 1215
Triflurothymidine
corneal effects, 1023
in neonatal herpes simplex virus keratoconjunctivitis, 794
toxic keratoconjunctivitis secondary to, 849
toxicity of, 849-850
Trifocal optical system, 2054
Trigeminal nerve
conjunctiva and, 45
eyelid and, 65
herpes simplex virus and, 641, 1193
herpes zoster ophthalmicus and, 1226
Trigeminal neuralgia, 675
Trimethoprim, 1174
Trimethoprim-sulfamethoxazole, *A268*
Tropheryma whippelii, 945-946
Troutman-Barraquer needle holder, 1577
Trypanosomiasis, 1312
Tuberculin skin test, 1389
Tuberculoid leprosy, 1006
Tuberculosis, 1009-1010
Cogan's syndrome *versus,* 1309
in Parinaud's oculoglandular syndrome, 801
Tularemia, 799-801
Tumor; *see* Neoplasm
Tumor necrosis factor-α, 79, 83
angiogenesis and, 152
lipopolysaccharide and, 132
Tumor necrosis factor-β, 83
Twist hook, 1578
Tylosis, 633
Tyndall's light/anterior chamber cells and flare, 252, 253
Tyndall's phenomenon, 290
Type-I hypersensitivity reaction, *A65*
Tyrosinemia II, 420-421, 912
Tyrosinosis type, 382
Tzanck smear
for herpes simplex virus, 308
in herpes zoster ophthalmicus, 1235
in herpetic blepharitis, 642
in varicella zoster virus infection, 645

U

Ulcer, 403-408, *A53*
after alkali burn, *A292*
Aspergillus in, *A195*
associated with photorefractive keratoplasty, 2203, 2204
bacterial, 398-399, 1148
in congenital corneal anesthesia, 1352
defined, 1816
diagnosis, 403-406, 407, 408
herpes simplex keratitis with, *A182, A290*
herpes zoster ophthalmicus with, *A193*
limbal, *A224*
metaherpetic, *A184*
Mooren's, 398, 399, 1397-1401, *A226*
conjunctival resection in, 1794
deep lamellar keratoplasty for, 1775
immune response in, 114
marginal staphylococcus keratitis *versus,* 1393
pellucid marginal degeneration *versus,* 1101
penetrating keratoplasty in, *A277*
Moraxella in, *A188*
phlyctenular lesion *versus,* 1391
protease inhibitors in, 192-193
Pseudomonas, A266
in rheumatoid arthritis, *A218*
from seventh nerve paralysis, *A214*
in Sjögren's syndrome, 677
surgery for, 1794-1797
with systemic lupus erythematosus, *A221*
from thermal injury, *A241*
treatment, 406-407
in vernal keratoconjunctivitis, 811
in vitamin A deficiency, 958-960
in Wegener's granulomatosis, 948-949
Ulcerative colitis, 943-945, 1519
Ulcerative keratitis, 2118-2120
Ultrasonic pachymeter, 2020
Ultrasonography
in ciliary body tumor, 1957
high resolution, 351-359
in corneal disease, 354-356, 357
in corneal surgery, 356-358
examination techniques, 352-353, 354

Ultrasonography—cont'd
  high resolution—cont'd
    instrumentation, 351-352, 353, 354
    of normal cornea, 353-354, 355
  in postoperative endophthalmitis, 1704
Ultrasound pachymeter, 279, 2065-2067
Ultraviolet radiation
  in corneal trauma, 1411-1414, *A228*
  for improving graft survival, 1765
  pterygium formation and, 1875-1876
Uncorrected visual acuity
  after photorefractive keratoplasty, 2192-2194
  to judge efficacy, 2243-2244
  in phototherapeutic keratectomy, 2220
Undercorrection
  in automated lamellar keratoplasty, 2177
  in radial keratotomy, 2105-2107, 2131-2132
Uniform Anatomical Gift Act of 1968, 531, 537
Unilateral epiphora, 696
United Network for Organ Sharing, 519
United Way, 545
Universal precautions, 532
Upper tarsal conjunctiva, 272
Urate deposits, 421
Urethritis
  Chlamydia trachomatis in, 784
  in Reiter's syndrome, 1518
Urokinase-plasminogen activator
  in epithelial wound healing, 184, 186, 205
  in sterile corneal ulceration, 206-207
Uronic acid, 32
Uvea
  herpes zoster ophthalmicus and, 1231
  leprosy and, 1008-1009
  syphilitic interstitial keratitis and, 1286
Uveitis
  after keratoprosthesis, 1860, 1861
  anterior, 1493-1503, *A269-272*
    classification, 1500-1501
    demography, 1494-1495
    diagnostic evaluation, 1501-1502
    HLA-B27 related, 1515-1521
    HLA-B27-related, *A272*
    idiopathic, 1505
    patient history, 1493-1494
    physical examination in, 1495-1500
    in sarcoidosis, 1524-1525
    symptoms, 1493
    treatment, 1502-1503
  herpes zoster, *A191*
  in herpes zoster ophthalmicus, 1231
  idiopathic, 1505-1513
    classification and previous occurrence, 1505, 1506
    consultation in, 1508
    laboratory evaluation, 1507-1508
    physical examination, 1506-1507
    treatment, 1508-1513
  in Kawasaki disease, 950
  in leprosy, 1008-1009
  in Reiter's syndrome, 1518
  in relapsing polychondritis, 1380
  in sarcoidosis, 1524, 1525-1526
  syphilitic, 1282, *A272*

V

Vaccine
  leprosy, 1009
  varicella zoster virus, 1238-1239
Vaccinia immune globulin, 649
Vaccinia virus
  cornea and, 1243
  eyelid and, 649
Vacuole in macular dystrophy, 1047
Valium, 2060
Valley fever, 654
Vancomycin, 1168
  in anterior segment trauma, 1934
  in corneal perforation, 1824
  in endophthalmitis, 1704
  in erysipelas, 637
  eye drops, 1176
  in infectious crystalline keratopathy, 1702
  in microbial keratitis, 433
  in postkeratoplasty keratitis, 1699
  postoperative, 1942
Vannas scissors, 1577
Variable frame analysis of cell size, 321-322
Varicella zoster virus, 1225-1242, *A109, A273*
  in acquired immunodeficiency syndrome, 1018
  in conjunctivitis, 777
  corticosteroids in, 1237
  definition, epidemiology, and prevalence, 1225
  in eyelid infection, 643-646
  herpes zoster ophthalmicus, 1226-1233, 1234-1236
  in immunocompromised patient, 1233-1234
  laboratory investigation, 308-309
  medical therapy, 1236-1237
  postherpetic neuralgia, 1237-1238
  prevention, 1238-1239
Varifocal optical system, 2055
Varifocality, 2054
Variola, 752, *A109*
  in corneal infection, 1243
  in eyelid infection, 648
Varix, eyelid, 589, *A13*
Vascular adhesion molecules, 86, 138
Vascular endothelial growth factor, 152
Vascular endothelium
  adhesion molecules on, 137-138
  angiogenesis and, 152
Vascular permeability factor, 152
Vascular system
  conjunctival, 44-45
  corneal, 3
  eyelid, 65-66
Vascular tissue tumor, 588-591
Vascularization
  after radial keratotomy, 2124-2125
  corneal, *A264-265*
  risk of allograft reaction, 1761-1762, 1768-1769
  stromal, *A264*
Vasculitis
  in Behçet disease, 1530
  in Churg-Strauss syndrome, 1384
  in Cogan's syndrome, 1308
  in giant cell arteritis, 1384
  in herpes zoster ophthalmicus, 1235
  polyarteritis nodosa, 1383-1384
  rheumatoid arthritis-associated, 1360
  Wegener's granulomatosis, 1381-1383
Vasoactive amines, 144
Vasodilation, 152
Vaughan study, 2088-2091, 2095
Vegetable foreign body, *A249*
Venereal Disease Research Laboratory test, 1298
Venous drainage of conjunctiva, 45
Vernal keratoconjunctivitis, 393, 750, 753, 811-813, *A66*
  giant papillary conjunctivitis *versus*, 323
  immunopathology of, 108-109
Verruca vulgaris, 647-648
Versatility of refractive surgery, 2244
Verticillata, *A115*
Vesicle
  corneal, *A81*
  in herpes zoster ophthalmicus, 1227
  in infectious epithelial keratitis, 1196-1197, 1198
  in posterior polymorphous dystrophy, 1063, 1065
  in varicella, 1226
Vestibuloauditory dysfunction, 1307
Vidarabine
  corneal effects, 1023
  in herpes simplex virus keratitis, 1214
  in infectious epithelial keratitis, 121[illegible]
  in neonatal conjunctivitis, 794
  in neonatal herpes simplex virus keratoconjunctivitis, 794
  toxicity of, 849-850
Video monitor, 2021
Videokeratography, 2039-2058
  in assessment of surgical result, 204[illegible]-2055, 2056
  challenges for future, 2055-2056
  in minimal visual loss, 450-451
  preoperative screening, 2042-2048
  videokeratoscope, 2039-2042
Videokeratoscopy, 226-234, 2039-2042
Vimentin, 9
Vinculin, 205
Viral infection, *A26*
  conjunctival, 773-777, 792, *A55-57*
  corneal
    flavivirus and bunyavirus, 1247
    herpesvirus, 1244-1245
    opacity in, 378-379
    orthomyxovirus, 1249
    papovavirus, 1245
    paramyxovirus, 1247-1248
    penetrating keratoplasty in, 1554
    perforation in, 1815-1816
    picornavirus, 1245-1246
    poxvirus, 1243-1244
    togavirus, 1246-1247
  Epstein-Barr, *A110*
  eyelid, 641-651
    herpes simplex virus, 641-643
    molluscum contagiosum, 646-647
    smallpox, 648-649
    varicella zoster virus, 643-646
    verruca vulgaris, 647-648
  herpes simplex, 1312-1313
Viroptic; *see* Triflurothymidine
Virulence, 1144
Viscoelastics, 1028
Vision loss
  after corneal trauma, 1947-1948
  in atopic keratoconjunctivitis, 814
  in Behçet syndrome, 1531
  minimal, 447-455
    conditions causing, 451-454
    examination techniques, 447-451
    patient history in, 447, 448
  in red eye, 439
Vision research, 339-343, 344, 345, 553-558
Visual acuity
  in *Acanthamoeba* keratitis, 1269-1270

after radial keratotomy, 2102, 2103, 2129
anterior segment surgery and, 1927
in corneal perforation, 1816
following lamellar keratoplasty, 1834
in minimal visual loss, 447
before penetrating keratoplasty, 1564-1565
before refractive surgery, 2008
Visual axis determination and marking, 2015, 2063-2064
coaxial light source, 2063-2064
miotic pupil centering, 2063
Visual rehabilitation
in alkali injury, 1449-1450
in anterior segment surgery, 1943
Visx excimer laser, 2183
Vital dyes
in photo slit lamp micrography, 301-303
in slit lamp examination, 261-263, 266, 267, 268
Vitamin A
deficiency, 955-963, *A100-101*
classification and clinical manifestations, 956-960
dry eye in, 675
epidemiology, 961, 963
historical considerations, 955-956
interactions with other factors, 960-961, 962
treatment, 961-963
in erythema multiforme, 843
to improve graft survival, 1785
metabolism of, 955, 956
ointment in superior limbic keratoconjunctivitis, 860
Vitamin B deficiency, 963
Vitamin C deficiency, 963-964
Vitrectomy, 1558
in diabetic patient, 981
before pediatric penetrating keratoplasty, 1745-1746
in penetrating keratoplasty with intraocular lens implantation
evaluation, 1620
technique, 1608-1609
in postoperative endophthalmitis, 1704
in torn posterior capsule, 1641
Vitreous
anterior segment surgery and, 1928, 1941-1942
anterior segment trauma and, 1952-1953
examination before penetrating keratoplasty, 1569
grading of opacities, 1507
Vitronectin, 35
Vogt-Koyanagi-Harada syndrome, *A271*
Vogt's limbal girdle, 1127, 1128, *A163*
Vogt's striae, *A150-152*
Voluntary tissue sharing, 523
Von Gierke syndrome, 903
Von Hippel's internal ulcer, 885
Vortex plume theory, 2206

W

Wagner syndrome, 935
Waiting list system for corneal tissue, 521-522
Waldenström macroglobulinemia, 975, *A104*
Waring study, 2086-2088, 2094-2095
Warm compress
in chalazion, 635
in cicatricial pemphigoid, 831
in meibomian gland dysfunction, 630
Wasp sting, 1419-1420
Wassermann test, 1276
Weck trephine, 1573, 1574
Wedge resection, 1631
Wegener's granulomatosis, 948-949, *A222-224*
corneal disease in, 1381-1383
macroulcerative peripheral keratitis and, 396-397
Welding arc exposure, 1414
Werblin study, 2084-2086, 2094
Werner syndrome, 938-939, 984-985, 998-999
Westcott scissors, 1577
Western blot, 1005
Whipple's disease, 945-946
White limbal girdle of Vogt, 389
White pulp, 85
White retrocorneal membrane, *A281*
White ring, *A246*
Wilson's disease, 390-391, 425, 915, *A95*
Wing cell, 6, 7, 183
With-the-rule astigmatism, 876, 2157-2158
World Health Organization trachoma classification, 781
Worst iris-claw minus powered anterior chamber intraocular lens, 2002
Wound
after astigmatic keratotomy, 2146
after penetrating keratoplasty, 1659, 1661, *A276*
for herpes simplex infection, 1809
pediatric, 1746, 1750-1751
perforating, *A230*
Wound healing, 183-198
after infection, 149-151
after phototherapeutic keratectomy, 2216, 2217
after radial keratotomy, 2121-2122
in child, 1767
endothelial, 193-195
epithelial, 183-190
in abrasion, 1406
extracellular matrix and, 18-20
migration in, 17
in ulceration, 205
excimer photoablation and, 179
in vivo four-dimensional analysis, 343, 344, 345
specular microscopy of, 318, 323
steroid delay of, 1024
stromal, 190-193
variations in, 177-178
Wright-Giemsa stain, 1159

X

X-linked ichthyosis, 426, 996-997, *A107*
X suture, 1589
Xanthelasma, 591, *A13*
Xanthogranuloma, *A7, A49*
Xanthoma, 591
Xenon arc photocoagulation, 1414
Xeroderma pigmentosum, 615-616, 914-915, 999
Xerophthalmia, 955-963, *A100-101*
classification and clinical manifestations, 956-960
dry eye in, 675
epidemiology, 961, 963
historical considerations, 955-956
interactions with other factors, 960-961, 962
metabolism of vitamin A, 955, 956
treatment, 961-963
Xerosis
conjunctival, 957-958
corneal, 958
in corneal perforation, 1815-1816
XYZ theory, 17

Y

YAG laser procedures, 1324-1325

Z

Zeis gland, 62, 63, 635
Ziehl-Neelsen stain
in bacterial keratitis, 1159
in microbial keratitis, 306
Zoster sine herpete, 1227, 1233